EQUINE
DERMATOLOGY

EQUINE DERMATOLOGY

Danny W. Scott, DVM
Diplomate, American College of Veterinary Dermatology
Professor of Medicine
Department of Clinical Sciences and Department of Biomedical Sciences
College of Veterinary Medicine
Cornell University
Ithaca, New York

William H. Miller, Jr., VMD
Diplomate, American College of Veterinary Dermatology
Professor of Medicine
Department of Clinical Sciences and Department of Biomedical Sciences
College of Veterinary Medicine
Cornell University
Ithaca, NY

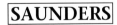

SAUNDERS

An Imprint of Elsevier Science

SAUNDERS

An Imprint of Elsevier Science

11830 Westline Industrial Drive
St. Louis, Missouri 63146

EQUINE DERMATOLOGY   ISBN 0-7216-2571-1
Copyright © 2003, Elsevier Science (USA). All rights reserved.

NOTICE

Veterinary Medicine is an ever-changing field. Standard safety precautions must be followed, but as new research and clinical experience broaden our knowledge, changes in treatment and drug therapy may become necessary or appropriate. Readers are advised to check the most current product information provided by the manufacturer of each drug to be administered to verify the recommended dose, the method and duration of administration, and contraindications. It is the responsibility of the treating veterinarian, relying on experience and knowledge of the patient, to determine dosages and the best treatment for each individual animal. Neither the publisher nor the editor assumes any liability for any injury and/or damage to animals or property arising from this publication.

International Standard Book Number 0-7216-2571-1

Acquisitions Editor: Ray Kersey
Developmental Editor: Denise LeMelledo
Publishing Services Manager: Linda McKinley
Project Manager: Jennifer Furey
Designer: Julia Dummitt
Cover Design: Sheilah Barrett

Printed in United States of America

Last digit is the print number: 9 8 7 6 5 4 3 2 1

Preface and Acknowledgments

Equine skin disorders are common and important. After dogs and cats, horses are the most common species presented to our Dermatology Service and telephone consultation service for evaluation. In general, the equine dermatoses seen worldwide are similar both in nature and frequency.[1-8]

Very little information is available concerning the demographics of equine skin disorders. A survey carried out by the British Equine Veterinary Association in 1962 and 1963 indicated that 2% of all cases seen by the membership were presented for skin disease.[9] A 1989 survey of the members of the American Association of Equine Practitioners revealed that skin disorders were the fourth most common medical problem encountered (following colic, viral respiratory tract disease, and endometritis).[10] The top 10 equine health problems as determined by a survey of horse owners included skin diseases, which ranked number 9.[11]

Panel reports of veterinary practitioners in 1975, 1981, and 1986 found that dermatophytosis, dermatophilosis, urticaria, insect hypersensitivities, onchocerciasis, eosinophilic granulomas ("nodular necrobiosis"), papillomas ("warts"), sarcoids, photodermatitis, and nutritional "seborrheas" were the most commonly encountered equine skin disorders.[4-6] In a 21-year (1979-2000) retrospective study of equine skin disorders at the College of Veterinary Medicine at Cornell University, 4.1% of all horses examined at the Large Animal Clinic were evaluated by a dermatologist for skin problems (Tables 1 and 2).[12] There was no breed predisposition for skin

● Table 1 **COMMON HORSE BREEDS PRESENTED FOR DERMATOLOGIC DIAGNOSIS**[12]

BREED	PERCENTAGE OF DERMATOLOGY CASES	PERCENTAGE OF TOTAL HOSPITAL POPULATION
Thoroughbred	23.9	22.9
Quarter Horse	16.5	14.6
Standardbred	15.8	24.2
Arabian	6.4	5.2
Appaloosa	5.8	5.4
Morgan	4.5	3.0
Belgian	3.9	2.1
American Paint	1.8	1.8
Percheron	1.1	0.7
American Saddle Horse	0.9	0.6
Clydesdale	0.6	0.4
All other breeds	18.8	19.1

● Table 2 **DERMATOLOGIC DIAGNOSES* FOR 900 HORSES OVER A 21- YEAR PERIOD (1979-2000)[12]**

DIAGNOSIS	# OF CASES	% OF CASES
Bacterial folliculitis	106	11.78
Dermatophytosis	80	8.89
Insect hypersensitivity	57	6.33
Dermatophilosis	50	5.56
Drug reaction	37	4.11
Eosinophilic granuloma	35	3.89
Atopy	35	3.89
Vasculitis	30	3.33
Chorioptic mange	24	2.67
Equine sarcoid	23	2.56
Urticaria, idiopathic	22	2.44
Idiopathic pruritus	19	2.11
Pemphigus foliaceus	17	1.89
Erythema multiforme	17	1.89
Onchocerciasis	15	1.67
Ear papillomas	13	1.44
Viral papillomatosis	12	1.33
Alopecia areata	12	1.33
Follicular dysplasia	12	1.33
Pediculosis	11	1.22
Idiopathic seborrhea	11	1.22
Unilateral papular dermatosis	11	1.22
Dermoid cysts	10	1.11
Bacterial pseudomycetoma	10	1.11
Telogen defluxion	10	1.11
Melanoma	9	1.00
Lymphoma	9	1.00
Anagen defluxion	9	1.00
Habronemiasis	9	1.00
Coronary band dysplasia	9	1.00
Ventral midline dermatitis	8	0.89
Cannon keratosis	7	0.78
Contact dermatitis†	7	0.78
Verrucous hemangioma	6	0.67
Linear keratosis	6	0.67
Trichorrhexis nodosa	6	0.67
Vitiligo	6	0.67
Bacterial cellulitis	6	0.67
Traumatic alopecia	5	0.56
Blackfly bites, pinna	5	0.56
Sterile eosinophilic folliculitis	5	0.56
Secondary seborrhea, hepatic	5	0.56
Pseudolymphoma	5	0.56
Epidermal nevus	5	0.56
Schwannoma	5	0.56
Sterile pyogranuloma	4	0.44
Sterile panniculitis	4	0.44
Sarcoidosis	4	0.44
Tick bite granuloma	4	0.44
Hyperadrenocorticism	4	0.44
Food hypersensitivity	4	0.44
Behavioral self-mutilation	4	0.44

● Table 2   **DERMATOLOGIC DIAGNOSES* FOR 900 HORSES OVER A 21- YEAR PERIOD (1979-2000)[12]—cont'd**

DIAGNOSIS	# OF CASES	% OF CASES
Mane and tail seborrhea	3	0.33
Idiopathic pastern dermatitis	3	0.33
Discoid lupus erythematosus	3	0.33
Epitrichial sweat gland neoplasm	3	0.33
Spotted leukotrichia	3	0.33
Amyloidosis	3	0.33
Barbering	3	0.33
Burns	2	0.22
Bullous pemphigoid	2	0.22
Lymphangitis, bacterial	2	0.22
Photodermatitis, hepatic	2	0.22
Systemic lupus erythematosus	2	0.22
Epitheliotropic lymphoma	2	0.22
Squamous cell carcinoma	2	0.22
Idiopathic delayed shedding	2	0.22
Sporotrichosis	2	0.22
Eumycotic mycetoma	2	0.22
Photic headshaking	2	0.22
Pressure sores	2	0.22
Multisystemic eosinophilic epitheliotropic disease	2	0.22
Aplasia cutis congenita	1	0.11
Malignant fibrous histiocytoma	1	0.11
Carcinosarcoma	1	0.11
Halicephalobiasis	1	0.11
Phaeohyphomycosis	1	0.11
Cutaneous asthenia	1	0.11
Mast cell tumor	1	0.11
Arsenic toxicosis	1	0.11
Hypotrichosis	1	0.11
Trichoepithelioma	1	0.11
Pili torti	1	0.11
Strawmite dermatitis	1	0.11
Organoid nevus	1	0.11
Lichenoid keratosis	1	0.11

*Where more than one dermatosis was present at the same time in one horse, only the most important are listed.
†Contact reactions associated with topical medicaments are included under Drug Reaction.

disease as a whole. Due to the referral nature of our practice, the types and frequencies of the various dermatoses documented would not be expected to be those seen in general equine practice. The "Top 10" equine dermatoses seen at our clinic were bacterial folliculitis, dermatophytosis, insect hypersensitivity, dermatophilosis, drug reaction, eosinophilic granuloma, atopy, vasculitis, chorioptic mange, and equine sarcoid. In a 16-year (1978-1994) retrospective study of biopsy specimens submitted to the Diagnostic Laboratory, College of Veterinary Medicine, at Cornell University, 23.4% of all equine submissions were skin lesions.[12]

Interest in equine dermatology has resulted in its being reviewed in a number of textbooks[13-36,46] and continuing education articles.[37-44] Of particular note is the special issue of Veterinary Dermatology dedicated to the late Dr. Tony Stannard.[45] Skin diseases are a source of animal suffering—through annoyance, irritability, pruritus, disfigurement, secondary infections, myiasis, and increased susceptibility to other diseases. In addition to compromising the animal's comfort and appearance, skin diseases can interfere with the horse's ability to function in riding, working, or show. Economic losses through the financial burdens of diagnostic, therapeutic, or preventive programs can be sizable. Rarely, zoonotic dermatoses may be a source of human disease and suffering.

We wholeheartedly echo the conclusion reached by the 1989 survey of the members of the American Association of Equine Practitioners: "Dermatologic disorders in horses are common problems that need emphasis in veterinary curricula and research endeavors."[8,10]

We cannot overstate our appreciation for those who have contributed to this text. We couldn't have done it without you! If we have failed to acknowledge anyone, please forgive us and send us your correction! Special thanks go out to Drs. Bill McMullen and Reg Pascoe for their many years of observation, investigation, and reporting. We remember and salute our greatest teacher in equine dermatology, the late Tony Stannard. We have purposely used many of Tony's slides that he so graciously donated to us over the years.

Held up for special praise and recognition are those who have given so much in terms of love, patience, and support during this endeavor: Kris, Travis, and Tracy (DWS) and Kathy, Steven, Julia, and Andrew (WHM). Yo Lexi (Alexis Wenski-Roberts) . . . thanx for your photomicrographic expertise! A big kiss for Denise LeMelledo, Jennifer Furey, Ray Kersey, and the whole W. B. Saunders gang.

I (DWS) first began working on the idea of an equine dermatology textbook in 1984. It has gone through many starts and stops, ups and downs, and incarnations in the subsequent 18 years. In the words of Sam Cooke, "It's been a long time comin'." Bill and I hope it's been worth the wait.

D.W. Scott

W.H. Miller, Jr.

● REFERENCES

1. Hutchins DR: Skin diseases of cattle and horses in New South Wales. N Z Vet J 8:85, 1960.
2. Pascoe RR: The nature and treatment of skin conditions observed in horses in Queensland. Aust Vet J 49:35, 1973.
3. Thomsett LR: Skin diseases of the horse. In Pract 1:16, 1979.
4. Panel Report: Skin conditions in horses. Mod Vet Pract 56:363, 1975.
5. Panel Report: Dermatologic problems in horses. Mod Vet Pract 62:75, 1981.
6. Panel Report: Skin diseases in horses. Mod Vet Pract 67:43, 1986.
7. von Tscharner C: Die wichtigsten Hautkrankheiten beim Pferd. Prakt Tierheilk 69:4, 1988.
8. Halldórsdóttir S: Hudlidelser hos hest. Norsk Veterinaer 102:19, 1990.
9. Hopes R: Skin diseases in horses. Vet Dermatol News 1(23):4, 1976.
10. Traub-Dargatz JL, et al: Medical problems of adult horses, as ranked by equine practitioners. J Am Vet Med Assoc 198:1745, 1991.
11. Underhill LJP, Showalter TL: The wellness movement. Equus, Nov. 1989, p 44.
12. Scott DW, Miller WH JR: Unpublished data.
13. Kral F, Novak BJ: Veterinary Dermatology. J.B. Lippincott Co., Philadelphia, 1953.
14. Kral F: Compendium of Veterinary Dermatology. Pfizer Laboratories, Exton, 1959.
15. Bone JF, et al (eds): Equine Medicine and Surgery I. American Veterinary Publications, Inc., Wheaton, 1963.
16. Kral F, Schwartzman RM: Veterinary and Comparative Dermatology. J.B. Lippincott Co., Philadelphia, 1964.
17. Stannard AA: The skin. In: Catcott EJ, Smithcors JF (eds): Equine Medicine and Surgery II. American Veterinary Publications, Inc., Wheaton, 1972, p 381.
18. Pascoe RR: Equine dermatoses. University of Sydney Post-Graduate Foundation in Veterinary Science, Vet Rev #14, 1974.
19. Pascoe RR: Equine dermatoses. University of Sydney Post-Graduate Foundation in Veterinary Sciences, Vet Rev #21, 1981.
20. McMullen WC: The skin. In: Mansmann RA, et al (eds): Equine Medicine and Surgery III, Vol II. American Veterinary Publications, Santa Barbara, 1982, p 789.
21. Robinson NE (ed): Current Therapy in Equine Medicine. W.B. Saunders Co., Philadelphia, 1983.
22. Montes LF, Vaughan JT: Atlas of Skin Diseases of the Horse. W.B. Saunders Co., Philadelphia, 1983.
23. Robinson NE (ed): Current Therapy in Equine Medicine II. W.B. Saunders Co., Philadelphia, 1987.
24. Scott DW: Large Animal Dermatology. W.B. Saunders Co., Philadelphia, 1988.
25. Chatterjee A: Skin Infections in Domestic Animals. Moitri Publication, Calcutta, 1989.

26. Ackerman LJ: Practical Equine Dermatology. American Veterinary Publications, Inc., Goleta, 1989.

27. Pascoe RR: A Colour Atlas of Equine Dermatology. Wolfe Publishing, Ltd., London, 1990.

28. Barbet JL, et al: Diseases of the skin. In: Colahan PT, et al (eds): Equine Medicine and Surgery IV, Vol II. American Veterinary Publications, Inc., Goleta, 1991, p 1569.

29. Robinson NE (ed): Current Therapy in Equine Medicine III. W.B. Saunders Co., Philadelphia, 1992.

30. Jubb KVF, et al: Pathology of Domestic Animals, IV. Academic Press, New York, 1993.

31. Radostits DM, et al: Veterinary Medicine. A Textbook of the Diseases of Cattle, Sheep, Pigs, Goats, and HorsesVIII. Baillière-Tindall, Philadelphia, 1994.

32. Kobluk CN, et al (eds): The Horse. Diseases and Clinical Management. W.B. Saunders Co., Philadelphia, 1995.

33. Robinson NE (ed): Current Therapy in Equine Medicine IV. W.B. Saunders Co., Philadelphia, 1997.

34. Fadok VA (ed): Dermatology. The Veterinary Clinics of North America: Equine Practice, April 1995.

35. Reed SM, Bayly WM (eds): Equine Internal Medicine. W.B. Saunders Co., Philadelphia, 1998.

36. Pascoe RRR, Knottenbelt DC: Manual of Equine Dermatology. W.B. Saunders Co., Philadelphia, 1999.

37. Fadok VA, Mullowney PC: Dermatologic diseases of horses part I. Parasitic dermatoses of the horse. Comp Cont Educ 5:S615, 1983.

38. Mullowney PC, Fadok VA: Dermatologic diseases of horses part II. Bacterial and viral skin diseases. Comp Cont Educ 6:S15, 1984.

39. Mullowney PC, Fadok VA: Dermatologic diseases of horses part III. Fungal skin diseases. Comp Cont Educ 6:S324, 1984.

40. Mullowney PC (ed): Symposium on Large Animal Dermatology. The Veterinary Clinics of North America: Large Animal Practice, March 1984.

41. Mullowney PC: Dermatologic diseases of horses part IV. Environmental, congenital, and neoplastic diseases. Comp Cont Educ 7:S22, 1985.

42. Mullowney PC: Dermatologic diseases of horses part V. Allergic, immune-mediated, and miscellaneous skin diseases. Comp Cont Educ 7:S217, 1985.

43. Vrins A, et al: Dermatologie équine. 1ère partie: les affections alopéciques et affections prurigineuses. Prat Vét Equine 24:73, 1992.

44. Vrins A, et al: Dermatologie équine 2 ème partie: les affections papuleuses et nodulaires et les boutons de chair. Prat Vét Equine 24:157, 1992.

45. von Tscharner C, et al (eds): Stannard's Illustrated Equine Dermatology Notes. Vet Dermatol 11:161, 2000.

46. Sloet van Oldruitenborgh-Oosterbaan MM, Knottenbelt DC: The Practitioner's Guide to Equine Dermatology. Uitgeverij Libre BV, Leeuwarden, 2001.

Contents

EQUINE
DERMATOLOGY

Chapter 1

Structure and Function of the Skin

The skin is the largest and most visible organ of the body and the anatomic and physiologic barrier between animal and environment. It provides protection from physical, chemical, and microbiologic injury, and its sensory components perceive heat, cold, pain, pruritus, touch, and pressure. In addition, the skin is synergistic with internal organ systems and thus reflects pathologic processes that are either primary elsewhere or shared with other tissues. Not only is the skin an organ with its own reaction patterns; it is also a mirror reflecting the milieu intérieur and, at the same time, the capricious world to which it is exposed.

● GENERAL FUNCTIONS AND PROPERTIES OF THE SKIN

The general functions of animal skin are as follows[*]:

1. Enclosing barrier. The most important function of skin is to make possible an internal environment for all other organs by maintaining an effective barrier to the loss of water, electrolytes, and macromolecules.
2. Environmental protection. A corollary function is the exclusion of external injurious agents—chemical, physical, and microbiologic—from entrance into the internal environment.
3. Motion and shape. The flexibility, elasticity, and toughness of the skin allow motion and provide shape and form.
4. Adnexa production. Skin produces glands and keratinized structures such as hair, hoof, and the horny layer of the epidermis.
5. Temperature regulation. Skin plays a role in the regulation of body temperature through its support of the hair coat, regulation of cutaneous blood supply, and sweat gland function.
6. Storage. The skin is a reservoir of electrolytes, water, vitamins, fat, carbohydrates, proteins, and other materials.
7. Indicator. The skin may be an important indicator of general health, internal disease, and the effects of substances applied topically or taken internally. It contributes to physical and sexual identity.
8. Immunoregulation. Keratinocytes, Langerhans' cells, lymphocytes, and dermal dendrocytes together provide the skin with an immunosurveillance capability that effectively protects against the development of cutaneous neoplasms and persistent infections.
9. Pigmentation. Processes in the skin (melanin formation, vascularity, and keratinization) help determine the color of the coat and skin. Pigmentation of the skin helps prevent damage from solar radiation.

---

[*]References 47, 63, 68, 103, 134, 152, 166, 169, 187, 202.

10. Antimicrobial action. The skin surface has antibacterial and antifungal properties.
11. Sensory perception. Skin is a primary sensory organ for touch, pressure, pain, itch, heat, and cold.
12. Secretion. Skin is a secretory organ by virtue of its epitrichial sweat glands, and sebaceous glands.
13. Excretion. The skin functions in a limited way as an excretory organ.
14. Vitamin D production. Vitamin D is produced in the skin through stimulation by solar radiation.[63,68,97] In the epidermis, vitamin D_3 (cholecalciferol) is formed from provitamin D_3 (7-dehydrocholesterol), via previtamin D_3 on exposure to sunlight. The vitamin D–binding protein in plasma translocates vitamin D_3 from the skin to the circulation. Vitamin D_3 is then hydroxylated in the liver to 25-hydroxyvitamin D_3 and again hydroxylated in the kidney to form 1,25-dihydroxyvitamin D_3, which is important in the regulation of epidermal proliferation and differentiation.

● ONTOGENY

Skin is a complex multicellular organ in which endoderm, neural crest, and ectoderm contribute to form a three-dimensional unit in a spatially and temporally defined manner. Skin morphogenesis involves the action of multiple genes in a coordinated fashion. Homeobox genes are a gene family that encode information critical for normal embryologic development and that likely play a very important role in the development of skin adnexa, pigment system, and stratified epithelium during embryogenesis.[172]

Epithelial-mesenchymal interactions regulate tissue homeostasis, the balanced regulation of proliferation and differentiation maintaining normal tissue architecture and function. Multiple circuits of reciprocal permissive and instructive effects exist between epithelial and mesenchymal cells and extracellular matrices.

To the authors' knowledge, the ontogeny of equine skin has not been reported. The following discussion is an amalgamation of information from other domestic mammals and humans.[63,68,166,169]

Initially, the embryonic skin consists of a single layer of ectodermal cells and a dermis containing loosely arranged mesenchymal cells embedded in an interstitial ground substance. The ectodermal covering progressively develops into two layers (the basal cell layer, or stratum germinativum, and the outer periderm), three layers (the stratum intermedium forms between the other two layers), and then into an adult-like structure. Melanocytes (neural crest origin) and Langerhans' cells (bone marrow origin) become identifiable during this period of ectodermal maturation.

Dermal development is characterized by an increase in the thickness and number of fibers, a decrease in ground substance, and the transition of mesenchymal cells to fibroblasts. This process of building a fiber-rich matrix has been referred to as a "ripening" of the dermis. Elastin fibers appear later than do collagen fibers. Histiocytes, Schwann cells, and dermal melanocytes also become recognizable. Fetal skin contains a large percentage of Type III collagen compared with the skin of an adult, which contains a large proportion of Type I collagen. Lipocytes (adipocytes, fat cells) begin to develop into the subcutis from spindle-shaped mesenchymal precursor cells (prelipoblasts) in the second half of gestation.

The embryonal stratum germinativum differentiates into hair germs (primary epithelial germs), which give rise to hair follicles, sebaceous glands, and epitrichial (apocrine) sweat glands. Hair germs initially consist of an area of crowding of deeply basophilic cells in the basal layer of the epidermis. Subsequently, the areas of crowding become buds that protrude into the dermis. Beneath each bud lies a group of mesenchymal cells, from which the dermal hair papilla is later formed.

As the hair peg lengthens and develops into a hair follicle and hair, three bulges appear. The lowest (deepest) of the bulges develops into the attachment for the arrector pili muscle; the middle bulge differentiates into the sebaceous gland; and the uppermost bulge evolves into the epitrichial sweat gland. In general, the first hairs to appear on the fetus are vibrissae and tactile or sinus hairs that develop on the chin, eye brows, and upper lip as white, slightly raised dots on otherwise smooth, bare skin. The general body hair appears first on the head and gradually progresses caudally.

Cell interaction plays a central role in the formation of skin appendages. Morphogens are substances that control the development of the hair follicle.[27,46] Adhesion molecules appear to be involved in recruiting cells and defining cell groups in the formation of skin appendages during the initiation stage, and homeoproteins (as determined by homeobox genes) appear to play a role in the determination stage in setting the phenotypes and orientation of skin appendages.[33,129] Several new adhesion molecule families that mediate cell-to-cell and cell-to-substrate adhesion have been identified: (1) neural cell adhesion molecules (N-CAM), which belong to the immunoglobulin gene superfamily; (2) cadherins, which mediate adhesion in the presence of calcium; (3) tenascin, which is a unique matrix molecule similar to epidermal cell growth factor; (4) fibronectin, fibrinogen, and syndecan; and (5) integrins, which serve as cellular receptors for fibronectin, collagen, and other extracellular matrix molecules.[32,46,68,114] Hair follicle proteoglycans (syndecan, perlecan, decorin) may be important in hair follicle morphogenesis, both with respect to the epithelium and dermal papilla cells.[40] Thus in each step of the morphogenesis of skin appendages, different adhesion molecules are expressed and are involved in different functions: induction, mesenchymal condensation, epithelial folding, and cell death.

All vessels in fetal skin develop first as capillaries. They have been suggested to organize *in situ* from dermal mesenchymal cells into single-layered endothelial tubes. Branches from large subcutaneous nerve trunks extend into the dermis and organize into deep and superficial plexuses related to the vascular plexuses.

• GROSS ANATOMY AND PHYSIOLOGY

At each body orifice, the skin is continuous with the mucous membrane located there (digestive, respiratory, ocular, urogenital). The skin and hair coat vary in quantity and quality among breeds and among individuals within a breed; they also vary from one area to another on the body, and in accordance with age and sex.

In general, skin thickness decreases dorsally to ventrally on the trunk and proximally to distally on the limbs.° The skin is thickest on the forehead, dorsal neck, dorsal thorax, rump, and base of the tail. It is thinnest on the pinnae and on the axillary, inguinal, and perianal areas. The reported average thickness of the general body skin is 3.8 mm, with a range of 1.7 to 6.3 mm[184,197,203] and was thickest over the lumbosacral and gluteal areas. The average skin thickness in the areas of the mane and tail was 6.2 mm, with a range of 3.8 to 10.7 mm.[197] The hair coat is usually thickest over the dorsolateral aspects of the body and thinnest ventrally, on the lateral surface of the pinnae, and on the undersurface of the tail.

The skin surfaces of haired mammals are, in general, acidic. The pH of normal equine skin has been reported to range from about 4.8 to 6.8, and to increase to as much as 7.9 with sweating.[44,103]

Skin temperature of horses was measured with an electronic thermometer.[206] The head and trunk were the warmest areas. Temperature decreased proximally to distally on the limbs. Temperature was lower over bony prominences.

°References 89, 103, 137, 166, 169, 175, 178, 184, 197.

Hair

Hair, which is characteristic of mammals, is important in thermal insulation and sensory perception and as a barrier against chemical, physical, actinic, and microbial injury to the skin.[68,124,169,187] The ability of a hair coat to regulate body temperature correlates closely with its length, thickness, and density per unit area and with the medullation of individual hair fibers. In general, hair coats composed of long, fine, poorly medullated fibers, with the coat depth increased by piloerection, are the most efficient for thermal insulation at low environmental temperatures. Coat color is also of some importance in thermal regulation; light-colored coats are more efficient in hot, sunny weather. The glossiness of the coat is important in reflecting sunlight. Transglutaminase is a marker of early anagen hair follicles, and it is important in the protein cross-linking that contributes to the shape and remarkable strength of hair.[68,116] The diameter of the hair shaft is largely determined by the volume of the hair matrix epithelium, and the final length of the hair shaft is determined by both the rate of hair growth and the duration of anagen.

Both primary (outercoat, guard) and secondary (undercoat) hairs are medullated. It has been reported that general body skin has from 2000 to 3000 primary hairs and from 3000 to 5000 secondary hairs, respectively, per cm² of skin.[184] In general, the shape of the hair fiber is determined by the shape of the hair follicle, with straight follicles producing straight hairs and curly follicles producing curly hairs.[166,169,170]

In general, no new hair follicles are formed after birth. The skin surface is smooth or contains grooves and ridges, and hairs emerge from the grooves.[197] Hair follicles and thus emerging hairs are oriented both obliquely and perpendicularly to the skin surface.[55,178,197] In general, the thinner the skin, the more acute the angle of the hair. The direction of the slope of the hairs, which varies from one region of the body to another, gives rise to the *hair tracts*.[170] The study of hair tract patterns is called *trichoglyphics*. The true significance and origin of hair tracts are unknown. With the hair slope generally running caudally and ventrally, benefits include minimal impediment to forward motion and the ability of water to flow off the body to the ground without soaking the hair coat, which would reduce its thermal-insulating properties. No ready explanation is apparent for either the hair coat pattern or the dermal cleavage lines in horses.[155a]

Hair Cycle

Analysis of the factors controlling or influencing hair growth is complicated by evolutionary history.[68,167] The pelage changes as a mammal grows, and that of the adult often differs markedly from that of the juvenile, reflecting different requirements for heat regulation, camouflage, and sexual and social communication. Exmoor and other mountain and moorland ponies that live outdoors in the United Kingdom are considered to have five characteristic hair coats during their lifetime: birth, foal, yearling, adult summer, and adult winter.[188] In addition, the cyclic activity of the hair follicles and the periodic molting of hairs have provided a mechanism by which the pelage can be adapted to seasonal changes in ambient temperature or environmental background. This mechanism is influenced by changes in the photoperiod, which acts through the hypothalamus, hypophysis, and pineal gland, altering levels of various hormones (including melatonin, prolactin, and those of gonadal, thyroidal, and adrenocortical origin) and modifying the inherent rhythms of the hair follicle anlagen and their concurrent downward growth and invasion through the dermis.[129,190,210] Signals controlling hair follicle induction, development, regression, and reactivation have not been identified; however, multiple growth factors or their receptors (e.g., epidermal growth factor [EGF], transforming growth factors [TGF-B_1, TFG-B_2], neurotrophin-3) have been localized to hair follicles and the surrounding mesenchyme. These control cellular proliferation and collagenase release from cultured hair follicles. In addition, an interplay among class I major histocompatibility complex (MHC) expression, chondroitin proteoglycans, and activated macrophages is involved in the regulation of hair growth, especially during the catagen phase.[3,66] Retinoic acid is important in hair shaft-follicular sheath interactions and processing.[214]

Neural mechanisms of hair growth control in mice have revealed that the sensory and autonomic innervation of hair follicles, the substance P content of the skin, and the cutaneous nerve-mast cell contacts show changes during the hair cycle.[150] The trophic effects of cutaneous nerves on follicular growth are exerted via regulation of vascular tone (nutrient and oxygen supply), neuropeptide stimulation of receptors on follicular keratinocytes and dermal papilla fibroblasts, and modulation of macrophage and mast cell activities.

Hairs do not grow continuously but rather in cycles (Fig. 1-1). Each cycle consists of a growing period (*anagen*), during which the follicle is actively producing hair, and a resting period (*telogen*), during which the hair is retained in the follicle as a dead (or *club*) hair that is subsequently lost. There is also a transitional period (*catagen*) between these two stages. The relative duration of the phases of the cycle varies with the age of the individual, the region of the body, the breed, and the sex, and it can be modified by a variety of physiologic or pathologic factors.

The hair cycle, and thus the hair coat, are controlled by photoperiod, ambient temperature, nutrition, hormones, general state of health, genetics, and poorly understood intrinsic factors.* Intrinsic factors include growth factors and cytokines produced by the follicle, the dermal papilla, and other cells (lymphocytes, macrophages, fibroblasts, mast cells) in the immediate environment. Hair replacement in horses is asynchronous (mosaic) in pattern because neighboring hair follicles are in different stages of the hair cycle at any one time. Replacement is unaffected by castration, and it responds predominantly to photoperiod and, to a lesser extent, to ambient temperature.[16,48,49,102]

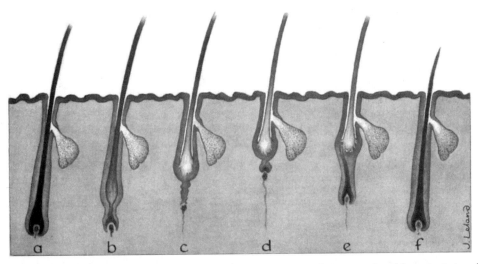

FIGURE 1-1. The hair cycle. *a,* Anagen: During this growing stage, hair is produced by mitosis in cells of the dermal papilla. *b,* Early catagen: In this transitional stage, a constriction occurs at the hair bulb. The hair above this will become a "club." *c,* Catagen: The distal follicle becomes thick and corrugated and pushes the hair outward. *d,* Telogen: This is the resting stage. The dermal papilla separates and an epithelial strand shortens to form a secondary germ. *e,* Early anagen: The secondary germ grows down to enclose the dermal papilla and a new hair bulb forms. The old "club" is lost. *f,* Anagen: The hair elongates as growth continues. *(From Scott DW, Miller WH, Jr, Griffin CE: Muller and Kirk's Small Animal Dermatology, 6th ed. WB Saunders Co, Philadelphia, 2001.)*

---

*References 3, 48, 49, 68, 95, 124, 129, 167, 170, 176, 202, 209.

An exception to this is the coarse permanent hairs of the mane, tail, and fetlock ("horse-hairs").[104,186,197] Mane hairs grow a mean of 0.059 cm/day.[213] Horses in temperate latitudes such as the northern United States, Canada, and the United Kingdom may shed noticeably in the spring.[167,170]

Exmoor and other mountain and moorland ponies living outdoors in the United Kingdom, as well as the Przewalski horse in Czechoslovakia shed once a year between March and May.[127,188] A cold, wet season may delay the shed. The spring shed takes as long as seven weeks, but the date of beginning the shed varies from individual to individual, and in the same individual from year to year. In general, the shed progresses from the limbs and ventral neck and finishes on the back. The short, fine summer coat lasts from June to August. Hair growth increases in autumn, resulting in an increased length and thickness of the hair coat. The long, thick winter coat lasts from September to May. Horses kept blanketed or in heated barns fail to develop a dense winter coat. It has been suggested that domestication and breeding schedules may be causing a shift from periodic to continuous shedding.[167]

Hair grows until it attains its preordained length, which varies according to body region and is genetically determined; it then enters the resting phase, which may last for a considerable amount of time. Each region of the body has its own ultimate length of hair beyond which no further growth occurs. This phenomenon is responsible for the distinctive coat lengths of various breeds and is genetically determined. Equine mane hairs are similar to human scalp hairs in that they grow to a greater length than the rest of the body hairs and have a long anagen growth phase.[214]

Because hair is predominantly protein, nutrition has a profound effect on its quantity and quality (see Chapter 10). Poor nutrition may produce a dull, dry, brittle, or thin hair coat with or without pigmentary disturbances and may result in the retention of the winter hair coat.

Under conditions of ill health or generalized disease, anagen may be considerably shortened; accordingly, a large percentage of body hairs may be in telogen at one time. Because telogen hairs tend to be more easily lost, the animal may shed excessively. Disease states may also lead to faulty formation of hair cuticle, which results in a dull, lusterless coat. Severe illness or systemic stress may cause many hair follicles to enter synchronously and precipitously into telogen. Shedding of these hairs (telogen defluxion; see Chapter 10) thus occurs simultaneously, often resulting in visible thinning of the coat or actual alopecia.

The hair cycle and hair coat are also affected by hormonal changes.[68,124] In general, anagen is initiated and advanced, and hair growth is accelerated, by thyroid hormones and growth hormones. Dermal papilla cells, which are a mesenchymal component of the hair bulb, are considered to play a fundamental role in the induction of epithelial differentiation. These cells are morphologically and functionally differentiated from dermal fibroblasts and are thought to be the primary target cells that respond to hormones and mediate growth-stimulating signals to the follicular epithelial cells.[84]

Obviously, the details of the regulation of hair follicle cycling and growth are extraordinarily complex and poorly understood. The factors that control the hair follicle cycle are, in general, different from the factors that control hair follicle structure. Alterations in factors (e.g., hormones) controlling hair follicle cycle result in *follicular atrophy*. Alterations in factors (e.g., morphogens) that control hair follicle structure result in *follicular dysplasia*.

Attention has been focused on the usefulness of *hair analysis* as a diagnostic tool.[25,174,223] It is well recognized by most dermatologists and nutritionists in human medicine that mineral and trace element analysis of hair samples is not a clinically useful tool in the assessment of nutritional status. For instance, coat color, age of animal, diet, corticosteroid therapy, and even month of the year have been shown to affect the mineral concentration of equine hair.[25] Until and unless adequate scientific documentation of the validity of such multi-element analysis is performed, it is necessary for health professionals and the public to be aware of the very limited value of hair analysis and of the potential to be confused and misled by it.[78b]

Hair has been analyzed for drug abuse in humans for years. A recent study showed a dose-time correlation for morphine concentration in equine mane hairs.[213] Hence, hair analysis may be of use in forensic investigations in horses.

Hair Coat Color

Coat color genetics in horses has been studied in some detail.[2,28,161,204] *Gene W* causes an inability to form pigment in skin and hair. Horses that possess the dominant allele W are typically "white" from birth (skin pink, eyes blue or brown, hair white). Such horses are sometimes called "albino." All nonwhite horses are ww.

Gene G determines exclusion of pigment from hair. The dominant allele G causes a progressive silvering of the hair with age. Such horses are GG or Gg and may be born any color but gradually become "gray" with age. G horses always have pigment in their skin and eyes. The first evidence of the G gene is often seen in foals as gray hairs around the eyes. All nongrays are gg.

Gene B determines black hair pigment. A horse possessing B has black hairs on its points (legs, tail, mane) and/or over most of its body. The b allele allows black pigment in skin but not in hair, resulting in "red" hair (chestnut to sorrel). A horse possessing no black hairs is bb.

Gene A determines the distribution of black hairs. Gene A in combination with B results in black hairs being confined to the points ("bay"). Thus any bay has A and B and is ww and gg.

Gene C determines pigment dilution. The allele C^{cr} causes pigment dilution. Fully pigmented horses are CC. Heterozygotes (Cc^{cr}) have red diluted to yellow, but black is not affected. Thus a bay becomes a "buckskin" and red becomes "palomino." Homozygotes ($c^{cr}c^{cr}$) are completely diluted to a very pale cream color (not white) and have pink skin and blue eyes. Such horses are often called "cremello," "perlino," or "albino."

Gene D determines the dun pattern and pigment dilution. D dilutes both black and red on the body but not on the points. This pigment dilution pattern is called "dun."

Gene To determines the tobiano spotting pattern. Gene To results in a variably restricted pattern of white hair with underlying pink skin in any coat color. The pattern is present at birth and is stable throughout life.

A horse with a mixture of white and dark hairs of any color is called a "roan." Roaning may be present at birth or may not be conspicuous until the first foal coat is shed. Several variable spotting patterns collectively known as "Appaloosa" can be found in any coat color. Besides white spotting, recognizable characteristics of Appaloosas include striped hooves, mottled skin (especially evident around muzzle and eyes), and prominent white sclera. A stable pattern of variable white spotting known as "overo" is characterized by white on the belly or sides of the midsections, which appears to extend upward to, but not including, the center line of the back.

White Camargue horses are black or dark gray at birth and lose their coloring during the course of their lives.[5,65] This process begins at 2 to 4 years of age, and the horses have a characteristic silver-gray coat by about 10 years of age. In one study, the degree of coat pigmentation in white Camargue horses correlated directly with α-MSH plasma levels.[5]

A number of cutaneous patterns or lines are evoked to explain certain distributions of skin lesions encountered clinically.[85] *Voight's lines* are the boundaries of the areas of distribution of the main cutaneous nerve stems. *Langer's lines* reflect the course of blood vessels or lymphatics. *Blaschko's lines* form the pattern assumed by many different nevoid and acquired skin diseases. Blaschko's lines reflect a mosaic condition deriving either from a single mutated clone of cells originating from a postzygotic mutation or from an x-linked mutation made evident by lyonization.[155] These lines follow a V-shape over the spine, an S-shape on the abdomen, an axial distribution on the limbs, and a wavy pattern down the forehead, over and below the eyes, over the upper lip, and behind the ear. *Tension lines* are determined by muscle action, connective tissue fiber orientation and traction, and gravity.

● MICROSCOPIC ANATOMY AND PHYSIOLOGY

The microscopic anatomy and physiology of the skin of horses have been the subjects of several studies (Fig. 1-2).[*]

Epidermis

The outer layer of the skin, or epidermis, is composed of multiple layers of cells defined by position, shape, polarity, morphology, and state of differentiation of the keratinocytes (Figs. 1-2 through 1-5). These are of four distinct types: keratinocytes (about 85% of the epidermal cells), melanocytes (about 5%), Langerhans' cells (3% to 8%), and Merkel's cells (about 2%), which are associated with tylotrich pads. For purposes of identification, certain areas of the epidermis are

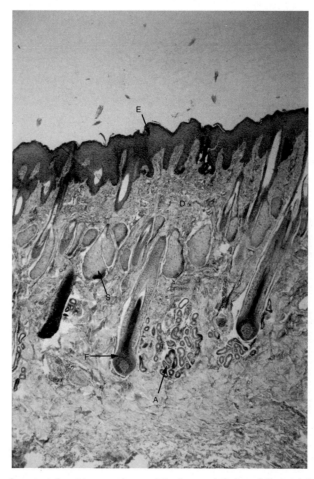

FIGURE 1-2. Normal equine skin. Note epidermis (*E*), dermis (*D*), hair follicles (*F*), sebaceous glands (*S*), and epitrichial sweat glands (*A*).

---

[*]References 20-23, 45, 55, 86, 105, 169, 178, 184, 192, 197, 203.

classified as layers and are named, from inner to outer, as follows: basal layer (stratum basale), spinous layer (stratum spinosum), granular layer (stratum granulosum), clear layer (stratum lucidum), and horny layer (stratum corneum). In general, the epidermis of the horse is 5 to 7 nucleated cell layers thick (not counting the horny layer) in haired general body skin (see Fig. 1-3), ranging from 30 to 95 μm in thickness (average 53 μm).[178,197] The epidermis is thicker in mane and

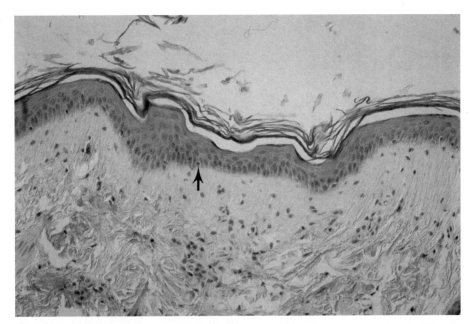

FIGURE 1-3. Appearance of epidermis in normal haired skin. Note melanocytes in basal cell layer (*arrow*).

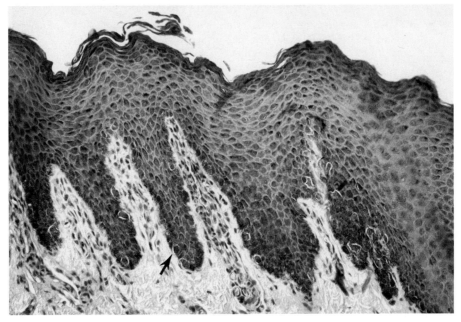

FIGURE 1-4. Appearance of epidermis in normal mucocutaneous junction (lip). Note melanocytes in basal cell layer (*arrow*) and more prominent intercellular spaces.

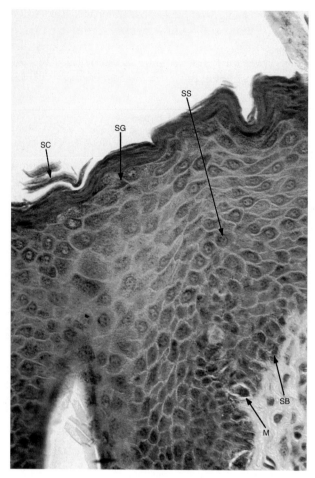

FIGURE 1-5. Close-up of lip epidermis. Note stratum corneum (*SC*), stratum granulosum (*SG*), stratum spinosum (*SS*), stratum basale (*SB*), and melanocytes (*M*).

tail regions (40 to 200 μm, average 91 μm) and near mucocutaneous junctions (40 to 1000 μm, average 238 μm) (see Fig. 1-4).[197] Rete ridges (projections of the epidermis into the underlying dermis) are not found in the normal hair-bearing skin of horses. Rete ridges, however, may be found in relatively glabrous areas (muzzle, mucocutaneous junctions) and the coronary band.

Basal layer. The stratum basale is a single row of columnar or cuboidal cells resting on the basement membrane zone that separates the epidermis from the dermis (see Fig. 1-5). Most of these cells are keratinocytes that are constantly reproducing and pushing upward to replenish the epidermal cells above. The daughter cells move into the outer layers of the epidermis and are ultimately shed as dead horny cells. Mitotic figures and apoptotic keratinocytes are occasionally seen, especially in areas of skin with thicker epidermis. There is morphologic and functional heterogenicity in basal keratinocytes;[45,68] some populations serve primarily to anchor the epidermis, and others serve a proliferative and reparative (stem cell) function. The tips of the deep epidermal rete ridges (in glabrous skin) and the bulb (Wulst) region of the hair follicle (site of attachment of the arrector pili muscle) are the presumed sites of the epidermal and hair follicle stem cells.[111,113] The basal cell layer not only serves as the progenitor cell layer, but also produces the basement membrane, which functions as the site of attachment of the epidermis to the dermis.

● Table 1-1   **COMPONENTS OF ADHESION STRUCTURES**

ADHESION STRUCTURE	TRANSMEMBRANE PROTEINS	PLAQUE PROTEINS	CYTOSKELETON FILAMENTS	FUNCTION AND LOCATION
Hemidesmosome	$\alpha_6\beta_4$ integrin, BPAGII° (collagen Type VII)	Plectin, BPAGI	Cytokeratin	Cell-substrate adhesion; basal cells and basal membrane
Focal adhesion	β_1 integrins ($\alpha_2\beta_1$, $\alpha_3\beta_1$, $\alpha_5\beta_1$)	Talin, vinculin, α-actinin, paxillin, zykin	Actin	Cell-substrate, basal cells
Desmosome	Desmosomal cadherins Dsg† I, II, III Dsc‡ I, II, III	Plakoglobin; desmoplakin I, II, IV; desmocalmin; plakophilin	Cytokeratin	Cell-cell adhesion; all keratinocytes
Adherens junction	Classical cadherins (E- and P-cadherins)	Plakoglobin, α- and β-catenin, α-actin, vinculin	Actin	Cell-cell adhesion; all keratinocytes (p-cadherin in basal cells only)

°BPAG, Bullous pemphigoid antigen.
†Dsg, Desmoglein.
‡Dsc, Desmocollin.

Hemidesmosomes are junctional complexes distributed along the inner aspect of basal keratinocytes, whose major role is epidermal-dermal adhesion.[68,152] The linkage of the keratin intermediate filament (cytokeratin) network to the hemidesmosome and basal keratinocyte plasma membrane involves several components, including the plaque proteins bullous pemphigoid antigen I (BPAG I or BP 230) and plectin, the transmembrane proteins $\alpha_6\beta_4$ integrin and BPAG II (BPAG 180 or collagen XVII), and laminin 5.[114,128,191] Various inherited or acquired defects in the hemidesmosome-anchoring filament components are known to produce various forms of epidermolysis bullosa and pemphigoid.[18,128]

Integrins are a large family of cell surface adhesive receptors.[114,191] These cell surface glycoproteins are important in cell-cell and cell-matrix interactions and also act as signal transducers through which extracellular and intracellular components can influence and modify each other. Each integrin consists of a heterodimer of an α and a β subunit, which are noncovalently associated. In the epidermis, integrin expression is normally confined to the basal layer. The integrin subunits that are most abundant in the epidermis are α_2, α_3, β_1, α_6, and β_4. Examples of keratinocyte integrin functions include $\alpha_5\beta_1$, which mediates keratinocyte adhesion to fibronectin; $\alpha_2\beta_1$, which mediates keratinocyte adhesion to collagens Type I and IV and laminin; $\alpha_3\beta_1$, which is a receptor for epiligrin and is involved in adhesion to laminin; $\alpha_1\beta_5$, which mediates keratinocyte adhesion to vitronectin; and $\alpha_6\beta_4$, which mediates keratinocyte adhesion to laminin (Table 1-1).[114]

Melanocytes and melanogenesis. Melanocytes, the second type of cell found in the basal layer of the epidermis (see Figs. 1-3 through 1-6), are also found in the outer root sheath and hair matrix of hair follicles, in the ducts of sebaceous and sweat glands, and perivascularly in the superficial dermis.° Traditionally, melanocytes are divided structurally and functionally into two compartments: epidermal and follicular.[68] Because melanocytes do not stain readily with hematoxylin and eosin (H & E) and because they undergo artifactual cytoplasmic shrinkage during tissue processing, they appear as clear cells. In general, there is one melanocyte per 10 to 20 keratinocytes in the basal layer. They are derived from the neural crest and migrate into the epidermis, adnexal epithelia, and superficial dermis in early fetal life. Although melanocytes are of nondescript appearance, with special stains (DOPA reaction, Fontana's ammoniacal silver nitrate)

°References 45, 53, 68, 115, 152, 197, 214, 219.

they can be seen to have long cytoplasmic extensions (dendrites) that weave among the keratinocytes. There is an intimate relationship between melanocytes and keratinocytes in which both cells interact and exist as epidermal symbionts—a functional and structural unit called the *epidermal melanin unit*.[68,115,152,202] The epidermal melanin unit is dynamic and highly responsive to endogenous and exogenous stimuli.[139] There is a complex communication among the melanocyte, its corresponding keratinocytes, and the surrounding epidermal environment that determines the constitutive level of melanocyte function. Ultrastructurally, melanocytes are characterized by typical intracytoplasmic melanosomes and premelanosomes and a cell membrane–associated basal lamina (Fig. 1-7). Most of the melanin pigment in the skin is located in the basal layer of the epidermis, but in dark-skinned animals melanin may be found throughout the entire epidermis, as well as within superficial dermal melanocytes. Melanin granules are often clustered as "caps" dorsal to keratinocyte nuclei, presumably a photoprotective localization.

Although the melanocyte accounts for only a small proportion of the epidermal cells, it serves a variety of important roles: (1) a cosmetic entity, participating in protective coloration and in sexual attraction; (2) a barrier against ionizing radiation, especially important in protection against ultraviolet light (UVL); (3) a scavenger of cytotoxic radicals and intermediates; and (4) a participant in developmental and inflammatory processes.[68,115,152] Although melanin absorbs UVL over a broad spectrum, including UVA and UVB, it is not a particularly efficient absorber of UVL. It probably photoprotects in other ways, possibly as a quencher of free radicals generated in response to UVL. In dark-skinned horses, melanin granules are present throughout all layers of the epidermis and are especially prominent in the stratum basale and the first cell layer of the stratum spinosum.

Melanin pigments are chiefly responsible for the coloration of skin and hair. Skin pigmentation is considered to consist of two components. *Constitutive* pigmentation is the pigmentation that is genetically determined in the absence of stimulatory influences. *Facultative* pigmentation is that which occurs with various stimuli (e.g., UVL, inflammation, hormones).

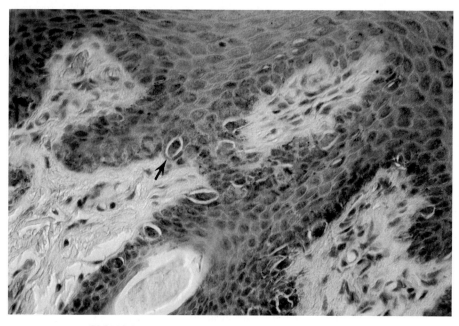

FIGURE 1-6. Melanocytes (*arrow*) in normal epidermis.

Melanins embrace a wide range of pigments, including the brown-black eumelanins, yellow or red-brown pheomelanins, and other pigments whose physicochemical natures are intermediate between the two. Pheomelanins differ from eumelanins by containing high proportion of sulfur. Despite the different properties of the various melanins, they all arise from a common metabolic pathway in which dopaquinone is the key intermediate.[68,129]

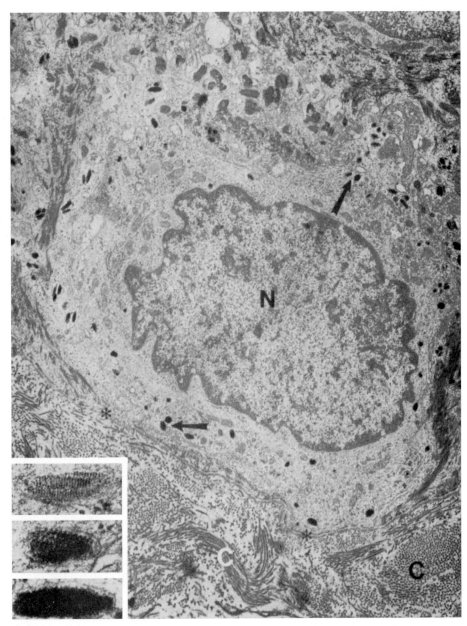

FIGURE 1-7. Melanocyte. *N*, Nucleus of melanocyte; *arrows*, melanosomes; *C*, collagen in the dermis; *asterisk*, basal lamina (× 10,000). Insets: Melanosomes in different stages of development: *upper inset*, Stage II; *middle inset*, Stage III; *lower inset*, Stage IV (× 75,000). (*From Lever WF, Schaumburg-Lever G: Histopathology of the Skin, 7th ed. JB Lippincott Co, Philadelphia, 1990.*)

Melanogenesis takes place exclusively within melanocytes and on the specialized organelle, the melanosome.[68,115,152] Here, the specific enzyme, tyrosinase, catalyzes the conversion of tyrosine to dopa. Tyrosinase is the rate-limiting enzyme in the melanin pathway. It is a copper-containing enzyme, is found exclusively in melanocytes, and is thus a good specific marker for these cells. Tyrosinase is an unusual enzyme in that it has three distinct catalytic activities. The most critical is its tyrosinase hydroxylase activity, converting tyrosine to dopa. However, it is also able to use dopa or 5,6-dihydroxyindole (DHI) as substrates for oxidase activities. Mutations in the tyrosine structural gene are responsible for several types of albinism.[152]

Once dopa is formed, it can spontaneously auto-oxidize to dopaquinone without tyrosinase (though at slower rates) and continue through the melanin pathway to dopachrome, 5,6-dihydroxy-indole-2-carboxylic acid (DHICA), DHI, and indole-5,6-quinone.[68,115,152] Another melanocyte-specific enzyme is dopachrome tautomerase, which converts dopachrome to DHICA.[115,152] This conversion requires the presence of iron.

The determination to produce eumelanins or pheomelanins is under genetic control.[24,68,115,152] If sulfhydryl groups are available, pheomelanins are produced. It has been proposed that the "switching" of melanin synthesis is mainly controlled by the levels of tyrosinase, with high levels producing eumelanins and low levels producing pheomelanins.[152]

Mammalian pigmentation is regulated at many different developmental, cellular, and subcellular levels, and is influenced by many genes.[68,115,152] Although melanocytes in the skin have characteristic basal levels of function that are particular to each individual, they are highly responsive cells that continually sample their environment and modulate their levels of proliferation and melanogenesis. Classically, melanin production was thought to be under the control of genetics and melanocyte-stimulating hormone (MSH) from the pituitary gland.[63,68,202] The main pigmenting hormones from the pituitary gland include α-MSH (α-melanocortin), adrenal cortical stimulating hormone (corticotropin), and β-lipotropic hormone (β-lipotropin).[115,152] These hormones are derived from a larger precursor molecule, proopiomelanocortin. However, the role of these hypophyseal origin hormones in physiologic and pathologic pigmentation in mammals is largely unknown. At present, interest focuses on the theory that melanogenesis and melanocyte proliferation and differentiation are most often regulated locally in paracrine and autocrine fashion.

Melanocytes express a number of cell surface receptors (e.g., intercellular adhesion molecule 1 [ICAM-1]) that allow interaction with other cells in their environment, including keratinocytes, Langerhans' cells, fibroblasts, lymphocytes, and macrophages.[115,152,214] They express receptors for and respond to (modifying their proliferation, differentiation, and melanogenesis) growth factor (e.g., β fibroblast growth factor), hormones, interferons, interleukins, eicosanoids, retinoic acid, vitamin D_3, and a host of other cytokines. In fact, melanocytes are able to produce some of these themselves, thus acting in an autocrine manner. Melanocytes themselves secrete several cytokines (e.g., interleukin-8 [IL-8]) and participate in inflammatory and immunologic reactions. Many of the precursors and intermediates of the melanin biosynthetic pathway are cytotoxic and could contribute to cellular injury and inflammation. It can be appreciated that a highly complex interaction exists between the cellular components of the epidermis, their respective immune cytokines, and the inflammatory mediators released in response to injury.

α-MSH is a neuroimmunomodulatory and anti-inflammatory peptide that is synthesized and released by keratinocytes, Langerhans' cells, fibroblasts, and endothelial cells, as well as melanocytes themselves.[115,123,152] α-MSH cell surface receptors can also be identified on these cells. α-MSH can, hence, modulate keratinocyte proliferation and differentiation, and endothelial cell and fibroblast cytokine and collagenase production. It also downregulates the production of proinflammatory cytokines and accessory molecules on antigen-presenting cells (monocytes and macrophages). α-MSH is an antagonist of IL-1, an important cytokine in the cutaneous immune response. Thus α-MSH is part of a mediator network that modulates cutaneous inflammation and hyperproliferative skin disorders. This may be far more important than any effect it has on skin pigmentation.

Melanogenesis takes place in membrane-bound organelles called *melanosomes*,[68,124] designated Stages I through IV according to maturation (see Fig. 1-7). It is often stated that the ultrastructural hallmark of the melanocyte is the melanosome. However, it is more accurate to say that Stage I melanosomes are melanocyte-specific, because later stage melanosomes may be found in keratinocytes and other phagocytic cells.[115] Melanosomes originate from the Golgi apparatus where the tyrosinase enzyme is formed. Stage I melanosomes contain no melanin and are electron-lucent. As melanin is progressively laid down on protein matrices, melanosomes become increasingly electron-dense. At the same time, they migrate to the periphery of the dendrites, where transfer of melanin to adjacent keratinocytes takes place. Transfer involves the endocytosis of the dendrite tips and the incorporated Stage IV melanosomes by the adjacent keratinocytes. Melanocytes eject melanosomes into keratinocytes by a unique biologic transfer process called *cytocrinia*.[68] Dermal melanocytes are often referred to as *continent* melanocytes, because they do not transfer melanosomes as do the epidermal or *secretory* melanocytes. Skin color is determined mainly by the number, size, type, and distribution of melanosomes.

At present, there are no histochemical stains that can be performed on routinely processed skin biopsy specimens that exclusively stain melanin.[115] *Argentaffin* stains rely on the ability of melanin to reduce silver from a silver solution (e.g., silver nitrate). Examples of argentaffin stains include Fontana-Masson and Gomori's methenamine silver. These agents also stain neurosecretory granules and formalin pigment. *Argyrophil* stains are similar to argentaffin stains but use an external silver reducer to produce elemental silver. An example of an argyrophil stain is Grimelius' stain. Argyrophil stains also stain nerves, reticulum, and elastic fibers.

Merkel's cells. Merkel's cells are dendritic epidermal clear cells confined to the basal cell layer, or just below, and occur in touch corpuscles (tylotrich pads) and the bulge region of the hair follicle (Fig. 1-8).[45,68,115,214] These specialized cells (slow-adapting mechanoreceptors) contain a large cytoplasmic vacuole that displaces the cell nucleus dorsally, and their long axis is usually parallel to the skin surface. They possess desmosomes and characteristic dense-core cytoplasmic granules and paranuclear whorls on electron microscopic examination (Fig. 1-9). Merkel's cells also contain cytokeratin, neurofilaments, and neuron-specific enolase, suggesting a dual epithelial and neural differentiation. Current evidence suggests that Merkel's cells are derived from a primitive epidermal stem cell.[45,68,114,158] Merkel's cells may have other functions, such as influencing cutaneous blood flow and sweat production (via the release of vasoactive intestinal peptide), coordinating keratinocyte proliferation, and maintaining and stimulating the stem cell population of the hair follicle (hence controlling the hair cycle).[68,214]

Spinous layer. The stratum spinosum (prickle cell layer) is composed of the daughter cells of the stratum basale (see Fig. 1-5).[68,197] In general body haired skin, this layer is 2 to 4 cells thick. The spinous layer becomes much thicker at mucocutaneous junctions, on the muzzle, and at the coronary band. The cells are lightly basophilic to eosinophilic, nucleated, and polyhedral to flattened cuboidal in shape. The keratinocytes of the stratum spinosum appear to be connected by intercellular bridges (prickles), which are more prominent in nonhaired skin.

Keratinocyte adhesion is mediated by four major types of adhesive and communicative structures: desmosomes, hemidesmosomes, adherens junctions, and focal adhesions (see Table 1-1).[68,114] Hemidesmosomes and focal adhesions are located on the basal surface of basal cells and mediate adhesion to the underlying extracellular matrix, whereas desmosomes and adherens junctions (containing the classic cadherins, E-cadherin and P-cadherin) mediate adhesion between keratinocytes in all epidermal layers. *Gap junctions* are formed by the protruding ends of many identical protein complexes that lie in the plasma membranes of apposed cells. These

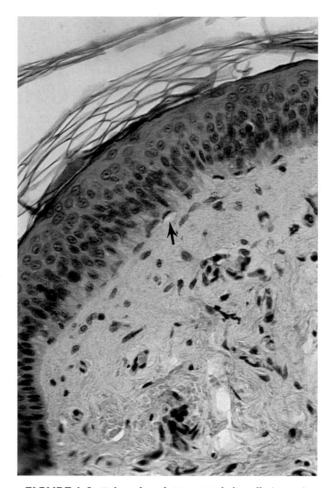

FIGURE 1-8. Tylotrich pad. Note Merkel's cells (*arrow*).

protein complexes are called *connexons*, and each connexon is made of 6 *connexins*. Gap junctions serve primarily as intercellular routes of chemical communication.[114,152]

Because of the research efforts directed at defining the pathomechanism of pemphigus, much has been learned concerning the structure and chemical composition of epidermal desmosomes.[68,114] Desmosomes are presently known to consist of keratin intermediate filaments and their attachment plaques, the keratinocyte plasma membrane, and the desmosomal core (desmoglea), which is interposed between two adjacent keratinocyte plasma membranes. Numerous desmosomal plaque proteins (desmoplakins I and II, plakoglobin, plakophilin, keratocalmin) and desmosomal core glycoproteins (which contain the desmosomal cadherins, desmogleins I, II, III and desmocollins I, II, III) have been characterized. The immunohistochemical staining pattern seen with human pemphigus foliaceus antibody is identical to that seen with an antibody directed at desmoglein I (desmosomal core glycoprotein).

Proteins of the plakoglobin (plakoglobin, β-catenin), vinculin (vinculin, α-catenin), and ezrin (talin, radixin) families are found at desmosomal and adherens junction attachments.[114]

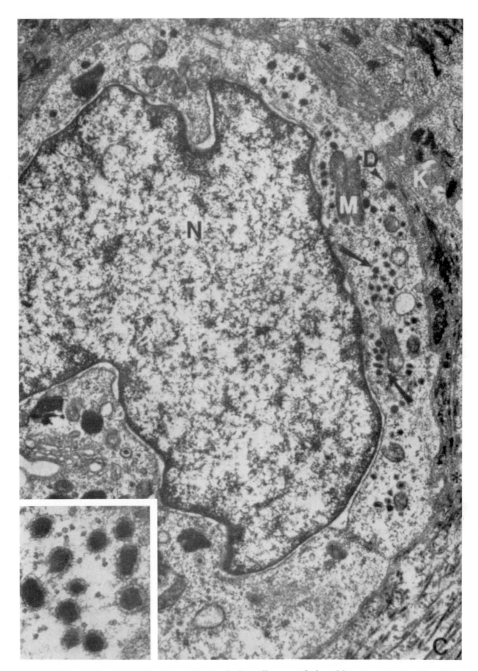

FIGURE 1-9. Merkel's cell. *N,* Nucleus of a Merkel's cell; *asterisk,* basal lamina; *M,* mitochondria; *arrows,* specific granules of the Merkel's cell; *D with pointer,* desmosome between the Merkel's cell and a keratinocyte, *K; C,* collagen with cross-striation (× 20,000). *Inset:* Specific membrane-bound granules at higher magnification (× 75,000). (*From Lever WF, Schaumburg-Lever G: Histopathology of the Skin, 7th ed. JB Lippincott Co, Philadelphia, 1990.*)

The keratinocyte cytoskeleton consists of three types of cytoplasmic filaments: cytokeratin, actin, and microtubules (tubulin).[114] These filaments function in the orientation, polarization, organelle sorting, motility, shape change, signal transduction, and structural resilience of keratinocytes.

Ultrastructurally, keratinocytes are characterized by tonofilaments and desmosomes (Fig. 1-10).[53,68,114] Calcium and calmodulin are crucial for desmosome and hemidesmosome formation. At least three keratinocyte-derived calmodulin-binding proteins participate in a flip-flop regulation (calcium concentration–dependent) of calcium-calmodulin interactions: caldesmon, desmocalmin, and spectrin.[68] Immunohistochemically, keratinocytes are characterized by the presence of cytokeratins.[68] All epithelia express a keratin pair: one keratin chain from the acidic subfamily (Type I keratins, cytokeratins 9-20) and one chain from the neutral-basic subfamily (Type II keratins, cytokeratins 1-8).[*] The keratin pairs change with different epithelia, and in the same epithelia at various stages of differentiation or proliferation. A number of workers have published electrophoretic patterns of proteins isolated from the keratins of a variety of animals and, on the basis of observed differences in banding patterns, have suggested that the technique might be useful as an aid to taxonomy, animal classification, and identification.[68] The keratinocytes of the stratum spinosum synthesize lamellar granules (keratinosomes, membrane-coating granules, Odland bodies), which are important in the barrier function of the epidermis (Fig. 1-11).[68] Keratinocytes are phagocytic (erythrocytes, melanin, melanosomes, cellular fragments, latex beads, inorganic substances) and play a role in the metabolism of potentially toxic compounds.[17,45,63] Culture techniques for equine keratinocytes have been described.[218]

The epidermis and the hair follicle epithelium have the capability to process and metabolize molecules in a manner similar to the liver.[45,63] The skin has a highly inducible cytochrome P-450–dependent microsomal mixed function oxidase system capable of metabolizing and conjugating a variety of compounds. The skin is believed to be a first line of metabolic defense against topical exposure to toxic compounds.

Langerhans' cells. Langerhans' cells are mononuclear, dendritic, antigen-presenting cells located in the suprabasal epidermis and the dermis.[45,68,74,214] They are epidermal clear cells that, like Merkel's cells, do not stain for melanin with DOPA. Langerhans' cells have characteristic intracytoplasmic organelles (Birbeck's or Langerhans' granules), which are observed by means of electron microscopy (Fig. 1-12).[45,68,73,107,214] Birbeck's granules are variously described as having an appearance similar to a zipper, rod, flask, or tennis racket. They form by invagination of the plasma membrane and bound antigen, thus providing the morphologic description of the mechanism by which Langerhans' cells internalize surface-bound antigen for processing and representation at the surface.[114] Langerhans' cells are aureophilic (i.e., they stain with gold chloride), and they contain membrane-associated adenosine triphosphatase, as well as vimentin, CD45 (common leukocyte antigen), and S-100 protein (immunohistochemical markers). They are most specifically identified by monoclonal antibodies to CD1. Langerhans' cells have Fc fragment (Fc)–IgG and complement 3 (C3) receptors, high-affinity receptors for IgE, and they synthesize and express antigens associated with the immune response gene. These cells are of bone marrow origin, of monocyte-macrophage lineage, and serve antigen-processing and alloantigen-stimulating functions. Following ultraviolet light exposure, epidermal Langerhans' cells are decreased in density and altered morphologically, resulting in an immunosuppressive environment and antigen-specific tolerance.[67,68] Topical or systemic glucocorticoids are known to depress Langerhans' cell numbers and function.[68] The number of Langerhans' cells per unit of skin varies from one area of skin to another in the same individual, emphasizing the need to use adjacent normal skin as a control when counting Langerhans' cells in skin lesions.[68]

---

[*]References 18, 68, 73, 114, 177, 209a.

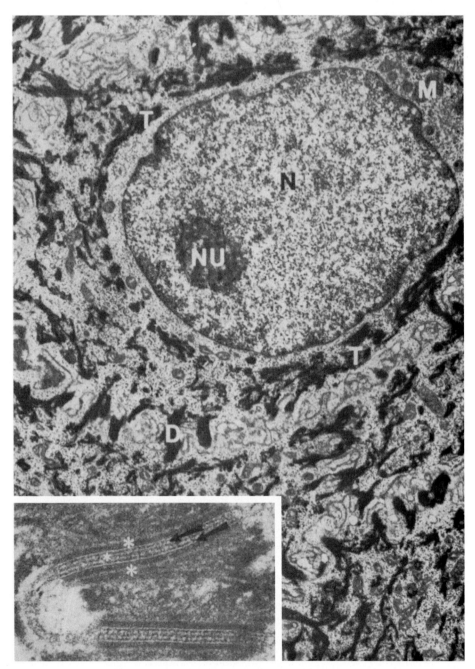

FIGURE 1-10. Squamous cell. *N*, Nucleus; *NU*, nucleolus; *T*, tonofilaments; *D*, desmosome; *M*, mito-chondria (× 12,500). *Inset*: Desmosomes at higher magnification (× 100,000). A desmosome connecting two adjoining keratinocytes consists of nine lines: five electron-dense lines and four electron-lucid lines. The two peripheral dense, thick lines (*large asterisks*) are the attachment plaques. The single electron-dense line in the center of the desmosome (*small asterisk*) is the intracellular contact layer. The two electron-dense lines between the intercellular contact layer and the two attachment plaques represent the cell surface coat together with the outer leaflet of the trilaminar plasma membrane of each keratinocytes (*arrows*). The two inner electron-lucid lines adjacent to the intercellular contact layer represent intercellular cement. The two outer electron-lucid lines are the central lamina of the trilaminar plasma membrane. (*From Lever WF, Schaumburg-Lever G: Histopathology of the Skin, 7th ed. JB Lippincott Co, Philadelphia, 1990.*)

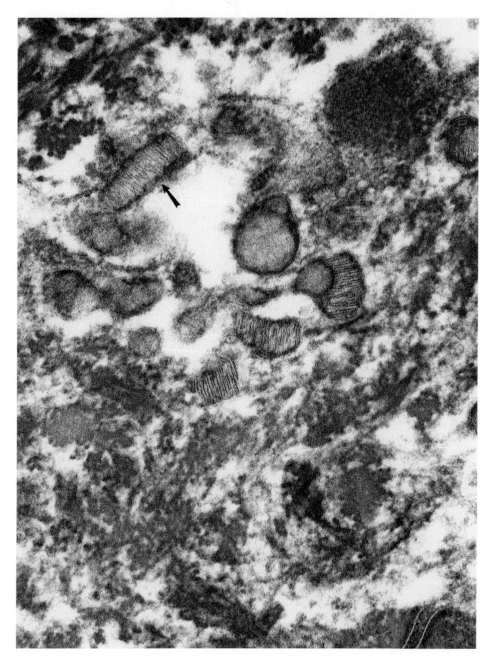

FIGURE 1-11. Electron micrograph of equine keratinocyte. Note lamellar granules (*arrow*).

The skin as an immunologic organ. The epidermis functions as the most peripheral outpost of the immune system. Langerhans' cells, keratinocytes, epidermotropic T lymphocytes, and draining peripheral lymph nodes are thought to form collectively an integrated system of *skin-associated lymphoid tissue (SALT)* or *skin immune system (SIS)* that mediates cutaneous immunosurveillance.[19,68,202,214,220] *Langerhans' cells* stimulate the proliferation of relevant helper T lymphocytes by the presentation of antigen; they also induce cytotoxic T lymphocytes directed to

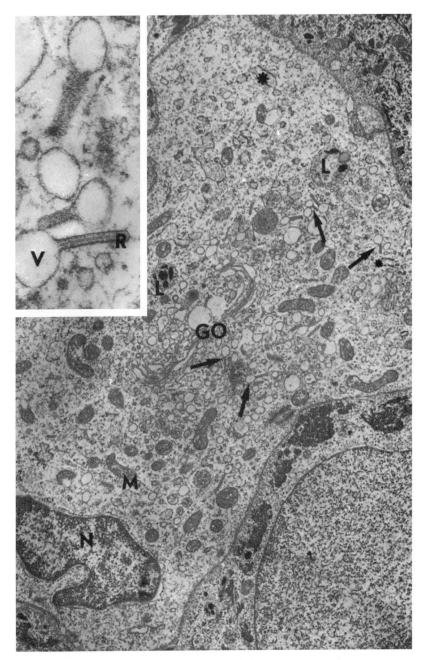

FIGURE 1-12. Electron micrograph of an epidermal Langerhans' cell. (*From Elder D, et al: Lever's Histopathology of the Skin, 8th ed. Lippincott-Raven, Philadelphia, 1998.*)

allogenic and modified self-determinants, produce interleukin (IL)-1 and other cytokines, contain numerous enzymes, and are phagocytic.[19,68,114,202,214]

Keratinocytes play an active role in epidermal immunity.[19,68,152] They (1) produce interleukins (IL-1, IL-2, IL-3, IL-8); (2) produce numerous other cytokines (e.g., prostaglandins, leukotrienes, interferon, colony-stimulating factors); (3) are phagocytic; and (4) can express antigens associated with the immune response gene in a variety of lymphocyte-mediated skin diseases (presumably as a result of interferon-γ secretion by activated lymphocytes).[19,68,75,114,202]

Granular layer. The stratum granulosum ranges from 1 to 2 cells thick in general body haired skin and is thicker at mucocutaneous junctions and at the infundibulum of hair follicles.[197] Cells in this layer are flattened and basophilic, and they contain shrunken nuclei and large, deeply basophilic keratohyalin granules in their cytoplasm (see Fig. 1-5). Keratohyalin granules are not true granules: they lack a membrane and are more accurately described as insoluble aggregates. Keratohyalin granules are the morphologic equivalents of the structural protein profilaggrin, which is the precursor of filaggrin and is synthesized in the stratum granulosum.[68,108,109] Keratohyalin granules are important in keratinization and barrier function. The sulfur-rich component of keratohyalin is a precursor to the cornified cell envelope. Filaggrin has two functions: (1) it aggregates, packs, and aligns keratin filaments and produces the matrix between keratin filaments in the corneocytes; and (2) it is a source of free amino acids which are essential for the normal hydration and barrier function of the stratum corneum ("natural moisturizing factor").

Loricrin is synthesized in the stratum granulosum in association with keratohyalin granules and is involved in the binding of keratin filaments together in the corneocyte and in anchoring them to the cross-linked envelope.[152] Another ultrastructural feature that characterizes granular cells are clustered lamellar granules at the margins of the cells.

In rodents, two morphologic forms of keratohyalin granules occur.[114] The P-F granule is irregularly shaped and contains profilaggrin, whereas the L-granule is smaller, rounded, and contains loricrin.

Clear layer. The stratum lucidum is a fully keratinized, compact layer of dead cells.[68] This layer is anuclear, homogeneous, and hyaline-like. The stratum lucidum apparently does not occur in equine skin.[197] The stratum lucidum has also been called the *stratum conjunctum*.

Horny layer. The stratum corneum is the outer layer of completely keratinized tissue that is constantly being shed.[68,197] It is a multilayered zone of corneocytes suspended in an extracellular lipid matrix, often likened to a series of bricks (corneocytes) bonded by mortar (lipids).[114] This layer, which consists of flattened, anuclear, eosinophilic cells called *corneocytes*, is thicker in lightly haired or glabrous skin (see Figs. 1-3 and 1-5). Its gradual desquamation is normally balanced by proliferation of the basal cells, which maintains a constant epidermal thickness. Corneocytes contain a variety of humectants and natural sunscreens that are synthesized from proteins.[152]

The terminally differentiated corneocyte has a highly specialized structure in the cell periphery, the *cell envelope*, which assumes protective functions.[68] It develops beneath the plasma membrane of stratified epidermal cells, and the cells of the inner root sheath and medulla of the hair follicle. The corneocyte has no true cell membrane because it contains no phospholipids. Cell envelope formation is associated with the increased activity of calcium-dependent epidermal or hair follicle transglutaminases that catalyze the cross-linking of soluble and particulate protein precursors into large, insoluble polymers. Major cytoplasmic protein precursors of the cell envelope synthesized in the stratum spinosum include involucrin, keratolinin, pancornulin, cornifin, and loricrin.° The impermeable cornified envelope provides structural support to the cell and resists invasion by microorganisms and deleterious environmental agents; however, it does not appear to have a significant role in regulating permeability. The stratum corneum has also been called the *stratum dysjunctum*.

In routinely processed sections, the stratum corneum in general body haired skin varies in thickness from 12 to 55 μm and is approximately one-half to equal the width of the subjacent

°References 51, 68, 108, 109, 114, 152, 177.

nucleated epidermis.[184] However, clipping and histologic preparation involving fixation, dehydration, and paraffin embedding result in the loss of about one-half of the stratum corneum. The loose, basket-weave appearance of the stratum corneum as seen in routinely processed sections is also an artifact of fixation and processing.[68]

Transglutaminases are a superfamily of enzymes that are important in apoptosis, keratinization, and hair follicle formation.[80] Two members of the superfamily—keratinocyte transglutaminase and epidermal transglutaminase—mediate the sequential cross-linking of the cornified cell envelope precursor proteins, such as involucrin, cytostan A, elafin, and loricrin. Transglutaminases are chiefly expressed in the stratum granulosum and upper stratum spinosum and require catalytic amino acids and calcium. Faulty keratinocyte transglutaminase expression is one cause of ichthyosis in humans.[80]

Lipids play an important role in barrier protection, stratum corneum water-holding, cohesion and desquamation of corneocytes, and control of epidermal proliferation and differentiation.[68,108,109,177] Epidermal lipid composition changes dramatically during keratinization, beginning with large amounts of phospholipids and ending with predominantly ceramides, cholesterol, and fatty acids. Epidermal surface lipids originate from maturing corneocytes, which contain about six times the amount of intracellular lipid as keratinocytes in the stratum basale. Skin surface lipids of horses were studied by thin-layer chromatography and found to contain more monoester sterols and waxes, diester waxes, and cholesterol, but fewer triglycerides and free fatty acids than those of humans.* No significant differences were found between individuals or breeds.[43] Equine sebum is unique in its content of giant ring lactones.[118] Surface lipids, unlike smegma, contained no squalene.[142,143] It was suggested that the surface lipids of horses are mainly of epidermal rather than sebaceous gland origin.

The stratum corneum contains antigenic or superantigenic material normally sequestered from the immune system that induces T lymphocyte activation when released following wounding and in disease.[72] This T lymphocyte activation and resultant inflammatory response may play a role in a range of skin pathologies.

Epidermopoiesis and keratogenesis. Normal epidermal homeostasis requires a finely tuned balance between growth and differentiation of keratinocytes. This balance must be greatly shifted in the direction of proliferation in response to injury and then must return to a state of homeostasis with healing. In addition, epidermal keratinocytes have important functions as regulators of cutaneous immunity and inflammation.

The most important product of the epidermis is keratin, a highly stable, disulfide bond–containing fibrous protein. The term *keratin* is derived from the Greek word *keratos*, meaning "horn." This substance is the major barrier between animal and environment, the so-called miracle wrap of the body. Prekeratin, a fibrous protein synthesized in the keratinocytes of the stratum basale and stratum spinosum, appears to be the precursor of the fully differentiated stratum corneum proteins.[68,202] Keratins have classically been divided into *soft* keratins (skin) and *hard* keratins (hair, hoof) or α-keratins (skin, hair) and β-keratins (scale, feather).[152,222]

The epidermis is ectodermal in origin and normally undergoes an orderly pattern of proliferation, differentiation, and keratinization.[68,108,109] The factors controlling this orderly epidermal pattern are incompletely understood, but the protein kinase C/phospholipase C second messenger system, the calcium/calmodulin second messenger system, the receptor-linked tyrosine kinases, and the adenylate cyclase/cyclic AMP–dependent protein kinases are important in coupling extracellular signals to essential biologic processes such as the immune response, inflammation, differentiation, and proliferation.[68] Among the intrinsic factors known to play a modulating role in these processes are the dermis, ECG, FGFs, insulin-like growth factors, colony-stimulating

---

*References 43, 68, 118, 142, 143, 211, 212.

factors, platelet-derived growth factor, TGFs, neuropeptides, interleukins, TNF, epidermal chalone, epibolin, tenascin, interferons, acid hydrolases, arachidonic acid metabolites, proteolytic enzymes (endopeptidases and exopeptidases or peptidases), and various hormones (particularly epinephrine, vitamin D_3, and cortisol).* In addition, there appears to be a host of hormones and enzymes that can induce, increase, or both induce and increase the activity of the enzyme ornithine decarboxylase.[68] This enzyme is essential for the biosynthesis of polyamines (putrescine, spermidine, and spermine), which encourage epidermal proliferation. Numerous nutritional factors are also known to be important for normal keratinization, including protein, fatty acids, zinc, copper, vitamin A, and the B vitamins.[68]

There are four distinct cellular events in the process of cornification: (1) keratinization (synthesis of the principal fibrous proteins of the keratinocyte); (2) keratohyalin synthesis (including the histidine-rich protein filaggrin); (3) the formation of the highly cross-linked, insoluble stratum corneum peripheral envelope (including the structural protein involucrin); and (4) the generation of neutral, lipid-enriched intercellular domains, resulting from the secretion of distinctive lamellar granules. The lamellar granules are synthesized primarily within the keratinocytes of the stratum spinosum and are then displaced to the apex and periphery of the cell as it reaches the stratum granulosum. They fuse with the plasma membrane and secrete their contents (phospholipids, ceramides, free fatty acids, hydrolytic enzymes, and sterols). Intercellular lipids then undergo substantial alterations and assume an integral role in the regulation of stratum corneum barrier function and desquamation.

Epidermal lipids directly or indirectly influence the proliferative and biochemical events in normal and diseased skin and mediate interactions between the "dead" stratum corneum and the "living" nucleated epidermal layers.[68,109,152] Dynamic transformations in lipid composition and structure occur as cells migrate through the epidermis. Ceramides are the most important lipid component for lamellar arrangement in the stratum corneum and barrier function. Polyunsaturated fatty acids are important because they are incorporated into the ceramides. Arachidonic acid is bound to the phospholipid in cell membranes and is the important precursor of eicosanoids. The eicosanoids are vital for epidermal homeostasis and the pathogenesis of inflammatory dermatoses. Lipids are important in barrier function, stratum corneum water-holding, cohesion and desquamation of corneocytes, and control of epidermal proliferation and differentiation.

The main changes in epidermal lipid composition are the replacement of phospholipids by ceramides, an increase in free sterols, and a large increase in free fatty acids at the expense of triglyceride and phospholipid.[109,152] This transformation of lipid provides the outer epidermal layers with a much more stable, waxy, impermeable lipid barrier. Ceramides play a crucial role in plasticizing the horny layer to allow stretching and bending by fluidizing the barrier lipids.

The clinical importance of epidermal lipids in disorders of keratinization is illustrated by the following examples: (1) the scaling and poor barrier function due to abnormal lamellar granules, defective ceramides, and deranged eicosanoid production associated with essential fatty acid deficiency; (2) the scaling and poor barrier function due to the loss of ceramides, cholesterol, fatty acids, waxes, and sterols associated with exposure to solvents and detergents; (3) the poor desquamation due to the steroid sulfatase defect and resultant increased accumulation of cholesterol sulfate associated with recessive X-linked ichthyosis of humans; (4) the scaling and abnormal lipid packing due to a defect in phytanic acid oxidase production in Refsum disease of humans; (5) the hyperkeratosis and defective lamellar granules in Harlequin ichthyosis of humans; and (6) the scaling and poor barrier function due to the inhibition of epidermal cholesterol synthesis seen with the administration of hypocholesterolemic agents in humans.[109,152]

---

*References 68, 108, 109, 117, 145, 151, 221.

Tritiated thymidine labeling techniques have shown that the turnover (cell renewal) time for the viable epidermis (stratum basale to stratum granulosum) of horses is approximately 17 days.[9]

Cutaneous ecology. The skin forms a protective barrier without which life would be impossible. This defense has three components: physical, chemical, and microbial.[68] Hair forms the first physical line of defense to prevent contact of pathogens with the skin and to minimize external physical or chemical insult to the skin. Hair also harbors microorganisms.

The stratum corneum forms the basic physical defense barrier. Its thick, tightly packed keratinized cells are permeated by an emulsion of sebum and sweat that is concentrated in the outer layers of keratin, where it also functions as a physical barrier. In addition to its physical properties, the emulsion provides a chemical barrier to potential pathogens. Water-soluble substances in the emulsion include inorganic salts and proteins that inhibit microorganisms. Sodium chloride, interferon, albumin, transferrin, complement, glucocorticoid, and immunoglobulins are in the emulsion.[45,63,68] Skin surface lipids are not constant in quantity or composition, and sebum is constantly being decomposed by resident flora into free fatty acids, some of which kill bacteria and fungi.[31] The polymeric immunoglobulin receptor, secretory component, is expressed and synthesized by keratinocytes and the secretory and ductal epithelium of sweat glands.[82] This receptor can interact with IgA and IgM; this interaction may be a mechanism for protecting the skin from microbial agents and foreign antigens.

A relationship exists between the acidity of the skin surface ("acid mantle" of the skin surface) and its antimicrobial activity.[31,132] The buffer capacity of the skin surface against external and internal acidifying and alkalinizing effects depends on several buffering systems, including lactic acid in sweat, ammonia in sweat, and amino acids. In general, inflammation causes the skin surface pH to switch from acid or neutral to alkaline.

The single factor with the greatest influence on the flora is the degree of hydration of the stratum corneum.[30,68] Increasing the quantity of water at the skin surface (increased ambient temperature, increased relative humidity, or occlusion) enormously increases the number of microorganisms. In general, the moist or greasy areas of the skin support the greatest population of microorganisms. In addition to the effects on microflora, epidermal water content appears to be important in the regulation of epidermal growth, keratinization, and permeability.[30]

The equilibrium between keratin and water is essential for keratinized tissues to fulfill their role correctly.[56] The stratum corneum can increase its thickness by over 100% by taking up water. By comparison, hairs can only increase their thickness by about 15%. This difference may be explained by the relatively low concentration of cystine in stratum corneum compared with that of hairs.[56] Transepidermal water loss (TEWL) represents the water vapor evaporating from the skin surface, and reflects the integrity of the stratum corneum.[12,56] A characteristic of healthy skin is that the relationship between TEWL and hydration (water-holding capacity) remains directly proportional. In pathologic skin, the correlation between TEWL and stratum corneum water content shows an inverse relationship as a result of damaged skin barrier function or alterations in keratinization (increased TEWL, decreased hydration).

The normal skin microflora also contributes to skin defense.[120,144] Bacteria and, occasionally, yeasts and filamentous fungi are located in the superficial epidermis (especially in the intercellular spaces) and in the infundibulum of hair follicles. The normal flora is a mixture of bacteria that live in symbiosis. The flora may change with different cutaneous environments, which include such factors as pH, salinity, moisture, albumin level, and fatty acid level. The close relationship between the host and the microorganisms enables bacteria to occupy microbial niches and inhibit colonization by invading organisms.

Interactions between cutaneous microbes may be classified as follows:[144]

1. Unilateral and reciprocal antagonism ("interference"). Production of growth conditions by one organism that are unfavorable for another. Proposed mechanisms include consumption of

nutrients, generation of unfavorable redox potential or pH, occupation of tissue receptors, or production of inhibitors (enzymes, antibiotics, or bacteriocins).

2. Reciprocal enhancement ("synergism"). Nutrients, such as amino acids, made available by the actions of one organism may allow "cross-feeding" by others. A possible example of this phenomenon is the frequent finding of increased populations of both *Staphylococcus intermedius* and *Malassezia pachydermatis* in lesional skin.

3. Neutral association.

The keratinocyte synthesizes various antimicrobial peptides (e.g., cathelicidins and b-defensins), which form a barrier for innate host protection against microbial pathogens (bacteria, fungi, viruses, protozoa).[64] These peptides also appear to function in regulating cell proliferation, extracellular matrix production, and cellular immune responses.

Some organisms are believed to live and multiply on the skin, forming a permanent population; these are known as *residents*, and they may be reduced in number but not eliminated by degerming methods.[68,144] The resident skin flora is not spread out evenly over the surface but is aggregated in microcolonies of various sizes. Other microorganisms, called *transients*, are merely contaminants acquired from the environment and can be removed by simple hygienic measures. A third class of organisms, whose behavior falls between that of residents and transients, has been called the *nomads*.[144] These are organisms that are readily able to take advantage of changes in the microenvironment of the skin surface and, thus, frequently become established and proliferate on the skin surface and deeper.

Most studies of the normal microbial flora of the skin of horses have been strictly qualitative. The skin is an exceedingly effective environmental sampler, providing a temporary haven and way station for all sorts of organisms. Thus only repeated quantitative studies allow the researcher to make a reliable distinction between resident and transient bacteria. Qualitative studies have shown that equine skin and hair coat are a veritable "cesspool" of bacteria and fungi (Box 1-1).[*] The most commonly isolated coagulase-negative staphylococci are *S. sciuri* and *S. xylosus*.[42] The most commonly isolated saprophytic fungi are *Alternaria* spp., *Aspergillus* spp., *Cladosporium* spp., *Fusarium* spp., *Mucor* spp., *Penicillium* spp., *Scopulariopsis* spp., *Trichoderma* spp., and *Trichothecium* spp.[1,83] Thus skin and hair must be adequately prepared prior to culturing for bacteria and fungi if meaningful results are to be obtained on a patient.

Epidermal histochemistry. The epidermis of equine skin has receptors for the lectins phytohemagglutinin, peanut agglutinin, and soybean agglutinin.[76]

Basement membrane zone. Basement membranes are dynamic structures that undergo constant remodeling and are the physicochemical interface between the epidermis and other skin structures (appendages, nerves, vessels, smooth muscle) and the underlying or adjacent connective tissue (dermis).[†] This zone is important in the following functions: (1) anchoring the epidermis to the dermis; (2) maintaining a functional and proliferative epidermis; (3) maintaining tissue architecture; (4) wound healing; (5) functioning as a barrier; and (6) regulating nutritional transport between epithelium and connective tissue. The basement membrane influences many aspects of cell and tissue behavior including adhesion, cytoskeletal organization, migration, and differentiation.[62,68] The basement membrane zone is well differentiated in H & E preparations, but even more nicely with period acid-Schiff (PAS) stain (Fig. 1-13).[197,198] It is most important in nonhaired areas of the skin and at mucocutaneous junctions. As observed by light microscopy, the basement membrane zone comprises only the fibrous zone of the sublamina densa area and is about 20 times thicker than the actual basal lamina.

---

*References 1, 29, 42, 57, 64a, 69, 83, 140, 168, 169, 195, 196.
†References 45, 62, 68, 152, 191, 202.

■ Box 1-1 **MICROORGANISMS ISOLATED FROM THE SKIN AND HAIR OF NORMAL HORSES**

BACTERIA

Acinetobacter sp.
Aerococcus sp.
Aeromonas sp.
Bacillus sp.
Corynebacterium sp.
Flavobacterium sp.
Micrococcus spp.
Nocardia sp.
Staphylococcus spp. (coagulase-negative)
Staphylococcus haemolyticus
Staphylococcus sciuri
Staphylococcus xylosus
Staphylococcus spp. (coagulase-positive)
Staphylococcus aureus
Staphylococcus hyicus hyicus (nonhemolytic)
Streptococcus spp. (nonhemolytic)

FUNGI

Absidia spp.
Acremonium spp.
Alternaria spp.
Aspergillus spp.
Aureobasidium sp.
Candida spp.
Cephalosporium spp.
Chaetomium spp.
Chrysosporium spp.
Cladosporium spp.
Cryptococcus spp.
Curvularia sp.
Diplosporium sp.
Doratomyces sp.
Epicoccum sp.
Fusarium sp.
Geomyces sp.
Helminthosporium spp.
Hormodendrum spp.
Malassezia sp.
Monotospora sp.
Mucor sp.
Nigrospora sp.
Paecilomyces sp.
Penicillium spp.
Phoma spp.
Rhodotorula spp.
Rhizopus spp.
Scopulariopsis sp.
Sordaria sp.
Stemphyllium spp.
Thamnidium sp.
Trichoderma sp.
Trichophyton equinum
Trichothecium sp.
Ulocladium spp.
Verticillium sp.

Ultrastructurally, the basement membrane zone can be divided into the following four components, proceeding from epidermis to dermis (Fig. 1-14): (1) the basal cell plasma membrane; (2) the lamina lucida (lamina rara); (3) the lamina densa (basal lamina); and (4) the sublamina densa area (lamina fibroreticularis), which includes the anchoring fibrils and the dermal microfibril bundles. The first three components are primarily of epidermal origin. The epidermal basement membrane is composed of a wide variety of glycoproteins and other macromolecules. Presently recognized basement membrane zone components, their localization, and their presumed functions are listed in Table 1-2.[62,68,152,191] It can be appreciated that the basement membrane is a veritable "soup" of interactive molecules with focal and regional variation that probably reflects functional differences. The involvement of the basement membrane zone in many important dermatologic disorders (pemphigoid, epidermolysis bullosa, and lupus erythematosus) and wound healing has prompted most of the current research interest.

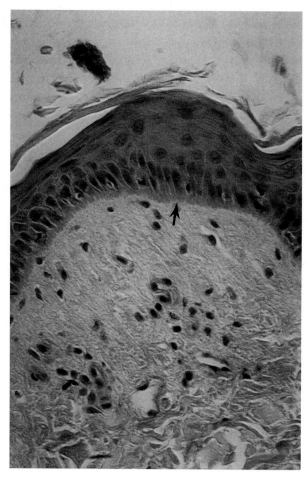

FIGURE 1-13. Epidermis from normal haired skin. Note prominent basement membrane zone (*arrow*).

Dermis

The dermis (corium) is an integral part of the body's connective tissue system and is of meso-dermal origin.[45,68,152] It is a composite system of insoluble fibers and soluble polymers that takes the stresses of movement and maintains shape. The insoluble fibers are collagens and elastin, and the major soluble macromolecules are proteoglycans and hyaluronan. The fibrous components resist tensile forces, whereas the soluble micromolecules resist or dissipate compressive forces.

In areas of thickly haired skin, the dermis accounts for most of the depth, whereas the epidermis is thin. In very thin skin, the decreased thickness results from the thinness of the dermis. In general body skin, the dermis ranges from 1.6 to 6.1 mm thick; in the mane and tail region, 3.7 to 10.5 mm.[184,197] The dermis is composed of fibers, ground substance, and cells. It also contains the epidermal appendages, arrector pili muscles, blood and lymph vessels, and nerves. Because the normal haired skin of horses does not have epidermal rete ridges, dermal papillae are not usually seen.[169,197] Thus a true papillary and reticular dermis, as described for humans, is not present in horses. The terms *superficial* and *deep* dermis are used. The dermis accounts for most of the tensile strength and elasticity of the skin; it is involved in the regulation of cell growth, proliferation, adhesion, migration, and differentiation, and it modulates wound healing and the structure and function of the epidermis.[68,152] Most of the dermal extracellular matrix (fibers and

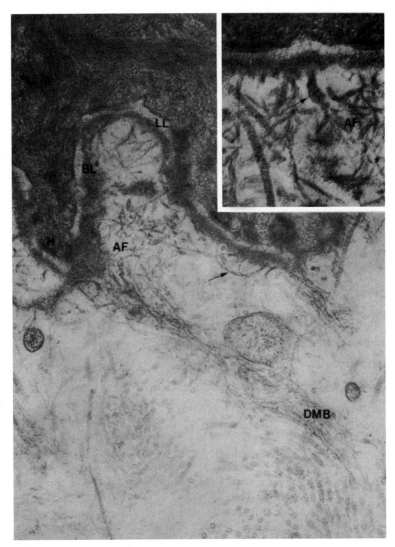

FIGURE I-I4. Epidermal-dermal junction. *H,* Hemidesmosome; *LL,* lamina lucida. Anchoring fibrils (*AF*) form a meshwork beneath the lamina densa. A dermal macrofibril bundle (*DMB*) extends from the basal lamina (*BL*) into the dermis (× 49,700). *Inset*: Sub-basal lamina fibrous components of the epidermal-dermal junction. Anchoring fibrils (*arrow*) with a central, asymmetric, cross-banded section. *AF,* Interlocking meshwork of anchoring fibrils (× 86,000). (*From Scott DW, Miller WH, Jr, Griffin CE: Muller and Kirk's Small Animal Dermatology, 6th ed. WB Saunders Co, Philadelphia, 2001.*)

ground substance) is synthesized by fibroblasts, which respond to a variety of stimuli such as growth factors elaborated by keratinocytes, inflammatory cells, and fibroblasts themselves.[13,152]

Dermal fibers. The dermal fibers are formed by fibroblasts and are collagenous, reticular, and elastic.[68] *Collagenous fibers* (collagen) have great tensile strength and are the largest and most numerous fibers (accounting for approximately 90% of all dermal fibers and 80% of the dermal extracellular matrix) (Fig. 1-15). They are thick bands composed of multiple protein fibrils and are differentially stained by Masson's trichrome. Collagen is a family of related molecules whose diverse biologic roles include morphogenesis, tissue repair, cellular adhesion, cellular migration,

● Table 1-2 **CHARACTERISTICS OF BASEMENT MEMBRANE ZONE COMPONENTS**

COMPONENT	LOCALIZATION	FUNCTION
Bullous pemphigoid antigens	Basal cell hemidesmosome and lamina lucida	Adherence
Cicatricial pemphigoid antigen	Lamina lucida	Adherence
Laminin I	Lamina lucida (partly lamina densa)	Adherence, promote keratinocyte proliferation and differentiation
Laminin 5 (nicein/kalinin/ epiligrin)	Basal cell hemidesmosome and lamina lucida	Adherence
Laminin 6	Lamina lucida	Adherence
Nidogen (entactin)	Lamina lucida (partly lamina densa)	Adherence (link laminin and type IV collagen)
Type IV collagen	Lamina densa and anchoring plaques	Adherence, networking
Type V collagen	Lamina densa (partly lamina lucida)	?
Heparan sulfate	Lamina densa	Networking, filtration
Chondroitin-6-sulfate	Lamina densa	Networking, filtration
Fibronectin	Lamina densa and lamina lucida	Networking
Epidermolysis bullosa acquisita antigen	Sublamina densa (partly lamina densa)	Adherence
Type IV collagen	Sublamina densa	Stabilization of connective tissue
Linkin	Sublamina densa	Stabilization of connective tissue
Fibrillin	Sublamina densa	Stabilization of connective tissue
Tenascin	Sublamina densa	Stabilization of connective tissue
Type VII collagen	Anchoring fibrils	Anchorage
AF1	Anchoring fibrils	Anchorage
AF2	Anchoring fibrils	Anchorage

chemotaxis, and platelet aggregation.[68] Collagen contains two unusual amino acids—hydroxylysine and 4-hydroxyproline—whose levels in urine have been used as indices of collagen turnover. *Reticular fibers* (reticulin) are fine, branching structures that closely approximate collagen with age. They can be detected best with special silver stains. *Elastin fibers* are composed of single, fine branches that possess great elasticity and account for about 4% of the dermal extracellular matrix. They are well visualized with Verhoeff's and van Gieson's elastin stains, and with acid orcein–Giemsa (Fig. 1-16). The two components of elastic fibers are amorphous elastin, which contains two unique cross-linked amino acids—desmosine and isodesmosine—that are not found in other mammalian proteins, and microfibrils, which are composed of fibrillin and Type VI collagen.[68,152] The remarkable strength of elastin is derived from the unusual cross-linking of desmosine and isodesmosine. The precursor to elastin is tropoelastin.

There are numerous (at least 17) genetically and structurally different types of collagen molecules.[68,152] Only three collagen types are fibrillar: Types I, III, and V collagen predominate in the dermis and account for approximately 87%, 10%, and 3%, respectively, of the dermal collagen. Type VI collagen is present as microfibrils and has presumed structural and communication functions. Types I, III, V, and VI collagen appear to be distributed uniformly throughout the dermis. Types III and V collagen are also concentrated around blood vessels. Types IV (lamina densa) and V (lamina lucida) collagen are found in the basement membrane zone, and Type VII collagen is found in the anchoring fibrils of the basement membrane zone. Types XII and XIV collagen are called *fibril-associated* collagens with interrupted triple helices (FACIT) collagens, and at present their function is unclear. The biosynthesis of collagen is a complex process of gene transposition and translation, intracellular modifications, packaging and secretion, extracellular modifications, and fibril assembly and cross-linking. Collagen abnormalities may result from

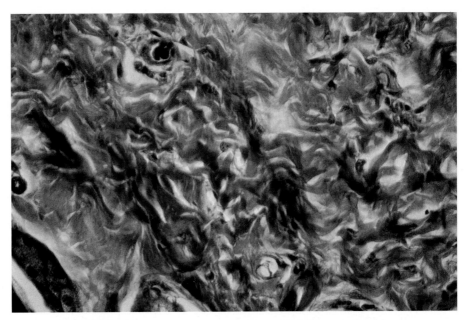

FIGURE 1-15. Appearance of middermal collagen in normal skin.

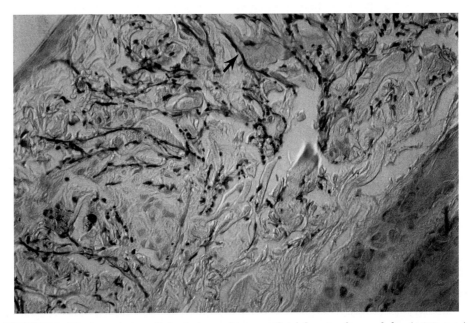

FIGURE 1-16. Appearance of elastin (*arrow*) in superficial dermis of normal skin (AOG stain).

genetic defects; from deficiencies of vitamin C, iron, and copper; and from β-aminopropionitrile poisoning (lathyrism). Collagen synthesis is stimulated by ascorbic acid (vitamin C), TGF-β, IL-1, insulin-like growth factor 1 (somatomedin C), insulin-like growth factor 2, superoxide generating systems, and bleomycin.[68] Collagen synthesis is inhibited by glucocorticoids, retinoids, vitamin D_3, parathormone, prostaglandin E_2, interferon-γ, D-penicillamine, and minoxidil.

Collagenases occupy a crucial position in both the normal and pathologic remodeling of collagen.[68,152] In the skin, a number of cell types contribute to connective tissue destruction by their capacity to synthesize and release collagenase. Dermal fibroblasts are the major source of skin collagenase under normal conditions of remodeling, as well as in many pathologic conditions. However, under certain conditions, keratinocytes, neutrophils, eosinophils, and macrophages can release a variety of proteolytic enzymes, including collagenase, and contribute to local connective tissue destruction in disease. Other degradative enzymes produced by fibroblasts, polymorphonuclear leukocytes, and macrophages include gelatinase (gelatin), stromelysins, and lysosomal hydrolases (fibronectin, proteoglycans, and glycosaminoglycans).

In general, the superficial dermis contains fine, loosely arranged collagen fibers that are irregularly distributed and a network of fine elastin fibers.[197] The deep dermis contains thick, densely arranged collagen fibers that tend to parallel the skin surface and elastin fibers that are thicker and less numerous than those in the superficial dermis. In the superficial dermis, thin elastic fibers, known as *elaunin* fibers, are organized in an arcade-like arrangement.[45,68,152] From these, still thinner elastic fibers, called *oxytalan* fibers, ascend almost vertically to terminate at the dermoepidermal junction and anchor to the basement membrane. Elaunin and oxytalan fibers are composed of microfibrils/elastin and microfibrils, respectively. Elastases are proteolytic enzymes capable of degrading elastic fibers, and a variety of tissues and cells (including fibroblasts) are capable of producing elastolytic enzymes. The elastases (serine proteinases) that are present in neutrophils and eosinophils are the most potent, and they readily degrade elastic fibers in disease states.

Horses have a third, special layer of collagen fibers in certain areas of their skin.[146,165,197,199] This third layer is immediately below the reticular dermis in the skin over the rump, the entire dorsal surface of the back, and the upper half of the chest. Because of the shiny gross appearance of this three-layered connective tissue structure, it has been called the "Ross-Spiegel" or "horse mirror." Microscopically, the collagen fibers of the deepest (third) layer are organized in a tree-like arrangement (Fig. 1-17).

Dermal ground substance. The ground (interstitial) substance is a viscoelastic gel-sol of fibroblast origin composed of glycosaminoglycans (formerly called *mucopolysaccharides*) usually linked *in vivo* to proteins (proteoglycans). These substances play vital roles in the epidermis, basement membrane, dermis, and hair follicle development and cycling.° The major proteoglycans and glycosaminoglycans include hyaluronate (synthesized by keratinocytes); heparin sulfate and chondroitin-6-sulfate in the basement membrane; and hyaluronic acid, dermatan sulfate, chondroitin-6-sulfate, chondroitin-4-sulfate, versican, syndecan, decorin, glypican, and serglycin in the dermis.

The ground substance fills the spaces and surrounds other structures of the dermis, but allows electrolytes, nutrients, and cells to traverse it, passing from the dermal vessels to the avascular epidermis. The proteoglycans and glycosaminoglycans are extracellular and membrane-associated macromolecules that function in water storage and homeostasis; in the selective screening of substances; in the support of dermal structure (resist compression); in lubrication; and in collagen fibrillogenesis, orientation, growth, and differentiation. Although glycosaminoglycans and proteoglycans account for only about 0.1% of the dry weight of skin, they can bind over 100 times their own weight in water.

Fibronectins are widespread extracellular matrix and body fluid glycoproteins capable of multiple interactions with cell surfaces and other matrix components.[38,39] They are produced by many cells, including keratinocytes, fibroblasts, endothelial cells, and histiocytes. The fibronectins moderate cell-to-cell interaction and cell adhesion to the substrate, and they modulate micro-

---

°References 39, 40, 45, 62, 68, 152.

vascular integrity, vascular permeability, basement membrane assembly, and wound healing. Fibronectins have been implicated in a variety of cell functions, including cell adhesion and morphology, opsonization, cytoskeletal organization, oncogenic transformation, cell migration, phagocytosis, hemostasis, and embryonic differentiation. Fibronectins are present in the dermis, especially perivascularly and perineurally and within the lamina lucida and lamina densa of the basement membrane.

Tenascin is a large glycoprotein that is prominently expressed at epithelial-mesenchymal interfaces.[117] It plays a significant role in epithelial morphogenesis and proliferation and wound healing.

Small amounts of *mucin* (a blue-staining, granular-to-stringy–appearing substance with H & E stain) can be seen in normal equine skin, especially around appendages and blood vessels.[169] Glycosaminoglycans are not easily visualized by H & E staining, but may be seen as translucent vaguely fibrillar material between collagen bundles in Alcian blue-stained sections.

Dermal cellular elements. The dermis is usually sparsely populated with cells.[68,169,197] *Fibroblasts* and *dermal dendrocytes* are present throughout. *Melanocytes* are commonly seen

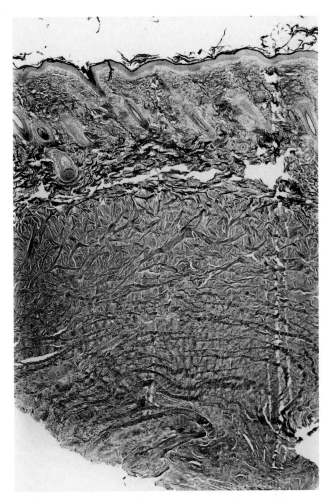

FIGURE 1-17. Appearance of third connective tissue layer ("horse mirror") in normal skin from croup area.

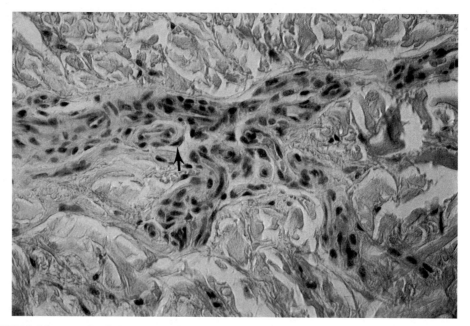

FIGURE 1-18. Superficial dermal blood vessel. Note associated lymphohistiocytic cells and pericytes (*arrow*).

under a heavily pigmented epidermis, and less commonly along blood vessels and epitrichial sweat ducts.[197]

Mast cells are present throughout the dermis but are most numerous in the adventitial dermis, especially along blood vessels.[197] Equine mast cells are often difficult to recognize in H & E stained sections, but their intracytoplasmic granules are nicely stained with toluidine blue or acid orcein–Giemsa. In a study of 10 normal horses, skin biopsies were performed at 10 different anatomic sites, and half of each biopsy specimen was fixed in 10% buffered formalin while the other half was fixed in Carnoy's fixative.[173] Microscopic examination of toluidine blue-stained sections revealed significantly fewer mast cells in formalin-fixed skin. In Carnoy's-fixed skin, the mean number of mast cells per high power microscopic field was 2.7 and 13.4 for the superficial dermis and dermoepidermal junction, respectively. Mast cells were not seen in the epidermis. There was little variation between different anatomic sites in a single horse, but there was significant variation at each anatomic site between different horses. Equine dermal mast cells are tryptase-positive, but negative for chymase.[205a]

Horses with clinically normal skin often have a mild perivascular accumulation of lymphocytes and histiocytes (Fig. 1-18).[169] In addition, small numbers of eosinophils are often seen in the clinically normal skin of horses.[169] This appears to be more common during the summer in the northeastern United States and presumably reflects exposure to biting insects and arthropods.

Dermal dendrocytes are bone marrow-derived, phagocytic (e.g., tattoo ink, melanin, hemosiderin), and antigen-presenting cells that express CD 1, common leukocyte antigen (CD 45), MHC class II molecules, and several adhesion molecules (e.g., ICAM-1).[71,77,141] These dermal dendritic cells are important members of the "dermal immune system."

Hair Follicles

Hair follicle morphogenesis is a complex process that occurs during the development of the skin, as part of the hair cycle, when skin repairs superficial wounds, and in response to certain

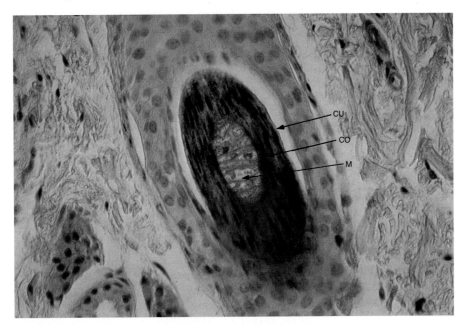

FIGURE I-19. Histologic section of hair shaft. Note cuticle (*CU*), cortex (*CO*), and medulla (*M*).

pharmacologic agents.[68,81] It is a complex, multistage process in which the epithelial cells of the hair follicle and the associated mesenchymal cells undergo a number of collaborative interactions. At each stage, the participating cells have different phenotypic properties and produce different products.

The hair shaft is divided into medulla, cortex, and cuticle (Fig. 1-19).[68,170,197] The *medulla*, the innermost region of the hair, is composed of longitudinal rows of cuboidal cells, or cells flattened from top to bottom. The *cortex*, the middle layer, consists of completely cornified, spindle-shaped cells, whose long axis is parallel to the hair shaft. These cells contain the pigment that gives the hair its color. In general, the cortex accounts for one-half of the width of the hair shaft, and it contributes the most to the mechanical properties of hair fibers. The *cuticle*, the outermost layer of the hair, is formed by flat, cornified, anuclear cells arranged like shingles on a roof, with the free edge of each cell facing the tip of the hair. Secondary hairs have a narrower medulla and a more prominent cuticle than do primary hairs. The epicuticle is an amorphous external layer derived from cuticular cells, as an exocellular secretion, or from the outer portion of cuticular cell membranes.[170]

Hair follicles may be oriented perpendicularly or obliquely to the skin surface.[55,178,197] In general, the thinner the skin, the more acute the angle of the follicle. Horses have a simple hair follicle arrangement, wherein hair follicles of different sizes occur singly and at random, displaying no obvious pattern of distribution (see Fig. 1-2).* Each hair follicle is accompanied by sebaceous and epitrichial sweat glands and an arrector pili muscle. Each hair emerges from a separate follicular opening. There are fewer follicles per unit area of skin in adults compared with neonates.

The hair follicle has five major components: the dermal hair papilla, the hair matrix, the hair itself, the inner root sheath, and the outer root sheath (Fig. 1-20).[45,169] The pluripotential cells of

---

*References 16, 27, 55, 89, 169, 170, 197, 203.

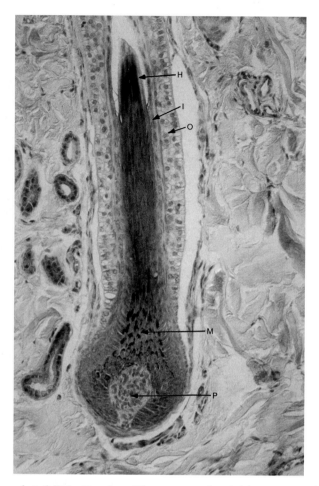

FIGURE 1-20. Anagen hair follicle. Note hair (*H*), inner root sheath (*I*), outer root sheath (*O*), hair matrix (*M*), and dermal papilla (*P*).

the hair matrix give rise to the hair and the inner root sheath. The outer root sheath represents a downward extension of the epidermis. Large hair follicles produce large hairs. The hair follicle is divided into three distinct anatomic segments (Fig. 1-21): (1) the *infundibulum*, or pilosebaceous region (the upper portion, from the entrance of the sebaceous duct to the skin surface); (2) the *isthmus* (the middle portion, between the entrance of the sebaceous duct and the attachment of the arrector pili muscle); and (3) the *inferior segment* (the lowest portion, which extends from the attachment of the arrector pili muscle to the dermal hair papilla).

The inner root sheath is composed of three concentric layers; from inside to outside, these include (1) the *inner root sheath cuticle* (a flattened, single layer of overlapping cells that point toward the hair bulb and interlock with the hair cuticle); (2) the *Huxley layer* (1 to 3 nucleated cells thick); and (3) the *Henle layer* (a single layer of nonnucleated cells) (Fig. 1-22). These layers contain eosinophilic cytoplasmic granules called *trichohyalin granules* (Fig. 1-23). Trichohyalin is a major protein component of these granules, which are morphologic hallmarks of the inner root sheath and medullary cells of the hair follicle and hair. Trichohyalin functions as a keratin-associated protein that promotes the lateral alignment and aggregation of parallel bundles of

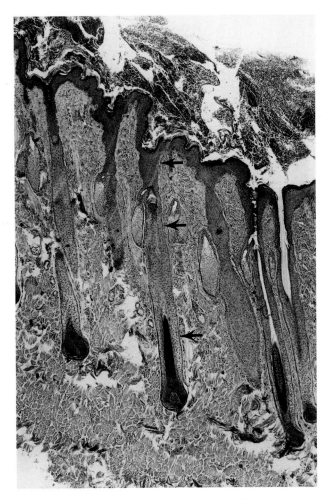

FIGURE 1-21. The anatomic segments of an anagen hair: infundibulum (*top arrow*), isthmus (*middle arrow*), inferior (*bottom arrow*).

intermediate filaments in inner root sheath cells.[68,147] The expression of trichohyalin is not unique to the hair follicle; it is found to occur normally in a number of other epithelial tissues (e.g., epidermis, filiform papilla of the tongue), where it is closely associated with the expression of filaggrin, the major keratohyalin granule protein.[148] The inner root sheath keratinizes and disintegrates when it reaches the level of the isthmus of the hair follicle. The prime function of the inner root sheath is to mold the hair within, which it accomplishes by hardening in advance of the hair. The amino acid citrulline occurs in high concentrations in hair and trichohyalin granules; it has been used as a marker for hair follicle differentiation.

The outer root sheath is thickest near the epidermis and gradually decreases in thickness toward the hair bulb. In the inferior segment of the hair follicle, the outer root sheath is covered by the inner root sheath. It does not undergo keratinization, and its cells have a clear, vacuolated (glycogen) cytoplasm. In the isthmus, the outer root sheath is no longer covered by the inner root sheath, and it does undergo trichilemmal keratinization (keratohyalin granules are not formed). In the infundibulum, the outer root sheath undergoes keratinization in the same fashion as does

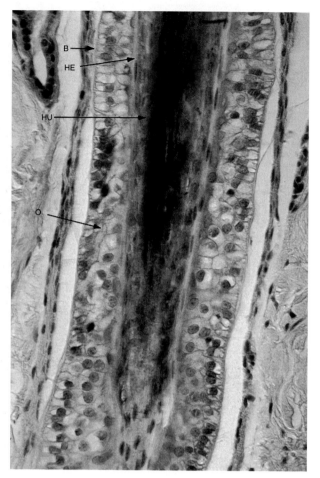

FIGURE 1-22. Anagen hair follicle: basement membrane zone (*B*), outer root sheath (*O*), Henle layer of inner root sheath (*HE*), Huxley layer of inner root sheath (*HU*).

the surface epidermis. The outer root sheath is surrounded by two prominent structures: a basement membrane zone, or glassy membrane (a downward reflection of the epidermal basement membrane zone), and a root sheath (a layer of dense connective tissue). The outer root sheath and hair matrix contain variable numbers of melanocytes.[68,197] Pigmentation is genetically determined and regulated by a *follicular melanin unit*, similar to that described for the epidermis.[68,149]

The dermal hair papilla is continuous with the dermal connective tissue and is covered by a thin continuation of the basement membrane (see Figs. 1-20 and 1-23).[35] The inner root sheath and hair grow from a layer of plump, nucleated epithelial cells that cover the papilla. These cells regularly show mitosis and are called the *hair matrix* (see Figs. 1-20 and 1-23). The importance of the papilla in the embryogenesis and subsequent cycling of hair follicles is well known.[39,68] Additionally, the morphology of the dermal papilla changes throughout the hair growth cycle, being maximal in volume in mature anagen and minimal at telogen. This is mostly a result of changes in the amount of extracellular matrix within the papilla. In the anagen hair follicle, dermal papilla volume is proportional to the volume of the hair.

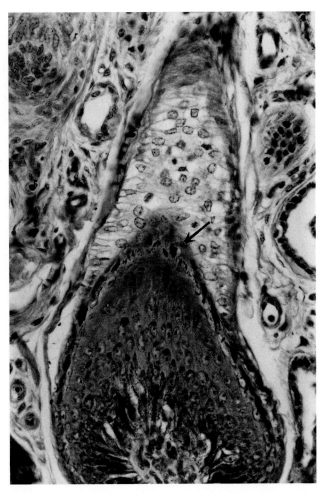

FIGURE 1-23. Anagen hair follicle. Note trichohyalin granules (*arrow*).

The hair follicles of animals with straight hair are straight, and those of animals with curly hair tend to be spiral in configuration. Follicular folds have been described.[170,197] These structures represent multiple corrugations of the inner root sheath, which project into the pilar canal immediately below the sebaceous duct opening. These folds are artifacts of fixation and processing.[170] Hair follicle epithelium is a major source of keratinocytes for wound healing.[45]

Two specialized types of tactile hairs are found: sinus hairs and tylotrich hairs.° *Sinus hairs* (vibrissae, whiskers) are found on the muzzle, lips, chin, and nares, as well as periocularly and over the zygomatic area.[157,197,208] These hairs are thick, stiff, and tapered distally. Sinus hairs are characterized by an endothelium-lined blood sinus interposed between the external root sheath of the follicle and an outer connective tissue capsule (Fig. 1-24). The sinus is divided into a superior, nontrabecular ring (or annular) sinus and an inferior, cavernous (or trabecular) sinus. A cushion-like thickening of mesenchyme (sinus pad) projects into the annular sinus. The cavernous sinuses are traversed by trabeculae containing many nerve fibers. Skeletal muscle fibers attach to the outer

°References 55, 68, 126, 169, 170, 197.

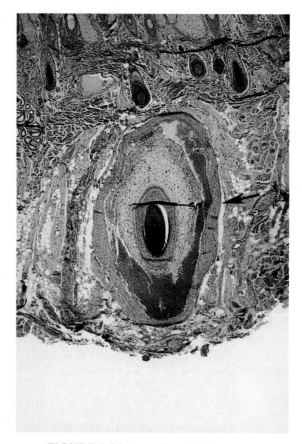

FIGURE 1-24. Sinus hair follicle (*arrow*).

layer of the follicle. Pacinian corpuscles are situated close to the sinus hair follicles. Sinus hairs function as slow-adapting mechanoreceptors.

Tylotrich hairs are scattered among ordinary body hairs. The hair follicles are larger than surrounding follicles and contain a single stout hair and an annular complex of neurovascular tissue that surrounds the follicle at the level of the sebaceous glands. Tylotrich hairs function as rapid-adapting mechanoreceptors. Each tylotrich follicle is associated with a touch corpuscle (tylotrich pad, Pinkus corpuscle, haarscheiben) (see Fig. 1-8). Touch corpuscles are composed of a thickened and distinctive epidermis underlaid by an area of fine connective tissue that is highly vascularized and innervated. Unmyelinated nerve fibers end as flat plaques in association with Merkel's cells (see Fig. 1-8), which serve as slow-adapting touch receptors.

The histologic appearance of hair follicles varies with the stage of the hair follicle cycle.[68,170,197] The *anagen* hair follicle is characterized by a well-developed, spindle-shaped dermal papilla, which is capped by the hair matrix (the ball-and-claw appearance) to form the hair follicle bulb (see Figs. 1-20 and 1-23). Hair matrix cells are usually heavily melanized and show mitotic activity. The anagen hair follicle extends into the deep dermis and even into the subcutis. Anagen has been divided into six stages: Stages I through IV, referred to as *proanagen* (differentiation); Stage V, referred to as *mesanagen* (transition to rapid growth); and Stage VI, referred to as *metanagen* (posteruptive hair elongation).[170]

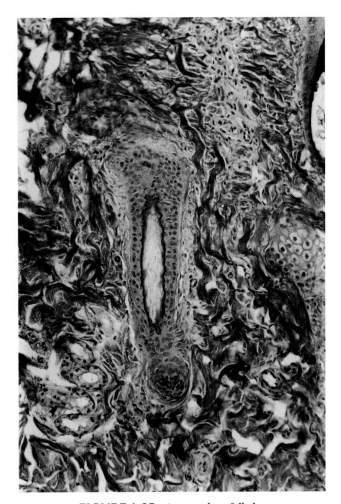

FIGURE 1-25. Catagen hair follicle.

The *catagen* hair follicle is characterized by a thickened, irregular, undulating basement membrane zone, a thickened basement membrane zone between the hair matrix and the dermal papilla, a smaller bulb, and an ovoid or round dermal papilla (Fig. 1-25).

The *telogen* hair follicle is characterized by the small dermal papilla that is separated from the bulb, by the lack of melanin and mitotic activity, and by the absence of the inner root sheath and the presence of club (brush-like) hair (Fig. 1-26).

A hair that is plucked in anagen shows a large expanded root that is moist and glistening, often pigmented and square at the proximal end, and surrounded by a root sheath (see Fig. 2-18). A hair plucked in telogen shows both a club root, with no root sheath or pigment, and a keratinized sac (see Fig. 2-19).

Studies on the amino acid content of equine hair and hoof have indicated that the content of threonine, serine, proline, and cysteine was greater in hair, while the content of alanine, glycine, isoleucine, leucine, tyrosine, phenylalanine, and aspartic acid was greater in the hoof.[162-164] The difference was greatest for cysteine, suggesting that this amino acid may play an important role in determining types of keratin.

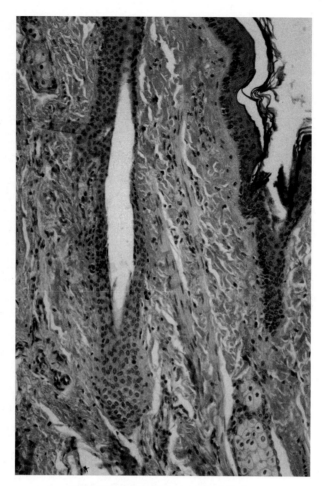

FIGURE I-26. Telogen hair follicle.

Sebaceous Glands

Sebaceous glands are simple or branched alveolar holocrine glands distributed throughout all haired skin (Fig. 1-27).° The glands usually open through a duct into the piliary canal in the infundibulum (pilosebaceous follicle). Sebaceous glands are largest and most numerous near mucocutaneous junctions, upper eyelids, mane, submandibular region, udder, teat, and near the coronet. In general, sebaceous glands are composed of 2 to 8 lobules, and range from 55 to 90 μm × 195 to 285 μm in size.[184]

Sebaceous lobules are bordered by a basement membrane zone, on which sits a single layer of deeply basophilic basal cells (called *reserve* cells). These cells become progressively more lipidized and eventually disintegrate to form sebum toward the center of the lobule. Ultrastructurally, nonmembrane-bound lipid vacuoles are the most prominent feature of sebocytes. Sebaceous ducts are lined with squamous epithelium, 2 to 4 cell layers thick, which is continuous with the outer root sheath of the hair follicle.

The oily secretion (*sebum*) produced by the sebaceous glands tends to keep the skin soft and pliable by forming a surface emulsion that spreads over the surface of the skin to retain moisture

---

°References 45, 54, 68, 92, 93, 169, 197.

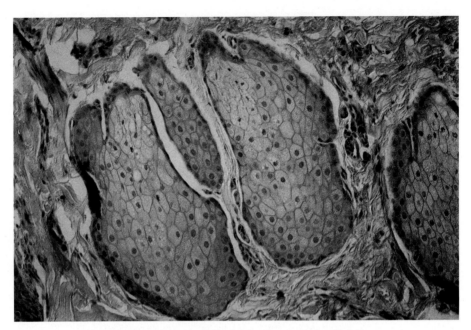

FIGURE 1-27. Normal equine sebaceous gland lobules.

and help maintain proper hydration.[36,37,68,152] The oil film also spreads over the hair shafts and gives them a glossy sheen. During periods of illness or malnutrition, the hair coat may become dull and dry, partly as a result of inadequate sebaceous gland function. In addition to its action as a physical barrier, the sebum-sweat emulsion forms a chemical barrier against potential pathogens. Freshly liberated sebum contains predominantly triglycerides and wax esters. In the hair follicle infundibulum, sebum becomes contaminated with lipase-producing bacteria (*Staphylococcus* spp.), which results in the production of fatty acids. Many of sebum's fatty acid constituents (linoleic, myristic, oleic, and palmitic acids) are known to have antimicrobial actions. Sebum may also have pheromonal properties.

One of the interesting aspects of sebaceous glands is that the lipid classes present in sebum and the structures of the sterols and fatty acids are extremely variable among species. Often the molecular structures of these lipids are so species-specific that knowledge of the weight percentage of mammalian skin surface lipids and their biochemical composition can function as a molecular fingerprint to identify the species. For example, to date, only the surface lipids of the Equidae contain lactones (47% of the total).[43,142,143] In addition, equine lipid contains sterol esters, cholesterol, and wax diesters.

Sebaceous glands have an abundant blood supply and appear to be innervated.[90,197] Their secretion is thought to be under hormonal control, with androgens causing hypertrophy and hyperplasia, and estrogens and glucocorticoids causing involution. The skin surface lipids of horses have been studied in some detail and are different from those of humans (see Horny Layer earlier in this chapter). Enzyme histochemical studies have indicated that sebaceous glands contain succinate acid dehydrogenase, cytochrome oxidase, monoamine oxidase, and a few esterases.[90,136,205]

Sweat Glands

Because of investigations into the physiology and ultrastructural aspects of sweat production by sweat glands, it has been suggested that the *apocrine* and *eccrine* sweat glands would be more

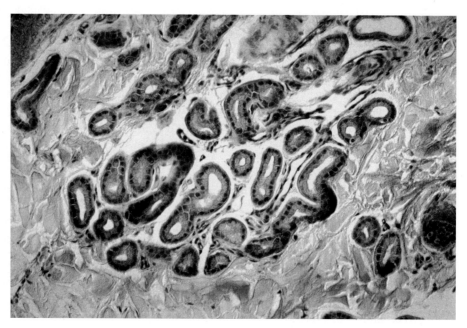

FIGURE 1-28. Normal equine epitrichial sweat gland coils.

accurately called the *epitrichial* and *atrichial* sweat glands, respectively.[93] This terminology has been adopted in this book. Atrichial sweat glands have not been described in the horse.

Epitrichial (apocrine) sweat glands. Epitrichial sweat glands are generally coiled and saccular or tubular and are distributed throughout all haired skin (Fig. 1-28).[*] These glands are located below the sebaceous glands, and they usually open through a duct into the piliary canal in the infundibulum, above the sebaceous duct opening. They are largest and most numerous near mucocutaneous junctions, the submandibular region, mane, and near the coronet. Glandular secretion is PAS-positive.[193,200]

The secretory portions of epitrichial sweat glands consist of a single row of cuboidal epithelial (secretory) cells and a single layer of fusiform myoepithelial cells. The epitrichial sweat gland excretory duct is lined by two cuboidal to flattened epithelial cell layers and a luminal cuticle, but no myoepithelial cells. Ultrastructurally, equine epitrichial sweat gland secretory cells have microvilli and their cytoplasm is filled with secretory vacuoles.[91] Equine epitrichial sweat glands appear to be innervated.[90,194] Epitrichial sweat probably has pheromonal and antimicrobial properties (IgA content).[45,93] They also serve as a minor avenue for waste product excretion.[45] Enzyme histochemical studies have demonstrated alkaline phosphatase and acid phosphatase in epitrichial sweat gland secretory epithelium.[136]

Studies in swine have shown that the sweat gland apparatus is capable of re-epithelializing the skin surface, although the resulting epidermis is not entirely normal.[133]

Sweating and thermoregulation. Horses sweat moderately to markedly in response to exercise, heat (high ambient temperature or fever), pain, and secretion of catecholamines (resulting from stress or pheochromocytoma), as well as when they have hyperadrenocorticism.[†] Because of the interest in racing, endurance riding, anhidrosis, and comparative physiology and

---

[*]References 45, 68, 93, 106, 193, 197, 200.
[†]References 7, 10, 14, 26, 61, 87, 89, 99, 100, 131, 134, 138, 156, 189.

pathophysiology, sweat and sweating have been extensively studied in the horse. Physiologic control of sweating in horses differs from that in other species. Horses have two mechanisms of control: humoral control by adrenergic agonists secreted from the adrenal medulla into the circulation, and nervous control by autonomic adrenergic nerves.[79] The main component of sweat control is neural, and the humoral component is activated during exercise.

In the horse, even though a rich supply of acetylcholine esterase has been reported in equine epitrichial sweat glands,[90] investigations have concluded that these glands are insensitive to cholinergic agonists and are predominantly under β_2-adrenergic control.* Nonspecific inhibition of nitric oxide synthase reduces the sweating response of exercising horses.[135] Decreased sweating rates seen during epinephrine infusion in horses suggest that the epitrichial sweat glands can become refractory ("fatigue") upon continuous exposure to adrenergic agonists. The average loss of body weight per hour during heat exposure and endurance exercise in horses was reported to be 0.8% and 1.5%, respectively.[156]

Sweat produced by all stimuli (prolonged epinephrine exposure, heat exposure, exercise) in horses is hypertonic (relative to plasma) for sodium, potassium, chloride, and urea.† Equine sweat protein (initially hypotonic), calcium (isotonic), and magnesium (initially hypertonic) concentrations decrease with time; urea levels (hypertonic) remain constant; and glucose is detectable only when plasma glucose levels increase. Equine sweat has been reported to be alkaline or acidic during sweating.[78,185] Horses have an extremely high concentration of protein (albumin, γ globulin, glycoproteins) in sweat compared with other species.‡

Other factors in thermoregulation include peripheral vasculature and arteriovenous anastomoses, which modify the effects of radiation, convection, and conduction in heat loss. Other proposed functions of epitrichial sweat glands include excretion of waste products, supplying moisture to assist the flow of sebum, immunity (IgA content), and scent signaling.§

Because of the interest in equine sweating, thermoregulation, and anhidrosis (see Chapter 15), equine epitrichial sweat gland cells have been cultured so that *in vitro* studies on stimulus-secretion coupling can be performed.[101,154,216,217]

Arrector Pili Muscles

Arrector pili muscles are of mesenchymal origin and consist of smooth muscle with intracellular and extracellular vacuoles (Fig. 1-29).[55,68,153,169,197] They are present in all haired skin and are largest in the dorsal neck, lumbar, and sacral regions as well as the base of the tail. They range from 15 to 60 μm in diameter.[184] Arrector pili muscles originate in the superficial dermis and insert approximately perpendicularly, via elastic tendons, on a bulge of the hair follicles. Branching of these muscles is often seen in the superficial dermis. The smooth muscle fibers of arrector pili muscles splay extensively between collagen bundles in the superficial dermis. The anchorage of the arrector pili muscle to the dermal extracellular matrix involves $\alpha_5\beta_1$ integrin-fibronectin interaction, and $\alpha_1\beta_1$ integrin functions in muscle cell-to-cell adhesion.[34a,130] Smooth muscle cells are characterized ultrastructurally by central nuclei, peripheral basement membrane, and intra-cytoplasmic myofilaments.[68] Arrector pili muscles are about one-sixth to one-fourth the diameter of the associated hair follicles.

These muscles receive cholinergic innervation and contract in response to epinephrine and norepinephrine, producing piloerection. Arrector pili muscles function in thermoregulation and in emptying sebaceous glands.

---

*References 14, 15, 26, 52, 58-61, 96, 99, 100, 112, 156, 180-182.
†References 26, 78, 94, 99, 131, 134, 138, 156, 182, 185.
‡References 50, 78, 88, 99, 156, 179.
§References 68, 99, 131, 134, 137, 187, 189.

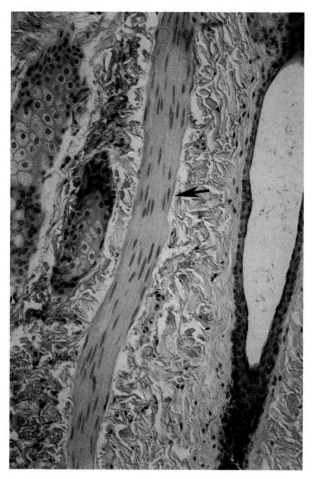

FIGURE 1-29. Normal equine arrector pili muscle (*arrow*) between hair follicle (*right*) and sebaceous gland lobules (*left*).

Blood Vessels

The microcirculation of skin is a rather complex and dynamic system that is important for skin metabolism and temperature regulation, and is an important part of the organ's defense system against invaders.

Cutaneous blood vessels are generally arranged in three intercommunicating plexuses of arteries and veins.° The deep plexus is found at the interface of the dermis and subcutis. Branches from this plexus descend into the subcutis and ascend to supply the lower portions of the hair follicles and the epitrichial sweat glands. These ascending vessels continue upward to feed the middle plexus, which lies at the level of the sebaceous glands. The middle plexus gives off branches to the arrector pili muscles, ascending and descending branches that supply the middle portions of the hair follicles and the sebaceous glands, and ascending branches to feed the superficial plexus. Capillary loops that are immediately below the epidermis emanate from the superficial plexus and supply the epidermis and upper portion of the hair follicles. The ability to accommodate a wide range of blood flow enables skin to conserve or eliminate heat rapidly. Blood vessels

---

°References 45, 68, 89, 119, 166, 169, 184.

are smaller and more numerous in the adventitial dermis. This location allows for rapid heat exchange.

The microcirculatory bed is composed of three segments: arterioles, arterial and venous capillaries, and venules.[11] Electron microscopy is necessary to identify these different segments of the microvasculature definitively.[11] The arterioles consist of endothelial cells surrounded by two layers of smooth muscle cells, and most likely function as part of the resistance vessels in skin. Arterial and venous capillaries lack surrounding smooth muscle cells. The majority of superficial dermal vessels are postcapillary venules, which are the most physiologically reactive segment of the microcirculation and are also the site where inflammatory cells migrate from the vascular space into tissues and where endothelial cells develop gaps that result in increased vascular permeability during inflammation.

Blood vessel endothelial cells are mesenchymal in origin and characterized: (1) ultra-structurally by a peripheral basement membrane and intracytoplasmic Weibel-Palade bodies (rod-shaped tubular structures enveloped in a continuous single membrane); (2) by their possession of factor VIII (von Willebrand) antigen, plasminogen activators, and prostaglandins; (3) by CD31 (platelet endothelial cell adhesion molecule [PECAM]); and (4) by being phagocytic.[8,68] Endothelial cells are strategically located between intravascular and tissue compartments and serve as key regulators of leukocyte trafficking.[98] Selectins (E- and P-selectin) and members of the immunoglobulin superfamily (ICAM-1, vascular cell adhesion molecule-1 [VCAM-1]) are upregulated on endothelial cells on inflammatory stimulation and mediate rolling, adhesion, and transmigration of leukocytes from the blood stream. Angiogenesis (new vessel formation) is controlled, at least in part by mast cells (histamine), macrophages (tumor necrosis factor-α [TNF-α]), and TGF-β.[8,98]

Arteriovenous anastomoses are normal connections between arteries and veins that allow arterial blood to enter the venous circulation without passing through capillary beds.[34,41,68,201] Because of the size and position of these anastomoses, they can alter circulation dynamics and blood supply to tissues. They occur in all areas of the skin, and are especially numerous in the pinna and coronary band. These anastomoses occur at all levels of the dermis, especially the deep dermis.

Arteriovenous anastomoses show considerable variation in structure, ranging from simple, slightly coiled vessels to such complex structures as the *glomus* (Hoyer-Grosser's organ), a special arteriovenous shunt localized within the deep dermis (Fig. 1-30).[122] Each glomus consists of an arterial segment and a venous segment. The arterial segment (Sucquet-Hoyer canal) branches from an arteriole. The wall shows a single layer of endothelium surrounded by a basement membrane and a tunica media that is densely packed with 4 to 6 layers of glomus cells. These cells are large and plump, have a clear cytoplasm, and resemble epithelioid cells. Glomus cells are generally regarded as modified smooth muscle cells. The venous segment is thin-walled and has a wide lumen.

Arteriovenous anastomoses are associated with thermoregulation. Constriction of the shunt restricts and dilatation enhances the blood flow to an area. Acetylcholine and histamine cause dilatation; epinephrine and norepinephrine cause constriction.

Pericytes, which vary from fusiform to club-like in appearance, are aligned parallel to blood vessels on their dermal side.[11,53,68] They are contractile cells, containing actin-like and myosin-like filaments, and they are important in regulating capillary flow. Pericytes are essential for micro-vessel stability and participate in the control of angiogenesis. The origin of pericytes is uncertain. In humans, 3G5 is a cell surface ganglioside antigen that appears to be specific for pericytes.[78a]

Veil cells are flat, adventitial, fibroblast-like cells that surround all dermal microvessels.[11,53,68] Although their exact function and nature are undetermined, the fact that they stain for factor XIIIa indicates that they are a component of the dermal dendrocyte system. Unlike pericytes, which are

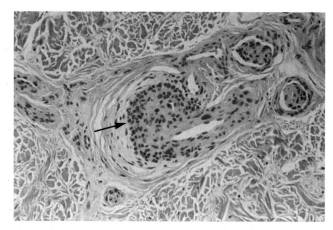

FIGURE 1-30. Glomus cells (*arrow*) surrounding vessel from acral skin. (*From Elder D, et al: Lever's Histopathology of the Skin, 8th ed. Lippincott-Raven, Philadelphia, 1998.*)

an integral component of the vascular wall and are enmeshed in the mural basement membrane material, veil cells are entirely external to the wall. The veil cell demarcates the vessel from the surrounding dermis. Perivascular mast cells are usually present in the space between the vascular wall and the surrounding veil cells.[11]

Microcirculatory measurements by cutaneous laser–Doppler velocimetry revealed significant differences in blood flow, velocity, and volume between different skin sites, but no correlation with skin thickness.[125]

Lymph Vessels

The skin is confronted by a specialized set of pathogenic organisms and environmental chemicals that represent a distinctive spectrum of antigenic specificities. It has a unique collection of lymphatics and lymphoid and dendritic cells to deal with these special demands.

Lymphatics arise from capillary networks that lie in the adventitial dermis and surround the adnexa.[45,68,166] The vessels arising from the networks drain into a subcutaneous lymphatic plexus. Lymph vessels are not usually seen above the middle dermis in routine histologic preparations of normal skin.

The lymphatics are essential for nutrition because they control the true microcirculation of the skin, the movement of interstitial tissue fluid. The supply, permeation, and removal of tissue fluid are important for proper function. The lymphatics are the drains that take away the debris and excess matter that result from daily wear and tear in the skin. They are essential channels for the return of protein and cells from the tissues to the blood stream and for linking the skin and regional lymph nodes in an immunoregulatory capacity. In skin, lymphatics carry material that has penetrated the epidermis and dermis, such as solvents, topical medicaments, injected vaccines and drugs, and products of inflammation.

Skin has a noncontractile initial lymphatic collector system that drains into contractile collector lymphatics.[159] Initial lymphatics have an attenuated endothelial layer, discontinuous basement membrane, and noncontiguous cell junctions. Lymph formation depends on the periodic expansion of the initial lymphatics, whereas compression leads to the emptying of the initial lymphatics into the contractile collector lymphatics, which have smooth muscle, exhibit peristalsis, and carry lymph toward the lymph nodes. Expansion and compression of collecting lymphatics is achieved by periodic tissue motions such as pressure, pulsations, arteriolar vaso-motion, skin massage, and muscle motion.

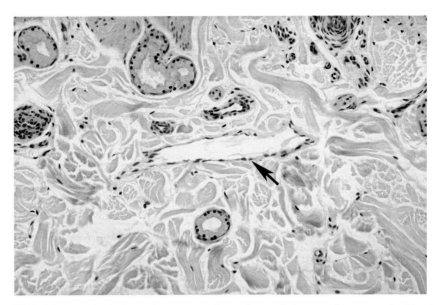

FIGURE 1-31. Lymphatic (*arrow*). Note angular outline and absence of intravascular blood cells.

In general, lymph vessels are distinguished from blood capillaries by: (1) possessing wider and more angular lumina; (2) having flatter and more attenuated endothelial cells; (3) having no pericytes; and (4) containing no blood (Fig. 1-31). However, even the slightest injury disrupts the wall of a lymphatic or blood vessel or the intervening connective tissue. Consequently, traumatic fistulae are commonplace. These account for the common observation of blood flow in the lymphatics in inflamed skin.

Nerves

Cutaneous nerve fibers have sensory functions, control the vasomotor tonus, and regulate the secretory activities of glands. They also exert a number of important functions, including the modulation of multiple inflammatory, proliferative, and reparative cutaneous processes.[6,150,207] Cutaneous nerves are in close contact with dermal vessels, mast cells, fibroblasts, keratinocytes, and Langerhans' cells. Neuropeptides released by cutaneous nerves can activate a number of target cells such as keratinocytes (inducing release of cytokines such as IL-1), mast cells (producing potent proinflammatory cytokines such as TNF-α), and endothelial cells (upregulating VCAM-1 expression and causing secretion of IL-8). Such neuropeptides include substance P, neurokinin A, calcitonin gene-related peptide, vasoactive intestinal peptide, neuropeptide Y, somatostatin, and pituitary adenylate cyclase activity peptide. In addition, skin epithelium can generate neurotrophins, thus influencing the development, sprouting, and survival of nerve fibers.

In general, cutaneous nerve fibers are associated with blood vessels (dual autonomic inneration of arteries) (Fig. 1-32), various cutaneous endorgans (tylotrich pad, Pacini's corpuscle, Meissner's corpuscle), sebaceous glands, epitrichial sweat glands, hair follicles, and arrector pili muscles.[68,90] The fibers occur as a subepidermal plexus. Some free nerve endings even penetrate the epidermis. The motor innervation of the skin is attributable to sympathetic fibers of the autonomic nervous system. Although ordinarily considered somatic sensory nerves, the cutaneous nerve trunks carry myelinated postganglionic sympathetic fibers. Under the light microscope, small cutaneous nerves and free nerve endings can be demonstrated satisfactorily only by methylene blue staining, metallic impregnation, or histochemical techniques.

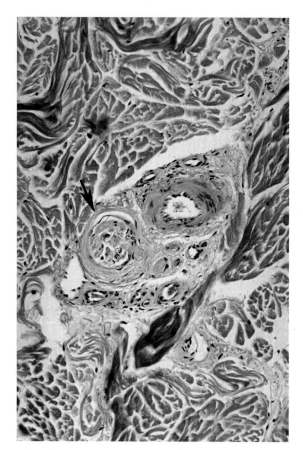

FIGURE 1-32. Large nerve fiber (*arrow*) to the left of a deep dermal arteriole.

In addition to the important function of sensory perception (touch, heat, cold, pressure, pain, and itch), the dermal nerves promote the survival and proper functioning of the epidermis (so-called trophic influences).

The area of skin supplied by the branches of one spinal nerve is known as its *dermatome.*

Overview of cutaneous sensation. The skin is a major sensory surface. Signals about external events and about the internal state of the skin are sent to the central nervous system by an array of receptor endings. *Thermoreceptors* fall into two categories: cold units, which are excited by falling skin temperatures, and warm units, which are excited by rising skin temperatures.[68] Cold units have C axons and A δ axons. Cold unit nerve terminals are branches of a small myelinated axon, ending in a small invagination in the basal cells of the epidermis.[68] Warm units also have C axons and A δ axons, but no morphologic nerve terminal has been identified.

Four types of sensitive *mechanoreceptor* units with A β axons are present in most skin regions.[68] Pacinian corpuscle units are extremely sensitive to small high-frequency vibrations and to very rapid transients.[68] Rapidly adapting units, which arise from Meissner's or other encapsulated corpuscles, are primarily sensitive to the velocity of skin movement.[68] In hairy skin, there are many afferent units that are excited by hair movement and have both A β and A δ axons. These provide the major tactile input from such regions. Guard and down hairs receive many nerve terminations of the lanceolate type. Such units can be subdivided into two major classes: (1) those excited only by movement of large guard or tylotrich hairs (G and T hair units); and (2) those excited by movement of all hairs, but especially by the fine down hairs (D hair units).[68] The units driven from large hairs nearly always have A β axons; those driven from down hairs have A δ axons. G and T hair units are activated by rapid hair movements, and D hair units respond to slow movements. An additional class of units activated by static deflection of hairs is associated with large sinus hairs such as vibrissae.[68] Slowly adapting Type I endings from Merkel's cell complexes signal about steady pressure.[68] Slowly adapting Type II units, which are associated with Ruffini's endings,[68] show directional sensitivity in response to skin stretch and may play a proprioceptive role.

Most *nociceptor* units fall into two categories: A δ high-threshold mechanoreceptor units with A δ axons, and polymodal nociceptor units with C axons.[68] The latter afferents are classic pain receptors, responding to intense mechanical and thermal stimuli and to irritant chemicals. C-polymodal nociceptor units are involved with hyperalgesia and itch. They are responsible, through the local release of vasoactive agents, for the flare around skin injuries.[68]

Pruritus. Pruritus, or itching, is an unpleasant sensation that provokes the desire to scratch.[68,202] It is the most common symptom in dermatology and may be due to specific dermatologic diseases or may be generalized without clinically evident skin disease. Pruritus may be sharp and well localized (epicritic), or it may be poorly localized and have a burning quality (protopathic).

The skin is richly endowed by a network of sensory nerves and receptors. The sensory nerves subserve hair follicles, as well as encapsulated structures such as Pacini's, Meissner's, and Ruffini's corpuscles.[68] In addition, sensory nerves may end as free nerve endings, referred to as *penicillate* nerve endings. The penicillate endings arise from the terminal Schwann cell in the dermis as tuft-like structures and give rise to an arborizing network of fine nerves, and they terminate either subepidermally or intraepidermally. These unmyelinated penicillate nerve endings are limited to the skin, mucous membranes, and cornea.

Although several morphologically distinct end organs have been described, a specific end organ for pruritus has not been found. There is a clear association between C-polymodal nociceptor activation and itch that appears to involve a subpopulation of specific itch afferent fibers.[68]

On the basis of the properties of afferent units, somatosensory activity can be subdivided into mechanoreceptors, thermoreceptors, and nociceptors. The nociceptors are involved in itch and pain. Nociceptors are supplied by A δ and C fibers. The A δ fibers (myelinated) conduct at about 10 to 20 m/sec and carry signals for spontaneous (physiologic), well-localized, pricking itch (epicritic itch). The C fibers (nonmyelinated) conduct more slowly (2 m/sec), subserve unpleasant, diffuse burning, and cross to the lateral spinothalamic tract. From there, they ascend to the thalamus and, via the internal capsule, to the sensory cortex. There, the itch sensation may be modified by emotional factors and competing cutaneous sensations.

At present, it has not been possible to isolate a universal mediator to explain pruritus, but a host of chemical mediators have been implicated (Box 1-2).[68,121] However, the pathophysiology of pruritus is complicated and poorly understood for most diseases in most species. The relative importance of these putative mediators and modulators of pruritus in any given species, disease, or individual is rarely known.

Central factors such as anxiety, boredom, or competing cutaneous sensations (e.g., pain, touch, heat, cold) can magnify or reduce the sensation of pruritus by selectively acting on the gate-control system.[68] For instance, pruritus is often worse at night because other sensory input is low. Although the mechanisms involved here are not clear, it has been suggested that stressful conditions may potentiate pruritus through the release of various opioid peptides (central opinergic pruritus).[68] Various neuropeptides, such as enkephalins, endorphins, and substance P, have been demonstrated to participate in the regulation of such cutaneous reactions as pruritus, pain, flushing, pigmentary changes, and inflammation.[68]

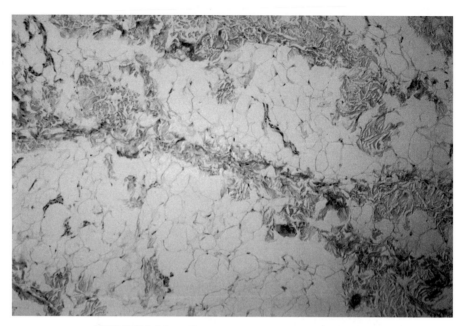

FIGURE 1-33. Subcutaneous fat in normal equine skin.

■ Box 1-2   **MEDIATORS AND MODULATORS OF PRURITUS**

Histamine
Eicosanoids
  Leukotrienes
  Prostaglandins
Serotonin
Platelet-activating factor
Proteases
  Kallikrein
  Cathepsins
  Trypsin
  Chymotrypsin
  Fibrinolysin
  Leukopeptidases
  Plasmin
  Microbial proteases

Peptides
  Bradykinin
  Neuropeptides (opioids)
    Substance P
    Vasoactive intestinal peptide

Subcutis

The subcutis (hypodermis) is of mesenchymal origin and is the deepest and usually thickest layer of the skin (Fig. 1-33).[45,68,166,169,197] However, for functional reasons, there is no subcutis in some areas (e.g., lip, cheek, eyelid, external ear, anus); in these areas, the dermis is in direct contact with musculature and fascia. Fibrous bands that are continuous with the fibrous structures of the dermis penetrate and lobulate the subcutaneous fat into lobules of lipocytes (adipocytes, fat cells) and form attachments of the skin to underlying fibrous skeletal components such as fascial sheets and periosteum. The superficial portion of the subcutis projects into the overlying dermis as papillae adiposae; these surround hair follicles, sweat glands, and vasculature to assist in protecting these structures from pressure and shearing forces. The subcutis is about 90% triglyceride by weight, and it functions (1) as an energy reserve; (2) in thermogenesis and insulation; (3) as a protective padding and support; and (4) in maintaining surface contours.[22] The subcutis is also important as a steroid reservoir, and as the site of steroid metabolism and estrogen production. The mature lipocyte is dominated by a large lipid droplet that leaves only a thin cytoplasmic rim and pushes the nucleus to one side.

The walls of arterial and venous capillaries present in fat are much thinner than those present in the dermis, and veil cells are not always present.[11] In addition, there are no lymphatics present in fat lobules.[160] The thickness of the subcutis is inversely proportional to blood flow, with slow circulation promoting lipogenesis and fast circulation promoting lipolysis.[160] As a result of these factors, fat is particularly susceptible to diseases and, with even minor injury, damage occurs in the absence of an efficient system for removing the damaged tissue.

● REFERENCES

1. Aho R: Saprophytic fungi isolated from the hair of domestic and laboratory animals with suspected dermatophytosis. Mycopathologia 83:65, 1983.
2. Al-Diwan MMA, et al: Coat colour inheritance of Arabian horses. Indian J Anim Sci 63:679, 1993.
3. Alhaidari Z, von Tscharner C: Anatomie et physiologie du follicule pileux chez les carnivores domestiques. Prat Méd Chir Anim Comp 32:181, 1997.
4. Allen TE, Bligh J: A comparative study of the temporal patterns of cutaneous water vapour loss from some domesticated animals with epitrichial sweat glands. Comp Biochem Physiol 31:347, 1969.
5. Altmeyer P, et al: The relationship between α-MSH level and coat color in white Camarque horses. J Invest Dermatol 82:199, 1984.
6. Ansel JC, et al: Interactions of the skin and nervous system. J Invest Dermatol Symp Proc 2:23, 1997.
7. Aoki T, et al: On the responsiveness of the sweat glands in the horse. J Invest Dermatol 33:441, 1959.
8. Arbiser JL: Angiogenesis and the skin: a primer. J Am Acad Dermatol 34:486, 1996.
9. Baker BB, et al: Epidermal cell renewal in the horse. Am J Vet Res 49:520, 1988.
10. Bell FR, Evans CL: The relation between sweating and the innervation of sweat glands in the horse. J Physiol 134:421, 1957.
11. Berardesca E, et al: Bioengineering of the skin: cutaneous blood flow and erythema. CRC Press, Boca Raton, FL, 1995.
12. Berardesca E, Borroni G: Instrumental evaluation of cutaneous hydration. Clin Dermatol 13:323, 1995.
13. Bernstein EF, Uitto J: The effect of photodamage in dermal extracellular matrix. Clin Dermatol 14:143, 1996.
14. Bijman J, Quinton PM: In vitro pharmacological stimulation of equine sweat glands shows equine sweating is predominantly under β-adrenergic control. Physiologist 25:279, 1982.
15. Bijman J, Quinton PM: Predominantly β-adrenergic control of equine sweating. Am J Physiol 246:R349, 1984.
16. Blackburn PS: The hair of cattle, horse, dog, and cat. In: Rook AJ, Walton GS (eds): Comparative physiology and pathology of the skin. Blackwell Scientific Publications, Oxford, UK, 1965, p 201.
17. Boiron G, et al: Phagocytosis of erythrocytes by human and animal epidermis. Dermatologica 165:158, 1982.
18. Borradori L, Sonnenberg A: Structure and function of hemidesmosomes: more than simple adhesion complexes. J Invest Dermatol 112:411, 1999.
19. Bos JD: Skin immune system (SIS). CRC Press, Boca Raton, FL, 1990.
20. Braun AA: Sravnitelny analiz mikrostruktury kozhnogo pokrova loshadi i krupnogo rogatogo skota. Topografiya Pokrova Loshadi, Vyp 1. Leningrad, 1935.
21. Braun A, Osterowskaja P: Beiträge zur topographischen Histologie des Integuments: III. Pferd. Arch Russ-Anat Histol Embryol 12:208, 1933.
22. Breidenbach A, et al: Studies on equine lipid metabolism. 1. A fluorometric method for the measurement of lipolytic activity in isolated adipocytes of rats and horses. J Vet Med A 45:635, 1998.
23. Bruni AC, Zimmerl U: Apparecchio Tegumentale. Anatomia degli Animali Domestici. Casa Editrice Dottor Francesco Vallardi, Milano, Italy, 1951.
24. Burchill SA: Regulation of tyrosine in hair follicular melanocytes of the mouse during the synthesis of eumelanin and pheomelanin. Ann NY Acad Sci 642:396, 1991.
25. Cape L, Hintz HF: Influence of month, color, age, corticosteroids, and dietary molybdenum on mineral concentration of equine hair. Am J Vet Res 43:1132, 1982.
26. Carlson GP, Ocen PO: Composition of equine sweat following exercise in high environmental temperatures and in response to intravenous epinephrine administration. J Equine Med Surg 3:27, 1979.
27. Carter HB: Variation in the hair follicle population of the mammalian skin. In: Lyne AG, Short BF (eds): Biology of the skin and hair growth. American Elsevier Publishing Co., New York, 1965, p 25.
28. Castle WE: Coat color inheritance in horses and other mammals. Genetics 39:33, 1954.
29. Chengappa MM, et al: Isolation and identification of yeasts and yeast-like organisms from clinical veterinary sources. J Clin Microbiol 19:427, 1984.
30. Chesney CJ: Water and the skin—the forgotten molecule. Vet Dermatol News 24:44, 1992.

31. Chikakane K, Takahashi H: Measurement of skin pH and its significance in cutaneous diseases. Clin Dermatol 13:299, 1995.

32. Chuong CM, et al: Adhesion molecules in skin development: morphogenesis of feather and hair. Ann NY Acad Sci 642:263, 1991.

33. Chuong CM, et al: Adhesion molecules and homeo-proteins in the phenotypic determination of skin appendages. J Invest Dermatol 101:105, 1993.

34. Clara M: Die arteriovenösen Anastomosen, 2nd ed. Springer-Verlag, Vienna, 1956.

34a. Clifton MM, et al: Immunofluorescent microscopic investigation of the distal arrector pili: a demonstration of the spatial relationship between $\alpha_5 \beta_1$ integrin and fibronectin. J Am Acad Dermatol 43:19, 2000.

35. Cohen J: The dermal papilla. In: Lyne AG, Short BF (eds): Biology of the skin and hair growth. American Elsevier Publishing Co, New York, 1965, p 183.

36. Colton SW, et al: Measure of the time between bio-synthesis and surface excretion of sebaceous lipids in the horse. Biochem Biophys Acta 835:98, 1985.

37. Colton SW, et al: The time course of lipid bio-synthesis in horse skin. Biochem Biophys Acta 836:306, 1985.

38. Couchman JR, et al: Fibronectin-cell interactions. J Invest Dermatol 94:75, 1990.

39. Couchman JR, et al: Proteoglycans and glyco-proteins in hair follicle development and cycling. Ann NY Acad Sci 642:243, 1991.

40. Couchman JR: Hair follicle proteoglycans. J Invest Dermatol 101:60S, 1993.

41. Daniel PM, Prichard MML: Arteriovenous anasto-mosis in external ear. Quart J Exptl Physiol 41:107, 1956.

42. Devriese LA: Identification and characteristics of staphylococci isolated from lesions and normal skin of horses. Vet Microbiol 10:269, 1985.

43. Downing DT, Cotton SW: Skin surface lipids of the horse. Lipids 15:323, 1980.

44. Draize HH: The determinations of the pH of the skin of man and common laboratory animals. J Invest Dermatol 5:77, 1942.

45. Dunstan RW, Henry GA: Pathophysiology and diag-nosis of skin diseases. In: Kobluk CN et al (eds): The horse. Diseases and clinical management, Vol. 1. WB Saunders, Philadelphia, 1995, p 487.

46. Dunstan RW: A pathomechanistic approach to diseases of the hair follicle. Br Vet Dermatol Study Grp 17:37, 1995.

47. Dyce KM, et al: Textbook of veterinary anatomy. WB Saunders, Philadelphia, 1987.

48. Ebling FJ: Comparative and evolutionary aspects of hair replacement. In: Rook AJ, Walton GS (eds): Comparative physiology and pathology of the skin. Blackwell Scientific Publications, Oxford, UK, 1965, p 87.

49. Ebling FJ: Systemic factors affecting the periodicity of hair follicles. In: Lyne AG, Short BF (eds): Bio-logy of the skin and hair growth. American Elsevier Publishing Co, New York, 1965, p 507.

50. Eckersall D, et al: An investigation into the proteins of equine sweat. Comp Biochem Physiol 73B:375, 1982.

51. Eckert RL, et al: Involucrin—structure and role in envelope assembly. J Invest Dermatol 100:613, 1993.

52. Ejima S, Muto K: On the secretory phenomenon in the sweat glands of horses. Jikken-Igaku-Zasshi 19:1735, 1935.

53. Elder D, et al: Lever's Histopathology of the skin VIII. Lippincott-Raven Publishers, Philadelphia, 1997.

54. Elder HY, et al: The use of computer-linked plani-metry in the image analysis of serial sections from horse sebaceous glands. J Physiol 343:21P, 1983.

55. Ellenberger W: Handbuch der Vergleichenden Mikroskopischen Anatomie der Haustiere. Paul Parey, Berlin, 1906.

56. Elsner P, et al: Bioengineering of the skin: water and the stratum corneum. CRC Press, Boca Raton, FL, 1994.

57. Euzeby J, et al: Investigations mycologiques. I. Recherches sur quelques pseudodermatophytes. Bull Soc Sci Vet Med Comp Lyon 75:355, 1973.

58. Evans CL, Smith DFG: Sweating response in the horse. Proc Roy Soc London B 145:61, 1956.

59. Evans CL, et al: A histological study of the sweat glands of normal and dry-coated horses. J Comp Pathol 67:397, 1957.

60. Evans CL, et al: Physiological factors in the condi-tion of "dry-coat" in horses. Vet Rec 69:1, 1957.

61. Evans LH, et al: Clinicopathologic conference. J Am Vet Med Assoc 159:209, 1971.

62. Fine JD: Structure and antigenicity of the skin basement membrane zone. J Cutan Pathol 18:401, 1991.

63. Freedberg IM, et al: Fitzpatrick's dermatology in general medicine IV. McGraw-Hill Book Co, New York, 1999.

64. Gallo RL, Huttner KM: Antimicrobial peptides: an emerging concept in cutaneous biology. J Invest Dermatol 111:739, 1998.

64a. Galuppo LD, et al: Evaluation of iodophor skin pre-paration techniques and factors influencing drainage from ventral midline incisions in horses. J Am Vet Med Assoc 215:963, 1999.

65. Gebhart W, Niebauer GW: Beziehungen Zwischen Pigmentschwund und Melanomatose am Beispiel des Lippizzanerschimmels. Arch Dermatol Res 259:39, 1977.

66. Gibson WT, et al: Immunology of the hair follicle. Ann NY Acad Sci 642:291, 1991.

67. Gillian AC, et al: The human hair follicle: A reservoir of CD40+ B7-deficient Langerhans' cells that repop-ulate epidermis after UVB exposure. J Invest Dermatol 110:422, 1998.

68. Goldsmith LA (ed): Physiology, biochemistry, and molecular biology of the skin, 2nd ed. Oxford University Press, New York, 1991.

69. Gravesen S, et al: Demonstration, isolation, and identification of culturable microfungi and bacteria in horse hair and dandruff. Allergy 33:89, 1978.

70. Gunson DE: Collagen in normal and abnormal tissue. Equine Vet J 11:97, 1979.

71. Nestle FO, Nickoloff BJ: A fresh morphological and functional look at dermal dendritic cells. J Cutan Pathol 22:385, 1995.

72. Hales JM, Camp RD: Potent T cell stimulatory material with antigenic properties in stratum corneum of normal human skin. J Invest Dermatol 110:725, 1998.

73. Hamada M, et al: Keratin expression in equine normal epidermis and cutaneous papillomas using monoclonal antibodies. J Comp Pathol 102:405, 1990.

74. Hamada M, et al: Langerhans' cells in equine cutaneous papillomas and normal skin. Vet Pathol 29:53, 1992.

75. Hargis AM, Liggitt HD: Cytokines and their role in cutaneous injury. In: Ihrke PJ et al (eds): Advances in veterinary dermatology II. Pergamon Press, New York, 1993, p 325.

76. Hashimoto Y, et al: Eine lectinhistochemische Untersuchung der Epidermis von Haut und Huf des Pferdes. Anat Histol Embryol 21:238, 1992.

77. Headington JT, Cerio R: Dendritic cells and the dermis: 1990. Am J Dermatopathol 12:217, 1990.

78. Hejlasz Z, et al: The role of sweat in maintaining the stimulation of effort homeostasis in horses. Arch Vet Polonicum 34:3, 1994.

78a. Helmbold P, et al: Human dermal pericytes express 3G5 ganglioside—A new approach for microvessel histology in the skin. J Cutan Pathol 28:206, 2001.

78b. Hintz HF: Hair analysis as an indicator of nutritional status. Equine J Vet Sci 21:199, 2001.

79. Hodgson DR, et al: Dissipation of metabolic heat in the horse during exercise. J Appl Physiol 74:1161, 1993.

80. Hotil D, et al: In vitro and rapid in situ transglutaminase assays for congenital ichthyoses—A comparative study. J Invest Dermatol 110:268, 1998.

81. Holbrook KA, Minami SI: Hair follicle embryogenesis in the human. Characterization of events in vivo and in vitro. Ann NY Acad Sci 642:167, 1991.

82. Huff JC: Epithelial polymeric immunoglobulin receptors. J Invest Dermatol 94:74S, 1990.

83. Ihrke PJ, et al: Cutaneous fungal flora in 20 horses free of skin or ocular disease. Am J Vet Res 49:770, 1988.

84. Itum S, et al: Mechanism of action of androgen in dermal papilla cells. Ann NY Acad Sci 642:385, 1991.

85. Jackson R: The lines of Blaschko: a review and reconsideration. Br J Dermatol 95:349, 1976.

86. Jadassohn J: Handbuch der Haut und Geschlechtskrankheiten I. Normale und pathologische Anatomie der Haut. Springer-Verlag, Berlin, 1968.

87. Jenkinson DM: Comparative physiology of sweating. Br J Dermatol 88:397, 1973.

88. Jenkinson DM, et al: Sweat protein. Br J Dermatol 90:175, 1974.

89. Jenkinson DM: The skin of domestic animals. In: Rook AJ, Walton GS (eds): Comparative physiology and pathology of the skin. Blackwell Scientific Publications, Oxford, UK, 1965, p 591.

90. Jenkinson DM, Blackburn PS: The distribution of nerves, monoamine oxidase, and cholinesterase in the skin of the horse. Res Vet Sci 9:165, 1968.

91. Jenkinson DM, et al: Ultrastructural variations in the sweat glands of anhidrotic horses. Equine Vet J 17:287, 1985.

92. Jenkinson DM: Anatomy and physiology of the mammalian sweat and sebaceous glands. Vet Dermatol News 12(2):8, 1990.

93. Jenkinson DM: Sweat and sebaceous glands and their function in domestic animals. In: von Tscharner C, Halliwell REW (eds): Advances in veterinary dermatology I. Ballière-Tindall, Philadelphia, 1990, p 229.

94. Jirka M, Kotas J: Some observations on the chemical composition of horse sweat. J Physiol 147:74, 1959.

95. Johnson E: Inherent rhythms of activity in the hair follicle and their control. In: Lyne AG, Short BF (eds): Biology of the skin and hair growth. American Elsevier Publishing Co, New York, 1965, p 491.

96. Johnson KG, Creed KE: Sweating in the intact horse and isolation perfused horse skin. Comp Biochem Physiol 73C:259, 1982.

97. Kang S, et al: Pharmacology and molecular action of retinoids and vitamin D in skin. J Invest Dermatol Symp Proc 1:15, 1996.

98. Karasek MA: Mechanisms of angiogenesis in normal and diseased skin. Int J Dermatol 30:831, 1991.

99. Kerr MG, Snow DH: Composition of sweat of the horse during prolonged epinephrine (adrenaline) infusion, heat exposure, and exercise. Am J Vet Res 44:1571, 1983.

100. Kerr MG, et al: Equine sweat composition during prolonged heat exposure. J Physiol 307:52P, 1980.

101. Ko WH, et al: Extracellular ATP can activate autonomic signal transduction pathways in cultured equine sweat gland epithelia cells. J Exptl Biol 190:239, 1994.

102. Kooistra LH, Ginther OJ: Effect of photoperiod on reproductive activity and hair in mares. Am J Vet Res 36:1413, 1975.

103. Kral F, Schwartzman RM: Veterinary and comparative dermatology. JB Lippincott Co, Philadelphia, 1964.

104. Kratochvil Z: Microscopic evaluation of hairs of the mane and tail of the wild horse (Equus prezewalskii) in comparison with the modern and domesticated horse (Equus prezewalskii f. caballus). Acta Vet Brno 40:23, 1971.

105. Krölling O, Grau H: Lehrbuch der Histologie und vergleichenden mikroscopischen Anatomie der Haustiere. Paul Parey, Berlin, 1960.

106. Kurosumi K, et al: Electron microscopic observations on the sweat glands of the horse. Arch Histol Jpn 23:294, 1963.

107. Kurotaki T, et al: Immunopathological study on equine insect hypersensitivity ("Kasen") in Japan. J Comp Pathol 110:145, 1994.

108. Kwochka KW: Keratinization abnormalities: understanding the mechanisms of scale formation. In: Ihrke PJ et al (eds): Advances in veterinary dermatology II. Pergamon Press, New York, 1993, p 91.

109. Kwochka KW: The structure and function of epidermal lipids. Vet Dermatol 4:151, 1993.

110. Lamar CH, et al: Equine endothelial cells in vitro. Am J Vet Res 47:956, 1986.

111. Lane EB, et al: Stem cells in hair follicles. Cytoskeletal studies. Ann NY Acad Sci 642:197, 1991.

112. Langley JN, Bennett S: Action of pilocarpine, arecoline, and adrenaline on sweating in the horse. J Physiol 57:1, 1923.

113. Lavker RM, et al: Stem cells of pelage, vibrissae, and eyelash follicles. The hair cycle and tumor formation. Ann NY Acad Sci 642:214, 1991.

114. Leigh IM, et al: The Keratinocyte Handbook. Cambridge University Press, New York, 1994.

115. Levine N: Pigmentation and Pigmentary Disorders. CRC Press, Boca Raton, 1993.

116. Lichti U: Hair follicle transglutaminases. Ann NY Acad Sci 642:82, 1991.

117. Lightner VA: Tenascin: does it play a role in epidermal morphogenesis and homeostasis? J Invest Dermatol 102:273, 1994.

118. Lindholm JS, et al: Variation of skin surface lipid composition among mammals. Comp Biochem Physiol B 69:75, 1981.

119. Lindsay WA: Blood supply to the skin of the equine fore- and hind limb: cutaneous arterial topography. Vet Surg 18:65, 1989.

120. Lloyd DH: The ecosystem of the epidermis. Vet Dermatol News 12(2):3, 1990.

121. Lloyd DH: Inflammatory mediators and skin disease. In: von Tscharner C, Halliwell REW (eds): Advances in Veterinary Dermatology I. Baillière-Tindall, Philadelphia, 1990, p 163.

122. Ludewig T: Occurrence and importance of glomus organs (Hoyer-Grosser's organs) in the skin of the equine and bovine mammary gland. Anat Histol Embryol 27:155, 1998.

123. Luger TA, et al: The role of α-melanocyte-stimulating hormone in cutaneous biology. J Invest Dermatol Symp Proc 2:87, 1997.

124. Lyne AG, Short BF: Biology of the Skin and Hair Growth. American Elsevier Publishing Co, New York, 1965.

125. Manning TO, et al: Cutaneous laser-Doppler velocimetry in 9 animal species. Am J Vet Res 52:1960, 1991.

126. Marshall FHA: On hair in the Equidae. Vet J 54:34, 1902.

127. Mazák V: Haarwechsel und Haarwuchs bei Przewalski-Pferd und onager im Prager Zoologischen Garten Während der Jahre 1958-1960. Mém Soc Zool Tchécosl 26:271, 1962.

128. McMillan JR, et al: Hemidesmosomes show abnormal association with keratin filament network in junctional forms of epidermolysis bullosa. J Invest Dermatol 110:132, 1998.

129. Messinger AG: The control of hair growth: an overview. J Invest Dermatol 101:4S, 1993.

130. Mendelson JK, et al: The microanatomy of the distal arrector pili: possible role for $\alpha_1\beta_1$ and $\alpha_5\beta_1$ integrins in mediating cell-cell adhesion and anchorage to the extracellular matrix. J Cutan Pathol 27:61, 2000.

131. Meyer H, et al: Untersuchungen uber Scheiffmenge und Schweiffzusammensetzung beim Pferd. Tierärztl Umsch 33:330, 1978.

132. Meyer W, et al: Der "Säureschutzmantel" der Haut unserer Haustiere. Deut Tierärztl Wschr 98:167, 1991.

133. Miller SJ, et al: Re-epithelialization of porcine skin by the sweat apparatus. J Invest Dermatol 110:13, 1998.

134. Meyer W, et al: Zur Bedeutung der apokrinen Hautdrusen der allgemeinen Korperdecke bei verschiedenen Haussaugetierarten. Dtsch Tierärztl Wochenschr 85:194, 1978.

135. Mills PC, et al: Nitric oxide and thermoregulation during exercise in the horse. J Appl Physiol 82:1035, 1997.

136. Montagna W: Comparative anatomy and physiology of the skin. Arch Dermatol 96:357, 1967.

137. Montagna W, Parakkal PF: The Structure and Function of Skin, 3rd ed. Academic Press, New York, 1974.

138. Montgomery I, et al: The effects of thermal stimulation on the ultrastructure of the fundus and duct of the equine sweat gland. J Anat 135:13, 1982.

139. Morelli JG, Norris DA: Influence of inflammatory mediators and cytokines on human melanocyte function. J Invest Dermatol 100:191S, 1993.

140. Nasser M, et al: Carrier-states of staphylococci in domestic animals and in contact persons. J Egypt Vet Med Assoc 40:23, 1980.

141. Nestle FO, Nicoloff BJ: A fresh morphological and functional look at dermal dendritic cells. J Cutan Pathol 22:385, 1995.

142. Nicolaides N, et al: The skin surface lipids of man compared with those of 18 species of animals. J Invest Dermatol 51:83, 1968.

143. Nicolaides N, et al: Diesterwaxes in surface lipids of animal skin. Lipids 5:299, 1970.

144. Noble WC: The Skin and Microflora in Health and Disease. Cambridge University Press, Cambridge, 1993.

145. Nozaki S, et al: Keratinocyte cytokines. Adv Dermatol 7:83, 1992.

146. Odoni E: Der Spiegel des Pferdes, eine modifizierte Hautpartie in der Kruppenund Oberschenkelgegend. Buchdruckerei, Zurich, 1951.

147. O'Guin WM, Manabe M: The role of trichohyalin in hair follicle differentiation and its expression in nonfollicular epithelia. Ann NY Acad Sci 642, 1991.

148. O'Keefe EJ, et al: Trichohyalin: a structural protein of hair, tongue, nail, and epidermis. J Invest Dermatol 101:65S, 1993.

149. Ortonne JP, Prota G: Hair melanins and hair color: ultrastructural and biochemical aspects. J Invest Dermatol 101:82S, 1993.

150. Paus R, et al: Neural mechanisms of hair growth control. J Invest Dermatol Symp Proc 2:61, 1997.

151. Pittelkow MR: Growth factors in cutaneous biology and disease. Adv Dermatol 7:55, 1992.

152. Priestley GC: Molecular Aspects of Dermatology. John Wiley & Sons, New York, 1993.

153. Rackow J: Beitrag zur Histologie und Physiologie des glatten Hautmuskels des Pferdes. Arch Tierheilk 24:273, 1898.

154. Rakhit S, et al: Persistent desensitisation of the β_2 adrenoreceptors expressed by cultured equine sweat gland epithelial cells. J Exp Biol 201:259, 1998.

155. Restano L, et al: Blaschko lines of the face: a step closer to completing the map. J Am Acad Dermatol 39:1028, 1998.

155a. Rooney JR: Hair patterns and dermal cleavage lines of the horse. J Equine Vet Sci 20:236, 2000.

156. Rose RJ, et al: Plasma and sweat electrolyte concentrations in the horse during long distance exercise. Equine Vet J 12:19, 1980.

157. Rotz A, Friess AE: A scanning electron-microscopic analysis of the morphology of equine lower lip sinus hair. Acta Anat 154:196, 1995.

158. Rutner D, et al: Merkel cell carcinoma. J Am Acad Dermatol 29:143, 1993.

159. Ryan TJ, Mortimor PS: Cutaneous lymphatic system. Clin Dermatol 13:417, 1995.

160. Ryan TJ, Mortimor PS: Lymphatics and adipose tissue. Clin Dermatol 13:493, 1995.

161. Salisbury GW: The inheritance of equine coat color. The basic colours and patterns. J Heredity 32:235, 1941.

162. Samata T: A biochemical study of keratin. I. Amino acid compositions of body hair and hoof of *Equidae*. J Fac Gen Educ Azabu Univ 18:17, 1985.

163. Samata T: A biochemical study of keratin. II. Solubilization of keratin in hair and hoof of Arab (*Equidae*) by oxidation. J Fac Gen Educ Azabu Univ 19:115, 1986.

164. Samata T, Matsuda M: Studies on the amino acid compositions of the equine body hair and the hoof. Jpn J Vet Sci 50:333, 1988.

165. Schönberg F: Der Ross-Spiegel. Eine Eigentümlichkeit des integumentum pelvis beim Pferde. Berl Munch Tierärztl Wchnschr 42:777, 1926.

166. Schummer A, et al: The Circulatory System, the Skin, and the Cutaneous Organs of the Domestic Mammals. Verlag, Paul Parey, Berlin, 1981.

167. Schwarz R: Haarwachstum und Haarwechsel-eine zusätzliche funktionelle Beanspruchung der Haut-am Beispiel markhaltiger Primärhaarfollikel. Kleintierpraxis 37:67, 1992.

168. Scott DW, Manning TO: Equine folliculitis and furunculosis. Equine Pract 6:11, 1980.

169. Scott DW: Large Animal Dermatology. WB Saunders Co, Philadelphia, 1988.

170. Scott DW: The biology of hair growth and its disturbances. In: von Tscharner C, Halliwell REW (eds): Advances in Veterinary Dermatology I. Baillière-Tindall, Philadelphia, 1990, p 3.

171. Scott DW: Autoimmune skin diseases: an update. Proc Eur Soc Vet Dermatol 12:36, 1995.

172. Scott GA, Goldsmith LA: Homeobox genes and skin development: A review. J Invest Dermatol 101:3, 1993.

173. Shearer DH, et al: A study of the number and distribution of cutaneous mast cells in the horse. Proc Eur Soc Vet Dermatol 12:250, 1995.

174. Sheretz EC: Misuse of hair analysis and a diagnostic tool. Arch Dermatol 121:1504, 1985.

175. Sisson S, Grossman JD: Anatomy of Domestic Animals. W.B. Saunders Co, Philadelphia, 1956.

176. Slee J: The genetics of hair growth. In: Rook AJ, Walton GS (eds): Comparative Physiology and Pathology of the Skin. Blackwell Scientific Publications, Oxford, 1965, p 103.

177. Smack DP, et al: Keratin and keratinization. J Am Acad Dermatol 30:85, 1994.

178. Smith F: The histology of the skin of the horse. Vet J 26:333, 1888.

179. Smith F: Note on the composition of the sweat of the horse. J Physiol 11:497, 1890.

180. Snow DH: Identification of the receptor involved in adrenaline-mediated sweating in the horse. Res Vet Sci 23:247, 1977.

181. Snow DH: Metabolic and physiological effects of adrenoreceptor agonists and antagonists in the horse. Res Vet Sci 27:372, 1979.

182. Snow DH, et al: Alterations in blood, sweat, urine, and muscle composition during prolonged exercise in the horse. Vet Rec 110:377, 1982.

183. Sobel H: Squalene in sebum and sebum-like materials. J Invest Dermatol 13:333, 1949.

184. Sokolov VE: Mammal Skin. University of California Press, Berkeley, 1982.

185. Soliman MK, Madim MA: Calcium, sodium, and potassium levels in the serum and sweat of horses after strenuous exercise. Zbl Vet Med A 14:53, 1967.

186. Song MD, et al: Hair follicle cycling in the mane and tail region of horses. Annu Memb Meet Am Acad Vet Dermatol Am Coll Vet Dermatol 7:18, 1991.

187. Spearman RIC: The Integument. Cambridge University Press, London, 1973.

188. Speed JG: The importance of the coat on Exmoor and other mountain and moorland ponies living out of doors. Brit Vet J 116:91, 1960.

189. Stephen E, Redecker R: Die Rolle der Haut beider Thermoregulation von Haustieren. Dtsch Tierärztl Wochenschr 77:628, 1970.

190. Straile WE: Root sheath-dermal papilla relationships and the control of hair growth. In: Lyne AG, Short BF (eds): Biology of the Skin and Hair Growth. American Elsevier Publishing Co, New York, 1965, p 35.

191. Suter MM, et al: Keratinocyte biology and pathology. Vet Dermatol 8:67, 1997.

192. Szeligowski E: Contribution to the histology of the skin of the horse. Folia Morphol (Warsaw) 13:531, 1962.

193. Tagaki S. Tagawa M: A cytological and cytochemical study of the sweat gland of the horse. Jpn J Physiol 9:153, 1959.

194. Tagaki S, Tagawa M: Nerve fibers supplying the horse sweat gland. Jpn J Physiol 11:158, 1961.

195. Takatori K, et al: Occurrence of equine dermatophytosis in Hokkaido. Jpn J Vet Sci 43:307, 1981.

196. Takatori K, et al: Fungal flora of equine skin with or without dermatophytosis. Jpn J Vet Med Assoc 34:580, 1981.

197. Talukdar AH, et al: Microscopic anatomy of the skin of the horse. Am J Vet Res 33:2365, 1972.

198. Talukdar AH: A histological study of the dermoepidermal junction in the skin of the horse. Res Vet Sci 15:328, 1973.

199. Talukdar AH, Calhoun ML: A modified dermal part in the skin of the croup region of the horse. Pak J Vet Sci 1:84, 1967.

200. Talukdar AH, et al: Sweat glands of the horse: A histologic study. Am J Vet Res 31:2179, 1970.

201. Talukdar AH, et al: Specialized vascular structures in the skin of the horse. Am J Vet Res 33:335, 1972.

202. Thoday AJ, Friedmann PS: Scientific Basis of Dermatology. A Physiological Approach. Churchill Livingstone, New York, 1986.

203. Trautman A, Fiebiger J: Fundamentals of Histology of Domestic Animals. Comstock Publishing Associates, Ithaca, 1957.

204. Trommershausen-Smith A: Positive horse identification, part 3: Coat color genetics. Equine Pract 1(6):24, 1979.

205. Tsukise A, Meyer W: Histochemical analysis of carbohydrates in the scrotal skin of the horse, with special reference to glandular appendages. Zool Anz 219:129, 1987.

205a. Van der Haegen, et al: Immunoglobulin E–bearing cells in skin biopsies of horses with insect bite hypersensitivity. Equine Vet J 33:699, 2001.

206. Verschooten F, Desmet P: Het klinisch belang van lokale temperatuurmeting bij paarden. Vlaams Diergeneesk Tijdsch 64:132, 1995.

207. Wallengren J: Vasoactive peptides in the skin. J Invest Dermatol Symp Proc 2:87, 1997.

208. Walter P: Sinneshaare im Bereich der Pferdelippe. Zbl Vet Med 3:599, 1956.

209. Walton GS: Abnormal hair growth in domestic animals. In: Rook AJ, Walton GS (eds): Comparative Physiology and Pathology of the Skin. Blackwell Scientific Publications, Oxford, 1965, p 211.

209a. Wattle O: Cytokeratins of the equine hoof wall, chestnut and skin: bio- and immunohisto- chemistry. Equine Vet J 26(suppl):66, 1998.

210. Weinberg WC, et al: Modulation of hair follicle cell proliferation and collagenolytic activity by specific growth factors. Ann NY Acad Sci 642:281, 1991.

211. Wertz PW, Downing DT: Glycolipids in mammalian epidermis: Structure and function of the water barrier. Science 217:1261, 1982.

212. Wertz PW, et al: Comparison of the hydroxyacids from the epidermis and from the sebaceous glands of the horse. Comp Biochem Physiol B 75:217, 1983.

213. Whittem T, et al: Detection of morphine in mane hair of horses. Aust Vet J 76:6, 1998.

214. White SD, Yager JA: Resident dendritic cells in the epidermis: Langerhans cells, Merkel cells, and melanocytes. Vet Dermatol 6:1, 1995.

215. Williams D, et al: 13-cis-retinoic acid affects sheath-shaft interactions of equine hair follicles *in vitro*. J Invest Dermatol 106:356, 1996.

216. Wilson SM, et al: Voltage-evoked currents in cultured equine sweat gland cells. J Physiol 446:433P, 1992.

217. Wilson SM, et al: Calcium-dependent regulation of membrane ion permeability in a cell line derived from the equine sweat gland epithelium. Comp Biochem Physiol A 111:215, 1995.

218. Wunn D, et al: Culture and characterization of equine terminal arch endothelial cells and hoof keratinocytes. Am J Vet Res 60:128, 1999.

219. Yaar M, Gilchrest BA: Human melanocyte growth and differentiation: A decade of new data. J Invest Dermatol 97:611, 1991.

220. Yager JA: The skin as an immune organ. In: Ihrke PJ, et al (eds): Advances in Veterinary Dermatology II. Pergamon Press, New York, 1993, p 3.

221. Yates RA, et al: Epidermal growth factor and related growth factors. Int J Dermatol 30:687, 1991.

222. Yu J, et al: Human hair keratins. J Invest Dermatol 101:56S, 1993.

223. Zlotkin SH: Hair analysis. A useful tool or waste of money? Int J Dermatol 24:161, 1985.

Chapter 2

Diagnostic Methods

● THE SYSTEMATIC APPROACH

Skin diseases are unique in medicine because the lesions and the symptoms are external and potentially visible to the owner and practitioner. This difference offers several unique opportunities for the practitioner. The progression of skin lesions and diseases can often be determined with a good history. Incomplete histories may eventually be amended because the chronic, recurrent nature of many diseases allows the practitioner to instruct clients in what observations they should try to make. The educated client may then add relevant information about the course of the disease. The physical examination reveals the gross pathologic lesions that are present for direct examination. With no other organ system is this great amount of information so readily available.

To benefit optimally from these opportunities, the clinician uses a systematic approach; this greatly increases the probability of determining the correct diagnosis in the most cost-effective manner. Ideally, a thorough examination and appropriate diagnostic procedures are accomplished the first time that the patient is seen and before any masking treatment has been initiated. However, in practice, many clients are reluctant to spend money on diagnostic tests, particularly for the initial occurrence of a problem. This makes a thorough history and physical examination even more important, because they often are the only tools available for arriving at a differential diagnosis.

At the first visit, it is important to establish the client's reliability as a historian and observer. The least expensive tool available to the practitioner is the education of the client about signs and symptoms to look for. The clinician can develop a better relationship with clients and gain valuable information by training clients in what they should observe and watch for, especially if there is a poor response to treatment or a recurrence. Spending some time educating the client in the value of this information often leads to better acceptance of the costs associated with future treatment.

A rational approach to the accurate diagnosis of dermatologic diseases is presented in Table 2-1.

● RECORDS

Recording historical facts, physical examination findings, and laboratory data in a systematic way is particularly important for patients with skin disease.[12,13,34,34a,42] Many dermatoses are chronic, and skin lesions may be slow to change. For this reason, many practitioners use outline sketches of the patient, which enable the clinician to draw the location and the extent of lesions.

Fig. 2-1 is a record form for noting physical examination and laboratory findings for dermatology cases. Most important, the form leads the clinician to consider the case in a systematic manner. It also enables one to apply pertinent descriptive terms, saves time, and ensures that no important information is omitted. This form details only dermatologic data and should be used as

59

● Table 2-1   **STEPS TO A DERMATOLOGIC DIAGNOSIS**

MAJOR STEP	KEY POINTS TO DETERMINE OR QUESTIONS TO ANSWER
Chief complaint	Why is the client seeking veterinary care?
Signalment	Record the animal's age, breed, sex, and weight.
Dermatologic history	Obtain data about the original lesion's location, appearance, onset, and rate of progression. Also determine the degree of pruritus, contagion to other animals or people, and possible seasonal incidence.
Previous medical history	Medical history that does not directly seem to relate should also be reviewed.
Client credibility	Determine what the clients initially noticed that indicated a problem. Repeat questions and ask in a different way to determine how certain the clients are and whether they understand the questions.
Physical examination	Determine the distribution pattern and the regional location of lesions. Certain patterns are diagnostically significant. Closely examine the skin to identify primary and secondary lesions. Determine skin and hair quality (e.g., thin, thick, turgid, elastic, dull, oily, or dry).
	Observe the configurations of specific skin lesions and their relationship to each other.
Differential diagnosis	Differential diagnosis is developed on the basis of the preceding data. The most likely diagnoses are recorded in order of probability.
Diagnostic or therapeutic plan	A plan is presented to the client. The client and the clinician then agree on a plan.
Diagnostic and laboratory aids	Simple and inexpensive office diagnostic procedures that confirm or rule out any of the most likely (first three or four) differential diagnostic possibilities should be done.
	More complex or expensive diagnostic tests or procedures are then recommended.
	Clients may elect to forgo these tests and pursue less likely differential diagnostic possiblities in attempts to save money. Often, this approach is not cost-effective when the expense of inefficient medications and repeated examination is considered.
Trial therapy	Clients may elect to pursue a therapeutical trial instead of diagnostic procedures. Trial therapies should be selected so that further diagnostic information is obtained. Generally, glucocorticoids are not acceptable because little diagnostic information is obtained.
Narrowing the differential diagnosis	Plan additional tests, observations of therapeutic trials, and re-evaluations of signs and symptoms to narrow the list and provide a definitive diagnosis.

a supplement to the general history and physical examination record. A special dermatologic history form is also useful, especially for patients with allergies and chronic diseases (Fig. 2-2).

The disadvantage of the forms is that many chronic cases have tremendous variations in the type of lesions and their distribution, making a map confusing. For example, how would one draw the following alopecia lesion? A 10-cm plaque in the flank fold has a central (8-cm) zone of lichenification, hyperpigmentation, alopecia, and crusts. The outer (2-cm) margin is alopecic and has a papular dermatitis with mild hyperpigmentation. Peripheral to the plaque are occasional tufted papules. Representing several different lesions on a small diagram is difficult or, if done, is often unreadable. This can make a diagram unsatisfactory to use. Therefore, the authors have found that brief written descriptions of lesions in various body regions are preferable to diagrams in complicated cases.

● HISTORY
General Concepts

The horse's disease is like an unsolved mystery in which the client is the witness to what has occurred and the veterinarian is the detective who must ascertain what the client observed. As this information is extracted, the veterinarian becomes the lawyer to determine whether the client is a

SKIN LESIONS (Check)

_____ Macule	_____ Patch	_____ Purpura	_____ Wheal
_____ Papule	_____ Nodule	_____ Plaque	_____ Tumor
_____ Pustule	_____ Vesicle	_____ Bulla	_____ Cyst
_____ Abscess	_____ Scale	_____ Erosion	_____ Erythema
_____ Hypotrichosis	_____ Alopecia	_____ Crust	_____ Ulcer
_____ Fissure	_____ Scar	_____ Excoriation	_____ Collarette
_____ Hyperpigmentation	_____ Hypopigmentation		
_____ Hyperkeratosis	_____ Callus	_____ Comedo	
_____ Lichenification	_____ Sinus	_____ Necrosis	
_____ Hyperhidrosis	_____ Nikolsky's sign		

SKIN CHANGES (Check)

_____ Normal	_____ Thick	_____ Thin	_____ Fragile
_____ Hypotonic	_____ Hyperextensible	_____ Increased laxity	

HAIR COAT CHANGES (Check)

_____ Hypotrichosis	_____ Alopecia	_____ Hypertrichosis	_____
_____ Leukotrichia	_____ Melanotrichia		
_____ Other color change	_____ Easy epilation		
_____ Dry coat	_____ Brittle coat	_____ Oily coat	
_____ Hair casts	_____ Color associated hair loss		

CONFIGURATION OF LESIONS (Check)

_____ Annular	_____ Follicular	_____ Grouped
_____ Linear	_____ Other	

CUTANEOUS PAIN (Check)

_____ Absent	_____ Mild	_____ Moderate	_____ Severe

PRURITUS (Check)

_____ Absent	_____ Mild	_____ Moderate	_____ Severe
_____ Lesional	_____ Nonlesional		

PARASITES (Check)

_____ Lice	_____ Ticks	_____ Chiggers	_____
_____ Other			

OTHER FINDINGS

Ears _____
Oral cavity _____
Mucocutaneous junctions _____
Coronets _____
Hooves _____

LABORATORY

Scrapings _____
Scotch tape _____
Trichography _____
Cytology _____
Culture _____

DIAGNOSIS/DIFFERENTIAL

_____
_____
_____

FIGURE 2-1. Dermatology examination sheet.

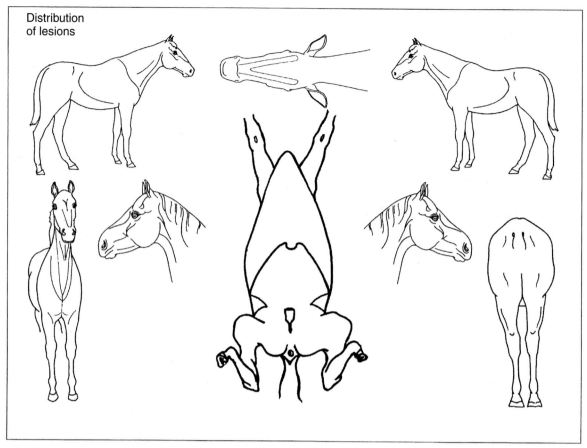

Distribution
of lesions

FIGURE 2-1, cont'd. Dermatology examination sheet. (*From Pascoe RRR, Knottenbelt DC: Manual of Equine Dermatology. W.B. Saunders Co. Philadelphia 1999.*)

credible or qualified witness. Obtaining a thorough history and being attentive to clues from the client are skills that must be practiced and developed by the clinician in order to develop a tentative diagnosis. A comprehensive history in conjunction with a thorough dermatologic examination is helpful for another practical reason: this is often when the veterinarian initially establishes her or his credibility as a professional with the client. In veterinary dermatology, the client-veterinarian relationship is often important for a successful outcome. Because many chronic diseases necessitate lifelong control and can be frustrating for client and veterinarian alike, it is critical for the client-veterinarian relationship to start well. If the veterinarian is thorough and obtains the most information possible from the history and the dermatologic examination, the client is more likely to recognize the effort and expertise of the veterinarian. These clients are often more agreeable to pursuing diagnostic tests or trial therapies if the information from the initial exhaustive examination is not sufficient for a diagnosis. Cursory examinations leave a sense of insecurity in some clients, making them reluctant to follow recommendations based on such examinations.

Owner's Chief Complaint

The owner's chief complaint, or chief cause of concern, is often one of the major signs initially used in establishing a differential diagnosis. Addressing the client's chief complaint is an important step in achieving satisfaction of clients and obtaining their confidence and often initiates a favorable

Owner name _____ Horse name _____ Date _____

Age when purchased _____

What is the horse's use? _____

What is your complaint about the horse's skin? _____

Age of horse? _____ Age when skin problem started? _____

Where on the body did the problem start? _____

What did the skin problem look like initially? _____

_____

How has it spread or changed? _____

Is the problem continual or intermittent? _____

If seasonal, what seasons is the disease present? _____

_____

Does the horse itch? _____ If so, where? _____

_____

Do any horses in contact with the affected horse have skin problems? _____

If so, are they similar or different from this horse's problem? _____

Do any people in contact with the horse have skin problems? _____

Do you use insect control? _____ If so, describe _____

_____

Do any relatives of this horse have skin problems? _____ If yes, explain _____

_____

Please list any injectable, oral, or topical medications that have been used to treat the problem (veterinary or "home remedies") _____

_____

Did any help the condition? _____ If yes, which ones? _____

Did any aggravate the condition? _____ If yes, which ones? _____

Describe the environment where the horse is kept: Indoors _____

_____ Outdoors _____

Does your horse travel? _____ If yes, where and when? _____

_____

What is the horse fed? _____

What feed additives do you use? _____

What is your deworming schedule? _____

Did the horse receive ivermectin? _____

List any other medical problems or drugs that the horse received _____

_____

List any additional information you feel is relevant to the skin disease _____

FIGURE 2-2. Dermatology history sheet.

client-veterinarian relationship. Other findings not directly related to the chief complaint may be uncovered. Although these additional findings are important to discuss, the client's chief complaint must always be addressed.

Age

Some dermatologic disorders are age-related, so age is important in the dermatologic history.[38] For example, hereditary disorders such as epidermolysis bullosa, cutaneous asthenia, and follicular dysplasia are usually apparent at birth or within the first 6 months of age. Allergies tend to appear in more mature animals, probably because repeated exposure to the antigen must occur and the immune response has to occur before clinical signs develop.

Breed

Breed predilection determines the incidence of some skin disorders (Table 2-2).[38]

Sex

Rarely, the sex of the patient is a key to diagnosis. Males are predisposed to mast cell tumors. Females with ovarian neoplasms may be predisposed to cutaneous lymphoma/pseudolymphoma.

Color

The color of an animal may also be related to certain problems—most notable is the association of solar dermatitis, actinic keratosis, and squamous cell carcinoma in white-skinned, thinly haired regions. Coat color may also relate to disease, as in lethal white and lavender foal syndromes and the frequency of melanocytic neoplasia in gray horses.

Medical History

The clinician should obtain a complete medical history in all cases.[12,13,34,34a,42] In practice, two levels of history are taken. The first level includes those questions that are always asked, and this level is often helped by having the client fill out a history questionnaire before the examination (see

● Table 2-2 **POSSIBLE BREED PREDILECTION FOR NON-NEOPLASTIC SKIN DISEASES**

BREED	DISEASE
Arabian	Atopy
	Hypotrichosis
	Lavender foal syndrome
	Spotted leukotrichia
	Vitiligo
Belgian	Epidermolysis bullosa
	Linear keratosis
Icelandic	*Culicoides* hypersensitivity
Quarter horse	Cutaneous asthenia
	Linear alopecia
	Linear keratosis
	Reticulated leukotrichia
	Unilateral papular dermatosis
Standardbred	Calcinosis circumscripta
	Reticulated leukotrichia
Thoroughbred	Atopy
	Reticulated leukotrichia

Fig. 2-2). Often, the answers on these forms will change if the client is questioned directly, so these form answers should be reviewed and not relied on as initially answered. The first level should initially include questions about previous illnesses and problems. The second level in history taking relates to more specific questions that relate to specific diseases. These more pertinent questions are usually asked once the practitioner has examined the animal and is developing a differential diagnosis or has at least established what some of the problems are. However, it is vital to use a systematic, detailed method of examination and history taking so that important information is not overlooked. A complete history takes a lot of time to obtain and usually is a major component of the initial examination period. In practice, most practitioners do not take the time to collect a thorough history for the problem. Learning which historical questions are most important for specific problems and being certain to collect this information becomes critical. Often, the history is completed during the examination and once the initial differential diagnosis is determined.

The clinician who can draw out a complete history in an unbiased form has a valuable skill. It is important that the questions presented to the client do not suggest answers or tend to shut off discussion. Some owners purposely or unconsciously withhold pertinent facts, especially about neglect, diet, previous medication, or other procedures they think may not be well received by the examining veterinarian. Other pertinent information may be left out because some owners are not aware of what is normal. Therefore, they may not supply valuable information because they do not perceive the information to be significant or abnormal. In other cases, they may recognize something as abnormal but attribute the observation to some other, unrelated cause.

The clinician must become skillful at extracting all the relevant history and observations, regardless of the client's perception of their importance. The skillful clinician is ever tuned to listen for side comments by the client or by the children. These may be veritable "pearls" of information in a mass of trivia. They also help to establish the client's accuracy and credibility.

Next, the following information about the skin lesions should be obtained from the owner: the date and age at onset, the original locations, the initial appearance, the tendency to progression or regression, factors affecting the course, and previous treatment (home or proprietary remedies used, as well as veterinary treatment). In addition, treatments of other problems should be determined and recorded. The relationships between all treatments and the onset of, or changes in, the disease should be recorded and a possible drug reaction considered. Drug reactions are diagnosed only when they are suspected, and because they may mimic any disease, the history aids in arriving at this diagnosis.

Almost all animals with skin disorders have been bathed, dipped, sprayed, or treated with one or more medications, and the owner may be reluctant or unable to disclose a complete list of previous treatments. It is important that the types of medication and the dates of application are completely divulged, because a modification of pertinent signs may have resulted.

Although the patient cannot relate subjective findings (symptoms such as itching, burning sensation, and pain), it is possible to determine the degree of pruritus reasonably well. The presence and severity of pain may also be evaluated in some cases by the patient's response to stimuli: exhibiting shyness, pulling away, exhibiting skin twitching, and responding with aggressiveness may be manifested when pain is provoked.

Pruritus is one of the most common presenting complaints and, in many cases, is a hallmark of allergy. The presence, location, and degree of itching are important criteria in the differential diagnosis of many skin diseases. The owner's idea of the intensity of itching, however, may vary considerably from that of the veterinarian. Consequently, it is helpful to ask questions, such as "How many times daily do you see your horse scratch or chew?" "Does it itch in many sites, or just a few?" "Does it shake its head?" "Does it stomp its feet?" "Does it lick the front legs or other areas?" "Does it rub parts of its body against things?" Because many diseases associated with pruritus are chronic, it is often helpful to have the client initially grade the itching on a scale of 0 to 10—0 being no itching at all, 1 being very mild, and 10 being as bad as the horse has ever itched. This level can be recorded and asked again as therapies or diagnostic procedures are tried to help determine how the horse's problem changes over time. Also, by obtaining answers to the previous questions about the pruritus, the practitioner establishes a record of the severity of the problem and the symptoms seen when the owner indicates a level of itching. Over time, the client's perceptions may change, and this approach allows any change to be determined and documented. It is also very helpful to determine, when possible, whether the pruritus involves initially normal-appearing skin (an itch that rashes, typical of allergy) or whether skin lesions precede or appear at the same time as the pruritus (a rash that itches).

The same types of specific questions are helpful when discussing diets, because the owner often states the typical feedings and leaves out treats and supplements. Specifically, the clinician asks whether any vitamins, supplements, or treats are given. The clinician also asks about changes in food sources throughout the year.

Because contact irritants or allergens are important contributors to or causes of skin disease, it is necessary to inquire about the animal's environment. Details about stables, paddocks, fields, bedding, grooming protocols, and so forth may be very important. Do the symptoms improve or resolve when the horse leaves its usual surroundings (travel, show, competition, boarding, and so forth)? Symptoms that resolve in a different environment are highly suggestive of a reaction to an environmental allergen or irritant. Other more organ-specific questions may also be asked, depending on the clinical suspicions of possible diseases.

In determining contagion, one should inquire about the skin health of other animals on the premises, and where the horse has been in the last 6 weeks. The presence of skin disease in the people living with the patient may also be highly significant in some disorders (e.g., dermatophytosis).

At this point, the clinician usually has a general idea of the problem and is ready to proceed with a careful physical examination. In some cases, the clinician may want to come back to the medical history if further examinations indicate a more serious or underlying systemic disease.

● PHYSICAL EXAMINATION
General Observations

A good examination necessitates adequate lighting. Normal daylight without glare is best, but any artificial light of adequate candlepower is sufficient if it produces bright, non–color-changing, uniform lighting. The lamp should be adjustable to illuminate all body areas. A combination loupe and light provides magnification of the field as well as good illumination.

Before the clinician concentrates on the individual lesions, the entire animal should always be observed from a distance of a couple of meters to obtain a general impression of abnormalities and to observe distribution patterns. Does the horse appear to be in good health? Is it fat or thin, unkempt or well groomed? Is the problem generalized or localized? What is the distribution and configuration of the lesions? Are they bilaterally symmetric or unilaterally irregular? Is the hair coat shiny or dull, and if it is dull, what is the pattern of those changes? Is it an appropriate color and pattern of colors for its breed? Are coat changes in quality or color lifelong, or did they develop before or after the symptoms for which the horse is presented?

To answer some of these questions, the clinician must examine the patient more closely. The dorsal aspect of the body should be inspected by viewing it from the rear, as elevated hairs and patchy alopecia may be more obvious from that angle. Then, the head, the lateral trunk, and the extremities should be observed. Next, the clinician should complete a thorough dermatologic examination.

Dermatologic Examination

After an impression is obtained from a distance, the skin should be examined more closely and palpated.[12,13,34,34a,42] It is important to examine every centimeter of skin and visible mucous membranes. Many subtle clues are located where the client is unaware of problems.

Many observations need to be made. What is the texture of the hair? Is it coarse or fine, dry or oily? Does it epilate easily? A change in the amount of hair is often a dramatic finding, although subtle thinning of the hair coat should also be noted. Alopecia is a partial or complete lack of hair in areas where it is normally present. Hypotrichosis implies partial hair loss and is a form of alopecia. Is the thinning diffuse, or are there numerous small focal areas of alopecia (the latter being often seen with folliculitis)? Hypertrichosis is excessive hair, and although the condition is uncommon, it usually has hormonal causes.

The texture, elasticity, and thickness of the skin should be determined and impressions of heat or coolness recorded. There is variation in an animal's coat density in different body areas, with skin lesions often being discerned more readily in sparsely haired regions. Therefore, the clinician must part or clip the hair in heavily haired areas to observe and palpate lesions that are present but obscured.

When abnormalities are discovered, it is important to establish their morphologic features, configuration, and general distribution. The clinician should try to appreciate the different lesions and their patterns. Together, they often represent the natural history of the skin disease.

Morphology of Skin Lesions

The morphologic characteristics of skin lesions, together with their history, are an essential feature of dermatologic diagnosis.[12,13,34,38,42] Morphologic features and the medical and dermatologic history are often the only guidelines if laboratory procedures cannot be performed or do not yield useful information. The clinician must learn to recognize primary and secondary lesions. A primary lesion is the initial eruption that develops spontaneously as a direct reflection of underlying disease. Secondary lesions evolve from primary lesions or are artifacts induced by the patients or by external factors such as trauma and medications. Primary lesions (pustules, vesicles, papules) may appear quickly and then disappear rapidly. However, they may leave behind secondary lesions (such as focal alopecia, epidermal collarettes, scaling, hyperpigmentation, and crusts), which may be more chronic and give clues about the presence of previous primary lesions. Therefore, the identification and the characterization of both primary and secondary lesions are important. Careful inspection of the diseased skin frequently reveals a primary lesion, which may suggest a limited differential diagnosis.

A primary lesion may vary slightly from its initial appearance to its full development. Later, through regression, degeneration, or traumatization, it may change in form and become a secondary lesion. Although classic descriptions and textbooks refer to lesions as primary or secondary, some lesions can be either (e.g., alopecia can be primary [from hereditary disorders] or secondary [from chewing because of pruritus]). Scales and pigment changes may also be primary or secondary.

Secondary lesions may also be informative. A ring of scaling usually follows a point source of inflammation, either a papule or a pustule. This is also true of small focal circular areas of alopecia. Yellow- to honey-colored crusts usually follow the rupture and drying of pustules. In many cases, however, the significant lesion must be differentiated from the mass of secondary debris. Variations of lesions and their configurations are common, because early and advanced stages coexist in most skin diseases. The ability to discover a characteristic lesion and understand its significance is an important aspect of mastering dermatologic diagnoses.

The following illustrations can help the clinician identify primary and secondary lesions. Also, the character of the lesions may vary, implying a different pathogenesis or cause. The definitions and examples in Figs. 2-3 to 2-17 explain the relationship of skin lesions to equine dermatoses.

- *Primary lesions*
  Macule or patch (Fig. 2-3)
  Papule or plaque (Fig. 2-4)
  Pustule (Fig. 2-5)
  Vesicle or bulla (Fig. 2-6)
  Wheal (Fig. 2-7)
  Nodule (Fig. 2-8)
  Tumor or cyst (Fig. 2-9)
- *Lesions that may be primary or secondary*
  Alopecia (Fig. 2-10)
  Scale (Fig. 2-11)
  Crust (Fig. 2-12)
  Hair casts (Fig. 2-13)

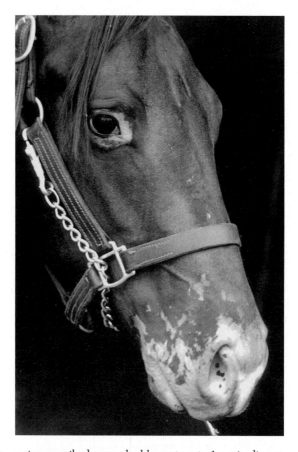

FIGURE 2-3. *Macule*—a circumscribed, nonpalpable spot up to 1 cm in diameter and caused by a change in the color of the skin. *Patch*—a macule larger than 1 cm in diameter. The discoloration can result from several processes: depigmentation, hyperpigmentation, erythema, or hemorrhage. Examples include postinflammatory hyperpigmentation and vitiligo (photograph illustrates vitiligo). Types of hemorrhagic macules and patches are as follows: purpura—bleeding into the skin (these are usually dark red but change to purple); petechiae—pinpoint macules that are much smaller than 1 cm in diameter; ecchymoses—patches of hemorrhage.

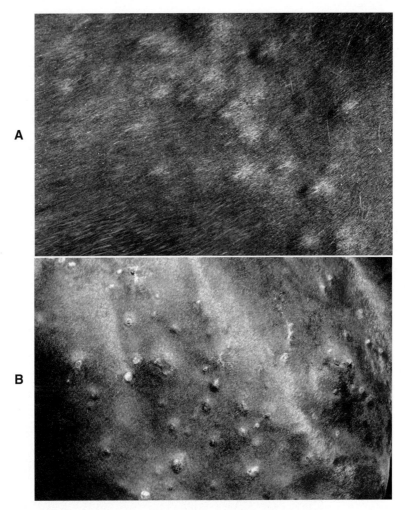

FIGURE 2-4. *Papule*—a small, firm, palpable mass in the skin that is up to 1 cm in diameter. Papules may be elevated, intradermal, or subcutaneous. Most papules are caused by inflammatory infiltrates and may or may not involve hair follicles. Most papules are caused by infectious agents (such as *Staphylococcus*, *Dermatophilus*, or dermatophyte) or ectoparasites. Papules caused by infectious agents typically involve hair follicles and begin as tufted papules (**A** illustrates early staphylococcal folliculitis), which then ooze, crust, lose hair, and may or may not result in erosions or ulcers (**B** illustrates bacterial pseudomycetoma or "botryomycosis").

Continued

Comedo—a dilated hair follicle filled with keratin and glandular secretion. Comedones are rarely seen in the horse, but could be associated with diseases of keratinization (e.g., seborrhea) or inflammatory disorders of the hair follicle.
Pigmentary abnormalities (Fig. 2-14)
• *Secondary lesions*
Epidermal collarette (Fig. 2-15)
Scar—an area of fibrous tissue that has replaced the damaged dermis or subcutaneous tissue
Excoriation (Fig. 2-16)
Erosion or ulcer (Fig. 2-16)

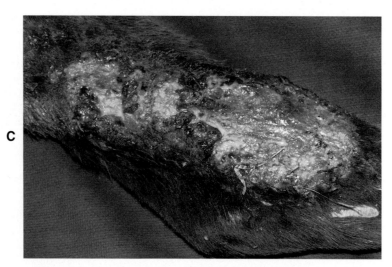

FIGURE 2-4, cont'd. *Plaque*—a larger, flat-topped elevation formed by the extension or coalescence of papules (**C** illustrates an ulcerated plaque caused by *Rhodococcus equi*).

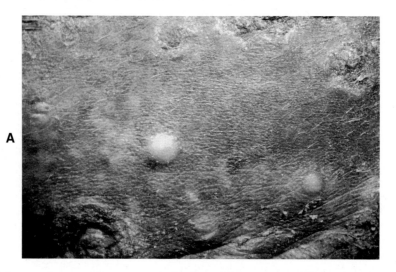

FIGURE 2-5. *Pustule*—a small, circumscribed, elevated lesion that is filled with pus. Pustules may be intraepidermal, follicular, or subepidermal in location. Their color is usually yellowish to whitish. Pustules are rarely seen in the horse, and are usually caused by bacterial infection or pemphigus foliaceus. **A**, Pemphigus foliaceus.

Fissure—a linear cleavage into the skin. Fissures occur when the skin is thick, dry, and inelastic.

Lichenification—a thickening and hardening of the skin by an exaggeration of the superficial skin markings. The most common cause is chronic inflammation.

Callus—a thickened, rough, hyperkeratotic, alopecic plaque that develops most commonly over bony prominences in response to pressure and low-grade friction.

Necrosis (Fig. 2-17)

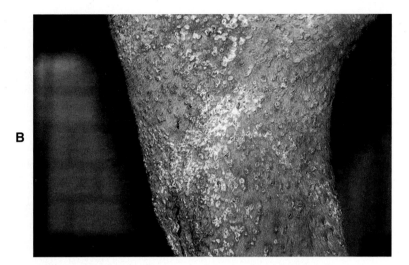

FIGURE 2-5, cont'd. B, Multiple pustules caused by a drug reaction (ivermectin). *Abscess*—a demarcated, fluctuant lesion resulting from the dermal or subcutaneous accumulation of pus. The pus is not visible on the surface of the skin until it drains to the surface. Abscesses are larger and deeper than pustules.

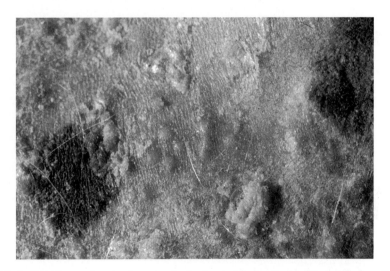

FIGURE 2-6. *Vesicle*—a sharply circumscribed, elevated lesion that is filled with clear fluid and is up to 1 cm in diameter. Vesicles are uncommonly seen in the horse and are caused by autoimmune dermatoses (photograph illustrates pemphigus foliaceus), epidermolysis bullosa, viral infections, drug reactions, photodermatitis, and burns (chemical, thermal). *Bulla*—a vesicle that is over 1 cm in diameter.

Two special techniques of close examination of the skin, although infrequently used, are noteworthy:
1. *Diascopy* is performed by pressing a clear piece of plastic or glass over an erythematous lesion. If the lesion blanches on pressure, the reddish color is due to vascular engorgement. If it does not, there is hemorrhage into the skin (petechia or ecchymosis).
2. *Nikolsky's sign* is elicited by applying pressure on a vesicle or at the edge of an ulcer or erosion or even on normal skin.[9a] It is positive when the outer layer of the skin is easily rubbed

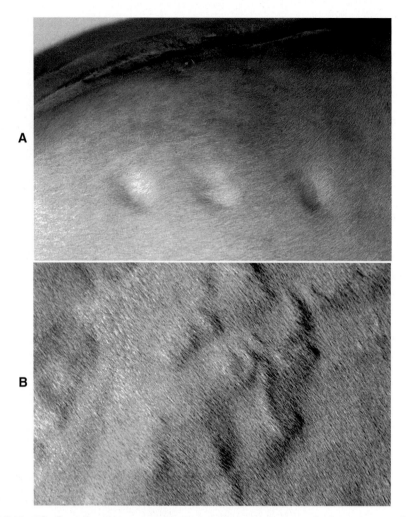

FIGURE 2-7. *Wheal*—a sharply circumscribed, raised lesion consisting of edema that usually appears and disappears within hours. Wheals usually produce no changes in the appearance of the overlying skin and hair coat, and disappear without leaving a trace. Wheals are very common on the horse, and are most commonly seen with hypersensitivity reactions (atopy, food hypersensitivity, contact reactions). Wheals may be annular and papular to flat-topped (**A** illustrates urticaria caused by penicillin drug reaction) or polycyclic (ring-like, arciform, serpiginous) in appearance (**B** illustrates urticaria in an atopic horse).

off or pushed away. It indicates poor cellular cohesion, as found in the pemphigus complex, bullous pemphigoid, erythema multiforme, and epidermolysis bullosa.

Configuration of Lesions[34,38]

The configuration of skin lesions may be helpful in establishing a differential diagnosis.[34,38,42] Some diseases often have lesions present in certain configurations, and although exceptions exist, recognizing the pattern of lesions adds information for decision making. Lesions may be single, such as the solitary dermatophytosis lesion, a foreign-body reaction, or a neoplasm. Multiple lesions are most commonly seen in skin diseases of horses.

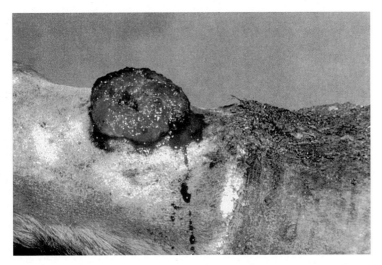

FIGURE 2-8. *Nodule*—a circumscribed, firm mass in the skin that is over 1 cm in diameter. Nodules may be elevated, intradermal, or subcutaneous in location. Nodules are very common in the horse, and are usually caused by granulomatous inflammation (infectious or sterile) or neoplasia. (Photograph illustrates an alopecic, ulcerated equine sarcoid.)

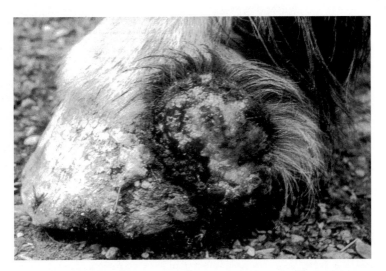

FIGURE 2-9. *Tumor*—a large mass that may arise from any cutaneous cell type. Tumors are very common in the horse; most are neoplastic or granulomatous in origin (Photograph illustrates bacterial pseudomycetoma.) *Cyst*—an epithelium-lined cavity containing fluid or solid material. It is a smooth, well-circumscribed, fluctuant to solid mass. Cutaneous cysts are usually lined by adnexal epithelium (hair follicle, sebaceous gland, epitrichial sweat gland) and filled with keratin, hair, and/or glandular secretion).

When lesions are linear, external forces such as scratching, being scratched by something, and having something applied to the skin are often responsible. In other cases, linear lesions may reflect the involvement of a blood or lymphatic vessel, a dermatome, or a congenital malformation. Diffuse areas of involvement tend to suggest a metabolic or systemic reaction, such as endocrine

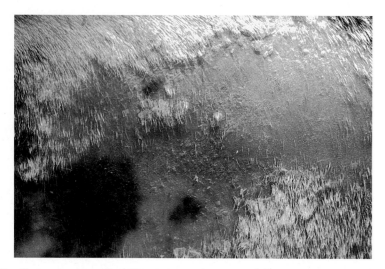

FIGURE 2-10. *Alopecia*—a loss of hair that may vary from partial (hypotrichosis) to complete. Alopecia is common in the horse and is most often associated with inflammation of hair follicles (infectious or sterile) or self-trauma in response to pruritus. (Photograph illustrates contact dermatitis.)

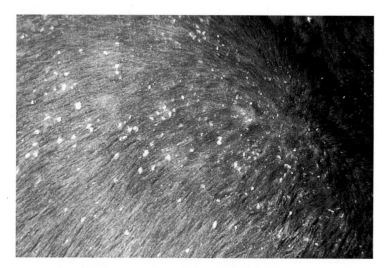

FIGURE 2-11. *Scale*—an accumulation of loose fragments of the stratum corneum. The corneocyte is the final product of epidermal keratinization. Normal loss occurs as individual cells or small clusters not visible to the eye. Abnormal scaling is caused by the shedding of larger clusters. Scales (flakes) vary in consistency from thin, nonadherent to thick, adherent, waxy. Color varies from white, yellowish, or grayish to brownish in color. Scales are common in the horse and are most often produced by inflammatory dermatoses. (Photograph illustrates seborrhea sicca in association with chronic liver disease.)

disorders, keratinization, and immunologic or hypersensitivity disorders. Annular lesions are often associated with peripheral spreading of a disease. Common examples of annular lesions are bacterial folliculitis, dermatophilosis, and dermatophytosis. Coalescing lesions occur when multiple lesions are present and spread so that they overlap.

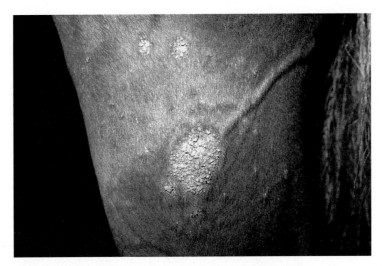

FIGURE 2-12. *Crust*—formed when dried exudate, serum, pus, blood, cells, scales, or medications adhere to the surface of the skin. Crusts are common in the horse and are usually annular and associated with infections (photograph illustrates dermatophytosis) and ectoparasites.

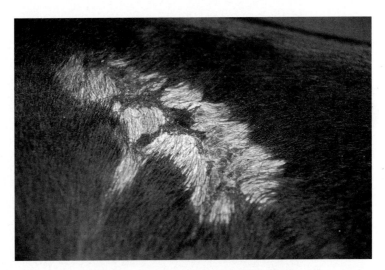

FIGURE 2-13. *Hair cast*—an accumulation of keratin and follicular material that adheres to the hair shaft. Hair casts indicate abnormalities in follicular keratinization and may be seen in primary seborrhea, dermatophytoses, staphylococcal folliculitis, and demodicosis. (Photograph illustrates hair casts in association with contact dermatitis; hair shafts are encircled by keratinous and medication-derived material.)

Different Stages

A skin disease and its individual lesions progress from its earliest appearance to a fully developed state and, in many cases, to a chronic or resolved stage. The distribution, the configuration, and the histologic appearance of lesions change. The evolution of lesions should be determined either by obtaining the history or by finding different stages of lesions on the patient. Papules may develop into vesicles and pustules, which may rupture to leave erosions or ulcers and finally crusts. An understanding of these progressions helps in the diagnostic process.

As lesions develop in specific patterns, they also involute in characteristic ways. The lesions change, along with their histologic appearance. For example, a macule may develop into a papule and then a crust or crusted erosion. It may then spread peripherally, occurring as a ring of lesions; the lesion then appears as a circular patch with multiple papules or crusts on the margins and central alopecia. The fully developed lesions could appear as a large alopecic patch with a central area of hyperpigmentation and multifocal erythematous macules, papules, or crusts intermittently along the leading margin; this lesion could then appear arciform. Scaling may also occur at the leading margins of inflammation. The healing phase of a chronic lesion may appear as a patch of alopecia and hyperpigmentation with no other primary or secondary lesions because they have spontaneously resolved or responded to therapy.

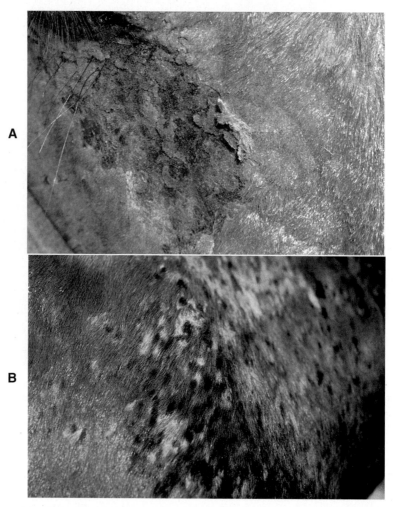

FIGURE 2-14. *Abnormal pigmentation*—usually caused by increased or decreased amounts of melanin. Increased melanization of skin and hair are referred to as *melanoderma* (hyperpigmentation) and *melanotrichia*, respectively. **A,** Alopecia and melanoderma caused by pemphigus foliaceus. **B,** Melanotrichia caused by *Culicoides* hypersensitivity. Decreased melanization of skin and hair are referred to as *leukoderma* (depigmentation) and *leukotrichia*, respectively. Fig. 2-3 illustrates leukoderma caused by vitiligo.

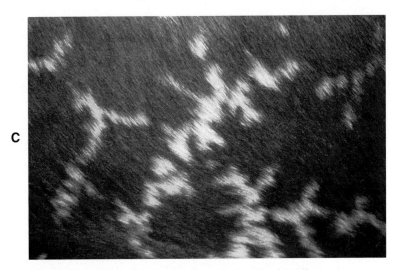

FIGURE 2-14, cont'd. C, Leukotrichia caused by reticulated leukotrichia.

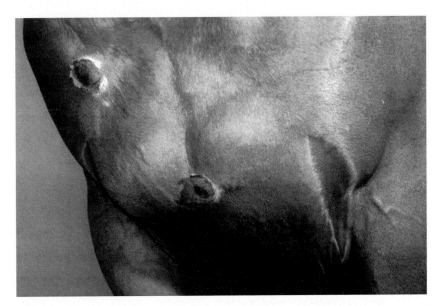

FIGURE 2-15. *Epidermal collarette*—a special type of scale arranged in an annular rim of separated ("peeling") epithelium or loose scales. Collarettes usually represent the remnants of the roof of a pustule, vesicle, or bulla, and hence the prior existence of a fluid-filled lesion. (Photograph illustrates epidermal collarettes in association with staphylococcal folliculitis.)

Because diseases and their lesions are evolutionary, the clinician must attempt to learn about all of the stages. The recognition of the different stages as well as the lesions becomes important when selecting areas to sample for diagnostic tests.

Distribution Patterns of Skin Lesions

The areas of skin involved with lesions or affected by symptoms of the disease help in determining the differential diagnosis because most skin diseases have a typical distribution.[34,38,42] It is important to emphasize that the accurate determination of the distribution necessitates detection

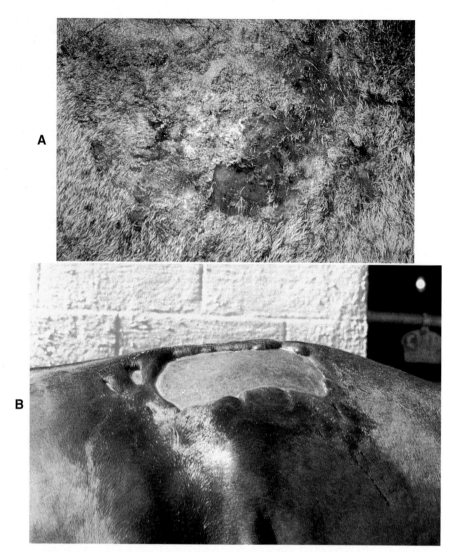

FIGURE 2-16. *Erosion*—a shallow epithelial defect that does not breech the basement membrane zone and consequently heals without scarring. Erosions usually result from the progression of papular, pustular, and vesicular diseases or self-trauma. **A**, Pemphigus foliaceus. *Ulcer*—a deeper defect that breeches the basement membrane and exposes the underlying dermal and possibly subcutaneous tissues. Scars may be left when ulcers heal. **B**, An ulcer resulting from a skin slough caused by clostridial cellulitis. *Excoriation*—self-induced erosions and ulcers caused by rubbing, biting, scratching, and so forth. Excoriations indicate the presence of pruritus, and are often linear in nature.

of all changes in the haircoat or the skin, the location of symptoms related to the disease, and the location of all primary and secondary lesions. An adequate determination of the distribution pattern can be achieved only by a thorough history and dermatologic examination; cursory examinations are often incomplete.

The study of skin diseases involves understanding the primary lesions that occur, as well as the typical distribution patterns. Diseases less commonly present with atypical patterns. The combination of the type of lesions present and their distribution is the basis for developing a

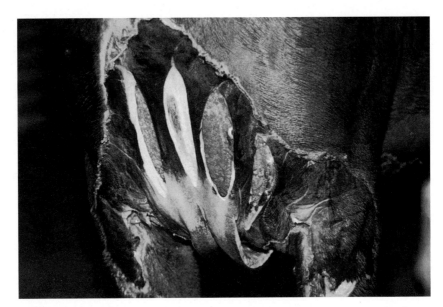

FIGURE 2-17. *Necrosis*—the death of skin due to ischemia or toxins. Necrotic skin becomes bluish, purplish, and black, and eventually dry and firm (leathery). Common causes include clostridial infection (photograph illustrates well-delineated necrosis and ulceration due to clostridial cellulitis), vasculitis, and pressure.

differential diagnosis. The distribution pattern may be very helpful by allowing clinicians to establish the differential diagnosis based on the region involved when animals have lesions and symptoms confined to certain regions (Table 2-3). In some instances, this regional pattern is such a major feature that it is a required aspect of the disease.

Table 2-3 lists areas or parts of the body along with the common skin diseases that are most frequently localized or especially severe in those areas. (Also see Tables 15-1 [nodules], 15-3 [pasterns], and 15-4 [coronary bands].) These charts are useful in the differential diagnosis. However, the clinician must also be aware that other diseases may occur in these regions and that diseases which often affect a certain region can also occur elsewhere and not involve the typical region. Therefore, regional evaluations aid in ranking differential diagnostic possibilities: they do not determine the diagnosis.

In many instances, the patterning that skin diseases take is unexplained. Recently, homeobox genes have received much attention.[7a] These genes are a family of regulatory proteins that influence pattern formation at many levels and may be fundamental to the development of the many patterns used to diagnose skin diseases.

Differential Diagnosis

A differential diagnosis is developed on the basis of a compilation of the preceding information. The possible diagnoses should be considered in their proposed likely order of occurrence. This point is important as the first step in developing a cost-effective plan.

Developing a Diagnostic or Therapeutic Plan

Laboratory tests or therapies can be recommended on the basis of tentative diagnosis and differential diagnosis. If a strong tentative diagnosis is not determined from the history and the physical examination, the approach should be directed at the two or three most likely diagnoses. Client-

● Table 2-3   **REGIONAL DIAGNOSIS OF NON-NEOPLASTIC DERMATOSES***

REGION	COMMON DISEASES	UNCOMMON TO RARE DISEASES
Face	Atopy	Alopecia areata
	Black fly bites	Amyloidosis
	Dermatophilosis	Bacterial pseudomycetoma
	Dermatophytosis	Besnoitiosis
	Insect hypersensitivity	Conidiobolomycosis
	Photodermatitis	Copper deficiency
	Staphylococcal folliculitis	Demodicosis
	Ticks	Discoid lupus erythematosus
	Trombiculosis	Eumycotic mycetoma
		Food hypersensitivity
		Forage mites
		Habronemiasis
		Halicephalobiasis
		Histoplasmosis
		Leishmaniasis
		Multisystemic eosinophilic exfoliative disease
		Oncocerciasis
		Pemphigus foliaceus
		Poultry mites
		Rhinosporidiosis
		Sarcoidosis
		Sarcoptic mange
		Snake bite
		Stachybotryotoxicosis
		Vaccinia
		Vitiligo
Ears	Atopy	Cryoglobulinemia
	Black fly bites	Ergotism
	Dermatophytosis	Food hypersensitivity
	Insect hypersensitivity	Leishmaniasis
	Photodermatitis	Psoroptic mange
	Ticks	Sarcoptic mange
	Trombiculosis	Vasculitis
Neck	Atopy	Alopecia areata
	Black fly bites	Amyloidosis
	Dermatophytosis	Demodicosis
	Horse fly bites	Erythema multiforme
	Insect hypersensitivity	Forage mites
	Stable fly bites	Histoplasmosis
	Staphylococcal folliculitis	Leishmaniasis
	Ticks	Linear alopecia
	Trombiculosis	Linear keratosis
	Urticaria	Molluscum contagiosum
		Onchocerciasis
		Panniculitis
		Parafilariasis
		Sarcoptic mange
		Snake bite
Trunk	Dermatophilosis	Amyloidosis
	Dermatophytosis	Axillary nodular necrosis
	Eosinophilic granuloma	Basidiobolomycosis
	Horse fly bites	Coccidioidomycosis
	Insect hypersensitivity	*Corynebacterium pseudotuberculosis* abscess

● Table 2-3   **REGIONAL DIAGNOSIS OF NON-NEOPLASTIC DERMATOSES*—cont'd**

REGION	COMMON DISEASES	UNCOMMON TO RARE DISEASES
	Pediculosis Staphylococcal folliculitis Urticaria	Demodicosis Fleas Hyperesthetic leukotrichia Hypodermiasis Linear alopecia Linear keratosis Molluscum contagiosum Panniculitis Parafilariasis Spotted leukotrichia Reticulated leukotrichia Unilateral papular dermatosis
Ventrum (abdomen, axillae, chest, groin)	Atopy Black fly bites Horn fly bites Horse fly bites Insect hypersensitivity Stable fly bites Ticks Trombiculosis	Besnoitiosis Bullous pemphigoid *Corynebacterium pseudotuberculosis* abscess Dracunculiasis Food hypersensitivity Habronemiasis Louse flies *Malassezia* dermatitis Onchocerciasis *Pelodera* dermatitis Poultry mites Pythiosis Tuberculosis
Legs	Atopy Black fly bites Chorioptic mange Dermatophilosis Dermatophytosis Horse fly bites Insect hypersensitivity Photodermatitis Stable fly bites Ticks Trombiculosis	Bacterial pseudomycetoma Besnoitiosis Cannon keratosis Dracunculiasis Epidermolysis bullosa Ergotism Eumycotic mycetoma Food hypersensitivity Forage mites Glanders Habronemiasis Histoplasmosis Hoary alyssum toxicosis Leishmaniasis Molluscum contagiosum *Mycobacterium avium* infection Onchocerciasis Pemphigus foliaceus Poultry mites *Rhodococcus equi* infection Pythiosis Snake bite Sporotrichosis Strongyloidosis Ulcerative lymphangitis Vasculitis Zinc-response dermatosis

Continued

● Table 2-3 **REGIONAL DIAGNOSIS OF NON-NEOPLASTIC DERMATOSES*—cont'd**

REGION	COMMON DISEASES	UNCOMMON TO RARE DISEASES
Mane and tail	Atopy Chorioptic mange Insect hypersensitivity Pediculosis Ticks	Alopecia areata Ergotism Food hypersensitivity Follicular dysplasia Mercurialism Mimosine toxicosis Oxyuriasis *Piedra* Psoroptic mange Seborrhea Selenosis Staphylococcal infection Trichorrhexis nodosa
Genital and perineal areas	Habronemiasis Herpes coital exanthema	Bacterial pseudomycetoma Besnoitiosis Candidiasis Dourine Halicephalobiasis Leishmaniasis Louse flies *Malassezia* dermatitis Sorghum toxicosis Tuberculosis
Mucocutaneous areas	Vesicular stomatitis Vitiligo	Bullous pemphigoid Epidermolysis bullosa Erythema multiforme Mucocutaneous pyoderma Pemphigus vulgaris Vasculitis Zinc-responsive dermatosis
Oral mucosa	Vesicular stomatitis	Bullous pemphigoid Candidiasis Epidermolysis bullosa Erythema multiforme Multisystemic eosinophilic exfoliative disease Pemphigus vulgaris Stachybotryotoxicosis Vaccinia Vasculitis

Drug reactions can mimic any dermatosis (see Chapter 9) and *contact dermatitis* can affect any body region (see Chapter 8).

veterinarian interaction is critical at this point. The client decides what is going to be done, but his or her decision is based on the clinician's recommendations. Therefore, the client needs to know the tentative or possible diagnoses, as well as expected costs and anticipated results of the diagnostic or therapeutic options proposed.

Diagnostic tests and laboratory procedures are useful whenever a definitive diagnosis cannot be made from the case history and clinical examination alone. Laboratory procedures may confirm many clinical diagnoses and provide a logical basis for successful therapeutic management. They should be recommended on the basis of the most likely diagnosis and should not be randomly suggested or recommended just to be comprehensive. The cost-effectiveness of each test should also be considered. In practice, it is often unacceptable to recommend numerous tests to screen for the long list of possible diagnoses in any given case. Instead, the results of recommended tests should confirm or rule out the diagnoses that the clinician deems most likely.

● LABORATORY PROCEDURES*

Surface Sampling

The lesions and pathologic changes of a skin disease are often readily available for study, and a variety of laboratory tests are based on this easy access to the skin's surface. A great deal of information may be obtained by studying microscopically materials collected from the hair and skin. Skin scraping and obtaining an acetate tape impression are techniques used to find microscopic ectoparasites. Hairs may be removed, and exudates may be collected and examined microscopically. Most of these techniques may be done in general clinical practice and rapidly add valuable information to a case work-up. However, practice and study may be necessary to maximize the benefits of many tests. The effort to learn these techniques is well worth the time. The alternatives are not to obtain this information, to do other more expensive and time-consuming tests, or to send samples to a laboratory, which adds cost and time delays.

SKIN SCRAPING

Skin scraping is used primarily for the demonstration of microscopic ectoparasites, especially mites. The procedure is quick, simple, and inexpensive, but is of limited value in the horse because mites are an uncommon cause of equine skin disease. It is important to realize that, although testing may accurately confirm diseases, its sensitivity for ruling out a diagnosis depends on the disease and the aggressiveness of sampling. The equipment needed to perform a skin scraping is mineral oil, a scalpel blade (with or without a handle) or a curet, microscope slides, coverslips, and a microscope.

Not all skin scrapings are made in the same way. Success in finding parasites is enhanced if the technique of scraping is adapted to the specific parasite that the clinician expects to find. No matter which type of scraping is made, a consistent, orderly examination of the collected material should be done until a diagnosis is made or all the collected material has been examined. It is easiest to start the examination at one end of the scraped material, which has been mixed with oil, and move the microscope stage straight across the slide in either a horizontal or a vertical direction. At the end of the slide, the examination moves over one field of vision and goes back in the opposite direction. This is continued back and forth until all the scraped material on the slide has been examined.

The following discussions elaborate on the special techniques needed to enhance the effectiveness of scraping for specific parasites.

DEEP SKIN SCRAPINGS

Deep skin scrapings are used to diagnose demodectic mange and *Pelodera* dermatitis. Generally, multiple scrapings from new lesions should be obtained. The affected skin should be squeezed between the thumb and the forefinger, if possible, to extrude the mites or nematodes from the hair follicles. The obtained material is scraped up and placed on a microscope slide. It is helpful to apply a drop of mineral oil to the skin site being scraped, or to the scalpel blade or curet, to facilitate the adherence of material to the blade. Then, additional material is obtained by scraping the skin more deeply, until capillary bleeding is produced. It is important that true capillary

---

*References 12, 13, 26, 34, 34a, 38, 47.

bleeding is obtained and not blood from laceration. Generally, two or three drops of mineral oil are added to the usual amount of scraped material on the microscope slide. The oil is mixed with the scraped material to obtain an even consistency. Placing a coverslip on the material to be examined ensures a uniform layer that is more readily examined. Lowering the condenser causes more light diffraction and contrast, resulting in easier recognition of the mites.

Diagnosis of demodicosis is made by demonstrating multiple adult mites, finding adult mites from multiple sites, or finding immature forms of mites (ova, larvae, and nymphs). Horses harbor two species of *Demodex* mites, *Demodex caballi* and *D. equi* (see Chapter 6). Scrapings taken from a normal horse, especially from the face, may contain an occasional adult mite. If one or two mites are observed, repeated scrapings should be done. Multiple positive results of scrapings from different sites should be considered abnormal. Observing whether the mites are alive (mouthparts or legs moving) or dead is of prognostic value while the animal is being treated. As a case of *Demodex* infestation responds to treatment, the ratio of live to dead mites decreases, as does the ratio of eggs and larvae to adults. If this is not occurring, the treatment regimen should be reevaluated.

Diagnosis of *Pelodera* dermatitis is made by demonstrating any *Pelodera strongyloides* nematodes (see Chapter 6).

SUPERFICIAL SKIN SCRAPINGS

Superficial skin scrapings are used to diagnose chorioptic mange, psoroptic mange, sarcoptic mange, trombiculosis, and forage and poultry mite infestations. It may be necessary to lightly clip long-haired areas (e.g., fetlock) prior to sampling. Multiple superficial scrapings are indicated. Skin that has not been excoriated, preferably skin with raised papules and crusts on top, should be scraped. The more scrapings are performed, the more likely is a diagnosis. However, even with numerous scrapings, sarcoptic mange cannot be ruled out because of negative results.

Extensive amounts of material should be accumulated in the scrapings and spread on microscope slides. Double-sized coverslips are sometimes useful. Alternatively, a second microscope glass slide may be used instead of a normal coverslip to compress the thick crusts. The clinician examines each field until a mite is found or all material has been examined; one mite is diagnostic. Dark brown, round or oval fecal pellets or ova from adult mites, if found, are also diagnostic. In difficult cases, it may be useful to accumulate an even larger amount of hair and keratin debris from scrapings. The material is placed in a warm solution of 10% potassium hydroxide (KOH) for 20 minutes to digest keratin, and the mixture is then stirred and centrifuged. Mites are thus concentrated and can often be picked off the surface film and identified with a microscope.

Chorioptes equi is a fast-moving mite, and it is a good idea to add an acaricidal or insecticidal agent to the mineral oil prior to sampling.[38]

The most common chigger mite is *Eutrombicula alfreddugèsi* (see Chapter 6). These mites can be seen with the naked eye. They appear as bright orange objects adhering tightly to the skin or centered in a papule. They are easily recognized by their large size, relatively intense color, and tight attachment to the skin. They should be covered with mineral oil and picked up with a scalpel blade. A true skin scraping is not needed. However, when removed from the host for microscopic examination, they should immediately be placed in mineral oil, or they may crawl away.[42] Only the larval form is pathogenic, and these have only six legs.

Dermanyssus gallinae is a mite that attacks poultry, wild and cage birds, and horses, as well as humans. It is red when engorged with blood; otherwise, it is white, gray, or black. When the animal shows evidence of itching and the history indicates exposure to bird or poultry housing, a skin scraping for this mite is indicated. The best place to find the mites is at excoriated sites. The clinician collects the debris, scales, and crusts that harbor the mites. The materials are placed on a microscope slide, and several drops of mineral oil are added. The slide is covered with another glass slide instead of a coverslip. The two slides are squeezed together firmly to crush any crusted material. The acetate tape method of collection may be used successfully.

Acetate Tape Impression

This alternative to skin scraping has been recommended to find superficial ectoparasites such as *Chorioptes* mites, poultry mites, forage mites, chiggers, and pinworms. Clear, pressure-sensitive acetate tape (Scotch No. 602 [3M Co.] is a good type) is pressed to the hair surface and to the skin adjacent to parted hairs or in shaved areas. Superficial scales and debris are also collected. The tape is then stuck with pressure on a microscope slide and examined.

To diagnose pinworms (*Oxyuris equi*), the acetate tape is pressed over several areas in the anal and perineal area and placed adhesive side down on a glass slide liberally coated with mineral oil.[12,13] The mineral oil helps clear debris and facilitate the examination. The finding of oval ova with an operculum (cap) on one end is diagnostic (see Chapter 6).

Hair Examination

Plucking hairs from the skin and examining them under the microscope is referred to as *trichography* and is helpful for diagnosing self-inflicted alopecia, dermatophytosis, piedra, nutritional or congenital hair dysplasias, trichorrhexis nodosa, anagen defluxion, telogen defluxion, endocrine alopecia, and pigmentary disturbances of hair growth. Trichography is performed by grasping a small number of hairs with the fingertips or rubber-covered hemostats, epilating them completely in the direction of their growth, laying them in the same orientation on a microscope slide with mineral oil, and examining them with the low-power objective of the microscope. If abnormalities are detected during scanning, closer examination will be necessary to categorize the defect.

Hairs will have either an anagen or telogen root (bulb). Anagen bulbs are rounded, smooth, shiny, glistening, often pigmented and soft, so the root may bend (Fig. 2-18). Telogen bulbs are club- or spear-shaped, rough-surfaced, nonpigmented, and generally straight (Fig. 2-19). A normal hair shaft is uniform in diameter and tapers gently to the tip. Straight-coated animals have straight hair shafts while curly- or wavy-coated animals have twisted hair shafts. All hairs should have a clearly discernible cuticle, and a sharply demarcated cortex and medulla. Hair pigmentation depends on the coat color and breed of horse but should not vary greatly from one hair to the next in regions where the coat color is the same.

Normal adult animals have an admixture of anagen and telogen hairs, the ratio of which varies with season, management factors, and a variety of other influences (see Chapter 1). The anagen to telogen ratio can be determined by categorizing the bulbs from approximately 100 hairs. Since no well-established normal values are available, the authors rarely compute this ratio. However, estimation of this ratio can be valuable. No normal animal should have all of its hairs in telogen (Fig. 2-20); therefore, this finding suggests a diagnosis of telogen defluxion or follicular arrest (see Chapter 10). Inappropriate numbers of telogen hairs (e.g., mostly telogen during the summer, when the ratio should be approximately 50:50) suggest a diagnosis of a nutritional or endocrine and metabolic disease (see Chapter 10).

Examination of the hair shaft follows bulbar evaluation. Hairs that are inappropriately curled, misshapen, and malformed suggest an underlying nutritional or metabolic disease (Fig. 2-21). Hairs with a normal shaft that are suddenly and cleanly broken (Fig. 2-22) or longitudinally split (trichoptilosis) indicate external trauma from excessive rubbing, chewing, licking or scratching or too vigorous grooming. Breakage of hairs with abnormal shafts can be seen in congenitohereditary disorders (see Chapter 11), trichorrhexis nodosa (see Chapter 14), anagen defluxion (see Chapter 10), alopecia areata (see Chapter 9), and dermatophytosis (Fig. 2-23; see Chapter 5). Abnormalities in hair pigmentation have not been well studied. When unusual pigmentation is observed, external sources (e.g., chemicals and topical medications, sun bleaching) or conditions that

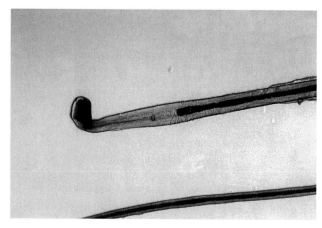

FIGURE 2-18. Anagen hair. Note rounded, pigmented bulb, which is bent dorsally.

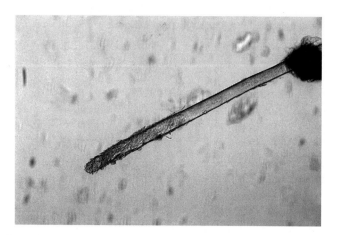

FIGURE 2-19. Telogen hair. Proximal end is rough-surfaced, nonpigmented, and pointed.

influence the transfer of pigment to the hair shaft (e.g., drugs, nutritional imbalances, endocrine disorders, and idiopathic pigmentary disorders) must be considered. Hair casts are usually seen in diseases associated with follicular keratinization abnormalities, such as primary seborrhea and follicular dysplasia. Hair casts should not be confused with louse nits (Fig. 2-24).

Cytologic Examination

An enormous amount of vital diagnostic data can be obtained by microscopic examination of stained material, such as smears of tissues or fluids, during a clinical examination. It is possible to accomplish this with minimal equipment and in less than 5 minutes.[4a,47a] The cost is much less than that for bacterial culture and susceptibility testing or biopsy. Although the same information as obtained by these more expensive tests is not really gathered, microscopic examination often supplies sufficient data to narrow a differential diagnosis and develop a diagnostic plan.

The type of inflammatory, neoplastic, or other cellular infiltrate; the relative amount of protein or mucin; and the presence of acantholytic keratinocytes, fungi, and bacteria can be determined by cytologic evaluation. It is the most common and most rewarding office test performed by the authors. The equipment includes a clean microscope slide, a coverslip, a stain, and a microscope.

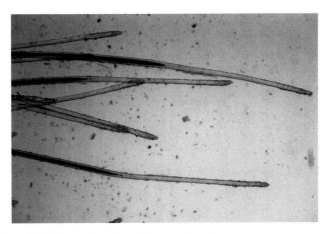

FIGURE 2-20. Telogen defluxion. All epilated hairs are in telogen.

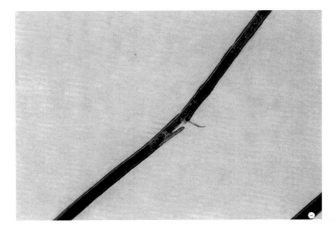

FIGURE 2-21. Drug reaction (ivermectin). Anatomy of hair shaft is focally obscured, and shaft is weakened resulting in breakage.

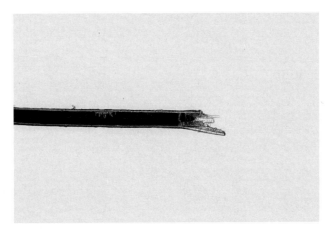

FIGURE 2-22. *Culicoides* hypersensitivity. Distal end of hair is fractured from rubbing.

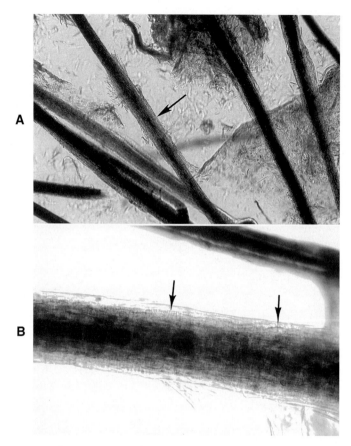

FIGURE 2-23. Dermatophytosis. **A**, Hair shaft is focally thickened and fuzzy (*arrow*). **B**, Arthroconidia and hyphae are seen within the hair (*arrows*).

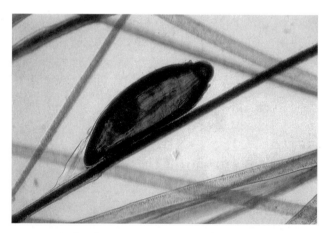

FIGURE 2-24. Louse nit attached to hair.

SPECIMEN COLLECTION

Materials for cytologic examination can be gathered by a variety of techniques. Those most commonly used by the authors include direct smears, impression smears, swab smears, and fine needle aspiration. In most situations, clipping the hair should be the only preparation of the surface. Scrubbing and applying alcohol or disinfectants are used only in areas where a fine needle aspirate of a mass lesion is to be done.

Direct smears are usually performed for fluid-containing lesions. A small amount of material is collected with the tip of a needle. The material is then smeared on the microscope slide.

Impression smears are often obtained when lesions are moist or greasy. This technique is also used after removing crusts, expressing fluid from lesions, or gently opening the surface of papules, pustules, or vesicles. The microscope slide is pressed directly against the site to be examined.

Swab smears are most often used to obtain specimens from draining tracts or sinuses, intertriginous areas, and ear canals. The cotton-tipped applicator is moistened and inserted into the tract, the sinus, the fold, or the ear canal. After the lesion has been sampled, the cotton tip is rolled over the surface of the microscope slide.

Fine needle aspiration is most commonly used to sample nodules, tumors, and cysts, although pustules, vesicles, or bullae may also be sampled this way. Fluid-filled lesions can be aspirated with 20- to 23-gauge needles and a 3-ml syringe. Firm lesions should be aspirated with 20-gauge needles and 6- or 10-ml syringes to obtain better suction. Fibrotic or dense masses may necessitate the use of an 18-gauge needle to get an adequate sample. For small lesions, a 25-gauge needle may be necessary. The needle is introduced into the lesion, and then suction is gently applied by withdrawing the plunger of the syringe. Little withdrawing is necessary for fluid-filled lesions, and the material within the needle is sufficient. In mass lesions, the plunger is withdrawn one-half to three-fourths of the syringe volume. Suction is then interrupted while the needle is redirected into another area of the mass. Suction is again applied, and this procedure is repeated for a total of three or four times. Suction is then released, and the needle is withdrawn from the lesion. The syringe and the needle are then separated, air is introduced into the syringe, the needle is reattached, and the contents of the needle and hub are expelled onto the surface of a glass slide. The material is then streaked across the surface with another glass slide or the needle.

STAINS

Collected materials are allowed to dry on the slide. Oily, waxy, or dry skin samples collected by direct impression or moistened cotton applicators may be heat-fixed before staining. After the specimens are heat-fixed and dried, the slide is stained and examined microscopically. The stains of choice in clinical practice are the modified Wright's stain (Diff Quik) and new methylene blue. Diff Quik is a quick and easy Romanovsky-type stain. It gives less nuclear detail than the supravital stains such as new methylene blue stain. However, it allows better differentiation of cytoplasmic structures and organisms. Because this is most commonly what the practitioner is interested in with non-neoplastic skin diseases, the Diff Quik stain is preferred by the authors. When a neoplasm is suspected, two slides may be made and both stains used. A Gram stain is occasionally used to acquire more information on the identity of bacteria.

CYTOLOGIC FINDINGS

Cytologic study is helpful to distinguish between bacterial skin infection and bacterial colonization, to determine the relative depth of infection, to determine whether the pustule contains bacteria or is sterile, to discover yeasts and fungi, to identify various cutaneous neoplasms, or to find the acantholytic cells of the pemphigus diseases.

Samples obtained by impression smears or swabs usually contain variable numbers of keratinocytes. Typically, the keratinocytes are anuclear corneocytes (Fig. 2-25). Many corneocytes

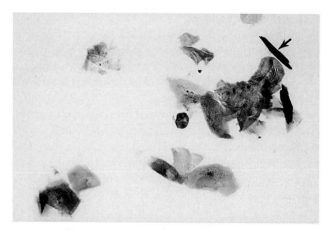

FIGURE 2-25. Normal skin. Corneocytes, which contain variable amounts of melanin, depending on the animal's normal pigmentation. Some corneocytes are rolled up, darkly stained, and spicule-like (*arrow*).

will be rolled-up, deeply basophilic, and spicule-like. Corneocytes contain variable amounts of melanin granules (brown or black in Diff Quik–stained specimens), reflecting the animal's normal pigmentation. If the skin is parakeratotic, nucleated corneocytes will be present. Occasionally, cells from the stratum granulosum are recognized by their keratohyalin granules (blue or purple in Diff Quik–stained specimens). Keratohyalin granules vary in size and shape, and should not be confused with bacteria.

Bacteria are a frequent finding in impression smears from skin and can be seen as basophilic-staining organisms in specimens stained with new methylene blue or Diff Quik. Although identification of the exact species of bacteria is not possible with a stain (as it is in a culture), it is possible to distinguish cocci from rods and often to institute appropriate and effective antibiotic therapy without performing a culture and antibiotic susceptibility testing. Generally, when cocci are seen, they are *Staphylococcus intermedius* or *S. aureus*. If no bacteria are found in the stained fluid, the clinical condition is probably not a bacterial pyoderma. If neither granulocytes nor intracellular bacteria are seen, even large numbers of bacteria are not likely to be of etiologic significance.

It is also possible to obtain some clues as to the type of bacterial pyoderma or the underlying condition. In general, deep infections have fewer bacteria present, with the vast majority being intracellular. In addition, deep infections have a mixed cellular infiltrate with large numbers of neutrophils, histiocytes, macrophages, lymphocytes, and plasma cells. The presence of these cells suggests that longer-term antibiotic therapy is necessary. Large numbers of intracellular and extracellular cocci are seen more commonly in superficial bacterial infections (Fig. 2-26, *A*), and the inflammatory cells are almost exclusively neutrophils.

Next, one looks for the cytologic response of the skin. Are there inflammatory cells? Are they eosinophils, neutrophils, or mononuclear cells? If eosinophils are present, any extracellular bacteria seen probably represent colonization, not infection, and most likely an ectoparasitic or allergic disease is the primary problem. If large numbers of eosinophils are seen in combination with degenerate neutrophils and intracellular bacteria, an allergic or ectoparasitic disease with secondary bacterial infection may be present, or furunculosis is present (free keratin and hair shafts serve as endogenous foreign bodies). It must be emphasized that eosinophils may be less numerous than expected or completely absent in inflammatory exudates from animals receiving glucocorticoids. Eosinophils are also prominent in eosinophilic granuloma (Fig. 2-26, *B*), axillary nodular necrosis, unilateral papular dermatosis, multisystemic epitheliotropic eosinophilic disease, and certain fungal infections (pythiosis, basidiobolomycosis, conidiobolomycosis).

If neutrophils are present, do they exhibit degenerative or toxic cytologic changes, which suggest infection (Figs. 2-26, *C*, and 2-26, *D*)? If bacteria and inflammatory cells are found in the same preparation, is there phagocytosis? Are the bacteria ingested by individual neutrophils, or are they engulfed by macrophages and multinucleate histiocytic giant cells? Are there many bacteria, but few or no inflammatory cells, none of which exhibit degenerative cytologic changes or phagocytosis? When macrophages containing numerous clear cytoplasmic vacuoles are present, one should consider the possibility of a lipophagic granuloma such as is seen with panniculitis and foreign-body reactions (Fig. 2-26, *E*).

Less commonly, cytologic examination allows the rapid recognition of (1) unusual infections (Fig. 2-26, *F*) (infections due to *Actinomycetes*, mycobacteria, *Leishmania*, and subcutaneous and deep mycoses); (2) autoimmune dermatoses (pemphigus) (Fig. 2-26, *G*); and (3) neoplastic conditions (Fig. 2-26, *H*).

A synopsis of cytologic findings and their interpretation is presented in Table 2-4. Cytomorphologic characteristics of neoplastic cells are presented in Table 2-5.

Culture and Examination for Fungi

Identification of fungi that have been isolated provides important information for case management and for public health decisions (see Chapter 5). When agents causing subcutaneous or deep mycoses are suspected, the samples should be sent to a veterinary laboratory with appropriate mycology skills. The propagation of many pathologic fungi, especially the agents of subcutaneous and deep mycoses, creates airborne health hazards. Additionally, examinations of the mycelial phase should be carried out in biologic safety cabinets. For these reasons, the authors recommend that, in the general practice setting, fungal assessments be limited to direct tissue microscopic examination and culturing for dermatophytes. For other suspected fungal infections, samples should be collected and sent to an appropriate laboratory.

In general, for subcutaneous and deep mycotic infections, punch biopsies from the lesion are the best way to obtain a culture specimen. Pieces from the margin and the center of lesions, as well as any different-appearing lesions, should be submitted for laboratory analysis. Tissue samples may be placed in a bacteriologic transport medium and should reach the laboratory within 12 hours, although up to 24 hours is permissible. Refrigeration may be helpful to preserve some fungi but *Aspergillus* spp. and *Zygomycetes* are sensitive to cold. When these organisms are suspected, the sample should be kept at room temperature.

Direct examination for most nondermatophyte fungal organisms is acceptable as described under Cytologic Examination in this chapter. In general, the Diff Quik stain is suitable for many fungi, especially yeasts and *Histoplasma capsulatum*. Periodic acid-Schiff stain is useful, but beyond the level of most general practice settings. India ink mixed with tissue fluid outlines the capsule of yeast and has been useful for identifying *Cryptococcus neoformans*. Clearing samples with 10% to 20% KOH, as discussed for dermatophytes under Direct Examination in this chapter, may help to identify hyphae of other fungi. When collecting samples for hyphal examination, one should not use gauze or cotton swabs because fibers may be mistaken for hyphae.

EXAMINATION FOR DERMATOPHYTES

In contrast to the case for other mycotic diseases, suspected cases of dermatophytosis can readily be tested for in a general practice situation. To ascertain the cause of a dermatophytosis, proper specimen collection and isolation and correct identification of dermatophytes are necessary.

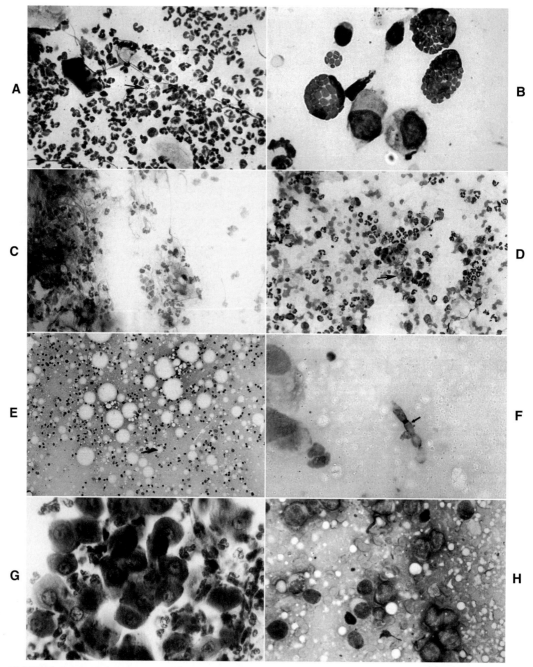

FIGURE 2-26. **A**, Staphylococcal folliculitis. Degenerative neutrophils, nuclear streaming, and intracellular cocci (*arrow*). **B**, Eosinophilic granuloma. Eosinophil and macrophage. **C**, Staphylococcal folliculitis. Degenerate neutrophils and nuclear streaming. **D**, Sterile pyogranuloma. Pyogranulomatous inflammation with nondegenerate neutrophils and neutrophagocytosis (*arrow*). **E**, Idiopathic sterile panniculitis. Granulomatous inflammation with numerous extracellular fat droplets. **F**, Phaeohyphomycosis. Dark, septate hypha (*arrow*) with macrophages. **G**, Pemphigus foliaceus. Nondegenerate neutrophils and acantholytic keratinocytes. **H**, Lymphoma. Malignant lymphocytes.

● Table 2-4 **CYTOLOGIC DIAGNOSIS FROM STAINED SMEARS**

FINDING	DIAGNOSTIC CONSIDERATIONS
Neutrophils	
Degenerate	Bacterial infection
Nondegenerate	Sterile inflammation (e.g., pemphigus), irritants, foreign-body reaction
Eosinophils	Ectoparasitism, endoparasitism, allergy, furunculosis, eosinophilic granuloma, mast cell tumor, pemphigus, sterile eosinophilic folliculitis
Basophils	Ectoparasitism, endoparasitism
Mast cells	Ectoparasitism, allergy, mast cell tumor
Lymphocytes, macrophages, and plasma cells	
Granulomatous	Infectious (especially furunculosis) versus sterile (e.g., foreign body, sterile granuloma syndrome, and sterile panniculitis)
Pyogranulomatous	Same as for granulomatous
Eosinophilic granulomatous	Furunculosis, ruptured keratinous cyst, eosinophilic granuloma
Acanthocytes	
Few	Any suppurative dermatosis
Many	Pemphigus, acantholytic dermatophytosis
Bacteria	
Intracellular	Infection
Extracellular only	Colonization
Yeast	
Peanut-shaped	*Malassezia* or rarely *Candida*
Fungi	
Spores, hyphae	Fungal infection
Atypical or monomorphous cell population	
Clumped and rounded	Epithelial neoplasm
Individual, rounded, and numerous	Lymphoreticular or mast cell neoplasm
Individual, rounded or elongated, and sparse	Mesenchymal neoplasm

● Table 2-5 **CYTOMORPHOLOGIC CHARACTERISTICS SUGGESTIVE OF MALIGNANCY**

GENERAL FINDINGS	NUCLEAR FINDINGS	CYTOPLASMIC FINDINGS
Pleomorphism (variable cell size and shape)	Marked variation in size (anisokaryosis)	Variable staining intensity, sometimes dark blue
Highly variable nucleus-to-cytoplasm ratios	Variation in shape (pleomorphism)	Discrete, punctate vacuoles
	Hyperchromatic chromatin with irregular distribution (clumping, uneven margination)	
	Coarsely clumped, sometimes jagged chromatin	
Variable staining intensity	Nuclear molding	Variable amounts
	Increased mitotic activity	
	Peripheral displacement by cytoplasmic secretions or vacuoles	
	Nucleoli that vary in size, shape, and number	
	Multinucleation	

Wood's Lamp Examination

A classic aid in specimen collection is the Wood's lamp examination. The Wood's lamp is an ultraviolet light with a light wave of 253.7 nm filtered through a cobalt or nickel filter. The Wood's lamp should be turned on and allowed to warm up for 5 to 10 minutes, because the stability of the light's wavelength and intensity is temperature dependent. The animal should be placed in a dark room and examined under the light of the Wood's lamp. When exposed to the ultraviolet light, hairs invaded by *M. canis* or *M. equinum* may result in a yellow-green fluorescence in 30% to 80% of the isolates. Hairs should be exposed for 3 to 5 minutes, as some strains are slow to show the obvious yellow-green color. The fluorescence is due to tryptophan metabolites produced by the fungus. These metabolites are produced only by fungi that have invaded actively growing hair and cannot be elicited from an in vitro infection of hair. To decrease the number of false-positive results, it is imperative that the individual hair shafts are seen to fluoresce. Fluorescence is not present in scales or crusts or in cultures of dermatophytes. Other less common dermatophytes that may fluoresce include *Microsporum distortum, M. audouinii,* and *Trichophyton schoenleinii.*

Many factors influence fluorescence. The use of medications such as iodine destroys it. Bacteria such as *Pseudomonas aeruginosa* and *Corynebacterium minutissimum* may fluoresce, but not with the apple green color of a dermatophyte-infected hair. Keratin, soap, petroleum, and other medication may fluoresce and give false-positive reactions. If the short stubs of hair produce fluorescence, the proximal end of hairs extracted from the follicles should fluoresce. These fluorescing hairs should be plucked with forceps and used for inoculation of fungal medium or for microscopic examination.

In the horse, the most common causes of dermatophytosis are *T. equinum, T. mentagrophytes, T. verrucosum,* and *M. gypseum,* and these do not produce fluorescence. Hence, the Wood's lamp is rarely useful in the horse.

Specimen Collection

Accurate specimen collection is necessary to isolate dermatophytes. Hair is most commonly collected for the isolation of dermatophytes. It is a good idea to pluck hairs from multiple lesions to increase the chance of success. Hair is collected from the margins of lesions. Whenever possible, one should select newly formed or actively expanding lesions that have not been recently medicated. The margins, as well as adjacent areas, are sampled. One should look for hairs that are broken or misshapen and associated with inflammation, scale, or crust. In long-haired areas, the hairs can be shaved so that only 0.5 to 1 cm protrudes above the skin. However, if hairs are to be sampled from a lesion for fungal culture, it is valuable to clip excessive hair and gently clean the area. Patting the lesion clean with 70% alcohol-impregnated gauze or cotton and then letting it air-dry decreases the occurrence of contaminants. The hairs obtained by these methods can be used for culture or microscopic examination. Some scales may also be collected, but one should avoid putting exudates or medications on the medium.

Direct Examination

The clinician should practice direct examination to become adept at identifying dermatophytes. Even the experienced clinician does not always obtain a diagnosis in cases of dermatophytosis. In addition, various filaments, fibers, cholesterol and KOH crystals, oil droplets, keratin fragments, and saprophytic fungal hyphae can be mistaken for pathogenic fungal elements. A negative direct examination finding does not rule out a diagnosis of dermatophytosis. Because most infections in animals are caused by ectothrix dermatophytes, clearing the hairs is not as necessary as it is for infections involving humans. The authors use only mineral oil to suspend hair with suspected dermatophytes. Others recommend clearing the keratin to visualize the hyphae and spores more effectively. Care must be taken not to get these clearing solutions on the microscope, because they can damage the lenses. The hair and scales may first be cleared by placing the specimens in several drops of 10% to 20% KOH on a microscope slide. A coverslip is added, and the slide is gently heated for 15 to 20 seconds. One should avoid overheating and boiling the sample. Alternatively, the preparation may be allowed to stand for 30 minutes at room temperature. An excellent result is obtained if the mount is placed on the microscope lamp for gentle heating. The preparation is ready for examination in 15 to 20 minutes, and the structures are better preserved. A more rapid method of clearing involves using a KOH-dimethyl sulfoxide (DMSO) solution (Dermassay Clearing Solution, Pitman-Moore), permitting immediate examination, but the specimen must be examined within 30 minutes of preparation or it will overclear.[12,42] Some authors have found the use of a chlorazol black E stain to be helpful.[12] Approximately 100 mg of chlorazol black E (Sigma Chemical) is dissolved in 10 ml of DMSO and is then added to 90 ml of water containing 5 g of KOH. A preparation made with this clearing solution should be heated gently before examination. The addition of the dye allows fungal elements to be identified more readily, as they will stain green against a light gray background.

The following formula called *chlorphenolac* has been recommended as a replacement for the KOH solution in the digestion process to clear keratin: 50 g of chloral hydrate is added to 25 ml of liquid phenol and 25 ml of liquid lactic acid. Several days may pass before the crystals go into solution, but when they do, no precipitate forms. The slide can be read almost immediately after hair and keratin are added to this chloral hydrate-phenol-lactic acid solution. Chlorphenolac-treated samples were of equal diagnostic value when compared with KOH-treated specimens.[2]

The use of calcafluor white solution and fluorescence microscopy has been reported to greatly increase the sensitivity of direct examination.[44] Calcafluor white is a textile brightener that binds specifically to the polysaccharide components of fungal cell walls and, when viewed under ultraviolet light, fluoresces strongly. The technique gave positive results in 76% of the samples examined, compared with 39% for the standard KOH prep. However, the need for fluorescence microscopy makes this procedure impractical in a practice setting.

Examination of cleared, mineral oil–suspended, or stained samples from mycotic lesions may reveal yeasts, conidia, hyphae, or pseudohyphae. To find dermatophyte-infected hairs, one should look for fragmented pieces of hair that are larger in diameter than most hairs present. Generally, it is best to look near the hair bulbs and watch for distorted hairs. Dermatophyte-infected hairs appear swollen and frayed, irregular, or fuzzy in outline, and the clear definition between cuticle, cortex, and medulla is lost (see Fig. 2-23). It is also important to remember that dermatophytes do not form macroconidia in tissue. Any macroconidia seen represent saprophytes and have no known clinical significance. The hyphae of the common dermatophytes are usually uniform in diameter (2 to 3 µm), septate, and variable in length and degree of branching. Older hyphae are usually wider and may be divided into bead-like chains of rounded cells (arthroconidia).

In haired skin and scales, the branched septate hyphae of different dermatophytes may be identical to one another and necessitate isolation and culture for identification.

In an ectothrix invasion of hair, hyphae may be seen within the hair shaft, but they grow outward and show a great propensity to form arthroconidia in a mosaic pattern on the surface of the hair. Large conidia (5 to 8 µm) in sparse chains outside the hairs are seen in *Microsporum gypseum* infections. Intermediate-sized conidia (3 to 7 µm) in dense chains are seen with *Trichophyton mentagrophytes*, *T. verrucosum*, and *T. equinum* infections. Small conidia (2 to 3 µm) in clusters are seen with *M. canis* infections.

An endothrix infection is characterized by conidia formation within the hair shaft; the hair cuticle is not broken, but the hairs break off or curl. Endothrix invasion is rarely seen in animals but is typical of *Trichophyton tonsurans* infections in humans. Endothrix invasion was seen in the hairs of a horse with *T. tonsurans* infection.[24] The clinician should practice to develop the technique of direct examination for fungi. The best way to learn this technique is to find a highly Wood's lamp–positive *M. canis* infection in the cat. A large volume of positive hairs should be collected and kept in a loosely closed pill vial. Every few days, some hairs should be removed and examined until the affected hairs are rapidly recognized. After this is done, affected hairs should be mixed with normal hairs and the process repeated several times during the succeeding weeks. This type of practice greatly improves one's ability to locate dermatophyte-infected hairs by microscopic examination. Even in the hands of an expert, direct examination of hairs is only positive in 54% (*T. equinum*) to 64% (*T. verrucosum*) of the animals wherein fungal culture is positive.[4]

FUNGAL CULTURE

Because the skin and hair of horses are veritable cesspools of saprophytic fungi and bacteria, it is essential to cleanse the skin and hair prior to taking samples for culture. This may be done by gently cleansing the area to be sampled with a mild soap and water, or 70% alcohol, and allowing it to air dry. Sabouraud's dextrose agar and dermatophyte test medium (DTM) are traditionally used in clinical veterinary mycology for isolation of fungi;[1,12,38,42] however, other media are available, although rarely used in general practice. DTM is essentially a Sabouraud's dextrose agar containing cycloheximide, gentamicin, and chlortetracycline as antifungal and antibacterial agents. The pH indicator phenol red has been added. Dermatophytes first use protein in the medium, with alkaline metabolites turning the medium from yellow to red. When the protein is exhausted, the dermatophytes use carbohydrates, giving off acid metabolites. The medium changes from red to yellow. Most other fungi use carbohydrates first and proteins only later; they too may produce a change to red in DTM—but only after a prolonged incubation (10 to 14 days or longer). Consequently, DTM cultures should be examined daily for the first 10 days. Fungi such as *Blastomyces dermatitidis*, *Sporothrix schenckii*, *H. capsulatum*, *Coccidioides immitis*, *Pseudoallescheria boydii*, and some *Aspergillus* species may cause a change to red in DTM, so microscopic examination is essential to avoid an erroneous presumptive diagnosis.

Because cycloheximide is present in DTM, fungi sensitive to it are not isolated. Organisms sensitive to cycloheximide include *Cryptococcus neoformans*, many members of the *Zygomycota*, some *Candida* species, *Aspergillus* species, *P. boydii*, and many agents of phaeohyphomycosis. DTM may depress the development of conidia, mask colony pigmentation, and inhibit the growth of some pathogens. Therefore, it is valuable to place part of the specimen on plain Sabouraud's dextrose agar. In some cases, identification is more readily obtainable from the sample inoculated onto Sabouraud's dextrose agar. For this reason, a double plate containing one side of DTM and one of Sabouraud's dextrose agar has gained favor among many dermatologists. When bottles containing DTM are used, it may be difficult to get a toothbrush onto the medium surface. When bottles are used, it is also important to put the lid on loosely.

Skin scrapings and hair should be inoculated onto Sabouraud's dextrose agar and DTM. Desiccation and exposure to ultraviolet light hinder growth. Therefore, cultures should be incubated in the dark at 30° C with 30% humidity. A pan of water in the incubator usually provides enough humidity. Cultures should be incubated for 10 to 14 days and should be checked daily for fungal growth. Proper interpretation of the DTM culture necessitates recognition of the red color change simultaneously with visible mycelial growth. False-positive results occur most commonly when the cultures are not observed frequently. As a saprophyte grows, it eventually turns the media red, thus emphasizing the importance of correlating the initial mycelial growth with the color change.

Studies indicate that DTM is clearly inferior to Sabouraud's dextrose agar for the isolation of dermatophytes from horses.[1,18a] Fewer dermatophytes are isolated on DTM, and false-positive and false-negative results are obtained. *T. verrucosum* does not grow on DTM.

IDENTIFICATION OF FUNGI

If a suspected dermatophyte is grown on culture, it should be identified. This necessitates collection of macroconidia from the mycelial surface. Generally, the colony needs to grow for 7 to 10 days before macroconidia are produced. Although colonies grown on DTM may provide adequate macroconidia, it is common that the colonies on the Sabouraud's dextrose agar may need to be sampled to find them. In occasional cases, especially with *Trichophyton* spp., no macroconidia are found. Subculturing these colonies on Sabouraud's dextrose agar or potato dextrose agar may facilitate sporulation. Alternatively, the sample may be sent to a diagnostic laboratory for identification.

The macroconidia are most readily collected by gently applying the sticky side of clear acetate tape (Scotch No. 602, [3M Co.]) to the aerial surface. The tape with sample is then placed onto several drops of lactophenol cotton blue that is on the surface of a microscope slide. A coverslip is placed over the tape and sample, and this is examined by microscopy.

Salient facts useful in identifying the four major dermatophytes are briefly described:

- *Microsporum gypseum.* No fluorescence is seen with Wood's lamp. The arthrospores on hair shafts are larger than those of *M. canis.*
  Colony Morphology. Colonies are rapid-growing with a flat to granular texture and a buff to cinnamon brown color. Sterile white mycelia may develop in time. The undersurface pigmentation is pale yellow to tan.
  Microscopic Morphology. Echinulate macroconidia contain up to six cells with relatively thin walls. The abundant ellipsoid macroconidia lack the terminal knob present in *M. canis.* One-celled microconidia may be present.
- *Trichophyton equinum.* No fluorescence is seen with Wood's lamp. Ectothrix chains of arthroconidia may be observed on hairs. There are two varieties of *T. equinum.* The common variety in North America, South America, and Europe is *T. equinum var. equinum.* In Australia and New Zealand the common variety is *T. equinum var. autotrophicum. T. equinum var. equinum* has an absolute growth requirement for nicotinic acid (niacin), whereas *T. equinum var. autotrophicum* does not.* As a result, *T. equinum var. equinum* (1) often does not grow on commercial mycologic media, such as DTM, unless nicotinic acid is added (usually accomplished by adding 2 drops of injectable vitamin B complex [not in alcohol!] to the media),[34,38,50] (2) does not penetrate human hair *in vitro* (*does* penetrate horse, cow, and dog hairs) unless nicotinic acid is added,[23,29] and (3) rarely cause dermatophytosis in humans (see Chapter 5).[29]
  Colony Morphology. A flat colony with a white to cream-colored, powdery surface is produced. The center of the colony is frequently reddish. The reverse pigmentation is usually deep yellow. The most common North American, South American, and European strains (*T. equinum var. equinum*) require nicotinic acid (niacin), while the Australian and New Zealand strains (*T. equinum var. autotrophicum*) do not. The optimum temperature for the growth of *T. equinum* is 26° to 28° C.[22]
  Microscopic Morphology. Typically, pyriform to spherical, stalked microconidia are seen along the hyphae. Less frequently, the microconidia are clustered with clavate macroconidia.
- *Trichophyton mentagrophytes.* No fluorescence is seen with Wood's light. Ectothrix chains of arthroconidia may be observed on hair.
  Colony Morphology. Colony morphologic characteristics are variable. Most zoophilic forms produce a flat colony with a white to cream-colored powdery surface. The color of the undersurface is usually brown to tan, but may be dark red. The anthropophilic form produces a colony with a white cottony surface.
  Microscopic Morphology. The zoophilic form of *T. mentagrophytes* produces globose microconidia that may be arranged singly along the hyphae or in grape-like clusters. Acroconidia, if present, are cigar-shaped with thin, smooth walls. Some strains produce spiral hyphae, which may also be seen in other dermatophytes but are most characteristic of *Trichophyton.* Samples that show this change should be submitted to a diagnostic laboratory for identification. When grown on potato dextrose agar, *T. mentagrophytes* does not produce a

*References 9, 16, 17, 22, 27, 29, 30, 37, 43.

dark red pigment like that formed by *T. rubrum*. Strains of *T. mentagrophytes* are more apt to be urease-positive than is *T. rubrum*. Because *T. rubrum* may be incorrectly identified as *T. mentagrophytes*, the above differential features are important.

- *Trichophyton verrucosum.* No fluorescence is seen with Wood's lamp. Ectothrix chains of arthroconidia may be observed on hairs.

  Colony Morphology. Usually, a white, very slow-growing glabrous colony is produced that is heaped-up and button-shaped in appearance. Two variants also occur: a flat, yellow, glabrous colony (*T. verrucosum var. ochraceum*), and a flat, slightly downy gray-white colony (*T. verrucosum var. discoides*). All strains require inositol and most grow best at 37° C. *T. verrucosum* does not grow on DTM.

  Microscopic Morphology. Tortuous hyphae with antler-like branching are seen. Tear-shaped microconidia and rat tail– or string bean–shaped macroconidia are characteristic.

  M. equinum was previously called *M. canis* in many reports.[21,38] However, *M. equinum* is distinguished from *M. canis* by having smaller macroconidia, failure to perforate hair in vitro, poor growth and sporulation on certain media, different antigenic composition, and incompatibility with *Nannizzia otae*, the telomorph of *M. canis*.[21,21a,35,46]

Examination for Bacteria

In general practice, cytologic examination is the primary method used to identify the presence of pathogenic bacteria. Unusual lesions, nodular granulomatous lesions, and draining nodules should also be cultured. Bacterial culture and susceptibility testing are not routinely cost-effective for the initial work-up of the case with a suspected bacterial pyoderma. Cytologic examination is the initial test of choice, and if intracellular cocci are seen, empirical antibiotic therapy for coagulase-positive staphylococci is warranted. When cytologic study reveals rod-shaped organisms, or when cocci are seen but appropriate empirical therapy is ineffective, bacterial culture and susceptibility testing are indicated. Veterinarians frequently take specimens for bacterial culture, but infrequently grow and identify the cultures in their own practice. Specimens should be collected for culture, properly prepared, and rapidly sent to a skilled microbiologist in a laboratory equipped to provide prompt, accurate identification and antibacterial susceptibilities.

The skin and hair of the horse is a veritable cesspool of bacteria (see Chapter 1); therefore, cultures must be carefully taken and interpreted. The selection of appropriate lesions for culturing is critical. Moist erosions and many crusts may be contaminated by bacteria, and cultures are not routinely recommended for these lesions. In cases with pustules, an intact pustule should be opened with a sterile needle. The pus collected on the needle should be transferred to the tip of a sterile swab. Papules may also be superficially punctured, and a relatively serous droplet of pus may be obtained. These superficial papular and pustular lesions should not be prepared at all, because false-negative cultures may result. With superficial cultures, a positive culture does not prove pathogenicity, and concurrent cytologic examination should be performed. This allows documentation of the intracellular location of bacteria, which confirms their role in eliciting an inflammatory response. In cases with furuncles, needle aspirates may be taken and cultured. When plaques, nodules, and fistulous tracts are to be cultured, the surface is disinfected and samples are taken aseptically by skin biopsy. The skin sample is placed in a culture transport medium and submitted to the laboratory, where it should be ground and cultured.

When unusual bacterial diseases such as mycobacteriosis, bacterial pseudomycetoma, actinomycosis, actinobacillosis, and nocardiosis are suspected, unstained direct smears and tissue biopsy specimens should be submitted. The laboratory should be informed of the suspected disorder.

Deep lesions, cellulitis, and nodular lesions may also be cultured for anaerobic bacteria. Again, tissue biopsy is preferred, and special transport media or equipment is necessary. A good diagnostic laboratory supplies material for sample transport.

Special Preparations

DERMATOPHILUS PREPARATION[12,26]

If stains of exudate are negative and/or only dry crusts are present, a *Dermatophilus* preparation can be performed. Crusts are removed and excess hair is carefully trimmed away with scissors. The crust is then minced with scissors and mixed with several drops of water on a glass slide. After the crust has softened in water for several minutes, it is crushed with the tip of a wooden applicator stick. Excess debris is removed, the slide is allowed to air dry, then heat-fixed, stained, and examined under the microscope. *Dermatophilus congolensis* is a gram-positive, branching, filamentous organism that divides horizontally and longitudinally to form parallel rows of cocci (zoopores). If the *Dermatophilus* prep is negative and the diagnosis is still suspected, the diagnosis should not be ruled out until crusts are cultured (see Chapter 4).

ONCHOCERCA PREPARATION[12,26,38]

If possible, select a lesion in an area where microfilariae are not usually recovered in high numbers (e.g., avoid the ventral midline). A 6-mm biopsy punch specimen is taken. One-half of the specimen is placed in formalin for routine histopathology, and the other half is placed on a dampened gauze sponge in a tightly closed container until the preparation can be performed. A small piece of this tissue is minced with a razor blade, and a few drops of nonbacteriostatic saline are added (bacteriostatic saline kills the microfilariae and makes identification more difficult). The specimen is incubated at room temperature for about 15 minutes, then scanned under the 4× objective of the microscope, paying particular attention to the margins of the tissue debris while looking for indications of motion in the saline. If the characteristic "whiplash" movement of the microfilariae is seen, go to higher power. If the sample is negative, a small amount of water is added to a Petri dish, the glass slide is rested on two wooden sticks above water level, and the preparation is covered for several hours or overnight and reexamined.

Biopsy and Dermatohistopathologic Examination

Skin biopsy is one of the most powerful tools in dermatology.* However, maximization of the potential benefits of this tool necessitates enthusiastic, skilled teamwork between a clinician who has carefully selected, procured, and preserved the specimens and a pathologist who has carefully processed, perused, and interpreted the specimens. When the clinician and the pathologist truly work together, the skin biopsy can correctly reflect the dermatologic diagnosis in more than 90% of cases.[40] However, despite this, skin biopsies are often not performed or are done relatively late in the diagnostic work-up. In other cases, the skin biopsy findings are unrewarding because of poor specimen selection, poor technique, or both. In many dermatologic cases, the differential diagnosis primarily includes diseases that can be diagnosed only by biopsy or other nonhematologic or serum laboratory tests.

When the condition presented is not readily recognized, the skin biopsy is often the most informative test. Skin biopsy should not be regarded as merely a diagnostic aid for the difficult case or for the case that can be diagnosed only by biopsy. It is also helpful in establishing the group of diseases to consider. Even without a definitive diagnosis, a biopsy usually helps to guide the clinician in the appropriate diagnostic direction. It provides a permanent record of the pathologic changes present at a particular time, and knowledge of this pathologic finding stimulates the clinician to think more deeply about the basic cellular changes underlying the disease. Symptomatic therapies may also be directed on the basis of cytologic findings.

Although biopsies are helpful, it is still important for the clinician to remember that they only add information. The diagnosis is usually made by the clinician who correlates all the relevant

---

*References 3, 6, 10-13, 19, 20, 26, 31, 33, 34a, 38, 40, 42, 48, 51.

findings of a case, not by the pathologist. The biopsy contributes to those findings; it does not replace a thorough history, physical examination, or other ancillary test results.

WHEN TO BIOPSY

There are no definite rules on when to perform a skin biopsy. The following suggestions are offered as general guidelines. Biopsy should be performed on (1) all obviously neoplastic or suspected neoplastic lesions; (2) all persistent ulcerations; (3) any case that is likely to have the major diseases that are most readily diagnosed by biopsy (e.g., follicular dysplasia, epidermolysis bullosa, eosinophilic granuloma, and immune-mediated skin disease); (4) a dermatosis that is not responding to apparently rational therapy; (5) any dermatosis that, in the experience of the clinician, is unusual or appears serious; (6) vesicular dermatitis; and (7) any suspected condition for which the therapy is expensive, dangerous, or sufficiently time-consuming to necessitate a definitive diagnosis before beginning treatment.

In general, skin biopsy should be performed within 3 weeks for any dermatosis that is not responding to what appears to be appropriate therapy. This early intervention (1) helps to obviate the nonspecific, masking, and misleading changes due to chronicity, the administration of topical and systemic medicaments, excoriation, and secondary infection and (2) allows more rapid institution of specific therapy, thus reducing permanent disease sequelae (scarring, alopecia), the patient's suffering, and needless cost to the owner. Anti-inflammatory agents can dramatically affect the histologic appearance of many dermatoses. The administration of such agents, especially glucocorticoids, should optimally be stopped for 2 to 3 weeks before biopsy. The histopathologic changes caused by secondary bacterial infection often obliterate the histopathologic features of any concurrent dermatoses. It is imperative to eliminate these secondary infections with appropriate systemic antibiotic therapy before biopsies are performed.

WHAT TO BIOPSY

The selection of appropriate biopsy sites is partly an art. Experienced clinicians often pick lesions and subtle changes that they suspect will show diagnostic changes. They are already aware of what histopathologic changes are helpful in making a diagnosis. They also know what types of changes may be expected to be found with certain clinical lesions. For example, pigmentary incontinence is a helpful histopathologic feature of lupus erythematosus. The clinician who knows this, and also knows that slate blue depigmenting lesions have that color because of dermal melanin (often from pigmentary incontinence), selects those sites for biopsy. One histologic criterion of lupus is likely to be present because the clinician knew the pathogenesis of that lesion.

If the disease is an unknown one or appears strange, a biopsy is important. If the distribution of lesions is unusual for the suspected disease, the clinician obtains biopsy specimens from the unusual areas, not just those typical of the suspected disease. It is also important to perform biopsy of areas representative of primary diseases and not just secondary complications. Many clinicians perform biopsy of secondary bacterial pyoderma lesions but not noninfected areas in cases with underlying allergy or keratinization disorders.

The histologic examination of the full spectrum of lesions present gives more information than does the examination of one lesion or stage. Therefore, the clinician should take multiple samples and obtain specimens from a variety of lesions. When primary lesions are present, a sample of at least one should be submitted to the laboratory. Fluid-filled lesions (pustules, vesicles) are often fragile and transient and, if present, should be sampled as soon as possible. If the suspected disease historically has pustules, having the patient return may allow sampling of the most appropriate lesions. In other cases, the patient may be hospitalized and be examined every 2 to 4 hours to find early intact lesions for biopsy. Most diseases that can be diagnosed by dermatopathologic examination have early, fully developed, and late changes. The greater the number of characteristic changes recognized, the more accurate the diagnoses are, and by selecting a variety of lesions, it is more likely that multiple characteristic changes are seen.

Multiple samples can document a pathologic continuum. Whenever possible, the clinician obtains biopsy specimens from the spontaneous primary lesions (macules, papules, pustules, vesicles, bullae, nodules, and tumors) and secondary lesions. Examination of crusts may sometimes add as much information as a biopsy of a papule. A greater number of biopsy specimens maximizes results. However, in practice, clinicians are usually limited to 3 to 5 samples. Most laboratories charge the same fee for one to three biopsy specimens submitted in the same container. Most important is that one learns from biopsy attempts. One should try to pay attention to what lesions are selected and what specimens give the best results. With practice, the clinician becomes more adept at selecting informative biopsy sites. Reading does not replace practice, attention to results, and experience, but it can help the clinician to achieve some proficiency in the art of maximizing the benefits of skin biopsy.

INSTRUMENTS REQUIRED

Biopsies are often performed simply and quickly with just local anesthesia. Equipment that is needed for most cases includes 2% lidocaine; a selection of punch biopsies of different sizes; Adson thumb forceps; iris or small, curved scissors; formalin vials; needles and suture material; needle holders; and gauze pads. Occasionally, scalpel handles, blades, and large formalin vials may also be necessary.

HOW TO BIOPSY

In general, a 6-mm biopsy punch provides an adequate specimen. It is imperative not to include any significant amount of normal skin margin with punch biopsy specimens. Unless the person obtaining the biopsy specimen personally supervises the processing of the specimen in the tissue block, rotation in the wrong direction may result in failure to section the pathologic portion of the specimen. In general, when a punch biopsy specimen is received at the laboratory, it is cut in half through the center. Therefore, a macule, pustule, papule or small lesions should be centered in the biopsy specimen. If the lesion is to one side, only the normal tissue may be examined. The sample is also generally cut parallel to the growth of the hair. In many laboratories, only half of the specimen is sectioned and processed; the other half is saved in case problems occur and new sections or blocks are needed. So even with deeper cuts, if the wrong half is blocked, the lesion may not be present. The clinician must also realize that, after fixation, erythema and color changes are not detectable by the pathologist who sections the sample. Small lesions such as papules and pustules may no longer be grossly visible. The biopsy punch should be rotated in only one direction so as to minimize shearing artifacts.

It is important for the clinician to compare the pathologist's report with the description of the clinical lesion. If a pustule was observed clinically and the pathologist's report does not describe a pustule, it may have been missed. If a biopsied lesion is missed or the tissue is interpreted as normal, the clinician should explain this to the pathologist and obtain deeper sections to find the lesion.

It is also important for the clinician to be aware of what changes occur in the specimen after the biopsy. Autolysis starts to occur almost immediately after removal of the biopsy specimen. Therefore, it is important to place the newly acquired samples into appropriate fixatives (10% neutral buffered formalin) immediately. This should be done for each sample; one should not wait until all samples are taken before placing them in formalin. Punch biopsy specimens left under a hot surgery light have microscopically observable damage in less than 5 minutes.

Secondary bacterial infections can complicate equine dermatoses. The histopathologic changes induced by bacterial infection can obliterate the changes associated with the underlying disease process. Thus, it is important to treat secondary infections before biopsies are performed.

Glucocorticoid therapy can drastically alter inflammatory conditions and can rapidly deplete tissue eosinophils. Thus, it is important to stop glucocorticoid therapy for 2 to 3 weeks (oral) or 6 to 8 weeks (repository injections) before biopsying.

Excisional biopsy with a scalpel is often indicated (1) for larger lesions; (2) for vesicles, bullae, and pustules (the rotary and shearing action of a punch may damage the lesion); and (3) for suspected disease of the subcutaneous fat (punches often fail to deliver diseased fat).

Because full-thickness biopsies of the coronary band may result in permanent hoof wall defects, superficial "shave" biopsies with a scalpel blade are preferred. A tangential incision is made to the level of the superficial dermis, and bleeding is controlled with pressure.

Skin biopsy is usually accomplished easily and rapidly using physical restraint and local anesthesia. If more restraint is needed, the combination of xylazine (0.5 to 1 mg/kg IV) and butorphenol (0.01 to 0.2 mg/kg IV) is usually satisfactory. The sites are gently clipped (if needed). Clippers should not touch the skin surface, because surface keratin and other substances can be removed. The veterinarian is careful not to remove surface keratin, and the surface is left untouched or gently cleaned by daubing or soaking with a solution of 70% alcohol. The sites should not be prepared with other antiseptics (e.g., iodophors). Under no circumstances should biopsy sites be scrubbed. Such endeavors remove important surface pathologic changes and create iatrogenic inflammatory lesions. Sites that are being traumatized by the horse may contain artifacts.

After the surface has air-dried, the desired lesion is undermined with an appropriate amount, usually 1 to 2 ml, of local anesthetic (1% to 2% lidocaine) injected subcutaneously through a 25-gauge needle. An exception to this procedure is made when disease of the fat is suspected, in which case regional or ring blocks or general anesthesia should be used, because injection into fat distorts the tissues. The local injection of lidocaine stings, and some animals object strenuously. The desired lesion is then punched or excised, including the underlying fat.

It is important to remember that lidocaine inhibits various gram-positive (including coagulase-positive *Staphylococcus*) and gram-negative (including *Pseudomonas*) bacteria, mycobacteria, and fungi.[49] Bicarbonate and epinephrine do the same.[49] Thus, if a culture is going to be obtained from the biopsy specimen, it is advisable to use a ring block, or regional or general anesthesia.

Great care should be exercised when manipulating the biopsy specimen, avoiding the use of forceps and instead using tiny mosquito hemostats, Adson thumb forceps, or the syringe needle through which the local anesthetic was injected. One cruciate (crisscross) suture effectively closes defects produced by 6-mm biopsy punches. One or two simple interrupted sutures may also be placed.

COMPLICATIONS OF SKIN BIOPSY

Complications after skin biopsy are rare. Caution should be exercised when performing biopsy on patients with bleeding disorders, including patients taking aspirin and anticoagulants. The administration of such medication should be stopped, if possible, for 1 to 2 weeks before biopsy. Problems with wound healing should be anticipated in patients with severe metabolic disorders, in patients with various collagen defects (such as cutaneous asthenia), and in patients taking glucocorticoids or antimitotic drugs. The administration of such drugs should be stopped 2 to 3 weeks before biopsy, if possible. Wound infections are rare. The veterinarian should make sure that tetanus prophylaxis is up to date. Fly repellents may be appropriate in some circumstances.

Caution should be exercised when injecting lidocaine, which may contain epinephrine, near extremities (ear tips, digits, and so forth); into patients with impaired circulation, cardiovascular disease, or hypertension; or into patients receiving phenothiazines, β-adrenergic receptor blockers, monoamine oxidase inhibitors, or tricyclic antidepressants. Full-thickness biopsies of the coronary band may result in permanent hoof wall defects.

WHAT TO DO WITH THE BIOPSY SPECIMEN

Skin biopsy specimens should be gently blotted to remove artifactual blood. In most instances, the fixative of choice is 10% neutral phosphate buffered formalin (100 ml of 40% formaldehyde, 900 ml of tap water, 4 gm of acid sodium phosphate monohydrate, and 6.5 gm of anhydrous disodium phosphate). It is not stable and oxidizes to formic acid, which can be seen histologically by the formation of acid hematin in blood cells. Also, the ratio of formalin to tissue is important, with a minimum of 10 parts formalin to 1 part tissue being necessary for adequate rapid fixation. Freezing should also be avoided; this sometimes occurs when samples are mailed in the winter months. This can be prevented by adding 95% ethyl alcohol as 10% of the fixative volume, or by allowing at least 12 hours of fixation before cold exposure.

Fixation in formalin also causes sample shrinkage, which is not a problem with 4-mm punch biopsy specimens. Larger punch biopsy specimens and elliptic excisions should be placed subcutis side down on a piece of wooden tongue depressor or cardboard to minimize the artifacts induced by shrinkage. They should be gently pressed flat for 30 to 60 seconds to facilitate adherence. Placing the specimens on a flat surface allows proper anatomic orientation and prevents potentially drastic artifacts associated with curling and folding. The specimen and its adherent splint are then immersed in fixative within 1 to 2 minutes, because artifactual changes develop rapidly in room air.

Also, formalin rapidly penetrates only about 1 cm of tissue. Samples larger than 1 cm should be partially transected at 1-cm intervals. This most commonly becomes important when large nodules and tumors are excised and submitted for histopathologic evaluation.

The last critical consideration is deciding where to send a skin biopsy specimen. Obviously, the clinician wants to send it to someone who can provide the most information. The choices should be ordered as follows: (1) a veterinary pathologist specializing in dermatopathology, (2) a veterinary dermatologist with a special interest and expertise in dermatohistopathology, (3) a general veterinary pathologist, and (4) a physician dermatopathologist with a special interest in comparative dermatopathology.

The clinician frequently does not provide adequate information concerning skin biopsy specimens. The clinician and the pathologist are a diagnostic team, and an accurate diagnosis is more likely (and the patient is best served) when both members of the team do their part. A concise description of the history, the physical examination findings, the results of laboratory examinations and therapeutic trials, and the clinician's differential diagnosis should always accompany the biopsy specimen.

TISSUE STAINS

Hematoxylin and eosin (H & E) stain is most widely used routinely for skin biopsies. In the laboratory of the authors, acid orcein–Giemsa (AOG) stain is also used regularly for skin biopsies. The routine use of AOG markedly reduces the need for ordering special stains (Table 2-6). Table 2-7 contains guidelines for the use of various special stains.

ARTIFACTS

Even the best dermatohistopathologist cannot read an inadequate, poorly preserved, poorly fixed, or poorly processed specimen.[10,38,42,51] Numerous artifacts can be produced by errors in site selection, preparation, technique in taking and handling and fixation and processing of skin biopsy specimens. It is important that the clinician and the pathologist be cognizant of these potentially disastrous distortions.

1. Artifacts due to improper site selection include excoriations and other physicochemical effects (e.g., maceration, inflammation, necrosis, and staining abnormalities caused by topical medicaments).

● **Table 2-6 STAINING CHARACTERISTICS OF VARIOUS CUTANEOUS COMPONENTS WITH ACID ORCEIN–GIEMSA STAIN**

TEST COMPONENT	COLOR
Nuclei	Dark blue
Cytoplasm of keratinocytes	Blue-purple
Cytoplasm of smooth muscle cells	Light blue
Keratin	Blue
Collagen	Pink
Elastin	Dark brown to black
Mast cell granules	Purple
Some acid mucopolysaccharides	Purple
Melanin	Dark green to black
Hemosiderin	Yellow-brown to green
Erythrocytes	Green-orange
Eosinophil granules	Red
Cytoplasm of histiocytes, lymphocytes, and fibrocytes	Light blue
Cytoplasm of neutrophils	Clear to light blue
Cytoplasm of plasma cells	Dark blue to gray-blue
Amyloid	Sky blue to gray-blue
Hyaline	Pink
Fibrin and fibrinoid	Green-blue
Keratohyalin	Dark blue
Trichohyalin	Red
Bacteria, fungal spores, and hyphae	Dark blue
Serum	Light blue

● **Table 2-7 STAINING CHARACTERISTICS OF VARIOUS SUBSTANCES WITH SPECIAL STAINS**

STAIN	TISSUE AND COLOR
van Gieson's	Mature collagen—red; immature collagen, muscle and nerves—yellow
Masson trichrome	Mature collagen—blue; immature collagen, keratin, muscle, and nerves—red
Verhoeff's	Elastin and nuclei—black
Gomori's aldehyde fuchsin	Elastin, sulfated acid mucopolysaccharides, and certain epithelial mucins—purple
Oil red O°	Lipids—dark red
Sudan black B°	Lipids—green-black
Scarlet red°	Lipids—red
Gomori's or Wilder's reticulin	Reticulin, melanin, and nerves—dark brown to black
Periodic acid–Schiff	Glycogen, neutral mucopolysaccharides, fungi, and tissue debris—red
Alcian blue	Acid mucopolysaccharides—blue
Hale's colloidal iron	Acid mucopolysaccharides—blue
Toluidine blue	Acid mucopolysaccharides and mast cell granules—purple
Gomori's methenamine silver	Fungi—black
Gram's or Brown-Brenn	Gram-positive bacteria—blue
	Gram-negative bacteria—red
Fite's modified acid-fast	Acid-fast bacteria—red
Fontana's ammoniacal silver nitrate	Premelanin and melanin—black (hemosiderin usually positive too, but less intense)

°Require frozen sections of formalin-fixed tissue.

2. Artifacts due to improper preparation include inflammation, staining abnormalities, and removal of surface pathologic changes (from surgical scrubbing and the use of antiseptics), as well as collagen separation pseudoedema and pseudosinus formation (due to intradermal injection of local anesthetic).

3. Artifacts due to improper technique in taking and handling include pseudovesicles, pseudoclefts, and shearing (caused by a dull punch or poor technique); pseudopapillomas or pseudonodules, pseudosclerosis, pseudosinuses, pseudocysts, and lobules of sebaceous glands within hair follicles, on the skin surface, or both (squeeze artifacts due to intervention with forceps); marked dehydration, elongation, and polarization of cells and cell nuclei (due to electrodesiccation [Fig. 2-27]); and intercellular edema, clefts, and vesicles (due to friction).

4. Artifacts caused by improper fixation and processing include dermoepidermal separation, intracellular edema, and fractures (due to autolysis); shrinkage, curling, and folding (due to failure to use wooden or cardboard splints); intracellular edema, vacuolar alteration, and multinucleate epidermal giant cells (from freezing); formalin pigment in blood vessels and extravascular phagocytes (due to the use of nonbuffered formalin); hardening, shrinkage, and loss of cellular detail (from too much alcohol in the fixative); poor staining and soft, easily displaced, and distorted tissue (with Bouin's solution); thick, fragmented sections (due to inadequate dehydration during tissue processing); pseudoacanthosis (in tangential sections associated with poor orientation of the specimen); and dermoepidermal separation and displacement of dermal tissues into epidermis (attributable to cutting sections from dermis to epidermis).

● THE VOCABULARY OF DERMATOHISTOPATHOLOGY

Dermatopathology is a specialty of medicine requiring many hours of training and many more of experience to master. It is beyond the scope of this book to train the student adequately in both dermatology and dermatopathology. However, because dermatopathologic examination is the single most valuable laboratory aid to the dermatologist, it is important to understand the vocabulary of the dermatopathologist.

Dermatohistopathology has a specialized vocabulary, because many of the histopathologic changes are unique to the skin. Unfortunately, as is true of most sciences, the dermatologic and general medical literature abounds with confusing and sometimes inappropriate dermatohistopathologic terms. The following discussion of terms is based on an amalgamation of such considerations as precision of definition, descriptive value, popular usage, historical precedent, and diagnostic significance in dermatohistopathology.[10,25,38,42,51]

Epidermal Changes

HYPERKERATOSIS

Hyperkeratosis is an increased thickness of the stratum corneum and may be *absolute* (an actual increase in thickness, which is most common) or *relative* (an apparent increase due to thinning of the underlying epidermis, which is rare). The types of hyperkeratosis are further specified by the adjectives *orthokeratotic* (anuclear) (Fig. 2-28) and *parakeratotic* (nucleated) (Fig. 2-29; also see Fig. 2-33). Orthokeratotic and parakeratotic hyperkeratoses are commonly, but less precisely, referred to as *orthokeratosis* and *parakeratosis*, respectively. Other adjectives commonly used to describe further the nature of hyperkeratosis include *basketweave* (e.g., dermatophytosis and endocrinopathic conditions), *compact* (e.g., chronic pruritus, lichenoid dermatoses, and cutaneous horns), and *laminated* (e.g., ichthyosis and follicular cysts).

Orthokeratotic and parakeratotic hyperkeratosis may be seen as alternating layers in the stratum corneum. This observation implies episodic changes in epidermopoiesis. If the changes

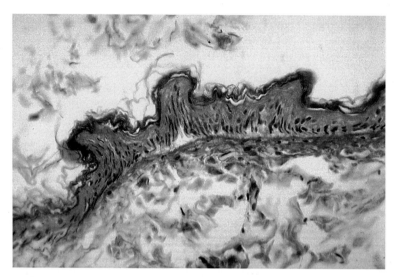

FIGURE 2-27. Electrodessication. Note how epidermal keratinocytes are vertically elongated, giving the appearance of standing at attention.

are *generalized*, the lesions appear as horizontal layers. If the changes are *focal*, the lesion is a vertical defect in the stratum corneum. Focal areas of orthokeratotic and parakeratotic hyperkeratosis are common, nondiagnostic findings in virtually any chronic dermatosis. They simply imply altered epidermopoiesis, whether inflammatory, hormonal, neoplastic, or developmental. *Diffuse parakeratotic hyperkeratosis* is occasionally seen with ectoparasitism, dermatophilosis, dermatophytosis, and necrolytic migratory erythema. *Focal parakeratotic hyperkeratosis overlying epidermal papillae* (parakeratotic "caps"), wherein the subjacent dermal papillae are edematous (papillary "squirting"), is seen in primary idiopathic seborrheic dermatitis. *Diffuse orthokeratotic hyperkeratosis* suggests endocrinopathies, nutritional deficiencies, secondary seborrheas, and developmental abnormalities (ichthyosis, follicular dysplasia, epidermal nevus).

HYPOKERATOSIS

Decreased thickness of the stratum corneum, called *hypokeratosis*, is much less common than hyperkeratosis and reflects an exceptionally rapid epidermal turnover time or decreased cohesion, or both, between cells of the stratum corneum. Hypokeratosis may be found in seborrheic and other exfoliative skin disorders. It may also be produced by excessive surgical preparation of the biopsy site, topical medicaments, or by friction and maceration in the intertriginous areas.

HYPERGRANULOSIS AND HYPOGRANULOSIS

The terms *hypergranulosis* and *hypogranulosis* indicate, respectively, an increase and a decrease in the thickness of the stratum granulosum. Both entities are common and nondiagnostic. *Hyper*granulosis (Fig. 2-30) may be seen in any dermatosis in which there is epidermal hyperplasia and orthokeratotic hyperkeratosis. *Hypo*granulosis is often seen in dermatoses in which there is parakeratotic hyperkeratosis.

HYPERPLASIA

An increased thickness of the noncornified epidermis due to an increased number of epidermal cells is called *hyperplasia*. The term *acanthosis* is often used interchangeably with hyperplasia. However, acanthosis specifically indicates an increased thickness of the stratum spinosum and may

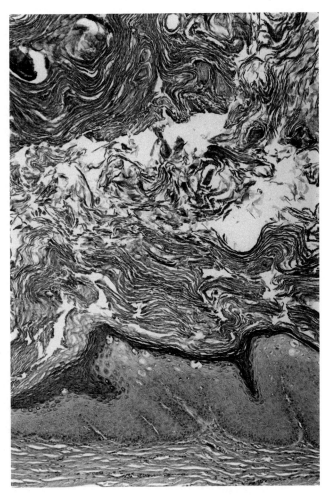

FIGURE 2-28. Orthokeratotic hyperkeratosis on surface of ear papilloma.

be due to hyperplasia (*true* acanthosis, which is the most common), or hypertrophy (*pseudo*acanthosis, which is uncommon). Epidermal hyperplasia is often accompanied by *rete ridge formation* (irregular hyperplasia resulting in "pegs" of epidermis that appear to project downward into the underlying dermis). Rete ridges are *not* found in normal *haired* skin of horses.

The following adjectives further specify the types of epidermal hyperplasia: (1) *irregular*—uneven, elongated, pointed rete ridges with an obliterated or preserved rete-papilla configuration (Fig. 2-31); (2) *regular*—more or less evenly thickened epidermis (Fig. 2-32); (3) *psoriasiform*—more or less evenly elongated rete ridges that are clubbed and/or fused at their bases; (4) *papillated*—digitate projections of the epidermis above the skin surface (Fig. 2-33); and (5) *pseudocarcinomatous (pseudoepitheliomatous)*—extreme, irregular hyperplasia, which may include increased mitoses, squamous eddies, and horn pearls, thus resembling squamous cell carcinoma (Fig. 2-34); however, cellular atypia is absent, and the basement membrane zone is not breached. These five forms of epidermal hyperplasia may be seen in various combinations in the same specimen.

Epidermal hyperplasia is a common, nondiagnostic feature of virtually any chronic inflammatory process. The five types are generally useful descriptive terms but have little specific diagnostic significance. Pseudocarcinomatous hyperplasia is most commonly associated with

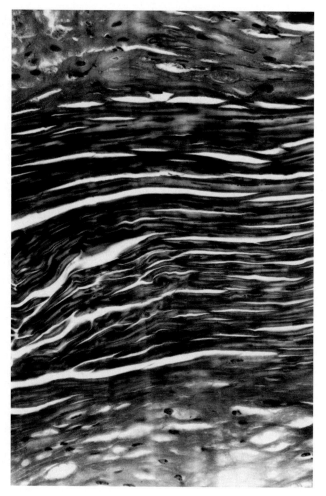

FIGURE 2-29. Parakeratotic hyperkeratosis associated with hepatocutaneous syndrome.

underlying dermal suppurative, granulomatous, or neoplastic processes and with chronic ulcers. Papillated hyperplasia is most commonly seen with neoplasia, callosities, epidermal nevi, and primary seborrhea.

HYPOPLASIA AND ATROPHY

Hypoplasia is a decreased thickness of the noncornified epidermis due to a decrease in the number of cells. *Atrophy* is a decreased thickness of the noncornified epidermis due to a decrease in the size of cells. An early sign of epidermal hypoplasia or atrophy is the loss of the rete ridges in areas of skin where they are normally present (i.e., in the nonhaired skin of horses).

Epidermal hypoplasia and atrophy are rare in skin diseases of horses but may be seen with hormonal (hypothyroidism), developmental (cutaneous asthenia), and inflammatory (discoid lupus erythematosus, vaccine-induced vasculitis) dermatoses.

NECROSIS, DYSKERATOSIS, AND APOPTOSIS

The term *necrosis* refers to the death of cells or tissues in a living organism and is judged to be present primarily on the basis of nuclear morphology. *Necrolysis* is often used synonymously with

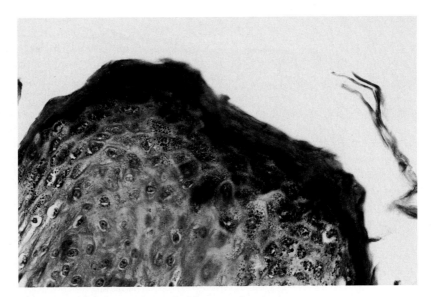

FIGURE 2-30. Hypergranulosis associated with atopic dermatitis.

necrosis, but actually implies a *separation* of tissue due to death of cells. Nuclear changes indicative of necrosis include *karyorrhexis* (nuclear fragmentation), *pyknosis* (nuclear shrinkage and consequent hyperchromasia), and *karyolysis* (nuclear "ghosts"). With all three necrotic nuclear changes, individual keratinocytes are characterized by loss of intercellular bridges, with resultant rounding of the cell, and a normal-sized or swollen eosinophilic cytoplasm. Necrosis is further specified by the adjectives *coagulation* (cell outlines preserved, but cell detail lost) or *caseation* (complete loss of all structural details, the tissue being placed by a granular material containing nuclear debris).

In fact, cell death and necrosis are different.[28,36] Cell death—defined functionally by the point of no return—occurs long before necrosis and is not detectable histologically. Necrosis is histologically visible and refers to changes that occur secondary to cell death by any mechanism (e.g., apoptosis, oncosis).

Epidermal necrosis may be focal as a result of drug eruptions, microbial infections, or lichenoid dermatoses, or may be generalized as a result of physicochemical trauma (primary irritant contact dermatitis, burns, photodermatitis), interference with blood supply (vasculitis, thromboembolism, subepidermal bullae, dense subepidermal cellular infiltrates), or an immunologic mechanism (erythema multiforme). So-called *satellite cell necrosis* (satellitosis) (Fig. 2-35) is a misnomer;[28,36] what actually occurs is satellite cell *apoptosis.* Individual apoptotic keratinocytes are seen in association with contiguous ("satellite") lymphoid cells. Satellitosis can be seen in a number of interface dermatitides, such as erythema multiforme, lupus erythematosus, drug reactions, and graft-versus-host disease.

The term *dyskeratosis* is used to indicate a premature and faulty keratinization of individual cells. The term is also used, although less commonly, to indicate a general fault in the keratinization process and, thus, in the state of the epidermis as a whole. Dyskeratotic cells are characterized by eosinophilic, swollen cytoplasm with normal or condensed, dark-staining nuclei. Such cells are difficult or impossible to distinguish from *necrotic* keratinocytes on light microscopic examination. The judgment usually depends on whether the rest of the epithelium is thought to be keratinizing or necrosing. Because no one has been able to define the term *dyskeratosis* consistently, and the original concepts upon which the term was based are now known to be wrong, it has been suggested this term be avoided.[45]

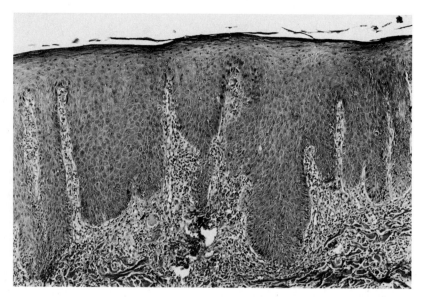

FIGURE 2-31. Irregular epidermal hyperplasia associated with staphylococcal dermatitis.

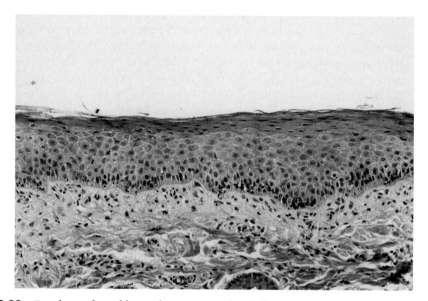

FIGURE 2-32. Regular epidermal hyperplasia associated with dermatophilosis.

Apoptosis (Figs. 2-35 and 2-36) is a form of intentional suicide based on a genetic mechanism.[28, 36] Programmed cell death and apoptosis are not identical, but genetic programming is involved in both. In programmed (spontaneous) cell death, there is an internal "clock" that specifies the fixed time for physiologic cell suicide. In apoptosis, genetic programming specifies the weapons (the means) to produce instant suicide. Apoptosis can be activated by many stimuli: growth factors, cytokines, hormones, immune system, viruses, and sublethal damage to cells. Apoptotic keratinocytes are common features of interface dermatoses, but they may be seen in small numbers (up to six in a section through a 6-mm punch specimen) in virtually any hyperplastic

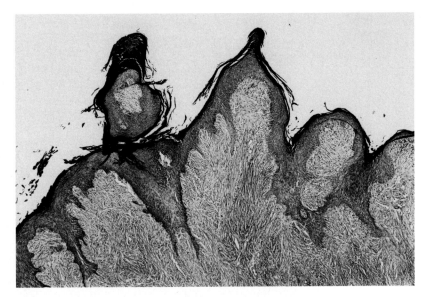

FIGURE 2-33. Papillated epidermal hyperplasia with equine sarcoid.

epidermis. Apoptotic keratinocytes are rarely seen (one or two in a section through a 6-mm punch specimen) in normal epidermis. However, apoptotic keratinocytes are numerous in the catagen and early telogen hair follicle epithelium. Cytotoxic drugs produce keratinocyte apoptosis, with phase-specific agents tending to target the basal cell layer and noncycle phase-specific agents affecting all epithelial layers.

Apoptotic keratinocytes undergo a series of morphologic changes: the cell shrinks, becomes denser and more eosinophilic, and loses its normal contacts; nuclear changes include pyknosis, margination of chromatin, and karyorrhexis; the cell emits processes ("buds") that often contain nuclear fragments and organelles and that do not swell; these buds often break off and become *apoptotic bodies*, which may be phagocytosed by macrophages or neighboring cells, or remain free. There is no swelling of mitochondria or other organelles. Synonyms for apoptotic keratinocytes include *Civatte bodies* (when in the stratum basale) and *sunburn cells* (when caused by ultraviolet radiation). Synonyms for apoptotic bodies include *colloid, hyaline, filamentous,* and *ovoid* bodies. Apoptosis may be more specifically detected in routinely processed and fixed skin specimens by the terminal uridinyl transferase nick end labeling (TUNEL) method.[5]

Oncosis is cell death as a result of overwhelming damage (e.g., ischemia, toxins, chemical injury) and is characterized by cellular swelling, organelle swelling, blebbing (blister-like cell membrane structures that do not contain cell organelles and that may swell and rupture) and increased membrane permeability.[28, 36] Oncosis and necrosis induce an inflammatory response, whereas apoptosis does not.

INTERCELLULAR EDEMA

Intercellular edema (*spongiosis*) (Fig. 2-37, A) of the epidermis is characterized by a widening of the intercellular spaces with accentuation of the intercellular bridges, giving the involved epidermis a "spongy" appearance. Severe intercellular edema may lead to rupture of the intercellular bridges and the formation of *spongiotic vesicles* within the epidermis. Some spongiotic vesicle formation may, in turn, "blow out" the basement membrane zone in some areas, giving the appearance of *sub*epidermal vesicles. Intercellular edema is a common, nondiagnostic

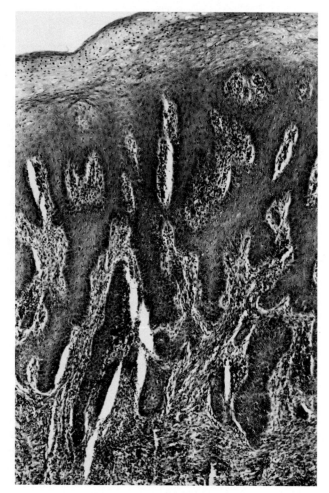

FIGURE 2-34. Pseudocarcinomatous epidermal hyperplasia with multisystemic epitheliotropic eosinophilic disease.

feature of any acute or subacute inflammatory dermatosis. Focal spongiosis of the superficial epidermis that is accompanied by lymphocytic (Fig. 2-37, *B*), eosinophilic (Fig. 2-37, *C*), or neutrophilic exocytosis with or without superficial epidermal necrosis suggests contact dermatitis. Spongiosis of the upper one-half of the epidermis, which is overlaid by marked parakeratotic hyperkeratosis, is seen in necrolytic migratory erythema.

INTRACELLULAR EDEMA

Intracellular edema (hydropic degeneration, vacuolar degeneration, ballooning degeneration) (Fig. 2-38) of the epidermis is characterized by increased size, cytoplasmic pallor, and displacement of the nucleus to the periphery of affected cells. Severe intracellular edema may result in *reticular degeneration* and intraepidermal vesicles.

Intracellular edema is a common, nondiagnostic feature of any acute or subacute inflammatory dermatosis. Caution must be exercised not to confuse intracellular edema with freezing artifact (Fig. 2-39), delayed fixation artifact, or the intracellular accumulation of glycogen seen in the outer root sheath of normal hair follicles and secondary to epidermal injury. In addition, one

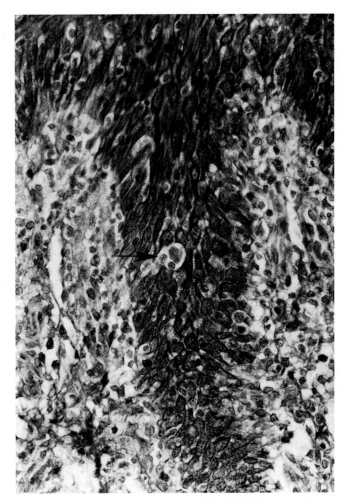

FIGURE 2-35. Satellitosis (*arrow*) associated with trimethoprim-sulfadiazine drug reaction.

can see individual keratinocytes with condensed, pyknotic nuclei surrounded by a clear vesicular space and a rim of homogeneous cytoplasm in a number of dermatoses.[32] These epidermal "clear cells" are artifacts due to occlusion, moisture in intertriginous areas, and other unknown factors.

RETICULAR DEGENERATION

This type of degeneration is caused by severe intracellular edema of epidermal cells in which the cells burst, resulting in multilocular intraepidermal vesicles in which septae are formed by resistant cell walls (see Fig. 2-38). It may be seen with any acute or subacute inflammatory dermatosis, but especially dermatophilosis and acute contact dermatitis.

BALLOONING DEGENERATION

Ballooning degeneration (koilocytosis) (Fig. 2-40) is a specific type of degenerative change seen in epidermal cells and characterized by swollen eosinophilic to lightly basophilic cytoplasm without vacuolization, by enlarged or condensed and occasionally multiple nuclei, and by a loss of cohesion resulting in acantholysis. Ballooning degeneration is a specific feature of viral infections.

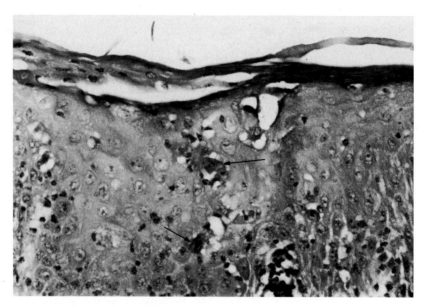

FIGURE 2-36. Apoptotic keratinocytes (*arrows*) in systemic lupus erythematosus.

HYDROPIC DEGENERATION OF BASAL CELLS

Hydropic degeneration (liquefaction degeneration, vacuolar alteration) of the basal epidermal cells (Fig. 2-41) is a term used to describe intracellular edema restricted to cells of the stratum basale. This process may also affect the basal cells of the outer root sheath of hair follicles. Hydropic degeneration of basal cells is usually focal but, if severe and extensive, may result in intrabasal or subepidermal clefts or vesicles owing to dermoepidermal separation. Hydropic degeneration of basal cells is an uncommon finding and is usually associated with drug eruptions, lupus erythematosus, erythema multiforme, and vasculopathies.

ACANTHOLYSIS

A loss of cohesion between epidermal cells, resulting in intraepidermal clefts, vesicles, and bullae, is known as acantholysis (dyshesion, desmolysis, desmorrhexis) (Fig. 2-42). Free epidermal cells in the vesicles are called *acantholytic keratinocytes*, or *acanthocytes*. This process may also involve the outer root sheath of hair follicles and glandular ductal epithelium. Acantholysis is further specified by reference to the level at which it occurs (i.e., *subcorneal*, *intragranular*, *intraepidermal*, or *suprabasilar*). Acantholytic keratinocytes are rounded, their nucleus is often morphologically normal, and their cytoplasm is normally stained or hypereosinophilic.

Acantholysis is most commonly associated with the pemphigus complex due to autoantibodies against various transmembrane desmosomal glycoproteins (e.g., desmogleins, desmocollins). However, other causes of acantholysis are severe spongiosis (any acute or subacute inflammatory dermatosis), ballooning degeneration (viral infection), proteolytic enzymes released by neutrophils (bacterial and fungal dermatoses), and neoplastic transformation (squamous cell carcinoma, actinic keratosis).

EXOCYTOSIS AND DIAPEDESIS

The term *exocytosis* refers to the migration of inflammatory cells or erythrocytes, or both, through the intercellular spaces of the epidermis (see Fig. 2-37, *B* and *C*). Exocytosis of inflammatory cells is a common, nondiagnostic feature of any inflammatory dermatosis. Exocytosis of erythrocytes

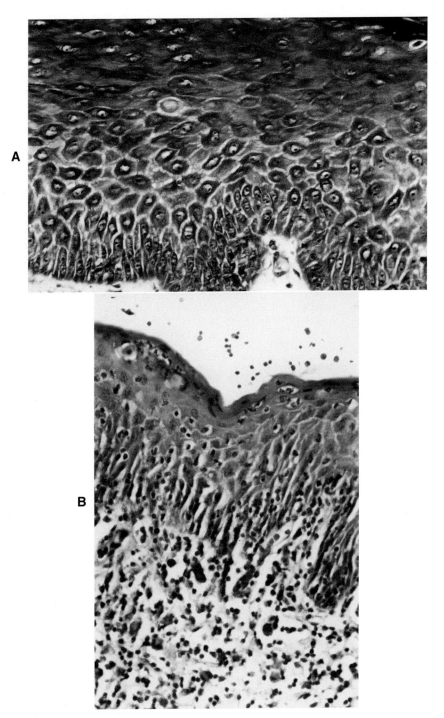

FIGURE 2-37. A, Intercellular edema with hepatic photosensitization. **B**, Exocytosis of lymphocytes with contact dermatitis.

Continued

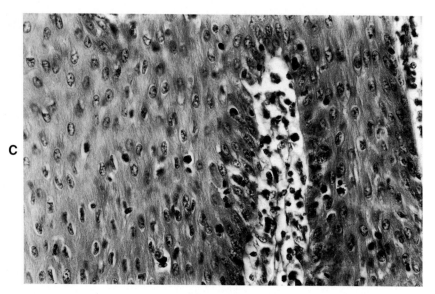

FIGURE 2-37, cont'd. C, Exocytosis of eosinophils associated with multisystemic epitheliotropic eosinophilic disease.

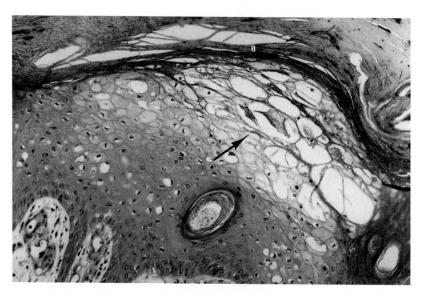

FIGURE 2-38. Intracellular edema and reticular degeneration (*arrow*) with dermatophilosis.

implies purpura (e.g., vasculitis, coagulation defect) and may be seen whenever superficial dermal inflammation, vascular dilatation, and engorgement are pronounced. When the condition involves eosinophils in combination with spongiosis, it is often referred to as *eosinophilic spongiosis* and may be seen in ectoparasitism, pemphigus, pemphigoid, eosinophilic granuloma, and multisystemic eosinophilic epitheliotropic disease.

    Diapedesis occurs when erythrocytes are present in the intercellular spaces of the epidermis. Diapedesis of erythrocytes implies loss of vascular integrity and may be seen whenever superficial

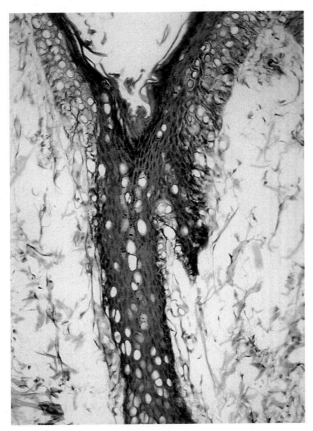

FIGURE 2-39. Freezing artifact. Note that keratinocytes are vacuolated at all levels of the epidermis and hair follicle outer root sheath with no accompanying intercellular edema, exocytosis of inflammatory cells, or dermal inflammation.

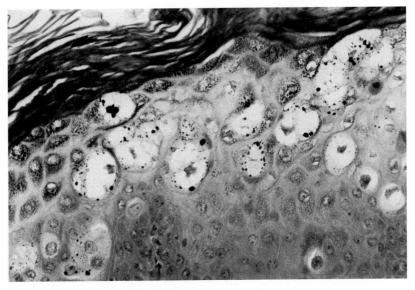

FIGURE 2-40. Koilocytosis (ballooning degeneration) associated with ear papilloma.

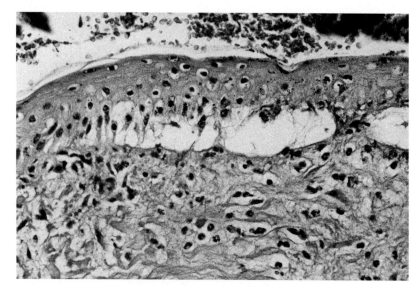

FIGURE 2-41. Hydropic degeneration of epidermal basal cells, with systemic lupus erythematosus.

dermal inflammation and vascular dilatation and engorgement are pronounced or when vasculitis or coagulation defects occur. These intraepidermal erythrocytes can be phagocytosed by keratinocytes.[7]

CLEFTS

The slit-like spaces known as *clefts* (lacunae), which do not contain fluid, occur within the epidermis or at the dermoepidermal junction. Clefts may be caused by acantholysis or hydropic degeneration of basal cells (Max Joseph spaces). However, they may also be caused by mechanical trauma and tissue retraction associated with the taking, fixation, and processing of biopsy specimens.

Artifactual dermoepidermal separation is fairly commonly observed at the margin of a biopsy specimen. In general, only tissue weakened through the dermoepidermal junction will separate in this manner during processing. Thus, this "usable artifact" may be valid evidence of basal cell or basement membrane damage. Spurious separation is characterized by clefting at different anatomic sites within the same specimen and evidence of tissue trauma (e.g., torn cytoplasm and fibers, bare cellular nuclei).

MICROVESICLES, VESICLES, AND BULLAE

Microvesicles, vesicles, and bullae are microscopic and macroscopic, fluid-filled, relatively acellular spaces within or below the epidermis. Such lesions are often loosely referred to as *blisters*. These lesions may be caused by severe intercellular or intracellular edema, ballooning degeneration, acantholysis, hydropic degeneration of basal cells, subepidermal edema, or other factors resulting in dermoepidermal separation (e.g., the autoantibodies in bullous pemphigoid). Microvesicles, vesicles, and bullae may thus be further described by their location as *subcorneal*, *intragranular*, *intraepidermal*, *suprabasilar*, *intrabasal*, or *subepidermal*. When these lesions contain larger numbers of inflammatory cells, they may be referred to as *vesicopustules*.

MICROABSCESSES AND PUSTULES

Microabscesses (Fig. 2-43) and pustules are microscopic or macroscopic intraepidermal and subepidermal cavities filled with inflammatory cells, which can be further described on the basis of location and cell type as follows.

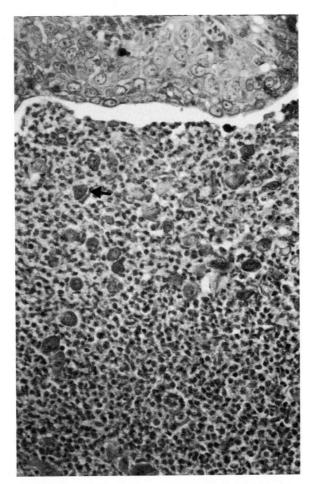

FIGURE 2-42. Acantholytic keratinocytes (*arrow*) with pemphigus foliaceus.

1. *Spongiform pustule of Kogoj*—a multilocular accumulation of neutrophils within and between keratinocytes, especially those of the stratum granulosum and stratum spinosum, in which cell boundaries form a sponge-like network. It is seen in microbial infections.
2. *Munro's microabscess*—a small, desiccated accumulation of neutrophils within or below the stratum corneum, which is seen in microbial infections and seborrheic disorders.
3. *Pautrier's microabscess*—a small, focal accumulation of abnormal lymphoid cells, which is seen in epitheliotropic lymphomas.
4. *Eosinophilic microabscess*—a lesion seen in ectoparasitism, eosinophilic granuloma, eosinophilic folliculitis, bullous pemphigoid, the pemphigus complex, and equine multisystemic epitheliotropic eosinophilic disease.
5. Small spongiotic foci containing normal mononuclear cells are occasionally seen in hypersensitive disorders. These cells may be lymphocytes, macrophages, or Langerhan's cells.

HYPERPIGMENTATION

Hyperpigmentation (hypermelanosis) refers to excessive amounts of melanin deposited within the epidermis and, often, concurrently in dermal melanophages. Hyperpigmentation may be focal or diffuse and may be confined to the stratum basale or present throughout all epidermal layers. It is

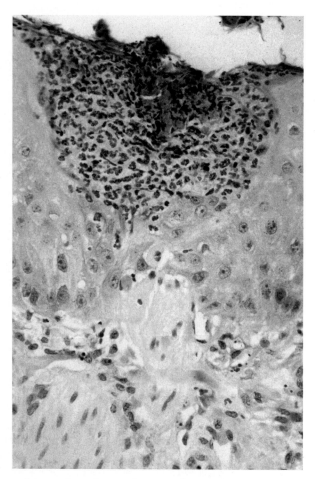

FIGURE 2-43. Neutrophilic epidermal microabscess with secondary staphylococcal dermatitis.

a common, nondiagnostic finding in chronic inflammatory and hormonal dermatoses, as well as in some developmental and neoplastic disorders. Postinflammatory hyperpigmentation is a common consequence of inflammatory insults. Increased melanin may be present in the epidermis (within keratinocytes) and/or dermis (within melanophages and melanocytes). The pathomechanism is unclear but could include epidermal injury and melanin fallout through a damaged basement membrane. Interferons stimulate melanin formation by melanocytes and may be a key mechanism in cutaneous postinflammatory hyperpigmentation. Hyperpigmentation must always be cautiously assessed with regard to the patient's *normal* pigmentation. Hyperpigmentation of sebaceous glands with extrusion of linear melanotic casts into hair follicle lumina is seen in follicular dysplasia.

HYPOPIGMENTATION

Hypopigmentation (hypomelanosis) (Fig. 2-44) refers to decreased amounts of melanin in the epidermis. The condition may be associated with congenital or acquired idiopathic defects in melanization (e.g., leukoderma, vitiligo), toxic effects of certain chemicals on melanocytes (e.g., monobenzyl ether of dihydroquinone in rubbers and plastics), inflammatory disorders that affect melanization or destroy melanocytes, and dermatoses featuring hydropic degeneration of basal

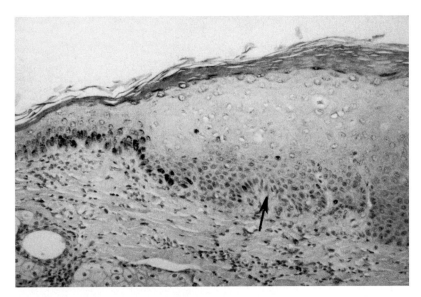

FIGURE 2-44. Hypomelanosis (*arrow*) with ear papilloma. Note melanization of normal epidermis to left.

cells (e.g., lupus erythematosus). In the hypopigmented dermatoses associated with hydropic degeneration of basal cells, the underlying superficial dermis usually reveals *pigmentary incontinence*.

CRUST

The consolidated, desiccated surface mass called crust is composed of varying combinations of keratin, serum, cellular debris, and often microorganisms. Crusts are further described on the basis of their composition: (1) *serous*—mostly serum; (2) *hemorrhagic*—mostly blood; (3) *cellular* —mostly inflammatory cells (Fig. 2-45); (4) *serocellular* (exudative)—a mixture of serum and inflammatory cells; and (5) *palisading*—alternating horizontal rows of orthokeratotic-to-para-keratotic hyperkeratosis and pus (e.g., dermatophilosis, dermatophytosis) (Fig. 2-46).

Crusts merely indicate a prior exudative process and are rarely of diagnostic significance. However, crusts should always be closely scrutinized, because they may contain the following important diagnostic clues: (1) dermatophyte spores and hyphae; (2) the filaments and coccoid elements of *Dermatophilus congolensis*; and (3) large numbers of acantholytic keratinocytes (pemphigus complex) (Fig. 2-47). Bacteria and bacterial colonies are common inhabitants of surface debris and are of no diagnostic significance. The presence of pigmented fungal elements in surface debris are occasionally seen and are of no diagnostic significance.

DELLS

These small depressions or hollows in the surface of the epidermis are usually associated with focal epidermal atrophy and orthokeratotic hyperkeratosis. Dells may be seen in lichenoid dermatoses, especially in lupus erythematosus.

EPIDERMAL COLLARETTE

The term *epidermal collarette* refers to the formation of elongated, hyperplastic rete ridges at the lateral margins of a pathologic process that appear to curve inward toward the center of the lesion. Epidermal collarettes may be seen with neoplastic, granulomatous, and suppurative dermatoses.

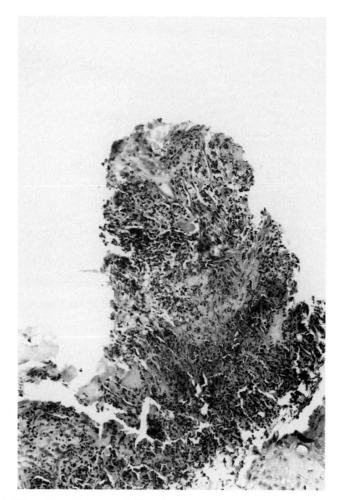

FIGURE 2-45. Cellular crust with bacterial folliculitis.

HORN CYSTS, PSEUDOHORN CYSTS, HORN PEARLS, AND SQUAMOUS EDDIES

Horn cysts (keratin cysts) are multiple, small, circular cystic structures that are surrounded by flattened epidermal cells and contain concentrically arranged lamellar keratin. Horn cysts are features of hair follicle neoplasms and basal cell tumors. *Pseudohorn cysts* are illusory cystic structures formed by the irregular invagination of a hyperplastic, hyperkeratotic epidermis. They are seen in numerous hyperplastic or neoplastic epidermal dermatoses. *Horn pearls* (squamous pearls) are focal, circular, concentric layers of squamous cells showing gradual keratinization toward the center, often accompanied by cellular atypia and dyskeratosis. Horn pearls are features of squamous cell carcinoma and pseudocarcinomatous hyperplasia. *Squamous eddies*, features of numerous neoplastic and hyperplastic epidermal disorders, are whorl-like patterns of squamoid cells with no atypia, dyskeratosis, or central keratinization.

EPIDERMOLYTIC HYPERKERATOSIS

Epidermolytic hyperkeratosis (granular degeneration) is characterized by (1) perinuclear clear spaces in the upper epidermis; (2) indistinct cell boundaries formed either by lightly staining material or by keratohyalin granules peripheral to the perinuclear clear spaces; (3) a markedly

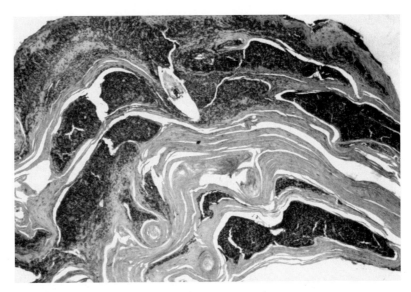

FIGURE 2-46. Palisading crust with dermatophilosis.

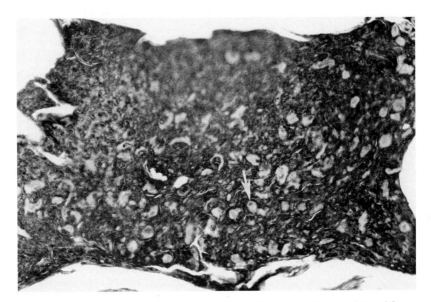

FIGURE 2-47. Numerous acantholytic keratinocytes (*arrow*) in crust with pemphigus foliaceus.

thickened stratum granulosum; and (4) orthokeratotic hyperkeratosis. It is seen in certain types of ichthyosis, epidermal nevi, actinic keratoses, papillomas, keratinous cysts, and squamous cell carcinoma.

Dermal Changes

COLLAGEN CHANGES

Dermal collagen is subject to a number of pathologic changes and may undergo the following: (1) *hyalinization*—a confluence and an increased eosinophilic, glassy, refractile appearance, as seen in chronic inflammation, vasculopathies, and connective tissue diseases; (2) *fibrinoid degeneration* —deposition on or replacement with a brightly eosinophilic fibrillar or granular substance resembling fibrin, as seen in connective tissue diseases; (3) *lysis*—a homogeneous, eosinophilic, complete loss of structural detail, as seen in microbial infections and ischemia; (4) *degeneration*— a structural and tinctorial change characterized by slight basophilia, granular appearance, and frayed edges of collagen fibers, rarely seen in equine dermatoses (Fig. 2-48); (5) *dystrophic mineralization*—deposition of calcium salts as basophilic, amorphous, granular material along collagen fibers, as seen with eosinophilic granuloma and percutaneous penetration of calcium (Fig. 2-49); (6) *atrophy*—thin collagen fibrils and decreased fibroblasts, with a resultant decrease in dermal thickness, as seen in severe malnutrition; and (7) *dysplasia*—disorganization and fragmentation of collagen bundles as seen in cutaneous asthenia.

A *flame figure* (Fig. 2-50) is an area of altered collagen surrounded by eosinophils and eosinophil granules.[14,15] Collagen fibers are surrounded totally or in part by eosinophilic material. This material is variable in shape, from annular to oval, to a radiating configuration resembling the spokes of a wheel ("starburst" appearance). Some collagen fibers within these areas appear normal, whereas others appear partially or wholly swollen, irregular or fuzzy in outline, and granular in consistency. The eosinophilic material itself varies from amorphous to granular. In the granular areas, one can see a transition from intact eosinophils, to eosinophil granules and nuclear debris, to completely amorphous material. Trichrome-stained sections show the collagen fibers to be normal in size, surface contour, and consistency.[14,15] Thus, the irregularities, granularity, and fuzziness seen in the H & E–stained sections are due to the coating of collagen fibers with the eosinophilic material. In humans, electron microscopic studies have revealed no collagen degeneration in flame figures. Immunofluorescence testing identifies eosinophil major basic protein in the amorphous material surrounding and coating collagen fibers. It is likely that all equine skin lesions previously described as containing "collagen degeneration," "necrobiotic collagen," or "collagenolysis" actually contained flame figures. Such conditions include eosinophilic granuloma, insect and arthropod reactions and axillary nodular necrosis.

SOLAR ELASTOSIS

Solar elastosis appears in H & E–stained sections as a tangle of indistinct amphophilic fibers, often in linear bands running approximately parallel to the surface epidermis, within the superficial dermis. With Verhoeff's or AOG stain, the tangled, thickened, elastotic material is clearly seen (Fig. 2-51). Solar elastosis is a rare manifestation of ultraviolet light–induced skin damage in horses.

DERMAL DEPOSITS

Amyloid appears in H & E–stained sections as a hyaline, amorphous, lightly eosinophilic material that tends to displace or obliterate normal structures.

Lipid deposits occur in the dermis in xanthomatosis. In H & E–stained sections, lightly eosinophilic, feathery deposits separate the collagen bundles to form small "lakes" of lipid.

Cholesterol clefts may be seen in xanthomatosis, panniculitis, and ruptured follicular cysts. They appear as clear spaces in needle or spicule shape.

FIBROPLASIA, DESMOPLASIA, FIBROSIS, AND SCLEROSIS

Fibroplasia refers to the formation and development of fibrous tissue in increased amounts and is often used synonymously with *granulation tissue*. The condition is characterized by a fibrovascular proliferation in which the blood vessels with prominent endothelial cells are oriented roughly perpendicular to the surface of the skin. The new collagen fibers, with prominent fibroblasts, are oriented roughly parallel to the surface of the skin. Edema and inflammatory cells are constant

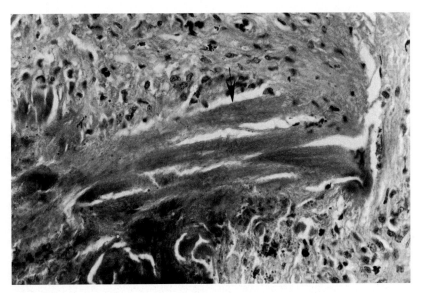

FIGURE 2-48. Collagen degeneration (*arrow*) with eosinophilic granuloma.

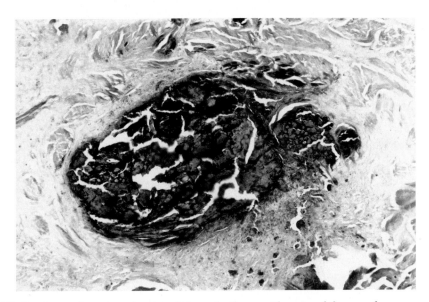

FIGURE 2-49. Dystrophic mineralization of dermal collagen with eosinophilic granuloma.

features of fibroplasia. *Desmoplasia* is the term usually used when referring to the fibroplasia induced by neoplastic processes.

Fibrosis is a later stage of fibroplasia in which increased numbers of fibroblasts and collagen fibers are the characteristic findings. Little or no inflammation is present. A subcategory of fibrosis wherein inflammation is typically still prominent is *alignment in vertical streaks*—elongated, thickened parallel strands of collagen in the superficial dermis, perpendicular to the epidermal surface, as seen in chronically rubbed, licked, or scratched skin. *Sclerosis* (scar formation) may be the endpoint of fibrosis, wherein the increased numbers of collagen fibers have a thick, eosinophilic, hyalinized appearance, and the number of fibroblasts is greatly reduced.

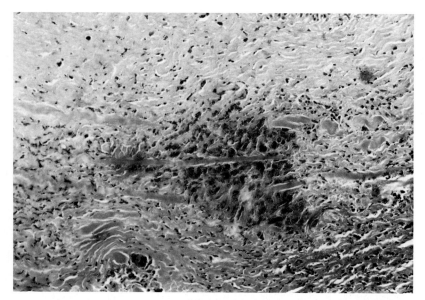

FIGURE 2-50. Collagen flame figure with eosinophilic granuloma.

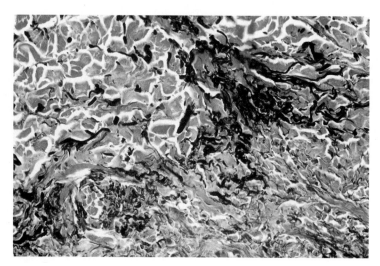

FIGURE 2-51. Solar elastosis. Note tangled, elastotic material in AOG-stained section.

PAPILLOMATOSIS, VILLI, AND FESTOONS

Papillomatosis refers to the projection of dermal papillae above the surface of the skin, resulting in an irregular undulating configuration of the epidermis. Often associated with epidermal hyperplasia, papillomatosis is also seen with chronic inflammatory and neoplastic dermatoses. *Villi* are dermal papillae, covered by 1 to 2 layers of epidermal cells, that project into a vesicle or bulla. Villi are occasionally seen in actinic keratosis and squamous cell carcinoma. *Festoons* are dermal papillae, devoid of attached epidermal cells, that project into the base of a vesicle or bulla. They are seen in bullous pemphigoid, epidermolysis bullosa, and drug-induced pemphigoid.

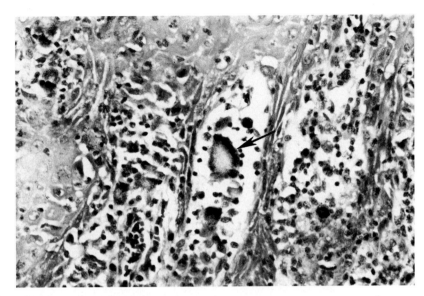

FIGURE 2-52. Pigmentary incontinence with systemic lupus erythematosus. Note melanin granules within macrophages and giant cells (*arrow*).

PIGMENTARY INCONTINENCE

Pigmentary incontinence refers to the presence of melanin granules that are free within the subepidermal and perifollicular dermis and within dermal macrophages (melanophages) (Figs. 2-52 and 2-57). Pigmentary incontinence may be seen with any process that damages the stratum basale and the basement membrane zone, especially with hydropic degeneration of basal cells (lupus erythematosus, erythema multiforme). In addition, melanophages may be seen, especially in a perivascular orientation, in chronic inflammatory conditions where melanin production is greatly increased.

EDEMA

Dermal *edema* is recognized by dilated lymphatics (not visible in normal skin), widened spaces between blood vessels and perivascular collagen (*perivascular* edema), or widened spaces between large areas of dermal collagen (*interstitial* edema) (Fig. 2-53). The dilated lymphatics and widened perivascular and interstitial spaces may or may not contain a lightly eosinophilic, homogeneous, frothy-appearing substance (serum). A scattering of vacuolated macrophages may be seen in the interstitium in chronic severe dermal edema.

Dermal edema is a common, nondiagnostic feature of any inflammatory dermatosis. Severe edema of the superficial dermis may result in subepidermal vesicles and bullae, necrosis of the overlying epidermis, and predisposition to artifactual dermoepidermal separation during handling and processing of biopsy specimens. Severe edema of the superficial dermis may result in a vertical orientation and stretching of collagen fibers, producing the "gossamer" (web-like) collagen effect seen with erythema multiforme and severe urticaria.

MUCINOSIS

Mucinosis (myxedema, mucoid degeneration, myxoid degeneration, mucinous degeneration) is characterized by increased amounts of an amorphous, stringy, granular, basophilic material that separates, thins, or replaces dermal collagen fibrils and surrounds blood vessels and appendages in

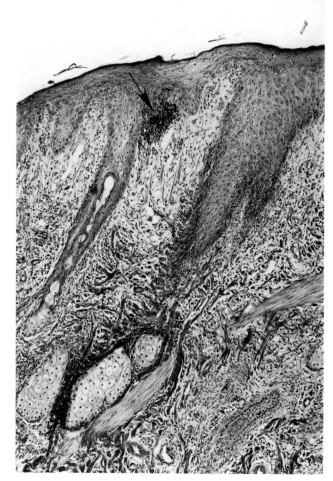

FIGURE 2-53. Interstitial dermal edema and extravasation of erythrocytes (*arrow*) with onchocerciasis.

H & E–stained sections. Only small amounts of mucin are ever visible in normal skin, mostly around appendages and blood vessels. Mucin is more easily demonstrated with stains for acid mucopolysaccharides, such as Hale's iron and Alcian blue stains. Mucinosis may be seen as a focal (usually perivascular) change in numerous inflammatory, neoplastic, and developmental dermatoses. Diffuse mucinosis may be seen with hypothyroidism and lupus erythematosus. Mucin may also be seen in the epidermis and hair follicle outer root sheath (Fig. 2-54) in dermatoses associated with numerous eosinophils (e.g., eosinophilic granuloma, unilateral papular dermatosis) and in lupus erythematosus.

GRENZ ZONE

This marginal zone of relatively normal collagen separates the epidermis from an underlying dermal alteration. A *grenz zone* may be seen in neoplastic and granulomatous disorders.

PAPILLARY MICROABSCESSES

Small neutrophilic microabscesses may occasionally be seen in the dermal papillae of biopsies from horses with vasculitis, bullous pemphigoid, and cutaneous adverse drug reaction (Fig. 2-55).

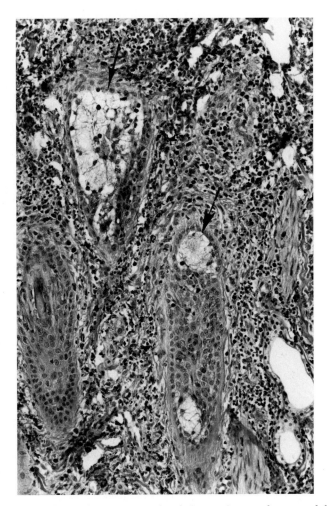

FIGURE 2-54. Mucinosis of follicular outer root sheath (*arrows*) in sterile eosinophilic folliculitis.

Follicular Changes

Follicular epithelium is affected by most of the histopathologic changes described for the epidermis. Follicular (poral) keratosis, plugging, and dilatation are common features of such diverse conditions as inflammatory, hormonal, and developmental dermatoses. Follicular hyperplasia and hypertrophy may be seen in chronic inflammatory dermatoses or in nevoid lesions. *Perifolliculitis*, *mural folliculitis*, *luminal folliculitis*, and *furunculosis* (penetrating or perforating folliculitis) refer to varying degrees of follicular inflammation. A cell-poor follicular necrosis may be seen in ischemic states and drug reactions. *Follicular atrophy* refers to the gradual involution, retraction, and occasionally miniaturization that may be seen with developmental and nutritional dermatoses.

Hair follicles should be examined closely to determine the phase of the growth cycle. *Telogenization*, a predominance of telogen hair follicles, is characteristic of hormonal dermatoses and states of telogen defluxion associated with stress, disease, and drugs. *Catagenization* ("catagen arrest") is seen with follicular dysplasias. *Follicular dysplasia* refers to the presence of incompletely or abnormally formed hair follicles and hair shafts and is seen in developmental abnormalities such as follicular dysplasia. Dysplastic hair follicles are primary hair follicles, wherein the infundibular region is dilated and filled with concentrically arranged orthokeratotic hyperkera-

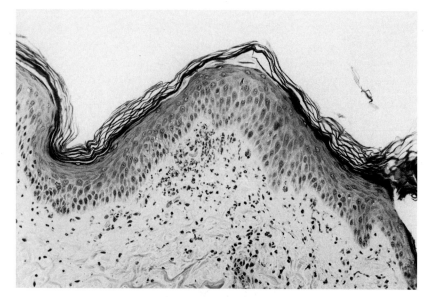

FIGURE 2-55. Papillary microabscess with trimethoprim-sulfadiazine drug reaction.

tosis.[42] The follicular shape is irregular and sebaceous ducts are filled with orthokeratotic hyperkeratosis. *Miniaturized* hair follicles may be seen in nutritional deficiencies and genetic hypotrichoses.

Perifollicular melanosis may be seen in various folliculitides, alopecia areata, and follicular dysplasia. *Perifollicular fibrosis* is seen in chronic folliculitides. Dystrophic mineralization of the basement membrane zone and subsequent transepithelial elimination of mineral is seen in the calcinosis cutis associated with percutaneous penetration of calcium.

Glandular Changes

Sebaceous and epitrichial sweat glands may be involved in various dermatoses. *Sebaceous glands* may rarely be involved in many suppurative and granulomatous inflammations (*sebaceous adenitis*) (Fig. 2-56). They may become *atrophic* (reduced in number and size, with pyknotic nuclei predominating) and *cystic* in developmental dermatoses and in occasional chronic inflammatory processes. Sebaceous glands may also become *hyperplastic* in chronic inflammatory dermatoses. Sebaceous gland atrophy and hyperplasia must always be cautiously assessed with regard to the area of the body from which the skin specimen was taken. Sebaceous gland melanosis may be seen with follicular dysplasia, alopecia areata, and demodicosis.[41]

Epitrichial sweat glands rarely are involved in suppurative and granulomatous dermatoses (*hidradenitis*). The epitrichial sweat glands may become dilated or cystic in many inflammatory dermatoses. The light microscopic recognition of epitrichial gland *atrophy* is a moot point, since dilated epitrichial secretory coils containing flattened epithelial cells are a feature of the normal postsecretory state.

Vascular Changes

Cutaneous blood vessels exhibit a number of histologic changes, including dilatation (ectasia), endothelial swelling, endothelial necrosis, hyalinization, fibrinoid degeneration, vasculitis, thromboembolism, and extravasation (diapedesis) of erythrocytes (purpura).

Subcutaneous Fat Changes

The subcutaneous fat (panniculus adiposus, hypodermis) is subject to the connective tissue and vascular changes described above. It is frequently involved in suppurative and granulomatous dermatoses. In addition, subcutaneous fat may exhibit its own inflammatory changes (*panniculitis, steatitis*) without any significant involvement of the overlying dermis and epidermis (sterile nodular panniculitis, infectious panniculitis).

Fat necrosis may develop whenever an inflammatory reaction involves a fat lobule. There are three different morphologic expressions of fat necrosis: (1) *microcystic fat necrosis*—the most common form, characterized by small, round microcysts that are often at the center of pyogranulomas, seen in many panniculitides; (2) *hyalinizing fat necrosis*—the lipocytes are converted into a feathery, eosinophilic amalgam trapping scattered fat microcysts, as seen in vasculopathies and vaccine reactions; and (3) *mineralizing fat necrosis*—the deposition of irregular, granular, basophilic material, often in the peripheral cytoplasm of necrotic lipocytes, as seen in some cases of traumatic panniculitis.

Miscellaneous Changes
Thickened Basement Membrane Zone

Thickening of the light microscopic basement membrane zone appears as focal, linear, often irregular, homogeneous, eosinophilic bands below the stratum basale (Fig. 2-57). The basement membrane zone is better demonstrated with periodic acid–Schiff (PAS) stain. Thickening of the basement membrane zone is a feature of lichenoid dermatoses, especially lupus erythematosus.

SUBEPIDERMAL VACUOLAR ALTERATION

Subepidermal vacuolar alteration is characterized by multiple small vacuoles within or immediately below the basement membrane zone, giving the appearance of "subepidermal bubbles" (Fig. 2-58). It is seen with bullous pemphigoid, lupus erythematosus, and occasionally overlying dermal fibrosis and scar. Subepidermal vacuoles may also be induced by improper fixation and by freezing artifact.

PAPILLARY SQUIRTING

Papillary squirting is present when superficial dermal papillae are edematous and contain dilated vessels and when the overlying dermis is also edematous and often contains exocytosing leukocytes and parakeratotic scale (Fig. 2-59). "Squirting" papillae are a feature of seborrheic dermatitis.

DYSPLASIA

Dysplasia refers to a faulty or abnormal development of individual cells, and it is also commonly used to describe abnormal development of the epidermis as a whole. Dysplasia may be a feature of neoplastic, hyperplastic, and developmental dermatoses. Epidermal dysplasia is characterized by keratinocytes that are atypical in size, shape, and staining characteristics, and whose polarity has been disrupted (Fig. 2-60).

ANAPLASIA

Anaplasia (atypia) is a feature of neoplastic cells, in which there is a loss of normal differentiation and organization.

METAPLASIA

Metaplasia occurs when the mature cells in a tissue change into a form that is not normal for that tissue. Through metaplasia, a given cell may exhibit epithelial, mesothelial, or mesenchymal characteristics, regardless of the tissue of origin.

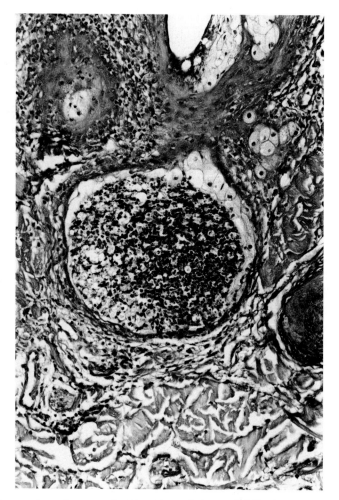

FIGURE 2-56. Suppurative sebaceous adenitis with staphylococcal folliculitis.

NESTS

Nests (theques) are well circumscribed clusters or groups of cells within the epidermis or the dermis. Nests are seen in some neoplastic and hamartomatous dermatoses, such as melanomas and melanocytomas.

LYMPHOID NODULES

Lymphoid nodules are rounded, discrete masses of primarily mature lymphocytes (Fig. 2-61). They are often found perivascularly in the deep dermis or subcutis, or both. Lymphoid nodules are most commonly recognized in association with immune-mediated dermatoses, dermatoses associated with tissue eosinophilia, and panniculitis.[39] They are also prominent in insect bite granuloma (pseudolymphoma) and postinjection panniculitis.

MULTINUCLEATED EPIDERMAL GIANT CELLS

Multinucleated epidermal giant cells (Fig. 2-62) are found in viral infections and in a number of nonviral and non-neoplastic dermatoses characterized by epidermal hyperplasia, abnormal keratinization, chronicity, or pruritus.

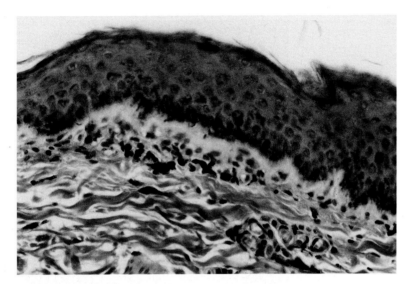

FIGURE 2-57. Thickened basement membrane zone and subjacent pigmentary incontinence with discoid lupus erythematosus.

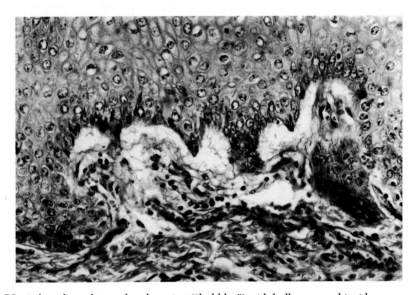

FIGURE 2-58. Subepidermal vacuolar alteration ("bubbles") with bullous pemphigoid.

SQUAMATIZATION

Squamatization refers to the replacement of the normally cuboidal or columnar, slightly basophilic basal epidermal cells by polygonal or flattened, eosinophilic keratinocytes. It may be seen in lichenoid tissue reactions.

TRANSEPIDERMAL ELIMINATION

Transepidermal elimination is a mechanism by which foreign or altered constituents can be removed from the dermis. The process involves unique morphologic alterations of the surface epidermis or hair follicle outer root sheath, which forms a channel and, therefore, facilitates

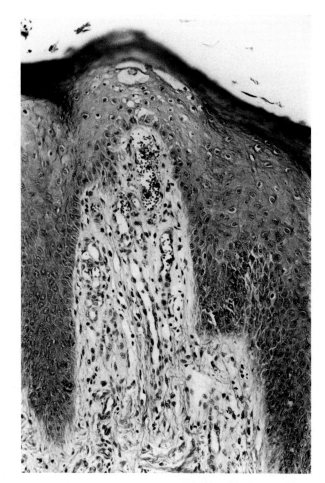

FIGURE 2-59. Papillary squirting associated with primary seborrhea.

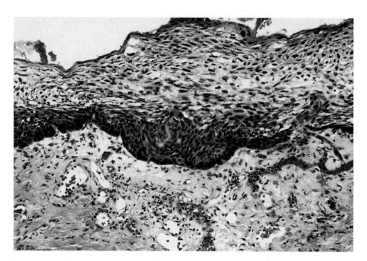

FIGURE 2-60. Epidermal dysplasia in actinic keratosis. Note how keratinocytes vary in staining intensity, size, and shape, and how their polarity is totally disrupted.

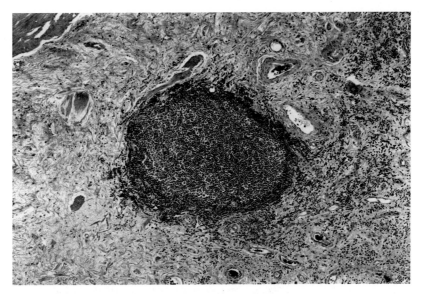

FIGURE 2-61. Lymphoid nodule associated with idiopathic sterile panniculitis.

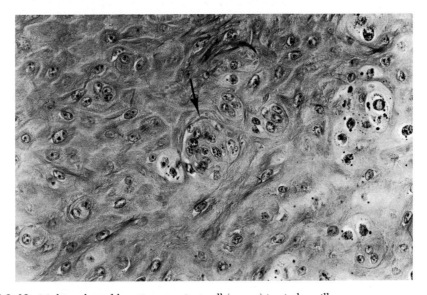

FIGURE 2-62. Multinucleated keratinocyte giant cell (*arrow*) in viral papilloma.

extrusion. Transepidermal elimination may be seen in foreign body reactions and calcinosis circumscripta.

Confusing Terms

NECROBIOSIS

Necrobiosis is the degeneration and death of cells or tissue followed by replacement. Examples of necrobiosis would be the constant degeneration and replacement of epidermal and hematopoietic cells. The term *necrobiosis* has been used in dermatohistopathology to describe various degenerative changes in collagen found in equine eosinophilic granuloma and human granuloma annulare, necrobiosis lipoidica, and rheumatoid and pseudorheumatoid nodules. The use of the term *necrobiosis* to describe a *pathologic* change is inappropriate and confusing, both histologically and etymologically, and should be discouraged. It is more accurate to use the more specific terms described previously in this chapter under Collagen Changes.

NEVUS AND HAMARTOMA

A *nevus* is a circumscribed developmental defect in the skin. Nevi may arise from any skin component or combination thereof. Nevi are hyperplastic in nature. The term *nevus* should never be used alone but always with a modifier such as epidermal, vascular, sebaceous, collagenous, and so on.

Hamartoma literally means "a tumor-like proliferation of normal or embryonal cells"; in other words, a hamartoma is a macroscopic hyperplasia of normal tissue elements and is often used synonymously with *nevus*. However, the term *hamartoma* may be applied to hyperplastic disorders in any tissue or organ system, whereas the term *nevus* is restricted to the skin.

Cellular Infiltrates

Dermal cellular infiltrates are described in terms of (1) the *types* of cells present and (2) the *pattern* of cellular infiltration. In general, cellular infiltrates are either *monomorphous* (one cell type) or *polymorphous* (more than one cell type). Further clarification of the predominant cells is accomplished by modifiers such as *lymphocytic, histiocytic, neutrophilic, eosinophilic,* and *plasmacytic.*

Patterns of cellular infiltration are usually made up of one or more of the following basic patterns: (1) *perivascular* (angiocentric—located around blood vessels); (2) *perifollicular and periglandular* (appendagocentric, periappendageal, periadnexal—located around follicles and glands); (3) *lichenoid* (assuming a band-like configuration that parallels and "hugs" the overlying epidermis and/or adnexae); (4) *nodular* (occurring in basically well-defined groups or clusters at any site); and (5) *interstitial or diffuse* (scattered lightly or solidly throughout the dermis). The types of cells and patterns of infiltration present are important diagnostic clues to the diagnosis of many dermatoses.

● DERMATOLOGIC DIAGNOSIS BY HISTOPATHOLOGIC PATTERNS

With pattern analysis, one first categorizes inflammatory dermatoses by their appearance (pattern) on the scanning objective of the light microscope and then zeroes in on a specific diagnosis, whenever possible, by the assimilation of fine details gathered by low- and high-power scrutiny. Pattern analysis has revolutionized veterinary dermatohistopathology and made the reading of skin biopsy specimens much simpler and more rewarding (for the pathologist, the clinician, and the patient).[38,40,51] However, as with any histologic method, pattern analysis works only when clinicians supply pathologists with adequate historical and clinical information and biopsy specimens most representative of the dermatoses being sampled.

In a retrospective study of skin biopsies from horses with inflammatory dermatoses,[40] pattern analysis was shown to be a useful technique. The specific clinical diagnosis was established in about 69% of the cases and was included in a reaction pattern–generated differential diagnosis in another 29% of the cases. A single reaction pattern was found in 84% of the cases, and mixed reaction patterns (two or three different patterns) were found in 16% of the cases. Mixed reaction patterns were usually caused by single etiologic factors or by a coexistence of two or three different dermatoses.

It is important to remember that many inflammatory dermatoses are characterized by a continuum of acute, subacute, and chronic pathologic changes. In other words, the lesions have "lives." For example, cellulitis begins as perivascular dermatitis, progresses to interstitial dermatitis, and eventuates as diffuse dermatitis. Thus, the histopathologic pattern seen in the biopsy specimen from this condition is, in part, dependent on the evolution or "age" of the lesion.

It is also important to realize that some patterns of inflammation are more important or more "powerful" than others. For example, perivascular dermatitis is present somewhere in virtually all inflammatory lesions: After all, the inflammatory cells usually have to exit the blood vessels in order to get to where the cutaneous action is! But the question is, Are those perivascular cells going somewhere more important, somewhere more diagnostic? Is there a more important inflammatory reaction pattern being formed? Hence, one can always find perivascular accumulations of inflammatory cells underlying an epidermal pustule or peripheral to a dermal nodule. However, the more important or the more diagnostic patterns are those of intraepidermal pustular dermatitis and the nodular dermatitis.

Perivascular Dermatitis

In perivascular dermatitis, the predominant inflammatory reaction is centered around the superficial and/or the deep dermal blood vessels (Fig. 2-63, *A* and *B*). Perivascular dermatitis is subdivided on the basis of accompanying epidermal changes into three types: (1) *pure perivascular dermatitis* (perivascular dermatitis without significant epidermal changes); (2) *spongiotic perivascular dermatitis* (perivascular dermatitis with prominent spongiosis); and (3) *hyperplastic perivascular dermatitis* (perivascular dermatitis with prominent epidermal hyperplasia).

In the horse, perivascular dermatitis is usually both superficial and deep. The usual causes are hypersensitivity reactions (inhalant, dietary, drug, contact, and so forth), ectoparasitisms, dermato-

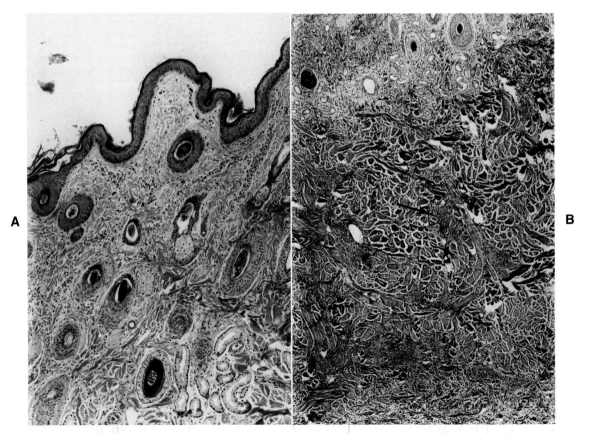

FIGURE 2-63. Perivascular dermatitis. **A,** Superficial perivascular dermatitis with atopy. **B,** Deep perivascular dermatitis (*arrow*) with insect hypersensitivity.

phytosis, dermatophilosis, seborrheic disorders, and contact dermatitis. *Deep* perivascular dermatitis, wherein the deep perivascular cellular accumulations are more prominent than those observed superficially, may be seen with systemic disorders (systemic lupus erythematosus, septicemia, viral infections, multisystemic eosinophilic epitheliotropic disease), or severe local reactions (vasculitis, discoid lupus erythematosus, cellulitis, and insect/arthropod-induced reactions).

Any perivascular dermatitis containing numerous eosinophils should be first suspected of representing ectoparasitism or endoparasitism. In the horse, tissue eosinophilia is also commonly seen with hypersensitivity disorders (inhalant, dietary). Focal areas of epidermal edema, eosinophilic exocytosis, and necrosis (epidermal "nibbles") are suggestive of ectoparasitism. Numerous eosinophils are also seen in equine multisystemic eosinophilic epitheliotropic disease. Perivascular dermatitides rich in neutrophils and/or plasma cells are usually associated with infections.

Diffuse orthokeratotic hyperkeratosis in combination with perivascular dermatitis suggests endocrinopathy, nutritional deficiencies, developmental abnormalities (follicular dysplasia, equine cannon keratosis, epidermal nevi), and secondary seborrheic disorders. *Diffuse parakeratotic hyperkeratosis* in combination with perivascular dermatitis may be seen with ectoparasitism, dermatophilosis, dermatophytosis, and necrolytic migratory erythema.

Focal parakeratotic hyperkeratosis (parakeratotic "caps") may be seen with ectoparasitism, seborrheic disorders, dermatophytosis, and dermatophilosis. When parakeratotic "caps" are combined with "papillary squirting," seborrheic dermatitis is likely. Perivascular dermatoses accompanied by *vertical streaking of collagen* and/or *sebaceous gland hyperplasia* suggest chronic pruritus (rubbing, licking, chewing), such as that seen with hypersensitivity reactions.

PURE PERIVASCULAR DERMATITIS

The cellular infiltrate in perivascular dermatitis may be monomorphous or polymorphous. The most likely diagnoses include hypersensitivity reactions (inhalant, dietary, drug), urticaria, and dermatophytosis.

SPONGIOTIC PERIVASCULAR DERMATITIS

Spongiotic perivascular dermatitis is characterized by prominent spongiosis and spongiotic vesicle formation. Severe spongiotic vesiculation may "blow out" the basement membrane zone, resulting in subepidermal vesicles. The epidermis frequently shows varying degrees of hyperplasia and hyperkeratosis. Spongiotic dermatitis may be *monomorphous* or *polymorphous*. The most likely diagnoses include hypersensitivity reactions, contact dermatitis, ectoparasitisms, dermatophytosis, dermatophilosis, and viral infection.[19a]

HYPERPLASTIC PERIVASCULAR DERMATITIS

Hyperplastic perivascular dermatitis is characterized by varying degrees of epidermal hyperplasia and hyperkeratosis with little or no spongiosis. This is a common, nondiagnostic, chronic dermatitis reaction. It is commonly seen with hypersensitivity reactions, contact dermatitis, diseases of altered keratinization, ectoparasitisms, viral dermatoses, dermatophilosis, and dermatophytosis.

Interface Dermatitis

In interface dermatitis, the dermoepidermal junction is the site of *hydropic degeneration*, *lichenoid cellular infiltrate*, or both (Fig. 2-64, *A* and *B*). Apoptotic keratinocytes, satellite cell apoptosis, and pigmentary incontinence are commonly seen. The *hydropic* type of interface dermatitis may be seen with drug eruptions, lupus erythematosus, erythema multiforme, graft-versus-host reactions, and occasionally vasculitis. The *lichenoid* type may be seen with drug eruptions, lupus erythematosus, pemphigus, erythema multiforme, and epitheliotropic lymphoma. The band-like cellular infiltration of lichenoid tissue reactions consists predominantly of lymphocytes and plasma cells. If nearby

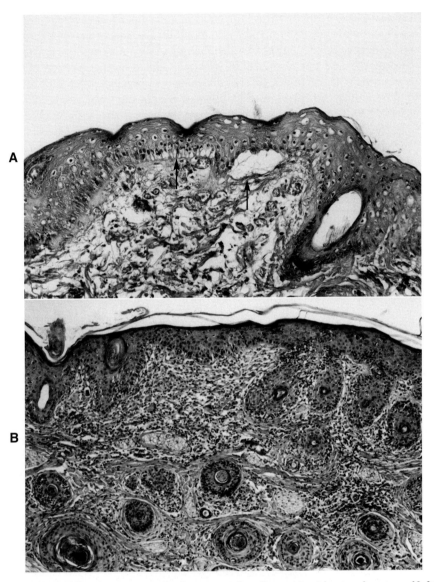

FIGURE 2-64. Interface dermatitis. **A**, Hydropic interface dermatitis with trimethoprim-sulfadiazine drug reaction. **B**, Lichenoid interface dermatitis with discoid lupus erythematosus.

ulceration or secondary infection exists, numerous neutrophils may be present. A lichenoid tissue reaction containing many eosinophils suggests an insect/arthropod bite reaction, multisystemic eosinophilic epitheliotropic disease, or drug eruption. A lichenoid tissue reaction containing multinucleated histiocytic giant cells suggests drug reaction but may be seen in discoid lupus erythematosus. Focal thickening or smudging of the basement membrane zone suggests lupus erythematosus.

Vasculitis

Vasculitis is an inflammatory process in which inflammatory cells are present within and around blood vessel walls and there are concomitant signs of damage to the blood vessels (e.g., degeneration and lysis of vascular and perivascular collagen, degeneration and swelling of endothelial cells, extravasation of erythrocytes, thrombosis, effacement of vascular architecture, and fibrinoid degeneration) (Fig. 2-65, *A* and *B*). Vasculitides are usually classified on the basis of the dominant inflammatory cell within vessel walls, the types being neutrophilic, eosinophilic, and lymphocytic. The appearance, of course, can be greatly modified by the duration of the lesion. Fibrinoid degeneration is inconsistently present in cutaneous vasculitides. Biopsies from animals with vasculitis will sometimes not reveal visually inflamed vessels, but rather, some of the signposts of vasculitis (Table 2-8). Serial sections or rebiopsy may be necessary to visualize the actual vasculitis.

Neutrophilic vasculitis, the most common type, may be *leukocytoclastic* (associated with karyorrhexis of neutrophils, resulting in "nuclear dust") or *nonleukocytoclastic*. Leukocytoclastic vasculitis is seen in connective tissue disorders (lupus erythematosus), allergic reactions (drug eruptions, infections, toxins), as an idiopathic disorder, and in equine purpura hemorrhagica. Nonleukocytoclastic vasculitis is seen with septicemia and thrombophlebitis from intravenous catheters causing thromboembolism.

Lymphocytic vasculitis is rare and may be seen in drug reactions, vaccine-induced vasculitis, equine viral arteritis, and ectoparasitism, or as an idiopathic disorder.

Eosinophilic vasculitis is rare and is seen as an idiopathic, presumably immune-mediated disorder of horses, and may be seen with insect/arthropod-induced lesions and mast cell tumors.

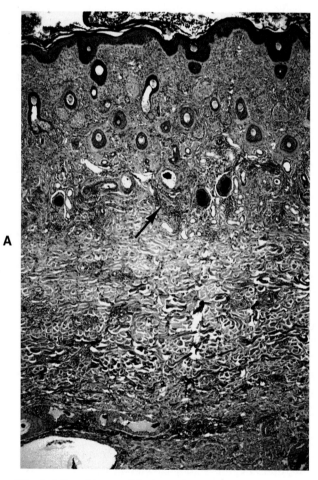

FIGURE 2-65. Vasculitis. **A**, Idiopathic vasculitis (*arrow*).

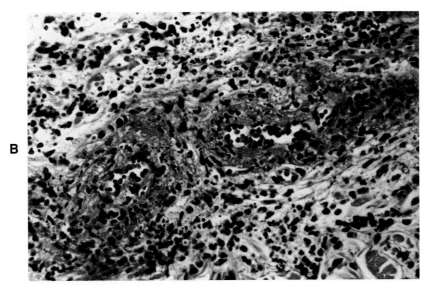

FIGURE 2-65, cont'd. B, Idiopathic necrotizing vasculitis.

● Table 2-8 **HISTOPATHOLOGIC SIGNPOSTS OF CUTANEOUS VASCULITIS**[42]

- Large numbers of leukocytes within the vessel wall, especially if the vessel is an arteriole or large venule.
- If the vessel is a postcapillary venule, there are disproportionately more leukocytes within the wall than in the adjacent dermis.
- Intramural or perivascular hemorrhage, intense edema, and fibrin deposition.
- The presence of leukocytoclasis within the vessel wall.
- Some evidence of damage to the vessel wall beyond edema and endothelial cell prominence.
- Evidence of cutaneous infarction.
- Atrophic changes in hair follicles, adnexal glands, and epidermis, reflecting chronic ischemia.

Equine photoactivated vasculopathy is characterized by thickening and hyalinization of superficial dermal blood vessels, extravasation of erythrocytes, thrombosis, and occasional karyorrhectic leukocytes.

Interstitial Dermatitis

Interstitial dermatitis is characterized by the infiltration of cells between collagen bundles (interstitial spaces) of the dermis (Fig. 2-66). The infiltrate is poorly circumscribed, mild to moderate in intensity, and does not obscure the anatomy of the skin. When the superficial dermis is primarily involved and the overlying epidermis is normal, urticaria is likely. When the superficial dermis is primarily involved and the epidermis is hyperplastic, the most likely causes are staphylococcal infection (numerous neutrophils), dermatophytosis (numerous neutrophils), and ectoparasitism (numerous eosinophils). When the superficial and deep dermis are involved, likely diagnoses include infection (bacterial, fungal) and early eosinophilic granuloma, onchocerciasis, or early habronemiasis.

Nodular and Diffuse Dermatitis

Nodular dermatitis denotes discrete clusters of cells (Fig. 2-67). Such dermal nodules are usually multiple but may occasionally be large and solitary. In contrast, *diffuse dermatitis* denotes a cellular infiltrate so dense that discrete cellular aggregates are no longer easily recognized and the anatomy of the skin is no longer easily visualized (Fig. 2-68, *A*).

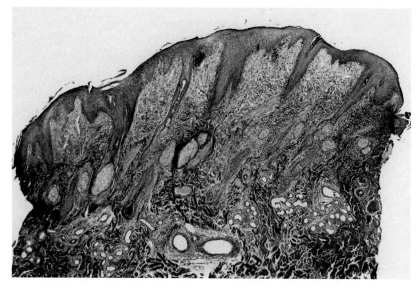

FIGURE 2-66. Interstitial dermatitis with onchocerciasis.

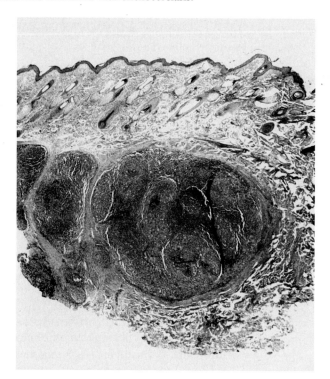

FIGURE 2-67. Nodular dermatitis with phaeohyphomycosis.

Granulomatous inflammation represents a heterogeneous pattern of tissue reactions in response to various stimuli. There is no simple, precise, universally accepted way to define granulomatous inflammation; however, a commonly proposed definition is as follows: a circumscribed tissue reaction that is subacute to chronic in nature and is located about one or more foci, wherein the histiocyte or macrophage is a predominant cell type. Thus, granulomatous dermatitis may be

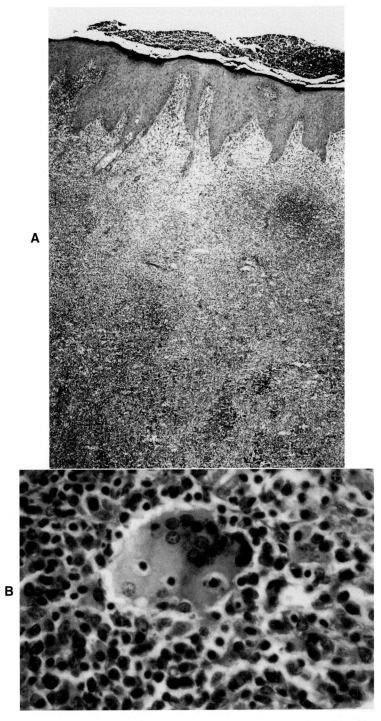

FIGURE 2-68. **A**, Diffuse dermatitis with *Rhodoccus equi* infection. **B**, Multinucleated histiocytic giant cell in bacterial pseudomycetoma.

nodular or diffuse, but not all nodular and diffuse dermatoses are granulomatous. Nongranulomatous diffuse dermatoses include cellulitis and habronemiasis. Pseudolymphoma (insect or arachnid bites; drug reactions; idiopathic disorder) is an example of a nongranulomatous nodular dermatitis. Granulomatous infiltrates that contain large numbers of neutrophils are frequently called *pyogranulomatous*.

CELL TYPES

Nodular dermatitis and diffuse dermatitis are often associated with certain unusual inflammatory cell types.

Foam cells are histiocytes with elongated or oval vesicular nuclei and abundant, finely granular, eosinophilic cytoplasm with ill-defined cell borders. They are called epithelioid because they appear to cluster and adjoin like epithelial cells.

Multinucleated histiocytic giant cells (Fig. 2-68, *B*) are histiocytic variants that assume three morphologic forms: (1) *Langerhans' cell* (nuclei form circle or semicircle at the periphery of the cell); (2) *foreign body cell* (nuclei are scattered throughout the cytoplasm); and (3) *Touton cell* (nuclei form a wreath that surrounds a central, homogeneous, amphophilic core of cytoplasm, which is in turn surrounded by abundant foamy cytoplasm). In general, these three forms of giant cells have no diagnostic specificity, although numerous Touton cells are usually seen with xanthomas.

Certain general principles apply to the examination of all nodular and diffuse dermatitides. The processes that should be used are (1) polarizing foreign material; (2) staining for bacteria and fungi; and (3) culturing. In general, microorganisms are most likely to be found near areas of suppuration and necrosis.

Nodular and diffuse dermatitis may be characterized by predominantly neutrophilic, histiocytic, eosinophilic, or mixed cellular infiltrates (Fig. 2-69). *Neutrophils* (dermal abscess) often predominate in dermatoses associated with bacteria, mycobacteria, actinomycetes, fungi, prototheca, protozoa, and foreign bodies. *Histiocytes* may predominate in the chronic stage of any of the entities just listed, in xanthomas (Fig. 2-70), myospherulosis, calcinosis circumscripta, and in the sterile pyogranuloma/granuloma syndrome. *Eosinophils* may predominate in equine eosinophilic granuloma, in certain parasitic dermatoses (habronemiasis, parafilariasis, tick and insect bites), certain fungal dermatoses (pythiosis, basidiobolomycosis, conidiobolomycosis), and where hair follicles have ruptured. *Mixed* cellular infiltrates are most commonly neutrophils and histiocytes (pyogranuloma), eosinophils and histiocytes (eosinophilic granuloma), or some combination thereof. *Plasma cells* are common components for nodular and diffuse dermatitis and are of no particular diagnostic significance. They are commonly seen around glands and follicles in chronic infections. Periepitrichial accumulations of plasma cells are also seen in lichenoid dermatoses. Hyperactive plasma cells (Mott cells) may contain eosinophilic intracytoplasmic inclusions (Russell's bodies) (Fig. 2-71). These accumulations of glycoprotein are largely globulin and may be large enough to push the cell nucleus eccentrically.

Granulomas may be subclassified as (1) *tuberculoid*—a central zone of neutrophils and necrosis surrounded by histiocytes and epithelioid cells, which are in turn surrounded by giant cells, followed by a layer of lymphocytes, and finally an outer layer of fibroblasts, as seen in tuberculosis and atypical mycobacteriosis; (2) *sarcoidal* (Fig. 2-72)—"naked" epithelioid cells, as seen in foreign body reactions, equine sarcoidosis; or (3) *palisading* (Fig. 2-73)—the alignment of histiocytes like staves around a central focus of collagen degeneration (equine eosinophilic granuloma, equine mastocytoma), lipids (xanthoma), parasite (habronemiasis), fungus (pythiosis, conidiobolomycosis, basidiobolomycosis), or other foreign material, such as calcium in dystrophic calcinosis cutis and calcinosis circumscripta. Granulomas and pyogranulomas, which track hair follicles resulting in large, vertically oriented (sausage-shaped) lesions, are typical of the sterile granuloma/pyogranuloma syndrome.

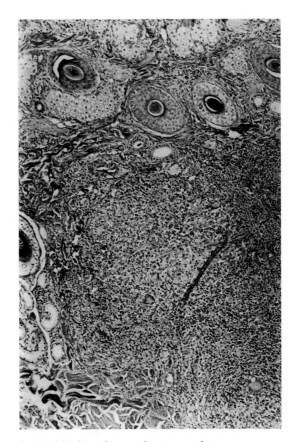

FIGURE 2-69. Pyogranuloma with idiopathic sterile pyogranuloma.

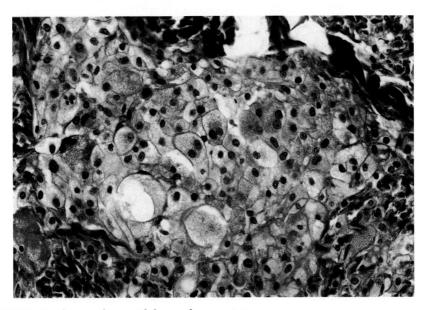

FIGURE 2-70. Xanthogranuloma with hyperadrenocorticism.

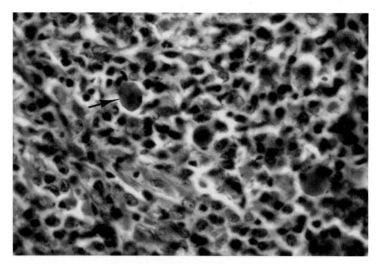

FIGURE 2-71. Mott cells (*arrow*) in bacterial pseudomycetoma.

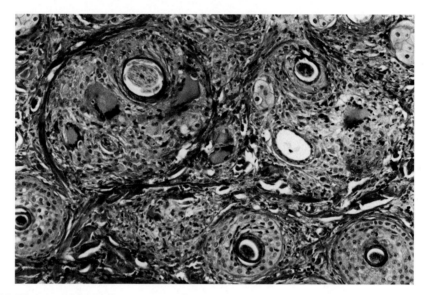

FIGURE 2-72. Sarcoidal granuloma in sarcoidosis.

Reactions to *ruptured hair follicles* are a cause of nodular and diffuse pyogranulomatous dermatitis, and any such dermal process should be carefully scrutinized for keratinous and epithelial debris and should be serially sectioned to rule out this possibility.

Nongranulomatous nodular and diffuse dermatitis can be caused by infectious agents, parasites (onchocerciasis), pseudolymphomas, and necrotizing dermatoses (e.g., photodermatoses, burns, spider bites).

Intraepidermal Vesicular and Pustular Dermatitis

Vesicular and pustular dermatitides show considerable microscopic and macroscopic overlap, because vesicles tend to accumulate leukocytes very early and rapidly. Thus, vesicular dermatitides

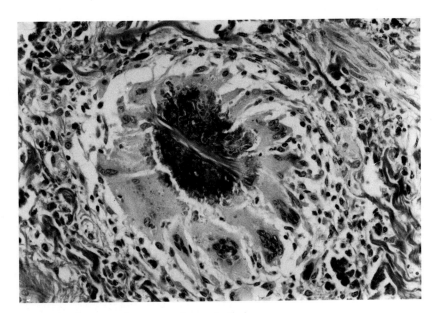

FIGURE 2-73. Palisading granuloma in onchocerciasis.

in horses frequently appear pustular or vesiculopustular, both macroscopically and microscopically (Fig. 2-74).

Intraepidermal vesicles and pustules may be produced by intercellular or intracellular edema (any acute-to-subacute dermatitis reaction), ballooning degeneration (viral infections), acantholysis (the autoantibodies of pemphigus; the proteolytic enzymes from neutrophils in microbial infections; the proteolytic enzymes from eosinophils in sterile eosinophilic folliculitides), and hydropic degeneration of basal cells (lupus erythematosus, erythema multiforme, drug eruptions). It is very useful to classify intraepidermal vesicular and pustular dermatitides by their anatomic level of occurrence within the epidermis (Table 2-9).

Subepidermal Vesicular and Pustular Dermatitis

Subepidermal vesicles (Fig. 2-75) and pustules may be formed through hydropic degeneration of basal cells (lupus erythematosus, erythema multiforme, drug eruption), dermoepidermal separation (bullous pemphigoid, drug eruption, photodermatitis, epidermolysis bullosa), severe subepidermal edema or cellular infiltration (especially urticaria, cellulitis, vasculitis, and ectoparasitism), and severe intercellular edema, with "blow out" of the basement membrane zone (spongiotic perivascular dermatitis). Concurrent epidermal and dermal inflammatory changes are important diagnostic clues (see Table 2-9). Caution is warranted when examining older lesions, because reepithelialization may result in subepidermal vesicles and pustules assuming an intraepidermal location. Such reepithelialization is usually recognized as a single layer of flattened, elongated basal epidermal cells at the base of the vesicle or pustule. Burns (physical or chemical) may produce subepidermal vesicles with necrosis of the epidermis *and* the superficial dermis.

Perifolliculitis, Folliculitis, and Furunculosis

Perifolliculitis denotes the accumulation of inflammatory cells around a hair follicle, wherein the follicular epithelium is not invaded.[18] Dense perifolliculitis may be seen in infectious hair follicle disorders.

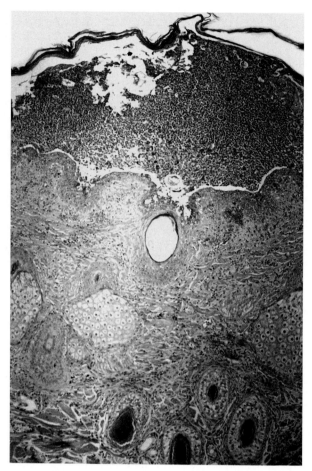

FIGURE 2-74. Intraepidermal pustular dermatitis (suppurative epidermitis) with pemphigus foliaceus.

Mural folliculitis occurs when the wall of the follicle is targeted and the lumen is spared.[18] Four major subdivisions of mural folliculitis are recognized.

1. *Interface mural folliculitis.* As in interface dermatitis, pathologic changes (hydropic degeneration, keratinocyte apoptosis, lymphocytic exocytosis) tend to target the outermost (basal) cell layer (Fig. 2-76).[18] Perifollicular inflammation may be cell-poor (hydropic) or cell-rich (lichenoid). Diseases to consider include lupus erythematosus, erythema multiforme, cutaneous adverse drug reaction, demodicosis, dermatophytosis, graft-versus-host disease, and various vasculitides and vasculopathies,

2. *Infiltrative mural folliculitis.* The follicle wall is infiltrated by lymphocytes and histiocytes in the absence of hydropic degeneration and apoptosis (Fig. 2-77).[18] The differential diagnosis includes cutaneous adverse drug reaction, cutaneous adverse food reaction, and early epitheliotropic lymphoma. A granulomatous degenerative folliculopathy, characterized by massive infiltration of lymphocytes, histiocytes, and multinucleate giant cells, is seen with linear alopecia and with drug reactions.

3. *Necrotizing mural folliculitis.* A usually eosinophil-dominated inflammation causes explosive rupture of follicles, with hemorrhage, and severe dermal mucinosis and edema (Fig. 2-78).[18]

● Table 2-9 **HISTOPATHOLOGIC CLASSIFICATION OF INTRAEPIDERMAL AND SUBEPIDERMAL PUSTULAR AND VESICULAR DISEASES**

ANATOMIC LOCATION*	OTHER HELPFUL FINDINGS
Intraepidermal	
Subcorneal	
Microbial infection	Neutrophilis, microorganisms (bacteria, fungi), ± mild acantholysis, focal necrosis of epidermis, ± follicular involvement
Pemphigus foliaceus	Marked acantholysis, neutrophils and/or eosinophilis, ± follicular involvement
Intragranular	
Pemphigus foliaceus	Marked acantholysis, granular "cling-ons," neutrophils and/or eosinophils, ± follicular involvement
Intraepidermal	
Epitheliotropic lymphoma	Atypical lymphoid cells, Pautrier's microabscesses
Viral dermatoses	Ballooning degeneration, ± inclusion bodies, ± acantholysis
Spongiotic dermatitis	Eosinophilic spongiosis suggests ectoparasitism, pemphigus, pemphigoid, multisystemic eosinophilic epitheliotropic disease
Intrabasal	
Lupus erythematosus	Interface dermatitis, ± thickened basement membrane zone, ± dermal mucinosis
Erythema multiforme	Interface dermatitis, marked single-cell apoptosis of keratinocytes
Graft-versus-host disease	Interface dermatitis
Subepidermal	
Bullous pemphigoid	Subepidermal vacuolar alteration, variable inflammation
Epidermolysis bullosa	Little or no inflammation
Lupus erythematosus	Interface dermatitis, ± thickened basement membrane zone, ± dermal mucinosis
Erythema multiforme	Interface dermatitis, marked single-cell apoptosis of keratinocytes
Severe subepidermal edema or cellular infiltration	
Severe spongiosis	Spongiotic vesicles
Burn	Necrosis of epidermis and superficial dermis

*Drug eruptions can mimic virtually all of these reaction patterns.

One often sees eosinophilic "molds" of destroyed follicle walls. The most common causes are arthropod/insect-related damage and unilateral papular dermatosis. Focal lesions can be seen in insect hypersensitivity, atopy, food hypersensitivity, onchocerciasis, and eosinophilic granuloma. Mucinosis of the hair follicle outer root sheath may be seen with these conditions. A relatively cell-poor or neutrophil-dominated necrotizing mural folliculitis may be a rare manifestation of cutaneous adverse drug reaction, and may also be seen in ischemic states.

4. *Pustular mural folliculitis*. Microabscesses and pustules form adjacent to the follicular stratum corneum, producing subcorneal or intragranular follicular pustules (Fig. 2-79).[18] The most common causes are pemphigus foliaceus (neutrophils or eosinophils with acantholytic keratinocytes) and sterile eosinophilic folliculitis.

Luminal folliculitis implies the accumulation of inflammatory cells within the superficial or deep aspects of the lumen (Fig. 2-80).[18] This is, by far, the most common histologic type and is

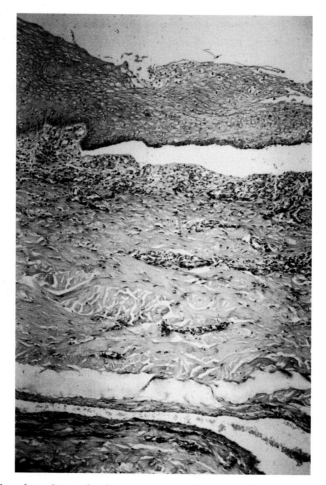

FIGURE 2-75. Subepidermal vesicular dermatitis with bullous pemphigoid.

usually associated with infectious agents: bacteria, dermatophytes, and *Demodex* mites. These folliculitides are dominated by neutrophils. Rare causes include *Pelodera* nematodes and sterile eosinophilic folliculitis. Focal areas of eosinophilic folliculitis may be seen in biopsy specimens from horses with atopy, food hypersensitivity, insect hypersensitivity, onchocerciasis, and eosinophilic granuloma.

Furunculosis (penetrating folliculitis) signifies follicular rupture (Fig. 2-81)[18] and most commonly occurs as a result of luminal folliculitis and less commonly as a result of necrotizing mural folliculitis. Furunculosis results in pyogranulomatous inflammation of the surrounding dermis and, occasionally, subcutis. When furunculosis is seen consecutively in three or more follicles (the "domino" effect), dermatophytosis (especially kerion) is the most likely diagnosis. Furunculosis is usually associated with moderate numbers of eosinophils, presumably a foreign body–type reaction to free keratin and hair shafts. When eosinophils are the dominant cell, an antecedent necrotizing (eosinophilic) mural folliculitis is the cause.

Bulbitis indicates a targeting of the inferior segment of the follicle (Fig. 2-82)[18] and is characteristically seen in alopecia areata. Lymphocytes surround the bulb of anagen hair follicles like "a swarm of bees." Histiocytes and eosinophils may be present in small numbers.

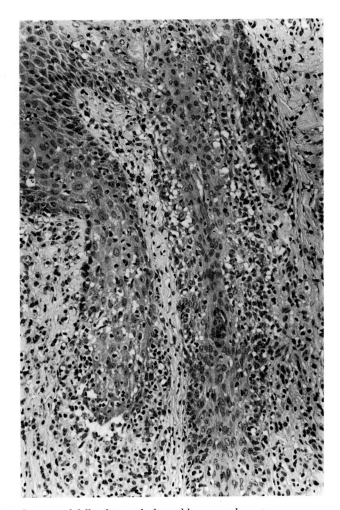

FIGURE 2-76. Interface mural folliculitis with discoid lupus erythematosus.

Perifollicular fibrosis is seen with chronic folliculitides. *Perifollicular melanosis* can occasionally be seen with numerous folliculitides, alopecia areata, and follicular dysplasia.

Follicular inflammation is a common microscopic finding, and one must always be cautious in assessing its importance. Because it is a common secondary complication in pruritic dermatoses (e.g., hypersensitivities and ectoparasitism) and disorders of keratinization, a thorough search (histologically and clinically) for underlying causes is mandatory.

Fibrosing Dermatitis

Fibrosis marks the resolving stage of an intense or insidious inflammatory process, and it occurs mainly as a consequence of collagen destruction. Fibrosis that is histologically recognizable does not necessarily produce a visible clinical scar. Ulcers that cause damage to collagen only in the superficial dermis do not usually result in scarring, whereas virtually all ulcers that extend into the deep dermis inexorably proceed to fibrosis and clinical scars.

Fibrosing dermatitis (Fig. 2-83) follows severe insults of many types to the dermis. Thus, fibrosing dermatitis alone is of minimal diagnostic value, other than for its testimony to severe

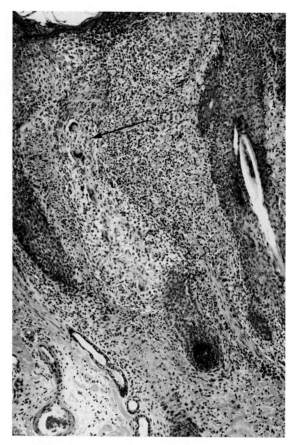

FIGURE 2-77. Infiltrative and granulomatous mural folliculitis in linear alopecia.

antecedent injury. The pathologist must look carefully for telltale signs of the antecedent process, such as furunculosis, vascular disease, foreign material, photodermatitis, lymphedema, lupus erythematosus, and exuberant granulation tissue.

Panniculitis

The panniculus is commonly involved as an extension of dermal inflammatory process, especially of suppurative and granulomatous dermatoses (Fig. 2-84). Likewise, there is usually *some* deep dermal involvement in virtually all panniculitides.

Panniculitis is conveniently divided on an anatomic basis into the *lobular* type (primarily involving fat lobules), the *septal* type (primarily involving interlobular connective tissue septae) (Fig. 2-85, *A*), and the *diffuse* type (both anatomic areas involved) (Fig. 2-85, *B*). Patterns of panniculitis presently appear to have little diagnostic or prognostic significance in horses; in fact, all three patterns may be seen in a single lesion from the same patient. Neither does the cytologic appearance (pyogranulomatous, granulomatous, suppurative, eosinophilic, lymphoplasmacytic, fibrosing) seem to have much diagnostic or prognostic significance. In fact, most panniculitides, regardless of the cause, look histologically similar. As with nodular and diffuse dermatitis, polarization, special stains, and cultures are usually indicated.

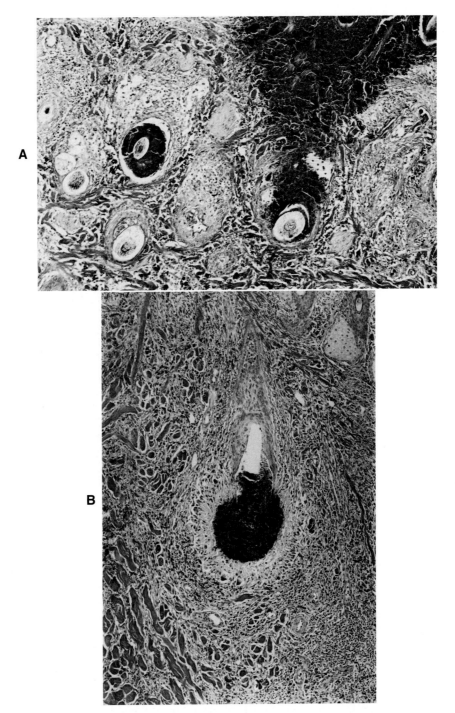

FIGURE 2-78. **A** and **B**, Necrotizing mural folliculitis with sterile eosinophilic folliculitis and furunculosis.

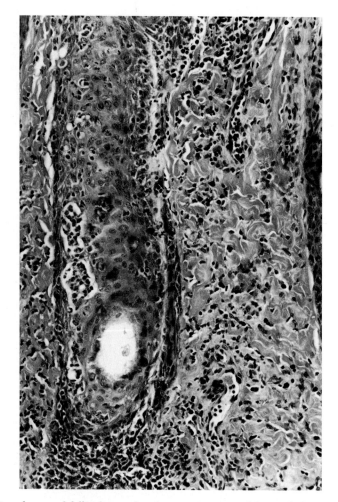

FIGURE 2-79. Pustular mural folliculitis and multisystemic eosinophilic epitheliotropic disease.

Atrophic Dermatosis

Atrophic dermatosis is characterized by varying degrees of epithelial and connective tissue atrophy. This is a rare reaction pattern in equine skin. The most common disorders in this category are endocrine, nutritional, and developmental dermatoses. Atrophic dermatoses show variable combinations of the following histopathologic changes: diffuse orthokeratotic hyperkeratosis, epidermal atrophy, follicular keratosis, follicular atrophy, telogenization of hair follicles, epithelial melanosis, and sebaceous gland atrophy.

Findings suggestive of nutritional disorders include misshapen, corkscrew hairs and small hairs. Developmental disorders such as follicular dysplasias are characterized by variable degrees of follicular dysplasia and anomalous deposition of melanin. The various follicular dysplasias produce dysplastic hair shafts, but endocrinopathies do not.[42] Dysplastic hair shafts may also be seen in alopecia areata and anagen defluxion. Eosinophilic, amorphous, "infarcted hairs" are seen with vasculopathies. Miniaturization of hair follicles and hair shafts may be seen in nutritional disorders and genetic hypotrichoses. Telogen defluxion is characterized by diffuse telogenization of hair follicles, with no other signs of cutaneous atrophy. In the chronic stage, alopecia areata may

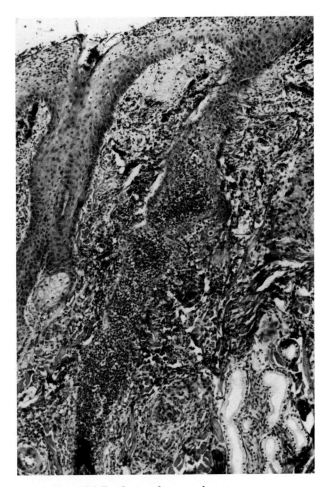

FIGURE 2-80. Suppurative luminal folliculitis in dermatophytosis.

be characterized by follicular atrophy, dysplastic hair shafts, or "orphaned" cutaneous glands and arrector pili muscles. Cutaneous asthenia may be associated with striking atrophy, attenuation, and disorganization of dermal collagen.

Mixed Reaction Patterns

Because diseases are a pathologic continuum, reflecting various combinations of acute, subacute, and chronic changes, and because animals can have more than one dermatosis at the same time, it is common to see one or two biopsies from the same animal that show two or more reaction patterns. For instance, it is common to see an overall pattern of perivascular dermatitis (due to hypersensitivity reactions or ectoparasitism) with a subordinate, focal pattern of folliculitis, furunculosis, or intraepidermal pustular dermatitis (due to secondary bacterial infection). Likewise, one can find multiple patterns from one or two biopsies from an animal with a single disease (e.g., vasculitis, diffuse necrotizing dermatitis, and fibrosing dermatitis in a patient with necrotizing vasculitis). In one study,[40] mixed reaction patterns (two or three) were found in about 16% of the biopsy specimens from horses with inflammatory dermatoses.

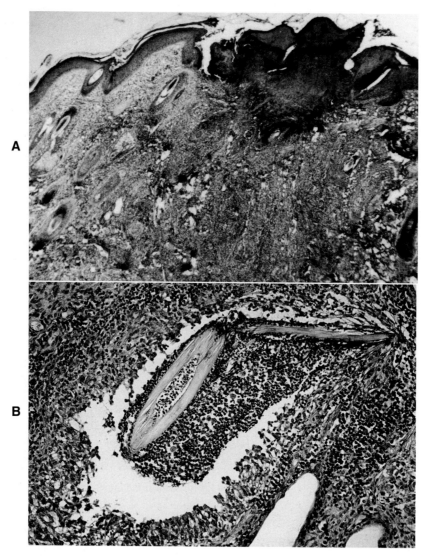

FIGURE 2-81. Furunculosis. **A,** Furunculosis in staphylococcal dermatitis. **B,** Free hair shafts in pyo-granuloma due to dermatophytic furunculosis.

Invisible Dermatoses

Generations of dermatohistopathologists have struggled with biopsy specimens from diseased skin that appear to be normal under the microscope. Since normal skin is rarely biopsied in clinical practice, one must assume that some evidence of disease is present. From the perspective of the dermatohistopathologist, the *invisible dermatoses* are clinically evident skin diseases that show a histologic picture resembling normal skin.[8] Technical problems must be eliminated, such as sampling errors that occur when normal skin on an edge of the biopsy specimen has been sectioned and the diseased tissue has been left in paraffin.

When confronted with an invisible dermatosis, the dermatohistopathologist should consider the following possible disorders and techniques for detecting them: dermatophytosis (special stain

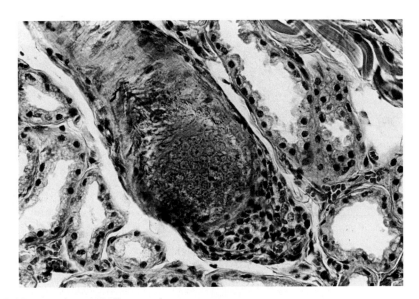

FIGURE 2-82. Lymphocytic bulbitis in alopecia areata.

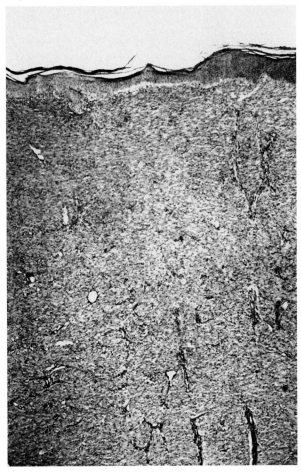

FIGURE 2-83. Fibrosing dermatitis with photodermatitis.

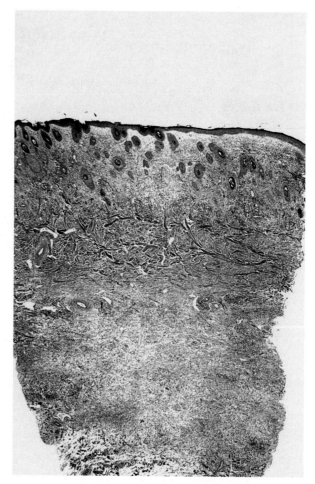

FIGURE 2-84. Panniculitis in sterile idiopathic panniculitis.

for fungi in keratin), ichthyosis (surface keratin removed?), psychogenic alopecia, pigmentary disturbances (hypermelanoses and hypomelanoses, such as lentigo and vitiligo), amorphous deposits in the superficial dermis (Congo red stain for amyloid deposits), urticaria, connective tissue disorder (cutaneous asthenia), and connective tissue nevi.

Conclusion

A skin biopsy can be diagnostic, confirmatory, and helpful, or it can be inconclusive—depending on the dermatosis; the selection, handling, and processing of the specimen; and the skill of the histopathologist.

The dermatopathologist has no right to make a diagnosis of nonspecific dermatitis or inflammation. Every biopsy specimen is a sample of some specific process, but the visible changes may be "noncharacteristic" and may not permit a diagnosis.

The clinician should never accept the terms *nonspecific changes* and *nonspecific dermatitis*. Many pathologic entities that are now well recognized were once regarded as nonspecific! Recourse to serial sections (the key pathologic changes may be very focal), special stains, second opinions, and further biopsies may be required.

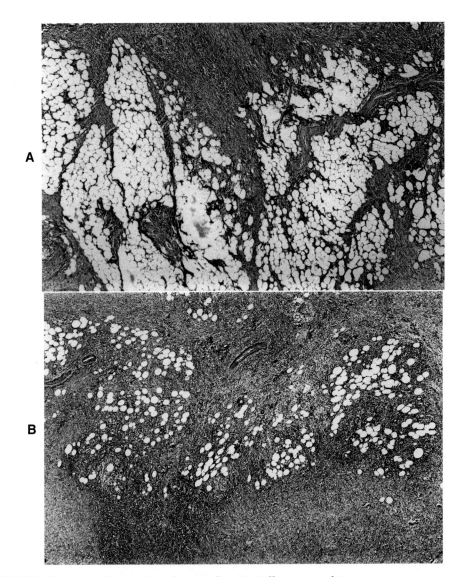

FIGURE 2-85. Panniculitis. **A**, Septal panniculitis. **B**, Diffuse panniculitis.

One study in human dermatopathology assessed the utility of deeper sections and special stains.[27a] Deeper sections provided diagnostic information in 37% of the cases in which they were ordered. Special stains contributed to the diagnosis in 21% of the cases for which they were ordered.

● SPECIAL PROCEDURES

In the past decade, a number of techniques have been developed for studying biopsy specimens. These techniques were usually advanced to allow the identification of special cell types. Examples of such procedures include immunofluorescence testing, electron microscopy, enzyme histochemistry, and immunocytochemistry.

● Table 2-10 **EXAMPLES OF MARKERS FOR THE IDENTIFICATION OF CELL TYPES**

MARKER	CELL TYPE
Enzyme Histochemical	
α-Naphthyl acetate esterase	Monocyte, histiocyte, Langerhans' cell, plasma cell
Chloroacetate esterase	Neutrophil, mast cell
Acid phosphatase	Monocyte, histiocyte, plasma cell
Alkaline phosphatase	Neutrophil, endothelial cell
β-Glucuronidase	Histiocyte, T lymphocyte, plasma cell
Adenosine triphophatase	Histiocyte, plasma cell, B lymphocyte, endothelial cell
5'-Nucleotidase	Endothelial cell
Nonspecific esterase	Monocyte, histiocyte, Langerhans' cell
Lysozyme	Monocyte, histiocyte
α_1-Antitrypsin	Monocyte, histiocyte, mast cell
Chymase	Mast cell
Tryptase	Mast cell
Dipeptidyl peptidase II	Mast cell
Immunohistochemical	
Cytokeratin	Squamous and glandular epithelium, Merkel's cell
Vimentin	Fibroblast, Schwann cell, endothelial cell, myoepithelial cell, lipocyte, smooth muscle, skeletal muscle, mast cell, plasma cell, melanocyte, lymphocyte, monocyte, histiocyte, Langerhans' cell
Desmin	Skeletal muscle, smooth muscle
Neurofilament	Axon cell bodies, dendrites
S100 protein	Melanocyte, Schwann cell, myoepithelial cell, sweat gland acini and ducts, lipocyte, macrophage
Myogloblin	Skeletal muscle
Factor VIII–related antigen	Endothelial cell
Peanut agglutinin	Histiocyte
Myelin basic protein	Schwann cell
Neuron-specific enolase	Schwann cell, Merkel's cell
Collagen IV	Basement membrane
Laminin	Basement membrane
CD1a	Langerhans' cell, dendritic cells
CD1b	Dendritic cells
CD1c	Dendritic cells
CD3	T lymphocytes
CD4	Helper T lymphocytes, dendritic cells, neutrophils
CD8	Cytotoxic T lymphocytes
CD11a	All leukocytes
CD11b	Monocytes, granulocytes
CD11c	Monocytes, macrophages, granulocytes, dendritic cells
CD18	All leukocytes
CD21	B lymphocytes
CD31	Endothelial cell
CD44	Lymphocytes, monocytes, granulocytes
CD45	All leukocytes
CD49	T lymphocytes, monocytes, granulocytes
CD54	ICAM-1
CD79	B lymphocytes

Immunofluorescence testing is not routinely done in veterinary medicine (see Chapter 9). Biopsy specimens for immunofluorescence testing must be carefully selected and either snap-frozen or placed in Michel's fixative. Electron microscopy is best performed on small specimens (1 to 2 mm in diameter) fixed in 3% glutaraldehyde. Enzyme histochemistry is performed on frozen sections or on tissues fixed in 2% paraformaldehyde, dehydrated in acetone, and imbedded in glycol methacrylate (Table 2-10). Immunocytochemistry may be performed on formalin-fixed, routinely processed tissues (e.g., immunoperoxidase methods) or on frozen sections (e.g., lymphocyte markers), depending on the substance being studied (Table 2-10).

Molecular biologic techniques (*in situ* hybridization, polymerase chain reaction) are having an impact on many different aspects of medicine. In the realm of infectious agents, these nucleic acid probes are enhancing diagnostic capabilities, avoiding the need of culturing infectious agents for the purpose of diagnosis, allowing earlier detection of infection, and permitting the detection of latent infections.

Immunohistochemical staining with anti-BCG antibodies has great potential for screening tissues for the presence of bacteria, mycobacteria, and fungi.[8a,8b] The anti-BCG antibodies do not react with normal skin structures or inflammatory cells. The technique is relatively fast, easy, and affordable and has advantages over specific immunohistochemical staining for individual organisms and PCR because it detects a wide variety of microorganisms with one stain.

● REFERENCES

1. Abdel-Hamlin MM, Kubsey AA: Evaluation of dermatophyte test medium for diagnosis of dermatophytosis among farm animals. J Egypt Vet Med Assoc 53:207, 1993.
2. Abdel-Hamlin MM, Kubsey AA: The practical application of chlor-phenolac solution for immediate diagnosis of animal dermatophytosis. J Egypt Vet Med Assoc 54:107, 1994.
3. Affolter VK, von Tscharner C: Malattie della pelle del cavallo. Biopsie della pelle. Ippologia 2:5, 1991.
4. Aho R, et al: Karvanäytteiden mikroskooppinen tutkimus. Suomen Eläinlääk 99:165, 1993.
4a. Alleman AR, Bain PJ: Diagnosing neoplasia: The cytologic criteria for malignancy. Vet Med 95:204, 2000.
5. Andreoletti O, et al: Identification de l'apoptose cutanée chez le chien et le chat par méthode TUNEL: étude préliminaire sur coupes histologiques après inclusion en paraffine. Rev Méd Vét 148:781, 1997.
6. Benhlarech S, Cadoré JL: Intérêt de la biopsie cutanée chez le cheval. Maghreb Vet 4:23, 1989.
7. Boiron G, et al: Phagocytosis of erythrocytes by human and animal epidermis. Dermatologica 165:158, 1982.
7a. Brown WM, Stenn KS: Homeobox genes and the patterning of skin diseases. J Cutan Pathol 20:289, 1993.
8. Brownstein AH, Rabinowitz AD: The invisible dermatoses. J Am Acad Dermatol 8:579, 1983.
8a. Bonenberger TE, et al: Rapid identification of tissue microorganisms in skin biopsy specimens from domestic animals using polyclonal BCG antibody. Vet Dermatol 12:41, 2001.
8b. Byrd J, et al: Utility of antibacillus Calmette-Guérin antibodies as a screen for organisms in sporotrichoid infections. J Am Acad Dermatol 44:261, 2001.
9. Connole MD, Pascoe RR: Recognition of *Trichophyton equinum var. equinum* infection of horses. Aust Vet J 61:94, 1984.
9a. Doubleday CW: Who is Nikolsky and what does his sign mean? J Am Acad Dermatol 16:1054, 1987.
10. Dunstan RW, Song MD: Skin biopsies in the diagnosis of inflammatory skin disease. In: Robinson NE (ed): Current Therapy in Equine Medicine, 3rd ed. W.B. Saunders Co, Philadelphia, 1992, p 683.
11. Dunstan RW, Henry GA: Pathophysiology and diagnosis of skin diseases. In: Kobluk CN, et al (eds): The Horse. Diseases and Clinical Management. W.B. Saunders Co, Philadelphia, 1995, p 487.
12. Evans AG, Stannard AA: Diagnostic approach to equine skin disease. Comp Cont Educ 8:652, 1986.
13. Fadok VA: Equine dermatology. Mod Vet Pract 66:A7, 1985.
14. Fairley RA: Collagenolysis: "It ain't easy being pink." Vet Pathol 28:96, 1991.
15. Fernandez CJ, et al: Staining abnormalities of dermal collagen in eosinophil or neutrophil rich inflammatory dermatoses of horses and cats as demonstrated with Masson's trichrome stain. Vet Dermatol 11:43, 2000.
16. Georg LK: Conversion of tryptophane to nicotinic acid by *Trichophyton equinum*. Proc Soc Exp Biol Med 72:653, 1949.
17. Georg LK, et al: *Trichophyton equinum*—A re-evaluation of its taxonomic status. J Invest Dermatol 29:27, 1957.
18. Gross TL, et al: An anatomical classification of folliculitis. Vet Dermatol 8:147, 1997.
18a. Haack D: Zum Nachweis von Hautpilzinfektionen des Pferdes mit dem Dermatophyten—Test-Medium Fungassay. Tierärztl Prax 15:269, 1987.
19. Hahn RA: Skin biopsy in horses. Mod Vet Pract 65:122, 1984.
19a. Hargis AM, et al: Spongiotic vesicular dermatitis as a cutaneous reaction pattern in seven horses. Vet Dermatol 12:291, 2001.
20. Head KW: Pathology of the skin. Vet Rec 87:460, 1970.

21. Kane J, et al: *Microsporum equinum* in North America. J Clin Microbiol 16:943, 1982.

21a. Kano R, et al: Chitin synthase 1 (Chs1) gene sequences of *Microsporum equinum and Trichophyton equinum*. Vet Microbiol 78:85, 2001.

22. Kostro K: Właściwości morfologiczne i hodowlane *Trichophyton equinum*. Polskie Arch Wet 29:15, 1989.

23. Kostro K: Własciwości biochemiczne krajowych i wzorcowych szczeow *Trichophyton equinum*. Polski Arch Wet 29:37, 1989.

24. Kulkarni VB, et al: Equine ringworm caused by *Trichophyton tonsurans var. sulfureum*. Indian Vet J 46:215, 1969.

25. Leider M, Rosenblum M: A Dictionary of Dermatological Words, Terms, and Phrases. McGraw-Hill Book Co, New York, 1968.

26. Littlewood JD: Diagnostic procedures in equine skin disease. Equine Vet Educ 9:174, 1997.

27. Londero AT, et al: An epizootic of *Trichophyton equinum* infection in horses in Brazil. Sabouraudia 3:14, 1963.

27a. Maingi CP, Helm KF: Utility of deeper sections and special stains for dermatopathology specimens. J Cutan Pathol 25:171, 1998.

28. Majno G, Joris I: Apoptosis, oncosis, and necrosis. An overview of cell death. Am J Pathol 146:3, 1995.

29. Mallet V, et al: Human dermatophytosis: relation to horses. In: Kwochka KW, et al (eds): Advances in Veterinary Dermatology III. Butterworth-Heinemann, Boston, 1998, p 537.

30. Maslen M, Thompson PG: Human infections due to *Trichophyton equinum var. autotrophicum* in Victoria. Aust J Dermatol 25:29, 1984.

31. McGavin MD, Fadok VA: Factors limiting the usefulness of histopathologic examination of skin biopsies in the diagnosis of large animal dermatoses. Vet Clin N Am Large Anim Pract 6:203, 1984.

32. Mehregan AH: Clear epidermal cells: an artifact. J Cutan Pathol 7:154, 1980.

33. Orr M: The histology of skin disease in large animals with particular reference to its role in diagnosis. Vet Dermatol News 3:26, 1978.

34. Pascoe RRR, Knottenbelt DC: Manual of Equine Dermatology. W.B. Saunders Co, Philadelphia, 1999.

34a. Paterson S: Investigation of skin disease and urticaria in the horse. In Pract 22:446, 2000.

35. Polonelli L, Morace G: Antigenic characterization of *Microsporum canis, M. distortum, M. equinum, M. ferrugineum*, and *Trichophyton soudanense* cultures. Mycopathologia 92:71, 1985.

36. Raskin CA: Apoptosis and cutaneous biology. J Am Acad Dermatol 36:885, 1997.

37. Schwayder T, et al: *Trichophyton equinum* from riding bareback: First reported U.S. case. J Am Acad Dermatol 29:785, 1994.

38. Scott DW: Large Animal Dermatology. W.B. Saunders Co, Philadelphia, 1988.

39. Scott DW: Lymphoid nodules in skin biopsies from dogs, cats, and horses with non-neoplastic dermatoses. Cornell Vet 79:267, 1989.

40. Scott DW: Diagnostic des dermatoses inflammatoires équines: analyse de la modalité de réaction histopathologique; étude personnelle portant sur 315 cas. Point Vét 24:245, 1992.

41. Scott DW: Sebaceous gland melanosis in the horse. Vet Dermatol 10:157, 1999.

42. Scott DW, et al: Muller & Kirk's Small Animal Dermatology, 6th ed. W.B. Saunders Co, Philadelphia, 2001.

43. Smith JMB, et al: *Trichophyton equinum var. autotrophicum*: Its characteristics and geographic distribution. Sabouraudia 6:296, 1968.

44. Sparkes AH, et al: Improved sensitivity in the diagnosis of dermatophytosis by fluorescence microscopy with calcafluor white. Vet Rec 134:307, 1994.

45. Steffen C: Dyskeratosis and the dyskeratoses. Am J Dermatopathol 10:356, 1988.

46. Takatori K, Hasegawa A: Mating experiment of *Microsporum canis* and *Microsporum equinum* isolated from animals with *Nannizzia otae*. Mycopathologia 90:59, 1985.

47. Thomsett LR: Diagnostic methods in equine dermatology. Equine Vet J 1:90, 1968.

47a. Thrall MA: Cytologic examination of cutaneous and subcutaneous lumps and lesions. Vet Med 95:224, 2000.

48. von Tscharner C, Hauser B: Pathologie der Haut. Kleintierpraxis 26:449, 1981.

49. Williams BJ, et al: Antimicrobial effects of lidocaine, bicarbonate, and epinephrine. J Am Acad Dermatol 37:662, 1997.

50. Williams MA, Angarano DW: Diseases of the skin. In: Kobluk CN, et al (eds): The Horse. Diseases and Clinical Management. W.B. Saunders Co, Philadelphia, 1995, p 541.

51. Yager JA, Scott DW: The skin and appendages. In: Jubb KVP, et al (eds): Pathology of Domestic Animals, 4th ed, Vol 1. Academic Press, New York, 1993, p 531.

Chapter 3

Dermatologic Therapy

Management of equine skin diseases has evolved in recent years to include a broader and more advanced selection of topical and systemic agents. Even so, there are only a limited number of products designed specifically for equine dermatoses. However, many products designed for companion animals and humans are very effective in the horse.

● BASIC NUTRITION AND THE SKIN

Nutritional factors that influence the skin are exceedingly complex (see Chapter 10). The skin and haircoat utilize a major part of the nutritional requirements of horses. Modifications of nutrition, therefore, may have visible effects on the skin and haircoat.

Nutritional modifications affect the skin and haircoat of horses in two ways. The first is the basic diet and additional supplements given to normal or diseased animals that are designed to produce a high-quality haircoat. The second is nutritional therapy or treatment wherein diets and supplements are given for a specific disease or problem. In many situations, these treatments entail high doses that most likely have metabolic or pharmacologic effects other than just meeting nutritional requirements. In most cases (other than those discussed in Chapter 10), the success of these treatments is probably not related to nutritional deficiency. The most common ingredients of the diet that seem to benefit the quality of the skin and haircoat are the protein level and fatty acids, with some effect coming from the vitamins and minerals.

The skin and hair are the organs that utilize the most protein from the diet. When there is a deficiency of protein, the haircoat is one of the first organs affected (see Chapter 10). However, protein deficiency is rare in horses, particularly if a good-to-excellent quality diet is used (see Chapter 10).

Fats are an important part of the diet and are valuable as a concentrated energy source. If there is too little total fat or linoleic acid, a dry scaly skin or poor haircoat could be the result. Fatty acids have been recommended for many years as dietary supplements to improve the sheen and luster of the hair (see Chapter 10). Fatty acids as therapeutic agents are discussed in Chapter 8.

Fatty acids are long carbon chains with a methyl group at one end. Polyunsaturated fatty acids have multiple double bonds. The numeric formulas used to identify fatty acids give the number of carbon atoms, followed by the number of double bonds, and then the location of the first double bond from the methyl group. Therefore, the formula for linoleic acid (18:2N-6) means there are 18 carbons and 2 double bonds, with the first occurring at the sixth carbon atom from the methyl end of the molecule.

The fatty acids that have the first double bond three carbon molecules away from the methyl group are the omega-3 (N-3) series. The omega-6 (N-6) series of polyunsaturated fatty acids have the first double bond six carbons from the methyl group. These two complete series of fatty acids cannot be synthesized by horses, and therefore the 18-carbon molecule (linoleic and linolenic acid) must be supplied in the diet. They are called *essential* fatty acids for this reason. The essential fatty acids most important in cutaneous homeostasis are linoleic acid (18:2N-6) and linolenic acid (18:3N-3). Dihomo-gamma-linolenic acid (DGLA) (20:3N-6) and eicosapentaenoic acid (EPA) (20:5N-3) can be synthesized in the animal from linoleic acid and linolenic acid, respectively.

The synthesis of fatty acids involves the action of various *desaturase* enzymes, which insert double bonds into the chain. Other enzymes called *elongases* add additional carbon molecules to the existing chain. The presence of these specific enzymes varies in different groups or species of animals and may differ among individuals with certain diseases.

The best example of this is Δ-6-desaturase deficiency in atopic humans and dogs.[71] Also, the skin is deficient in desaturase enzymes. Therefore, when linoleic acid, γ-linolenic acid (18:3N-6), or DGLA accumulates locally, it cannot be metabolized to arachidonic acid locally. DGLA competes with arachidonic acid for cyclooxygenase and lipoxygenase enzymes. This competitive inhibition, in addition to the effects of their metabolic byproducts, is thought to be the mechanism for anti-inflammatory action of fatty acid therapy, which generally involves modification of leukotriene and prostaglandin synthesis and activity. Fatty acids are also important for other reasons, however.

Fatty acids are valuable components of cell membranes but also have an extracellular function in the skin. They are responsible for the luster of the normal haircoat and the smoothness of the skin. Linoleic acid is particularly important because only it supplies the proper conditions for the water permeability functions of the intercellular lipid bilayer of the skin (see Chapter 1).

Metabolic byproducts are important in promoting or inhibiting inflammation. This is especially true of arachidonic acid metabolites. Arachidonic acid is stored in cells in an unavailable form until it is released by the action of phospholipase A_2. Arachidonic acid metabolites have been identified in many cell types that participate in hypersensitivity reactions (mast cells, neutrophils, eosinophils, lymphocytes, monocytes, macrophages, keratinocytes, and vascular endothelial cells).

The effects of prostaglandins on the skin include alteration of vascular permeability, potentiation of vasoactive substances such as histamine, modulation of lymphocyte function, and potentiation of pain and itch. Prostaglandins and leukotrienes potentiate each other. The effects of leukotrienes on the skin are to alter vascular permeability, activate neutrophils, modify lymphocyte function, and cause potent neutrophil and eosinophil chemotaxis. Manipulation of fatty acid metabolism by using the shared enzyme system to competitively inhibit formation of some of these substances seems possible.

Many owners inquire about vitamin and mineral supplements. It appears that most good-to-excellent quality foods have adequate levels. Vitamins A, C, and E have all been recommended to treat a number of diseases, but these vitamins have not been shown to improve haircoat quality in normal animals. Little is known about what level is required for optimal skin and hair quality. This has led to many anecdotal claims and products on the market. Mineral therapy is also often recommended to clients, again with only anecdotal benefits.

• CLEANING THE SKIN

The normal skin surface film contains excretory products of skin glands and keratinocytes, corneocytes, bacteria and dirt, pollen, grains, and mold spores. Excessive amounts of these, together with altered or abnormal fatty acids, serum, red blood cells, proteinaceous exudates, degenerating inflammatory cells, and the byproducts of their degradation, as well as bacterial degradation, are found in the surface film of abnormal skin. The skin and coat should be groomed to minimize these accumulations and to promote health. If proper skin and coat care is neglected, skin irritation may result or accumulations of debris may adversely affect a skin disease that is already present.

Hair Care Products

SHAMPOOS

Shampoos should remove external dirt, grime, and sebum and leave the hair soft, shiny, and easy to comb. To accomplish this, shampoos should lather well, rinse freely, and leave no residue. Optimally, they would remove soil rather than natural oils, but the natural oils are removed to varying degrees. For some animals, this may require the use of oil or conditioning rinses. Some shampoos have a soap base, but most shampoos are surfactants or detergents with a variety of additives that function as thickeners, conditioners, lime soap dispersants, protein hydrolysates, and perfumes. Dozens of products are available on the market.

Many clients are familiar with pH-balanced shampoos for human use. The same promotion of pH adjusting for equine shampoos has been recommended. The equine skin is approximately neutral, with a pH of 7 to 7.4, which is different from that of human skin. Therefore, human pH-adjusted shampoos are not optimal for equine use. Theoretically, pH products temporarily affect the electrostatic charges in the surface lipid bilayer and could alter the normal barrier effect. However, the clinical relevance or the documentation of alterations in barrier function related to the pH of a shampoo is lacking in veterinary medicine.

Soap shampoos work well in soft water. In hard water, they leave a dulling film of calcium and magnesium soap on the hair unless special lime-dispersing agents are added to bind calcium, magnesium, and heavy metal ions.

Detergent shampoos are synthetic surfactants or emulsifying agents, usually salts of lauryl sulfate. Sodium lauryl ether sulfate (sodium laureth sulfate) is less irritating than sodium lauryl sulfate. If a horse seems to be irritated by most shampoos, trying a shampoo with sodium laureth sulfate may prove worthwhile. Such shampoos do not react with hard water, but they tend to be harsher cleaning agents than soap. This disadvantage is partially overcome by various additives.

Satisfactory detergents to use as shampoos for normal coats tend to dry the coat and contain few additives to counter the detergent effect. Conditioners should be used after detergents. Glycol, glycerol esters, lanolin derivatives, oils, and fatty alcohols are considered superfattening or emollient additives that prevent the complete removal of natural oils or tend to replace them. They also give the hair more luster and, as lubricants, make it easier to comb.

CONDITIONERS

Hair conditioners have four main purposes: (1) to reduce static electricity so that coarse hair does not snarl or become flyaway, (2) to give body to limp or thin hair, (3) to supply fatty acids or oil to coat the hair and skin, and (4) to deliver medication to the skin and hair surface in a vehicle that will not be completely rinsed away or removed. Normal hair maintains relative electric neutrality with a slight negative charge. However, if clean, dry hair is in a low-humidity environment or is brushed excessively, it picks up increased negative electric charges. Adjacent hairs that are similarly charged repel one another and produce the condition known as "flyaway."

Conditioners or cream rinses are cationic (positively charged) surfactants or amphoteric materials that neutralize the charge and eliminate flyaway. They are slightly acidic, which hardens keratin and removes hard water residues. They also contain a fatty or oily component that adds a film to provide luster. Thus, these products make hair lie flat and comb easily, but they do not provide the body or fluff that some coats require.

Protein conditioners, or body builders, contain oil and protein hydrolysates. Oils add luster, whereas protein hydrolysates coat the hair and make it seem thicker. This may be a slight advantage in hair with a dried, cracked, outer cuticle layer, but the effect is actually minimal. Only a thin film is added, so hair is not strengthened. If the protein is added to a shampoo rather than used separately, most of it is washed away during rinsing, further reducing the effect.

OIL RINSES

Oil rinses are used after a bath to replenish and restore the natural oils removed by the shampooing. These products are emollients that add luster and improve the combability of the haircoat. They may decrease dry, flaky skin and dry flakes within the haircoat. Oil rinses are primarily oils that require dilution (otherwise, they will leave the haircoat too greasy), or they are oil-in-water emulsions that may be diluted or sprayed directly on the haircoat. The essential fatty acids are often incorporated into these products and are absorbed percutaneously.

Clipping

Clipping is beneficial when topical treatment will be used. Clipping permits thorough cleaning, adequate skin contact, and a more economical application of the desired medicament. In many cases, complete removal of the coat may be preferred, but usually, clipping the local area suffices. This should be done neatly to avoid disfigurement. If the hair over the involved area is clipped closely (against the grain with a No. 40 clipper), whereas a border around this is clipped less closely (with the grain), the regrowth of hair more quickly blends the area into the normal coat pattern.

Clipping should always be discussed with the owner to obtain approval. This contact is especially important when treating show animals or those with long coats. All needless clipping should be avoided. During clipping, a vacuum cleaner can be used to remove all loose hair and debris. Shampoo therapy may be an acceptable alternative to clipping in some cases. It may remove surface lipids and clean the skin and hair enough that topical dips are able to be effectively applied to the skin surface. In other cases, the desired active ingredients may be incorporated into the shampoo formulation.

• CLIENT COMPLIANCE

The successful treatment of skin disorders depends to a large extent on the client. In addition to supplying the historical information needed for diagnosis, the client administers most prescribed therapies. The successful management of many dermatologic diseases necessitates long-term or lifelong therapy, often involving more than one medicament. The client must also give the medications correctly at the proper intervals and for the proper duration.

Many animals have been referred to us after the correct diagnosis was made, appropriate treatment was recommended, but treatment failed because of improper execution by the owner. Excellent diagnosticians often have poor results if they are not able to interact with clients effectively, because this often leads to failure in compliance. These failures may occur for a variety of reasons. Understanding the possible reasons for poor compliance, recognizing when treatment failures occur, and developing corrective measures is an art that the successful clinician develops.

The reasons for poor client compliance include the following:

1. Failure of the client to understand the importance of giving the treatment.
2. Lack of education of the client regarding the proper treatment.
3. Improper frequency of or interval between medication applications.
4. Faulty application, which can take multiple forms.
5. Inadequate duration of therapy.
6. Client's lack of time or labor-intensive treatment.
7. Disagreeable cosmetic appearance or odor of treatment.
8. Perceived danger of treatment.
9. Premature discontinuation of treatment because of perceived lack of efficacy.
10. Discontinuation of treatment because it was too difficult or not tolerated by the horse.

Many of these problems are avoidable if the clinician or the veterinary assistants adequately explain the treatment plan.

It is important to make the client aware of potential problems, and these possible difficulties should be thoroughly discussed. We encounter numerous cases wherein the clients have unused treatments at home. Because the treatment was too labor-intensive or the treatment appeared ineffective, the client discontinued it. The successful clinician tries to prevent these treatment failures. Some clients may not readily admit that a treatment will be too difficult or unacceptable, and therefore alternatives may not be offered.

Another major factor influencing client compliance is the use of multiple therapeutic agents. Often, the best management of a dermatologic disease, particularly a chronic one, is a therapeutic regimen or plan that entails the use of multiple products. This makes education of the client more difficult and time-consuming, as well as potentially more confusing. Despite these problems, the best long-term control is often achieved by using multiple agents rather than a single medicament.

Particularly with chronic skin problems, the education of the client regarding the horse's disease becomes critical. Over the life of the horse, many different therapies may be required and changes in the disease or secondary manifestations are likely. The client needs to be educated about the likely course of the disease, as well as the need for follow-up and therapeutic modifications. The importance of maintenance therapy must be emphasized.

● TOPICAL THERAPY

Topical therapy has always played a large role in dermatology because of the obvious access to the affected tissue.[4,38,63,71,97] In the past, topical therapy was used for treating localized lesions and ectoparasite infestations. In the last 15 years, topical applications have become even more prominent and continue to flourish in treating skin disease. Undoubtedly, this growth in topical therapy reflects multiple factors, which may include (1) the development of more products, better delivery systems, and active ingredients; (2) the reduction in systemic absorption or effects and adverse reactions; and (3) the recognition of the adjunctive and synergistic effects in the overall management of numerous skin diseases. These factors are also the advantages that topical therapy offers to the clinician and the horse owner.

However, this therapy also entails some disadvantages. In general, topical therapy is much more time-consuming and labor-intensive than systemic therapy. Understanding the proper use and application of topical therapy is also important, and therefore client education and compliance become more difficult to achieve. Localized adverse reactions not seen with systemic therapy may occur, most commonly irritant reactions.

Topical therapy is often adjunctive, and it may significantly increase the cost of the overall therapeutic plan. Some topical agents may be so costly that their use is limited to localized lesions. On the other hand, appropriate topical therapy may greatly reduce the need for systemic therapy. The clinician needs to consider the potential benefits and disadvantages, the client's preferences, and the patient's needs when deciding on the use of topical therapy.

When a clinician elects to use topical therapy, several factors must be considered. First and foremost is, What is the purpose or desired result of the topical therapy? Is this the sole therapy, or is it adjunctive to other nontopical therapies? What type of delivery system best facilitates obtaining the desired result? What active ingredients are used for this purpose? As previously discussed, patient and client considerations are paramount. Table 3-1 lists the most common delivery systems and formulations of active ingredients used in veterinary dermatology. The amount of use for each type of product relative to the others is based solely on the authors' opinions and clinical impressions.

Factors That Influence Drug Effects on the Skin

Topical medications consist of active ingredients incorporated in a vehicle that facilitates application to the skin. In selecting a vehicle, one must consider the solubility of the drug in the vehicle, the

● Table 3-1 **TOPICAL FORMULATIONS AND RELATIVE EFFICACY OF INCORPORATED ACTIVE AGENTS***

TOPICAL FORMULA-TIONS	ASTRINGENT	EMOLLIENT	ANTI-SEBORRHEIC	ANTI-PRURITIC	ANTI-BACTERIAL	ANTI-MYCOTIC	ANTI-PARASITIC	ANTI-INFLAM-MATORY	ULTRA-VIOLET SCREEN
Shampoo	X	XX	XXX	XX	XXX	X	XX	X	—
Rinse	X	XXX	—	XX	X	XXX	XXXX	X	—
Leave-on conditioners	—	XXX	—	XXX	XXX	XX	—	X	—
Powder	—	—	—	X	X	?	X	X	X
Lotion	XXX	X	X	XXX	XX	XX	—	XXX	XXX
Spray	XX	XXX	XX	XXX	X	X	XXX	XX	XXX
Cream or ointment	—	X	X	XX	XXX	X	—	XXX	XXX
Gels	—	—	X	—	XX	X	—	—	—

*Relative use based on authors' opinions and clinical impressions: — = not used; X = infrequently used or use associated with lower frequency; XX = occasionally used; XXX = commonly used and tend to be efficacious; and XXXX = preferred formulation for that class of active ingredients.

rate of release from the vehicle, the ability of the vehicle to hydrate the stratum corneum, the stability of the active agent in the vehicle, and the interactions (chemical and physical) among the vehicle, the active agent, and the stratum corneum. The vehicle is not always inert and many have important therapeutic effects.

When topical medications are used, one basic question is whether the drug penetrates the skin and, if so, how deeply. Absorption varies highly, and most drugs penetrate only 1% to 2% after 16 to 24 hours.[3,27] However, even in the same vehicle, similar drugs may vary dramatically in their absorption.[26] This was exemplified in a study with three organophosphate insecticides applied topically in three different vehicles.[31] With only one organophosphate (parathion) of the three tested, the vehicle dimethyl sulfoxide (DMSO) increased absorption from 4% to 5% up to 15% to 30%. In some cases (e.g., insecticides), the absorbability greatly influences the potential for side effects.

Clinical efficacy and absorption are not synonymous; absorption is only one factor in efficacy. Some drugs in an insoluble form in the vehicle have only a surface effect. Once absorbed, a drug must also interact with specific receptors before an action will result. The drug's affinity for the receptors, as well as local factors that effect this drug-receptor interaction, are also important.[71] Absorption of drugs through the skin involves many variables. There are physicochemical factors related to the topical formulation and biologic factors.[4] The physicochemical factors involve the interactions between the drug and the vehicle, the drug and the skin, and the vehicle and the skin. Some of these factors are determined by the concentration of the drug, the drug's movement between the vehicle and the skin, the diffusion coefficient, and the local pH.

1. The concentration of the drug and its solubility in the vehicle affects absorption. The package label gives the percentage of drug concentration, not the percentage of solubility. In addition to concentration, the solubility of the drug and the solubilizing capacity of the vehicle affect drug absorption. In general, poor solubility and excessive solubilizing capacity decrease the rate of absorption.[4] Usually, ointment vehicles for topical corticosteroids increase solubility and drug delivery, so systemic effects after topical use are more common—and potentially dangerous.

2. The drug must move from the vehicle through the skin barrier to be effective. The solubility of the drug in the horny layer relative to its solubility in the vehicle is described by the partition coefficient. The concentration of the drug in the barrier, not in the vehicle, is what determines the diffusion force. Increased lipid solubility favors drug penetration because the stratum corneum is lipophilic.

3. The diffusion coefficient is a measure of the extent to which the barrier interferes with the drug's mobility. The stratum corneum is unsurpassed as an unfavorable environment for drug penetration. Physical disruption of the epidermal barrier by the use of lipid solvents, keratolytic agents, or cellulose-tape stripping of the top layers of cells increases the potential for absorption. In some cases, the vehicle itself may be able to diffuse through the stratum corneum and carries any dissolved drug with it. DMSO facilitates cutaneous penetration of some substances. Moisture and occlusive dressings enhance percutaneous absorption as well. Large molecular size results in poor mobility and poor absorption.

4. The pH of the drug's local environment may also affect absorption by altering the amount of drug in its unionized form. Many drugs are either weak acids or bases and occur in an ionized and unionized form. In general, the unionized form is more readily absorbed; this amount may change as the local pH is altered.[71]

The active ingredient of the drug may interact with all other components in the formulation. In practice, the addition of other ingredients or the mixing of ingredients on the skin may alter the drug's effect. Drug effects may be altered by interactions between the drug and the new drug or its vehicle, or by interactions between the new drug or vehicle and the original vehicle. Changes that may occur include inactivation of the drug by chemical bonding or precipitation, changes in pH, allowing decomposition of the drugs by altering the stabilizing effects of the vehicle, and altering the concentration of the drug.

Temperature and hydration of the skin can affect the interaction among the drug, the vehicle, and the skin. Hydration probably plays a greater role than temperature in affecting absorption. In general, permeability to drugs increases as the hydration of the stratum corneum increases.[3,4]

Biologic factors also affect drug absorption. The body region treated greatly influences absorption. In humans, the amount of hydrocortisone being absorbed varied tremendously, in descending order, on the scrotum, the forehead, the forearm, and the plantar foot.[27] Age is an important factor, with newborns experiencing greater absorption than adolescents, who in turn experience greater absorption than adults. Obviously, the health and condition of the skin is important because inflamed, abraded, or otherwise damaged skin often absorbs more drug. Blood flow also affects absorption. Greater blood flow favors increased systemic absorption.

Hydrotherapy

Water is often overlooked as a therapeutic agent, especially when it is applied with a shampoo, as a rinse, or as a component of many lotions.[63,71] Hydrotherapy may be used to moisten the stratum corneum, to dry out the epidermis, to cool or heat the skin, to soften surface crusts, and to clean the skin. Increased effects occur by the addition of other agents.

Water may be applied as a wet dressing or in baths. Frequent periodic renewal of wet dressings (15 minutes on, several hours off) prolongs the effect, but if more continuous therapy or occlusive coverings are used, the skin becomes overly moistened, the skin temperature rises, and undesirable maceration occurs. This is less likely if the wet dressings are left open.

Hydrotherapy can hydrate or dehydrate the skin, depending on how it is managed. The application of loose, damp gauze compresses for 15 minutes followed by the removal for 1 hour promotes evaporation of water from the gauze and from the subadjacent skin surface and is drying to the underlying tissues. If water is maintained on the skin surface constantly by wet towels, soaks, or baths, the skin hydrates as water is taken up by keratin and hair. If a film of oil is applied immediately after soaking (occlusive rinses), evaporation of water (transpiration) is hindered and the skin retains moisture.

The water may be cool or above body temperature. These treatments may be used to remove crusts and scales, to clean wounds and fistulae, to rehydrate skin, to reduce pain and pruritus, and to provide prophylaxis for patients prone to decubital problems, urine scalds, and other ills. Therapeutic treatment once or twice daily (each treatment lasting 10 to 15 minutes) is adequate. The patients should be toweled and placed in an air stream drier to dry. Other topical medications can be applied later, if needed.

In hydrotherapy, moisture is the specific agent; various additives change the actions of moisture only slightly but add their own effects. Astringents, antipruritics, moisturizers, parasiticides, and antibiotics are common additives. In general, water treatment removes crusts, bacteria, and other debris and greatly reduces the possibility of secondary infection. It promotes epithelialization and allays the symptoms of pain and burning. Cool water is antipruritic. It also softens keratin. The suppleness and softness of the skin are due to its water content, not to the oils on the surface.[71] Dryness of the skin is recognized when any one of the following is present: roughness of the surface, scaliness, inflexibility of the horny layer, and fissuring with possible inflammation.

Cold applications cause capillary constriction and decreased blood flow.[84] They are often used to retard swelling, prevent hematoma formation, and allay pain and itch. *Warm* applications cause vasodilation, increased blood flow, increased tissue oxygenation, and increased lymph flow.[84]

Normal skin is not a waterproof covering but is constantly losing water to the environment by transpiration. The extent of this loss depends on body temperature, environmental temperature, and relative humidity. The stratum corneum, composed of corneocytes and an intercellular matrix lipid bilayer, is the major deterrent to water loss. The lipids of this layer are derived from phospholipids and lipids secreted by the keratinocytes as they migrate to the stratum corneum and from sebum. Dry skin may result from excessive transpiration of water.

Sebum on the skin or externally applied lipid films tend to make the surface feel smoother. The flexibility of keratin is directly related to its moisture content. Major factors determining moisture content are the amount of water that the horny layer receives from the epidermis and the transepidermal loss. The transepidermal loss from the stratum corneum partially depends on the environment, especially the relative humidity. Water content of the horny layer can be increased by applying occlusive dressings or agents to prevent loss, by adding water with baths or wet dressings, or by using hygroscopic medications to attract water.

Topical Formulations

Active medications may be applied to the skin by a variety of delivery systems.[4,63,71] These different delivery systems include, but are not limited to, the following formulations: shampoos; rinses; powders; lotions; sprays; creams, emulsions, and ointments; and gels. Each type of formulation has advantages and disadvantages that the clinician should consider when selecting a topical medication. Besides incorporating active ingredients, each type of formulation contains ingredients that act as the vehicle for delivering the active agents. These vehicles may also have certain therapeutic, irritant, or cosmetic effects, making the overall formulation more or less desirable.

In general, vehicles contain ingredients to adjust the pH, stabilize the active agents, prolong the effects of the active ingredients, promote the delivery of the active agents to the skin surface or into or through the stratum corneum, and make the product cosmetically pleasing (e.g., fragrance). The selection of the topical formulation depends on a variety of factors, most notably the surface area to be treated, the need for residual activity, the presence of hair in the area to be treated, and the nature of the lesion (e.g., moist or dry).

The active ingredients are often available in a variety of different formulations and delivery systems. In general, they have the same basic activity regardless of the formulation, but their ease of use, cost, and efficacy for the desired purpose are affected by the formulation and the method of application. The following categories of active agents are used: astringents, or drying agents; emollients and moisturizers; antiseborrheics; antipruritics; antibacterials; antifungals; antiparasitics; anti-inflammatory agents; and ultraviolet screens. The following discussion describes first the different delivery systems and then the types of active ingredients.

SHAMPOOS

Medicated shampoos contain additional ingredients that enhance the action of the shampoo or add other actions to that of the shampoo.[97] With most shampoo formulations, the active drugs have a limited contact time because they are removed during the rinsing of the shampoo base. Some medicaments may have enough opportunity for effect or for limited absorption during a prolonged shampoo, and their addition may be justified (e.g., insecticides, salicylic acid, sulfur, tar, and antiseptics). Medicated shampoos are valuable in that they may be used for diseases involving large areas of the body or localized lesions.

Newer formulations of shampoos have been developed that utilize sustained-release microvesicle technology. In one type, the microvesicles have an outer lipid membrane and contain water (Novasomes, EVSCO). The lipid membrane binds to hair and skin and has a long-term moisturizing effect as the microvesicles break down (Fig. 3-1, *A* and *B*). This counteracts the drying that may occur with some medications and is therapeutic for dry skin. However, the active medication is not incorporated and will still be rinsed away. The authors prefer the EVSCO products.

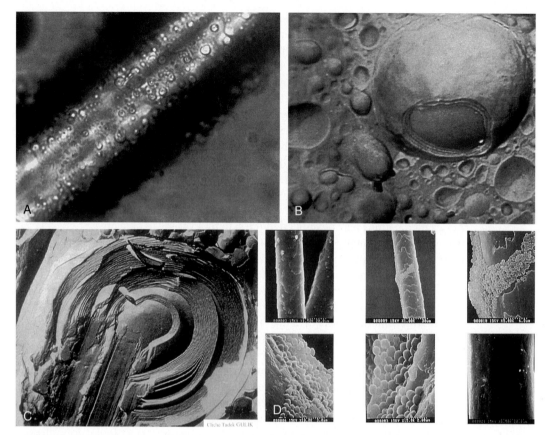

FIGURE 3-1. A, Novasome attached to canine hair shaft. **B,** Scanning electron micrograph of a novasome showing the multiple layers and large cargo hold. **C,** Scanning electron micrograph of a spherulite showing the multiple layers. **D,** Scanning electron micrographs showing spherulites attached to hair shafts. (Courtesy EVSCO and Virbac.)

The second microvesicle technology (Spherulites, Virbac) actually incorporates different ingredients, such as salicylic acid and sulfur, chlorhexidine, ethyl lactate, benzalkonium chloride, oatmeal extract, glycerin, and urea, into multiple layers of these microvesicles. Also, these microvesicles have multiple (10 to 1,000) layers that slowly break down (Fig. 3-1, *C*). With the breakdown of each layer, the active ingredients and the surfactants that make up these layers are released onto the hair and skin. The microvesicles can be made with different charges on the exterior; making them positively charged causes them to bind with the negatively charged hair and skin (Fig. 3-1, *D*). Chitosanide has been used to make the microvesicles called *spherulites*. Besides supplying the outer cationic surface, chitosanide is an active moisturizing agent and is hygroscopic.

Efficacy of these shampoos is determined by proper use, as well as by active ingredients. It is imperative that products be applied properly, allowed to remain on for sufficient contact time, and then properly rinsed. Education of the client regarding the use of these products is an important element and time well spent. The client should be instructed to use a clock to determine the correct contact time because subjective assessments are often inadequate. Contact time starts after the shampoo is applied, not when the bath begins. More severely affected regions should be the first areas shampooed. Sometimes, problem areas benefit from a second lathering before the final rinse.

Pharmaceutical companies provide a multitude of medicated shampoos, which often have specific indications and contraindications. It is important to become familiar with a few (perhaps one of each type) and to thoroughly understand the ingredients and their concentration and actions. Choosing the mildest or most client-pleasing shampoo that produces the desired actions often increases compliance. Strong shampoos can be harmful as well as helpful.

The clinician must evaluate the whole animal when selecting active ingredients, and some animals may benefit from the simultaneous use of different products. Although one shampoo may be recommended for the whole body, another shampoo may be applied to a more localized region.

Certain principles should be kept in mind when using medicated shampoos:

1. *Clipping the haircoat.* Clipping the haircoat and keeping the haircoat short may be critical to the proper use and maximal benefit of the product.
2. *Premedicated shampoo bathing.* It is often a good idea to remove grease, debris, and dirt with a nonmedicated shampoo, such as baby shampoo, or a dishwashing detergent. In this way, the medicated shampoo is better able to contact the skin, less product is used, and less expense is incurred.
3. *Contact time.* The shampoo should be allowed to remain in contact with the skin for 10 to 15 minutes. This allows the active ingredients to be effective and allows for the hydration of the stratum corneum. This time should be counted from the time lathering is finished and, for some owners, may be best measured with an actual timer.
4. *Explanation/demonstration.* It is important to explain, and perhaps demonstrate, the entire process of shampooing. This includes application *and* removal of the product.

Medicated shampoos are often classified on the basis of their primary activity or function.

1. Emollients and moisturizers are often present in hypoallergenic shampoos and many better-quality cleansing shampoos for normal skin and haircoat. They are used when horses will be bathed frequently (weekly or more often) or for horses with slightly dry or scaly haircoats. Ingredients that moisturize are fatty acids and lipids, urea, glycerin, colloidal oatmeal, and chitosanide.
2. Antiparasitic shampoos are commonly used, but they are generally not as efficacious as antiparasitic rinses (see Chapter 6). Their main use is for quick removal of ectoparasites in foals and debilitated animals. Antiparasitic shampoos are often ineffective for adequate long-term ectoparasite control. The most common ingredients are pyrethrins and synthetic pyrethroids.
3. Antiseborrheic shampoos usually contain salicylic acid, sulfur, tar, and selenium sulfide in various combinations and strengths. These shampoos are indicated in keratinization defects (for details, see Chapter 11). They are also indicated in any other disorder associated with excessive scaling of the skin.
4. Antibacterial shampoos contain disinfectants or antibiotics such as chlorhexidine, benzoyl peroxide, iodine, ethyl lactate, benzalkonium chloride, triclosan, and sulfur. Other ingredients with less effect include quaternary ammonium compounds and phenols, alcohols, and parabens. These products are indicated whenever there is superficial bacterial infection (see Chapter 4 for discussions of their specific use). An indication for long-term use is in the allergic horse that is still prone to recurrent folliculitis even though the pruritus is controlled with the allergy therapy. In these situations, nonirritating, nondrying shampoos with antibacterial agents are often beneficial if used regularly.
5. Antimycotic shampoos contain disinfectants or antifungal agents such as chlorhexidine, sulfur, selenium sulfide, miconazole, and ketoconazole (see Chapter 5). They are used mainly as adjunctive therapy for dermatophytosis (to achieve a quick decrease of contagion) and

Malassezia dermatitis. These shampoos are not effective as single agent therapy for dermatophytosis.[71] They have been recommended as sole therapy for *Malassezia* dermatitis. Antimycotic shampoos may be used alone, as adjunctive therapy, or as a preventive to decrease the recurrence rate.

6. Antipruritic or anti-inflammatory agents, such as 1% hydrocortisone, 0.01% fluocinolone, 2% diphenhydramine, 1% pramoxine, colloidal oatmeal, and moisturizers, are found in a variety of shampoo formulations (see Chapter 8). In general, they are adjunctive treatments and are not effective as the sole therapy unless they are used every 1 to 3 days. This high frequency of use is usually not acceptable to owners. The topical glucocorticoid shampoos have been shown not to be systemically absorbed in the dog.[71,83] Controlled studies of their use and efficacy in horses are lacking.

RINSES

Rinses are made by mixing concentrated solutions or soluble powders with water. They are usually poured, sponged, or sprayed onto the animal's body. Similar to the case with shampoos, they may be used to treat large areas of the body. Rinses are generally a cost-effective and efficacious method to deliver topical active ingredients such as moisturizers, antipruritic agents, parasiticides, and anti-fungal agents.

Rinses that dry on the horse's skin leave a residual layer of active ingredients and therefore have more prolonged effects than application by shampoo therapy. Rinses are often used after a medicated or cleaning shampoo. If the active ingredient to be applied is lipid-dispersed, shampooing may remove the normal surface lipids and decrease the longevity of the active ingredients. In these situations, adding a small amount of safflower oil or lipid-containing moisturizer may help to prolong the effect. This is most commonly recommended for lipid-soluble (petroleum distillate–based) parasiticidal agents.

Rinses are our preferred method of delivery for most topical medications other than antibacterials and antiseborrheics, which require whole-body coverage.

POWDERS

Powders are pulverized organic or inorganic solids that are applied to the skin in a thin film. In some cases, they are made to be added to water for use as a rinse, to liquids to form "shake lotions," or to ointments to form pastes. Some powders (talc, starch, zinc oxide) are inert and have a physical effect; other powders (sulfur) are active ingredients that have a chemical or antimicrobial effect. Powders are used to dry the skin and to cool and lubricate intertriginous areas. Most often, powders are used with parasiticidal agents and locally with anti-inflammatory agents (Neo-Predef Powder, Pharmacia & Upjohn). Some powders may contain antimicrobials for use on localized lesions and, although not yet available in the United States, an enilconazole powder has shown promise for the treatment of dermatophytosis.

The affected skin should be cleaned and dried before the powder is applied. Powder buildup or caking should be avoided, but if it occurs, wet compresses or soaks can gently remove the excess. On long-coated animals, a fine powder is used as a retention vehicle for insecticides and fungicides. Powders dry the coat and skin and may accumulate in the environment, making them less desirable for whole-body use. Some owners find powders irritating to their own respiratory mucosa. We use powders infrequently and prefer other delivery systems.

LOTIONS

Lotions are liquids in which medicinal agents are dissolved or suspended. Some are essentially liquid powders because a thin film of powder is left on the skin when the liquid evaporates. Lotions tend to be more drying (because of their water or alcohol base) than are liniments, which have an oily base. Newer lotions tend to use more propylene glycol and water, with less or no alcohol. Drying, cooling lotions contain alcohol, whereas soothing, moisturizing lotions usually do not. Lotions tend to be cooling, antipruritic, and drying (depending on the base).

Lotions are vehicles for active ingredients such as 1% hydrocortisone with aluminum acetate (Hydro-B 1020, Butler; Hydro-Plus, Phoenix), 0.1% betamethasone valerate (Betatrex, Savage), 1% hydrocortisone (Corticalm, DVM), 1% pramoxine (Relief, DVM), 1% diphenhydramine with calamine and camphor (Caladryl, Parke-Davis), melaleuca, and aloe vera. The liquid preparations can be applied repeatedly, but they should not be allowed to build up. In general, lotions are indicated for acute oozing dermatoses and are contraindicated in dry, chronic conditions. They are most often used to deliver localized treatment with astringents and antipruritic, anti-inflammatory, and antifungal agents. They occasionally carry ultraviolet screens and antiseborrheic agents.

SPRAYS

A variety of topical lotions are available in pump spray bottles. Most commonly, they are used when relatively larger body areas are to be treated and when the product needs to be applied to only the haircoat or small, nonhaired areas. Rinses may also be applied by pump spray bottles, but if skin contact is needed, thorough soaking through the haircoat is required. Sprays are most commonly used with emollients or moisturizers that are lightly applied and then rubbed into the coat, antiparasitic agents (particularly those with repellent activity), and antipruritic agents for local lesions. Newer sprays have antimicrobial activity, such as 4% chlorhexidine.

Antipruritic sprays contain agents such as 1% hydrocortisone (Cortispray, DVM), 2% diphenhydramine (Histacalm, Virbac), 1% pramoxine (Relief, DVM; Dermal Soothe, EVSCO), hamamelis extract with menthol (Dermacool, Virbac), and tar (LyTar, DVM). Sprays are also frequently used to apply astringents and anti-inflammatory agents, such as 1% hydrocortisone with aluminum acetate.

CREAMS, EMULSIONS, AND OINTMENTS

Creams and ointments lubricate and smooth skin that is roughened. They form a protective covering that reduces contact with the environment. Certain occlusive types may reduce water loss. They also transport medicinal agents into follicular orifices and keep drugs in intimate contact with the horny layer. Creams and ointments are mixtures of grease or oil and water that are emulsified with high-speed blenders. Emulsifiers, coloring agents, and perfumes are added to improve the physical characteristics of the product. Pastes are highly viscous ointments into which large amounts of powder are incorporated. Although pastes may be tolerated on slightly exudative skin (the powder takes up water), in general, creams and ointments are contraindicated in oozing areas.

A wide variation in characteristics of the products is determined by the relative amount and melting point of the oils used. This can be illustrated by comparing cold cream and vanishing cream. Cold cream is mostly oil with a little water. The oils have a low melting point, so when the water evaporates a thick, greasy film is left on the skin. A vanishing cream, on the other hand, is mostly water with oils that have a high melting point. When the water evaporates, a thin film of fat is left on the skin. This wax-like film does not feel greasy. Urea added to creams also decreases the greasy feel and, as a hygroscopic agent, helps to moisturize the stratum corneum.

Emulsions are oily or fatty substances that have been dispersed in water. As a group, they have a composition between that of lotions and ointments. Emulsions are thicker than lotions but thinner than ointments. They are similar to creams, which for the most part have replaced the use of emulsions in small animal practice. Emulsions are of two types: oil dispersed in water and water dispersed in oil. Although both types are used as vehicles, the former dilutes with water, loses water rapidly, and therefore is cooling. The latter type dilutes with oil and loses its water slowly.

In both cases, after the water evaporates, the action of the vehicle on the skin is no different from that of the oil and emulsifying agent alone. Thus, the characteristics of the residual film are those of the oily phase of the vehicle.

These bases are commonly used as vehicles for other agents. They have the advantage of easy application, give mechanical protection, and are soothing, antipruritic, and softening. The more oily creams and ointments tend to be occlusive, which facilitates hydration of the stratum corneum and often increases penetration of incorporated active ingredients. The disadvantage of their use in the hairy skin of animals is that they are occlusive, greasy, heat-retaining, and messy, and they may produce a folliculitis because of occlusion of pilosebaceous orifices. These types of medication should be applied with gentle massage several times daily to maintain a thin film on the skin. Thick films are wasteful, occlusive, and messy to surroundings. An obvious film of ointment left on the skin surface means that too much has been applied.

Water-washable ointment bases such as polyethylene glycol (Carbowax 1500) can be readily removed with water. Oily bases are not freely water-washable. It is important for the clinician to understand the uses and advantages of these types of bases because the total effect on the skin is caused by the vehicle as well as its active ingredient.

Hydrophobic oils (e.g., mineral oil and sesame oil) mix poorly with water. They contain few polar groups (—OH, —COOH, and so on). These oils contact the skin, spread easily, and are often incorporated into emulsion-type vehicles. Because they are hydrophobic, it is difficult for water to pass through a film of these oils, and they are occlusive. These oils retain heat and water, and thick films of the more viscid forms are messy and may get on articles in contact with the horse.

Hydrophilic oils are miscible with water. They contain many polar groups, and those oils with the greatest number are most soluble in water. Although they are ointments only in terms of their physical characteristics, the polyethylene glycols are alcohols that are readily miscible with water. Polymers with a molecular weight greater than 1000 are solid at room temperature, but a slight rise in body temperature causes melting to form an oily film. Carbowax 1500 is such a product. It mixes with skin exudates well, is easily washed off with water, and is less occlusive than other bases.

The use of creams, emulsions, and ointments is limited to localized, relatively small lesions. Most commonly, they are used with antimicrobial, anti-inflammatory, and ultraviolet radiation–blocking agents. They are often the most efficacious delivery system for areas needing moisturization or keratolytic effects, but their application is usually limited to localized areas.

GELS

Gels are topical formulations composed of combinations of propylene glycol, propylene gallate, disodiumethylenediamine tetra-acetate, and carboxypolymethylene, with additives to adjust the pH. They act as a clear, colorless, thixotropic base and are greaseless and water-miscible. The active ingredients incorporated in commercially used bases of this type are completely in solution.

Gels are being more widely used because, despite their oily appearance, they can be rubbed into the skin completely and do not leave the skin with a sticky feeling. Gels are relatively preferable to creams and ointments because they pass through the haircoat to the skin and are not messy. Most commonly, they are used for localized lesions for which antimicrobial or antiseborrheic effects are desired.

The most common ingredient of gels is benzoyl peroxide for areas of bacterial pyoderma and follicular hyperkeratosis or areas of comedones. (Examples of gels used in veterinary medicine with benzoyl peroxide are OxyDex, DVM; Pyoben, Virbac). However, because gels are cosmetically tolerated better than are creams and ointments, their use is expanding to include virtually any ingredient that can be stabilized in a gel form. KeraSolv (DVM) is a keratolytic, humectant gel for hyperkeratotic conditions (e.g., linear keratosis, cannon keratosis).

Topical Active Agents

ASTRINGENTS

Astringents precipitate proteins and generally do not penetrate deeply. These agents are drying and decrease exudations. They are indicated in acute, subacute, and some chronic exudative dermatoses.

Vegetable astringents include tannins from oak trees, sumac, or blackberries. They are especially recommended for more potent action. Tan Sal (Tanni-Gel, Vet-A-Mix—4% tannic acid, 4% salicylic acid, and 1% benzocaine in 70% alcohol) is a potent astringent and should not be used more than once on the same lesion (it may cause irritation or sloughing). Witch hazel (hamamelis) contains tannins that are astringent and anti-inflammatory and that decrease bleeding.

Aluminum acetate solution (Burow's solution) is available commercially as Domeboro (Bayer). It is drying, astringent, antipruritic, acidifying, and mildly antiseptic. The solution is usually diluted 1:40 in cool water, and soaks are repeated three times daily for 30 minutes. (One packet of powder, or one tablet, is added to 0.5 L [1 pt] or 1 L [1 qt] of water.) It is tolerated better than tannins and does not stain. It tends to be used more frequently than other astringents.

Acetic acid in a 0.25% to 0.5% solution (e.g., 1 part vinegar with 9 parts water) is also an effective astringent, acidifying, and drying agent.

Silver nitrate 0.25% solution may be applied to moist, weeping, denuded areas as an antiseptic, coagulant, and stimulating agent. This solution should be used frequently and sparingly. It stains the skin.

Potassium permanganate 1:1,000 to 1:30,000 solution (1-grain tablet or 5 ml [1 tsp] to 15 ml [1 tbsp] of crystals per 1 L [1 qt] of water) may be applied in fresh preparations for soaks or irrigations. It is astringent, antiseptic, and antimicrobial and toughens and stains the skin.

EMOLLIENTS AND MOISTURIZERS

Emollients are agents that soften, lubricate, or soothe the skin; moisturizers increase the water content of the stratum corneum. Both types of drugs are useful in hydrating and softening the skin. Demulcents are high-molecular substances in aqueous solution that coat and protect the skin (e.g., glycerin, propylene glycol).

Many of the occlusive emollients are actually oils (safflower, sesame, and mineral oil) or contain lanolin. These emollients decrease transepidermal water loss and cause moisturization. These agents work best if applied immediately after saturation of the stratum corneum with water. For maximal softening, the skin should be hydrated in wet dressings, dried, and covered with an occlusive hydrophobic oil. The barrier to water loss can be further strengthened by covering the local lesion with plastic wrap under a bandage. Nonocclusive emollients are relatively ineffective in retaining moisture.

1. Vegetable oils—olive, cottonseed, corn, and peanut oil
2. Animal oils—lard, whale oil, anhydrous lanolin (wool fat), and lanolin with 25% to 30% water (hydrous wool fat)
3. Hydrocarbons—paraffin and petrolatum (mineral oil)
4. Waxes—white wax (bleached beeswax), yellow wax (beeswax), and spermaceti

Hygroscopic agents (humectants) are moisturizers that work by being incorporated into the stratum corneum and attracting water. These agents, such as propylene glycol, glycerin, colloidal oatmeal, urea, sodium lactate, carboxylic acid, and lactic acid, may also be applied between baths. Both occlusive and hygroscopic agents are found in a variety of veterinary spray and rinse formulations, which are more effective than shampoo bases. A liposome-based humectant technology (Hydra-Pearls cream rinse, Evsco) was shown to be superior to a traditional humectant emollient (Humilac, Virbac) for the treatment of dry skin in dogs.[71]

ANTISEBORRHEICS

The seborrheic complex comprises important and variably common skin diseases, such as primary seborrhea, mane and tail seborrhea, secondary seborrhea (accompanying hypersensitivities, ectoparasitisms, and so forth), linear keratosis, and cannon keratosis. Topical antiseborrheic therapy is useful for these diseases.

Antiseborrheics can be applied as ointments, creams, gels, and lotions, but the most popular form for hairy skin is the antiseborrheic shampoo or the humectant rinse. Antiseborrheics are commercially available in various combinations. The clinician must decide which combination of drugs to use and needs to know each drug's actions and concentrations. Ideal therapeutic response depends on the correct choice, but individual patient variation does occur. For dry and scaly seborrhea (seborrhea sicca), a different preparation is needed than for oily and greasy seborrhea (seborrhea oleosa). Emollients, for instance, are useful in dry seborrhea but are not effective degreasers. Benzoyl peroxide, on the other hand, degreases well but can be too keratolytic and drying for dry, brittle skin (see Chapter 11 for details).

ANTIPRURITICS

Antipruritic agents attempt to provide temporary relief from itching but are not usually satisfactory as sole therapy because of their short duration of effect. Pruritus is a symptom of many diseases, and most antipruritic topical therapies are directed at the sensation, not the cause. As such, they are still useful symptomatic treatments while waiting to alleviate the primary disease or when the cause cannot be determined. As adjunctive therapy or for small localized areas of pruritus, they can be more beneficial. Some antipruritic agents listed here have other actions and are discussed elsewhere in this chapter. Table 3-2 lists some veterinary nonsteroidal, topical, antipruritic agents. In general, antipruritics give relief from itching by means of six methods:

1. Decreasing the pruritic load by depleting, removing, or inactivating pruritic mediators. For example, astringents denature proteins and high-potency corticosteroids deplete cutaneous mast cells. Shampoos or cleaners can also remove surface irritants, bacteria, pruritogenic substances, and allergens that are on the surface of the skin waiting to be absorbed and to contribute to the pruritic load.
2. Substituting some other sensation, such as heat and cold, for the itch. This may also help by raising the pruritic threshold. Heat initially lowers the pruritic threshold, but if the heat is high enough and is applied for a sufficient duration, the increased itching or burning sensation abates and induces a short-term antipruritic effect. Cooling tends to decrease pruritus. Examples of such agents are menthol 0.12% to 1%, camphor 0.12% to 5%, thymol 0.5% to 1%, heat (warm soaks or baths), and cold (ice packs) or cool wet dressings.
3. Protecting the skin from external influences such as scratching, biting, trauma, temperature changes, humidity changes, pressure, and irritants. This can be done with bandages or any impermeable protective agents.
4. Anesthetizing the peripheral nerves by using local anesthetics such as pramoxine, benzocaine, tetracaine, lidocaine, benzoyl peroxide, and tars. These products generally have short actions, and in cases of chronic pruritus, resistance often occurs. Pramoxine has antipruritic effects that appear to be from a mechanism other than its anesthetic effect.[98] Pramoxine has also been added to hydrocortisone for additive antipruritic effects in people; in veterinary medicine it is available with colloidal oatmeal (Relief shampoo and cream rinse, DVM; Dermal Soothe shampoo and cream rinse, EVSCO; Resiprox leave-on lotion, Virbac).
5. Raising the pruritic threshold by cooling or moisturizing the skin. Dry skin lowers the pruritic threshold, and the effective use of emollients and moisturizing agents, such as fatty acids, glycerin, urea, and colloidal oatmeal, partially alleviates pruritus by reducing the dry skin.

● Table 3-2 **USEFUL NONSTEROIDAL TOPICAL AGENTS FOR PRURITIC HORSES**

PRODUCT	ACTIVE INGREDIENTS OR ACTION	FORM	MANUFACTURER
Spot Application			
Caladryl	1% diphenhydramine hydrochloride, 8% calamine, camphor	Lotion	Parke-Davis
Dermacool with Lidocaine	*Hamamelis* extract, lidocaine, menthol	Spray	Virbac
Domeboro	Aluminium sulfate, calcium acetate	Soak	Miles
Histacalm Spray	2% diphenhydramine	Spray	Virbac
Ice	Water—cold	Pack	Nature!
†Micro Pearls Advantage Dermal-Soothe Spray	1% pramoxine	Spray	EVSCO
†Micro Pearls Advantage Hydra-Pearls Spray	Moisturizing, hypoallergenic	Spray	EVSCO
PTD Lotion	2% benzoyl alcohol, 0.05% benzalkonium chloride, *Hamamelis* distillate	Lotion	Veterinary Prescription
Relief Spray	1% pramoxine	Spray	DVM
Total Body Application			
Allergroom Shampoo	Moisturizing, hypoallergenic	Shampoo	Virbac
HyLy°efa Shampoo	Moisturizing, hypoallergenic	Shampoo	Virbac
†Hy-Ly°efa Creme Rinse	Moisturizing, hypoallergenic	Shampoo	DVM
Epi-Soothe Shampoo	Colloidal oatmeal	Shampoo	Virbac
Histacalm Shampoo	2% diphenhydramine, colloidal oatmeal	Shampoo	Virbac
†Hy-Ly°efa Creme Rinse	Moisturizing, hypoallergenic	Rinse	DVM
†Micro Pearls Advantage Dermal-Soothe Shampoo	1% pramoxine	Shampoo	EVSCO
†Micro Pearls Advantage Dermal-Soothe Creme Rinse	1% pramoxine	Rinse	EVSCO
†Micro Pearls Advantage Hydra-Pearls Shampoo	Moisturizing, hypoallergenic	Shampoo	EVSCO
†Micro Pearls Advantage Hydra-Pearls Cream Rinse	Moisturizing, hypoallergenic	Rinse	EVSCO
Water	Water	Soak	Nature!
Aveeno	Colloidal oatmeal	Soak	Rydelle
Epi-Soothe Creme Rinse	Colloidal oatmeal	Rinse	Virbac
Relief Shampoo	1% pramoxine	Shampoo	DVM
†Relief Creme Rinse	1% pramoxine	Rinse	DVM

†Labeled for horses.

6. Using specific biochemical agents, such as topical glucocorticoids, antihistamines, and moisturizers.

   Most potent glucocorticoids, administered systemically and topically, are helpful because of their anti-inflammatory effect, but they are not without risk.[71,78] Hydrocortisone 0.5% to 2% is safest for topical use and could be considered an antipruritic agent because it has mild anti-inflammatory effects at these concentrations. The fluorinated corticosteroids are more potent and penetrate better but with greater risk for systemic absorption and local or systemic adverse effects. Antihistamines administered systemically are occasionally useful, but when applied topically, they have even less efficacy. They may be helpful as a component of a combination product, such as 1% diphenhydramine with calamine and camphor (Caladryl, Parke-Davis). Some topical antihistamines have been shown to cross the stratum corneum and may exert their antihistaminic effect after topical application.[6,33]

Topical anesthetics may be partially effective, but they may also be toxic (causing methemoglobinemia) or have sensitizing potentials (phenol 0.5%; tetracaine and lidocaine 0.5%).[71] Also, their duration of effect is short and becomes even shorter when used frequently and repetitively. Veterinary products with these types of agents are Histacalm shampoo, Resihist leave-on lotion, and Histacalm spray (Virbac—2% diphenhydramine); 1% pramoxine shampoos, sprays, rinses, and leave-on lotions (DVM, EVSCO, and Virbac); Dermal Soothe shampoo and cream rinse (EVSCO—1% pramoxine); and Dermacool (Virbac—hamamelis extract and menthol).

Pramoxine is a local anesthetic that is chemically different from traditional "caines" (benzocaine, lidocaine, procaine).[71] It has low sensitization and irritation potentials and does not produce the methemoglobinemia and the severe side effects that can be noted with the misuse of "caines" in dogs and cats.[71] Pramoxine was shown to be useful in the management of pruritus in dogs and horses with atopic conditions.[70,71]

Cool wet dressings are often helpful, and in general, any volatile agent provides a cooling sensation that might be palliative. This is the basis for using menthol (1%), thymol (1%), and alcohol (70%) in antipruritic medications. In addition, menthol has a specific action on local sensory nerve endings. Cool water baths alone or accompanied by Burow's solution (aluminum acetate) soaks (Domeboro, Bayer) or colloidal oatmeal (Aveeno, Rydelle; Epi-Soothe, Virbac) may be helpful for hours to days.

ANTIMICROBIAL AGENTS

No group of drugs is employed more widely than antimicrobial agents. Anytime the skin is abnormal, the potential develops for secondary microbial infections or overgrowth. These agents are therefore often used as prophylaxes even when pyoderma is not present. The terminology used to describe the actions of drugs on microbes is somewhat confusing because of discrepancies between strict definitions of terms and their general usage. *Antiseptics* are substances that kill or prevent growth of microbes (the term is used especially for preparations applied to living tissue). *Disinfectants* are agents that prevent infection by destruction of microbes (the term is used especially for substances applied to inanimate objects). Antiseptics and disinfectants are types of germicides, which are agents that destroy microbes. Germicides may be further defined by the appropriate use of terms such as *bactericide*, *fungicide*, and *virucide*.

In a discussion of such heterogeneous compounds as antimicrobials, some method of classification is desirable. Because the compounds are so varied with respect to chemical structure, mechanism of action, and use, too strict a classification may be more confusing than elucidating. The following discussion represents a compromise.

The antiseptic agents are listed with brief comments so that their purposes can be appreciated when they are recognized as ingredients in proprietary formulations. The use of some of these agents is described elsewhere in the text (see Chapters 4 and 5).

• **Alcohols.** These act by precipitating proteins and dehydrating protoplasm. They are bactericidal (not sporicidal), astringent, cooling, and rubefacient. However, they are irritating to denuded surfaces and are generally contraindicated in acute inflammatory disorders. The most effective concentrations are 70% ethyl alcohol and 70% to 90% isopropyl alcohol; these concentrations are bactericidal within 1 to 2 minutes at 30° C.

• **Propylene Glycol.** This is a fairly active antibacterial and antifungal agent. A 40% to 50% concentration is best. Propylene glycol and polyethylene glycol are primarily used at concentrations of less than 50% as vehicles for other powerful antimicrobial agents. In dilute solution, propylene glycol has few humectant properties because it is hygroscopic. In a 60% to 75% solution, it denatures and solubilizes protein and is keratolytic.

● **Phenols and Cresols.** Agents such as hexachlorophene, resorcinol, hexylresorcinol, thymol, and picric acid act by denaturing microbial proteins. They are also antipruritic and somewhat antifungal. These agents may be added at low levels as preservatives in some products. At higher antimicrobial levels, they are irritating, toxic (hexachlorophene), and currently have few legitimate uses on the skin.

● **Chlorhexidine.** Chlorhexidine is a phenol-related biguanide antiseptic and disinfectant that has excellent properties. It is highly effective against many fungi, viruses, and most bacteria, except perhaps some *Pseudomonas* and *Serratia* strains.[11] A 2% to 4% concentration of chlorhexidine is needed for an effective anti-*Malassezia* effect. Chlorhexidine is nonirritating, rarely sensitizing, not inactivated by organic matter, and persistent in action; furthermore, it is effective in shampoo, ointment, surgical scrub, and solution formulations containing 1% to 4% concentrations of chlorhexidine diacetate or gluconate. A 0.05% dilution in water is an effective, nonirritating solution for wound irrigation.

● **Halogenated Agents.** *Iodine.* This is one of the oldest antimicrobials. Elemental iodine is the active agent (its mechanism is unknown). It is rapidly bactericidal, fungicidal, virucidal, and sporicidal. Older products such as tincture of iodine (2% iodine and 2% sodium iodide in alcohol) and Lugol's iodine solution (5% to 7% iodine and 10% potassium iodide in water) are irritating and sensitizing and should no longer be used.

Currently, the only commonly used iodines are the "tamed" iodines (iodophors) because of their lower level of irritation or sensitization. Povidone-iodine (Betadine, Purdue-Frederick)—iodine with polyvinylpyrrolidone, which slowly releases iodine to tissues—has a prolonged action (4 to 6 hours), is nonstinging and nonstaining, and is not impaired by blood, serum, necrotic debris, or pus. A study using a povidone-iodine shampoo showed efficacy, although less than that of benzoyl peroxide as a prophylactic agent against *Staphylococcus intermedius*.[71] Polyhydroxydine (Xenodine, VPL) at 1% is reportedly superior in efficacy to povidone-iodine solutions or tincture of iodine against gram-positive and gram-negative organisms. Even tamed iodines can be drying to the skin, staining to light-colored haircoats, and especially irritating to scrotal skin and the external ear.

Sodium Hypochlorite and Chloramines. These are effective bactericidal, fungicidal, sporicidal, and virucidal agents. Their action is thought to be due to liberation of hypochlorous acid. Fresh preparations are required. Sodium hypochlorite 5.25% (Clorox) diluted 1:10 with water (modified Dakin's solution) is usually well tolerated. The presence of organic material greatly reduces the solution's antimicrobial activity. This solution is most often recommended as an antifungal agent or disinfectant.

● **Oxidizing Agents.** *Hydrogen peroxide* is a weak germicide that acts through the liberation of nascent oxygen (e.g., 3% hydrogen peroxide used in dilute water solution). It has limited usefulness for skin disease, although it is used as an ear-flushing agent and for cleaning minor skin wounds, partly for its effervescent activity.

Potassium permanganate acts as a bactericidal, astringent, and fungicidal agent (especially against *Candida* spp.). Its action is thought to involve liberation of nascent oxygen. This agent stings and stains, and it is inhibited by organic material. The staining is particularly a problem.

Benzoyl peroxide is a potent, broad-spectrum antibacterial agent that has keratolytic, keratoplastic, antipruritic, degreasing, and follicular flushing action.[71] It is a potent oxidizing agent that reacts with biologic materials. The resultant benzoyl peroxy radicals interact with hydroxy and sulfoxy groups, double bonds, and other substances. This allows the benzoyl peroxide to disrupt microbial cell membranes. Benzoyl peroxide is metabolized in the skin to benzoic acid, which lyses intercellular substance in the stratum corneum to account for its keratolytic effect. It is irritating in about 10% of horses treated.

Benzoyl peroxide is available as a 5% gel and a 2.5% or 3% shampoo (OxyDex, DVM; SulfOxydex, DVM; Pyoben, Virbac; Benzoyl-Plus, EVSCO), which is an excellent adjunct to antibiotic therapy for superficial and deep bacterial pyodermas. In a shampoo formulation, it was superior to chlorhexidine, complexed iodine, and triclosan for prophylaxis against *S. intermedius*.[71] It is often recommended in seborrheic disorders, particularly cases that are greasy or have follicular plugs, follicular casts, or comedones.

One should not use generic or more concentrated benzoyl peroxide formulations (e.g., 5% shampoo or 10% gel) on animals because stability may be compromised and the higher concentrations are more often irritating. Even at 2.5% or 3% concentrations, benzoyl peroxide is drying and occasionally irritating, especially in horses with dry skin and/or allergic skin disease. Repackaging should be avoided because improper packaging may affect stability of the product. A commercial benzoyl peroxide shampoo containing liposome-based humectant technology (Benzoyl-Plus benzoyl peroxide shampoo, EVSCO) can be used even on horses with dry skin without exacerbating the dryness. Controlled release of benzoyl peroxide from a microsphere system reduces topical irritation in humans.[71]

Other side effects of 2.5% to 3% benzoyl peroxide include bleaching of hair and clothing. It has skin tumor–promoting activity in laboratory rodents, but no skin tumor–initiating activity has been documented in any other species.[71]

• **Surface-Acting Agents.** Surface-acting agents, in the form of emulsifiers, wetting agents, or detergents, act by altering energy relationships at interfaces, thus disrupting or damaging cell membranes. They also denature proteins and inactivate enzymes. The most commonly used examples are the cationic detergents (quaternary ammonium compounds), especially benzalkonium chloride.

Benzalkonium chloride is a broad-spectrum antibacterial agent (not effective against *Pseudomonas* spp.). However, anionic soaps inactivate it.

Silver salts precipitate proteins and interfere with bacterial metabolic activities. They are antibacterial and astringent but irritating, staining, stinging, and escharotic (e.g., silver nitrate 0.5%). Silver sulfadiazine is useful to treat superficial burns and has also been shown to be effective *in vitro* at 0.1%, allowing for the dilution of the thick cream to a much more liquid lotion.[71]

ANTI-INFLAMMATORY AGENTS

Cold dressings are among the simplest and safest agents that reduce inflammation. However, topical glucocorticoid preparations are used most commonly and effectively to reduce inflammation. There is little evidence to suggest that they have caused dissemination of cutaneous infections, but if they are used in the presence of known infections, specific antibacterial or antifungal agents should be added to the preparation. The basic hydrocortisone molecule or synthetic analogs thereof are modified by halogenation, methylation, acetylation, esterification, and/or double-bond induction in an effort to enhance the therapeutic effect and reduce side effects. Generic products may not always be equivalent to proprietary products (Table 3-3).[21]

In high concentration, in abraded and inflamed skin, or under occlusive dressings, these corticosteroids are absorbed. They rarely produce serious untoward clinical effects if used in the short term. In normal dogs, adrenocortical suppression was produced by topical applications of various glucocorticoids to the skin, ear canal, or eye.[71] In the normal horse, topical application of a dexamethasone ophthalmic ointment for 8 days produced low blood concentrations of dexamethasone.[77] Clearly, topical glucocorticoids should not be considered to be innocuous drugs.

Local effects of glucocorticoids, including atrophy, scaling, comedones, alopecia, poor healing, and pyoderma, may occur even without systemic effects. Glucocorticoid-induced cutaneous atrophy is most likely to occur on the lower legs of the horse.[62,63] A subepidermal bullous dermatosis has been reported from the topical application of triamcinolone acetonide, fluocinolone acetonide,

● Table 3-3 **RELATIVE ANTI-INFLAMMATORY POTENCIES OF SELECTED TOPICAL GLUCOCORTICOIDS***

AGENT	BRAND NAME	MANUFACTURER
Group I		
Betamethasone dipropionate, 0.5% cream, ointment	Diprolene	Schering-Plough
Clobetasol propionate, 0.05% cream, ointment	Temovate	Glaxo Derm
Diflorasone diacetate, 0.5% ointment	Psorcon	Dermik
Group II		
Betamethasone dipropionate, 0.5% ointment	Diprosone	Schering-Plough
Desoximetasone, 0.25% cream, ointment	Topicort	Hoechst-Roussel
Flucoinonide, 0.05% cream, ointment	Lidex	Dermik
Group III		
Betamethasone valerate, 0.1% ointment	Valisone	Schering-Plough
Triamincolone acetonide, 0.5% cream	Kenalog	Westwood-Squibb
Group IV		
Fluocinolone acetonide, 0.025% ointment	Synalar	Syntex
Fluocinolone acetonide, 0.1% solution	Synotic†	Fort Dodge
Triamcinolone acetonide, 0.1% ointment	Vetalog†	Fort Dodge
Group V		
Betamethasone valerate, 0.1% cream, lotion	Valisone	Schering-Plough
Fluocinolone acetonide, 0.025% cream	Synalar†	Syntex
Triamcinolone acetonide, 0.1% cream, lotion	Kenalog	Westwood-Squibb
Group VI		
Desonide, 0.05% cream	Tridesilon	Miles
Fluocinolone acetonide, 0.01% shampoo	FS shampoo	Hill
Group VII		
Dexamethasone, 0.1% cream	Decaderm	MSD
Dexamethasone, 0.04% spray	Decaspray	MSD
Hydrocortisone, 1% and 2.5% cream, ointment	Hytone	Dermik
Hydrocortisone, 1% spray	Cortispray†	DVM
Hydrocortisone, 1% spray	Dermacool-HC†	Allerderm/Virbac
Hydrocortisone, 1% spray	Hydro-Plus†	Phoenix
Hydrocortisone, 1% spray	Hydro-10 mist†	Butler
Hydrocortisone, 1% spray	PTD-HC†	VRx
Hydrocortisone, 1% shampoo	Cortisoothe†	Allerderm/Virbac

*Group 1 is most potent. Group VII is least potent.
†Veterinary label.

and betamethasone valerate. These solutions maintain a "reservoir" pool in the skin, enough that a once-daily application may suffice to continue the topical effect. Topical glucocorticoid therapy should follow principles similar to those used for systemic therapy. That is, potent drugs should be administered twice daily to stop inflammation, then tapered to once daily; finally, if the drugs are still effective and long-term treatment is expected, the treatment is changed to less potent topical agents for maintenance therapy, and alternate-day administration is used whenever possible. Twice-weekly applications may suffice in some cases. People handling these medications should wear gloves to prevent exposure and toxic effects.

The fluorinated steroids are more potent, penetrate better, and thus are more effective. Table 3-3 lists therapeutic concentrations of several topical glucocorticoids and provides brand name examples.

MISCELLANEOUS TOPICAL AGENTS

• **Sulfur.** Medicinal use of sulfur is as old as Hippocrates.[46] Lime sulfur (sulfurated lime) is prepared by boiling a suspension of sublimated sulfur, lime (Ca [OH]$_2$), and water, thus producing calcium pentasulfide and calcium thiosulfate. Sulfur is a degreasing agent. At low concentrations, it is keratoplastic, whereas higher concentrations are keratolytic (H$_2$S breaks down keratin). In this respect sulfur is synergistic with salicylic acid. Sulfur is antifungal and antibacterial, presumably by conversion to pentathionic acid and H$_2$S (this conversion can be accomplished by cutaneous bacteria and by keratinocytes).

Lime sulfur was more effective than chlorhexidine, captan, povidone iodine, and ketoconazole shampoo in inhibiting *Microsporum canis* growth from infected cat hairs.[95] Its parasiticidal activity is thought to be due to H$_2$S and polythionic acid. Lime sulfur is inexpensive and nontoxic (Lym Dyp, DVM). Side effects include occasional excessive drying and/or irritation of the skin. Cosmetic drawbacks include a disagreeable odor (rotten eggs), temporary yellow staining of light haircoats and skins, staining of clothing and other materials, and tarnishing of jewelry.

• **Vitamin A Acid.** A 0.05% concentration of retinoic acid (tretinoin [Retin-A, Roche]) is popular in human dermatology (used for treating acne, decreasing wrinkles, and treating ichthyosis). It is relatively expensive but has been used in dogs and cats for acne and some localized keratinization disorders.[71] Topical retinoids may also be useful in equine disorders of keratinization (e.g., linear keratosis, cannon keratosis), but no published information exists at this time.

The effectiveness of topical tretinoin for the treatment of the effects of photoaging is well documented. The gel form at 0.01% concentration is initially used because it is less irritating than the 0.025% concentration. It increases the epidermal turnover time, reduces the cohesiveness of keratinocytes, normalizes maturation of follicular epithelium, and is comedolytic.[88] In animal models it prevents corticosteroid-induced skin atrophy.[69] Local irritation is a significant problem for many people and cats (e.g., with Retin-A). A microsphere formulation (Retin-A-MICRO) is now available that is much less irritating in humans.

Synthetic retinoids are also becoming available as topical formulations. Adapalene (Differin, Galderma) is a new topical retinoid with specific receptor activity for intranuclear retinoic acid receptors and causes less irritation than retinoic acid. It also inhibits neutrophil activation and lipoxygenase enzymes.[73,89] Tazarotene (Tazorac, Allergan) is a new topical formulation. It is a novel acetylenic retinoid that is being evaluated as a 0.1% and 0.05% gel formulation.[13] As a topical therapy it appears to have minimal systemic absorption, with no adverse systemic signs yet reported.

Tazarotene acts on retinoic acid receptors and results in downregulation of keratinocyte proliferation, differentiation, and inflammation.[22,50] It does this by a combination of effects, including the induction and activation of new genes, downregulation of AP1 (a proinflammatory genetic factor), and antagonizing the effects of interferon-γ. Tazarotene has been shown to be effective for acne and psoriasis while having no adverse systemic reactions.

• **Urea.** Urea has hygroscopic and keratolytic actions that aid in normalizing the epidermis, especially the quality of the stratum corneum.[94] The application of urea in a cream or an ointment base has a softening and moisturizing effect on the stratum corneum and makes the vehicle feel less greasy. It acts as a humectant in concentrations of 2% to 20%; however, in concentrations above that level, it is keratolytic. That action is a result of the solubilization of prekeratin and keratin and the possible breakage of hydrogen bonds that keep the stratum corneum intact. It also promotes desquamation by dissolving the "intercellular substance."

A hypoallergenic, moisturizing shampoo (Allergroom, Virbac) contains 5% urea free and in spherulites. Humilac (Virbac) contains both urea and lactic acid, and it can be used as a spray or rinse. To make a rinse, five capfuls of Humilac are added to 1 L (1 qt) of water. The mixture is rinsed over the horse's coat and allowed to dry. KeraSolv (DVM) contains 6% salicylic acid, 5% urea, and 5% sodium lactate. It is a potent keratolytic used to treat focal hyperkeratoses (e.g., linear keratosis, cannon keratosis).

• **αHydroxyacids 2% to 10%.** These include lactic, malic, citric, pyruvic, glutamic, glycolic, and tartaric acids. They are effective in modulating keratinization, being keratoplastic, and being able to delay terminal differentiation and to reduce the intercellular cohesion forces of the stratum corneum. Lactic acid and sodium lactate can absorb up to 30 times their weight in water.[20]

• **Fatty Acids.** These acids are keratolytic and fungistatic. Examples are caprylic, propionic, and undecylenic acids. The best of these (although it is weak) is undecylenic acid (e.g., Desenex). Topical fatty acids are also used to treat essential fatty-acid deficiency. Topical sunflower oil, which is high in linoleic acid, decreases transepidermal water loss in seborrheic dogs.[71]

• **Propylene Glycol.** This agent is primarily used as a solvent and a vehicle.[29,37] At higher concentrations (>75%), it occasionally causes irritation or sensitization. Propylene glycol is an excellent lipid solvent and defats the skin; however, its chief value is probably the ability to enhance percutaneous penetration of drugs. Propylene glycol is also a potent and reliable antibacterial agent and has antidermatophyte and anticandidal properties. For most dermatologic cases, it can be used in concentrations of 30% to 40%. Propylene glycol is a superior humectant (hygroscopic) and can induce keratolysis. Thus, higher concentrations are particularly helpful in hyperkeratotic conditions (e.g., linear keratosis, canine keratosis).

• **Dimethyl Sulfoxide (DMSO).** DMSO is a simple, hygroscopic, organic solvent.[8] Because it is freely miscible with lipids, organic solvents, and water, it is an excellent vehicle. When exposed to the air, concentrated solutions take in water to become hydrated at 67%. Stronger concentrations tend to cross the skin barrier better. DMSO penetrates skin (within 5 minutes), mucous membranes, and the blood-brain barrier, as well as cell, organelle, and microbial membranes. Unlike most solvents, DMSO achieves penetration without membrane damage. It facilitates absorption of many other substances across membranes, especially corticosteroids. On a cellular level, DMSO and steroids exert a synergistic effect.

DMSO has properties of its own as a cryoprotective, radioprotective, anti-ischemic, anti-inflammatory (free-radical scavenger, decreases prostaglandin synthesis, stabilizes lysosomal membranes), and analgesic (blocks C fibers) agent. It also has variable antibacterial, antifungal, and antiviral properties, depending on the concentration (usually 5% to 50%) and the organism involved. DMSO decreases fibroplasia.

Although its mechanism of action is incompletely understood, the systemic toxicity and teratogenicity of DMSO in its pure form are considered low. Toxicity may be of concern, depending on the dose, the route of administration, the species, and the individual animal's reaction. Impurities or combinations with other agents may make DMSO dangerous as a result of its ability to enhance transepidermal absorption. Industrial forms of DMSO should never be used for medical purposes because the contained impurities are absorbed and may be toxic. Well-known minor side effects include a garlic-like odor, increased warmth and/or pruritus (histamine release, exothermic with water), and dehydration (too hygroscopic).

Potential uses might include topical application to cutaneous ulcers, burns, insect bites, and sterile granulomas. One formula shown to be safe and useful contains Burow's solution, hydrocortisone, and 90% DMSO.[71] Equal parts of 90% DMSO and Hydro-B 1020 (1% hydrocortisone and 2% Burow's solution in a water and propylene glycol base) are mixed. The formulation is applied daily to benefit patients with dermatoses that are moist, pruritic, and noninfected.

• **Aloe Vera.** Much of the information on aloe vera is anecdotal.[2,72] Over 300 species of Aloe plants exist, and chemical composition differs with the species, climate, and growing conditions. The terms *aloe, aloe vera, aloin,* and *aloe extract* refer to the end products of different methods of extracting juice from Aloe plants. The result of this nonuniformity of collection or extraction is a wide difference in the contents, consistency, and appearance of various products. Likewise, interpreting and comparing various studies is often impossible.

Aloe vera contains a large number of organic compounds and inorganic elements: anthraquinones (e.g., anthracene, emodin), saccharides (e.g., glucose, cellulose, mannose), enzymes (e.g., oxidase, lipase), vitamins (e.g., niacinamide, C, E, A), amino acids, and minerals (e.g., copper, zinc). Anti-inflammatory properties include salicylic acid, bradykininase activity (reduction of pain, swelling, and erythema), magnesium lactate (reduction of histamine production), antiprostaglandin activity, and protease inhibitor activity. *In vitro* studies indicate that aloe vera inhibits the growth of *Staphylococcus aureus, Pseudomonas aeruginosa,* and *Trichophyton mentagrophytes.*

Anecdotal reports indicate that aloe vera is useful for the treatment of pain, pruritus, fungal infections, bacterial infections, insect bites, burns, and exuberant granulation tissue.[2,54,72]

• **Acetic Acid.** Acetic acid is a potent antibacterial agent: A 5% solution (e.g., vinegar) kills coagulase-positive staphylococci in 5 minutes, and a 2.5% solution (e.g., one part vinegar, one part water) kills *P. aeruginosa* in 1 minute. A 2.5% solution kills *Malassezia pachydermatis* (see Chapter 5). Acetic acid may also be used in ears (0.25% to 0.5% solution) as a ceruminolytic, astringent, and acidifier.

• **Melaleuca Oil.** Melaleuca oil ("tea tree oil") is extracted from the leaves of the tea tree (genus *Melaleuca*).[86] It has proven antibacterial properties (e.g., against coagulase-positive staphylococci) and fungicidal properties (e.g., against *Candida albicans, T. mentagrophytes*). Melaleuca oil is marketed for use on dogs, cats, and ferrets in skin care products for cleaning, healing, and relieving pruritus. Claims are also made that it is a deodorizer, detangler, and external parasite repellent. The inappropriate or excessive application of melaleuca oil to the skin may result in toxicosis: hypersalivation, incoordination, weakness, hypothermia, and hepatic injury.

• **Colloidal Oatmeal.** Colloidal oatmeal is useful in the management of dry skin and pruritus by virtue of its demulcent, humectant, and antipruritic properties. It is incorporated into a number of veterinary shampoos. It may also be used as a rinse or soak by adding 1 to 2 tablespoons (15 to 30 ml) of the powder (Epi-Soothe, Virbac; Aveeno, Rydelle Laboratories) to 1 gallon (4 L) of water. Colloidal oatmeal can leave a residue in the haircoat.

• **Topical Sunscreens.** A dense haircoat protects most horses from excessive exposure to sunlight. In many horses, the skin is pigmented, which also protects from ultraviolet radiation damage. However, whenever nonpigmented, unhaired skin is exposed to sunlight, solar damage may occur. Some animals respond with hyperpigmentation, whereas other animals do not experience hyperpigmentation but may incur sunburn or solar dermatitis.

Protection from the sun can be attained by staying indoors from 10 AM to 4 PM, by tanning the skin (a process of building up pigmentation and mild acanthosis and hyperkeratosis), and by using topical or oral sunscreens.[55] Topical sunscreens may act physically or chemically. In chemical screens, aminobenzoic acid or benzophenone derivatives act to absorb ultraviolet rays. They are clear, cosmetically acceptable lotions or gels.

Physical (barrier) sunscreens include chemicals such as zinc oxide and titanium dioxide, which reflect and scatter light by forming an opaque barrier. These agents tend to be messy, especially in long haircoats. They also are water-resistant and are not as easily removed by the horse. Topical sunscreens are rated for efficiency by a sun protective factor (SPF) number. Numbers 2 to 4 are mild blockers, 8 to 10 give moderate protection, and 15 or higher gives blockage. For use in animals, water-resistant sunscreens with an SPF of 15 or greater should be used. These numbers are only guides, because the frequency and thickness of application, temperature, humidity, potency of light exposure, patient's sensitivity, and many other factors modify results.

Usually, sunscreen needs to be applied three or four times a day for greatest effectiveness. Photodecomposition is a problem, and titanium dioxide or zinc oxide sunscreens tend to resist this and are preferred if repeat application is not possible.[85] A common misconception is that if the animal licks the area after application, the sunscreen is removed. Although this is true for the physical blockers (e.g., zinc oxide), it is a minimal problem with chemical blockers because these products are absorbed into the skin and pool within the stratum corneum to produce a reservoir of protection. Chemical blockers are not effective if no epithelium is present (e.g., on ulcers).

•**Combination Products.** Maxi/Guard Zn7 Equine Wound Care Formula (Addison Biological Laboratory) is a spray containing zinc gluconate complexed with L-lysine and taurine, glycerin, carboxymethylcellulose, methylparaben, and propyparaben. The manufacturer claims that the product is antimicrobial, antipruritic, humectant, protective, insect-repellent, nonirritating, and nonstaining, that it does not stimulate exuberant granulation ("proud flesh"), and that it causes enhanced hair follicle regeneration. We wait impatiently for peer-reviewed documentation of any or all of these amazing claims!

Dermacloth (Vet Medics Corp) is a cotton/cellulose acetate/polyester fabric containing water, surfactants, vitamin E, dexpanthenol, biguanide, and fragrance. The manufacturer claims that the product is quite effective as an aid in the treatment of bacterial and fungal infections, as well as "scaly, crusty, and flaky skin." Again, independent documentation of same is eagerly awaited!

• PHYSICAL THERAPY

The use of heat, cold, light, and radiation therapy for the treatment of skin disorders is not new, but advances have made the therapies more specific and more effective. Freezing, heat, electricity, and laser light are presented as surgical techniques at the end of this chapter.

Photochemotherapy

Photochemotherapy uses light waves to excite or increase the energy of a photosensitive drug that causes a selective cytotoxic effect on tumors. The initial drug used in veterinary medicine is a hematoporphyrin derivative porfimer sodium (Photofrin-V, QLT Phototherapeutics).[71,79] The drug has a much greater affinity for tumor tissue than for surrounding normal cells. A newer-generation photosensitizer is chloroaluminum sulfonated phthalocyanine (Porphyrin products). It is reported to have the advantages of less cutaneous photosensitization and better light absorption for the wavelengths commonly used in this therapy.[71] Light is effective on only a few layers of surface cells, except red-range lights, which can penetrate as much as 1 to 2 cm. The light source is a laser system that produces a red laser beam, which passes through low-attenuation fiberoptic tracts. The laser beam is directed through 19-gauge needles into the appropriate areas of tumor. Treatment takes about 20 minutes, and repeated exposures are no problem. Patients should be kept out of sunlight for 3 to 4 weeks, because they are systemically photosensitized. The indications for photochemotherapy in horses remain to be documented.

Hyperthermia

Local current-field radiofrequency is used to produce enough heat in a local superficial area to cause tissue necrosis. This technique has been used in the treatment of cutaneous neoplasms in dogs and cats.[71] Heat is controlled to affect only the tumor and 2 to 3 mm of surrounding normal tissue. Results are much better with lesions less than 5 mm in diameter by 2 mm deep. The indications for hypothermia in equine dermatology remain to be documented.

Radiation Therapy

Radiation therapy has important benefits in the treatment of cutaneous neoplasms (see Chapter 16). Because not all cells are equally sensitive to radiation, these rays act selectively. Cells that divide rapidly, such as carcinoma cells, basal cells of the hair papilla, and vascular endothelial cells, are damaged more easily than those of the remaining skin. X-ray beams that are filtered through aluminum or copper sheets to remove soft rays penetrate deeply into the tissues because of their short wavelengths. Radiation delivered at about 80 kV with little or no filtration (0.5 mm of aluminum) has longer wavelengths, and its energy is dissipated superficially.

Before considering radiation therapy for a patient, the clinician must be certain of the following:
1. The treatment has clear potential for benefit and little potential for harm.
2. Safer forms of therapy were not effective or radiation therapy is considered a therapy of choice.
3. Relative cost of this therapy is acceptable.
4. The number and frequency of treatments is acceptable.
5. Proper, safe equipment and facilities are available so that:
   a. The exact dose can be administered.
   b. The patient can be anesthetized or restrained for therapy without exposure of personnel.
   c. Proper shielding of unaffected parts is provided.
6. Adequate records are kept for future reference.

If these criteria can be accomplished, radiation therapy may be considered. Such cases should be referred to a radiologist who specializes in radiation therapy.

Miscellaneous Modalities

Biomagnets (magnetic therapy) are purported to produce local warming, vasodilation, increased blood circulation, and a variety of potential benefits. However, magnetic therapy produced no effects on cutaneous circulation in horses.[84]

Ultrasound is purported to cause local warming, vasodilation, increased blood circulation, increased tissue oxygenation and nutrition, protein synthesis, fibroblast activation, and increased wound healing. Ultrasound exposure did cause local warming of equine skin.[84]

• BROAD-SPECTRUM SYSTEMIC THERAPIES

Systemic Nonsteroidal Antipruritic or Nonsteroidal Anti-Inflammatory Agents

In practice, one is often presented with a pruritic or inflammatory dermatosis that is not microbial or parasitic. In other cases, even though a specific cause is determined, symptomatic antipruritic or anti-inflammatory therapy may be desired. Systemic glucocorticoids are most commonly prescribed. However, although glucocorticoids are highly effective in managing these cases and many hypersensitivity disorders, the desire to avoid these agents and their side effects stimulates continual investigations for alternative drugs or methods that will allow an avoidance or reduction in the dose of glucocorticoid.

Reasons for electing nonsteroidal agents include (1) unacceptable acute or chronic glucocorticoid side effects, (2) immunosuppressed patients, (3) patients with infectious diseases (viral, fungal, and bacterial), (4) patients with other diseases in which glucocorticoids may be contraindicated, and (5) horse owners who do not want to use glucocorticoids in their animals. A variety of unrelated nonsteroidal drugs may be used.[70] Because antihistamines are used primarily in allergic diseases, they are covered in Chapter 8.

Fatty Acids

Fatty acids, as previously discussed, are an important part of the normal diet. By controlling the relative levels of omega-6 to omega-3 in the total diet, the development of inflammatory mediators in neutrophils and other organs may be modified.[71] The use of supplements for treating pruritic inflammatory diseases and crusting diseases in dogs and cats has been the subject of multiple open and controlled studies. In general, this method has shown success for the management of pruritus and inflammation associated with a variety of diseases, though predominantly allergic.

The proposed mechanism, besides the inhibition of arachidonic acid metabolism, relates to metabolic byproducts of fatty acid metabolism. Supplements used for pruritus usually contain γ-linolenic acid or EPA, or both. γ-Linolenic acid is found in relatively high concentrations in evening primrose, borage, and black currant oils. It is elongated to DGLA, which directly competes with arachidonic acid as a substrate for cyclooxygenase and 15-lipoxygenase. The result of DGLA metabolism is the formation of prostaglandin E1 and 15-hydroxy-8,11,13-eicosatetraenoic acid, both of which are thought to have anti-inflammatory effects.[71]

EPA, which is usually supplied by using cold water marine fish oils, also competes as a substrate for cyclooxygenase and 5- and 15-lipoxygenase. The metabolism of EPA by the lipoxygenase enzymes results in the formation of leukotriene B5 and 15-hydroxyeicosapentaenoic acid. These two products are thought to inhibit leukotriene B4, which is a potent proinflammatory mediator. Fig. 3-2 demonstrates the interactions of γ-linolenic acid, EPA, and arachidonic acid.

Few studies on the effects of these fatty acids in horses have been published. Nonetheless, these agents appear to be useful in some equine dermatoses (see Chapter 8).

Pentoxifylline

Pentoxifylline (Trental, Hoechst-Roussel) is a methylxanthine derivative that produces a variety of physiologic changes at the cellular level.[65] Immunomodulatory and rheologic effects include increased leukocyte deformability and chemotaxis, decreased platelet aggregation, decreased leukocyte responsiveness to interleukin-1 (IL-1) and tumor necrosis factor (TNF)-α, decreased production of TNF-α from macrophages, decreased production of IL-1, IL-4, and IL-12, inhibition of T- and B-lymphocyte activation, and decreased natural killer cell activity. It also has been shown to inhibit T-cell adherence to keratinocytes.[10] Pentoxifylline may be useful in some horses with allergic and immune-mediated dermatoses (see Chapters 8 and 9).

Synthetic Retinoids

Retinoids refer to all the chemicals, natural or synthetic, that have vitamin A activity. Synthetic retinoids are primarily retinol, retinoic acid, or retinal derivatives or analogs. They have been developed with the intent of amplifying certain biologic effects while being less toxic than their natural precursors. More than 1,500 synthetic retinoids have been developed and evaluated. Retinoids are usually classified as being first generation (e.g., tretinoin, isotretinoin); second generation or monoaromatic (e.g., etretinate, acitretin); or third generation or polyaromatic (e.g., adapalene, tazarotene).[94]

Different synthetic drugs, all classed as synthetic retinoids, may have profoundly different pharmacologic effects, side effects, and disease indications. The existence of different types of receptors, dimers, response elements, and intermediary proteins means that retinoid physiology is mediated by multiple pathways. Nonselective retinoids that activate multiple pathways are likely to be associated with a high incidence of adverse effects.[12] With all the retinoid research being conducted, there will undoubtedly be many new discoveries and uses in the near future. To date, the biggest deterrent to their use is expense.

Naturally occurring vitamin A is an alcohol, all-trans retinol. It is oxidized in the body to retinal and retinoic acid. Each of these compounds has variable metabolic and biologic activities, although both are important in the induction and maintenance of normal growth and differentiation of keratinocytes. Only retinol has all the known functions of vitamin A.

Two compounds have been used most in clinical veterinary dermatology: isotretinoin (13-cis-retinoic acid [Accutane, Roche]), synthesized as a natural metabolite of retinol, and etretinate (Tegison, Roche), a synthetic retinoid. Etretinate is no longer available in the United States. It has

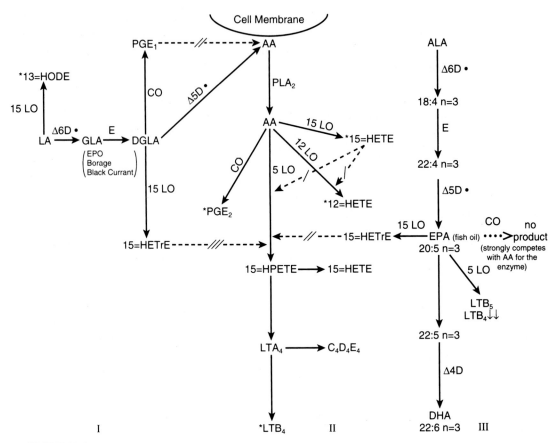

FIGURE 3-2. *I*, N-6 fatty acid metabolism with production of anti-inflammatory eicosanoids. *II*, Arachidonic acid cascade with production of proinflammatory eicosanoids. *III*, N-3 fatty acid metabolism with production of anti-inflammatory eicosanoids. *13-HODE*, 13-hydroxyoctadecadienoic acid; *PG*, prostaglandin; *E*, elongase; *D-6-D*, D-6-desaturase; *LA*, linoleic acid; *GLA*, γ-linolenic acid; *EPO*, evening primrose oil; *DGLA*, dihomo-γ-linolenic acid; *AA*, arachidonic acid; *ALA*, α-linolenic acid; *EPA*, eicosapentaenoic acid; *DHA*, docosahexaenoic acid; *DES*, desaturase; *PLA2*, phospholipase A2; *CO*, cyclooxygenase; *LO*, lipoxygenase; *HETE*, hydroxyeicosatetraenoic acid; *HPETE*, hydroperoxyeicosatetraenoic acid; *HEPE*, hydroxyeicosapentaenoic acid; *15-HETrE*, 15-hydroxy-8,11,13-eicosatriaenoic acid; *LT*, leukotriene.
^cIndicates arachidonic acid–derived eicosanoids identified in inflammatory skin disease. ° Indicates inhibitory or anti-inflammatory eicosanoid (number of *slash lines* indicates degree of inhibition). (From White P: Essential fatty acids: Use in management of canine atopy. Comp Cont Educ 15:451, 1993.)

been replaced by acitretin (Soriatane, Roche), which is a carboxylic acid, metabolically active metabolite of etretinate. Acitretin is less toxic, owing to a shorter terminal elimination half-life of 2 days versus etretinate's 100 days. Etretinate is stored in body fat and has been found in trace amounts up to 3 years after cessation of therapy.[56]

Retinoids function by entering cells and being transported to the nuclei, where they interact with specific gene regulatory receptors. The natural vitamin A works at the cellular level by binding first to the cell membrane, then transferring through the cellular cytoplasm by specific proteins, cellular retinol binding protein, and cellular retinoic acid binding protein. Nuclear retinoid receptor molecules transfer the retinoids through the nucleus.

There are two main nuclear receptor families: the retinoic acid receptors and the retinoid X receptors.[49] Both families have at least three members for a minimum of six different nuclear receptors. These receptors can function as heterodimers, homodimers, or in conjunction with other nuclear receptors such as those for vitamin D_3 and thyroid hormone. The nuclear receptor(s) and retinoid complex then bind with specific areas of target genes and alter gene transcription. A new class of retinoids that may act by a unique mechanism is being investigated and has been called *inverse agonists*. Retinoids may also function by suppression of other nuclear transcription factors, which results in less production of other proteins. This is thought to be a mechanism responsible for some of the anti-inflammatory effects.

Some of the different tissue and individual sensitivity for toxic effects may relate to the relative and absolute levels of the cellular and nuclear binding proteins present in the target cells. Once these genetic changes are made, the cells may alter their growth and differentiation by altering the expression of growth factors, keratins, and transglutaminases.[56] Another method of action relates to an anti-inflammatory effect in epithelial structures by the downregulation of nitrites and TNF–α.[5]

All retinoids have variable antiproliferative, anti-inflammatory, and immunomodulatory effects. Because of their numerous pharmacologic effects, retinoids are being used in the management of numerous diseases in humans. The long list includes such diverse diseases as acne, gram-negative folliculitis, hidradenitis suppurativa, the ichthyoses, multiple forms of psoriasis, a variety of cutaneous neoplasms, epidermal nevi, subcorneal pustular dermatosis, discoid lupus erythematosus, lichen planus, cutaneous sarcoidosis, Darier's disease, and acanthosis nigricans.[56] The biologic effects of retinoids are numerous, but their ability to regulate proliferation, growth, and differentiation of epithelial tissues is their major benefit in dermatology.[5] However, retinoids also affect proteases, prostaglandins, humoral and cellular immunity, and cellular adhesion and communication.[56] In general, the response of established skin cancers to retinoids is disappointing, with remissions being uncommon, incomplete, and of short duration.[43] Retinoids enhance wound healing by stimulating fibroblasts to produce various chemicals (e.g., TGF-β).[24]

In companion animals, isotretinoin is usually dosed at 1 to 3 mg/kg q24h and appears to be indicated in diseases that require alteration or normalization of adnexal structures, although some epidermal diseases respond.[71] Isotretinoin must be administered with food or absorption is quite variable.[91]

Acitretin is indicated for disorders of epithelial or follicular development or keratinization.[71] It must be given with food or absorption is highly variable.[92] In companion animals, acitretin is usually dosed at 0.5 to 1 mg/kg q 24 hr.[71]

Toxicities that may be seen with oral retinoids include cutaneous, mucocutaneous, gastrointestinal, ocular, and skeletal abnormalities.[56,71] All retinoids are teratogenic.

The authors are not aware of any publications concerning the use of oral retinoids in horses. At current prices, these agents would be prohibitively expensive for use in horses.

Cyclosporine

Cyclosporine (Sandimmune, Novartis) is a fat-soluble cyclic polypeptide metabolite of the fungus *Tolypocladium inflatum gams*. It is effective in preventing human organ transplantation rejection. In animal models, this agent has been used with similar excellent results.[71] Cyclosporine is being used for a wide variety of dermatologic diseases in humans such as atopic dermatitis, psoriasis, lichen planus, pyoderma gangrenosum, epidermolysis bullosa acquisita, actinic dermatitis, and chronic hand eczema.[30,45] It has also been evaluated for the treatment of immune-mediated skin diseases and epitheliotropic lymphoma in animals.[71] Most clinicians use the microemulsified capsule or solution forms of cyclosporine (Neoral, Novartis), because these products are absorbed better and produce more stable blood levels.

Cyclosporine has low cytotoxicity relative to its immunosuppressive potency. Cyclosporine blocks IL-2 transcription and T cell responsiveness to IL-2, leading to impaired T-helper and

T-cytotoxic lymphocytes. It also inhibits IFN-α transcription, thus diminishing amplification signals for macrophage and monocyte activation. The production of other cytokines, including IL-3, IL-4, IL-5, TNF-α, and IFN-α, may be impaired. In these ways, cyclosporine inhibits mononuclear cell function, antigen presentation, mast cell and eosinophil production, histamine and prostaglandin release from mast cells, neutrophil adherence, natural killer cell activity, and growth and differentiation of B cells. It has also been suggested that a mechanism of action in the treatment of atopic dermatitis involves the inhibition of mast cell degranulation by affecting the interaction between mast cells and nerves.[82]

Humans using cyclosporine have experienced a high incidence of nephrotoxicity and hepatic toxicity. Dogs (on daily doses of 20 to 30 mg/kg) may experience gingival hyperplasia and papillomatosis, vomiting, diarrhea, bacteriuria, bacterial skin infection, anorexia, hirsutism, involuntary shaking, nephropathy, bone marrow suppression, and lymphoplasmacytoid dermatosis.[71] These effects appear to be rare with daily doses of 5 to 10 mg/kg. Cats are reported to have only minor side effects (primarily soft feces), although they may be more susceptible to viral infections.[71] Cyclosporine should probably be stopped at least 4 weeks prior to intradermal skin testing.[71]

The oral dosage for dogs and cats is 5 to 10 mg/kg q 24h.[71] Blood concentrations achieved after a specific dose vary from patient to patient and within each patient over time. These variabilities are largely determined by differences in absorption, distribution, and metabolism. Absorption may be enhanced by administration with a fatty meal. Frequent drug monitoring may be needed to maintain blood cyclosporine concentrations in an effective range yet avoid toxicities. After a response occurs, tapering to as low as 10 mg/kg every 48 hours may be effective. Because this is an expensive drug, the reduction to the lowest effective levels is usually important. Additionally, the expense and marginal efficacy usually limit its use to cases of treatment failure with, or adverse reaction to, alternative treatments.

Drugs that inhibit cytochrome P-450 microsomal enzyme activity (e.g., ketoconazole, itraconazole, fluconazole, erythromycin, methylprednisolone, and allopurinol) potentiate cyclosporine toxicity. When ketoconazole was given to normal dogs (average dose 13.6 mg/kg/day) that had targeted blood levels of cyclosporine (average daily dose 14.5 mg/kg), the cyclosporine doses could be reduced by an average of 75%, resulting in a 57.8% savings in the cost of therapy.[71] The authors are not aware of any publications on the use of cyclosporine in equine dermatoses. Treatment would be prohibitively expensive at current drug cost.

Glucocorticoid Hormones

Glucocorticoid hormones have potent effects on the skin, and they profoundly affect immunologic and inflammatory activity.[16,60,67,90] They directly or indirectly affect leukocyte kinetics, phagocytic defenses, cell-mediated immunity, humoral immunity, and the production of inflammatory mediators. The major effects thought to be important in counteracting allergic inflammatory reactions are presented in Table 3-4 and have been reviewed.[16,90] In addition, fibroblastic activity is reduced, synthesis of histamine is delayed, and complement is inhibited. Antibody production is not stopped but may be decreased, especially autoantibody titers.

At pharmacologic levels, glucocorticoids increase the production of lipocortin-1. This is thought to cause a reduction in the action of phospholipase A_2 on cell membranes, which results in inhibition of the arachidonic acid cycle.[17] This action is probably one of the more clinically relevant actions in decreasing inflammation. High doses of glucocorticoids may suppress antibody production.[16,90] There is circumstantial evidence that in some allergic dogs glucocorticoids may suppress IgE production at therapeutic protocols used by some veterinarians.[71]

Glucocorticoid response to inflammatory stimuli is nonspecific: it is the same whether it is a response to infection, trauma, toxin, or immune complex deposition. The drug must reach the local site of inflammation to be effective, and the degree of response and cellular protection from injury

● Table 3-4	ANTI-INFLAMMATORY ACTIONS OF GLUCOCORTICOIDS
Effects on eosinophils	Decrease formation in bone marrow
	Induce apoptosis and inhibit prolongation of eosinophil survival and function from IL-3 and IL-5
Effects on lymphocytes and monocytes	Reduce number of lymphocytes and monocytes that bear low-affinity of IgE and IgG receptors
	Decrease serum immunoglobulin levels
	Decrease all lymphocyte subpopulations
	Decrease lymphocyte production of IL-1, -2, -3, -4, -5, -6, and IFN-γ
	Inhibit release of IL-1 and TNF-α from monocytes
Effects on mast cells	May decrease number of mast cells
Inhibition of phospholipase A_2	Decrease production of arachidonic acid metabolites
	Decrease production of platelet-activating factor
Decreased vascular permeability	Mechanism unknown
Reversal of reduced β-adrenergic responsiveness	Part of this effect is by increasing the number of β-adrenergic receptors expressed on cell surface

is proportionate to the concentration of glucocorticoid in the inflamed tissue. Thus, dosages and dose intervals should vary with the patient's specific needs.

Several other factors influence the tissue glucocorticoid effect. One is the relative potency of the drug. Synthetic compounds made by adding methyl or fluoride groups to the basic steroid molecule increase the potency and the duration of action. Another factor is the effect of protein binding. Only free glucocorticoid is metabolically active. Many synthetics are poorly protein-bound, which partly explains their relatively high potency at low doses.

Corticosteroid-binding globulin is a specific glycoprotein that binds glucocorticoids, but it has a relatively low binding capacity. When large doses of glucocorticoids are administered, its capacity is exceeded, and albumin becomes the protein used for binding. Animals with low serum albumin levels have a lower binding capacity, and the excessive unbound glucocorticoid becomes freely available, increasing toxicity. In addition, the route of administration and water solubility affect the duration of action. Oral glucocorticoids, given as the free base or as esters, are rapidly absorbed. Parenteral glucocorticoids are usually esters of acetate, diacetate, phosphate, or succinate. Acetate and diacetate are relatively insoluble, resulting in slow release and prolonged absorption. The phosphates and succinates are water-soluble and rapidly absorbed. As a result, parenteral glucocorticoids produce continuous low levels of glucocorticoid for days (water-soluble) or weeks (water-insoluble). The effect produces significant adrenal suppression, a problem that can be diminished by giving short-acting glucocorticoids orally every other day.

Many of the desirable properties of glucocorticoids can be responsible for adverse effects if present in excess or at the wrong time. In addition, adverse effects may relate to the numerous other effects that glucocorticoids have on carbohydrate, protein, and lipid metabolism. It is imperative to make an accurate diagnosis so that the need for, type, duration, and level of glucocorticoid therapy can be determined. Except in the case of hypoadrenocorticism, glucocorticoids do not correct a primary deficiency but act symptomatically or palliatively. The anti-inflammatory and immunosuppressive actions desired for one therapeutic need may facilitate the establishment or spread of concomitant infections or parasitic diseases.

Animals treated with glucocorticoids tend to experience bacterial infections of the skin and the urinary and respiratory systems.[60,63] Because of the profound effects of glucocorticoids on phagocytosis and cell-mediated immunity, increased susceptibility to fungal infections and intracellular pathogens is to be expected.[16,60]

INDICATIONS

The major indications for glucocorticoid therapy are hypersensitivity dermatoses (insect hypersensitivity, atopy, and food hypersensitivity), contact dermatitis (irritant or hypersensitivity reactions), urticaria (numerous causes), and immune-mediated dermatoses (pemphigus, pemphigoid, lupus erythematosus, vasculitis, erythema multiforme, and drug reactions). They are occasionally used in other inflammatory skin diseases such as many diseases listed in Chapter 15 (e.g., eosinophilic granuloma, sterile pyogranuloma). Whenever possible, their use should be short-term (less than 3 months).

Glucocorticoids are usually only part of the management employed for most dermatoses, and the clinician must control or minimize other predisposing, precipitating, and complicating factors to keep the glucocorticoids in their proper perspective, which is to use them (1) as infrequently as possible, (2) at as low a dose as possible, (3) in alternate-day regimens whenever possible, and (4) only when other less hazardous forms of therapy have failed or could not be employed.

ADMINISTRATION

For dermatoses, glucocorticoids are usually administered orally, by injection (intramuscularly, subcutaneously, intralesionally, and intravenously), topically, or in some combination thereof. In any given patient, the decision as to which route or routes to employ depends on various factors.

Of the systemic routes, oral administration is preferred because (1) it can be more closely regulated (a daily dose is more precise than with a repository injection; the drug can be rapidly withdrawn if undesirable side effects occur) and (2) it is the only safe, therapeutic, physiologic way to administer glucocorticoids for more long-term therapy.

Injectable glucocorticoids are usually administered intramuscularly or subcutaneously. Although most injectable glucocorticoids are licensed for only intramuscular use, some clinicians administer them subcutaneously. The reasons purported for choosing the subcutaneous route are (1) there are few patient objections and (2) it is clinically as effective as intramuscular administration.

A theoretical preference exists for using the intramuscular route in the obese patient, because subcutaneous deliveries could be sequestered in fat tissue. However, the major reason for using the intramuscular route (other than the liability or legal issue) is to decrease the occurrence of local atrophy. Although this problem may be more common in humans, it also occurs in the horse. Local areas of alopecia, pigmentary changes, and epidermal and dermal atrophy are more commonly induced by subcutaneous injection. These reactions are noninflammatory and atrophic in contrast with most other injection reactions.

An excellent injectable anti-inflammatory glucocorticoid is methylprednisolone acetate (Depo-Medrol, Pharmacia & Upjohn). Horses are usually given 200 mg intramuscularly, and the effect may last for 1 to 3 weeks. Another commonly used injectable glucocorticoid is triamcinolone (Vetalog Parenteral, Fort Dodge), 0.02 to 0.04 mg/kg IM.

Intralesional injections of glucocorticoids are often thought of as local, intracutaneous therapy, devoid of any systemic effect. Intralesional therapy is employed for solitary or multiple cutaneous lesions, but it has systemic effects, some of which can be serious. The major indications for intralesional use are eosinophilic granulomas, sterile granulomas, pseudolymphomas (e.g., insect bite reactions) and axillary nodular necrosis. Intralesional (or sublesional) glucocorticoid therapy is typically performed with triamcinolone (3 to 5 mg/lesion) or methlyprednisolone (5 to 10 mg/lesion) and repeated every 1 to 2 weeks to effect.

CHOOSING A GLUCOCORTICOID

The choice of a glucocorticoid may be difficult. One cannot establish a single rule or set of rules that applies to all patients with a given glucocorticoid-responsive dermatosis. Factors that must be considered include the duration of therapy, the personality of the patient, the personality and reliability of the owner, the response of the patient to the drug, the response of the patient's disease to the drug, and other considerations specific to the patient or the disease.

Although many horses respond well to oral prednisone, some do not. The horses that do not respond to prednisone usually respond well to oral prednisolone or oral dexamethasone at equipotent doses. In studies of small numbers of horses with chronic obstructive pulmonary disease ("heaves"), prednisone and prednisolone could not be detected in blood following oral administration of prednisone.[56a,61] However, prednisolone was detected in the blood of these horses after the oral administration of prednisolone. It appears that some horses do not respond to oral prednisone because of poor absorption, rapid excretion, failure of hepatic conversion to prednisolone, or some combination of these. It is recommended, therefore, to always use prednisolone initially.

Dexamethasone can be administered orally in horses, either as tablets, powder, or using the injectable liquid.[62,63] Some horses will not accept the powder mixed with feed. The oral bioavailability of dexamethasone powder is incomplete and variable in horses.[18,75,80] Because dexamethasone is a longer-acting glucocorticoid than prednisolone or prednisone, it is not as safe for alternate-morning maintenance protocols.[18,75,80] If dexamethasone can be used every third morning, it is safer.

The clinician learns, by history or personal experience, that some glucocorticoids do not seem to work as well as others in certain patients. However, the claim that injectable glucocorticoids are needed in some cases and that oral glucocorticoids are not effective is rarely accurate. In the majority of these cases, ineffective oral dosages were used or oral agents were tapered too fast. A common mistake is to give an injection, then go immediately to a low alternate-day oral dose. In some cases, the problem probably reflects dosage, absorption, and metabolic differences.

As a corollary, the clinician notes that, in some patients, a glucocorticoid that was previously satisfactory apparently loses its effectiveness. For example, in an atopic horse that initially did well when given prednisolone, the prednisolone seemed to lose its effect. Subsequently, the horse responded well to equipotent doses of orally administered dexamethasone. In most cases, after a variable length of time, the clinician is able to return to managing the atopy successfully with prednisolone. This well-recognized but poorly understood phenomenon is called *steroid tachyphylaxis*.[23,71] However, in most clinical cases referred to dermatology specialists for the development of steroid resistance or steroid tachyphylaxis, the real problem is the development of concurrent disorders. In such cases, secondary bacterial pyoderma, *Malassezia* dermatitis, increased exposure to ectoparasites, or reactions to ongoing topical therapy are often the reasons for failure of previously effective glucocorticoid regimens.

Finally, the clinician may discover, by history or personal experience, that a patient can receive certain glucocorticoids without significant adverse effects but not other glucocorticoids.

THERAPEUTIC DOSAGE

Optimal therapeutic doses have not been scientifically determined for any equine dermatosis. Presently espoused anti-inflammatory, antipruritic, antiallergic, or immunosuppressive glucocorticoid doses have been determined through years of clinical experience. Moreover, it is imperative to remember that every patient is unique and that glucocorticoid therapy must be individualized. Recommended glucocorticoid doses are only guidelines.

The two most commonly used oral glucocorticoids are prednisolone and prednisone. For all practical purposes, these two drugs are identical. However, prednisone must be converted in the liver to prednisolone, the active form. As previously discussed, some horses do not respond to oral prednisone, and prednisolone is the oral glucocorticoid of choice. Dosage recommendations in this text are based on prednisolone (prednisone) equivalents. Table 3-5 contains information on approximate equipotent dosages of other oral glucocorticoids.

DRUG	EQUIVALENT DOSE (mg)	DURATION OF EFFECT (H)	ALTERNATE-DAY THERAPY*
Short-Acting			
Cortisone	25	8-12	NAS
Hydrocortisone	20	8-12	NAS
Intermediate-Acting			
Prednisone	5	24-36	P
Prednisolone	5	24-36	P
Methylprednisolone	4	24-36	P
Long-Acting			
Flumethasone	1.3	36-48	A[‡]
Triamcinolone	0.5[†]	36-48	A[‡]
Dexamethasone	0.5	36-54	A[‡]
Betamethasone	0.4	36-54	

● Table 3-5 **RELATIVE POTENCY AND ACTIVITY OF ORAL GLUCOCORTICOIDS**

*NAS = Not accepted for short duration; *P* = preferred; *A* = alternative selection for alternate-day therapy.
[†]Previous publications stated dosages often equivalent to those of methylprednisolone. No studies on clinical effects are available.
[‡]May be useful on every-third-day regimen.

Physiologic doses of glucocorticoids are those that approximate the daily cortisol (hydrocortisone) production by normal individuals. Pharmacologic doses of glucocorticoids exceed physiologic requirements. Significantly, any pharmacologic dose of glucocorticoid, no matter how large or small, may suppress the hypothalamic-pituitary-adrenal axis.

Clinicians usually talk in terms of anti-inflammatory versus immunosuppressive doses of glucocorticoids. A commonly used anti-inflammatory (as in allergic dermatoses) induction dosage of oral prednisolone in horses is 2.2 mg/kg q24h. However, in severe allergy, such as the horse with insect hypersensitivity that is exposed to numerous insects, a higher dosage of 3 to 4.4 mg/kg/day may be needed. For maintenance, the dosage should be lowered as much as possible and optimally ends up at less than 0.5 mg/kg q48h. For immune-mediated diseases, the initial dosage is usually 4.4 mg/kg q24h. If there is no response, this may be raised to as high as 6.6 mg/kg q24h.

The authors administer oral glucocorticoids only once daily and find no loss of clinical efficacy. A commonly used immunosuppressive maintenance dosage for horses is 1.1 mg of prednisolone per kilogram every other morning.

In the horse, blood cortisol concentrations are highest in the morning and lowest at night.* There are also endogenous rhythmic and episodic fluctuations, as well as exogenously provoked fluctuations in blood cortisol concentrations throughout the day (see Chapter 10). It is thus important to administer maintenance doses of oral glucocorticoids no more frequently than every other morning so that adrenal suppression and chronic side effects are minimized.

REGIMEN

Glucocorticoid regimens vary with the nature of the dermatosis, the specific glucocorticoid being administered, and the use of induction versus maintenance therapy.

*References 7, 25, 32, 34-36, 41, 42, 81, 99.

In general, dermatoses necessitating anti-inflammatory doses of oral glucocorticoid need smaller doses and shorter periods of daily induction therapy to bring about remission compared with dermatoses necessitating immunosuppressive doses. Anti-inflammatory induction doses are usually given for 2 to 6 days, whereas immunosuppressive induction doses are often administered for 4 to 10 days. Initially, the doses are given every 24 hours until the dermatosis is in remission. Then, the total daily dose is given every 48 hours. After this point, tapering to maintenance therapy begins.

Maintenance therapy with oral glucocorticoid is best accomplished with prednisolone or prednisone on alternate days. Because dexamethasone suppresses the hypothalamic-pituitary-adrenal axis for 24 to 48 hours, it is best given every 72 hours.

With alternate-day therapy, the daily dose of glucocorticoid used for successful induction therapy is given as a single massive dose, every other morning. Alternate-day therapy is begun as soon as remission is achieved with induction therapy. For maintenance therapy, the alternate-day dose is reduced by 50%, every 1 to 2 weeks, until the lowest satisfactory maintenance dose is achieved. This regimen does not eliminate adrenal atrophy, but the atrophy is less severe and its onset is delayed. It is the only dosage system that should be used for long-term therapy of steroid-responsive diseases.

In some animals, alternate-day glucocorticoid therapy can be extended to every third or fourth day. Rarely, anti-inflammatory alternate-day glucocorticoid therapy with the preferred prednisolone or prednisone is unsuccessful. In these cases, the clinician has two therapeutic options (assuming that glucocorticoid therapy is all that can be done):

1. Administer prednisolone or prednisone daily, informing the owner of the inevitability of side effects.
2. Switch to a more potent oral glucocorticoid on an alternate-day basis.

Although the more potent oral glucocorticoids are clinically effective for alternate-day therapy, they do not spare the hypothalamic-pituitary-adrenal axis (because of potency and duration of effect). They may occasionally be employed with few or no significant side effects. Clinically, the most satisfactory agent in this respect appears to be dexamethasone. Although not always clinically effective, dexamethasone is safer when administered every 72 hours in maintenance protocols. Some clinicians consider dexamethasone to be the glucocorticoid of choice in urticaria.[62,63]

Intramuscular or subcutaneous glucocorticoid therapy is usually fine for acute, short-term diseases that necessitate a single injection. Additionally, animals that need only three or four injections per year probably do not experience significant side effects. However, for dermatoses that need long-term maintenance therapy, injectable glucocorticoids are not satisfactory. It has been shown that a single intramuscular injection of methylprednisolone acetate (Depo-Medrol, Pharmacia & Upjohn) is capable of altering adrenocortical function in dogs for at least 5, and up to 10, weeks. In other studies, a single intramuscular injection of triamcinolone acetonide (Vetalog, Fort Dodge) was capable of altering adrenocortical function in dogs for up to 4 weeks.

Intralesional injections of glucocorticoids are usually repeated every 7 to 10 days until the dermatosis is in remission (usually two to four treatments) and then given as needed.

SIDE EFFECTS

Glucocorticoids are, in general, well-tolerated by horses.[62,63,70] Possible side effects include increased susceptibility to infections, polydipsia, polyuria, poor wound healing, decreased muscle mass, weight loss, behavioral changes, and diabetes mellitus.[15,60] However, these are rarely seen. Although the risk of laminitis in horses treated with glucocorticoids is always mentioned as an anecdote in textbooks and review articles, the authors are not aware of a single reported case of this happening following the use of the clinical protocols discussed herein. One horse developed laminitis and hepatopathy following a massive overdose of injectable triamcinolone.[15] Intramuscular injections of dexamethasone did not affect blood histamine levels in normal horses.[59]

Iatrogenic secondary adrenocortical insufficiency ("hypoadrenocorticism," "adrenal insufficiency," "steroid letdown syndrome") is poorly documented in horses.[60] It is most commonly thought to occur as a result of the sudden discontinuation of prolonged glucocorticoid administration. Affected horses may exhibit some combination of depression, anorexia, weight loss, muscle weakness, lameness, dull/dry haircoat, mild abdominal discomfort, and hypoglycemia.

It must be remembered that adrenocortical suppression is produced by topical, intralesional, intraarticular, oral, intramuscular, and subcutaneous administration of glucocorticoids. The duration of adrenocortical suppression with even short-term treatment may be 24 hours to 14 days, depending on the glucocorticoid and the route of administration.[60]

EVALUATION

Evaluation of the results during glucocorticoid therapy is important. When appropriate systemic anti-inflammatory glucocorticoid therapy is given to an otherwise healthy horse, the risks are minimal. The risks associated with immunosuppressive doses are of greater concern, especially because the medication is usually prescribed for serious or life-threatening diseases, which will probably be treated for the rest of the animal's life. Significant concurrent dysfunction of major organ systems also increases the risks.

When long-term systemic therapy is started, owners should be instructed to observe their animals closely and to immediately report any significant side effects. A physical check-up is advised every 6 to 12 months. Periodic urinalysis and urine cultures may be needed to recognize urinary tract infections that are not clinically apparent. Serum chemistry screens are advised every 12 to 24 months before more medication is dispensed. The ACTH response test is useful in animals with suspected iatrogenic Cushing's disease. Marked suppression indicates that other attempts at lowering the dosage should be made because major problems are inevitable. Horses receiving appropriate long-term, alternate-day steroid therapy usually have mildly to moderately suppressed adrenocortical responses to ACTH but are otherwise clinically normal.

● ORAL SUNSCREENS

Oral sunscreens are chemicals such as β-carotene and chloroquine that quench free radicals and stabilize membranes. They have not been proved to prevent sunburn in humans but have been useful in cases of light-induced dermatosis.[47,66] A β-carotene derivative has been used in cats and dogs to reduce phototoxicity.[71] Canthaxanthin (β,β-carotene-4,′-dione) is a red-orange pigment found in plants and other sources. The safety of this product has been challenged. Side effects include orange-brown skin, brick-red stools, crystalline gold deposits on the retinae, orange plasma, and lowered amplitudes on electroretinograms. The usual maximal dosage for humans is 25 mg/kg daily, but some companies recommend four 30-mg capsules once daily (Golden Tan, Orobronze). Whether such products would be useful in the management of various equine photodermatoses is unclear.

● SKIN SURGERY

Skin surgery can be an important part of equine dermatology. Many new developments have arisen, from skin biopsies for diagnosis to cryosurgery for specialized procedures. It is essential to know what equipment is needed and to be able to use the equipment properly. Cold steel surgery, cryosurgery, laser surgery, and electrosurgery are mentioned in this chapter. Biopsy techniques are covered in Chapter 2.

Cold Steel Surgery

Excision of small tumors and other lesions is a minor procedure that can often be performed on an outpatient basis but is usually better performed if the animal is held in the hospital for several hours. This enables the practitioner to use tranquilization, sedation, or general anesthesia as needed to promote control and relaxation of the patient. Cases requiring extensive surgery with plastic repair procedures and grafts need an operating room with complete aseptic routine. Even minor cases, however, must be handled with proper preparation, sterile instruments, and other measures to accomplish a scrupulously clean operation.

The dermatologist who employs surgical treatment of human diseases usually performs minor techniques on skin that is relatively hairless; therefore, the cosmetic effects are crucial. Most procedures appear complex because avoidance of scarring is a primary consideration. In veterinary dermatology, the clinician should, of course, avoid disfigurement, but because of the dense pelage, small scars are relatively unimportant.

With any surgical procedure, it is necessary to clip the hair closely, wash the unbroken skin surface carefully until it is clean using a surgical scrub solution such as 1% chlorhexidine diacetate (Nolvasan, Fort Dodge) or 0.75% povidone-iodine (Betadine, Purdue Frederick), and rinse thoroughly. The skin is defatted by wiping the surface in a circular fashion from the center outward, using sterile swabs soaked in 70% alcohol. The skin can then be sprayed or swabbed with 0.5% solution of chlorhexidine diacetate or, as a second choice, 1% solution of povidone-iodine. The surgical site is then ready to drape.

The lesions should be outlined by elliptic scalpel incisions that extend through the skin. The specimen or lesion is dissected free from the underlying tissue with scissors, hemostats, or both. Healing and final results are better if the long-axis incisions are oriented parallel to the tension lines.

Cryosurgery

Cryosurgery is the controlled use of freezing temperatures to destroy undesirable tissue while doing minimal damage to surrounding healthy tissue.[57,93] In general, cryosurgery is the most useful for small, localized skin lesions (see Chapter 16) treated on an outpatient basis. Liquid nitrogen and nitrous oxide are the most commonly used agents.

The lethal effect of subzero temperatures on cells depends on five factors:
1. Type of cell being frozen
2. Rate of freezing
3. Final temperature (must be at least –20° C)
4. Rate of thawing
5. Repetition of the freeze-thaw cycle

Cell damage is more severe with rapid freezing, slow thawing, and three freeze-thaw cycles. A final temperature of –70° C is reached at the surface of the probe with nitrous oxide equipment so that it can cool only a limited mass of tissue below the required –20° C, thereby restricting its application to small, superficial lesions. A final temperature of –185° C can be reached at the tissue junction using liquid nitrogen. This enables the forming of a larger ice ball of tissue and allows larger areas to be effectively frozen.

It has been speculated that useful immunologic effects are possible with cryosurgery. When a cell mass is frozen and left to die in situ, membrane lipoprotein complexes, and hence antigen-antibody complexing and receptor sites, are inevitably disrupted or altered. They are probably not totally destroyed. The nucleus may remain relatively intact. Thus, for a short time, antigenicity may be enhanced. Enough antigen is released systemically to produce a strong specific immunologic response that may kill escaped cells of the same tumor species.

Cryosurgery has the following advantages:

1. Lesions can be removed in areas where the skin is so tight or the lesion so large that closure with sutures is impossible. Tumors on the lower portions of the leg are examples.
2. In cases in which conventional excision surgery would produce shock or excessive blood loss, cryosurgery results in minimal hemorrhage. This is particularly effective in old or debilitated patients. Scarring is slight, and the cosmetic effect is good.
3. Selective destruction of diseased or neoplastic skin is possible with little damage to normal tissue. Chances of tumor cells spreading from premalignant lesions are reduced.
4. Cryosurgery has a possible immunotherapeutic effect on malignant neoplasms.

Cryosurgery has the following disadvantages:

1. The surgeon performing cryosurgery must be experienced and needs postgraduate training. Without specialized knowledge and skill, undesirable sequelae can result.
2. The necrosis and sloughing of frozen tissue are visually unpleasant and malodorous for 2 to 3 weeks after cryosurgery.
3. Regrowth of depigmented, white hair on the surgery site leaves a cosmetic defect.
4. Vital structures surrounding the frozen lesion may be damaged. This applies especially to blood vessels, nerves, tendons, ligaments, and joint capsules.
5. Large blood vessels frozen during cryosurgery for tumor removal may start bleeding 30 to 60 minutes later, when postoperative attention has been relaxed, or several hours later when the animal is at home. Air embolism is possible if sprays are used on open vessels.
6. Cryosurgery is contraindicated for mast cell tumors.

Laser Surgery

Laser surgery is highly successful in some branches of medicine[76] and is rapidly finding a place in veterinary dermatology (see Chapter 16). The word *laser* is an acronym for *light amplification by the stimulated emission of radiation*. Laser light, in contrast with regular light, is characterized in three different ways. It is monochromatic, meaning it is a wavelength of one color. It is coherent, meaning all the light waves are traveling in the same parallel direction and in phase. It is intense, which means the number of photons delivered to a surface area is great.

Multiple types of lasers are available and usually named for the dye or mineral used to elicit the light, but only two are being reported with any frequency in the United States. The argon pumped dye laser is more versatile in the wavelength of light that may be emitted and has been used to activate the photosensitizing agents in photochemotherapy. This type of laser has limited availability at certain specialty centers. The carbon dioxide (CO_2) laser is the most widely used type of laser in medicine worldwide. The CO_2 laser is gaining acceptance in the veterinary field, and a model for veterinarians has been developed (Accuvet, Luxar). Its cost is low enough that some moderate- to high-volume practices are justifying the expense.

When a laser light is directed at a tissue, it is either absorbed, reflected, scattered, or transmitted. The absorbed light is the goal, which results in transfer of energy to the molecules in the absorbing tissue. This results in the majority of uses in the creation of heat. The tissue destruction that results from the rapid and high heat formation is called *photothermolysis*. The CO_2 laser emits a beam of light at 10,600 nm, which is the wavelength that water maximally absorbs the light energy. Because water is a major component of cells, they are heated and removed layer by layer. When the temperature of the tissue rises, different effects occur. At 43° to 45° C, cells heat up and die; at 60° C, there is protein denaturation and coagulation; at 80° C, collagen denaturation and membrane permeabilization occur; at 90° to 100° C, carbonization and tissue burning occur; and at 100° C, vaporization and ablation occur.[53]

Advantages of laser surgery are less pain (the nerve endings are sealed during the cutting), less bleeding (due to sealing of small vessels and the ability to cause coagulation by defocusing and lower power emission), and less tissue destruction. The laser light also sterilizes the surgical incision site except for viral particles, and the surgical field can be sterilized by defocusing the beam, an advantage in contaminated lesions such as foreign body removal. These advantages result in less postoperative swelling and inflammation. Disadvantages are limited to the cost of the equipment and safety requirements. The disadvantages of the safety requirements are readily overcome with training.

Electrosurgery

Just as heat cautery was replaced by electrocautery, the latter has been improved on by modern electrosurgery. However, electrocautery equipment is still used to destroy tissue and to control hemorrhage by means of specialized tips that are heated to a bright cherry-red, producing incandescent heat. The healing of tissue after the use of electrocautery is like that after a third-degree burn. This is not discussed further because the newest electrosurgical units are more efficient. High-frequency electrosurgical units are capable of cutting, cutting and coagulation, desiccation, fulguration, and coagulation.

The main advantages of electrosurgery are (1) reduction of surgery time, (2) reduction of total blood loss, (3) ease of coagulation when ligature application is difficult, and (4) reduction of foreign material left in the wound. The disadvantages are (1) the possibility of improper use, leading to greater tissue damage, (2) presence of necrotic tissue within a wound, (3) delay in wound healing, (4) reduced early tensile strength of the wound up to 40 days after surgery, (5) decreased resistance to infection, (6) greater scar width on the skin, and (7) inability to suture most electrosurgical wounds.

Broad-based tumors are best removed with a blade. Next in value is hemostasis during both conventional surgery and electrosurgery. The newest electrosurgical units generate currents that perform cutting and coagulation functions simultaneously.

Electrosurgery uses electric currents to destroy tissues selectively. Electrosurgery is possible because electric current of greater than 10,000 Hz passes through the body without causing pain or muscle contractions, whereas the tissues and fluid of the body have electric impedance. Low frequencies (3000 Hz) result in pain and muscle contractions. At moderate frequencies (3000 to 5000 Hz), heat is produced, which causes tissue damage. Heat production is directly related to the power and concentration of the current delivered, the duration of application to the tissue, and the resistance of the tissue.

Radiosurgery

The next generation beyond electrosurgery is radiowave surgery, or radiosurgery. This form of surgery utilizes high-frequency radiowaves around 4 million hertz (4 MHz) and does not require a grounding plate (Ellman Surgitron, Ellman). However, a passive electrode is placed beneath the patient in the area of the surgery to act as an antenna to focus the radiowaves.[1] This plate does not require skin contact to function.

Multiple settings for different types of current allow some selection in the tissue effects produced. Also, the power setting is variable and needs to be set so that there is smoothest cutting with no sparking. Tissue damage is minimized when fully rectified and fully filtered current is utilized because there is little lateral heat spread to adjacent tissue. However, for better hemostasis, only fully rectified current may be used and will cause coagulation as well as cutting. Partially rectified current is mainly used for coagulation and hemostasis.

Advantages over cold steel surgery are that cutting is accomplished without pressure being required, hemostasis with fully filtered current effectively seals vessels under 2 mm in diameter, and the incision site and electrode tip are sterilized. Radiosurgery equipment is available at lower costs than laser equipment. Practice is required to develop a technique that minimizes lateral tissue damage, but with experience the advantages of radiosurgery over cold steel surgery become obtainable.

Disadvantages of this type of surgery include the risk for combustion of volatile gases and liquids (thus alcohol is contraindicated as a prepping solution or near the antennae). Radiosurgery should not be used to cut cartilage or bone, and there is risk if this technique is used near an unshielded pacemaker. Smoke and an unpleasant odor may be produced, but this is minimized with the use of a vacuum smoke evacuator. Tissue burning is possible, especially if the equipment is improperly used. However, adequate training and practice make this a useful surgical option.

Indications described for veterinary dermatology include cutaneous biopsy (but samples should be taken only with the fully rectified and fully filtered current) and removal of cutaneous neoplasms.

• ALTERNATIVE THERAPIES

Interest in so-called alternative therapies is increasing among horse owners. Unfortunately, little in the way of scientific evaluation is available in the veterinary dermatology literature. We encourage clinicians who use these modalities to design, perform, and publish meaningful clinical trials. We have so much to learn about these "natural" remedies.

Current veterinary literature contains much misinformation on the nature of both modern and ancient Chinese medical practices and acupuncutre.[58] For instance:

1. A basic misconception is that Chinese medicine, as currently practiced in the West, reflects the type of medicine most commonly practiced in China and, furthermore, that current medical practice in China truly reflects age-old customs.
2. Contrary to what appears to be popular belief, acupuncture is not and never was the primary therapeutic method used by the Chinese.

Today, science-based medicine has largely supplanted traditional practices in China.[58] It is curious that interest in Chinese medicine is rising in the West and waning in the East![58]

Acupuncture

Acupuncture can be defined as the insertion of very fine needles into specific, predetermined points on the body to produce physiologic responses.[58,68] In addition to needles, many other methods are used to stimulate acupuncture points, including acupressure, moxibustion, cupping, applying heat or cold, ultrasound, aquapuncture, electrostimulation, implantation, and laser use. The International Veterinary Acupuncture Society (IVAS, PO Box 2074, Nederland, CO 80466-2074) conducts courses, seminars, and international veterinary acupuncture congresses, and it is responsible for the accreditation of veterinary acupuncturists throughout the world.

Holistic Medicine (Herbal Medicine, Homeopathy)

Holistic health involves the use of herbs and other natural substances.[19,68a,96] A list of holistic veterinarians can be obtained from the American Holistic Veterinary Medical Association (2214 Old Emmerton Road, Bel Air, MD 21015), which also publishes a veterinary journal. We are aware of no well-designed clinical studies using this modality in veterinary dermatology.

In Asian and some European countries, many herbal products are in routine use for various dermatoses in humans.[9,39] Examples include Calendula (from *Calendula officinalis*, the marigold flower, which contains flavonoids and saponins that have anti-inflammatory, immunomodulatory, wound-healing properties)—available in ointment or cream for burns, diaper rash, minor wounds, leg ulcers; chamomile (from *Matricaria recutita*, the daisy flower family, containing oxides, flavonoids, and matricin that inhibit cyclooxygenase, lipoxygenase, and histamine release)—available in ointment or cream for various dermatitides, including atopic dermatitis and a 10-herb product ("decoction") taken by mouth and shown to be effective for atopic dermatitis in double-blinded, placebo-controlled studies.[9,39]

There have been a number of anecdotal reports on the use of a multiaction herbal skin gel (Phytogel, Ayuvet) in companion animals.[71,74] The product contains *Pongamia glabra, Cedrus deodara, Azadirachta indica*, and *Eucalyptus globus*. These are claimed to have antibacterial, antifungal, antiparasitic, anti-inflammatory, antipruritic, and wound-healing properties. The product is recommended for bacterial pyoderma, dermatophytosis, scabies, demodicosis, insect bites, pyotraumatic dermatitis, wounds, maggots, burns, solar dermatitis, papillomatosis, and so forth. Unfortunately, published trials are not interpretable.

Homeopathic medicine is based on the principle of similars; that is, the symptoms or syndromes a substance causes experimentally (at pharmacologic or toxic doses) are those that it may clinically resolve when given in specially prepared, exceedingly small doses to individuals who experienced similar symptoms and syndromes.[68a] Homeopathic remedies are specially prepared small doses that undergo a specific process of consecutive dilution and succussion (vigorous shaking); this process is called "potentization." The efficacy of homeopathic remedies in equine dermatology is largely unproven and quite controversial.

• GENE THERAPY

Gene therapy may someday be used to treat skin diseases in horses. Skin gene therapy can be defined as insertion or introduction of a desired gene into the skin in order to express the gene product.[87] The goal is to treat a specific disease process with the protein product of the introduced gene. There are potentially large numbers of diseases that could be treated in this manner, including diseases without a clear genetic basis (polygenic diseases).

Generally, there are two gene therapy approaches: (1) the in vivo approach, wherein the genes are directly introduced into the skin, and (2) the ex vivo approach, wherein target cells (e.g., keratinocytes) are cultured from biopsy specimens, the desired gene is inserted into the cultured cells, and the genetically modified cells are then grafted back onto the donor.[87] Genes may be introduced by chemical (DNA transfection), physical (microprojectiles, direct injection), or biologic (retrovirus, adenovirus) techniques.

• REFERENCES

1. Ackerman LJ: Dermatologic applications of radiowave surgery (radiosurgery). Comp Cont Educ 19:463, 1997.
2. Anderson BC: Aloe vera juice: a veterinary medicament? Comp Cont Educ 5:S364, 1983.
3. Andreassi L: Bioengineering of the skin. Clin Dermatol 13:289, 1995.
4. Arndt KA, et al: The pharmacology of topical therapy. In: Fitzpatrick TB, et al (eds): Dermatology in General Medicine, 4th ed. McGraw-Hill Book Co., New York, 1993, p 2837.
5. Becheral PA, et al: CD23 mediated nitric oxide synthase pathway induction in human keratinocytes is inhibited by retinoic acid derivatives. J Invest Dermatol 106:1182, 1996.
6. Bernstein JE, et al: Inhibition of histamine induced pruritus by topical tricyclic antidepressants. J Am Acad Dermatol 5:582, 1981.
7. Bottoms GD, et al: Circadian variation in plasma cortisol and corticosterone in pigs and mares. Am J Vet Res 33:785, 1972.
8. Brayton CF: Dimethyl sulfoxide (DMSO), a review. Cornell Vet 76:61, 1986.
9. Brown DJ, Dattner AM: Phytotherapeutic approaches to common dermatologic conditions. Arch Dermatol 134:1401, 1998.
10. Bruynzeel I, et al: Pentoxifylline inhibits T-cell adherence to keratinocytes. J Invest Dermatol 104:1004, 1995.
11. Carlotti DN, Maffart P: La chlorhexidine, revue bibliographique. Prat Méd Chir Anim Comp 31:553, 1996.
12. Chandraratna RAS: Rational design of receptor-selective retinoids. J Am Acad Dermatol 39(part 2): S124, 1998.
13. Chandraratna RAS: Tazarotene: the first receptor-selective topical retinoid for the treatment of psoriasis. J Am Acad Dermatol 37(Suppl 2, Part 3):S12, 1997.
14. Clark TP: Pharmacodynamics drug action and interaction. In: Dowling PM, et al (eds): Clinical Pharmacology: Principles and Practice. Western Veterinary Conference, Las Vegas, 1998, p 5.

15. Cohen ND, Carter GK: Steroid hepatopathy in a horse with glycocorticoid-induced hypoadrenocorticism. J Am Vet Med Assoc 200:1682, 1992.

16. Cohn LA: Glucocorticoids as immunosuppressive agents. Semin Vet Med Surg 12:150, 1997.

17. Croxtall JD, et al: Lipocortin 1 and the control of cPLA2 activity in A459 cells: glucocorticoids block EGF stimulation of cPLA2 phosphorylation. Biochem Pharmacol 52:351, 1996.

18. Cunningham FE, et al: The pharmacokinetics of dexamethasone in the Thoroughbred racehorse. J Vet Pharmacol Ther 19:68, 1996.

19. De-Hui S, et al: Manual of Dermatology in Chinese Medicine. Eastland Press, Seattle, 1995.

20. Draelos ZD: New developments in cosmetics and skin care products. Adv Dermatol 12:3, 1997.

21. Drake LA, et al: Guidelines of care for the use of topical glucocorticoids. J Am Acad Dermatol 35:615, 1996.

22. Duvic M, et al: Molecular mechanisms of tazarotene action in psoriasis. J Am Acad Dermatol 37(Suppl 2, Part 3):S18, 1997.

23. duVivier A, Stoughton RB: Tachyphylaxis to the action of topically applied corticosteroids. Arch Dermatol 111:581, 1975.

24. Elson ML: The role of retinoids in wound healing. J Am Acad Dermatol 39(Part 3):S79, 1998.

25. Evans JW, et al: Rhythmic cortisol secretion in the equine: analysis and physiological mechanisms. J Interdiscipl Cycle Res 8:11, 1977.

26. Fledman RJ, Maibach HI: Regional variation in percutaneous penetration of C14 cortisol in man. J Invest Dermatol 48:181, 1967.

27. Franz TJ: Kinetics of cutaneous drug penetration. Int J Dermatol 22:499, 1983.

28. Goette DK, Odom RB: Adverse effects of corticosteroids. Cutis 23:477, 1979.

29. Goldsmith LA: Propylene glycol. Int J Dermatol 17:703, 1978.

30. Granlund H, et al: Long-term follow-up of eczema patients treated with cyclosporine. Acta Dermatol Venereol 78:40, 1998.

31. Gyrd-Hansen N, et al: Percutaneous absorption of organophosphorus insecticides in pigs—the influence of different vehicles. J Vet Pharmacol Ther 16:174, 1993.

32. Hoffsis GF, et al: Plasma concentration of cortisol and corticosterone in the normal horse. Am J Vet Res 31:1379, 1970.

33. Humphreys F, Shuster S: The effect of topical dimethindene maleate on wheal reactions. Br J Clin Pharmacol 23:234, 1987.

34. Irvine CHG, Alexander SL: Factors affecting the circadian rhythm in plasma cortisol concentrations in the horse. Dom Anim Endocrinol 11:227, 1994.

35. James VHT, et al: Adrenocortical function in the horse. J Endocrinol 48:319, 1970.

36. Johnson AL, Malinowski K: Daily rhythm of cortisol and evidence for a photo-inducible phase for prolactin secretion in nonpregnant mares housed under non-interrupted and skeleton photoperiods. J Anim Sci 63:169, 1986.

37. Kinnunen T, Koskela M: Antibacterial and antifungal properties of propylene glycol, kexylene glycol, and 1,3-butylene glycol in vitro. Acta Dermatol Venereol 71:148, 1991.

38. Koch HJ, Vercelli A: Workshop report 3: Shampoos and other topical therapies. In: Ihrke PJ, et al (eds): Advances in Veterinary Dermatology, Vol 2. Pergamon Press, Oxford, 1993, p 409.

39. Koo J, Arain S: Traditional Chinese medicine for the treatment of dermatologic disorders. Arch Dermatol 134:1388, 1998.

40. Koo J, et al: Advances in psoriasis therapy. Adv Dermatol 12:47, 1997.

41. Kumar MKSA, et al: Diurnal variation in serum cortisol in ponies. J Anim Sci 42:1360, 1976.

42. Larsson M, et al: Plasma cortisol in the horse, diurnal rhythm and effects of exogenous ACTH. Acta Vet Scand 20:16, 1979.

43. Levine N: Role of retinoids in skin cancer treatment and prevention. J Am Acad Dermatol 39(Part 3):S62, 1998.

44. Lichtenstein J, et al: Nonsteroidal anti-inflammatory drugs: their use in dermatology. Int J Dermatol 26:80, 1987.

45. Lim KK, et al: Cyclosporine in the treatment of dermatologic disease: an update. Mayo Clin Proc 71:1183, 1996.

46. Lin AN, et al: Sulfur revisited. J Am Acad Dermatol 18:553, 1988.

47. Lober CW: Canthaxanthin: the "tanning" pill. J Am Acad Dermatol 13:660, 1985.

48. Maibach HI, Stoughton RB: Topical corticosteroids. Med Clin North Am 57:1253, 1973.

49. Manglesdorf DJ, et al: The retinoid receptors. In: Span HG, et al (eds): The Retinoids: Biology, Chemistry, and Medicine. New York, Raven Press, 1994, p 319.

50. Marks R: Pharmacokinetics and safety review of tazarotene. J Am Acad Dermatol 39(Part 2):S134, 1998.

51. Mason KV: Clinical and pathophysiologic aspects of parasitic skin diseases. In: Ihrke PJ, et al (eds): Advances in Veterinary Dermatology, Vol 2. Pergamon Press, New York, 1993, p 177.

52. Mukhtar H, et al: Green tea and skin: anticarcinogenic effects. J Invest Dermatol 102:3, 1994.

53. Nelson JS, Berns MW: Basic laser physics and tissue interactions. Contemp Dermatol 2:3, 1998.

54. Northway RB: Experimental use of aloe vera extract in clinical practice. Vet Med Small Anim Clin 71:196, 1975.

55. Pathak MA: Sunscreens, topical and systemic approaches for protection of human skin against harmful effects of solar radiation. J Am Acad Dermatol 7:285, 1982.

56. Peck GL, DiGiovanna JJ: The retinoids. In: Freedberg IM, et al (eds): Fitzpatrick's Dermatology in General Medicine V. McGraw-Hill, New York, 1999, p 2810.

56a. Peroni DL, et al: Prednisone per os is likely to have limited efficacy in horses. Equine Vet J 34:283, 2002.

57. Podkonjak KR: Veterinary cryotherapy—2. Vet Med (Small Animal Clinician) 77:183, 1982.

58. Ramey DW, et al: Veterinary acupuncture and traditional Chinese medicine: facts and fallacies. Comp Cont Educ :188, 2001.

59. Rautschka R, et al: Plasma histamine levels in laminitic horses and in horses treated with a corticosteroid. J Vet Med A 38:716, 1991.

60. Reed SM, Bayly WM: Equine Internal Medicine. W.B. Saunders Co, Philadelphia, 1998.

61. Robinson NE, et al: Why is oral prednisone ineffective for treating heaves? Proc Am Assoc Equine Practit 46:266, 2000.

62. Rosenkrantz WS, Frank LA: Therapy of equine pruritus. In: Ihrke PJ, et al (eds). Advances in Veterinary Dermatology II. Pergamon Press, New York, 1993, p 433.

63. Rosenkrantz WS: Systemic/topical therapy. Vet Clin N Am Equine Pract 11:127, 1995.

64. Ruszczak Z, Schwartz RA: Interferons in dermatology. Adv Dermatol 13:235, 1998.

65. Samlaska CP, et al: Pentoxifylline. J Am Acad Dermatol, 30:603, 1994.

66. Schauder S, Ippen H: Photodermatoses and light protection. Int J Dermatol 21:241, 1982.

67. Schleimer RP: Glucocorticosteroids. In: Middleton E, et al (eds): Allergy Principles and Practice. Mosby Year Book, St. Louis, 1993.

68. Schoen AM: Veterinary Acupuncture: Ancient Art to Modern Medicine. American Veterinary Publications, Goleta, California, 1994.

68a. Schoen AM, Wynn SG: Complementary and Alternative Veterinary Medicine. Principles and Practice. Mosby, St. Louis, 1998.

69. Schwartz E, et al: *In vivo* prevention of corticosteroid-induced skin atrophy by tretinoin in the hairless mouse is accompanied by modulation of collagen, glycosaminoglycans, and fibronectin. J Invest Dermatol 102:241, 1994.

70. Scott DW: La dermatite atopique du cheval. Méd Vét Québec 30:82, 2000.

71. Scott DW, et al: Muller & Kirk's Small Animal Dermatology VI. W.B. Saunders Co., Philadelphia, 2001.

72. Shelton RM: Aloe vera: Its chemical and therapeutic properties. Int J Dermatol 30:679, 1991.

73. Shroot B: Pharmacodynamics and pharmacokinetics of topical adapalene. J Am Acad Dermatol 39(Part 3):S17, 1998.

74. Silver RJ, et al: Multi-center clinical evaluation of an ayurvedic topical herbal formulation for veterinary dermatopathies. J Am Holistic Vet Med Assoc 17:33, 1998.

75. Skrabalak DS, Maylin GA: Dexamethasone metabolism in the horse. Steroids 39:233, 1982.

76. Spicer MS, Goldberg DJ: Lasers in dermatology. J Am Acad Dermatol 34:1, 1996.

77. Spiess BM, et al: Systemic dexamethasone concentrations in horses after continued topical treatment with an ophthalmic preparation of dexamethasone. Am J Vet Res 60:571, 1999.

78. Surber C, et al: Topical corticosteroids. J Am Acad Dermatol 32:1025, 1995.

79. Thoma RE, et al: Phototherapy: a promising cancer therapy. Vet Med Small Anim Clin 78:1693, 1983.

80. Tontain PL, et al: Dexamethasone and prednisolone in the horse: pharmacokinetics and action on the adrenal gland. Am J Vet Res 45:1750, 1984.

81. Toutain PL, et al: Diurnal and episodic variations of plasma hydrocortisone concentrations in horses. Dom Anim Endocrinol 5:55, 1988.

82. Toyoda M, Morohashi M: Morphological assessment of the effects of cyclosporine A on mast cell–nerve relationship in atopic dermatitis. Acta Dermatol Venerol 78:321, 1998.

83. Trettien A: Workshop Report 13: shampoos and other topical therapy. In: Von Tscharner C, Halliwell REW (eds): Advances in Veterinary Dermatology, Vol 1. Baillière-Tindall, Philadelphia, 1990, p 434.

84. Turner TA, et al: Effects of heat, cold, biomagnets and ultrasound on skin circulation in the horse. Proc Am Assoc Equine Practit 37:249, 1991.

85. Vaughan C, et al: Photoinstability of UVA sun protection products. Am J Cosmetic Surg 14:1423, 1997.

86. Villar D, et al: Toxicity of melaleuca oil and related essential oils applied topically on dogs and cats. Vet Hum Toxicol 36:139, 1994.

87. Vogel JC, et al: Gene therapy for skin diseases. Adv Dermatol 11:383, 1996.

88. Webster GF: Topical tretinoin in acne therapy. J Am Acad Dermatol 39(Part 3):S38, 1998.

89. Weiss JS, Shavin JS: Adapalene for the treatment of acne vulgaris. J Am Acad Dermatol 39(Part 3):S50, 1998.

90. Werth VP, Lazarus GS: Systemic glucocorticoids. In: Freedberg IM, et al (eds): Fitzpatrick's Dermatology in General Medicine V. McGraw-Hill, New York, 1999, p 2783.

91. Wiegand UW, Chou RC: Pharmacokinetics of oral isotretinoin. J Am Acad Dermatol 39(Part 3):S8, 1998.

92. Wiegand UW, Chou RC: Pharmacokinetics of acitretin and etretinate. J Am Acad Dermatol 39(Part 3):S25, 1998.

93. Withrow SJ (ed): Symposium on cryosurgery. Vet Clin N Am Small Anim Pract 10:753, 1980.

94. White GM: Acne therapy. Adv Dermatol 14:29, 1999.

95. White-Weiterhs N, Medleau L: Evaluation of topical therapies for the treatment of dermatophyte-infected hair from dogs and cats. J Am Anim Hosp Assoc 31:250, 1995.

96. Winter WG: The Holistic Veterinary Handbook. Galde Press, Lakeville, MN, 1997.

97. Wolf R: Soaps, shampoos, and detergents: a scientific soap opera. Clin Dermatol 14:1, 1996.

98. Yosipovitch G, Maibach HI: Effect of pramoxine on experimentally induced pruritus in humans. J Am Acad Dermatol 37:278, 1997.

99. Zokolovick A, et al: Diurnal variation in plasma glucocorticosteroid levels in the horse (*Equus caballus*). J Endocrinol 35:249, 1966.

Chapter 4

Bacterial Skin Diseases

● CUTANEOUS BACTERIOLOGY AND NORMAL DEFENSE MECHANISMS

The skin forms a protective barrier without which life would be impossible. The defense has three components: physical, chemical, and microbial (see Chapter 1).

Hair forms the first line of physical defense to protect against the contact of pathogens with the skin. Hair may also harbor bacteria, especially staphylococci. However, the relatively inert stratum corneum forms the basic physical defense layer. Its tightly packed keratinized cells are permeated by an emulsion of sebum, sweat, and intercellular cement substance. The emulsion is concentrated in the outer layers of keratin, where some of the volatile fatty acids vaporize, leaving a fairly impermeable superficial sebaceous crust. Together, the cells and the emulsion function as an effective physical barrier. The emulsion provides a chemical barrier to potential pathogens in addition to its physical properties. Fatty acids, especially linoleic acid, have potent antibacterial properties. Water-soluble substances in the emulsion include inorganic salts and proteins that inhibit bacteria.

The skin is viewed as an immune organ that plays an active role in the induction and maintenance of immune responses, which can be beneficial or detrimental (see Chapter 8). Specific components include epidermal Langerhans' cells, dermal dendrocytes, keratinocytes, skin-seeking T lymphocytes, mast cells, and the endothelium of postcapillary venules. Various cytokines, complement, and immunoglobulins are found in the emulsion layer and contribute to the skin's immunologic function. Many individual components of this complicated system have antimicrobial effects, so the normal skin should be viewed as an organ that is resistant to infection.

The normal skin microflora also contributes to skin defense mechanisms. Bacteria are located in the superficial epidermis and in the infundibulum of the hair follicles, where sweat and sebum provide nutrients. The normal flora is a mixture of bacteria that live in symbiosis, probably exchanging growth factors. The flora may change with different cutaneous environments. These are affected by factors such as heat, pH, salinity, moisture, albumin level, and fatty acid level. The close relationship between the host and the microorganisms enables bacteria to occupy microbial niches and to inhibit colonization by invading organisms. In addition, many bacteria (*Bacillus* spp., *Streptococcus* spp., and *Staphylococcus* spp.) are capable of producing antibiotic substances, and some bacteria can produce enzymes (e.g., β-lactamase) that inhibit antibiotics.

Bacteria cultured from normal skin are called *normal inhabitants* and are classified as resident or transient, depending on their ability to multiply in that habitat (see Chapter 1).[35,36] Residents successfully multiply on normal skin, thus forming a permanent population that can be reduced in number by degerming methods, but not eliminated. Transients are cutaneous contaminants acquired from the environment and can be removed by simple hygienic measures.

Studies on the microbial flora of normal equine skin have been strictly qualitative (see Chapter 1).[35] It is clear that skin and hair coat are exceedingly effective environmental samplers, providing a temporary haven and way station for all sorts of organisms. Thus, only repetitive quantitative studies will allow reliable distinction between equine cutaneous residents and transients.

There has been speculation about the means by which only a small number of a vast array of bacteria in the environment are able to colonize or infect the skin. The potent cleaning forces of dilution, washout, drying, and desquamation of surface cells prevent many organisms from colonizing the skin. It is now recognized that bacterial adhesion is a prerequisite to colonization and infection.[27,36] Bacterial adhesion is a complex process influenced by both the host and the organism. Bacteria possess surface adhesion molecules, which influence their ability to bind to keratinocytes. For staphylococci, teichoic acid and protein A appear to be most important surface adhesion molecules. These molecules bind to host surface receptors (e.g., fibronectin and vitronectin) to prevent the bacteria from being brushed from the skin. Adhesion is increased with increasing time, temperature, and concentration of bacteria, as well as in certain diseases. In hyperproliferative disorders, more bacteria adhere to the skin because more binding sites are available. Organisms from the transient group are pathogenic in rare cases. Gram-negative organisms tend to flourish in moist, warm areas and to predominate when medications depress the gram-positive flora.

Anaerobic bacteria are usually abundant in gastrointestinal secretions; therefore, fecal contamination is a cause of soft tissue infections due to these organisms. Anaerobic bacteria isolated from horse infections include *Clostridium* spp., *Bacteroides* spp., and *Fusobacterium* spp. These bacteria are usually found in granulomas, cellulitis, abscesses, fistulae, and other soft tissue wounds.

The numbers of resident bacteria on the skin tend to vary among individuals; some animals have many organisms, whereas others have few. The number per individual may remain constant, unless disturbed by antibacterial treatment or changes in climate. More bacteria are found on the skin in warm, wet weather than in cold, dry weather. Moist, intertriginous areas tend to have large numbers, and individuals with oily skin have higher counts.

• SKIN INFECTIONS

The normal skin of healthy individuals is highly resistant to invasion by the wide variety of bacteria to which it is constantly exposed. Pathogenic organisms such as coagulase-positive staphylococci may produce characteristic lesions of folliculitis, furunculosis, and cellulitis in the absence of any obvious impairment of host defenses. However, localized disruption of normal host defenses as produced by maceration (water, friction from skin folds, and topical treatments), physical trauma (abrasions, cuts, punctures, biting insects and arthropods, scratching, and rubbing), or the introduction of a foreign body (plant awns) may facilitate development of overt infection. Treatment with immunosuppressive agents and immunosuppressive diseases can predispose patients to infections.

The host-bacteria relationship in infections of the skin involves three major elements: (1) the pathogenic properties of the organism (particularly the invasive potential and the toxigenic properties), (2) the portal of entry, and (3) the host defense and inflammatory responses to bacterial invasion.[27] Bacterial infection involving the skin may manifest itself in either of two major forms: (1) as a primary cutaneous process or (2) as a secondary manifestation of infection elsewhere in the body. The cutaneous changes associated with systemic infection are not necessarily suppurative but may represent those of vasculitis or a hypersensitivity response.[35]

Microorganisms isolated from an intact lesion such as a pustule are evidence of infection, not colonization. Colonization means that a potential pathogen is living on the skin or in a lesion but that its presence is causing no reaction in the host. The problem in evaluating a pyoderma culture is to separate secondary colonization from secondary infection. The presence of many degenerate neutrophils and phagocytosed bacteria is direct evidence of a host reaction and is compatible with infection. Infection can be determined by direct smears of lesion exudates, which may be more informative than cultures.

Staphylococcal organisms, common isolates from skin infections in horses, are not particularly virulent; thus, any skin infection should be considered a sign of some underlying cutaneous, metabolic, or immunologic abnormality. Traditionally, skin infections are classified as either primary or secondary to reflect the absence or the presence of an underlying cause.

Secondary infections are by far the most common and result from some cutaneous, immunologic, or metabolic abnormality. Secondary infections may involve organisms other than staphylococci, tend to respond slowly or poorly to treatment if the underlying problem is ignored, and recur unless the cause is resolved. Virtually any skin condition described in this text can predispose to infection, but allergic, ectoparasitic, seborrheic, or follicular disorders are the most common causes of infection.

Allergic horses are prone to infections because of the damage they do to their skin while itching, the corticosteroids that they often receive, and possibly some immunologic abnormalities associated with their allergic predisposition. When their skin becomes infected, the level of pruritus increases quickly and does not respond well to corticosteroid administration. Antibiotic treatment resolves the lesions of infection and reduces, but does not eliminate, the pruritus.

Seborrheic animals have greatly increased numbers of bacteria on their skin surface, which can colonize an epidermal or follicular defect and cause infection. They also contribute to the alteration of the surface lipid layer to one that can induce inflammation. In this situation, the patches of seborrheic dermatitis cause the animal to itch and induce true infection in these areas. Superficial infections result in significant scaling during their development and resolution. It can sometimes be difficult to decide whether the seborrhea induced the infection or vice versa. Scaling caused by infection decreases quickly with antibiotic therapy. If seborrheic signs are still pronounced after 14 to 21 days of antibiotic treatment, the animal should be evaluated for an underlying seborrheic disorder.

Follicular inflammation, obstruction, degeneration, or a combination of these predisposes the follicle to bacterial infection. Inflammatory causes are numerous, but dermatophytosis is most commonly implicated. Follicular obstruction occurs as part of generalized seborrhea, in focal seborrheic disorders, follicular dysplasias, and other congenital disorders of the follicle. Follicular degeneration can be caused by all of these conditions, as well as by alopecia areata. In cases of follicular infection, examination of skin scrapings, cytology, and evaluations for dermatophytes (e.g., trichogram and fungal culture) are always recommended. After those tests, the skin biopsy is most useful because pathologic changes are too deep to be appreciated with the naked eye. The inflammation associated with the secondary bacterial infection can mask some of the histologic features of the predisposing disease; thus, it is best to resolve the infection first and then perform the skin biopsy.

The most common metabolic cause of skin infection is hyperadrenocorticism (iatrogenic or spontaneous), but diabetes mellitus, and other systemic metabolic problems must also be considered. These disorders predispose to infection by their impact on the animal's immune system and the changes they induce in the hair follicle.

Acquired immunodeficiencies are common complications of many serious illnesses. The best-known examples of acquired immunodeficiency disease are associated with viral and protozoal infections.

The classification of primary infection is more problematic. *Primary infections* are described as those that occur in otherwise healthy skin, are staphylococcal with rare exception, and are cured by appropriate antibiotic therapy. This definition overlooks the tendency for the infection to recur. For instance, a horse is examined for a skin infection and no historical or physical abnormality to explain the infection is found. Is this a primary infection, an infection secondary to some transient insult to the skin, or an infection secondary to some as yet undefined underlying problem? The key to the primacy of the infection is its tendency to recur. Infections that resolve with no residual skin disease and do not recur with regularity or within a reasonable period (e.g., 3 to 6 months) could be considered primary infections. If the infection recurs early, the animal has some subclinical skin disease or an immunologic abnormality.

Identification of bacteria from skin lesions may provide important information as to the cause of cutaneous infections, whether primary or secondary to systemic processes. The presence of normal skin flora may confuse interpretation of these studies. All too often, the finding on culture of a potential pathogen, such as a coagulase-positive *Staphylococcus* sp., is equated with the presence of infection. It is essential to remember that damaged skin provides a medium for proliferation of many bacteria. Only by correlating the clinical appearance of the lesion with cytologic and bacteriologic data can one reach the proper decision concerning the presence of bacterial disease.

Samples of pus or exudates from intact pustules, nodules, abscesses, draining tracts, or ulcers can be smeared on glass slides, air-dried, and stained with new methylene blue, Gram's stain, or Diff Quik for light microscopic examination. Important observations to be made include (1) type(s) of bacteria present (cocci versus rods; gram-positive or gram-negative) and (2) the associated inflammatory response. Skin contaminants are usually recognized by being extracellular and being often clumped in microcolonies. Pathogenic bacteria are found intracellularly within neutrophils and macrophages. Thus, direct smears often provide the first clue to the specific cause of the infection and also serve as a guide in selecting appropriate culture media and antibiotic therapy.

Because the skin of large animals is a veritable cesspool of bacteria, cultures must be carefully taken and interpreted (see Chapter 1). Intact pustules, nodules, and abscesses are preferred lesions for culture and may be aspirated with a needle and syringe or punctured and swabbed with a culturette, after the overlying epithelium has been gently swabbed with alcohol and allowed to air-dry. Cultures of open sores (erosions, ulcers, and sinuses) and exudative surfaces often generate confusing, if not misleading, bacteriologic data.

When intact, pus-containing lesions are not available for sampling, the culturing of surgical biopsy specimens is preferred. Papules, plaques, nodules, and areas of diffuse swelling may be surgically prepared (e.g., povidone-iodine or chlorhexidine scrub) and punch or excision biopsies taken with aseptic techniques. The epidermis must be removed with a sterile scalpel blade, as topical antiseptics may be retained in this layer and affect culture results. These biopsy specimens can then be delivered to the laboratory in various transport media for culture and antibiotic susceptibility testing.

• TREATMENT OF SKIN INFECTIONS

Satisfactory resolution of a skin infection necessitates that the cause of the infection be identified and corrected and that the infection receive proper treatment.* If the cause of the infection persists, either the response to treatment is poor or the infection recurs shortly after treatment is discontinued. If the cause is resolved but inappropriate treatment for the infection is given, the infection persists and worsens.

Skin infections can be treated topically, systemically, surgically, or by some combination of these. Some equine infections are too widespread or too deep to be resolved with topical treatment alone, but judicious topical therapy can make the patient more comfortable and hasten its response to antibiotics. Topical treatment can take considerable time and effort on the owner's part

---

*References 4-6, 13, 26, 29, 35.

and can irritate the skin if the products are too harsh. Surgery alone can be useful with focal lesions or can be performed as an adjunct to other treatments. Management must be individualized.

Topical Treatment

Topical treatments are used to reduce or eliminate the bacterial population in and around an area of infection and to remove tissue debris (see Chapter 3).[6,36] Debris removal is of paramount importance because it allows direct contact of the active ingredient with the organism and promotes drainage. Agents commonly used include chlorhexidine, povidone-iodine, benzoyl peroxide, and various antibiotics, especially fusidic acid, mupirocin, and bacitracin.

Infections restricted to the skin surface or intact hair follicles may be effectively treated with topical agents alone. When the number of lesions is small and they are confined to a limited area, antiseptics or antibiotics in a cream, ointment, or gel formulation may be sufficient to resolve the infection (see Chapter 3). Benzoyl peroxide gels or antibiotic formulations receive widest use. The benzoyl peroxide gels marketed to veterinarians contain 5% active ingredient, which can be irritating, especially with repeated application. In most instances, antibiotic preparations are nonirritating. In most cases, transdermal absorption of the agent is limited, but frequent application over wide areas should be avoided.

Many potent antibacterial agents are available in topical form (see Chapter 3). The most commonly used are mupirocin (Bactoderm, Pfizer), fusidic acid, neomycin, gentamicin, bacitracin, polymyxin B, and thiostrepton. Important considerations for some of these agents are as follows: (1) mupirocin and fusidic acid are more effective than other topical agents for treatment staphylococcal pyodermas; (2) mupirocin has poor activity against gram-negative infections; (3) neomycin has more potential for allergic sensitization than do most topicals, and susceptibility is variable for gram-negative organisms; and (4) polymyxin B and bacitracin in combination may be effective for gram-negative as well as gram-positive organisms; however, they are rapidly inactivated by purulent exudates and do not penetrate well. Mupirocin is particularly useful because of its ability to penetrate the skin and its very low incidence of adverse reactions.[6,15,36] It is inactivated by exudates and debris, so the surface of lesions must be cleaned prior to application.

Often, topical antibiotics are formulated with other ingredients, most commonly glucocorticoids. There are numerous antibiotic-steroid combinations (Gentocin spray, Otomax, Tresaderm, and Animax). These are occasionally indicated in chronic, dry, lichenified, secondarily infected dermatoses (seborrhea complex and allergic dermatoses) and pyotraumatic dermatitis. Several clinical and bacteriologic trials in humans and dogs showed that these antibiotic-steroid combinations were superior to either agent alone.[36]

Widespread superficial infections are best treated with antibacterial shampoos (see Chapter 3).[6,35,36] The manipulation of the skin during its application and the vehicle of the shampoo removes tissue debris, which allows better contact between the antiseptic and the bacteria. When four commercial antibacterial shampoos were studied on dog skin, none could completely sterilize the skin, but all significantly reduced the bacterial population.[36] Benzoyl peroxide was the most effective, followed by chlorhexidine acetate. Mixtures of acetic and boric acid are also effective.

Product selection depends on the preferences of the owner and the clinician and the condition of the animal's skin. Animals with underlying hypersensitivity disorders or "sensitive" skin should be bathed with nonirritating or minimally irritating agents such as chlorhexidine (see Chapter 3). Benzoyl peroxide products should be reserved for greasy horses or horses with deep crusted infections (see Chapter 3). In this latter group, shampoo selection should be reevaluated in 10 to 14 days because the skin will be much different then.

Iodophors have been popular topical antimicrobial agents in equine practice.* Povidone-

---

*References 4-6, 17, 18, 24, 29, 35, 53, 64.

iodine is available as a 5% solution (Betadine, Purdue Frederick; Poviderm, Vetus; Povidone-Iodine, Equicare), a 5% shampoo (Poviderm, Vetus; Povidone, Butler), and a 10% ointment (Povidone Iodine, First Priority). Polyhydroxydine complex iodine is available as a 1% solution and a 1% spray (Xenodine, V.P.L.). Although these products are excellent antimicrobial agents, their propensity for causing dry, scaly skin and haircoat, as well as irritation, and possible staining of skin and haircoat makes them less desirable than chlorhexidine or benzoyl peroxide.

A thorough bath with a 10- to 15-minute shampoo contact time is indicated at the beginning of treatment. The timing to the next bath depends on the severity of the infection, the cause of the infection, and the speed of the animal's response to the antibiotics used. Some clinicians request that the client bathe the animal at a set interval, typically every third to seventh day, whereas other clinicians give the client guidelines for when a bath is indicated and let the client decide when to bathe. If the client is not overzealous, the latter method is most appropriate because it treats the animal on the basis of its needs.

In the case of deep draining infections, the hair in the area must be clipped to prevent the formation of a sealing crust and to allow the topical agents to contact the diseased tissues. Although shampooing is beneficial, soaks are more appropriate at the onset of treatment. Hydrotherapy loosens and removes crusts, decreases the number of surface bacteria, promotes epithelialization, and helps to lessen the discomfort associated with the lesions. With warm-water soaks, the vascular plexus opens, which may allow better distribution of the systemic antibiotic. Antiseptics such as chlorhexidine and povidone-iodine are added for additional antibacterial activity.

If there are draining lesions on a distal limb, the area can be soaked in a bucket. For lesions higher up on the limb, a newborn disposable baby diaper is a useful aid. The outer plastic layer protects the environment while the high absorbency pad holds the soaking solution next to the skin. For these lesions, a hypertonic drawing solution of magnesium sulfate (Epsom salts) (2 tbsp/qt or 30 ml/L of warm water) can be beneficial. Soaks are typically done for 15 to 20 minutes, once or twice daily. Because hydrotherapy hydrates the epithelium, excessively soaked skin macerates easily and may become infected more easily. As the antibiotic therapy progresses, drainage should decrease. When drainage is slight after a soak, the frequency of soaking should be decreased or stopped entirely. Typically, soaking is continued for 3 to 7 days.

Systemic Antibiotics

Systemic antibiotic agents are used for bacterial skin diseases that are not treatable with topical therapy.* Because the majority of equine skin infections are caused by coagulase-positive staphylococci and *Dermatophilus congolensis*, antibiotics that affect these bacteria and concentrate in the skin are of primary interest.

Because each antibiotic has its own unique features, the drugs used in equine dermatology, namely the penicillins, potentiated sulfonamides, macrolides, and fluoroquinolones, should be studied before they are used. Proper antibiotic use necessitates that the antibiotic inhibit the specific bacteria, preferably in a bactericidal manner. Bacteriostatic drugs may also be effective as long as the host is not immunocompromised. The drug should have a narrow spectrum so that it produces little effect on organisms of the natural flora of the skin or the intestinal tract (for oral medications). The antibiotic should be inexpensive, should be easily given (orally, if it is to be prescribed for home use) and absorbed, and should have no adverse effects.

The most important factors influencing the effectiveness of antibiotics are the susceptibility of the bacteria and the distribution to the skin in effective levels of activity at the infection site. Only about 4% of the cardiac output of blood reaches the skin, compared with 33% that reaches muscle.[36] This variation is reflected in the relative distribution of antibiotics among organs.

---

*References 4-6, 13, 26, 29, 35, 44, 49, 62, 65.

Although the epidermis is relatively avascular, studies of skin infections showed that the systemic route of therapy is better than the topical route for all but the most superficial infections. The stratum corneum is a major permeability barrier to effective topical drug penetration. These facts led to the inescapable conclusion that the skin is one of the most difficult tissues in which to obtain high antibiotic levels. Factors that may reduce the effectiveness of a therapeutic plan are the following:

1. The organism is resistant to the antibiotic, and because most coagulase-positive staphylococci organisms produce β-lactamase, antibiotics resistant to this substance should be selected.
2. The dosage is inadequate to attain and then maintain inhibitory concentrations in the skin.
3. The organism may be surviving inside macrophages, where it is not exposed to the effect of most antibiotics.
4. The organism is within a necrotic center or protected by a foreign body such as a hair fragment.
5. The organism is walled off by dense scar tissue.
6. The duration of therapy is inadequate to eradicate the infection.

In addition to the susceptibility of the organism, various owner and animal factors enter into the equation during antibiotic selection. Antibiotics are either time-dependent or concentration-dependent in their action. Time-dependent drugs must be given at their specified interval of administration for maximal efficacy. The total dose administered is more important for the concentration-dependent drugs. The route of administration (oral versus intramuscular) and frequency of administration (q8h versus q24h) are also often important for owner and patient compliance.

The depth of the infection also influences drug selection. Deep infections require protracted courses of treatment, can respond less favorably to certain drugs than more superficial infections, and tend to become fibrotic. Twelve-week courses of antibiotics are not unusual in treating some infections.

Antibiotic selection is not so straightforward when the empirically selected antibiotic is not effective or when the infection recurs shortly after treatment is discontinued. If the empirically selected antibiotic has only good susceptibility, most clinicians empirically select another drug with excellent susceptibility. If this new drug fails to be effective, one must carefully evaluate whether the owner is complying with the treatment regimen and whether the skin is truly infected. If no reason for this poor response can be found, susceptibility testing is mandatory.

If cytologic study shows a mixed infection, susceptibility testing is mandatory because the sensitivity of nonstaphylococcal organisms is not always predictable. If all organisms are susceptible to a safe, reasonably inexpensive drug, that drug should be used. Occasionally, no one drug fits the susceptibility profile of all organisms or the singular drug is too toxic or expensive for long-term use. If the infection contains coagulase-positive staphylococci, as many do, the initial antibiotic selection should be aimed at that organism. Eradication of the staphylococcal component may make the microenvironment unfavorable for the growth of the other organisms. If the antistaphylococcal antibiotic improves but does not resolve the infection, alternative drugs must be used.

After an antibiotic has been selected, it should be dispensed at the correct dosage, administered at the appropriate dosage interval, and be used for a sufficient period of time.

Systemic treatment of bacterial dermatoses in horses can be challenging. Factors to consider include the size of the patient (and, thus, the cost of medication), bioavailability of orally administered agents, ability to achieve adequate cutaneous concentrations of drug, the compliance of the patient and owner, the limited number of antibiotics approved for use in the horse, the limited number of antibiotics that are practical and/or safe to use in the horse, and the duration of therapy required (and, hence, the cost of treatment).

Penicillins are a good choice when bacteria are susceptible. They are bactericidal, narrow-spectrum, and have a low incidence of severe side effects. They are a common cause of drug-induced urticaria (see Chapter 8). Most streptococci, *Corynebacterium pseudotuberculosis,* many anaerobes, many actinomycetes (*Dermatophilus, Actinomyces*), and *Actinobacillus* spp. are susceptible. Most coagulase-positive staphylococci are resistant. Potassium penicillin G seems to be interchangeable with procaine penicillin G.[69] Since most racing jurisdictions in North America consider *any* concentration of procaine in urine to be a violation, potassium penicillin G is a useful alternative. Amoxicillin has poor oral bioavailability in the horse.[51]

Trimethoprim-potentiated sulfonamides are effective and popular antibiotics in equine dermatology. They are broad-spectrum and generally well-tolerated, but they are a common cause of drug-induced urticaria, erythema multiforme, exfoliative dermatitis, and allergy-like pruritus (see Chapters 8 and 9). Some clinicians have occasionally seen anemia and/or leukopenia in horses treated with long-term trimethoprim-potentiated sulfonamides and recommend monthly hemograms during prolonged therapy.[15] Most coagulase-positive staphylococci, streptococci, *Dermatophilus congolensis,* and many *Actinobacillus* spp., *Rhodococcus equi,* and *Corynebacterium pseudotuberculosis* are susceptible. Published therapeutic protocols vary from 15 to 35 mg/kg, given orally q12-24h.* The authors routinely use 15 mg/kg q12h and use 30 mg/kg q12h for particularly chronic, fibrosed, pyogranulomatous lesions.

Erythromycin is a macrolide, narrow-spectrum, bacteriostatic antibiotic that is useful in equine dermatology. It enters phagocytic cells and can be particularly effective for intracellular bacteria and in pyogranulomatous lesions. Most coagulase-positive staphylococci, streptococci, *Clostridium* spp., *Actinobacillus* spp., and *R. equi* are susceptible. In foals with *R. equi* pneumonia that are treated with erythromycin, there is an increased risk for diarrhea, hyperthermia, and respiratory distress as compared with foals treated with trimethoprim-potentiated sulfonamides or penicillin.[67] In spite of this, erythromycin, with or without concurrent rifampin, is the treatment of choice for *R. equi* infections. Erythromycin estolate is often referred to as the erythromycin of choice,[44] although one study indicated that erythromycin phosphate or erythromycin stearate should be just as effective.[52] Published treatment protocols vary from 25 mg/kg given orally q6-8h, to 37.5 mg/kg q12h.† Erythromycin ethylsuccinate caused severe colitis in a small number of adult horses.[58a] Some authors have actually indicated that the use of erythromycin in horses is associated with significant and unacceptable risks.[37] However, the majority of authors and clinicians do not share this opinion, at least as concerns erythromycin base, phosphate, stearate, or estolate.[15]

Enrofloxacin is increasingly used in equine dermatology. It is broad-spectrum, bactericidal, enters phagocytic cells, penetrates pyogranulomatous and fibrosed lesions, has few side effects, and is user-friendly. Serum levels may be higher when feed is withheld.[55] Coagulase-positive staphylococci, streptococci, and *Actinobacillus* spp. are susceptible. Therapeutic protocols vary from 2.5 to 5 mg/kg given orally q12-24h.‡ The major concern with enrofloxacin is the production of chondrotoxicity and lameness, especially in foals. Results of published studies are contradictory, partially because of different doses and frequencies of administration. In some studies, 5 to 15 mg/kg/day for up to 3 weeks in adult horses produced no side effects.[46,54-56] In one study, 1 of 4 adult horses given 5 mg/kg/day developed lameness and joint swelling after 19 days.[61] Foals are more susceptible to chondrotoxicity.[45,47,48,61] The authors use 5 mg/kg PO q24h in adults and have not seen side effects. Many clinicians administer the bovine injectable enrofloxacin (Baytril 100, Bayer) orally in horses. Because of the uncertain incidence of side effects in adult horses, enrofloxacin should be used when other antibiotics fail or are inappropriate.

---

*References 4-6, 13, 26, 29, 49, 58, 62, 65, 70, 71.
†References 4-6, 13, 26, 29, 44, 49, 52, 62, 65.
‡References 4, 5, 29, 46, 54-56.

Rifampin enters phagocytic cells and is effective for intracellular bacteria and in pyogranulomatous, abscessed, fibrosed lesions. Coagulase-positive staphylococci, streptococci, *R. equi*, and *C. pseudotuberculosis* are susceptible. Recommended therapeutic protocols vary from 10 mg/kg given orally q12h to 10 to 20 mg/kg q24h.* Because resistance to rifampin monotherapy can occur frequently and rapidly, it is usually given in conjunction with other antimicrobial agents (e.g., erythromycin, penicillin, trimethoprim-potentiated sulfonamides).

Gentamicin is occasionally used in equine dermatology. Coagulase-positive staphylococci, *Actinobacillus* spp., and *R. equi* are usually susceptible. Pharmacokinetic data[63] and clinical experience indicate that 6.6 mg/kg given IM q24h is as effective and safe as previously recommended protocols (2 to 4 mg q6-12h).[6,44,62]

Metronidazole has been used for anaerobic infections, but often in combination with other antibiotics (e.g., penicillins, aminoglycosides, trimethoprim-potentiated sulfonamides). Recommended treatment protocols vary from 7.5 to 25 mg/kg given orally q6-8h,[6,62] to 20 to 25 mg/kg q12h.[43,68] Side effects are rare, the most common being appetite depression.[68]

Cephalosporins are excellent broad-spectrum, bactericidal antibiotics that are very effective against coagulase-positive staphylococci, streptococci, and anaerobes. However, current products and protocols are, for the most part, impractical and very expensive.†

The most commonly recognized cause of the inability to resolve a skin infection, or of its relapse days after the treatment is discontinued, is an insufficient course of treatment. Although textbooks and clinical experience can suggest appropriate courses of treatment, each animal responds at its own rate and must be treated until its infection is resolved. Resolution means that all lesions have healed both on the surface and in the deeper tissues. Surface healing is easy to determine by visual inspection, but deep healing is much more difficult to assess and necessitates palpation of the lesions and regional lymph nodes.

Intercurrent corticosteroid administration confounds the problem greatly. Corticosteroids decrease visual and palpable inflammation, which is the key sign in determining when an infection is resolved. An inflamed hair follicle is still infected, whereas one that looks and feels normal is probably healed. With concurrent corticosteroid use, it is impossible to determine whether the antibiotic resolved the inflammation, and therefore the infection, or whether the corticosteroid is masking the infection. If an individual animal requires both antibiotics and corticosteroids, the corticosteroid administration should be discontinued at least 7 days before the final evaluation of the infection.

In infections of the intact hair follicle, deep tissues rarely become inflamed enough to be detected by palpation, so infection could still be present when the surface has healed. To prevent relapses because of this inapparent infection, it is recommended that antibiotic treatment be continued for 7 to 10 days after surface healing. In deeper infections, surface healing is misleading and antibiotic treatment must be continued after the dermal inflammation is gone. Deep lesions always heal on the surface well before the deep infection is resolved. Because some small, nonpalpable nidi of infection can persist even when the tissues feel normal by palpation, antibiotic treatment should be continued for 14 to 21 days after the tissues return to apparent normalcy. The time to resolution dictates the length of postnormalcy treatment.

Ideally, the clinician should reexamine all animals to determine when true healing has occurred. This is impractical in many instances and is not absolutely necessary in the case of more superficial infections. As long as the owner is an astute observer and treats the animal after clinical normalcy is present, most infections can be resolved without reexamination. Reexamination is

---

*References 4-6, 13, 26, 29, 42, 60, 72.
†References 4-6, 13, 26, 29, 49, 62.

mandatory for animals with deep infections. Owners cannot tell when the deep infection is resolved and almost always underestimate the need for antibiotics. Some clinicians schedule examinations every 14 days, whereas other clinicians examine the animal only when the owner reports that the lesions have healed. The approach is individualized for best results.

Deep infections are problematic for both the client and the clinician. With follicular rupture and damage to the dermal tissues, the inflammation tends to be pyogranulomatous and endogenous foreign bodies (keratin, hair shafts, and damaged collagen) are usually found in the dermis. During the first 2 to 4 weeks of antibiotic treatment, the lesion improves dramatically and then apparently stops responding. If treatment is stopped at this point, any ground gained is lost because it is unlikely that the deep infection is resolved. The rapid initial improvement is due to the resolution of the pyogenic component of the infection, but the granulomatous component remains and responds much more slowly. As long as there is slow, steady improvement, the antibiotic administration should be continued, even if the course of treatment approaches 12 weeks or longer. With long-term treatment, most lesions resolve completely, but the healing of some lesions reaches a certain point and improves no further. In these cases, the tissues never return to palpable normalcy because of resultant fibrosis, the presence of sterile endogenous foreign bodies in the dermis, or walled-off nidi of infection.

Skin biopsies can be both helpful and misleading. If infection is apparent, the need for additional treatment is documented. If no infection is visible, the question remains as to whether some infection is present in areas that do not undergo biopsy. If the lesion does not improve at all with 2 to 3 weeks of additional antibiotic treatment, one must assume that the infection is resolved and stop treatment. If infection is present, the lesion begins to worsen again in 2 to 21 days.

Relapses usually occur because the current infection was not treated appropriately or because the underlying cause of the infection was not identified or resolved. The timing to relapse is important. If new lesions appear within 7 days of the termination of treatment, it is likely that the infection was not resolved. More intense treatment is necessary. If the relapse occurs weeks to months after the last treatment, the animal has some underlying problem that must be resolved.

No discussion of antibiotics would be complete without mentioning some of the anti-inflammatory and immunomodulatory properties inherent to some of these agents: macrolides (inhibit leukocyte chemotaxis, IL-1, and lymphocyte blastogenesis), trimethoprim (inhibits leukocyte chemotaxis), and fluoroquinolones (inhibit IL-1, leukotriene, and TNF-α synthesis; inhibit granulomatous inflammation).[36] These effects can be beneficial but may also be misleading.

Immunomodulatory Agents

Recurrent bacterial skin infections in an otherwise clinically normal horse are rare.[35] Recurrent bacterial dermatoses are usually associated with recurrent or persistent predisposing conditions such as hypersensitivities (atopic, insect, food, contact), ectoparasitisms, environmental triggers (weather, filth, trauma, etc.), and systemic or metabolic disorders.

Horses with recurrent, unexplained skin infections, wherein clinical and laboratory findings are normal when the infections are eliminated with antibiotic therapy, pose a difficult therapeutic problem. Weekly or biweekly antibacterial shampoos and/or rinses may help reduce the frequency of relapses.[23,35] If topical treatments are ineffective, and recurrences are not too frequent (e.g., twice or thrice a year), appropriate systemic antibiotic therapy may be satisfactory. More frequent episodes of infection, or inability to use antibiotics, may cause the veterinarian to consider immunomodulatory therapy.

There is growing interest in developing preparations that augment innate immune defenses to prevent and treat infectious diseases.[66] Immunostimulant preparations produce nonantigen-specific enhancement of cellular and humoral defense mechanisms, presumably through T lymphocyte and macrophage activation and subsequent immunoenhancing cytokine release. In equine medicine,

● Table 4-1   **IMMUNOMODULATORY AGENTS USED IN EQUINE MEDICINE[66]**

Levamisole (Levasole, Schering-Plough); PO; not labeled for horses
Inactivated *Propionibacterium acnes* (EqStim, Neogen); 1 ml/foal or 1 ml/250-lb adult IV on day 1, 3, 7, and weekly as needed
Mycobacterial cell wall fraction (Equimune I.V., Vetrepharm); 1.5 ml IV; may repeat in 1 to 3 weeks
Mannan polymer extract (Acemannan Immunostimulant, Veterinary Product Labs); IV; not labeled for horses; serious adverse effects reported (hypotension, tachycardia, syncope)
Recombinant interferon-α (Roferon-A, Roche; Intron-A, Schering); 50 to 150 IU PO; not labeled for horses
°Purified *Parapoxvirus ovis* (Baypamune, Bayer AG)

°Germany.

immunostimulant preparations are used predominantly for treatment of chronic respiratory disease and sarcoids (Table 4-1).[66] These preparations are also being used in horses with various dermatoses, infectious and noninfectious, on a completely empirical and anecdotal basis. The authors have used none of these products for treating bacterial dermatoses in horses.

Autogenous bacterins have reported to be helpful in recurrent bacterial dermatoses in horses.[23,35,83] All such reports are anecdotal. The use of autogenous bacterins is controversial and *unproven* in small animal dermatology.[36]

● STAPHYLOCOCCAL INFECTIONS

Staphylococcus species are versatile pathogens of animals and humans. The organisms are gram-positive cocci, have a worldwide distribution, are prevalent in nature, and may gain entry to the animal host through any natural orifice and contaminated wounds. Coagulase-positive staphylococci are common equine pathogens.

Prior to 1980, all coagulase-positive staphylococci isolated from horses were identified as *Staphylococcus aureus.* Currently, three coagulase-positive staphylococci are known to be associated with equine skin infections: *S. aureus, S. hyicus subsp. hyicus,* and *S. intermedius.*° It is not presently clear whether or not the different staphylococci vary in frequency of isolation from equine pyogenic dermatoses, or are always associated with particular clinical syndromes and epidemiologic scenarios. For instance, some authors state that *S. aureus* is the major staphylococcus isolated from equine dermatoses, and that *S. intermedius* is rarely isolated.[15] Other authors report that *S. aureus* and *S. intermedius*[73,74] or *S. aureus* and *S. hyicus*[91] are isolated with about equal frequency.

The coagulase-positive staphylococci produce various combinations of enterotoxins (A, B, C, D), protein A, hemolysins, leukocidins, and dermonecrotoxins that may be involved in the pathogenesis of infections.[27,35,36] Protein A and enterotoxin C, in particular, are capable of acting as superantigens (see Chapter 8) and triggering local cutaneous and immunologic responses.[36] *S. aureus* strains isolated from three horses with cellulitis in Japan did not produce enterotoxins A, B, and C.[89] An *S. aureus* strain isolated from a horse with cellulitis in Japan produced an exfoliative toxin ("exfoliatin"), which produced generalized exfoliation when injected into 3-day-old mice and 1-day-old chicks.[87] The toxin was, thus, similar to that associated with so-called staphylococcal scalded skin syndrome in humans. However, the horse from which the exfoliation-producing *S. aureus* was isolated had no clinical exfoliation. Ribotyping of *S. intermedius* isolates from horses and dogs showed similarities and differences.[81] The following is a discussion of some of the clinical syndromes associated with staphylococcal infection in equine dermatology.

°References 35, 57, 73-80, 84-86, 88-93.

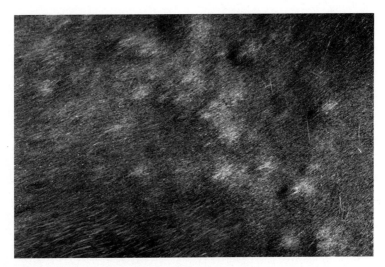

FIGURE 4-1. Early staphylococcal folliculitis. Note tufted papules.

Folliculitis and Furunculosis

Staphylococcal folliculitis and furunculosis are usually secondary to cutaneous trauma and various physiologic stresses.[20,35] Folliculitis is an inflammation, with or without infection, of hair follicles. When the inflammatory process breaks through the hair follicles and extends into the surrounding dermis and subcutis, the process is called *furunculosis.* When multiple areas of furunculosis coalesce, the resultant focal area of induration and fistulous tracts is called a carbuncle (boil).

The primary skin lesion of folliculitis is a follicular papule. Pustules may arise from these papules. However, pustules are rarely seen in bacterial folliculitis. Frequently, one first notices erect hairs over a 2- to 3-mm papule that is more easily felt than seen (Fig. 4-1). These lesions can regress spontaneously but often progressively enlarge. Some lesions enlarge to 6 to 10 mm in diameter, develop a central ulcer that discharges a purulent or serosanguineous material, and then become encrusted. The chronic or healing phase is characterized by progressive flattening of the lesion and a static or gradually expanding circular area of alopecia and scaling. Hairs at the periphery of these lesions are often easily epilated. Epidermal collarettes are uncommonly seen (Fig. 4-2). It is extremely important to remember that in the chronic or healing stage, all folliculitides, regardless of cause, are often characterized by circular areas of alopecia and scaling (so-called classic ringworm lesion).

Some lesions progress to furunculosis. This stage is distinguished by varying combinations of nodules, draining tracts, ulcers, and crusts (Fig. 4-3, *A*). Large lesions are often associated with severe inflammatory edema and may assume an edematous plaque or urticarial appearance. Cellulitis may occur. Scarring, leukoderma, and leukotrichia may follow.

The incidence of staphylococcal folliculitis and furunculosis (acne, heat rash, summer rash, summer scab, sweating eczema of the saddle region, saddle scab, saddle boils) is controversial. Some clinicians believe the entities are common,* while others consider them to be rare.[6,15] Bacterial folliculitis (cocci phagocytosed by neutrophils seen on cytology, cultures usually not done) accounts for 11.78% of the equine dermatology cases seen at the Cornell University Clinic. No age, breed, or sex predilections are evident. About 90% of the cases begin in spring and early

*References 3, 7, 10, 14, 17, 18, 22-24, 26, 34, 35, 39.

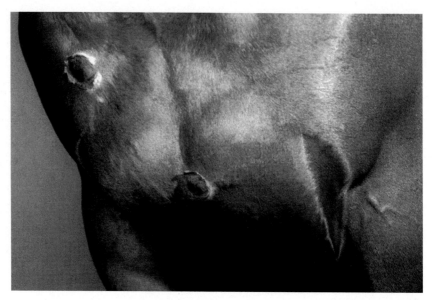

FIGURE 4-2. Staphylococcal folliculitis. Annular areas of alopecia bordered by epidermal collarettes.

summer. This period coincides with shedding, heavy riding and work schedules, higher environmental temperature and humidity, and increased insect population densities. Poorly groomed horses may be at risk. Lesions can, of course, occur at any time of year, and on any part of the body, reflecting the many predisposing causes (hypersensitivities, ectoparasites, trauma, filth, etc.).

Skin lesions initially affect the saddle and tack areas in about 90% of cases (Fig. 4-4). The lesions are painful in up to 70% of cases, rendering the horse unfit for riding or work, but they are rarely pruritic. Whether or not immunity develops is unclear, but cases of chronically recurrent lesions are well known.

Although all coagulase-positive staphylococci have been isolated from folliculitis-furunculosis lesions, there is conflicting information as to which species is most common. Some clinicians indicate that *S. aureus* is most common,[15] while others find *S. hyicus subsp. hyicus* most common.[91]

Pastern Folliculitis

Bacterial infections may uncommonly be restricted to the caudal aspect of the pastern and fetlock regions, with involvement of one or more limbs (Fig. 4-5).* This disorder must be considered in the differential diagnosis of "grease heel" or "scratches" (see Pastern Dermatitis, Chapter 15). Bacterial infections may, of course, be superimposed on other dermatoses of the pastern (vasculitis, dermatophytosis, dermatophilosis, chorioptic mange, contact dermatitis, etc.). Although all coagulase-positive staphylococci have been isolated from pastern folliculitis—sometimes more than one species simultaneously—there is conflicting information concerning the most commonly isolated species. A Japanese study[91] found that *S. aureus* was most commonly isolated, while a Belgian study[77] found *S. hyicus subsp. hyicus* most commonly. Infections were produced in normal horses by scarifying skin and applying *S. hyicus* inocula from clinical cases.[77]

Tail Pyoderma

So-called tail pyoderma—actually folliculitis and furunculosis of the tail (see Fig. 8-4, *F*)—usually follows the cutaneous trauma produced by tail rubbing provoked by insect bite hypersensitivity,

*References 18, 26, 30, 35, 37, 41.

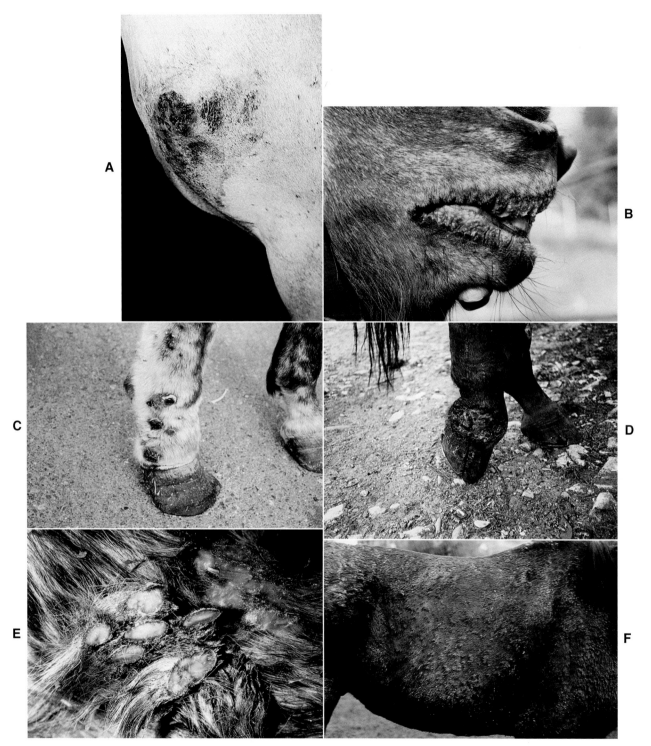

FIGURE 4-3. A, Staphylococcal furunculosis. Papules, nodules, ulcers, and multiple draining tracts over the chest. **B,** Mucocutaneous staphylococcal pyoderma. Exudation, swelling, erosion, ulceration, and crusts on lips. **C,** Ulcerative lymphangitis due to *C. pseudotuberculosis* infection (Courtesy A. Stannard). **D,** Ulcerative lymphangitis due to mixed bacterial infection. **E,** Dermatophilosis. In active infection, avulsed "paintbrush-like" crusts reveal a yellowish to greenish pus and eroded, oozing underlying skin. **F,** Dermatophilosis. Generalized tufted papules and crusts. (*Courtesy J. Baird.*)

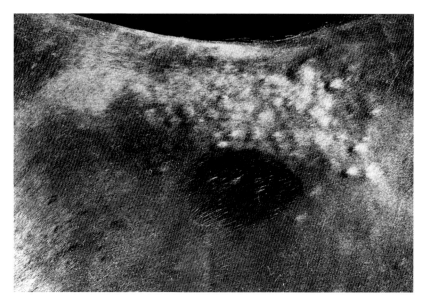

FIGURE 4-4. Staphylococcal folliculitis. Multiple papules over saddle area.

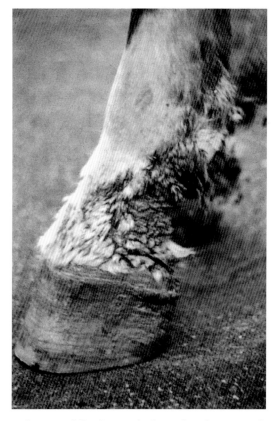

FIGURE 4-5. Staphylococcal pastern folliculitis. Tufted papules, alopecia, and crusts on pastern. (*Courtesy W. McMullen.*)

atopy, food hypersensitivity, chorioptic mange, psoroptic mange, pediculosis, oxyuriasis, and behavioral abnormalities (vice).[17,18,23,35,37]

Cellulitis

Cellulitis (phlegmon) is a severe, deep, suppurative infection wherein the process spreads along tissue planes. The infection may extend to the skin surface, producing draining tracts, and/or involve the subcutaneous fat. Depending on the cause of the cellulitis, there may be extensive edema. The overlying skin may be friable, darkly discolored, and devitalized. Affected tissues may slough.

Staphylococcal cellulitis is rarely reported in Thoroughbred racehorses.[84,89] Affected animals presented with acute-onset swelling and lameness of a leg with no known antecedent trauma or infections. Typically, one leg—front or hind—was affected, though some animals had bilateral hind leg involvement. Severe swelling and cellulitis often progressed to necrosis, sloughing, and ulceration. Affected horses were febrile and usually had leukocytosis, neutrophilia, and hyper-fibrinogenemia. About one-half of the horses developed laminitis in the contralateral leg. When the isolated coagulase-positive staphylococci were speciated (one-third of the cases), *S. aureus* was identified.

Subcutaneous Abscess

Subcutaneous abscesses are occasionally associated with staphylococcal infection.[26,37,73,74,92a] *S. aureus* and *S. intermedius* have been isolated with about equal frequency.

Wound Infections

Staphylococcal wound infections are probably common. *S. aureus* and *S. intermedius* have been isolated with about equal frequency.[73,74]

Postoperative wound infections associated with methicillin-resistant staphylococci (*S. aureus, S. epidermidis*) have been reported.[80,87a,90a,92] Methicillin-resistant staphylococci are a component of the resident bacterial microflora on human skin and are believed to be an opportunistic pathogen in humans. The epidemiology of methicillin-resistant staphylococcal infections in horses is not clear. In one study,[87a] molecular analyses of methicillin-resistant staphylococcal isolates from horses were closely related to isolates from the veterinarians providing treatment. However, in another study,[90a] molecular typing of methicillin-resistant staphylococci from horses and humans indicated that the equine and human isolates were different. Nearly one-third of healthy horses sampled at riding clubs in Japan harbored methicillin-resistant coagulase-negative staphylococci (*S. epidermidis, S. xylosus, S. saprophyticus, S. lentus, S. haemolyticus, S. sciuri*) on their skin and/ or nares.[93]

A peculiar staphylococcal wound infection was reported in 2- to 5-day-old suckling foals in Germany.[78] Cutaneous necrosis occurred on the lateral aspects of both hind legs and appeared to follow the caudal branch of the lateral saphenous vein. *S. aureus* was isolated from the wounds. Traumatic wounds and pressure sores in the region of the malleolus of the lateral tibia were thought to be the entry point for ascending staphylococcal infections. The condition was only seen in boxes with hard floors where straw bedding had been pushed aside, never in boxes with deep and permanent straw bedding or sawdust.

Impetigo

Staphylococcal impetigo is commonly seen in horses with pruritic skin diseases (especially hypersensitivities). Areas of exudation, matting of hairs, crusts, alopecia, and scaling develop in areas of pruritus (Fig. 4-6). This secondary impetiginization may dramatically increase the animal's level of pruritus.

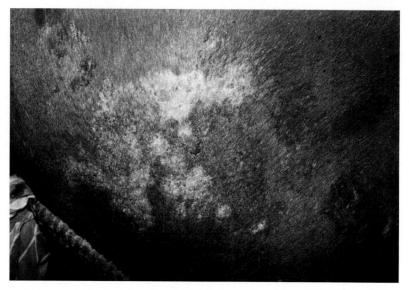

FIGURE 4-6. Staphylococcal impetigo in an atopic horse. Areas of alopecia, crusts, scale, and exudation over rump area.

Mucocutaneous Pyoderma

Staphylococcal infections are rarely isolated to mucocutaneous areas, especially the lips (Fig. 4-3, B) and/or eyelids. Initiating factors are usually not documented, but presumably include various forms of local trauma.

DIAGNOSIS

The differential diagnosis of staphylococcal skin diseases varies with the clinical syndrome.

1. Folliculitis and furunculosis can also be produced by dermatophytes, *Dermatophilus congolensis*, *Demodex* mites, *Pelodera strongyloides*, *Corynebacterium pseudotuberculosis*, and streptococci.[35,37] Sterile folliculitides may be seen with pemphigus foliaceus and eosinophilic folliculitis (associated with hypersensitivities, unilateral papular dermatosis, or idiopathy) (see Chapters 8, 9, and 15). Alopecia areata causes annular areas of alopecia, but the skin surface appears normal (see Chapter 9). Annular areas of scale, crust, and alopecia is seen with occult sarcoids.
2. Pastern folliculitis must be differentiated from the myriad of conditions producing dermatitis of the caudal aspect of the pastern (see Pastern Dermatitis, Chapter 15).
3. Tail pyoderma is usually associated with conditions that produce tail rubbing (see previous discussion).
4. Cellulitis and subcutaneous abscesses can also be produced by streptococci, *C. pseudotuberculosis*, *Rhodococcus equi*, various anaerobic bacteria (especially *Clostridium* spp.), and various fungi (see Chapter 5). Abscesses can also be sterile (injections, foreign bodies).
5. Staphylococcal impetigo is typically seen in horses with hypersensitivity disorders (insect hypersensitivity, atopy, food hypersensitivity).
6. Mucocutaneous pyoderma must be differentiated from yeast infections (*Malassezia, Candida*) (see Chapter 5) and immune-mediated disorders (pemphigus, vasculitis, drug reaction, etc.) (see Chapter 9).

The diagnosis of staphylococcal dermatitis may be confirmed by cytology, culture, and/or biopsy. *Cytology* is quick, inexpensive, and practical for the clinician (see Chapter 2). Exudate from super-

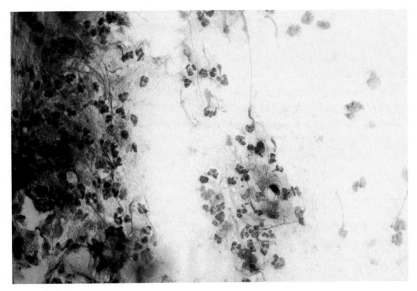

FIGURE 4-7. Staphylococcal folliculitis. Degenerate neutrophils and nuclear streaming.

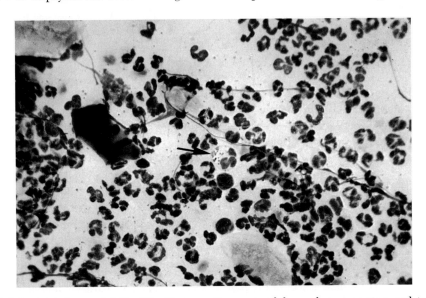

FIGURE 4-8. Staphylococcal folliculitis. Degenerative neutrophils, nuclear streaming, and intracellular cocci (*arrow*).

ficial infections contains predominantly neutrophils, many of which are degenerative, and variable amounts of nuclear streaming (suppurative inflammation) (Fig. 4-7). Cocci (about 1 μm in diameter) occur intra- and extracellularly in groups of 2 and 4 and in irregular clusters (Fig. 4-8). In deep infections, especially where furunculosis is present, the above findings are accompanied by variable numbers of macrophages, plasma cells, lymphocytes, and eosinophils (pyogranulomatous inflammation).

Some horses with clinical staphylococcal impetigo do not have pus and cocci on the samples taken. These horses may, however, have large numbers of cocci, many of which are adherent to keratinocytes (Fig. 4-9). Although cytologic evidence of infection is not present, antibiotic therapy

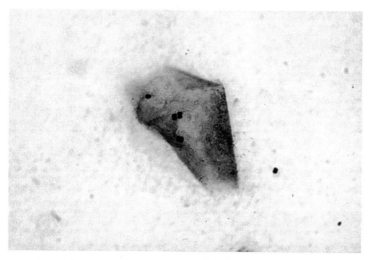

FIGURE 4-9. Cytologic specimen from horse with atopy and clinical impetiginization. Many cocci are found adherent to keratinocytes.

usually produces significant improvement. Perhaps, in these horses, the staphylococci are functioning predominantly as superantigens, rather than infectious agents per se.

Because of the predictable antibiotic susceptibility of coagulase-positive staphylococci, *culture and susceptibility testing* are not usually performed. However, if cytology reveals other than the expected cocci, or if appropriate empirical antibiotic therapy is ineffective, culture and susceptibility testing are indicated (see Chapter 2). The in vitro antibiotic susceptibility of S. aureus, S. hyicus, and S. intermedius are usually identical, with reports from around the world generally showing >90% susceptibility to cephalosporins, enrofloxacin, erythromycin, gentamicin, methicillin (oxacillin), and trimethoprim-potentiated sulfonamides.* Susceptibility to penicillin, ampicillin (amoxicillin), tetracycline, and nonpotentiated sulfonamides is typically poor. Regional differences may be seen.

Skin biopsy is not commonly performed. Histopathologic findings vary with the type of infection. *Classical folliculitis and furunculosis* are characterized by suppurative luminal folliculitis (Fig. 4-10) and pyogranulomatous furunculosis (Fig. 4-11), respectively. Cocci may or may not be seen with routine and special (Gram, Brown and Brenn) staining. *Cellulitis* is characterized by diffuse suppurative-to-pyogranulomatous dermatitis with variable degrees of edema, hemorrhage and necrosis. *Staphylococcal impetigo* is characterized by large areas of suppurative epidermitis (Fig. 4-12) wherein cocci are easily visible (Fig. 4-13). *Mucocutaneous pyoderma* is characterized by variable degrees of suppurative epidermitis and suppurative luminal folliculitis accompanied by a superficial interstitial-to-lichenoid accumulation of neutrophils, lymphocytes, and plasma cells and variable pigmentary incontinence.

CLINICAL MANAGEMENT

Treatment of staphylococcal dermatitis varies with the severity, depth, and stage of the infection, the natural course of the infection, owner and patient compliance considerations, and economic factors. Management always includes recognition and treatment/elimination of underlying or associated disorders. Clipping of hair may be indicated to (1) remove matted hairs and debris, (2) establish drainage, and (3) provide access for topical agents. It may be necessary to keep tack, blankets, and so forth off the animal until healing is complete.

---

*References 34, 42, 44, 50, 57, 73, 77, 84.

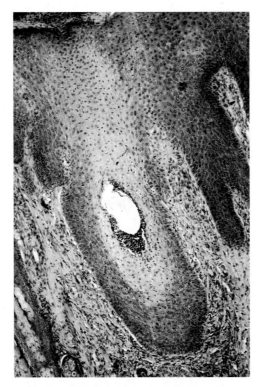

FIGURE 4-10. Staphylococcal folliculitis. Suppurative luminal folliculitis.

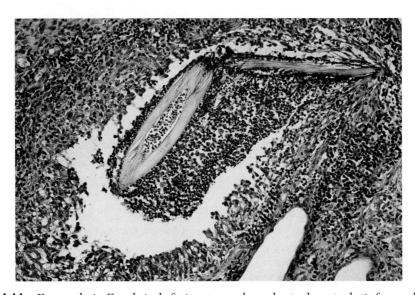

FIGURE 4-11. Furunculosis. Free hair shafts in pyogranuloma due to dermatophytic furunculosis.

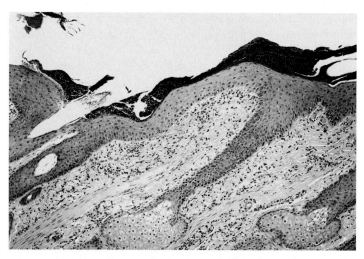

FIGURE 4-12. Staphylococcal impetigo in an atopic horse. Suppurative epidermitis. Hair follicles are not involved.

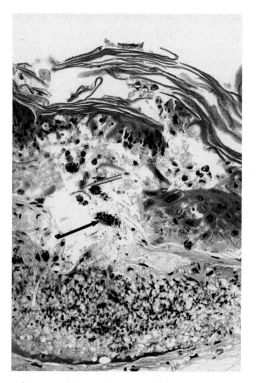

FIGURE 4-13. Close-up of Fig. 4-12. Note clusters of cocci (*arrow*) within pustule.

Mild, superficial infections may resolve spontaneously.[35] Other superficial infections may be successfully managed with topical cleansing, drying, and antibacterial therapy (see Treatment of Skin Infections).* Topical applications of chlorhexidine or benzoyl peroxide, daily for 5 to 7 days, then twice weekly until the infection is resolved, are usually effective. Shampoos or rinses are used for localized or widespread infections, and gels (benzoyl peroxide) and sprays (chlorhexidine) can

---

*References 4-6, 13, 23, 26, 29, 34, 35, 37.

be used for localized infections. Mupirocin ointment is particularly useful for localized infections, superficial or deep (e.g., pastern folliculitis, mucocutaneous pyoderma, focal folliculitis and furunculosis).[6,15]

Severe (widespread superficial and/or deep) infections usually require combined topical and systemic antibiotic therapy (see Treatment of Skin Infections). Trimethoprim-potentiated sulfonamides are the most commonly used systemic antibiotics, with enrofloxacin, erythromycin, gentamicin, and rifampin reserved for the most difficult cases (failure to respond; known resistance; or adverse reactions to first-line antibiotics; deep granulomatous, fibrosing infections).* Antibiotic therapy is continued until the infection is visually and palpably healed, plus an additional 7 to 10 days (superficial infections) or 14 to 21 days (deep infections) of treatment. Systemic antibiotics are typically given for 3 weeks (superficial infections) to 6 to 8 weeks (deep infections).

Subcutaneous abscesses usually require hot compresses or poulticing and surgical drainage.[26] Cellulitis may require surgical intervention where necrosis and sloughing occur.[84]

Tail pyoderma is reported to carry a poor prognosis.[17,18,37] This may, in part, reflect failure to (1) employ aggressive systemic antibiotic therapy and (2) control underlying or associated diseases.

• STREPTOCOCCAL INFECTIONS

Streptococcus species are numerous and associated with variable clinical manifestations.[†] The organisms are gram-positive cocci, worldwide in distribution, and prevalent in nature and may gain entry to the animal host through any natural orifice and contaminated wounds.

In horses, streptococci (especially *Streptococcus equi, S. zooepidemicus,* and *S. equisimilis*) have been isolated from individuals with ulcerative lymphangitis,[‡] folliculitis and furunculosis,[14,26,35] and abscesses (especially in foals)[26,35,94,95] (Fig. 4-14). *Streptococcus equi* is the cause of equine strangles, an acute contagious upper respiratory disease characterized by pyrexia, mucopurulent nasorrhea, and abscess formation in mandibular or retropharyngeal lymph nodes. Streptococcal hypersensitivity associated with *S. equi* infection has been the alleged pathologic mechanism of urticaria, dermatitis, and purpura hemorrhagica (see Chapter 9, discussion on Vasculitis) seen in conjunction with equine strangles.

Diagnosis is based on cytology and culture. Cytologic findings in superficial infections include neutrophils, most of which are degenerate, nuclear streaming, and intra- and extracellular cocci (about 1 μm in diameter) tending to occur in chains. Because of the predictable antibiotic susceptibility of streptococci, culture and susceptibility testing are often not performed. Over 90% of equine streptococcal isolates are susceptible to penicillin, ampicillin (amoxicillin), erythromycin, enrofloxacin, cephalosporins, and trimethoprim-potentiated sulfonamides.[42,44,50] Initial empirical systemic antibiotic therapy might include penicillin (for short courses, due to IM administration) or trimethoprim-potentiated sulfonamides or erythromycin for longer courses of treatment. Abscesses may require hot compresses or poulticing and surgical drainage.

In general, streptococcal cross-infections in animals and humans have been poorly studied. At present, the major concerns are *S. pyogenes* and *S. equisimilis* infections, which may produce sore throats or scarlet fever in humans.[§]

*References 4-6, 13, 15, 26, 29, 37.
†References 4, 5, 13, 27-29.
‡References 14, 19, 26, 30, 35, 39, 96.

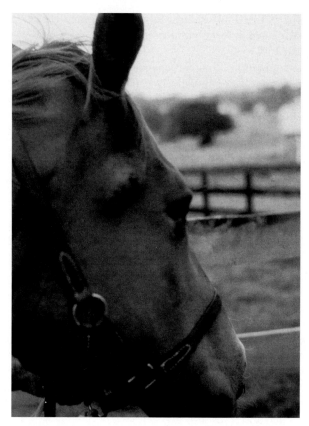

FIGURE 4-14. Streptococcal abscess in temporal region. (*Courtesy R. Pascoe.*)

● CORYNEBACTERIAL INFECTIONS

Corynebacterium species are gram-positive, pleomorphic bacteria. In general, (1) these bacteria require various predisposing factors to become established as an infection, (2) manipulation of the immune response by natural or artificial methods is not adequate for producing resistance to these bacteria, and (3) good management practices may be the most important means of controlling infections with these bacteria.° *Corynebacterium pseudotuberculosis* (*C. ovis*, Preisz-Nocard bacillus) causes deep-seated subcutaneous abscesses, folliculitis and furunculosis, and ulcerative lymphangitis in horses.[34,35,100,105,106] *C. pseudotuberculosis* is capable of producing infections in humans.[8,35]

C. pseudotuberculosis is a facultative intracellular pathogen which survives and replicates in phagocytes.[27] Virulence is related to the organism's cell wall lipid content (antiphagocytic) and elaboration of exotoxins, especially phospholipase D.[27,29] Phospholipase D hydrolyzes lysophosphatidylcholine and sphingomyelin, thus degrading endothelium and increasing vascular permeability, which in turn produces edema. Phospholipase D also inhibits neutrophil chemotaxis and degranulation of phagocytic cells, and activates complement by the alternate pathway.

Corynebacterium pseudotuberculosis Abscesses in the Horse

C. pseudotuberculosis is a cause of deep subcutaneous abscesses ("Wyoming strangles," false strangles, bastard strangles, "pigeon breast") in horses.† Most of the reports of this disorder have

---

°References 2, 4, 5, 13, 28, 29, 35, 100.
†References 2, 4, 5, 13, 17, 25, 26, 28, 29, 35, 99, 103, 104, 107, 108, 113-115, 121, 122.

come from the western United States, especially California, although the condition has also been recognized in Brazil. Two biotypes of the organism have been described, and isolates from horses are a nitrate-positive biotype.[27,35]

C. pseudotuberculosis is believed to be spread by biting flies, especially horn flies, and inoculated through fly bites during the summer. Subsequent lymphatic spread and abscess formation occur. Fly bites seem uniquely susceptible, as *C. pseudotuberculosis* rarely contaminates lacerations, wire cuts, abrasions, and so forth. Although *C. pseudotuberculosis* is capable of living in soil and fomites for long periods of time (up to 55 days),[35] it has usually not been isolated from the soil on premises where infected horses are kept. However, ticks can harbor the organism, and dipterids have been experimentally contaminated and were mechanical vectors for three days. In addition, the seasonal patterns of ventral midline dermatitis (see Chapter 6, discussion on equine ventral midline dermatitis) and *C. pseudotuberculosis* are similar. An evaluation of temporal and spatial clustering of affected horses indicated that the disease was directly or indirectly (short distance and time) transmitted, and the incubation period was 3 to 4 weeks.[102]

There are no apparent age, breed, or sex predilections, although infection is rare in horses younger than 1 year of age. Neither do husbandry practices appear to be important. The condition has a seasonal occurrence, with peak incidences in late summer, fall, and early winter. The highest incidence of disease is seen following winters of above average rainfall, which result in optimal breeding conditions for insects in the following summer and fall.[102]

Clinically, the condition is characterized by single or multiple slowly or rapidly developing deep subcutaneous abscesses. About 70% of the horses with an external abscess have a single lesion.[99,105,121] About 50% of these abscesses occur in the pectoral, ventral abdominal, axillary, and inguinal areas. Additionally, abscesses can occur on the thorax, shoulder, neck, back, head, and genital area. The purulent discharge is usually creamy to caseous and whitish to greenish. These abscesses are often associated with pitting edema and ventral midline dermatitis. About 24% of the horses with external abscesses are febrile, compared with 45% of those with internal abscesses. Weight loss and depression are more likely to be seen in horses with internal abscesses. Pain, lameness, and gait abnormalities may be seen with axillary and inguinal abscesses. Occasional horses will have concurrent ulcerative lymphangitis. Untoward sequelae, consisting of prolonged or chronic suppurative discharge, multiple abscesses, internal abscesses, and abortion, were not uncommon in cases of marked or prolonged fever and in cases of cutaneous abscesses in areas other than the typical pectoral or ventral abdominal regions.[35,99,100,115,119] Purpura hemorrhagica may be a sequela in some long-standing refractory cases.[35]

The differential diagnosis includes other bacterial, fungal, and foreign body abscesses, as well as hematoma. Definitive diagnosis is based on direct smears and culture. In smears, *C. pseudotuberculosis* appears as small gram-positive, pleomorphic (coccoid, club, and rod forms) organisms which may be arranged in single cells, palisades of parallel cells, or in angular clusters resembling "Chinese letters." However, the organisms are often present in too small a number to be detected in smears. Ultrasound guided needle aspiration has been used to confirm the diagnosis with deep-seated masses.[101] Serologic techniques have value as epidemiologic tools, but titers are not accurate for detecting active clinical disease.[99,110,111] Normochromic, nonregenerative anemia, leukocytosis with neutrophilia, hyperfibrinogenemia, and hyperproteinemia are seen in 45%, 36%, 40% and 38%, respectively, of the horses with external abscesses.

Treatment is best accomplished by allowing the subcutaneous abscesses to come to a head (mature) and then surgically incising, draining, and lavaging them. Healing is usually complete within 2 to 3 months. Hot compresses, warm soaks, and poultices may help bring slowly developing abscesses to a head. Using systemic antibiotics before the abscesses have come to a head is usually ineffective and is commonly followed by exacerbations when the drugs are stopped.[35,99,105,115,121] When drainage is not feasible, high doses of penicillin (22,000 to 50,000 IU/

kg/IM q12h) for prolonged periods (up to 6 months) may be effective.[35,119] *C. pseudotuberculosis* is also susceptible to erythromycin, trimethoprim-potentiated sulfonamides, cephalosporins, and rifampin.[99] About 91% of affected horses have a single episode of infection.[99]

Attempts to use bacterins and toxoids for prevention have not been successful.[110] Any immunity produced by natural or artificial means is very transitory. Good sanitation and fly control should help to decrease the incidence of disease. In one study, affected horses were not able to be used for a mean of 13 days (range 0 to 75 days), and the cost of treatment per horse was a mean of $139 (range $100 to $850).

C. pseudotuberculosis is also capable of producing infections in humans.[8,35] The sudden onset of a mildly painful regional lymphadenopathy that proceeds to rupture and drain a greenish, creamy, odorless pus is the typical clinical picture. Thus, caution should be exercised when handling infected materials.

Ulcerative Lymphangitis

Ulcerative lymphangitis is a bacterial infection of the cutaneous lymphatics.* The condition, most commonly associated with poor hygiene and management and insect transmission, is infrequently seen today. Ulcerative lymphangitis accounts for only 0.22% of the equine dermatoses seen at the Cornell University Clinic. Interestingly, although abscesses associated with *C. pseudotuberculosis* infection are geographically restricted, ulcerative lymphangitis is not.

The most commonly isolated organism is *C. pseudotuberculosis,* with staphylococci, streptococci, *Actinomyces pyogenes, Rhodococcus equi, Pasteurella haemolytica, Pseudomonas aeruginosa, Fusobacterium necrophorum (Fusiformis necrophorus),* and *Actinobacillus equuli* being

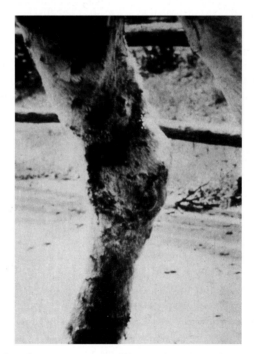

FIGURE 4-15. Ulcerative lymphangitis. Severe swelling with multiple draining tracts and ulcers.

---

*References 3-6, 13, 14, 17, 18, 23-26, 28, 29, 35, 98.

less frequently found.* Mixed infections, as well as negative cultures, have been described. These infections are thought to arise from wound contamination.

Cases are sporadic, with no apparent age, breed, or sex predilections.† Lesions are most commonly found on a hind limb, especially the fetlock, and rarely above the hock (Figs. 4-3, *C* and *D*, and 4-15). Lesions consist of hard to fluctuant nodules, which abscess, ulcerate, and develop draining tracts. Individual ulcers tend to heal within 1 to 2 weeks, but new lesions continue to develop. The regional lymphatics are often corded. In *C. pseudotuberculosis* infections, edema and fibrosis are usually striking. Lameness and debilitation may be seen. Rarely, lymph node involvement or systemic spread may occur.

The differential diagnosis includes glanders, sporotrichosis, histoplasmosis farciminosi, and mycobacterial infections. Definitive diagnosis is based on direct smears and culture. Histopathologic findings include diffuse or nodular, suppurative to pyogranulomatous dermatitis (Fig. 4-16). Edema and/or fibrosis are often marked. Actual lymphangitis is uncommonly seen (Fig. 4-17). The organism(s) may or may not be seen with special stains.

Although ulcerative lymphangitis is rarely fatal, debilitation and disfigurement can occur. In early cases, hydrotherapy, exercise, surgical drainage, and high doses of procaine penicillin (22,000 to 80,000 IU/kg IM q12h) for prolonged periods (over 30 days) may be effective.‡ However, once significant fibrosis occurs, the prognosis worsens. *C. pseudotuberculosis* is also susceptible to erythromycin, trimethoprim-potentiated sulfonamides, and rifampin.

Although early workers[14,112] claimed success with bacterins in the treatment of *C. pseudotuberculosis* ulcerative lymphangitis, more recent investigators have not had good results. Good

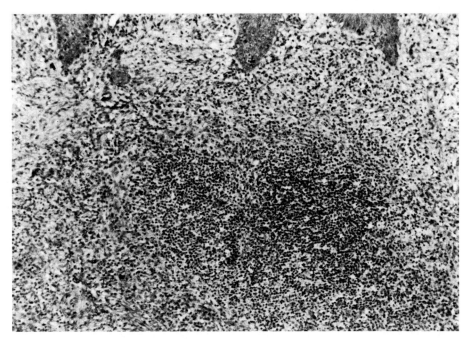

FIGURE 4-16. Ulcerative lymphangitis due to mixed bacterial infection. Diffuse pyogranulomatous dermatitis.

*References 2-6, 13, 14, 17-19, 23-26, 28-30, 35, 37, 116.
†References 2-6, 13, 14, 17-19, 22-26, 28-30, 35, 37, 97, 117, 120.
‡References 2, 4-6, 13, 18, 24, 28-30, 35, 99.

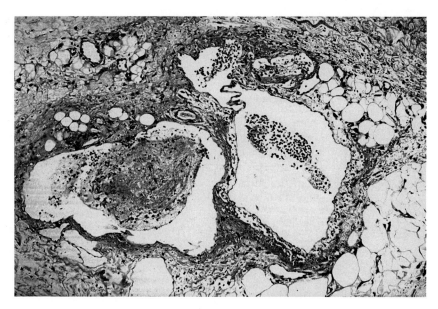

FIGURE 4-17. Ulcerative lymphangitis due to mixed bacterial infection. Pyogranulomatous lymphangitis.

hygiene and management practices, as well as early wound treatment and fly control, should be helpful control measures.

Equine Folliculitis and Furunculosis

Bacterial hair follicle infection is common in horses. *C. pseudotuberculosis* (Canadian horsepox, contagious acne, contagious pustular dermatitis) is a rare cause of this condition.[*] There are no apparent age, breed, or sex predilections.

C. pseudotuberculosis folliculitis and furunculosis are most commonly seen in spring and summer and may be precipitated by various forms of cutaneous trauma (riding, work, heat, moisture). Lesions consist of follicular papules and nodules, which are often painful and occur most commonly over the saddle and tack areas. These lesions tend to ulcerate and drain a creamy, greenish-white pus.

Diagnosis and treatment of equine folliculitis and furunculosis are discussed in the section on staphylococcal infections.

● RHODOCOCCAL INFECTIONS

Rhodococcus (Corynebacterium) equi is an important cause of pneumonia and lymphadenitis, especially in foals less than 6 months of age.[†] *R. equi* is a gram-positive, coccoid-to-rod-shaped, opportunistic soil and intestinal saprophyte.[27] Exposure of foals to large numbers of bacteria at a time when maternal antibody levels are waning (4 to 6 weeks of age) is thought to be a major factor in the development of infection. Cell-mediated immunity appears important in the prevention or clearing of infection. *R. equi* virulence factors include polysaccharide capsule (inhibits leukocyte phagocytic function), cholesterol oxidases (affect lysosomal and cell membrane stability), and mycolic acid cell wall components (induce granuloma formation).

---

[*]References 2, 10, 14, 17, 23-26, 30, 34, 35, 106.
[†]References 4, 5, 13, 28, 29, 35, 123, 127-131.

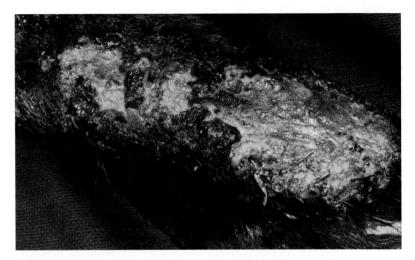

FIGURE 4-18. *R. equi* cellulitis. Ulcerated plaque on hind leg.

Cutaneous involvement is not uncommon in *R. equi* infections, and may or may not be associated with extracutaneous disease (pneumonia, enteritis, and so forth).* Single subcutaneous abscesses may be seen, especially in the chest, axillary, or hind leg areas. Cellulitis with or without multiple abscesses, draining tracts, and ulcerated nodules and plaques occur, especially on the hind leg (Fig. 4-18). Rarely, ulcerative lymphangitis may be seen.

Diagnosis is based on cytology and culture. Cytologic examination reveals suppurative to pyogranulomatous inflammation, in which coccoid-to-rod-shaped organisms may or may not be seen. Histopathologic examination usually reveals modular-to-diffuse pyogranulomatous dermatitis wherein the organisms may or may not be found (Fig. 4-19). Serologic tests are not useful for the diagnosis of active infection in individual animals.[123]

Treatment includes the administration of erythromycin (base, phosphate, or stearate) and rifampin, and surgical drainage where indicated[123,129,131,132] (see Treatment of Skin Infections). Initial pharmacokinetic and field usage suggest that azithromycin (10 mg/kg given orally q24h) may be superior to erythromycin.[109,129] *R. equi* is also susceptible to gentamicin.[50] Certain measures are useful in the prevention and control of *R. equi* infections:[123] removal of manure and contaminated soil from paddocks; elimination of dusty areas; maintaining small numbers of mares and foals within bands; isolating mares and foals that have returned from farms with *R. equi* infections.

R. equi also produces disease in humans.[8,35] Its ability to produce pneumonia and lung abscesses in immunocompromised persons (e.g., HIV infection) is of particular concern.[123,125]

• ACTINOMYCETIC INFECTIONS

Horses are susceptible to infection with a number of actinomycetes (filamentous or fungus-like bacteria). Examples of such infections include dermatophilosis, actinomycosis, and nocardiosis.

With many of these infections, except dermatophilosis, the resultant lesions are often called actinomycotic mycetomas ("fungal" tumors). Clinically, the triad of tumefaction, draining tracts, and "grains" always suggests mycetoma (actinomycotic or eumycotic, see Chapter 5). The grains, or granules, are pinpoint in size and variable in color and represent microorganisms coated with host immunoglobulin and fibrin.

---

*References 35, 124, 126-128, 131-136.

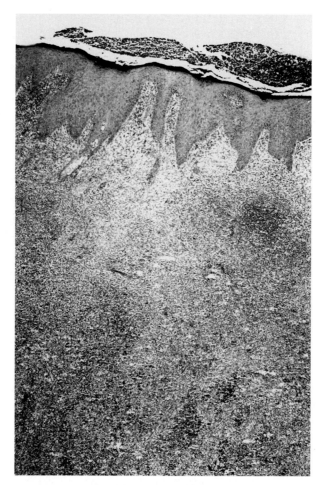

FIGURE 4-19. Diffuse dermatitis with *Rhodoccus equi* infection.

● DERMATOPHILOSIS

Dermatophilosis is a common infectious, superficial, pustular, and crusting dermatitis caused by *Dermatophilus congolensis.*

CAUSE AND PATHOGENESIS

Dermatophilus congolensis is a gram-positive, facultative anaerobic actinomycete.[12,16,27,28,35] Prior incorrect synonyms for the organism include *Actinomyces dermatonomus, Nocardia dermatonomus, Dermatophilus dermatonomus, D. pedis, Polysepta pedis,* and *Rhizopus.* The disease itself has also been branded with numerous names, some reflecting obsolete conceptions of the etiologic agent, others being descriptive of the clinical appearance: streptothricosis, mycotic dermatitis, cutaneous actinomycosis, cutaneous nocardiosis, aphis, Senkobo skin disease, rain scald, rain rot, and mud fever.

The natural habitat of *D. congolensis* is unknown.* Most attempts to isolate it from soil have been unsuccessful.† Experiments have shown that the organism's survival in soil is dependent on the type of soil and the water content, but not the pH.[40,154] This suggests that soil could act as a

---

*References 12, 16, 35, 137, 148, 161, 166.
†References 12, 16, 137, 148, 161, 166.

temporary reservoir of the organism. *D. congolensis* has been isolated from the integument and crusts of various animals and is thought to exist in quiescent form in clinically inevident but chronically infected carrier animals until climatic conditions are favorable for its infectivity.*

There is probably a multiplicity of factors in operation for the initiation, development, and propagation of dermatophilosis, and to consider one factor in isolation is probably unrealistic.† Research workers have failed to produce the disease as it is seen in nature, and field work in different parts of the world aimed at elucidating the reasons for the pronounced seasonal variations in occurrence and for the disease's various manifestations has led to apparently conflicting results.

The two most important factors in the initiation and development of dermatophilosis are skin damage and moisture.‡ It is virtually impossible to establish infection and lesions on intact, undamaged skin, even with very heavy, pure cultures of *D. congolensis*. Moisture causes the release of the infective, motile, flagellated zoospore form of the organism. These zoospores are attracted to low concentrations of carbon dioxide but repelled by high concentrations.[28,35,166] The high concentrations of carbon dioxide produced in wet crusts by dense populations of zoospores accelerate their escape to the skin surface, whereas the respiratory efflux of low concentrations of carbon dioxide from the skin attracts zoospores to susceptible areas on the skin surface.

Important sources of skin damage include biting flies and arthropods, prickly vegetation, and maceration.§ The distribution of clinical lesions often mirrors these environmental insults. *D. congolensis* can survive on the mouthparts of ticks for many months and can be transmitted by biting and nonbiting flies for up to 24 hours after they have fed on donor lesions.¶ The importance of moisture is evidenced by the markedly increased incidence of disease during periods of heavy rainfall.# The intensity of the rainfall is probably more important than the total amount. Thus, severe wetting or saturation for several days is associated with greater disease prevalence than intermittent and evenly distributed rainfall.[166]

Other, more controversial proposed predisposing factors in the pathogenesis of dermatophilosis include high ambient temperature, high relative humidity, poor nutrition, poor hygiene, and various debilitating or stressful conditions.Π In mice with experimentally induced dermatophilosis, concurrent administration of glucocorticoids increased the severity of the lesions.[35] Chronic dermatophilosis has been associated with a wide range of circumstances that all produce a reduction of the host's immune responses, such as poor nutrition, heavy intestinal parasite burden, viral disease, hyperadrenocorticism, lymphoma, and localized reductions in immunity in the area of an arthropod bite.◊ The thickness of the skin and stratum corneum were not found to be important predisposing factors.[35,158] In any particular herd or group of animals, all the animals are presumably exposed, yet often only one or a few become infected. Additionally, of those that do become clinically affected, some have a very mild disease, whereas others are severely diseased. This has caused investigators to postulate an intrinsic factor(s) that favors or hinders the development of dermatophilosis.[16] By the same token, apparent breed differences in susceptibility to disease have raised the question of genetic factors in resistance.[16]

It has been hypothesized that *D. congolensis* can be eliminated from normal skin, but if the processes involved in elimination are inhibited, the lesion produced by the bacterium becomes

---

*References 12, 16, 18, 35, 137, 161, 166.
†References 12, 16, 18, 31, 35, 137, 161, 166.
‡References 12, 16, 18, 28, 31, 35, 137, 161, 166.
§References 16, 23, 24, 28, 30, 35, 137, 152, 161, 166.
¶References 16, 28, 35, 137, 152, 161, 166.
#References 12, 16, 23-28, 35, 137, 161, 166.
ΠReferences 12, 16, 28, 35, 137, 144, 161, 166.
◊References 6, 16, 35, 49, 161, 166.

chronic.[35] Guinea pigs were sensitized to dinitrochlorobenzene and infected with *D. congolensis* at the site of a subsequent application of this chemical.[35] The bacterium was recovered from the skin over a longer period of time in sensitized individuals than in nonsensitized control subjects. However, the lesions produced at the site of infection did not become chronic.

Studies have shown that zoospores can remain viable within crusts, at a temperature of 28° to 31° C, for up to 42 months.[16,35,166] In addition, zoospores within crusts can resist drying and can withstand heating at 100° C when dried.[16,35,166] Therefore, crusts on animals and in the environment are important potential sources of infection and reinfection.[16,35,166] Organisms preserved in freeze-dried isolates or crusts were still viable for up to 26 years and 13 years, respectively.[153] Dermatophilosis is a contagious disease. The incubation period averages about 2 weeks but may be as short as 24 hours or as long as 34 days.[12,16,35,166]

Seven biotypes of *D. congolensis* have been identified,[143] and significant variation in virulence and antigenicity exists between isolates.[141] Such factors may be important in epidemiology, clinical syndromes, disease severity, and vaccine development.

Certain bacteria on normal skin, mainly *Bacillus* spp. and *Staphylococcus* spp., can inhibit the growth of *D. congolensis in vitro*.[149,165] Perhaps one of the important effects of rainfall and moisture is to dilute the antimicrobial components of these bacteria.

CLINICAL FEATURES

Dermatophilosis is a common disease of horses worldwide.[*] It is more severe in tropical and subtropical climates. Dermatophilosis accounts for 5.56% of the equine dermatoses seen at the Cornell University Clinic. In general, there are no age, breed, or sex predilections. Infections in any one group of animals may involve a single individual or up to 80% of the herd.

The primary lesions in dermatophilosis are follicular and nonfollicular tufted papules. Pustules are rarely seen. These lesions rapidly coalesce and become exudative, which often results in large (up to 5 cm in diameter) ovoid groups of hairs becoming matted together (paintbrush effect). Close examination shows the proximal portions of these hairs to be embedded in thick crusts (dried exudate). When these paintbrushes are plucked off, ovoid areas of erythematous to eroded to ulcerated, often bleeding and pustular skin are revealed (see Fig. 4-3, *E*). Active lesions contain a thick, creamy, whitish, yellowish, or greenish pus, which adheres to the skin surface and to the undersurface of the crusts. The undersurface of the crusts is usually concave, with the roots of the hairs protruding. In some animals, the lesions are smaller (2 to 4 mm in diameter) and annular. Lesions are often polycyclic and follow a "run-off," "dribbling" or "scald line" pattern. Horses with shorter, summer coats tend to have less exudative lesions.[25,26,37] Acute, active lesions of dermatophilosis are often painful, but the disease is rarely pruritic. The healing or chronic stage of the disease is characterized by dry crusts, scaling, and alopecia (ringworm-like lesions).

In horses, these exudative, crusted lesions are commonly found over the (1) rump and topline (rain scald), typically associated with rainfall (Figs. 4-20 and 4-21), (2) saddle area, (3) face and neck (Fig. 4-22), and (4) pasterns, coronets, and heels (grease heel, scratches, mud fever), typically associated with poorly drained pastures and muddy paddocks (Fig. 4-23).[†] Lesions of the distal limbs may be associated with edema, pain, and lameness. Infections on white-skinned and haired areas, especially the muzzle and distal limbs, are often associated with severe erythema (dew poisoning) and may represent a type of photodermatitis caused by *D. congolensis*.[‡] In other horses, the infection may be isolated to the cranial aspect of the hind cannon bones (resembling cannon

*References 3-7, 12, 13, 17, 18, 21, 23-26, 28, 29, 34, 35, 37-39, 41, 137, 140, 142, 144, 147, 148, 151, 152, 156-162, 164, 166.
†References 3-6, 12, 16-18, 23-26, 28, 34, 35, 37, 38, 140, 142, 144, 148, 152, 156-162, 164.
‡References 6, 18, 24-26, 35, 144.

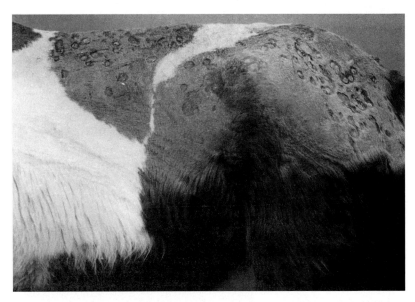

FIGURE 4-20. Dermatophilosis. Large, thick, polycyclic crusts ("scald lines," "dribbles") over the rump and topline (area has been clipped).

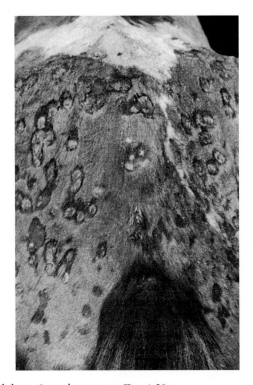

FIGURE 4-21. Dermatophilosis. Same horse as in Fig. 4-20.

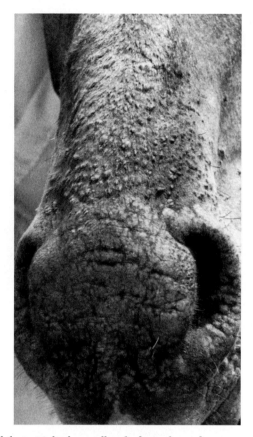

FIGURE 4-22. Dermatophilosis. Multiple, small, tufted papules and crusts on the muzzle and bridge of the nose.

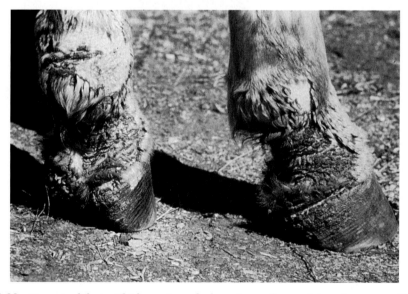

FIGURE 4-23. Dermatophilosis. Thick crusts and alopecia on the caudal pastern area. (*Courtesy W. McMullen.*)

keratosis), especially in race horses exercised in long, wet grass or on cinder tracks,[25,26,37] or may become generalized (see Fig. 4-3, *F*).° Severely affected animals may show depression, lethargy, poor appetite, weight loss, fever, and lymphadenopathy.

Dermatophilosis is a rare zoonosis. Human infections are characterized by pitted keratolysis, erythematous, pruritic or painful, pustular folliculitis in contact areas; intertrigo; subcutaneous nodules (in immunosuppressed individuals).[8,35,144,147,163]

DIAGNOSIS

The differential diagnosis includes dermatophytosis, staphylococcal folliculitis, demodicosis, and pemphigus foliaceus. In horses with lower leg lesions, cranial cannon bone lesions, or highly erythematous lesions in white haired/skinned areas, the differential includes other causes of pastern dermatitis (see Chapter 15), cannon keratosis, and photodermatitis, respectively. Definitive diagnosis is based on cytology, skin biopsy, and culture. Direct smears of pus or saline-soaked and minced crusts may be stained with new methylene blue, Diff Quik, or Gram's stains. *D. congolensis* appears as fine, branching, and multiseptate hyphae, which divide transversely and longitudinally to form cuboidal packets of coccoid cells arranged in two to eight parallel rows within branching filaments (railroad track appearance) (Fig. 4-24). Neutrophils are the predominant inflammatory cell. In the healing or dry chronic stages of the disease, direct smears are rarely positive.

Skin biopsy usually reveals varying degrees of suppurative luminal folliculitis, intraepidermal pustular dermatitis, and superficial perivascular dermatitis.[11,16,34,35,42] Intracellular edema and reticular degeneration of keratinocytes is often striking (Fig. 4-25). Surface crust is characterized by alternating layers of keratin (orthokeratotic or parakeratotic) and leukocytic debris (palisading crust) (Figs. 4-26 and 4-27). *D. congolensis* is usually seen in the keratinous debris on the surface of the skin and within hair follicles (Fig. 4-28). The organism can be seen in sections stained with

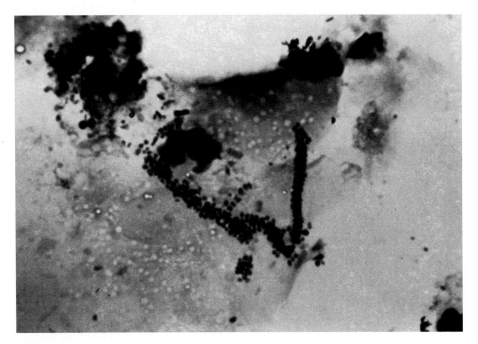

FIGURE 4-24. Dermatophilosis. Coccoid organisms are present as branching filaments ("railroad tracks").

°References 18, 24-26, 35, 144.

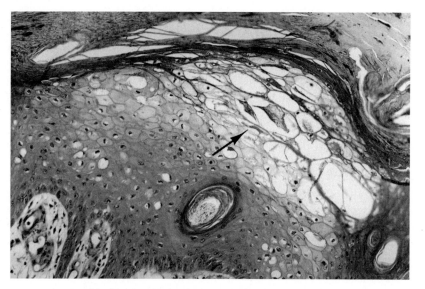

FIGURE 4-25. Intracellular edema and reticular degeneration (*arrow*) with dermatophilosis.

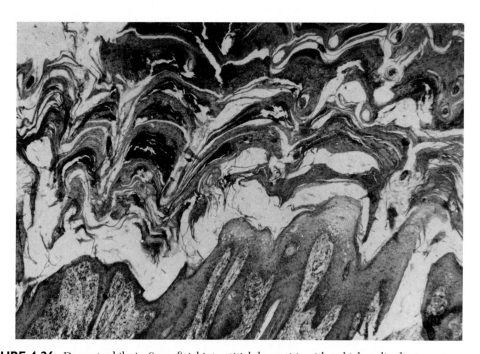

FIGURE 4-26. Dermatophilosis. Superficial interstitial dermatitis with a thick, palisading crust.

H & E but is better visualized with Giemsa's, Brown and Brenn's, or acid orcein–Giemsa (AOG) stains. When active lesions are not present, the clinician can submit avulsed thick crusts in formalin for histopathologic evaluation, wherein the organism is usually easily found.

D. congolensis grows well on blood agar, brain heart infusion agar, and tryptone broth when incubated in a microaerophilic atmosphere with increased carbon dioxide at 37° C.[12,16,27,166] However, the culture can be unsatisfactory as a result of rapid overgrowth of secondary invaders and

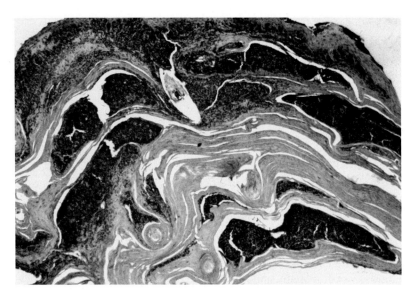

FIGURE 4-27. Palisading crust with dermatophilosis.

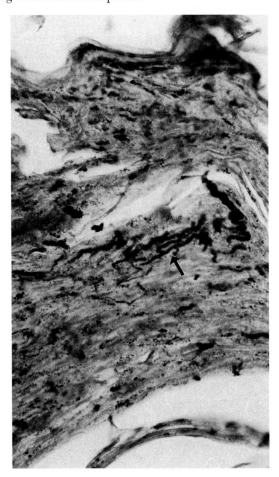

FIGURE 4-28. Dermatophilosis. Organisms are found in the keratinous layers of crust (*arrow*).

contaminating saprophytes and in the chronic nonexudative stage.* In such instances, special, often complicated isolation techniques may be helpful.[16,138] On blood agar, *D. congolensis* is dry, filamentous, whitish, and hemolytic in a microaerophilic atmosphere at 37° C and is moist, coccoid, nonhemolytic, and generally bright orange at 22° C.

Serologically, there are no cross-reactions between *D. congolensis* and *Actinomyces* or *Nocardia* species,[16] and agar gel precipitin and passive hemagglutination tests were found to be inaccurate for the diagnosis of active disease.[16,35] A specific fluorescent antibody technique was reported to be rapid and specific for the diagnosis of dermatophilosis.[16,146]

CLINICAL MANAGEMENT

Differences in management practices, climate, and economic considerations make a standard therapeutic protocol unrealistic and make "doing the best we can under the circumstances" mandatory. For example, treatment regimens recommended for temperate areas of the world are often unsuccessful in subtropical and tropical regions.[16,35] General therapeutic guidelines are as follows: (1) most cases spontaneously regress within 4 weeks if the animals can be kept dry; (2) keeping the animals dry is very important; (3) crust removal and disposal and topical treatments are also very important; and (4) systemic therapy is often needed for severe, generalized, or chronic infections.†

In temperate regions of the world, commonly used topical solutions include iodophors, 2% to 5% lime sulfur, and 1% to 4% chlorhexidine.‡ In general, the topical solutions are applied as total body shampoos or rinses (dips) for 3 to 5 consecutive days, then weekly until healing has occurred. It must be remembered that iodophors and lime sulfur can stain hair. For focal lesions, the daily topical application of iodophors or chlorhexidine in ointment or spray form is effective.

In vitro, *D. congolensis* is usually susceptible to penicillin, erythromycin, trimethoprim-potentiated sulfonamides, and gentamicin.[16,145,150,164] The most commonly used antibiotics are penicillin (short-term) and trimethoprim-potentiated sulfonamides (long-term).§ Treatment is continued until resolution of all active lesions. Crust removal is often painful, and may require sedation.

Other recommendations for therapy and control of dermatophilosis include improved hygiene, nutrition, and management practices; biting insect and arthropod control measures; avoidance of mechanical trauma to skin.¶

Previously infected animals do not develop a significant immunity to reinfection.[16,35,137,166]

Actinomycosis

Actinomycosis is an infectious, suppurative to pyogranulomatous disease caused by *Actinomyces* species.

CAUSE AND PATHOGENESIS

Actinomycosis is worldwide in distribution. *Actinomyces* species are normal inhabitants of the oral cavity, upper respiratory tract, and digestive tract of domestic animals and humans.[27,35] Although the exact pathogenesis of actinomycosis is not clear, these gram-positive, filamentous anaerobes are probably opportunistic invaders of damaged oral mucosa and skin. Predilection factors include mucosal damage done by dietary roughage (thorns, awns), exposure of dental alveoli when deciduous teeth are shed, and penetrating wounds of the skin, with or without an associated foreign body.

---

*References 12, 16, 35, 137, 138, 148, 159.
†References 4-6, 12, 13, 16-18, 23-26, 28-30, 34, 35, 37, 41, 142, 144, 157, 159, 162, 164, 166.
‡References 4-6, 13, 16-18, 23-26, 28, 29, 35, 37, 142, 151.
§References 4-6, 13, 16-18, 23-26, 28, 29, 35, 37, 41, 142, 159, 162, 164.
¶References 4-6, 13, 16-18, 23-26, 28, 29, 35.

CLINICAL FEATURES

Actinomycosis is very rare in horses, with most infections being associated with mandibular lymphadenitis and abscessation, fistulous withers, and poll evil.*

One horse had multiple pyogranulomas, abscesses, and draining tracts on the head and neck, as well as involvement of multiple internal organs.[168] The exudate was honey-like and contained hard yellowish-white granules (sulfur granules) that were the size and consistency of sand. Another horse had pustules, nodules, and draining tracts in the right lumbar area.[169] The area was painful, and the exudate was whitish and flocculent.

DIAGNOSIS

The differential diagnosis includes other bacterial, fungal, and foreign body granulomatous diseases. Definitive diagnosis is made by cytology, biopsy, and culture. Cytologic examination reveals suppurative-to-pyogranulomatous inflammation wherein the organism may or may not have been seen as long filaments (<1 μm in diameter) and as shorter V, Y, or T forms. The sulfur granules may be squashed on a glass slide and shown to consist of gram-positive filamentous organisms. Skin biopsy reveals a nodular to diffuse suppurative or pyogranulomatous dermatitis and panniculitis, in which the organisms may be seen individually or in granules (grains). These granules contain masses of the organism, usually surrounded by an eosinophilic covering of material that has a radiating or club-like appearance (Splendore-Hoeppli phenomenon). The organisms are best visualized in sections stained with Gram's or Grocott's methenamine silver stain.

The sulfur granules may also be collected, rinsed with sterile saline, and used for culture (anaerobic), which may require 2 to 4 weeks. The simple swabbing of a fistula often results in other organisms being cultured as well, especially *Corynebacterium* and coagulase-positive staphylococci. Many *Actinomyces* spp. exist.[27] Older literature indicates that *A. bovis* was the cause of equine infections, while the most recent report involved *A. viscosus.*[169]

CLINICAL MANAGEMENT

In horses, reports of therapy for actinomycosis are few, sketchy, and difficult to evaluate. In two horses, surgical drainage and parenteral therapy with penicillin and streptomycin were curative.[9] Another horse was treated with isoniazid (8 mg/kg given orally q24h), trimethoprim-potentiated sulfonamide (30 mg/kg given orally q24h), and sodium iodide (66 mg/kg IV q1-2wk) for 12 weeks, with no relapse 1 year later.[169]

Miscellaneous *Actinomycete* Infections

Arcanobacterium (Corynebacterium, Actinomyces) pyogenes is an occasional cause of wound infections and abscesses in the horse.[27,28,35,171] Human infections have been reported.[8,171] The organism is susceptible to penicillin, cephalosporin, gentamicin, erythromycin, and rifampin.[171]

An *Actinomyces suis*-like organism has rarely been reported to cause pustules, abscesses, and draining tracts in horses.[170,172] The organism is susceptible to cephalosporin, gentamicin, and trimethoprim-potentiated sulfonamide.

Nocardiosis

Nocardiosis is an infectious, suppurative to pyogranulomatous disease caused by *Nocardia* spp.

CAUSE AND PATHOGENESIS

These organisms are environmental saprophytes that gain entry to the host via wound contamination.[27,28,35] *Nocardia* spp. are gram-positive, partially acid-fast, filamentous bacterial. Some

---

*References 9, 11, 14, 27, 28, 167.

Nocardia asteroides can survive intracellularly, and produce superoxide dismutase, catalase, and a thick peptidoglycan layer in the cell wall that resists phagocytosis. Immunosuppression appears to be important in the development of most equine infections.

CLINICAL FEATURES

Nocardiosis is very rare in horses. Most animals have had immunosuppressive disorders (combined immunodeficiency disease, hyperadrenocorticism, lymphoma, and fatal nocardial pneumonia and/or disseminated disease).[173-176] Such animals occasionally have concurrent solitary or widespread cutaneous pyogranulomas, abscesses, and draining tracts. Rarely, apparently healthy horses develop solitary lesions as a result of wound contamination.[173-175]

DIAGNOSIS

The differential diagnosis includes other bacterial, fungal, and foreign body granulomatous diseases. Definitive diagnosis is made by cytology, biopsy, and culture (aerobic). Cytologic examination reveals suppurative to pyogranulomatous inflammation wherein the organism may or may not be seen as long, slender, branching filaments that tend to fragment into rod and coccoid forms. When branched and beaded, the organisms can resemble "Chinese letters." Skin biopsy reveals a nodular to diffuse suppurative or pyogranulomatous dermatitis and panniculitis in which the organisms may be seen individually or in granules (grains) (see Actinomycosis).

CLINICAL MANAGEMENT

Information on the treatment of equine nocardiosis is virtually nonexistent. One horse with a wound infection was reported to be cured with penicillin and streptomycin.[174] In other species, trimethoprim-potentiated sulfonamides, enrofloxacin, cephalosporins, and erythromycin are often used, and treatment requires several weeks.[36]

● ACTINOBACILLOSIS

Actinobacillosis is an infectious, suppurative to pyogranulomatous disease caused by *Actinobacillus lignieresii*.

Cause and Pathogenesis

Although the exact pathogenesis of actinobacillosis is not clear, these gram-negative, aerobic to facultatively anaerobic commensals of the oral and upper respiratory mucosa apparently cannot invade healthy tissues and require antecedent trauma (sharp awns, stickers, or oral and cutaneous wounds).[27,28,35]

Clinical Features

In horses, actinobacillosis (*A. equuli*) is usually a highly fatal septicemic disease in newborn foals (shigellosis).[13,28,29] *A. equuli* was isolated in pure culture from two horses with bacterial pseudomycetoma (botryomycosis).[35] *A. lignieresii* is a rare cause of equine disease. One horse had a pyogranulomatous glossitis;[35] another had a warm, painful pyogranuloma in the udder region;[177] another had a firm, warm, papulonodular pyogranulomatous dermatitis of the muzzle.[177] The classic "sulfur granules" (grains) seen in bovine actinobacillosis[28,35] were not seen.

Diagnosis

The differential diagnosis includes other bacterial, fungal, and foreign body granulomatous diseases. Definitive diagnosis is made by cytology, biopsy, and culture. Cytologic examination reveals suppurative to pyogranulomatous inflammation wherein the organism may or may not be seen in the form of rods or coccobacilli (0.3 to 0.5 μm × 0.6 to 1.4 μm). Skin biopsy reveals a nodular to diffuse suppurative or pyogranulomatous dermatitis and panniculitis, in which the organisms may be seen individually or in granules. These granules contain masses of the organism, usually surrounded by an eosinophilic covering of material that has a radiating or club-like appearance (Splendore-Hoeppli phenomenon). The organisms are best visualized in sections stained with Gram's stain or Grocott's methenamine silver stain.

Clinical Management

Information on the treatment of equine cutaneous actinobacillosis is skeletal. One horse was successfully treated with trimethoprim-potentiated sulfonamide and potassium iodide given orally for 4 weeks.[177] Another was successfully treated with trimethoprim-potentiated sulfonamide and rifampin given orally.[177] *Actinobacillus* spp. are usually sensitive to penicillin, erythromycin, gentamicin, enrofloxacin, and trimethoprim-potentiated sulfonamides.[42,44,50]

Human infections, some as a result of bite wounds from horses, have been reported.[8,177]

● ABSCESSES

Abscesses, circumscribed subcutaneous accumulations of pus, are seen commonly in horses. They usually follow bacterial contamination of skin wounds (from accidents, fighting, surgery, infections, foreign bodies, or ectoparasites). Abscesses are also a problem in cushingoid horses.

In horses, subcutaneous abscesses are usually caused by *Corynebacterium pseudotuberculosis* and, less commonly, *Clostridium* spp., various anaerobes, coagulase-positive staphylococci, streptococci, *A. pyogenes*, *Actinomyces* spp., *Nocardia* spp., *Actinobacillus* spp., and *R. equi* (see appropriate sections of this chapter).[26,28,35] Abscesses may also be sterile, as with injection and foreign body reactions.

The therapy for subcutaneous abscesses in all animals includes hot compresses and/or poulticing to bring lesions to a head (mature), surgical drainage and débridement, flushing or packing with topical antimicrobials, and, occasionally, appropriate systemic antibiotics.

● BACTERIAL PSEUDOMYCETOMA

Bacterial pseudomycetoma (botryomycosis) is a bacterial granulomatous disorder of the skin and, rarely, viscera.

Cause and Pathogenesis

The term *botryomycosis* is technically erroneous.[35] It comes from the Greek word *botrys*, which means "a bunch of grapes"; the original misinterpretation was that the disease was caused by a fungus (mycosis). The pathogenesis of bacterial pseudomycetoma is unclear.[37,179] Most cases are initiated by local trauma, with or without an associated foreign body. The granulomatous reaction presumably develops because a delicate balance exists between the virulence of the organism and the response of the host. The host is able to isolate and contain the infection but is unable to eradicate it.

Clinical Features

Bacterial pseudomycetoma is uncommon in horses° and has most frequently followed wound contamination on the limbs, lips, and scrotum. It accounts for 1.11% of the equine dermatoses

---

°References 4-6, 17, 18, 25, 26, 28, 29, 35, 37, 178, 179.

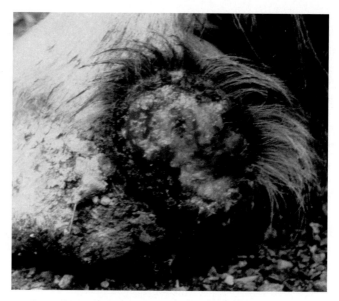

FIGURE 4-29. Bacterial pseudomycetoma. Ulcerated mass with draining tracts near the hoof.

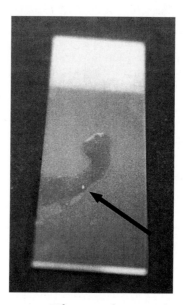

FIGURE 4-30. Bacterial pseudomycetoma. White granules in purulent exudate on glass slide (*arrow*).

seen at the Cornell University Clinic. The lesions are usually solitary, well to poorly circumscribed, firm, nonpruritic nodular to tumorous growths (Fig. 4-29). Draining tracts and ulcerations are often present. Small whitish to yellowish granules (grains) may be visible in the purulent discharge (Fig. 4-30).

Less commonly, multiple papules, pustules, nodules, and draining tracts are seen over large areas of the body (Fig. 4-31). In some of these widespread cases, some lesions appear to follow lymphatic vessels. Affected horses are typically otherwise healthy.

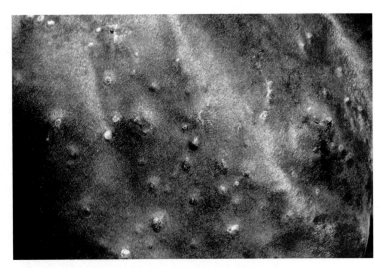

FIGURE 4-31. Bacterial pseudomycetoma or "botryomycosis."

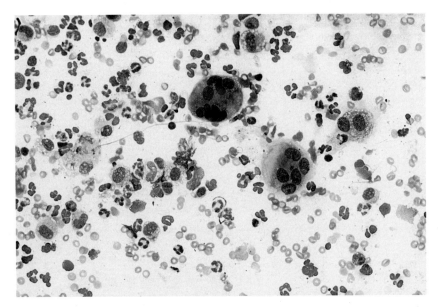

FIGURE 4-32. Bacterial pseudomycetoma. Pyogranulomatous inflammation with multinucleated histiocytic giant cells.

Diagnosis

The differential diagnosis includes other bacterial, fungal, and foreign body granulomas, habronemiasis, granulation tissue, and neoplasia. Definitive diagnosis is based on cytology, skin biopsy, and culture. Cytologic examination reveals pyogranulomatous inflammation with numerous multinucleated histiocytic giant cells (Fig. 4-32). Microorganisms may or may not be seen. Coagulase-positive staphylococci are most commonly isolated; however, other bacterial and mixed infections can occur.[35,179]

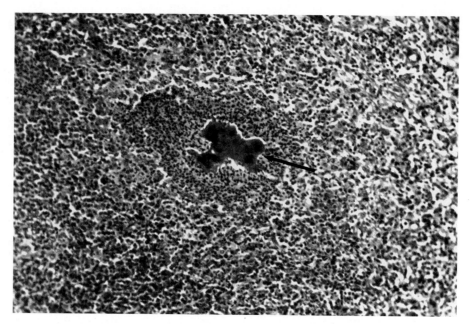

FIGURE 4-33. Bacterial pseudomycetoma. Pyogranulomatous dermatitis with an angular ("stag horn") tissue grain (*arrow*).

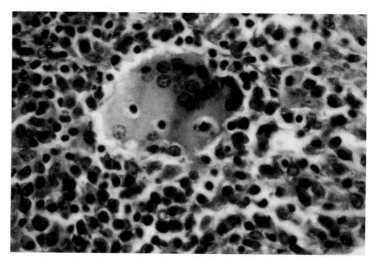

FIGURE 4-34. Multinucleated histiocytic giant cell in bacterial pseudomycetoma.

Histopathologically, there is a nodular to diffuse dermatitis or panniculitis, or both, with pleomorphic ("stag horn–like") tissue granules surrounded by a granulomatous to pyogranulomatous cellular infiltrate (Fig. 4-33). Multinucleated histiocytic giant cells and plasma cells containing Russell's bodies (Mott cells) are prominent (Figs. 4-34 and 4-35). The edges of the granules (masses of bacteria) may show clubbing and may be eosinophilic with H & E stain (Splendore-Hoeppli phenomenon). Bacteria within the tissue granules are best demonstrated with tissue Gram's or Brown and Brenn's stain (Fig. 4-36).

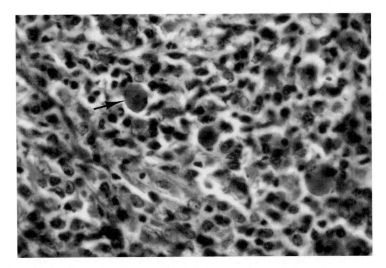

FIGURE 4-35. Mott cells (*arrow*) in bacterial pseudomycetoma.

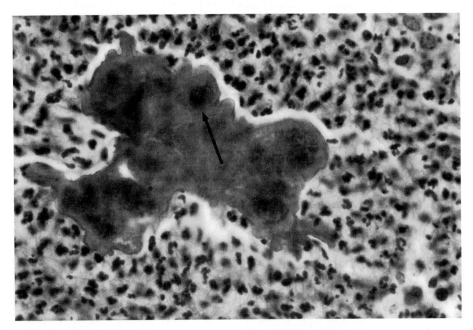

FIGURE 4-36. Bacterial pseudomycetoma. Angular ("stag horn") tissue grain containing clusters of cocci (*arrow*).

Clinical Management

Surgical excision is usually curative for solitary lesions.[179] For solitary lesions that cannot be totally excised, surgical debulking and appropriate systemic antibiotic therapy is often curative.[179] Horses with widespread lesions are very difficult to treat. The authors have seen complete clinical resolution after several weeks of systemic antibiotic therapy (trimethoprim-potentiated sulfonamides), only to have the condition relapse when therapy was stopped. As these horses are typically healthy and the skin lesions are not pruritic or painful, observation without treatment may be an alternative approach.

● CLOSTRIDIAL INFECTIONS

Clostridium species are ubiquitous, anaerobic, spore-forming, gram-positive rods.[27,28,35] They produce a wide variety of toxins (hemolytic, necrotizing, and lethal) and diseases.

Malignant edema (gas gangrene) is an acute wound infection (from trauma, injections, or surgery) of horses caused by *Clostridium* species, including *C. septicum, C. chauvoei,* and *C. perfringens (welchii).*° *Clostridium* spp. are gram-positive, anaerobic, spore-forming rods present as saprophytes in soil and water. These three clostridial organisms produce identical clinical syndromes. All three organisms produce toxins that are important in the pathogenesis: α-toxin is a lecithinase that is necrotizing, leukocidal, and hemolytic; β-toxin is a deoxyribonuclease that is toxic to leukocytes; γ-toxin is a hyaluronidase that promotes spreading of infection.[27,190]

Clinical Signs

Clinical signs are typically noted 12 to 48 hours after the inciting factor, typically an IM injection.[180-195] The lesion is initially a warm, painful, pitting, poorly circumscribed, deep swelling. Crepitus (gas formation) may be present, but is usually absent. The swelling may extend, slowly or rapidly, to progressively involve more of the skin and muscle. Drainage is typically sero-sanguineous and foul-smelling. Later the swelling becomes cool and hypoesthetic or anesthetic, the skin becomes bluish to purplish, taut, necrotic, and sloughs (Figs. 4-37 through 4-39). Animals are typically febrile, depressed, tachycardic, and have congested mucous membranes. Toxemia and death often occur within a week in untreated animals.

Diagnosis

The differential diagnosis includes other bacterial (especially anaerobic) and fungal causes of cellulitis and abscessation. Diagnosis is typically based on clinical signs and cytology. Cytologic

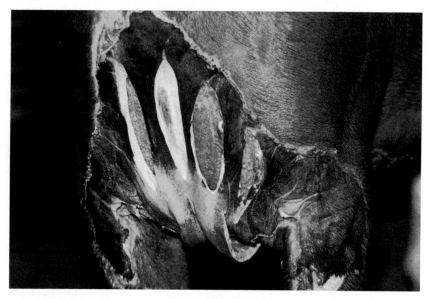

FIGURE 4-37. Clostridial infection. Note the well-delineated area of necrosis (black skin). Several vertical fenestrations have been created surgically.

°References 4, 5, 13, 27-29, 180-195.

examination reveals suppurative inflammation with numerous gram-positive straight or slightly curved rods. Although culture (anaerobic) and fluorescent antibody techniques provide the definitive diagnosis, these take too long to be of practical benefit to the clinician and patient.[27,188,190]

Clinical Management

The keys to successful treatment are early recognition, appropriate systemic antibiotic therapy, and proper wound management.[188,190,191] Intravenous administration of potassium penicillin appears to be more effective than IM injections, and does not contribute to increasing muscle pain. Wound management includes fenestration (often possible without anesthesia) to disrupt the anaerobic environment, and débridement to remove necrotic tissue and organisms. Because pain is usually

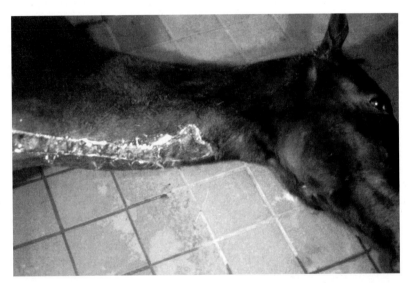

FIGURE 4-38. Clostridial infection. Well-delineated, linear area of necrosis and slough on neck.

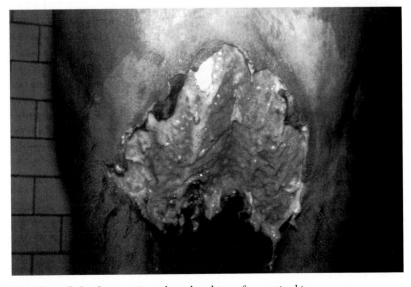

FIGURE 4-39. Clostridial infection. Complete sloughing of necrotic skin.

profound, the use of analgesics is indicated. About 50% of all reported cases have died or been euthanized, often despite treatment.

● ANAEROBIC INFECTIONS

Anaerobic bacteria produce cellulitis, abscesses, and draining tracts.[28,35,59,196] Infection typically follows traumatic puncture wounds, injections, or foreign body introduction, but can also be a sequela to trauma, surgery, and burns. Most clinically important anaerobic bacteria are commensals on mucous membranes or skin surfaces. Anaerobic infections are characterized by rapid progression, poor demarcation, marked edema and swelling, and necrosis. The wounds often, but not uniformly, have a putrid smell and are crepitant if the organism is a gas producer.

A presumptive diagnosis of anaerobic infection is based on history and physical examination. Cytologic examination that yields suppurative inflammation and polybacterial findings is supportive. Multiple morphologic forms of bacteria are suggestive of an anaerobic infection. The most commonly isolated anaerobes are *Bacteroides* spp. (pleomorphic gram-negative bacilli that may be beaded, coccoid, or slender), *Fusobacterium* spp. (thin gram-negative bacilli with tapered ends and a cigar shape), and *Clostridium* spp. (large gram-positive, spore-forming rods).[59,196] Diagnosis is confirmed by anaerobic culture.

Therapy includes surgical drainage and débridement and appropriate systemic antibiotics. Most anaerobic bacteria are susceptible to penicillin, cephalosporin, and metronidazole. Penicillin is the antibiotic of choice.

● MYCOBACTERIAL INFECTIONS

Mycobacteria can be divided into three groups: obligate pathogens such as *Mycobacterium tuberculosis* and *M. lepraemurium,* which do not multiply outside vertebrate hosts; facultative pathogens, which normally exist as saprophytes in the environment but sporadically cause disease; and environmental saprophytes, which almost never cause disease. Mycobacteria and the disease syndromes they cause can be further classified as follows:

1. True tuberculosis mycobacteria. *M. tuberculosis*, both bovine and human types, cause equine tuberculosis in endemic areas. They are photochromogenic and slow-growing and, if injected into guinea pigs, cause death in 6 to 8 weeks; opportunistic mycobacteria do not.
2. Leprosy mycobacteria. *M. lepraemurium* causes rat leprosy, which is possibly transmitted to small animals. It is scotochromogenic and grows with great difficulty in the laboratory. Many acid-fast organisms are usually found in histologic sections.
3. Opportunistic mycobacteria. These can be divided into groups according to their rate of growth and pigment production. One group of slow-growing organisms (longer than 7 days) is nonchromogenic and pathogenic only to cold-blooded animals. Another slow-growing mycobacteria group is the facultative pathogens, including *M. kansasii, M. marinum, M. ulcerans,* and *M. avium.* The fast-growing (2 to 3 days, or less than 7 days) mycobacteria in the atypical, or opportunistic, group include *M. fortuitum, M. chelonei, M. thermoresistible, M. xenopi, M. phlei,* and *M. smegmatis.* Organisms may be scattered through tissues, necessitating a careful search. They are often found in small vacuoles in the granulomatous tissue.

Tuberculosis: *M. tuberculosis* and *M. bovis*

"True" tuberculosis is rarely reported in horses. Tuberculosis typically produces systemic disease, with skin lesions rarely seen.[28] Reports of cutaneous tuberculosis in the horse are few, old, and difficult to interpret.[197,200,201,203-205] Diagnosis was based on the "tuberculous" and "pachydermatous" appearance of the lesions. Lesions consisted of nodules, plaques, and draining tracts on the ventral thorax, ventral abdomen, medial thighs, and perineum. *M. bovis* was isolated in only one case,[200] and organisms were not seen in skin biopsy specimens from any case. Some lesions were characterized microscopically as tuberculoid granulomatous dermatitis, others were not.

Tuberculosis: *M. avium*

M. avium is a slow-growing environmental saprophyte. *M. avium* was isolated from one horse with a granulomatous disorder of the udder.[198] Histologically there were no tubercles, caseation, or necrosis, and no organisms were seen. Another horse had widespread exfoliative dermatitis and ulcers (especially on the head, neck, forelimbs, and ventral thorax), and severe systemic disease.[202] Culture was positive and a few intracellular acid-fast bacilli were seen. *M. avium* has been isolated from skin lesions in horses in Mexico.[206] Initial localized swelling of one or more legs is seen, often following an injury to the site. Eventually the entire limb is swollen and painful, with multiple crusted ulcers. A light yellowish-green exudate underlies the crust.

Opportunistic Mycobacterial Granulomas

These mycobacteria are ubiquitous, free-living organisms that are usually harmless and are commonly found in nature. They are found in the soil, but they especially favor water tanks, swimming pools, and sources of natural water. After injury or injection, animals can experience chronic subcutaneous abscesses and fistulae due to these organisms. The history of cases of these granulomas in humans commonly cites instances of the disease after a contaminated injection or an infected wound. *M. smegmatis* was isolated from a firm, painful, subcutaneous abscess in the stifle region.[199]

● ANTHRAX

Anthrax is an acute infectious disease characterized by septicemia, sudden death, and the exudation of tarry blood from body orifices. The specific cause is *Bacillus anthracis*, a large (up to 10 mm in length) gram-positive spore-forming bacillus that appears as cells in singles, pairs, or long chains in cytologic specimens.[2,17,27,28] In horses, hot, painful rapidly developing inflammatory edema is seen on the neck, sternum, abdomen, prepuce, and udder.[14,30,35] Dermatohistopathologic findings include diffuse subcutaneous and dermal edema with numerous extravasated erythrocytes, but few inflammatory cells. Bacteria can usually be identified with Gram's stain, and blood vessel walls may show degenerative changes.

In humans, anthrax is considered an occupational disease, being more commonly recognized in people handling animal products and having close contact with infected animals (e.g., veterinarians, farmers, and butchers).[8,28,35]

Humans develop cutaneous, respiratory, and intestinal forms of anthrax. The cutaneous lesions occur in exposed skin (wound contamination) and are characterized by variably pruritic, erythematous macules and papules, which become edematous and vesicular and develop central necrosis and a characteristic black eschar.

● GLANDERS

Glanders (farcy) is an infectious, contagious, highly fatal disease characterized by the formation of nodules of the skin, lung and other internal organs, and ulcers of the upper respiratory mucosae.

Cause and Pathogenesis

Glanders is caused by *Burkholderia* (*Pseudomonas, Actinobacillus, Malleomyces, Bacillus, Pfeifferella, Loefflerella*) *mallei*, a gram-negative rod.[27,210,213] The organism is an aerobic obligate parasite, and infected equines and carriers that have made an apparent recovery are the natural reservoir. *B. mallei* has little resistance to drying, heat, light, and chemicals, and is unlikely to survive more than 2 weeks outside the body.[214] Close contact between horses facilitates transmission by infective discharges from the upper respiratory tract and skin. Transmission may also occur by ingestion of contaminated feed and via communal water sources. Fomites, such as contaminated grooming tools or harnesses, may result in inoculation of infected material. The minimum incubation period is 2 weeks but may be several months. Horses kept in poor environments, given poor nutrition, or subjected to exhausting work are more susceptible.

Clinical Signs

Glanders occurs in Asia, Africa, and eastern Europe.* There are no age, breed, or sex predilections. The disease occurs in acute and chronic forms. In many horses, chronic lesions do not produce clinical signs, and the disease may be occult.

In the acute form of the disease, there is a high fever, cough, nasal discharge, painful enlargement of the submaxillary lymph nodes, epistaxis, and dyspnea. Rapid spread of ulcers in the nasal mucosa and nodules of the lower leg or abdomen may be seen. Death due to septicemia occurs in a few days.

The majority of horses have the chronic form of the disease. The onset may be insidious, with general malaise, unthriftiness, intermittent fever, coughing, and epistaxis. Skin lesions can occur anywhere but are more common on sites predisposed to trauma, especially the medial hock. There is nodule (1 to 2 cm in diameter) formation, ulceration, an exudate that is yellowish or dark honey-like in color and consistency, healing, and scarring. Draining lymphatic vessels ("corded") and lymph nodes become enlarged and may abscess ("farcy buds"). Deep seated nodules may fistulate and, in some cases, gross enlargement of the hind legs may occur. A mucopurulent nasal discharge often begins unilaterally, then becomes bilateral with a green-yellow pus that is sometimes flecked with blood and flakes of necrotic epithelium. The nasal septum and ventral turbinates may contain military yellowish nodules that later ulcerate with raised granular edges and peripheral hyperemia. Characteristic stellate scars may be seen. Horses with chronic glanders may die after several months or make a partial recovery and continue to shed infection as carrier animals.

Humans are susceptible to glanders, and the infection is usually fatal.[8,35,214] Humans are infected by inhalation, ingestion, and wound contamination, and develop acute respiratory disease, septicemia, and multiple cutaneous eruptions.

Diagnosis

The differential diagnosis consists mainly of histoplasmosis farcinimosi (epizootic lymphangitis). Other causes of lymphangitis (sporotrichosis, various bacteria) are rarely, if ever, associated with respiratory disease and severe systemic signs. *B. mallei* is usually plentiful in cytologic (suppurative to pyogranulomatous inflammation) and histologic (nodular to diffuse suppurative to pyogranulomatous dermatitis and panniculitis) specimens.[208] Diagnosis is confirmed by the mallein test, various serologic tests (complement fixation, IFA, ELISA) and culture.[207-216] Mallein is a derivative of heat-extracted *B. mallei* which is injected intradermally in the lower eyelid. A positive reaction occurs in 24 to 48 hours and is characterized by marked edematous swelling of the eyelid with blepharospasm. False-negative (in as many as 54% of the cases in one study)[213] and false positive (especially in *Streptococcus equi* infections)[209] reactions occur.[213,214] The preferred culture media are brain heart infusion agar alone or with 2% to 3% glycerol, or potato-dextrose agar.[210]

Clinical Management

Because of the risk to humans and animals, glanders is a reportable disease in most of the world, and treatment is forbidden.[28,213,214] Quarantine, slaughter and appropriate carcass disposal, and

---

*References 28, 207-210, 212-214.

environmental disinfection are indicated. In one study,[213] all *B. mallei* isolates were susceptible to chloramphenicol, fluoroquinolones, and trimethoprim-potentiated sulfonamide. Three-week courses of treatment with these agents resulted in marked improvement, but immediate relapse.

MISCELLANEOUS INFECTIONS

An exfoliative dermatitis was described in two horses wherein *Bacillus cereus* was isolated in culture.[217] A 5-day course of treatment with enrofloxacin (5 mg/kg given IV q24h) was curative.

Proliferative masses on the caudal pastern area of three legs of a horse were associated with the demonstration of spirochetes, gram-negative rods, and small nematodes.[218] Histologic findings included papillomatous hyperplasia, spongiosus, necrosis, suppurative inflammation, and surface spirochetes, rods, and nematodes. Transmission electron microscopic examination revealed spirochetes within the cytoplasm of keratinocytes. The condition was likened to papillomatous digital dermatitis of cattle.

● REFERENCES

General

1. Bone JF, et al (eds): Equine Medicine and Surgery I. American Veterinary Publications, Wheaton, 1963.
2. Catcott EJ, Smithcors JF: Equine Medicine and Surgery II. American Veterinary Publications, Wheaton, 1972.
3. Chatterjee A: Skin Infections in Domestic Animals. Moitri Publication, Calcutta, 1989.
4. Colahan PT, et al (eds): Equine Medicine and Surgery IV. American Veterinary Publications, Goleta, 1991.
5. Colahan PT, et al (eds): Equine Medicine and Surgery V. American Veterinary Publications, Goleta, 1999.
6. Fadok VA (ed): Dermatology. Vet Clin N Am Equine Pract 11(1), 1995.
7. Hopes R: Skin diseases in horses. Vet Dermatol News 1:4, 1976.
8. Hubbert WT, et al: Diseases Transmitted from Animals to Man VI. Charles C. Thomas Publishers, Springfield, 1975.
9. Hutchins DR: Skin diseases of cattle and horses in New South Wales. N Z Vet J 8:85, 1960.
10. Hutyra F, et al: Special Pathology and Therapeutics of the Diseases of Domestic Animals V. Alexander Eger, Chicago, 1946.
11. Jubb KVF, et al (eds): Pathology of Domestic Animals IV. Academic Press, New York 1993.
12. Jungerman PF, Schwartzman RM: Veterinary Medical Mycology. Lea & Febiger, Philadelphia, 1972.
13. Kobluk CN, et al (eds): The Horse. Diseases and Clinical Management. W.B. Saunders Co, Philadelphia, 1995.
14. Kral F, Schwartzman RM: Veterinary and Comparative Dermatology. J.B. Lippincott Co, Philadelphia, 1964.
15. Kwochka KW, et al (eds): Advances in Veterinary Dermatology III. Butterworth-Heinemann, Boston, 1998.
16. Lloyd DH, Sellers KC: Dermatophilus Infection in Animals and Man. Academic Press, New York, 1976.
17. Mansmann RA, et al: Equine Medicine and Surgery III. American Veterinary Publications, Santa Barbara, 1982.
18. Mullowney PC, Fadok VA: Dermatologic diseases of horses. Part II. Bacterial and viral skin diseases. Comp Cont Educ 6:S16, 1984.
19. Page EH: Common skin diseases of the horse. Proc Am Assoc Equine Practit 18:385, 1972.
20. Panel Report: Skin conditions in horses. Mod Vet Pract 56:363, 1975.
21. Panel Report: Skin diseases in horses. Mod Vet Pract 67:43, 1986.
22. Pascoe RR: The nature and treatment of skin conditions observed in horses in Queensland. Aust Vet J 49:35, 1973.
23. Pascoe RR: Equine Dermatoses. University of Sydney Post-Graduate Foundation in Veterinary Science, Veterinary Review No. 22, Sydney, 1981.
24. Pascoe RR: Infectious skin diseases of horses. Vet Clin N Am Large Anim Pract 6:27, 1984.
25. Pascoe RR: A Colour Atlas of Equine Dermatology. Wolfe Publishing Ltd, London, 1990.
26. Pascoe RRR, Knottenbelt DC: Manual of Equine Dermatology. W.B. Saunders Co, Philadelphia, 1999.
27. Quinn PJ, et al: Veterinary Microbiology and Microbial Disease. Blackwell Science, Ltd., Oxford, 2002.
28. Radositits OM, et al: Veterinary Medicine. A Textbook of the Diseases of Cattle, Sheep, Pigs, Goats, and Horses VIII. Baillière-Tindall, Philadelphia, 1994.
29. Reed SM, Bayly WM (eds): Equine Internal Medicine. W.B. Saunders Co., Philadelphia, 1998.
30. Robinson NE (ed): Current Therapy in Equine Medicine. W.B. Saunders Co., Philadelphia, 1983.
31. Robinson NE (ed): Current Therapy in Equine Medicine II. W.B. Saunders Co., Philadelphia, 1987.
32. Robinson NE (ed): Current Therapy in Equine Medicine III. W.B. Saunders Co., Philadelphia, 1992.
33. Robinson NE (ed): Current Therapy in Equine Medicine IV. W.B. Saunders Co., Philadelphia, 1997.
34. Scott DW, Manning TO: Equine folliculitis and furunculosis. Equine Pract 2:11, 1980.

35. Scott DW: Large Animal Dermatology. W.B. Saunders Co., Philadelphia, 1988.
36. Scott DW, et al: Muller & Kirk's Small Animal Dermatology VI. W.B. Saunders Co., Philadelphia, 2001.
37. Sloet van Oldruitenborgh-Oosterbaan MM, Knottenbelt DC: The Practitioners Guide to Equine Dermatology. Uitgeverij Libre BV, Leeuwarden, 2001.
38. Stannard AA: Equine dermatology. Proc Am Assoc Equine Practit 22:273, 1976.
39. Thomsett LR: Skin diseases of the horse. In Pract 1:15, 1979.
40. von Tscharner C, Halliwell REW (eds): Advances in Veterinary Dermatology I. Baillière Tindall, Philadelphia, 1990.
41. von Tscharner C, et al: Stannard's illustrated equine dermatology notes. Vet Dermatol 11:200, 2000.

Therapy

42. Adamson PJW, et al: Susceptibility of equine bacterial isolates to antimicrobial agents. Am J Vet Res 46:447, 1985.
43. Baggot JD, et al: Clinical pharmacokinetics of metronidazole in horses. J Vet Pharmacol Therap 11:417, 1988.
44. Baggot JD, Prescott JF: Antimicrobial selection and dosage in the treatment of equine bacterial infections. Equine Vet J 19:92, 1987.
45. Beluche LA, et al: In vitro dose-dependent effects of enrofloxacin on equine articular cartilage. Am J Vet Res 60:577, 1999.
46. Bertone AL, et al: Effect of long-term administration of an injectable enrofloxacin solution on physical and musculoskeletal variables in adult horses. J Am Vet Med Assoc 217:1514, 2000.
47. Davenport CLM, et al: Effects of enrofloxacin and magnesium deficiency on matrix metabolism in equine articular cartilage. Am J Vet Res 62:160, 2001.
48. Egerbacher M, et al: Effects of enrofloxacin and ciprofloxacin hydrochloride on canine and equine chondrocytes in culture. Am J Vet Res 62:704, 2001.
49. English PB, et al: Antimicrobial chemotherapy in the horse: I. Pharmacological considerations. Equine Vet. J 3:259, 1979.
50. Ensink JM, et al: In vitro susceptibility to antimicrobial drugs of bacterial isolates from horses in the Netherlands. Equine Vet J 25:309, 1993.
51. Ensink JM, et al: Oral bioavailability and in vitro stability of pivampicillin, bacampicillin, talampicillin, and ampicillin in horses. Am J Vet Res 57:1021, 1996.
52. Ewing PJ, et al: Comparison of oral erythromycin formulations in the horse using pharmacokinetic profiles. J Vet Pharmacol Therap 17:17, 1994.
53. Galuppo LD, et al: Evaluation of iodophor skin preparation techniques and factors influencing drainage from ventral midline incisions in horses. J Am Vet Med Assoc 215:963, 1999.
54. Guaguère S, Belanger M: Concentration of enrofloxacin in equine tissues after long term oral administration. J Vet Pharmacol Therap 20:402, 1997.
55. Guaguère S, et al: Pharmacokinetics of enrofloxacin in adult horses and concentration of the drug in serum, body fluids, and endometrial tissues after repeated intragastrically administered doses. Am J Vet Res 57:1025, 1996.

56. Guaguère S, et al: Tolerability of orally administered enrofloxacin in adult horses: A pilot study. J Vet Pharmacol Therap 22:343, 1999.
57. Goyette G, Higgins R: Résistance des isolats de Staphylococcus hyicus spp. hyicus d'origine porcine et équine, envers différents agents antimicrobiens. Méd Vét Québec 18:199, 1998.
58. Gustafsson A, et al: Repeated administration of trimethoprim/sulfadiazine in the horse. Pharmacokinetics, plasma protein binding and influence on the intestinal microflora. J Vet Pharmacol Therap 22:20, 1999.
58a. Gustafsson A, et al: The association of erythromycin ethylsuccinate with acute colitis in horses in Sweden. Equine Vet J 29:314, 1997.
59. Hirsh DC, et al: Changes in prevalence and susceptibility of obligate anaerobes in clinical veterinary practice. J Am Vet Med Assoc 186:1086, 1985.
60. Kohn CW, et al: Pharmacokinetics of single intravenous and single and multiple dose oral administration of rifampin in mares. J Vet Pharmacol Therap 16:119, 1993.
61. Langston VC, et al: Disposition of single-dose oral enrofloxacin in the horse. J Vet Pharmacol Therap 19:316, 1996.
62. Lundin CM: Antimicrobial therapy for soft tissue infections in the horse. Equine Pract 12:35, 1990.
63. Magdesian KG, et al: Pharmacokinetics of a high dose of gentamicin administered intravenously or intramuscularly to horses. J Am Vet Med. Assoc 213:1007, 1998.
64. Merchant SR: The use of iodine in small animal and equine topical therapy. Vet Rep 2(3):8, 1989.
65. Roberts MC, et al: Antimicrobial chemotherapy in the horse: II. The application of antimicrobial therapy. Equine Vet J 3:308, 1979.
66. Rush BR: Clinical use of immunomodulatory agents. Equine Vet Educ 13:45, 2001.
67. Stratton-Phelps M, et al: Risk of adverse effects in pneumonic foals treated with erythromycin versus other antibiotics: 143 cases (1986-1996). J Am Vet Med Assoc 217:68, 2000.
68. Sweeney RW, et al: Clinical use of metronidazole in horses. 200 cases (1984-1989). J Am Vet Med Assoc 198:1045, 1991.
69. Uboh CE, et al: Pharmacokinetics of penicillin G procaine versus penicillin G potassium and procaine hydrochloride in horses. Am J Vet Res 61:811, 2000.
70. van Duijkeren E, et al: Trimethoprim/sulfonamide combinations in the horse: a review. J Vet Pharmacol Therap 17:64, 1994.
71. van Duijkeren E, et al: Pharmacokinetics of trimethoprim/sulfachlorpyridazine in horses after oral, nasogastric and intravenous administration. J Vet Pharmacol Therap 18:47, 1995.
72. Wilson WD, et al: Pharmacokinetics, bioavailability, and in vitro antibacterial activity of rifampin in the horse. Am J Vet Res 49:2041, 1988.

Staphylococcal Infections

73. Biberstein EL, et al: Species distribution of coagulase-positive staphylococci in animals. J Clin Microbiol 19:610, 1984.
74. Cox HU, et al: Species of Staphylococcus isolated from animal infections. Cornell Vet 74:124, 1984.
75. Devriese LA, Oeding P: Characteristics of Staphylococcus aureus strains isolated from different animal species. Res Vet Sci 21:284, 1976.

76. Devriese LA, et al: Identification and characterizing of staphylococci isolated from lesions and normal skin of horses. Vet Microbiol 10:269, 1985.

77. Devriese LA, et al: *Staphylococcus hyicus* in skin lesions of horses. Equine Vet J 15:263, 1983.

78. Elze K, et al: Dermonekrose in Verlauf des Ramus caudalis der Vena saphena lateralis beim Fohlen infolge einer *Staphylococcus aureus* Infektion. Tierärztl Prax 22:55, 1994.

79. Hajek VA: *Staphylococcus intermedius*, a new species isolated from animals. Int J Syst Bacteriol 26:401, 1976.

80. Hartmann FA, et al: Isolation of methicillin-resistant *Staphylococcus aureus* from a postoperative wound infection in a horse. J Am Vet Med Assoc 211:590, 1997.

81. Hesselbarth J, Schwarz S: Comparative ribotyping of *Staphylococcus intermedius* from dogs, pigeons, horses, and mink. Vet Microbiol 45:11, 1995.

82. Kawano J, et al: Isolation of phages for typing of *Staphylococcus intermedius* isolated from horses. Jpn J Vet Sci 43:933, 1981.

83. Lynch JA: Successful bacterin therapy in a case of chronic equine staphylococcal infection. Can Vet J 24:224, 1983.

84. Markel MD, et al: Cellulitis associated with coagulase-positive staphylococci (1975-1984). J Am Vet Med Assoc 189:1600, 1986.

85. Oeding P, et al: A comparison of antigenic structure and phage pattern with biochemical properties of *Staphylococcus aureus* strains isolated from horses. Acta Pathol Microbiol Scand B 82:899, 1974.

86. Sanchez-Negbrete M, et al: Ulcera estafilococica en piel de equinos. Vet Argentina 3:43, 1986.

87. Sato et al: A new type of staphylococcal exfoliative toxin from a *Staphylococcus aureus* strain isolated from a horse with phlegmon. Infect Immunity 62:3780, 1994.

87a. Seguin JC, et al: Methicillin-resistant *Staphylococcus aureus* outbreak in a veterinary teaching hospital: potential human-to-animal transmission. J Clin Microbiol 37:1459, 1999.

88. Shimizu A, Kato E: Bacteriophage typing of *Staphylococcus aureus* isolated from horses in Japan. Jpn J Vet Sci 41:409, 1979.

89. Shimizu A, et al: Characteristics of *Staphylococcus aureus* isolated from lesions of horses. J Vet Med Sci 53:601, 1991.

90. Shimizu A, et al: Distribution of *Staphylococcus* species on animal skin. J Vet Med Sci 54:355, 1992.

90a. Shimizu A, et al: Genetic analysis of equine methicillin-resistant *Staphylococcus aureus* by pulse-field gel electrophoresis. J Vet Med Sci 59:935, 1997.

91. Shimozawa K, et al: Fungal and bacterial isolation from race horses with infectious dermatoses. J Equine Sci 8:89, 1997.

92. Trostle SS, et al: Treatment of methicillin-resistant *Staphylococcus epidermidis* infection following repair of an ulnar infection and humeroradial joint luxation in a horse. J Am Vet Med Assoc 218:554, 2001.

92a. West JE, et al: Postparturient pectoral abscess in a mare. Mod Vet Pract 67:531, 1986.

93. Yasuda R, et al: Methicillin-resistant coagulase-negative staphylococci isolated from healthy horses in Japan. Am J Vet Res 61:1451, 2000.

Streptococcal Infections

94. Bain AM: Common bacterial infections of foetuses and foals and association of the infection with the dam. Aust Vet J 39:413, 1963.

95. Sweeney CR, et al: Complications associated with *Streptococcus equi* infection on a horse farm. J Am Vet Med Assoc 191:1446, 1987.

96. Wegmann E: Lymphangitis from *Streptococcus pyogenes* infection in a foal. Mod Vet Pract 67:735, 1986.

Corynebacterial Infections

97. Abu-Samra MT, et al: Ulcerative lymphangitis in a horse. Equine Vet J 12:149, 1980.

98. Addo PB: Role of the common housefly (*Musca domestica*) in the spread of ulcerative lymphangitis. Vet Rec 113:496, 1983.

99. Aleman M, et al: *Corynebacterium pseudotuberculosis* infection in horses: 538 cases (1982–1993). J Am Vet Med Assoc 209:804, 1996.

100. Benham CL, et al: *Corynebacterium pseudotuberculosis* and its role in disease of animal. Vet Bull 32:645, 1962.

101. Chaffin MK, et al: What is your diagnosis? J Am Vet Med Assoc 200:377, 1992.

102. Doherr MG, et al: Evaluation of temporal and spatial clustering of horses with *Corynebacterium pseudotuberculosis* infection. Am J Vet Res 60:284, 1999.

103. Hall IC, Stone RV: The diphtheroid bacillus of Preisz-Nocard from equine, bovine, and ovine abscesses. J Infect Dis 18:195, 1916.

104. Hall IC, fisher CW: Suppurative lesions in horses and a calf of California due to the diphtheroid bacillus of Preisz-Nocard. J Am Vet Med Assoc 48:18, 1915.

105. Hall K, et al: *Corynebacterium pseudotuberculosis* infections (pigeon fever) in horses in western Colorado: an epidemiological investigation. J Equine Vet Sci 21:284, 2001.

106. Heffner KA, et al: *Corynebacterium* folliculitis in a horse. J Am Vet Med Assoc 193:89, 1988.

107. Hughes JP, Biberstein EL: Chronic equine abscesses associated with *Corynebacterium pseudotuberculosis*. J Am Vet Med Assoc 135:559, 1959.

108. Hughes JP, et al: Two cases of generalized *Corynebacterium pseudotuberculosis* infections in mares. Cornell Vet 52:51, 1962.

109. Jacks S, et al: Pharmacokinetics of azithromycin and concentration in body fluids and bronchoalveolar cells in foals. Am J Vet Res 62:1870, 2001.

110. Knight HD: Corynebacterial infections in the horse: problems of prevention. J Am Vet Med Assoc 155:146, 1969.

111. Knight HD: A serologic method for the detection of *Corynebacterium pseudotuberculosis* infection in horses. Cornell Vet 68:220, 1978.

112. Knowles RH: Treatment of ulcerative lymphangitis by vaccines made from the Preisz Nocard bacillus prepared with ethyl chloride. J Comp Pathol Therap 31:262, 1918.

113. Maddy KT: *Corynebacterium pseudotuberculosis* infection in a horse. J Am Vet Med Assoc 122:387, 1953.

114. Mayfield MA, Martin MT: *Corynebacterium pseudotuberculosis* in Texas horses. Southwest Vet 32:133, 1979.

115. Miers KC, Levy WB: *Corynebacterium pseudo-tuberculosis* infection in the horse: study of 117 clinical cases and consideration of etiopathogenesis. J Am Vet Med Assoc 117:250, 1980.

116. Miller RM, Dresher LK: Equine ulcerative lymph-angitis caused by *Pasteurella hemolytica* (2 case reports). Vet Med Small Anim Clin 76:1335, 1981.

117. Mitchell CA, Walker RVL: Preisz-Nocard disease: study of a small occurring among horses. Can J Comp Med Vet Sci 8:3, 1944.

118. Reid CH: Habronemiasis and *Corynebacterium* "chest" abscess in California horses. Vet Med Small Anim Clin 60:233, 1965.

119. Rumbaugh GE: Internal abdominal abscesses in the horses: a study of 25 cases. J Am Vet Med Assoc 172:304, 1978.

120. Simmons J: A case of ulcerative lymphangitis. Southwest Vet 19:235, 1965.

121. Welsh RD: *Corynebacterium pseudotuberculosis* in the horse. Equine Pract 12:7, 1990.

122. Wisecup WB, et al: *Corynebacterium pseudo-tuberculosis* associated with rapidly occurring equine abscesses. J Am Vet Med Assoc 144:152, 1964.

Rhodococcal Infections

123. Ainsworth DM: Rhodococcal infections in foals. Equine Vet Educ 11:191, 1999.

124. Bain AM: *Corynebacterium equi* infections. Aust Vet J 39:116, 1963.

125. Bern, D, Lammler C: Biochemical and serological characteristics of *Rhodococcus equi* isolates from animals and humans. J Vet Med B 41:161, 1994.

126. Dewes HF: *Strongyloides westeri* and *Corynebacterium equi* in foals. N Z Vet J 20:82, 1972.

127. Ellenberger MA, Genetzky RM: *Rhodococcus equi* infections: literature review. Comp Cont Educ 8:S414, 1986.

128. Etherington WS, Prescott JF: *Corynebacterium equi* cellulitis associated with *Strongyloides* penetration in a foal. J Am Vet Med Assoc 177:1025, 1980.

129. Lakritz J, Wilson WD: Erythromycin and other macrolide antibiotics for treating *Rhodococcus equi* pneumonia in foals. Comp Cont Educ 24: 256, 2002.

130. Martens RJ, et al: Association of disease with isola-tion and virulence of *Rhodococcus equi* from farm soil and foals with pneumonia. J Am Vet Med Assoc 217:220, 2000.

131. Paradis MR: Cutaneous and musculoskeletal manifestations of *Rhodococcus equi* infection in foals. Equine Vet Educ 9:266, 1997.

132. Perdrizet JA, Scott DW: Cellulitis and subcutaneous abscesses caused by *Rhodococcus equi* infection in a foal. J Am Vet Med Assoc 190:1559, 1987.

133. Rooney JR: Corynebacterial infections in foals. Mod Vet Pract 47:43, 1966.

134. Simpson R: *Corynebacterium equi* in adult horses in Kenya. Bull Epizoot Dis Afr 12:303, 1964.

135. Smith BP, Jang S: Isolation of *Corynebacterium equi* from a foal with an ulcerated leg wound and a pectoral abscess. J Am Vet Med Assoc 177:623, 1980.

136. Zink MC, et al: *Corynebacterium equi* infections in horses, 1958-1984: a review of 131 cases. Can Vet J 27:213, 1986.

Dermatophilosis

137. Abu-Samra MT: *Dermatophilus* infection: the clinical disease and diagnosis. Zbl Vet Med B 25:641, 1978.

138. Abu-Samra MT, Walton GS: Modified techniques for the isolation of *Dermatophilus* spp. from infected material. Sabouraudia 15:23, 1977.

139. Abu-Samra MT, Imbabi SE: Experimental infection of domesticated animals and fowl with *Dermato-philus congolensis*. J Comp Pathol 86:157, 1976.

140. Bussieras J, et al: La dermatophilose équine en Normandie. Rec Méd Vét 157:415, 1981.

141. Ellis TM, et al: Strain variation in *Dermatophilus congolensis* demonstrated by cross protection studies. Vet Microbiol 28:377, 1991.

142. Evans AG: Dermatophilosis: Diagnostic approach to nonpruritic crusting dermatitis in horses. Comp Cont Educ 14:1618, 1992.

143. Faibra DT: Heterogeneity among *Dermatophilus congolensis* isolates demonstrated by restriction fragment length polymorphisms. Rev Élev Méd Vét Pays Trop 46:253, 1993.

144. Ford RB, et al: Equine dermatophilosis: a two-year clinicopathologic study. Vet Med Small Anim Clin 69:1557, 1974.

145. Hermoso De Mendoza J, et al: *In vitro* studies of *Dermatophilus congolensis* antimicrobial susceptibility by determining minimal inhibitory and bacteriocidal concentrations. Brit Vet J 150:189, 1994.

146. How SJ, Lloyd DH: Use of a monoclonal antibody in the diagnosis of infection by *Dermatophilus congo-lensis*. Res Vet Sci 45:416, 1988.

147. Hyslop NG: Dermatophilosis (streptothricosis) in animals and man. Comp Immunol Microbiol Infect Dis 2:39, 1980.

148. Kaplan W, Johnston WJ: Equine dermatophilosis (cutaneous streptothricosis) in Georgia. J Am Vet Med Assoc 149:1162, 1966.

149. Kingali JM, et al: Inhibition of *Dermatophilus congolensis* by substances produced by bacteria found in the skin. Vet. Microbiol 22:237, 1990.

150. Krüger B, et al: Phänotypische Charakterisierung von equinen *Dermatophilus congolensis* Feldisolaten. Berl Münch Tierärztl Wschr 111:374, 1998.

151. Kuranen H, et al: *Dermatophilus congolensis*-bakteerin aiheuttama ihotulehdus hevosilla tapausselostus. Suomen Eläin 106:359, 2000.

152. Macadam I: Streptothricosis in Nigerian horses. Vet Rec 76:420, 1964.

153. Makinde AA, et al: Survival of *Dermatophilus congo-lensis* under laboratory conditions in Nigeria. Vet Rec 149:154, 2001.

154. Martinez D, Prior P: Survival of *Dermatophilus congolensis* in tropical clay soils submitted to differ-ent water potentials. Vet Microbiol 29:135, 1991.

155. McCaig J: "Mud fever" in horses. Vet Rec 81:173, 1967.

156. Pascoe RR: An outbreak of mycotic dermatitis in horses in Southeastern Queensland. Aust Vet J 47:112, 1971.

157. Pascoe RR: Further observations on *Dermatophilus* infection in horses. Aust Vet J 48:32, 1972.

158. Searcy GP, Hulland TJ: *Dermatophilus* dermatitis (streptothricosis) in Ontario. I. Clinical observations. Can Vet J. 9:7, 1968.

159. Searcy GP, Hulland TJ: *Dermatophilus* dermatitis (streptothricosis) in Ontario. II. Laboratory findings. Can Vet J. 9:16, 1968.

160. Shores SA: Dermatitis in a colt. Southwest Vet 18:68, 1964.

161. Stewart GH: Dermatophilosis: a skin disease of animals and man. Part I. Vet Rec 91:537, 1972.

162. Stewart GH: Dermatophilosis: a skin disease of animals and man. Part II. Vet Rec 91:555, 1972.

163. Towersey L, et al: *Dermatophilus congolensis* human infection. J Am Acad Dermatol 29:351, 1993.

164. Yeruham I, et al: Outbreak of dermatophilosis in a horse herd in Israel. J Vet Med A 43:393, 1996.

165. Zaria LT: *In vitro* and *in vivo* inhibition of *Dermatophilus congolensis* by coagulase negative antibiotic-producing staphylococci from pigs. Res Vet Sci 50:243, 1991.

166. Zaria LT: *Dermatophilus congolensis* infection (dermatophilosis) in animals and man: an update. Comp Immun Microbiol Infect Dis 16:179, 1993.

Actinomycosis

167. Burns RHG, Simmons GC: A case of actinomycotic infection in a horse. Aust Vet J 28:34, 1952.

168. Guard WG: Actinomycosis in a horse. J Am Vet Med Assoc 93:198, 1938.

169. Specht TE, et al: Skin pustules and nodules caused by *Actinomyces viscosus* in a horse. J Am Vet Med Assoc 198:457, 1991.

Miscellaneous Actinomycete Infections

170. Elad D, et al: *Actinobacillus suis*-like organism in a mare—first report in Israel and a brief review of the literature. Isr J Vet Med 46:102, 1991.

171. Guérin-Faublée V, et al: *Actinomyces pyogenes*: susceptibility of 103 clinical animal isolates to 22 antimicrobial agents. Vet Res 24:251, 1993.

172. Jang SS, et al: *Actinobacillus suis*-like organisms in horses. Am J Vet Res 48:1036, 1987.

173. Andreatta JN, Fernandez EJ: Dermatitis equine causada par *Nocardia* sp. Rev Agron Vet Argentina 2:16, 1978.

174. Biberstein EL, et al: *Nocardia asteroides* infection in horses: a review. J Am Vet Med Assoc 186:273, 1985.

175. Otcensek M, et al: *Nocardia asteroides* vyvolavatelem superficiání dermatózy kon?. Veterinarstvi 25:29, 1975.

176. Rodriguez IG: Aportacion al estudio de las nocardiosis del caballo. Una enzootia de nocardiosis equina. Biol Inf Cons Gen Colegios Vet Espana 8:747, 1961.

Actinobacillosis

177. Carmalt JL, et al: *Actinobacillus lignieresii* infection in two horses. J Am Vet Med Assoc 215:826, 1998.

Bacterial Pseudomycetoma

178. Bollinger O: Mycosis der Lunge beim Pferde. Virchows Arch Pathol Anat 49:583, 1870.

179. Scott DW: Bacterial pseudomycosis (botryomycosis) in the horse. Equine Pract 10:15, 1988.

Clostridial Infections

180. Breuhas BA, et al: Clostridial muscle infections following intramuscular injections in the horse. J Equine Vet Sci 3:42, 1983.

181. Coloe PJ, et al: *Clostridium fallax* as a cause of gas-oedema disease in a horse. J Comp Pathol 93:595, 1983.

182. Erid CH: Malignant edema infection in a horse. Calif Vet 8:30, 1955.

183. Estola T, Stenberg H: On the occurrence of *Clostridia* in domestic animals and animal products. Nord Vet Med 15:35, 1963.

184. Hagemoser WA, et al: *Clostridium chauvoei* infection in a horse. J Am Vet Med Assoc 176:631, 1980.

185. Horner RF: Malignant oedema caused by *Clostridium perfringens* type A in a horse. Tdskr S Afr Vet Ver 53:122, 1982.

186. McKay RJ, et al: *Clostridium perfringens* associated with a focal abscess in a horse. J Am Vet Med Assoc 175:71, 1979.

187. McLaughlin SA, et al: *Clostridium septicum* infection in the horse. Equine Pract 1:17, 1979.

188. Moore AK: Malignant edema in the horse. Oklahoma Vet Med Assoc 40:90, 1988.

189. Murphy DB: *Clostridium chauvoei* as the cause of malignant edema in a horse. Vet Med Small Anim Clin 75:1152, 1980.

190. Perdrizet JA, et al: Successful management of malignant edema caused by *Clostridium septicum* in a horse. Cornell Vet 77:328, 1987.

191. Rebhun WC, et al: Malignant edema in horses. J Am Vet Med Assoc 187:732, 1985.

192. Reef VG: *Clostridium perfringens* cellulitis and immune-mediated hemolytic anemia in a horse. J AM Vet Med Assoc 182:251, 1983.

193. Valberg SJ, McKinnar AO: Clostridial cellulitis in the horse: a report of five cases. Can Vet J 25:67, 1984.

194. Van Heerden J, Botha WS: Clostridial myositis in a horse. J S Afr Vet Assoc 53:211, 1982.

195. Westman CW, et al: Clostridial infection in a horse. J Am Vet Med Assoc 174:725, 1979.

Anaerobic Infections

196. Moore RM: Diagnosis and treatment of obligate anaerobic bacterial infections in horses. Comp Cont Educ 15:989, 1993.

Mycobacterial Infections

197. Antepioglu H: Skin tuberculosis in a horse. Ank Univ Fak Vet Derg 10:399, 1963.

198. Baker JR: A case of generalized avian tuberculosis in a horse. Vet Rec 93:105, 1973.

199. Booth TM, Wattret A: Stifle abscess in a pony associated with *Mycobacterium smegmatis*. Vet Rec 147:452, 2000.

200. Buss W: Hauttuberkulose des Pferdes als Ursache menschlicher Hauttuberkulose. Tierärztl Umsch 9:164, 1954.

201. Dukie B, Putrik M: Tuberculosis of the skin of the abdomen in a horse. Acta Vet (Belgr) 21:13, 1971.

202. Flores JM, et al: Avian tuberculosis dermatitis in a young horse. Vet Rec 128:407, 1991.

203. Laszlo F: Beitrag zur Hauttuberkulose. Dtsch Tierärztl Wschr 43:196, 1935.

204. Nieland H: Haut und Nasenscheide-wand-tuberkulose beim Pferd. Dtsch Tierärztl Wschr 46:98, 1938.

205. Pinkiewicz A, et al: Skin tuberculosis in a horse. Med Wet 19:692, 1963.

206. Sevilla HC, et al: Micobacteriosis cutánea en mulas y burros. Vet Méx 26:283, 1995.

Glanders

207. Al-Ani FK, et al: Glanders in horses: clinical and epidemiological studies in Iraq. Pakistan Vet J 7:126, 1987.

208. Al-Ani FK, et al: Glanders in horses: histopathological and electron microscopic studies. Pakistan Vet J 12:1, 1992.

209. Al-Ani FK, et al: A micro-enzyme-linked immunosorbent assay (ELISA) for detection of antibodies to *Pseudomonas mallei* infection in horses. Pakistan Vet J 13:70, 1993.
210. Al-Ani FK, et al: Glanders in horses: clinical, biochemical, and serological studies in Iraq. Vet Archiv 68:155, 1998.
211. Jana AM, et al: Rapid diagnosis of glanders in equines by counter-immunoelectrophoresis. Indian Vet J 59:5, 1982.
212. Ma CL, et al: Diagnosis of glanders in horses by the indirect fluorescent antibody (IFA) technique. Chinese J Vet Sci Technol 19:3, 1986.
213. Muhammed G, et al: Clinico-microbiological and therapeutic aspects of glanders in equines. J Equine Sci 9:93, 1998.
214. Pritchard DG: Glanders. Equine Vet Educ 7:29, 1995.
215. Verma RD: A micro-complement fixation test for identification of *Pseudomonas mallei*. J Remount Vet Corps 29:1, 1990.
216. Verma RD, et al: Development of an avidin-biotin dot enzyme-linked immunosorbent assay and its comparison with other serological tests for diagnosis of glanders in equines. Vet Microbiol 25:77, 1990.

Miscellaneous Infections

217. Frölich T: Abszedierende desquamierende B.-cereus-Dermatitis bei zwei Pferden. Tierärztl Umsch 46:390, 1991.
218. Black SS, et al: Papillomatous pastern dermatitis with spirochetes in a horse. Vet Pathol 34:506, 1997.

Chapter 5

Fungal Skin Diseases

● CUTANEOUS MYCOLOGY

Fungi are omnipresent in our environment. Of the thousands of different species of fungi, only a few have the ability to cause disease in animals. The great majority of fungi are either soil organisms or plant pathogens; however, more than 300 species have been reported to be animal pathogens. A *mycosis* (pl. *mycoses*) is a disease caused by a fungus. A *dermatophytosis* is an infection of the keratinized tissues, hair, and stratum corneum that is caused by a species of *Microsporum, Trichophyton,* or *Epidermophyton.* These organisms—dermatophytes—are unique fungi that are able to invade and maintain themselves in keratinized tissues. A *dermatomycosis* is a fungal infection of hair, claw, or skin that is caused by a nondermatophyte, a fungus not classified in the genera *Microsporum, Trichophyton,* or *Epidermophyton.* Dermatophytosis and dermato-mycosis are different clinical entities. Fungi, however, are not nearly as common a cause of skin disease as supposed; many dermatoses are misdiagnosed as "fungus infections" on the basis of clinical presentation. On the other hand, many true fungal infections are probably not diagnosed because of the variability of clinical presentations.

General Characteristics of Fungi

The term *fungus* includes yeasts and molds. The kingdom of *Fungi* is recognized as one of the five kingdoms of organisms. The other four kingdoms are *Monera* (bacteria and blue-green algae), *Protista* (protozoa), *Plantae* (plants), and *Animalia* (animals).[5-7,10,13,26] Fungi are eukaryotic achlorophyllous organisms that may grow in the form of a yeast (unicellular), a mold (multicellular-filamentous), or both. The cell walls of fungi consist of chitin, chitosan, glucan, and mannan and are used to distinguish the fungi from the Protista. Unlike plants, fungi do not have chlorophyll. The kingdom of Fungi contains five divisions: *Chytridomycota, Zygomycota, Basidiomycota, Ascomycota,* and *Fungi Imperfecti* or *Deuteromycota.*

Fungi have traditionally been identified and classified (1) by their method of producing conidia and spores; (2) by the size, shape, and color of the conidia; and (3) by the type of hyphae and their macroscopic appearance (e.g., by the color and texture of the colony and sometimes by physiologic characteristics). Therefore, it is important to understand the terms that describe these characteristics. A single vegetative filament of a fungus is a *hypha.* A number of vegetative filaments are called *hyphae,* and a mass of hyphae is known as a *mycelium.* Hyphae are *septate,* if they have divisions between cells, or *sparsely septate,* if they have many nuclei within a cell. This latter condition is known as *coenocytic.* The term *conidium* (pl. *conidia*) should be used only for an asexual *propagule* or unit that gives rise to genetically identical organisms. A *conidiophore* is a simple or branched mycelium bearing conidia or conidiogenous cells. A *conidiogenous cell* is any fungal cell that gives rise to a conidium. (Modern taxonomists also may use sexual reproduction characteristics and biochemical and immunologic methods for identification.) There are six major types of conidia: blastoconidia, arthroconidia, annelloconidia, phialoconidia, poroconidia, and aleuriconidia. More detailed information about fungal taxonomy can be found in other texts.[5-7,13,26]

Changes in the scientific names resulting from recent taxonomic studies have caused some confusion regarding the names of pathogenic fungi. Some disease names have been based on geographic distribution or have been created by the indiscriminate lumping together of dissimilar diseases. The authors here attempt to name diseases on the basis of a single etiologic agent and common usage, tempered by contemporary knowledge of geographic distribution and current taxonomy. Mycotic diseases are divided into three categories: superficial, subcutaneous, and systemic. The first category contains the most common fungal diseases in veterinary dermatology.

Characterization of Pathogenic Fungi

Fungi that are pathogenic to plants are distributed throughout all divisions of fungi, but those that are pathogenic to animals are found primarily in the Fungi Imperfecti and the Ascomycota.[5-7,13,26]

A yeast is a unicellular budding fungus that forms blastoconidia, whereas a mold is a filamentous fungus. Some pathogenic fungi, such as *Coccidioides immitis*, *Sporothrix schenckii*, and *Blastomyces dermatitidis*, are *dimorphic*. Dimorphic fungi are capable of existing in two different morphologic forms. For example, at 37° C (98.6° F) in enriched media or *in vitro*, *B. dermatitidis* exists as a yeast, but at 30° C (86° F) it grows as a mold. *C. immitis* is unique in that at 37° C (98.6° F) or in tissue, spherules containing endospores are formed. Some fungi such as *Aspergillus* form true hyphae in tissue and are a mold at either 30° C or 37° C (86° F or 98.6° F). Another manifestation of fungal growth in tissue is the presence of granules (grains) that are organized masses of hyphae in a crystalline or amorphous matrix. These granules are characteristic of the mycotic infection mycetoma and are the result of interaction between the host tissue and the fungus.

At one time, numerous fungi were thought to be pathogens. Today, with the increased use of broad-spectrum antibiotics and immunosuppressive therapy, the presence of chronic immunosuppressive diseases, and improved mycologic techniques, many fungi that were considered contaminants have, in fact, been found to be pathogenic. The following criteria can be helpful in differentiating pathogenic from contaminant fungi: (1) source, (2) number of colonies isolated, (3) species, (4) whether the fungus can be repeatedly isolated, and most important, (5) the presence of fungal elements in the tissue. A fungus isolated from a normal sterile site, such as a biopsy specimen, warrants greater credence as a pathogen than that same fungus isolated from the surface of the skin, where it may be an airborne contaminant. The number of colonies isolated should influence the decision as to whether an organism is a contaminant or a pathogen. One isolated colony of *Aspergillus* may have resulted from an airborne conidium that floated into a plate, whereas a petri dish filled with *Aspergillus fumigatus* could represent a pathogen. Colonies that are not seen on the streak line of the agar should be considered contaminants. Certain species of fungi are definitely recognized as pathogens, however, so if even only one colony is isolated, it should be reported. Such organisms include *B. dermatitidis*, *C. immitis*, and *Cryptococcus neoformans*. Another indication of fungal pathogenicity is that the same fungus can be repeatedly isolated from the lesion. In order to confirm that a fungus is a cause of a mycosis, the fungal structures observed in tissue or a direct smear must correlate with the fungus identified in culture.

When these interpretational guidelines are not followed, erroneous conclusions can be drawn and reported. For instance, *Scopulariopsis brevicaulis* was reported to be the cause of skin disease in horses in Brazil.[107] The organism was seen in skin scrapings and grown in culture. However, hair or tissue invasion was never demonstrated. Neither were therapeutic trials reported. We know that *S. brevicaulis* is a common, widespread saprophytic fungus that can be isolated from the skin and haircoat of perfectly normal horses (see Table 1-2).

Although gross colonies of dermatophytes are never black, brown, or green, the proper identification of organisms in fungal cultures should be made by medical laboratory clinicians who have expertise in such matters. Detailed information on the cultural growth of four common dermatophytes (*Trichophyton equinum*, *Microsporum equinum*, *Microsporum gypseum*, *Trichophyton mentagrophytes*) and commonly isolated fungal contaminants is available in other texts (see Chapter 2).[5,6,13,26]

Normal Fungal Microflora

Horses harbor many saprophytic molds and yeasts on their haircoats and skin (see Table 1-2). The most commonly isolated fungi from horses are species of *Alternaria*, *Aspergillus*, *Cladosporium*, *Fusarium*, *Penicillium*, and *Scopulariopsis* (see Chapter 1).[28,33,96,131,132] Most of these saprophytic isolates probably represent repeated transient contamination by airborne fungi or by fungi in soil.

Dermatophytes are also isolated from the haircoats and skin of normal horses (see Chapter 1).[27,132] It is likely that dermatophytes isolated from normal horses—such as *M. gypseum*, *T. mentagrophytes*, *T. rubrum*, *T. terrestre*—simply represent recent contamination from the environment. For instance, it is not unheard of to isolate a geophilic dermatophyte, such as *M. gypseum*, from normal horses or from a horse presented for a skin disease wherein these dermatophytes are playing no pathogenic role.

Culture and Examination of Fungi

Proper specimen collection, isolation, culture, and identification are necessary to determine the cause of a fungal infection. Detailed information on these important techniques is in Chapter 2.

• SUPERFICIAL MYCOSES

The superficial mycoses are fungal infections that involve superficial layers of the skin, hair, and claws. The organisms may be dermatophytes such as *Microsporum* and *Trichophyton*, which are able to use keratin. However, other fungi such as *Candida* (*Monilia*), *Malassezia* (*Pityrosporum*), and *Trichosporon* (piedra) may also produce superficial mycoses.

Dermatophytosis

CAUSE AND PATHOGENESIS

The dermatophytes that most frequently infect animals are *Microsporum* and *Trichophyton*. These genera can be divided into three groups on the basis of natural habitat: geophilic, zoophilic, and anthropophilic. Geophilic dermatophytes, such as *M. gypseum*, normally inhabit soil, in which they decompose keratinous debris. Zoophilic dermatophytes, such as *M. canis*, *M. equinum*, *M. distortum*, and *T. equinum*, have become adapted to animals and are only rarely found in soil. Anthropophilic dermatophytes, such as *M. audouinii*, have become adapted to humans and do not survive in soil.

Trichophyton equinum is the most common cause of dermatophytosis in horses throughout the world.° Other less frequently isolated dermatophytes include *T. mentagrophytes*,[†] *T. verrucosum*,[‡] *M. equinum*,[§] and *M. gypseum*.[Π] There is considerable variation in the frequency of isolation of these less common dermatophytes in different parts of the world. Rare causes of equine dermatophytosis include *M. canis*[¶] and *Keratinomyces ajelloi*.[8,33,112,117] Extremely rare

---

°References 8, 33-37, 39, 42, 43, 47, 53-55a, 57, 59-61, 63, 72, 73, 75, 91, 96, 98, 99, 106, 108, 111, 113, 118, 119, 121, 122, 125, 130, 131, 139, 141, 142.
†References 8, 33, 36, 40, 42, 49, 96, 106, 108, 113, 122.
‡References 8, 37, 53, 72-74, 76, 106, 108, 125, 143, 144.
§References 36, 42, 44, 49, 72, 73, 79, 100, 108, 113, 125, 138.
ΠReferences 8, 33, 42, 45, 48, 49, 53, 72, 73, 78, 80, 81, 83, 88, 103, 104, 106, 108, 113, 125, 135, 137.
¶References 33, 35, 49, 53, 56, 67, 101, 108, 122, 131.

isolates include *T. tonsurans*,[89,90] *T. rubrum*,[27,33] *M. nanum*,[33] *M. audouinii*,[33] *M. cookei*,[27] *T. terrestre*,[27] *T. schoenleinii*,[8,27] *M. distortum*,[8] and *Epidermophyton floccosum*.[33] Rarely, infections with more than one dermatophyte have been reported.[33,35,39,67]

The incidence and prevalence of dermatophytosis vary with the climate, natural reservoirs, and living conditions.[27] A higher incidence is seen in hot, humid climates than in cold, dry climates.[27] Although dermatophytosis is seen at all times of the year, it is especially common in fall and winter, particularly in confined animals, in temperate climates.* In topical or subtropical climates, dermatophytosis is more common during moist, warm weather, when there are large populations of biting insects.[22-24,108] Frequent outbreaks of dermatophytosis are seen when horses are brought together for training, racing, and breeding purposes.†

Dermatophytes are transmitted by contact with infected hair and scale or fungal elements on animals, in the environment, or on fomites.† Combs, brushes, clippers, bedding, blankets, tack, fencing, transport vehicles, and other paraphernalia associated with the grooming, movement, and housing of animals are all potential sources of infection and reinfection. The sources of *M. equinum* or *M. canis* infections are usually an infected horse or cat, respectively. *Trichophyton* spp. infections are usually acquired directly or indirectly by exposure to typical reservoir hosts, which may be determined by specific identification of the fungal species or subspecies. For example, most *T. mentagrophytes* infections are associated with exposure to rodents or their immediate environment. *M. gypseum* is a geophilic dermatophyte that inhabits rich soil. Infections with anthropophilic species are extremely rare; they are acquired as reverse zoonoses by contact with infected humans. Hair shafts containing infectious arthrospores may remain infectious in the environment for many months to years.§

When an animal is exposed to a dermatophyte, an infection may be established. Mechanical disruption of the stratum corneum appears to be important in facilitating the penetration and invasion of anagen hair follicles.[9,27,28] Hair is invaded in both ectothrix and endothrix infections. The ectothrix fungi produce masses of arthrospores on the surface of hair shafts, whereas endothrix fungi do not. Fungal hyphae invade the ostium of hair follicles, proliferate on the surface of hairs, and migrate downward (proximally) to the hair bulb, during which time the fungus produces its own keratinolytic enzymes (keratinases) that allow penetration of the hair cuticle and growth within the hair shaft until the keratogenous zone (Adamson's fringe) is reached. At this point, the fungus either establishes an equilibrium between its downward growth and the production of keratin or it is expelled. Spontaneous resolution occurs when infected hairs enter the telogen phase or if an inflammatory reaction is incited. When a hair enters telogen, keratin production slows and stops; because the dermatophyte requires actively growing hairs for survival, fungal growth also slows and stops. Infectious arthrospores may remain on the hair shaft, but reinfection of that particular hair follicle does not occur until it reenters anagen. In humans, it has been shown that dermatophytes may be isolated from normal-looking skin up to 6 cm from the margins of clinical lesions.[82] There may be differences in the pathogenicity of various strains of a dermatophyte.[103]

In experimental models of *T. equinum* or *M. gypseum* infection in horses,[103,112,119] the incubation period between inoculation and development of clinical lesions was 6 to 17 days. Lesions enlarged until 3 to 10 weeks postinoculation, then decreased in size and healed by 5 to 14 weeks postinoculation. With natural infections, incubation periods vary from 1 to 6 weeks.[27,108]

---

*References 10, 14, 16, 17, 27, 29, 94, 108.
†References 22-24, 71, 73, 104, 105, 108, 111, 131, 134, 138.
‡References 8, 10, 12, 14, 16, 24, 27, 29.
§References 24, 25, 27, 28, 105, 108.

Cutaneous inflammation is due to toxins produced in the stratum corneum that provoke a sort of biologic contact dermatitis.[9,27,28] Host factors are poorly documented, but the host's ability to mount an inflammatory response plays a critical role in determining the type of clinical lesions produced and in terminating the infection. Dermatophyte infections in healthy horses are usually self-limiting.[*] Dermatophytes have shared and specific antigens.[85,114] It has been shown that *T. rubrum* and *T. mentagrophytes* produce substances (especially mannans) that diminish cell-mediated immune responses and indirectly inhibit stratum corneum turnover.[51] These effects could predispose the animal to persistent or recurrent infections. *Trichophyton* equinum and *T. mentagrophytes* produce urease, gelatinase, protease, hemolysins, and keratinases.[86] In addition, *T. equinum* produces lipase.[86] These substances can have a variety of proinflammatory and pathologic consequences. *Trichophyton* spp. can produce proteolytic enzymes that induce keratinocyte acantholysis *in vitro* and *in vivo*.[124] It has been shown that dermatophytes can elaborate penicillin-like substances, which can result in the isolation of penicillin-resistant bacteria from affected skin.[27]

Although dermatophytosis may be seen in horses of any age, young animals (<2 years old) are predisposed to acquiring symptomatic dermatophyte infections.[†] This is partly due to a delay in development of adequate host immunity. However, differences in biochemical properties of the skin and skin secretions (especially sebum), the growth and replacement of hair, and the physiologic status of the host as related to age may also be factors. Local factors, such as the mechanical barrier of intact skin and the fungistatic activity of sebum caused by its fatty acid content, are deterrents to fungal invasion.

Natural and experimental infections have been shown to incite various forms of hypersensitivity in their hosts.[9,27,28] Horses having recovered from *T. equinum* or *M. gypseum* infections show enhanced resistance to reinfection.[22-24,103,120] There is no correlation between circulating antibodies and protection. It is believed that the cell-mediated immune response is the mainstay of the body against fungal infection. This is corroborated by the increased incidence of fungal infections in patients with various acquired or inherited forms of immunosuppression.[9,28] The presence of ectoparasites, lice, are probably important in the establishment and spread of dermatophytosis. It is unusual for a healthy horse to get dermatophytosis a second time, unless a different genus or species of dermatophyte is involved. Horses suffering from severe, chronic, or recurrent dermatophytosis usually have concurrent immunosuppressive disorders, are being treated with glucocorticoids, or inhabit filthy, moist, crowded environments.[24,27,49,96]

CLINICAL FINDINGS

Dermatophytosis is common in horses.[†] It was reported to be the most common equine skin disease in the Netherlands.[126a] However, when clinicians rely on clinical signs alone, dermatophytosis (ringworm, tinea) is greatly overdiagnosed. Over a 21-year period, dermatophytosis has accounted for 8.89% of the equine dermatology cases seen at our university practice. The analysis of cultures submitted from suspected dermatophytosis cases in horses generally reveals that between 10% and 23.1% are positive.[42,121] Several other dermatoses, especially staphylococcal folliculitis, dermatophilosis, pemphigus foliaceus, and sterile eosinophilic folliculitis mimic the classic ringworm lesion. On the other hand, dermatophytosis is a diagnosis that is often missed because of the protean nature of the dermatologic findings.[27]

Because the infection is almost always follicular in horses, the most consistent clinical sign is one or many circular patches of alopecia with variable scaling and crusting.[13,34] Some patients may

---

*References 10, 14, 16, 17, 24, 27, 29, 49, 97, 103, 112, 123.
†References 10, 12, 14, 16, 17, 22-25, 27, 29, 94, 108.
‡References 1-4, 8, 10, 12, 14, 16, 17, 19-24, 27, 29, 47, 59, 63, 69, 87, 88, 108, 123, 131.

develop the classic ring lesion with central healing and fine follicular papules and crusts at the periphery. However, signs and symptoms are highly variable and depend on the host-fungus interaction and, therefore, the degree of inflammation. Pruritus is usually minimal or absent; however, it is occasionally marked and suggests an ectoparasitism or allergy. In addition, dermatophytosis may be complicated by secondary bacterial (usually staphylococcal) infection. *In vitro* studies have shown that dermatophytes can produce antibiotic substances and encourage the development of penicillin-resistant staphylococci.[16,41]

The initial lesions are often tufted papules, 2-5 mm in diameter (Fig. 5-1, *A*). Early lesions may also appear as erect hairs in annular areas of 5-20 mm diameter. Occasionally, an urticarial-like eruption will precede the more obvious follicular dermatosis by 24 to 72 hours.[27] Unlike true urticaria (hives), the lesions do not pit with digital pressure. Hair can easily be plucked from lesions within 4 to 6 days. Crusts may be thin or thick. Alopecia and a prominent silvery scaling are seen in older lesions. Lesions typically expand peripherally and may coalesce to form polycyclic shapes. Erythema is only seen in white horses. Pruritus is usually minimal to absent and, if present, is most noticeable in the early stages of infection. However, pruritus is occasionally severe and suggestive of an ectoparasitism or an allergy.[24,27,91] Variable degrees of pain are often present in early lesions. In horses with acantholytic dermatophytosis or those with secondary bacterial infections, erosions, epidermal collarettes, suppurative exudate, or rare pustules may be present.

Lesions are most commonly present on the face (Fig. 5-1, *B* and *C*), neck, dorsolateral thorax (Fig. 5-2), and girth ("girth itch") (Fig. 5-1, *D*).[27] The legs are less commonly affected (Figs. 5-1, *E*, and 5-3). The mane and tail are rarely, if ever, affected. Lesions may be limited to the caudal pastern region ("scratches," "mud fever," "grease heel") (Fig. 5-1, *F*) and may wax and wane (analogous to "athlete's foot" in humans) with stress, local irritation, moisture, and unsanitary conditions.[27] Dermatophytosis may also manifest as multifocal to generalized scaling ("seborrhea sicca") with only irregular ill-defined areas of hair loss, or widespread well-circumscribed alopecia (Fig. 5-4, *A*).[27] Rarely, dermatophytic pseudomycetoma is seen in the horse.[116] It is characterized by one or more subcutaneous to dermal nodules than may be ulcerated and discharging. These nodules are usually present over the dorsal thoracic area and have been caused by *T. equinum.*

Lesions are usually multiple, and may be very asymmetric or more-or-less symmetric in distribution. Solitary lesions are rarely seen. Generalized dermatophytosis is uncommon and usually seen in immunosuppressed horses or in foals.

In general, the nature of the dermatophyte cannot be determined from the clinical presentation. Some authors have suggested that *M. gypseum* infections occur most commonly on the face, legs, and dorsal neck and rump (reflecting spread by biting insects), but not on the girth or saddle region.[24,45,103,104] Others suggest that *M. equinum* infections do not involve the girth and saddle regions,[49,104] and that *T. equinum* infections rarely affected the head, flank, and rump.[49] *T. equinum equinum* and *T. equinum autotrophicum* produce identical clinical disease in horses.[104] *T. verrucosum* infections may produce thicker, gray crusts.[72,74,143,144]

Zoonotic Aspects

In most areas of the world, dermatophytosis is rarely transmitted from horses to humans. This is because the most commonly isolated equine dermatophyte is *T. equinum equinum* (see Chapter 2).* Transmission from horse to human is more likely with *T. verruscosum*[27,144] and where *T. equinum autotrophicum* is prevalent (Australia and New Zealand) (see Chapter 2).[24,93] *M. canis* was reported to be transmitted from a horse to a human.[101] When contracted from horses, human dermatophytosis is characterized by a pruritic, papulopustular (rarely vesicular) dermatitis. Lesions are most commonly seen on the legs (bareback horseriding!) or arms.[93,101, 126,134,144]

---

*References 46, 91, 92, 126, 132a, 134.

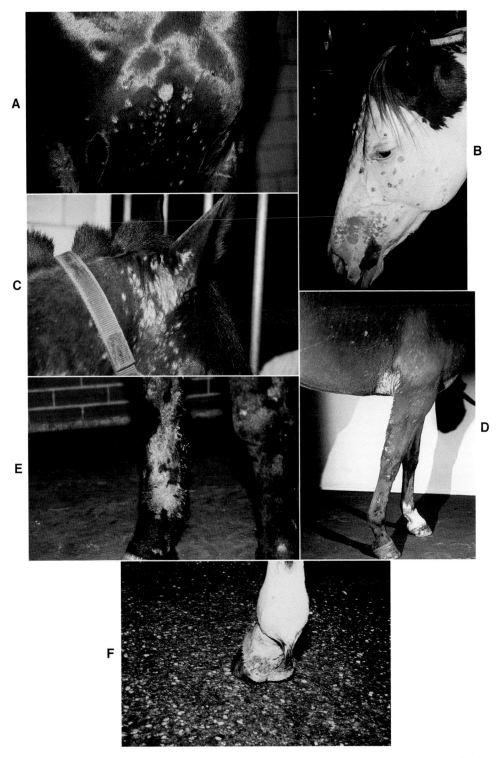

FIGURE 5-1. Dermatophytosis. **A,** Tufted papules and annular areas of crust and alopecia on brisket. **B,** Annular areas of alopecia, scaling, and erythema on the face. **C,** Annular areas of alopecia, scale, and crust near base of ear. **D,** Alopecia and scaling in the girth area. **E,** Alopecia, scaling, and crusting on leg. **F,** Crusting and alopecia on caudal pastern. (*Courtesy Dr. W. McMullen.*)

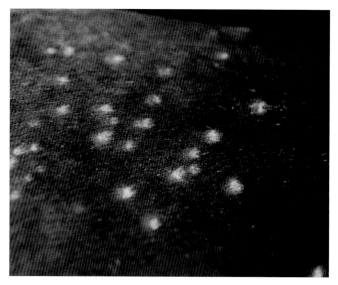

FIGURE 5-2. Dermatophytosis. Multiple annular areas of alopecia and crust over saddle area.

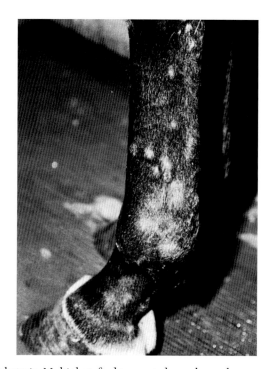

FIGURE 5-3. Dermatophytosis. Multiple tufted to crusted papules on leg.

DIAGNOSIS

Because most infections are follicular, the primary differential diagnoses are staphylococcal folliculitis, dermatophilosis, pemphigus foliaceus, and eosinophilic folliculitis. Demodicosis is extremely rare in horses. Although alopecia areata produces annular areas of alopecia, the alopecic skin appears otherwise normal. Dermatophytic pseudomycetoma must be differentiated from other infectious or foreign-body granulomas, sterile panniculitis, and various neoplasms. When the

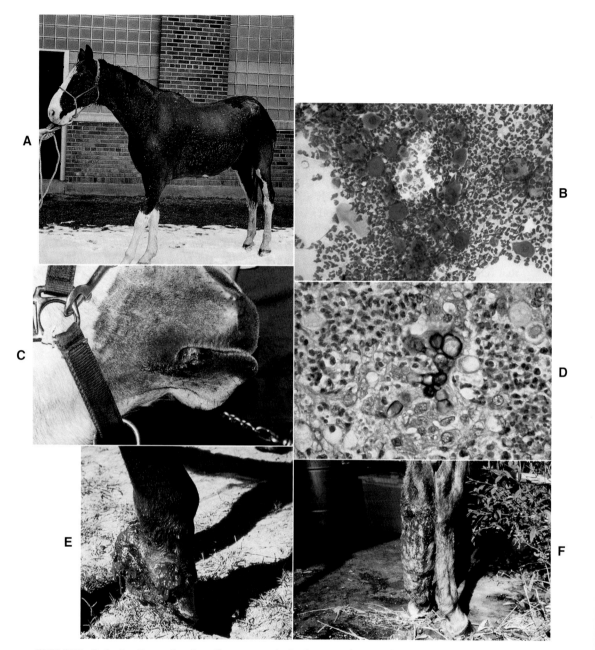

FIGURE 5-4. A, Generalized well-circumscribed alopecia due to dermatophytosis. **B,** Acantholytic dermatophytosis. Cytologic examination of direct smear reveals nondegenerate neutrophils and numerous acantholytic keratinocytes. **C,** Eumycotic mycetoma at commissure of lips. **D,** Phaeohyphomycosis. Brown fungal elements in pyogranuloma. **E,** Ulcerative granuloma on pastern in pythiosis (Courtesy Dr. R. Miller). **F,** Ulcerative granuloma involving entire metatarsal area in pythiosis (Courtesy Dr. R. Miller).

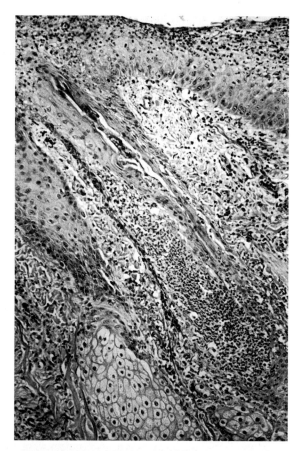

FIGURE 5-7. Dermatophytosis. Suppurative luminal folliculitis.

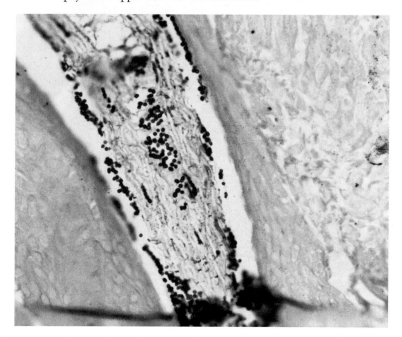

FIGURE 5-8. Dermatophytosis. Special stain reveals numerous arthroconidia and hyphae (GMS stain).

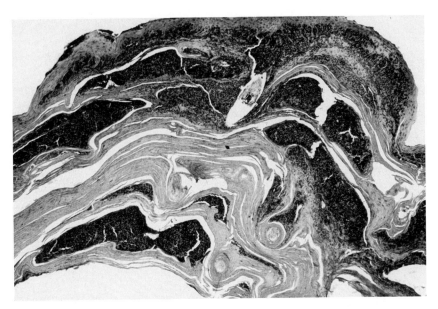

FIGURE 5-9. Dermatophytosis. Palisading crust.

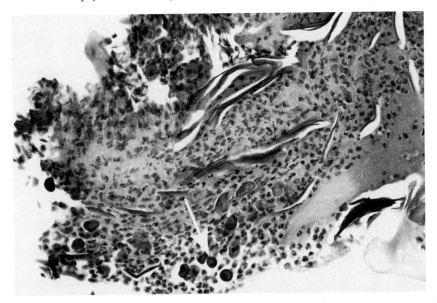

FIGURE 5-10. Acantholytic dermatophytosis. Numerous acantholytic keratinocytes (*arrow*) in surface crust.

arthroconidia may be present in and around infected hairs (Fig. 5-11), in hair follicles, and within the stratum corneum of the surface epidermis. The number of fungal elements present is often inversely proportional to the severity of the inflammatory response.

CLINICAL MANAGEMENT

Dermatophytosis in healthy horses usually undergoes spontaneous remission within 3 months.° Some authors believe that exposure to sunshine is beneficial.[24] Because of this, a veritable plethora of "therapeutic agents" have been espoused as ringworm cures.[27] Controlled studies documenting

---

°References 10, 14, 16, 17, 24, 27, 29, 49, 97, 103, 112, 123.

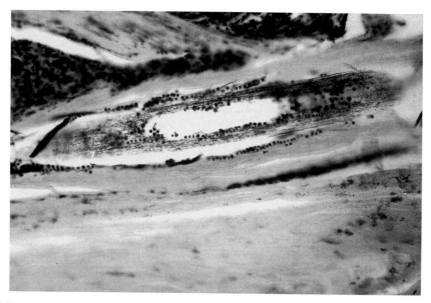

FIGURE 5-11. Acantholytic dermatophytosis. Special stain reveals numerous arthroconidia on hair in crust (AOG stain).

the efficacy of this "sea of antifungal agents" in equine dermatophytosis are virtually nonexistent. The goals of therapy are (1) to maximize the patient's ability to respond to the dermatophyte infection (by the correction of any nutritional imbalances and concurrent disease states and by the termination of systemic anti-inflammatory and immunosuppressive drugs), (2) to reduce contagion (to the environment, other animals, and humans), and (3) to hasten resolution of the infection.[16,24,27,29] A critical feature of clinical management is the treatment of all horses in contact with the infected horse and treatment of the environment.[16,24,27,29] It is advisable to stop riding, training, or working animals until they are recovered, as continued trauma and exercise may lead to more lesions, worse lesions, and a prolonged recovery.[24,49,104,106]

Topical Therapy

Every confirmed case of dermatophytosis should receive topical therapy.[16,24,27,29] Creams and lotions are available for use on focal lesions, and these are typically applied every 12 hours. There is a wide variety of topical antifungals available, and there is no particular advantage of one product over another (Table 5-1). For highly inflamed lesions, a product containing glucocorticoid in combination with antifungal agents may hasten resolution of clinical disease. For horses with multifocal or generalized skin involvement, antifungal rinses (dips) are indicated. Rinses are preferred because the entire body surface can be treated, rubbing of the haircoat is minimized, and the antifungal agent can be allowed to dry on the skin. Rinses are usually applied daily for 5 to 7 days, then once or twice weekly until clinical cure. Lime sulfur 2% (Lym Dyp) and enilconazole 0.2 % (Imaverol) are the most effective (see page 307).° Rinses of 0.2% enilconazole (not approved for horses in the United States) applied once or twice weekly were reported to be effective for the treatment of equine dermatophytosis (see page 307).[50,106] A spray of 100 ppm natamycin (not approved for horses in the United States) applied twice weekly was also reported to be effective for the treatment of equine dermatophytosis (see page 308).[97,144]

°References 24c, 24d, 31b, 32b, 57, 70.

● Table 5-1 **PRODUCTS FOR THE TOPICAL TREATMENT OF SUPERFICIAL MYCOSES**

PRODUCT		INDICATION*
Spot Treatment		
Amphotericin B 3% cream, lotion	Fungizone (Apothecin)	C,M
Chlorhexidine 4% spray[‡]	ChlorhexiDerm Maximum (DVM)	C,D,M
Clotrimazole 1% cream, lotion	Lotrimin (Schering)	C,D,M
Clotrimazole 1%/bethamethasone 0.1% cream	Lotrisone (Schering)	C,D,M
Clotrimazole 1%/bethamethasone 0.3% gentamicin ointment	Otomax (Schering)	C,D,M
Miconazole 2% cream, 1% lotion, 1% spray	Conofite (Schering)	C,D,M
Miconazole 2% spray[‡]	Miconazole Spray (EVSCO)	C,D,M
Naftifine 1% cream, gel	Naftin (Allergan)	C,D
Nystatin cream	Mycostatin (Squibb)	C,M
Nystatin/triamcinolone cream, ointment	Animax (Pharmaderm)	C,M
Terbinafine 1% cream	Lamisil (Novartis)	C,D
Thiabendazole 4% dexamethasone	Tresaderm (Merck Ag Vet)	C,D,M
Shampoos[†]		
Chlorhexidine 2%[‡]	ChlorhexiDerm (DVM)	C,M
Chlorhexidine 2%	Seba-Hex (EVSCO)	C,M
Chlorhexidine 3%	Hexadene (Allerderm/Virbac)	C,M
Chlorhexidine 4%[‡]	ChlorhexiDerm Maxi (DVM)	C,M
Miconazole 2%	Dermazole (Allerderm/Virbac)	C,M
Miconazole 2%	Miconazole (EVSCO)	C,M
Chlorhexidine 2% and miconazole 2%[‡]	Malaseb (DVM)	C,D,M
Rinses		
Acetic acid 2.5%	(Vinegar: Water)	C.M
Enilconazole 0.2%	Imaverol (Janssen)	C,D,M
Lime sulfur 2%	LymDyp (DVM)	C,D,M

*C = candidiasis; D = dermatophytosis; M = malasseziasis.
[†]Shampooing may disperse more arthrospores into the haircoat and environment and may not be the most effective or the safest way to treat dermatophytosis.
[‡]Labeled for horses.

Shampoos are less desirable because (a) they have no residual action and (b) the physical act of their application and removal may macerate fragile hairs and increase the release and dispersal infective spores into the coat, thus increasing the likelihood of spreading the infection and of human exposure.[28] Nonetheless, it has been reported that the use of 2% chlorhexidine/2% miconazole shampoo (Malaseb, DVM), twice weekly, resulted in the resolution of clinical signs of dermatophytosis (*T. equinum*) in horses within 6 weeks (see page 307).[106] Other shampoos used on horses with dermatophytosis include 4% chlorhexidine (ChlorhexiDerm Maximum, DVM) and 2% miconazole (Miconazole, EVSCO).

Systemic Therapy

Griseofulvin (Fulvicin U/F) has been recommended for the systemic treatment of equine dermatophytosis.* Dosage and frequency protocols vary widely. In fact, there are no published

---

*References 14, 17, 20, 22-25, 27, 66, 68, 136.

data on the pharmacokinetics of griseofulvin in horses, and published clinical trials in equine dermatophytosis are flawed (see page 309). When oral griseofulvin powder is administered according to the manufacturer's recommendations, it is of doubtful therapeutic efficacy (see page 309). Many investigators, including the authors, cannot endorse the use of currently recommended therapeutic protocols for griseofulvin in horses.[16,27,29,71] See page 308 concerning the use of griseofulvin.

Ketoconazole (Nizoral), *itraconazole* (Sporonox), *fluconazole* (Diflucan), and *terbinafine* (Lamisil) are effective for the systemic treatment of dermatophytosis in humans, dogs, and cats.[9,28] These agents are not presently approved for use in horses in the United States, and would be cost-prohibitive. In addition, no information is currently available on the pharmacokinetics or clinical efficacy of these agents in horses (see page 309).

Dermatophytic pseudomycetoma is difficult to treat in dogs and cats, requiring surgical excision and long-term itraconazole therapy.[28] Two horses seen by the authors had solitary lesions and were cured by surgical excision.

Vaccination

Fungal vaccines (lyophilized, modified live fungus) have been successful in Europe in the management of endemic dermatophytoses in cattle and foxes.[27,28]

In eastern Europe, a modified live fungal (*T. equinum*) vaccine was reported to be very effective.[109,119] The vaccine was administered intramuscularly twice at 14-day intervals. Vaccinated horses developed either no lesions or only a few, short-lived lesions when challenged naturally or experimentally. In the United States, an experimental inactivated (killed) fungal (*T. equinum*) vaccine was also given intramuscularly twice at 10- to 14-day intervals.[112] Of the vaccinated horses, 87% did not develop dermatophytosis under natural conditions, while 52% of the nonvaccinated horses did develop disease. Over a 3-year period, the vaccine protocol reduced the frequency of equine dermatophytosis from 40% to 0%.

Environmental Decontamination

The critical role of premise disinfection in eradication of dermatophytes from a premise cannot be overemphasized.

1. Dermatophyte spores can remain viable in the environment (corrals, stalls, tack, grooming equipment, etc) for months to years.[27,28,105,108] Sodium hypochlorite 0.5%, when added to *M. canis* infected cat hairs for 5 minutes twice weekly, prevented fungal growth only after 8 "treatments."[28] When 10 disinfectants were tested at various dilutions as single applications to a surface contaminated with *M. canis* infected cats hairs and spores, only undiluted bleach (5.25% sodium hypochlorite) or 1% formalin were able to inactivate infected cat hairs within 2 hours.[28] Enilconazole was effective within 8 hours.[28] When 14 disinfectants were repeatedly applied to isolated *M. canis* infected cats hairs, the most effective were stabilized chlorine dioxide (Oxygene, Oxyfresh USA, Spokane, WA), glutaraldehyde and quaternary ammonium chloride (GPC 8, Solomon Industries, Cocoa, FL), potassium monoperoxysulfate (Virkon, S. Durvet, Blue Springs, MO), and a 0.525% sodium hypochlorite.[28] Undiluted bleach is corrosive and irritating. Because of its human health hazards, formalin solution is not recommended for routine use in disinfecting premises. Enilconazole sprays and "foggers" have been used successfully in Europe.[28] In one study on equine dermatophytosis,[106] potassium monopersulfate (Virkon) spray was used on stables, walls, buckets, and so forth, while enilconazole foggers were used twice at 10-day intervals for tack, blankets, grooming equipment, and so forth.
2. Destroy all bedding, rugs, brushes, combs, and the like.

Candidiasis

CAUSE AND PATHOGENESIS

Candida spp. (especially *C. albicans*) yeasts are normal inhabitants of the alimentary, upper respiratory, and genital mucosa of mammals.[5-7,27,28,145] *Candida* species cause opportunistic infections of skin, mucocutaneous areas, and external ear canal. Factors that upset the normal endogenous microflora (prolonged antibiotic therapy) or disrupt normal cutaneous or mucosal barriers (maceration, burns, indwelling catheters) provide a pathway for *Candida* spp. to enter the body.[28] Once in the body, further spread of infection correlates with cell-mediated immuno-competence and neutrophil function.[28] Immunosuppressive disease states (diabetes mellitus, hyperadrenocorticism, hypothyroidism, viral infections, cancer, inherited immunologic defects) or immunosuppressive drug therapy predispose some animals to candidiasis.[28] Vulvovaginal candidiasis was reported in horses following the oral administration of altrenogest (synthetic progestogen).[146a] *Candida* spp. produce acid proteinases and keratinases (degrade stratum corneum), and phospholipases (penetration of tissues).[28]

Candidiasis has been reported under the following names in earlier literature: *candidosis*, *moniliasis*, and *thrush*.

CLINICAL FINDINGS

Candidiasis is an extremely rarely reported disease in horses. A 5-year-old Freiberg mare had multiple cutaneous nodules (especially over neck, shoulder, and thorax) that were firm, painful, and covered by normal skin and haircoat.[147] The horse also had ventral edema, mastitis, and pyrexia. Histopathologic findings in skin biopsy specimens include nodular granulomatous dermatitis with numerous yeasts (2 to 6 µm diameter) and blastoconidia (budding yeast cells) within macrophages and multinucleated histiocytic giant cells. Culture and fluorescent antibody testing were positive for *C. guilliermondii*. Treatment with sodium iodide was curative.

Oral candidiasis (white, pseudomembranous plaques and ulcers on tongue and gingiva) was reported in immunodeficient foals.[146] Candidal arthritis (*C. tropicalis*, *C. parapsilosis*) has also been reported in horses.[145a]

Vulvovaginal candidiasis was reported in six thoroughbred mares following the oral administration of altrenogest.[146a] The perivulvar and perineal skin was erythematous, pustular, eroded, and variably hyper- or hypopigmented.

DIAGNOSIS

The differential diagnosis for nodular forms of candidiasis includes infectious and sterile granulomatous disorders. Mucocutaneous candidiasis must be differentiated from immunologic diseases (e.g., pemphigus vulgaris, bullous pemphigoid, systemic lupus erythematosus, erythema multiforme, vasculitis), drug eruptions, and epidermolysis bullosa. Cytologic examination of direct smears reveals suppurative inflammation and numerous yeasts (2 to 6 µm in diameter) and blastoconidia (budding cells).[5-7,28] Pseudohyphae may occasionally be seen. In contrast to *Malassezia pachydermatis*, *Candida* spp. show narrow-based and multilateral budding. *Candida* species grow on Sabouraud's dextrose agar at 25 to 30° C. The API 20C system is a convenient and reliable system for identification.

CLINICAL MANAGEMENT

Correction of predisposing causes is fundamental. Excessive moisture must be avoided. For localized lesions, clipping, drying, and topical antifungal agents are usually effective. Useful topical agents include nystatin (100,000 U/gm), azoles (2% miconazole, 1% clotrimazole), 3% amphotericin B, gentian violet (1:10,000 in 10% alcohol), and potassium permanganate (1:3000 in water).[9,28] These agents should be applied 2 to 3 times daily until lesions are completely healed (1 to 4 weeks).

Oral, widespread mucocutaneous, and generalized lesions require systemic antifungal therapy.[9,28] Vulvovaginal candidiasis in mares was cured by the intravaginal insertion of 500 mg clotrimazole per day for 5 consecutive days.[146a] Although intravenous amphotericin B is effective,[145a] ketoconazole or itraconazole administered orally are the drugs of choice in other species. These agents have not been evaluated in equine candidiasis. Therapy should be continued for 7 to 10 days beyond clinical cure (2 to 4 weeks). One horse with nodular cutaneous candidiasis was cured with the administration of sodium iodide (see page 311).[147]

Malassezia Dermatitis

CAUSE AND PATHOGENESIS

Malassezia pachydermatis (*M. canis, Pityrosporum pachydermatis, P. canis*) is a lipophilic, nonlipid-dependent, nonmycelial saprophytic yeast that is commonly found on normal and abnormal skin, in normal and abnormal ear canals, on mucosal surfaces (oral, anal), and in the anal sacs and vagina of many mammals.[28,147a,147c]

Recent advances in electrophoretic karyotyping have shown that the genus *Malassezia* contains six lipid-dependent species (*M. furfur* [*P. ovale*], *M. globosa, M. obtusa, M. restricta, M. slooffiae,* and *M. sympodialis*) and one nonlipid-dependent species (*M. pachydermatis*).[28,147c] *M. pachydermatis* is the most common species isolated from horses.[147c] In one study of normal horses, a novel *Malassezia* sp., most closely related to *M. sympodialis*, was isolated.[147b]

The diversity of *M. pachydermatis* isolates from a wide variety of hosts was investigated, and seven types or strains (sequevars), Ia through Ig, were identified.[28] The predominant sequevar, type Ia, appeared to be ubiquitous. None of the seven sequevars correlated with isolation from healthy skin or a particular lesion (otitis externa or dermatitis). In addition, this study indicated that the skin of a given animal may be colonized by more than one type of *M. pachydermatis*.

Trypsin-sensitive proteins or glycoproteins on yeast cell walls are important for adherence of *M. pachydermatis* to canine corneocytes,[28] and mannosyl-bearing carbohydrate residues on canine corneocytes serve as ligands for adhesions expressed by *M. pachydermatis*.[28] There is, however, variability among strains of the organism.[28] Enhanced adherence of *M. pachydermatis* to corneocytes does not appear to be important in the pathogenesis of *Malassezia* dermatitis in dogs.[28]

Because *M. pachydermatis* does not invade subcorneally, dermatitis is hypothesized to result from inflammatory and/or hypersensitivity reactions to yeast products and antigens.[28] Virulence factors for *M. pachydermatis* have not been characterized. It has been shown that *M. pachydermatis* isolated from dogs with otitis externa produce proteases, lipases, lipoxygenases, phosphatases, phosphohydralases, glucosidase, galactosidase, urease, and zymosan.[28] These substances could contribute to the pathogenesis, inflammation, and pruritus of *Malassezia* dermatitis through proteolysis, lipolysis, alteration of local pH, eicosanoid release, and complement activation.

Histologically, *Malassezia* dermatitis in dogs is often characterized by prominent exocytosis of lymphocytes (CD3-positive) and a subepithelial accumulation of mast cells, which suggest a hypersensitivity reaction.[28] Immediate intradermal skin test reactivity to *M. pachydermatis* antigens was reported in all atopic dogs with concurrent *Malassezia* dermatitis,[28] while all normal dogs and atopic dogs without concurrent *Malassezia* dermatitis did not react. Hypersensitivity to *Malassezia* antigens is also thought to be important in atopic humans.[28] The levels of *M. pachydermatis*–specific IgG (by ELISA) were significantly greater in dogs with *Malassezia* dermatitis than in normal dogs.[28]

Many predisposing factors have been hypothesized to allow the commensal *M. pachydermatis* to become a pathogen.[28] Increased humidity is probably important, as *Malassezia* dermatitis seems to be more common in humid climates (e.g., summer) and in certain anatomical locations (e.g., ear canals, skin folds). Increased availability of yeast nutrients and growth factors are also probably important: hormonal alterations of the quantity and quality of sebum, "seborrheic" skin (keratinization disorders), increased populations of commensal symbiotic staphylococci.

Immunologic dysfunction—especially as concerns cell-mediated immunity—could play a role in the pathogenesis of *M. pachydermatis* infection.[28] Chronic glucocorticoid therapy could have a precipitating role here. Widespread *Malassezia* dermatitis in cats has been associated with concurrent FIV infection, thymoma, and pancreatic adenocarcinoma.[28] As mentioned previously, hypersensitivity to *M. pachydermatis* antigens likely plays an important role in many dogs.

It has been suggested that canine *Malassezia* dermatitis is often associated with prior antibiotic therapy.[13,101b,106,108,113] This has not been sufficiently corroborated. In fact, unlike *Candida* spp., *Malassezia* populations are not subject to the inhibitory effects of bacteria.

CLINICAL FINDINGS

Malassezia dermatitis is only anecdotally recognized in horses, but may be more common than the absence of published reports would indicate. The authors have seen *Malassezia* dermatitis in horses characterized by variably pruritic, greasy-to-waxy, foul-smelling dermatoses in intertriginous areas: axillae, groin, udder, and prepuce.

Zoonotic Aspects

Malassezia pachydermatis has been cultured from the blood, urine, and cerebrospinal fluid of low-birth-weight neonates that were receiving intravenous lipid emulsions in an intensive care facility.[28] An identical strain of *M. pachydermatis* was cultured from one health worker and from pet dogs. These problems were terminated when handwashing procedures were enforced.

DIAGNOSIS

Malassezia dermatitis should be considered a factor in any scaly, erythematous, greasy to waxy, pruritic dermatitis in which other differentials have been eliminated by diagnostic tests and there is a lack of response to treatment (e.g., glucocorticoids, antibiotics, antiseborrheic shampoos, insecticides, miticides).

The most useful and readily available tool for the clinician presented with a suspected case of *Malassezia* dermatitis is cytologic examination.[28] Samples of surface scale or grease are gathered by making a superficial skin scraping, vigorously rubbing a cotton swab on the skin surface, pressing a piece of clear cellophane tape onto lesional skin several times, or pressing a section of a clean glass microscope slide on the skin.[28] It is not clear which of these methods is the best, and each has its own benefits and shortcomings. *Superficial scrapings* are reliable, but can be difficult to perform in certain areas. *Tape strips* are good where the skin surface is flat and not overly waxy or greasy. *Direct impression with a glass slide* is good for flat surfaces and where grease and wax are plentiful. *Cotton swab (Q-Tip) smears* are good for ears and folds. In normal dogs, impression smears, skin scrapings, and swabs gave similar results.[28] Other investigators found scrapings and tape strippings to be superior to swabs.[28] Still others have found tape stripping to be unsatisfactory.[28] Results of a recent study on dogs with Malassezia pododermatitis[28] indicated no statistically significant difference between the numbers of yeasts recovered with superficial scrapings, tape strippings, and direct impressions. However, swabs were significantly inferior to the other three techniques. Whichever method is used, all material is transferred to a glass slide, heat fixed (not if cellophane tape has been used!), and stained for cytologic examination. Heat fixing can be avoided by using a direct stain like New Methylene Blue. One looks for round to oval, to the classic peanut-shaped yeasts. *Malassezia pachydermatis* is characterized by monopolar budding of daughter cells from one site on the cell wall, formation of a prominent bud scar or collar at the site of daughter cell development, a peanut-shape, and a diameter of 3 to 8 μm.[28] Yeasts are often seen in clusters or adhered to keratinocytes (Fig. 5-12).

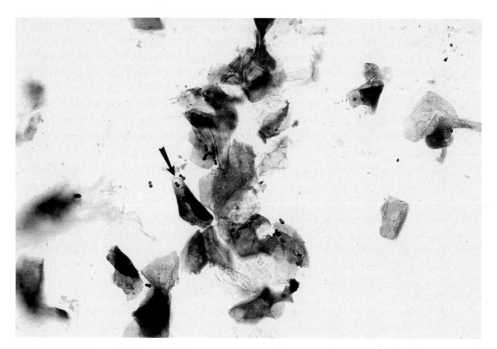

FIGURE 5-12. *Malassezia* dermatitis. Direct impression smear reveals numerous budding yeast adherent to keratinocytes (*arrow*).

The full diagnostic value of cytologic examination in any species remains to be determined, and only one study has been conducted on normal equine skin. An extensive study of normal dog skin sampled by impression smears, skin scrapings, and swabs revealed that most specimens contained less than 10 organisms/1.25 cm^2 (0.5 in^2) of sample (median value of 1 organism per sample).[28] Another study of normal and affected skin of dogs with various dermatoses, sampled by impression smears, revealed that normal skin had <1 organism/HPF, whereas affected skin had <1 organism/HPF (80% of samples) or 1 to 3 organisms/HPF (20% of samples).[28] In dogs, *Malassezia* dermatitis is more likely when >10 organisms are seen in 15 randomly chosen oil-immersion microscopic fields (1000×) using tape strip samples, when an average of ≥4 organisms are seen per oil-immersion microscopic fields, when an average of ≥1 organisms is seen in 10 oil-immersion microscopic fields, or when >2 organisms/HPF (400×) are found with any of the commonly used sampling techniques.[28]

In one study of 12 normal horses,[147b] yeasts were found in one or more cutaneous sites (especially the groin) in 7 horses (from <1 to >10 yeasts per 1000× microscopic field).

Skin biopsy findings in dogs are characterized by a superficial perivascular-to-interstitial dermatitis with irregular hyperplasia, diffuse spongiosis, and diffuse lymphocytic exocytosis of the epidermis and follicular infundibulum.[28] Parakeratosis is prominent, and dermal inflammatory cells are dominated by lymphocytes, histiocytes, and plasma cells. Eosinophils, neutrophils, and mast cells are frequently seen. Yeasts are seen in surface and/or infundibular keratin in about 70% of the cases. They are randomly distributed. Eosinophilic epidermal microabscesses may be seen in about 14% of the cases, and mast cells are linearly aligned at the dermoepidermal junction in about 47% of the cases. Signs of concurrent bacterial infection (suppurative epidermitis and folliculitis) are commonly seen. Yeasts can occasionally be seen on the surface of biopsies from numerous canine and feline dermatoses and yet play no known role in their pathogenesis or treatment. We can assume that the same thing applies to horses. Yeasts present in hair follicles, however, are always assumed to be possibly pathogenic. No histopathologic studies of equine *Malassezia* dermatitis have been published.

Malassezia pachydermatis is usually easy to culture.[28] Because it is not lipid-dependent, it grows well on routine Sabouraud's dextrose agar at 32 to 37° C. However, some strains of *M. pachydermatis* do show poor growth on unsupplemented media. An atmosphere containing 5% to 10% carbon dioxide significantly increased the frequency of isolation and colony counts on Sabouraud's dextrose agar, but not on modified Dixon's agar. The lipid-dependent *Malassezia* spp. will not grow on Sabouraud's dextrose agar, and require alternative, supplemented media. Modified Dixon's agar will grow all *Malassezia* spp. The novel *Malassezia* sp. isolated from horses did not grow on Sabouraud's dextrose or modified Dixon's agar, but growth was obtained on Sabouraud's dextrose agar enriched with oleic acid and incubated at 30° C.[147b] Because *Malassezia* spp. are commensal organisms, their isolation in culture is of little or no practical diagnostic value.

Ultimately, the diagnosis of *Malassezia* dermatitis rests on the response to antiyeast treatment.[28]

CLINICAL MANAGEMENT

The treatment of *Malassezia* dermatitis is individualized according to severity and various horse and owner considerations. Focal areas of *Malassezia* dermatitis (e.g., skin fold) may be easily treated with the daily spot application of an antifungal cream, ointment, lotion, or spray (see Antifungal Therapy).[28] Multifocal or more generalized cases are treated with total body applications of shampoos and/or rinses.[28] Miconazole 2% (Dermazole, Miconazole Shampoo), chlorhexidine 4% (ChlorhexiDerm Maximum), and combinations of 2% miconazole and 2% chlorhexidine (Malaseb) are excellent shampoos. If the animal is very greasy, waxy, and scaly, these shampoos should be preceded by a keratolytic degreasing shampoo. Alternatively, selenium sulfide 1% shampoo is keratolytic, degreasing, and antiyeast all in one. For stubborn cases, twice weekly shampoos can be followed by leave-on rinses such as lime sulfur 2% (LymDyp), acetic acid 2.5% (1 part water: 1 part vinegar), or enilconazole 0.2% (Imaverol).[28,147a] Enilconazole is not licensed for use in the United States. The authors have used shampoos (4% chlorhexidine, 1% selenium sulfide) and rinses (2% lime sulfur) successfully in horses.

In dogs and cats, when topical therapy is unsuccessful or undesirable, the oral azoles are very effective (see Antifungal Therapy). The most commonly used drug is ketoconazole (Nizoral) at 10 mg/kg, q24h, per os.[28] No information exists as to the usefulness of oral azoles in the horse. Griseofulvin and the allylamine antifungals are not effective.

Dramatic clinical improvement is seen within 7 to 14 days with topical therapy. Therapy should be continued for 7 to 10 days beyond clinical cure. An average duration of treatment would be 4 weeks.

Piedra

CAUSE AND PATHOGENESIS

Piedra is an asymptomatic fungal infection of the extrafollicular portion of the hair shaft caused by *Piedraia hortae* ("black piedra") and *Trichosporon beigelii* ("white piedra").[9,27] White piedra has been described in horses.[27] White piedra is most commonly seen in the temperate and subtropical climates of South America, Europe, Asia, Japan, and the southern United States. The source of the infection is unknown, although the fungus has been isolated from a variety of natural substrates (e.g., soil and vegetation) and direct transmission is thought to be rare. These fungi invade beneath the hair cuticle, proliferate, and break out to surround the hair shaft. "Nodules" (black or white) are thus formed on the hair shaft; they are composed of tightly packed septate hyphae held together by a cement-like substance.

CLINICAL FINDINGS

White piedra affects only the long hairs of the mane, tail, and distal limbs.[12,17,27,148] Whitish nodules and thickenings along the hair shafts result in splitting and breakage.

DIAGNOSIS

The differential diagnosis includes trichorrhexis nodosa, hair casts, and various developmental defects of hair shafts. Microscopic examination of affected hairs shows nodules up to a few millimeters in diameter on and encircling the hairs shafts. (Fig. 5-13). These nodules may result in a weakening and breakage of infected hair shafts. Microscopic examination of infected hairs reveals extra- and intrapilar hyphae arranged perpendicularly to the hair surface. Septate hyphae and arthroconidia (3 to 7 µm in diameter) may be seen. *Trichosporon beigelii* (*T. cutaneum*) grows readily on Sabouraud's dextrose agar at 25° C, but is inhibited by cycloheximide.

CLINICAL MANAGEMENT

The condition is cured by shaving off the hair.[9,27,28] Spontaneous remissions occur frequently in humans.

● SUBCUTANEOUS MYCOSES

The subcutaneous (intermediate) mycoses are fungal infections that have invaded the viable tissues of the skin.[5-7,13,26,28] These infections are usually acquired by traumatic implantation of saprophytic organisms that normally exist in soil or vegetation. The lesions are chronic and, in most cases, remain localized. The terms used to refer to the subcutaneous mycoses have been contradictory, confusing, and frequently changing. The term *chromomycosis* includes subcutaneous and systemic diseases caused by fungi that develop in the host tissue in the form of dark-walled (pigmented, dematiaceous) fungal elements.[5-7,13,26,28] Chromomycosis is separated into two forms, depending on the appearance of the fungus in tissues. In *phaeohyphomycosis*, the organism appears as septate hyphae and yeast-like cells. In *chromoblastomycosis*, the fungus is present as large (4 to 15 µm in diameter), rounded, dark-walled cells (sclerotic bodies, chromo bodies, Medlar bodies).

A *mycetoma* is a unique infection wherein the organism is present in tissues as granules or grains.[5-7,13,26] Mycetomas may be *eumycotic* or *actinomycotic*. The etiologic agents of eumycotic mycetomas are fungi, whereas actinomycotic mycetomas are caused by members of the Actinomycetales order, such as *Actinomyces* and *Nocardia*, which are bacteria (see Chapter 4).

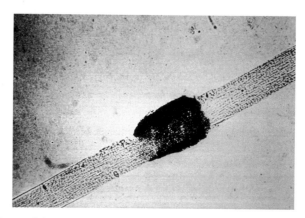

FIGURE 5-13. *Piedra.* Nodule encircles hair shaft (Courtesy Dr. A. Stannard).

Eumycotic mycetomas may be caused by dematiaceous fungi (black-grained mycetomas) or nonpigmented fungi (white-grained mycetoma). Pseudomycetomas have differences in granule formation and are caused by dermatophytes (dermatophytic pseudomycetoma) or bacteria, such as *Staphylococcus* (bacterial pseudomycetoma or botryomycosis).

The term *hyalohyphomycosis* has been proposed to encompass all opportunistic infections caused by nondematiaceous fungi (at least 19 genera), the basic tissue forms of these being hyaline hyphal elements that are septate, branched or unbranched, and nonpigmented in tissues.[26,28]

Another term that creates confusion is *phycomycosis*.[5-7,13,26,28] The class *Phycomycetes* no longer exists. *Pythiosis* (oomycosis) and *zygomycosis* are now the preferred terms for phycomycosis. Members of the genus *Pythium* are properly classified in the kingdom *Protista* and in the phylum *Oomycetes*. The phylum *Zygomycota* includes the orders *Mucorales* and *Entomophthorales*. The term *zygomycosis* is used to include both *mucormycosis* and *entomophthoromycosis*.

Eumycotic Mycetoma

CAUSE AND PATHOGENESIS

The fungi causing eumycotic mycetoma in horses are ubiquitous soil saprophytes that cause disease via wound contamination.* The condition occurs most frequently near the Tropic of Cancer between the latitudes 10° S and 30° N, including Africa, South and Central America, India, and southern Asia. The disease is rare in the United States and Europe. It accounted for only 0.22% of the equine dermatoses seen at the Cornell University Clinic. The most commonly reported fungus causing eumycotic mycetoma in the United States is *Pseudallescheria boydii*. Many previously reported cases of eumycotic ("maduromycotic") mycetoma in horses were actually phaeohyphomycosis.[156,157,159,162a]

CLINICAL FINDINGS

The three cardinal features of eumycotic mycetoma (maduromycosis) are tumefaction, draining tracts (sinuses), and grains (granules) in the discharge.[9,27,28] Draining tracts are not always present in equine eumycotic mycetomas.[149-154] Lesions are usually solitary and occur most commonly on the distal limbs (including the coronary band) and face (especially around the nostrils and commissures of the lips) (Fig. 5-4, *C*). Rarely, multiple lesions are present.[149] Early papules evolve into nodules (1 to 10 cm diameter) that are usually firm and asymptomatic. As lesions enlarge, they may become alopecic, hyperpigmented, ulcerated, and/or develop draining tracts that exude a serous, purulent, or hemorrhagic discharge. As some fistulas heal, scar tissue develops and forms the hard, tumor-like mass that characterizes mycetoma. Grains present in discharge vary in color, size, shape, and texture, depending on the particular fungus involved. Black- or dark-grain mycetomas are usually associated with *Curvularia geniculata*.[149,150,153] White-grain mycetomas are usually caused by *Pseudallescheria (Allescheria, Petriellidium) boydii*[152,154] and, rarely, *Aspergillus versicolor*.[151] Chronic infections can extend into underlying muscle, joint, or bone. There are no apparent age (5 to 15 years), breed, or sex predilections.

DIAGNOSIS

The differential diagnosis includes infectious and foreign-body granulomas and neoplasms (especially sarcoid and melanoma). Cytologic examination of aspirates or direct smears reveals pyogranulomatous inflammation with occasional fungal elements. Fungi are easily seen by squashing and examining grains. Biopsy findings include nodular to diffuse pyogranulomatous to

*References 5-7, 9, 13, 26, 28.

granulomatous dermatitis and panniculitis. Fungal elements are present as a grain (granule, thallus) within the inflammatory reaction (Fig. 5-14). The grains (0.2 to 5 mm in diameter) are irregularly shaped, often taking a scalloped or scroll-like appearance, and consist of broad (2 to 7 μm in diameter), septate, branching (infrequent and dichotomous) hyphae, which often form chlamydoconidia (terminal cystic dilatations, 5 to 20 μm diameter), and a cementing substance.[4] The center of the grains consist of densely tangled hyphae, whereas the outer rim contains the chlamydoconidia. The fungal elements may be pigmented or nonpigmented. In white-grain

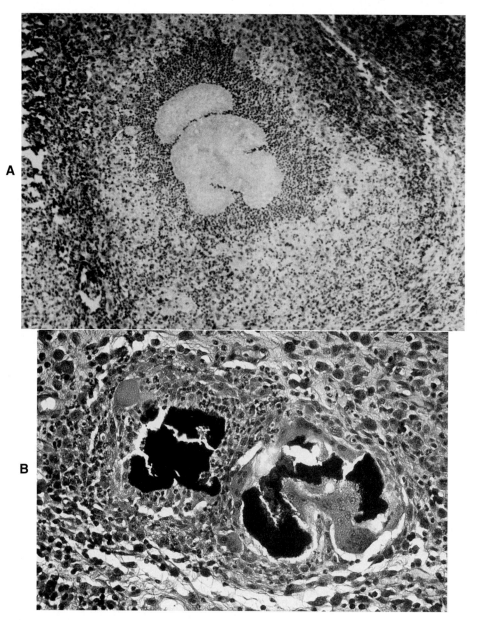

FIGURE 5-14. Eumycotic mycetoma. **A,** "White grain" in pyogranuloma due to *P. boydii*. **B,** "Black grain" in pyogranuloma due to *C. geniculata*.

mycetomas, the hyphae and chlamydoconidia are indistinct and faintly eosinophilic in H & E stained sections. Typically, the grains are surrounded by an inner zone of karyorrhectic neutrophils, a middle zone of macrophages and variable numbers of multinucleated histiocytic giant cells, and an outer zone of fibroplasia. The fungi grow on Sabouraud's dextrose agar at 25° C. Either tissue grains or punch biopsies are the preferred material for culture (see Chapter 2).

CLINICAL MANAGEMENT

Wide surgical excision is the treatment of choice and can be curative.[9,28,151,152] Any attempt at antifungal chemotherapy should be based on *in vitro* susceptibility testing of the isolate.[9,28] In humans, dogs, and cats, medical therapy is often unsuccessful. Ketoconazole and itraconazole have enjoyed erratic success.[9,28] Treatment must be continued for 2 to 3 months past clinical cure.

Phaeohyphomycosis

CAUSE AND PATHOGENESIS

Phaeohyphomycosis (chromomycosis) is caused by a number of ubiquitous saprophytic fungi found in various soils and organic materials.[5-7,13,26,28] Infection occurs via wound contamination. These fungi have the characteristic of forming pigmented (dematiaceous) hyphal elements (but not grains) in tissues.

CLINICAL FEATURES

Phaeohyphomycosis is rare in horses in the United States, and accounted for only 0.11% of the equine dermatoses seen at the Cornell University Clinic.

Most horses have multiple lesions that can be localized to the face or widely scattered on the body (Fig. 5-15).[155-163] Lesions are typically asymptomatic firm (rarely fluctuant), well-circumscribed, dermal nodules (1 to 3 cm diameter), with the overlying skin and hair coat appearing normal. Occasional lesions may be alopecic, hyperpigmented, ulcerated, draining, or studded with papules and pustules. There are no apparent age (5 months to 27 years), breed, or sex predilections.

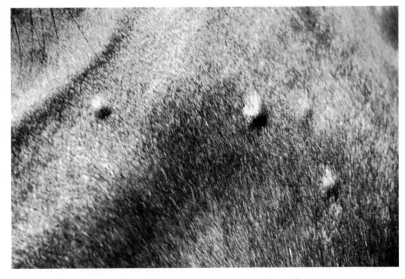

FIGURE 5-15. Phaeohyphomycosis. Multiple firm nodules over shoulder.

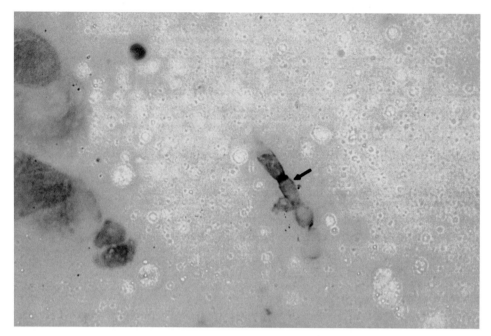

FIGURE 5-16. Phaeohyphomycosis. Dark, septate hypha (*arrow*) with macrophages.

DIAGNOSIS

The differential diagnosis includes infectious granulomas, sterile granulomas, foreign-body granulomas, and neoplasms.

Cytologic examination of aspirates or direct smears reveals granulomatous to pyogranulomatous inflammation. Pigmented fungal hyphae may be seen (Fig. 5-16). Biopsy findings include nodular to diffuse pyogranulomatous to granulomatous dermatitis and panniculitis (Fig. 5-17). Numerous fungal elements are present as broad (2 to 6 μm in diameter), often irregular, pigmented, septate, branched or unbranched hyphae with occasional chlamydoconidia and numerous round to oval, pigmented yeast forms (Medlar bodies, so-called copper pennies) (see Fig. 5-4, *D*). Some specimens are characterized by remarkable lymphoid follicle formation.[158a] The fungi grow on Sabouraud's dextrose agar at 25° to 35° C, and punch biopsies are the preferred material for culture. Fungi isolated from horses with cutaneous phaeohyphomycosis include *Bipolaris speciferum* (*Drechslera speciferum, Helminthosporium speciferum, Brachycladium speciferum*),[156,159,160] *Alternaria alternata*,[158,158a,162] *Exserohilum rostratum*,[161] and *Cladosporium* sp. (*Hormodendrum* sp.).[163]

CLINICAL MANAGEMENT

Wide surgical excision of solitary lesions may be curative.[155,158a,162a] Horses with multiple lesions may heal spontaneously within 3 months after the diagnosis is made,[156] or be "cured" within several weeks with the topical application of iodophors or gentian violet.[158,160,162] These apparent responses to topical therapy are illogical and probably also represent spontaneous resolution.

In humans, dogs, and cats, chemotherapy may be curative, depending on the agent, but the response is unpredictable. This may be due to differing susceptibilities of the fungi involved and differences in the therapeutic protocols that have been used to date. Drugs should be chosen on the basis of *in vitro* susceptibility testing. The preferred treatment would be surgical excision

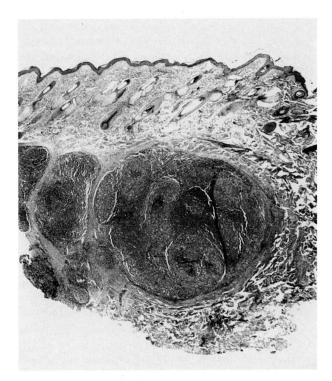

FIGURE 5-17. Nodular dermatitis with phaeohyphomycosis.

followed by chemotherapy.[28] Ketoconazole has been used successfully and unsuccessfully, alone or in combination with flucytosine.[28] Flucytosine has been used successfully and unsuccessfully, alone or in combination with ketoconazole or amphotericin B.[28] Amphotericin B has been used successfully or unsuccessfully, alone or in combination with flucytosine.[28] In humans, itraconazole, cryosurgery, and local application of heat have also been curative in some cases.[9]

Pythiosis

CAUSE AND PATHOGENESIS

Pythium spp. are aquatic organisms that rely on aquatic plant or organic substance for their normal life cycle.[5,6,27,28,191] They are not true fungi. The motile zoospore stage shows chemotaxis toward damaged plant or animal tissues. Once in the vicinity of their host, the zoospores become sluggish, lose their flagella, and become encysted on the tissue. The organisms then develop germ tubes in the direction of the affected tissues, which allow for penetration and invasion. Animals become infected by standing in or drinking stagnant water, and damaged skin appears to be a prerequisite for infection. Environmental conditions are probably the most influential factors governing the occurrence of pythiosis. *P. insidiosum* requires an aquatic environment and organic substrate (e.g., moist, decaying vegetation) for maintenance of its normal life cycle and temperatures between 30° C to 40° C for reproduction.[172,191] Thus, most cases are seen during the summer and fall in tropical and subtropical areas of the world (especially Australia, India, Thailand, Brazil, and Costa Rica).* In North America, cases are reported from the southern United States exclusively, particularly from the Gulf Coast region.[14,27,168,181,200]

---

*References 27, 173a, 174, 178, 180, 182, 183, 185, 186.

Pythium insidiosum (*P. gracile*, *Hyphomyces destruens*, *H. equi*) is the species isolated from horses.[*] Pythiosis has been reported under other names in the literature: swamp cancer, summer sores, espundia, bursatti, Florida horse leeches, Gulf Coast fungus, phycomycosis, hyphomycosis, and oomycosis.

CLINICAL FINDINGS

There are no apparent age, breed, or sex predilections.[†] Commonly, affected horses have had prolonged contact with water in lakes, ponds, swamps, and flooded areas.[200a] Frequently, minor and even undetectable wounds become infected. Lesions are most commonly found on the distal limbs (below the carpus and hock) and ventral abdomen and thorax, because these are the body parts most often in prolonged contact with water. Occasionally, lesions are seen on the lips, nostrils, external genitalia, face, neck, trunk, or dorsal midline.[24,172,172a] Lesions are usually single and unilateral, but may rarely be multiple and bilateral.[172,172a,207]

Early lesions are characterized by a focal swelling, which subsequently exudes serum through small sinuses. Lesions are capable of expanding in size at a very rapid rate. Within days, the lesion may be characterized by rapid enlargement, ulceration, granulomatous appearance, and draining tracts that discharge serosanguineous, hemorrhagic, or sometimes mucopurulent fluid (Figs. 5-4, E and F, and 5-18, A). Characteristic sticky, stringy discharge mats the hair coat and hangs from the body wall in thick strands. Lesions are deep and routinely involve the subcutis. Tissue necrosis results in a foul odor. The lesions are usually very pruritic, which often leads to self-mutilation of the lesion and surrounding tissues. Irregularly shaped, yellow-tan to gray, gritty, coral-like masses ("kunkers," "leeches," "roots") are present within the sinuses (Fig. 5-18, B). These kunkers range from 2 to 10 mm in size, and are composed of vessels and tissue that have undergone coagulative necrosis, necrotic eosinophils, and *Pythium* hyphae. Lesions may rarely be covered by non-ulcerated skin, exhibit little or no secretion, or be pedunculated.[193a]

Lesions are usually circular and vary in size according to location and duration. Lesions on the ventrum can attain a diameter of 50 cm. Lesions on the extremities may encircle the limb. Lymphangitis and edematous swellings may develop on the limbs with chronic skin lesions.

Pythiosis is typically confined to the skin, but in chronically affected horses, deeper structures can be affected.[27,172a] The infection can spread via fascial planes or through lymphatics. The organism may invade the intestinal tract,[27,165,169,172a,197] bone,[164,172a,176,188,195] lungs,[27,172a,177] trachea,[27,172a] lymph nodes,[27,172a,194] joints,[164,172a,186] and tendon sheaths,[164,172a,188] causing gastroenteritis, periostitis, osteomyelitis, pneumonia, lymphadenitis, arthritis, laminitis, tenosynovitis, and septicemia.

In chronically affected (more than 2 months) horses, *P. insidiosum* may invade underlying bone.[‡] The age of the lesion is an important factor in the development of bone involvement. Osseous involvement is not seen in lesions ≤4 weeks old.[164] In addition to signs associated with cutaneous lesions, horses with osseous involvement exhibit lameness. Osseous involvement of the third metatarsal and metacarpal bones, the proximal sesamoid bones, and all three of the phalanges has been described.

DIAGNOSIS

The differential diagnosis includes infectious granulomas, habronemiasis, foreign-body granulomas, and neoplasms (especially sarcoid and squamous cell carcinoma). Cytologic examination of aspirates or direct smears reveals granulomatous to pyogranulomatous inflammation wherein eosinophils are numerous; however, fungal elements are only occasionally seen. Biopsy findings

---

[*]References 171, 173, 187a, 189, 191, 199.
[†]References 8, 14, 16, 27, 29, 172a, 174.
[‡]References 164, 172a, 176, 188, 196, 201.

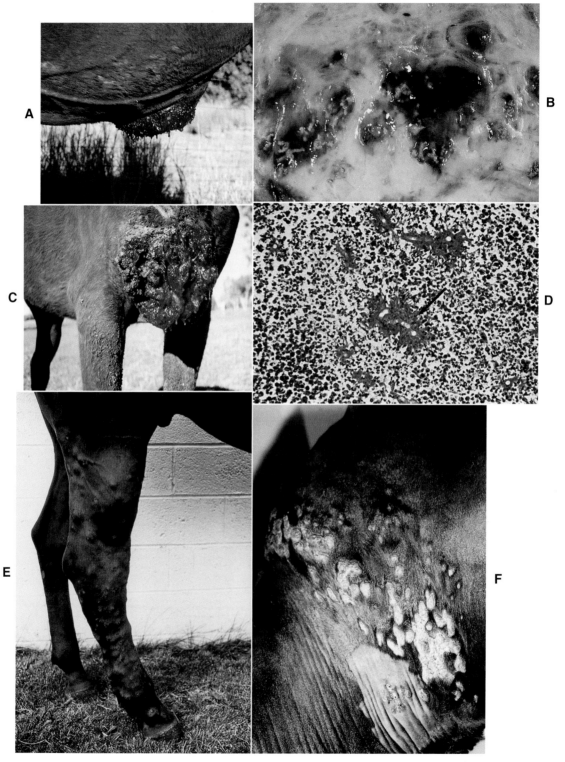

FIGURE 5-18. **A,** Ulcerative granuloma on ventral abdomen in pythiosis (Courtesy Dr. R. Miller). **B,** Numerous cord-like "leeches" in necrotic sinuses in pythiosis (Courtesy Dr. R. Miller). **C,** Ulcerative granuloma on brisket in basidiobolomycosis (Courtesy Dr. R. Miller). **D,** Biopsy of basidiobolomycosis reveals eosinophils and "ghost" hyphal spaces within necrotic areas (Courtesy Dr. R. Miller). **E,** Multiple nodules and draining tracts on leg in sporotrichosis. **F,** Multiple nodules and crusted plaques over shoulder in sporotrichosis.

include nodular to diffuse pyogranulomatous to granulomatous dermatitis and panniculitis with numerous eosinophils (Fig. 5-19, *A* and *B*). Inflammation is centered on foci of necrosis and amorphous eosinophilic material. Hyphae are difficult to see in H & E stained sections, and often appear as clear spaces (hyphal "ghosts") or slightly basophilic granular material.[167a,174,210] Hyphae are 3 to 8 μm in diameter, occasionally septate, irregularly branching, with nonparallel sides (Fig. 5-19, *C*). Fungal elements are most commonly found, and are most numerous, within foci of necrosis. Hyphae are often surrounded by eosinophilic "sleeves" of Splendore-Hoeppli phenomenon. Fungal elements stain very well with GMS, but not with PAS. Hyphae occasionally invade blood vessels (especially arteries), whereupon thrombosed vessels may be prominent. Histologic studies may not be definitive because the appearances of pythiosis, basidiobolomycosis, and conidiobolomycosis are similar. However, the hyphae of *B. haptosporus* and *C. coronatus* are usually larger and more commonly septate than those of *P. insidiosum*.[210]

Pythium antigen can be detected in sections of formalin-fixed, paraffin-embedded tissues by an indirect immunoperoxidase technique (Louisiana State University Veterinary Medical Diagnostic Laboratory, Baton Rouge, Louisiana).[170,172a,201] This technique is rapid and specific, allowing the early institution of aggressive therapy and an improved prognosis.[172a]

Pythium spp. grow rapidly at 25° to 37° C on blood agar and Sabouraud's dextrose agar, and wedge biopsies are the preferred material for culture. In addition, kunkers can be collected from lesions and submitted to the laboratory.[27,172a] Selective culture media (e.g., V8 agar with streptomycin and ampicillin, Campy blood agar) may be more effective.[179a] To increase the likelihood of growing *P. insidiosum*, it has been recommended that specimens should *not* be refrigerated or transported on ice. However, for samples that were stored or shipped for 1 to 3 days prior to culturing on nonselective media, isolation rates were higher for samples stored at 4° C or on cold packs.[179a] Special water culture techniques which induce diagnostic zoospore formation are time-consuming and somewhat unreliable.[170,172a,189] It is advisable to submit specimens to veterinary diagnostic laboratories, where the microbiologist is more likely to be familiar with *Pythium* spp.[146]

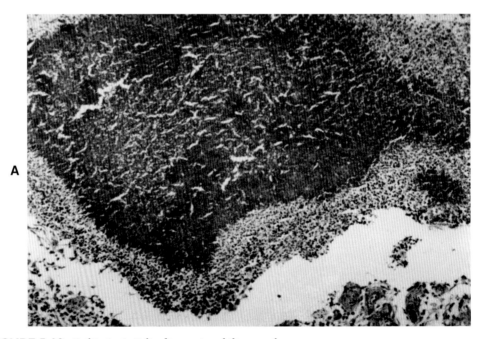

FIGURE 5-19. Pythiosis. **A,** Palisading eosinophilic granuloma.

Immunologic studies on horses with pythiosis showed that 64% of clinically affected horses, 100% of recovered horses, and 31% of normal in-contact horses had evidence of cellular immunity to *Pythium* as assessed by delayed-type hypersensitivity reactions to the intradermal injection of a *Pythium* antigen.[192] Serologic diagnosis by precipitin, complement fixation, and immunodiffusion tests has not been satisfactory.[186,187] PCR is very reliable when performed on skin specimens frozen at −70° C or stored at ambient temperature in 95% ethanol.[201a]

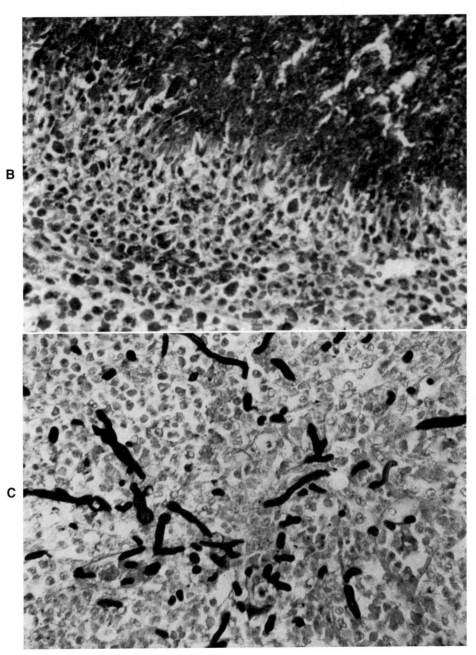

FIGURE 5-19, cont'd. B, Eosinophilic palisading granuloma bordering central area of necrosis. **C,** *Pythium* hyphae (GMS stain).

Hematologic studies of horses with pythiosis revealed a frequent occurrence of microcytic, hypochromic anemia (presumably due to iron deficiency resulting from the long-term loss of blood through copious cutaneous discharges) or normocytic, normochromic anemia, moderate leukocytosis, neutrophilia and eosinophilia.[172a,175,193,201]

CLINICAL MANAGEMENT

There are no reported instances of spontaneous remission of pythiosis. Without treatment, mortality is 100%—by death (toxic shock due to gram-negative bacteria, and so forth) or by euthanasia.[190] Treatment of pythiosis should be instituted as soon as possible because chronic lesions have a poorer prognosis.* Because lesions of pythiosis have the potential to expand rapidly, surgical intervention should be undertaken prior to laboratory confirmation of the diagnosis in typical clinical cases. Surgery is curative if all diseased tissue is removed. When possible, a 2-cm portion of skin surrounding the lesion should be removed. However, even with radical surgical excision, recurrence is frequent (up to 30% of cases). Surgical success is greatly influenced by the size and site of the lesion and the duration of infection. Lesions on the trunk can usually be successfully excised, but those on the legs are difficult. Repeat surgery is indicated as soon as new foci of infection are noted. These are first recognized as dark red to black, hemorrhagic spots, 1 to 5 mm in diameter, in the new granulation bed. One major surgical procedure and two or three minor "retrims" are customary in cases treated in referral centers.[14,184a] Because treatment is often difficult and expensive, severely affected horses are often euthanized.

Prognosis becomes increasingly guarded with leg lesions of over 1 to 2 months in duration, as these are more likely to have osseous involvement.† Only one horse with osseous involvement has been successfully treated: by surgical excision of affected bone and intraarterial perfusion with miconazole (1.2 mg/kg q48h for 3 treatments), then skin grafting.[201]

Some lesions may be heavily contaminated by bacteria.[190] Thus, systemic antibiotic therapy may be very important.

Topical and fungal agents have been used and recommended, but "successes" are anecdotal.‡ Both iodophors and amphotericin B (gauze dressing pads soaked in a solution of 50 mg of amphotericin B in 10 ml of sterile water and 10 ml of dimethyl sulfoxide [DMSO]) have been recommended. Other more elaborate topical concoctions, such as ketoconazole-rifampin-iodophor-DMSO-hydrochloric acid[176] and ketoconazole-rifampin-DMSO-ammonium chloride,[201] are of equally dubious value. Metalaxyl, a fungicide used to kill Oomycetes pathogenic to plants, was used topically in dogs and horses without success.[28,172a]

Systemic antifungal agents (amphotericin B, sodium iodide, see page 311) have also been used and recommended, but again, reports are anecdotal.§ Because *Pythium* spp. do not share cell wall characteristics with true fungi, antifungal chemotherapeutic agents (amphotericin B, ketoconazole, flucytosine) have been disappointing in the treatment of this disease in other species.[9,28]

Immunotherapy has been effective for the treatment of some horses with pythiosis.[27,172a,190,196,206] One vaccine was a crude, killed, phenolized, ultrasonicated, whole-cell hyphal extract from *P. insidiosum* cultures.[206] The vaccine was injected subcutaneously, in 2 ml doses, weekly for at least 3 treatments. The vaccine lost its efficacy after 8 weeks of refrigeration.

Two other vaccines—a cell-mass antigen (CMA) and a soluble concentrated antigen (SCA)—were also given subcutaneously and were effective for 3 weeks and 18 months, respectively, postpreparation.[190]

---

*References 14, 23, 24, 27, 172, 172a, 175, 184a, 209.
†References 24, 164, 172a, 176, 188, 201.
‡References 14, 22-24, 27, 172a, 184, 184a, 209.
§References 14, 23, 24, 27, 172a, 179, 184, 184a.

All vaccines were often curative if administered to horses with lesions ≤2 weeks in duration. Likewise, all vaccines were usually ineffective if administered to horses with lesions ≥2 months in duration. In one study,[190] age of the horse had no influence on response to vaccine, while in another study[206] old horses did not respond. Immunotherapy may be more effective for large lesions when administered following surgical debulking.[172a,206]

Vaccine injection sites became painful and swollen, and sterile abscesses formed within 5 to 10 days postinjection in about 30% of treated horses. For this reason, vaccines were given over the superficial pectoral muscles so as to facilitate drainage. The initial signs indicating a positive response to vaccination usually occurred 1 to 2 weeks after initial vaccination and included cessation of pruritus, stabilization of lesion size, decrease in the amount of exudate, and expulsion of kunkers. Lesions then slowly regressed over a 1-month period. Some horses cured by immunotherapy were reinfected the following year, indicating that immunity is short-term.[190]

No *Pythium* vaccine is commercially available, and a permit from the United States Department of Agriculture is required to manufacturer and distribute vaccine against pythiosis.[196]

Two horses with ventral abdominal *Pythium* granulomas were successfully treated by photo-ablation with a neodymium:yttrium-aluminum-garnet laser.[198] Resultant wounds were allowed to heal by secondary intervention and no recurrence were seen after a 1-year follow-up period.

Zygomycosis

Zygomycetes are ubiquitous saprophytes of soil and decaying vegetation and a component of the normal flora of skin and haircoat.° The portal of entry may be gastrointestinal, respiratory, or cutaneous via wound contamination. In humans, a compromised immune system is generally necessary for invasion to occur. However, in horses, such factors have not been identified in most instances.

Zygomycosis occurs most commonly in tropical and subtropical areas.[27,209] In the United States, these disorders are seen most commonly in states along the Gulf of Mexico ("Gulf Coast fungus").[27]

There are two orders of *Zygomycetes* that cause disease: (1) *Mucorales*, which includes the genera *Rhizopus, Mucor, Absidia, Mortierella*, and (2) *Entomophthorales*, which includes the genera *Conidiobolus* and *Basidiobolus*. Infections caused by fungi from the order *Mucorales* were previously called *mucormycosis* and those associated with the order *Entomophthorales* were called *entomophthoromycosis*. In addition, many of the older reports of phycomycosis in horses could have been zygomycosis.

CLINICAL FINDINGS

Basidiobolomycosis is an ulcerative granulomatous equine skin disease caused by *Basidiobolus haptosporus*.[203-205,207-209,211,212] There are no apparent age, breed, or sex predilections, and cases occur regularly throughout the year. Most lesions are found on the chest, trunk, head, and neck, where they are often located on the more lateral aspects of the body. Large (up to 50 cm diameter), circular, ulcerative granulomas with a serosanguineous discharge are characteristic (Fig. 5-18, *C*). Solitary lesions are the rule, and pruritus is usually moderate to severe. The "leeches" that characterize pythiosis are not always seen in basidiobolomycosis but, if present, are smaller and of no characteristic shape.

Conidiobolomycosis (entomophthoromycosis, rhinophycomycosis) is an ulcerative granulomatous equine disease caused by *Conidiobolus coronatus* (*Entomophthora coronata*).[24,207-209,212-220] There are no apparent age, breed, or sex predilections, and cases occur regularly throughout the year. Most lesions are found on the external nares and/or in the nasal passages. Lesions may be

---

°References 5-7, 13, 26-28, 208, 209.

single or multiple and unilateral or bilateral, and those of the external nares appear grossly similar to those of basidiobolomycosis. Lesions in the nasal passages are firm nodules covered by an edematous, focally ulcerated mucosa. "Leeches" are often present, but are often smaller than 0.5 mm. Horses often develop a hemorrhagic nasal discharge and dyspnea due to nasal passage blockage.

Mucormycosis due to *Absidia corymbifera* infection was diagnosed in one horse with a large, pruritic, ulcerative granuloma on a leg,[221] and in another horse with erythematous, necrotic, ulcerative lesions on the muzzle, nostrils, lips, carpi, and tarsi.[220a]

DIAGNOSIS

The differential diagnosis includes numerous infectious granulomas, habronemiasis, foreign-body granulomas, exuberant granulation tissue, and neoplasms (especially sarcoid and squamous cell carcinoma). Cytologic examination of aspirates or direct smears reveals pyogranulomatous to granulomatous inflammation with numerous eosinophils, wherein fungal elements may be visualized. Biopsy findings include nodular to diffuse, pyogranulomatous to granulomatous dermatitis and panniculitis containing numerous eosinophils (Fig. 5-20, *A*). Inflammation is centered on amorphous eosinophil material, which occasionally contains either clear spaces representing poorly stained hyphae (hyphal "ghosts") (Fig. 5-18, *D*) or slightly basophilic granular material representing hyphal protoplasm.[210] Vascular invasion and hematogenous spread is more common in mucormycosis than in entomophthoromycosis. The hyphae of *B. haptosporus* are broad (6 to 20 μm in diameter) as are those of *C. coronatus* (5 to 13 μm in diameter). The hyphae of both fungi are occasionally septate, irregularly branching, with nonparallel sides.[210] Hyphae are often surrounded by eosinophilic "sleeves" of Splendore-Hoeppli phenomenon. Fungal elements are most commonly found, and are most abundant, within foci of necrosis (Fig. 5-20, *B*). Fungal elements stain well with GMS, but variably with PAS. *Zygomycetes* grow on Sabouraud's dextrose agar at 25° to 37° C, and punch or wedge biopsies are the preferred material for culture. Biopsy specimens submitted for culture should not be ground or macerated, as this may destroy the organism. "Leeches" are collected from the lesions, vigorously washed in water, and implanted into the agar. Cycloheximide may inhibit fungal growth.

A serum agar gel immunoprecipitation test is useful for the diagnosis of conidiobolomycosis.[218a,219a] Horses infected with *C. coronatus* have 1 to 5 precipitins of identity, whereas control horses have no bands. Immunohistochemical identification of *A. corymbifera* in biopsy specimens was reported.[22a]

CLINICAL MANAGEMENT

The susceptibility of the *Zygomycetes* to antimycotic agents is quite variable and largely unknown.[9,28,202] Treatment of equine zygomycosis should be attempted as soon as possible after diagnosis, as chronic lesions have a poorer prognosis. Solitary lesions may be surgically excised.[*] In other cases, surgical excision or debulking may be followed by chemotherapy as dictated by *in vitro* susceptibility tests (amphotericin B, azoles, potassium iodide).[9,28,202] Systemic antifungal therapy is expensive and has not been carefully evaluated. In general, systemic iodides are used as a first-line agent to treat basidiobolomycosis and conidiobolomycosis (see page 311).[†] Iodide therapy should be preceded by surgical debulking where feasible. Iodides are not effective for other zygomycoses, such as those caused by *Mucor*, *Rhizopus*, and *Absidia*.[271] Surgery and amphotericin B (IV and topical) were unsuccessful in a horse with *Absidia corymbifera* infection.[221]

---

[*]References 14, 24, 27, 184a, 207, 209, 211.
[†]References 14, 24, 184a, 209, 299, 218, 271.

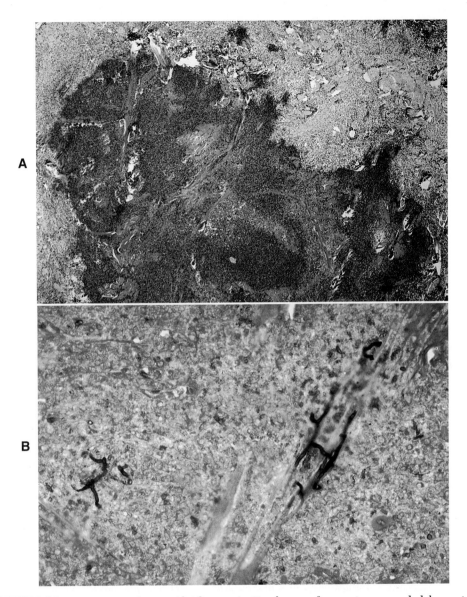

FIGURE 5-20. Zygomycosis due to *Absidia* sp. **A,** Focal area of necrosis surrounded by eosinophilic granulomatous inflammation. **B,** Numerous branching hyphae in necrotic area (GMS stain).

Itraconazole (3 mg/kg PO q12h for 4½ months was ineffective in one horse with conidiobolomycosis.[218b] Another horse with *A. corymbifera* infection was reported to be cured with 3 weeks of amphotericin B (40 mg/kg/day PO).[220a] Because amphotericin B is usually not absorbed from the gastrointestinal tract, the authors hypothesized that intestinal lesions may have allowed partial absorption of the drug. Immunotherapy utilizing a phenolized vaccine prepared from *Pythium insidiosum* cultures was of no benefit in horses with basidiobolomycosis and conidiobolomycosis.[190,206]

Sporotrichosis

CAUSE AND PATHOGENESIS

Sporotrichosis is caused by the ubiquitous dimorphic fungus *Sporothrix schenckii*, which exists as a saprophyte in soil and organic debris.[5-7,11,13,26,28] Infection occurs as a result of wound contamination. Glucocorticoids and other immunosuppressive drugs are contraindicated in animals with sporotrichosis.[28] These drugs should be avoided both during and after treatment of the disease, as immunosuppressive doses of glucocorticoids have been reported to cause a recurrence of clinical sporotrichosis as long as 4 to 6 months after apparent clinical cure.[28]

CLINICAL FINDINGS

Sporotrichosis is uncommon in the horse.* It accounted for only 0.22% of the equine dermatoses seen at the Cornell University Clinic. The cutaneolymphatic form is the most common presentation. After inoculation of the fungus into the skin—usually following puncture wounds from thorns and wood splinters—a primary lesion occurs on an exposed part of the body, usually a distal limb (often begins around fetlock region) (Fig. 5-18, *E*) and less commonly a part of the upper body, such as the shoulder, hip, or perineal region. Progressively, hard dermal and subcutaneous nodules develop along the lymphatics draining the region (lateral or medial aspect of limb). The lymphatics may become enlarged and thickened ("corded"), and larger nodules may abscess, ulcerate, and discharge a small amount of thick, red-brown to yellowish exudate or serosanguineous fluid. The lesions are usually nonpainful and nonpruritic. Regional lymph nodes are usually not involved. Occasionally, a primary cutaneous form is seen with no lymphatic involvement (Fig. 5-18, *F*). There are no apparent age, breed, or sex predilections.

Zoonotic Aspects

Humans are susceptible to sporotrichosis.[9] There have been several reports documenting transmission of sporotrichosis to humans through contact with an ulcerated wound or the exudate from an infected cat,[28] but never from an infected horse. This is presumably because large numbers of organisms are found in contaminated feline tissues, exudates, and feces.[28] In infected horses, organisms are sparse in skin lesions. Veterinarians, veterinary technicians, veterinary students, and owners of infected cats have a higher risk for infection.[28]

The most common form of sporotrichosis in humans is cutaneolymphatic.[9] A primary lesion—which may be a papule, pustule, nodule, abscess, or verrucous growth—develops at the site of injury. This lesion may be painful. Most lesions are on an extremity (finger, hand, foot) or the face. Secondary lesions then ascend proximally via lymphatic vessels. The cutaneous (fixed) form is less common.

DIAGNOSIS

The differential diagnosis includes other infectious granulomas, foreign-body granulomas, and neoplasms. Because of the zoonotic potential of sporotrichosis, precautions must be taken. All people handling animals suspected of having sporotrichosis should wear gloves. Gloves should also be worn when samples are taken of exudates or tissues. The gloves should then be carefully removed and disposed of. Forearms, wrists, and hands should be washed in chlorhexidine or povidone-iodine.

Cytologic examination of aspirates or direct smears reveals suppurative to pyogranulomatous to granulomatous inflammation. The organism is difficult to impossible to find in the exudates of horses. *S. schenckii* is a pleomorphic yeast that is round, oval, or cigar-shaped, 2 to 10 μm in length.

---

*References 3, 4, 8, 10, 12, 14, 16, 17, 19, 22-25, 27, 29, 222-229.

Biopsy findings include nodular to diffuse pyogranulomatous to granulomatous dermatitis (Fig. 5-21, *A*). Multinucleated histologic giant cells are commonly seen. Fungal elements are usually sparse and difficult to impossible to find (Fig. 5-21, *B* and *C*). The fungi have a refractile cell wall from which the cytoplasm may shrink, giving the impression that the organism has a capsule. When this occurs, the organisms may be confused with *Cryptococcus neoformans*. *S. schenckii* grows on Sabouraud's dextrose agar at 30° C; samples submitted for culture should include both a sample of the exudate (from deep within a draining tract) and a piece of tissue (removed surgically) for a macerated tissue culture.

CLINICAL MANAGEMENT

The treatment of choice is the administration of iodides (see page 311).[14,24,27,228] Sodium iodide is often used as a 20% solution and slowly administered intravenously (20 to 40 mg/kg/day) for 2 to 5 days, then orally at the same dose daily, until cured. A supersaturated solution of potassium iodide has been given orally at 1 to 2 mg/kg q12h or q24h for 1 week, then 0.5 to 1 mg/kg q24h until cured. The organic iodide, ethylenediamine dihydroiodide (EDDI) has been given orally in a fashion identical to that for potassium iodide. The oral iodides are usually administered with sweet feed or mixed with molasses and administered by syringe. Treatment must be continued for 30 days beyond clinical cure (4 to 8 weeks).

Tolerance to iodides is variable, and some horses may show signs of iodism: scaling and alopecia, depression, anorexia, fever, coughing, lacrimation, serous nasal discharge, salivation,

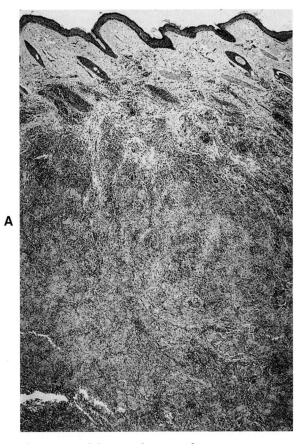

FIGURE 5-21. Sporotrichosis. **A,** Nodular granulomatous dermatitis.

Continued

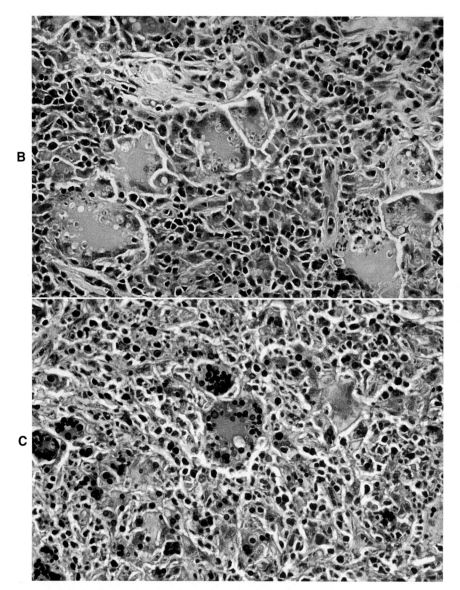

FIGURE 5-21, cont'd. B, Close-up of A. Numerous organisms within multinucleated histiocytic giant cells. **C,** Special stain reveals "cigar-shaped" appearance of *S. schenckii* (GMS stain).

nervousness, or cardiovascular abnormalities.[27] If iodism is observed, medication should be stopped for 1 week. The drug may then be reinstituted at the same or a lower dose. If iodism becomes a recurrent problem or if side-effects are severe, alternative treatment should be considered. In addition, systemic iodides may cause abortion in mares and should not be used during pregnancy.[27]

The imidazole and triazole classes of drugs may be considered for horses that do not tolerate iodides, are refractory to them, or relapse after apparent clinical cure.[6,154,155] Ketoconazole or itraconazole may be used successfully, and are continued for 30 days beyond clinical cure. Side-effects are usually mild.

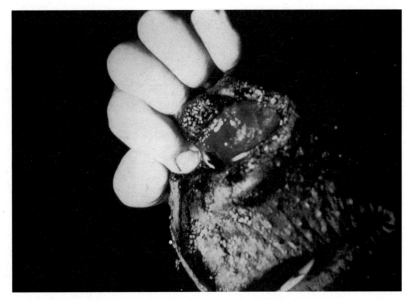

FIGURE 5-22. Rhinosporidiosis. Ulcerated nodule on nostril. (*Courtesy Dr. J. Bentinck-Smith.*)

Rhinosporidiosis

CAUSE AND PATHOGENESIS

Rhinosporidium seeberi is a fungal organism of uncertain classification.[5-7,13,26,28] Attempts to culture it using conventional fungal culture media were unsuccessful; however, the organism has been grown in tissue culture. The disease is endemic in India and Argentina, but North American reports have come almost exclusively from the southern United States. It is thought that infection is acquired by mucosal contact with stagnant water or dust and that trauma is a predisposing factor.

CLINICAL FINDINGS

The disease appears to be rare in horses.* There appears to be no age, breed, or sex predilections. Affected horses typically present for wheezing, sneezing, unilateral seropurulent nasal discharge, and epistaxis. Nasal polyps may be visible in the nares (Fig. 5-22) or may be visualized by rhinoscopy. Single or multiple polyps varying in size from a few millimeters up to 3 cm are pink, red, or grayish and are covered with numerous pinpoint, white foci (fungal sporangia). Polyps may be sessile or pedunculated, and may protrude out of, or involve, the mucocutaneous area of the nostril.

DIAGNOSIS

The differential diagnosis includes numerous infectious granulomas and neoplasms. Cytologic examination of nasal exudate or histologic examination of the polyp should be diagnostic. Biopsy findings include a fibrovascular polyp containing numerous sporangia (spherules) having a thick, double outer membrane (Fig. 5-23). The sporangia vary from 100 to 400 μm in diameter, and contain a variable number of sporangiospores (endospores). A variable number of lymphocytes, plasma cells, and neutrophils are often found where sporangiospores (2 to 10 μm in diameter) have been released into the surrounding connective tissue.

---

*References 3, 4, 10, 14, 25, 230, 231.

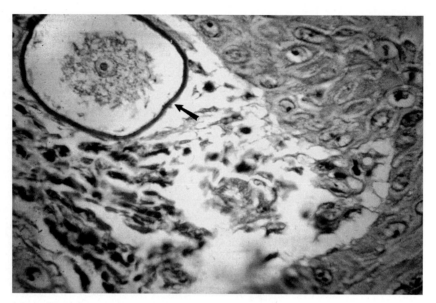

FIGURE 5-23. Rhinosporidiosis. Sporangium in dermis (*arrow*). (*Courtesy Dr. J. Bentinck-Smith.*)

CLINICAL MANAGEMENT

Surgical excision is the treatment of choice, although recurrence 6 to 12 months following surgery has been reported. In dogs, successes have been reported with dapsone or ketoconazole administered orally; however, the utility of medical therapy in equine rhinosporidiosis requires further evaluation.

Alternaria Dermatitis

CAUSE AND PATHOGENESIS

Alternaria spp. are ubiquitous saprophytic fungi in soil and organic debris and a common component of the flora of the equine integument.[5-7,13,26,27]

CLINICAL FINDINGS

Alternaria spp. are rarely reported to cause skin diseases in horses. A 7-year-old quarter horse mix had randomly distributed cutaneous nodules on the head, chest, and limbs.[232] The nodules were firm, 1 to 2 cm diameter, dermal in location, and variably alopecic and crusted.

DIAGNOSIS

The differential diagnosis for nodules includes infectious and foreign-body granulomas and neoplasms. Cytologic examination of aspirates or direct smears from nodular lesions reveals pyogranulomatous inflammation and numerous fungal elements. Biopsy findings include nodular to diffuse pyogranulomatous dermatitis (Fig. 5-24, *A* and *B*) with numerous broad (3 to 12 μm in diameter), septate, branched or unbranched hyphae (Fig. 5-24, *C*), and occasional chlamydoconidia. *Alternaria* spp. grow on Sabouraud's dextrose agar. Punch biopsies are the preferred culture material.

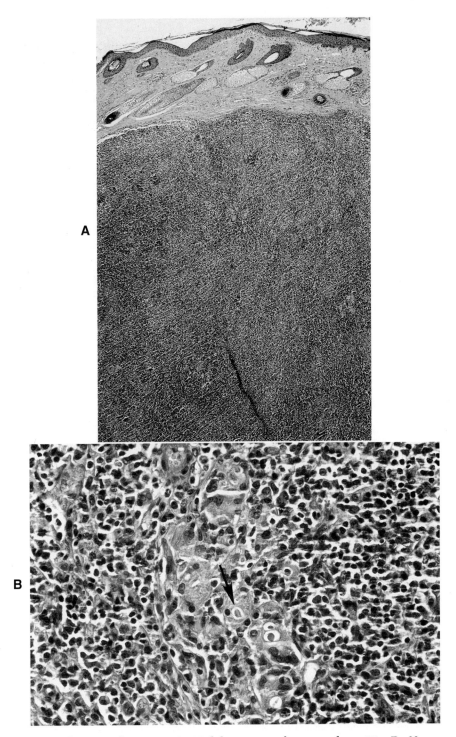

FIGURE 5-24. *Alternaria* dermatitis. **A,** Nodular pyogranulomatous dermatitis. **B,** Numerous multi-nucleated histiocytic giant cells containing fungal elements (*arrow*).

Continued

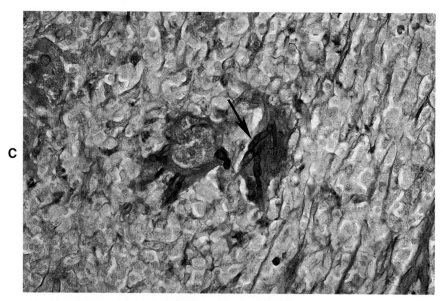

FIGURE 5-24, cont'd. C, Special stain reveals numerous fungal elements (*arrow*) (PAS stain).

CLINICAL MANAGEMENT

Surgical excision of nodules may be curative. Antifungal chemotherapy should be based on *in vitro* susceptibility tests. Successful medical therapy has not been reported in horses.

● SYSTEMIC MYCOSES

Deep mycoses are fungal infections of internal organs that may secondarily disseminate by hematogenous spread to the skin. Fungi that cause deep mycoses exist as saprophytes in soil or vegetation. These infections are usually not contagious because the animal inhales conidia from a specific ecologic niche. Skin lesions that occur via primary cutaneous inoculation are very rare, and animals with skin lesions are assumed to have systemic infection until proven otherwise. The deep mycoses are discussed only briefly here. The reader is referred to texts on mycology and infectious diseases for additional information.

Blastomycosis

CAUSE AND PATHOGENESIS

Blastomyces dermatitidis is a dimorphic saprophytic fungus.[5-7,13,26] Four elements—moisture, soil type (sandy, acid), presence of wildlife, and soil disruption—make up the "microfocus model" which helps explain where *B. dermatitidis* is most likely to be found.[28] Even within endemic areas, the fungus does not seem to be widely distributed. Rarely has the organism been successfully isolated from the environment. Most people and dogs living in such areas show no serologic or skin test evidence of exposure. A point source where the exposure occurs within an enzootic area is more likely. Blastomycosis (Gilchrist's disease, Chicago disease) is principally a disease of North America, but it has been identified in Africa and Central America. In North America, blastomycosis has a well-defined endemic distribution that includes the Mississippi, Missouri, New York, Ohio, and St. Lawrence River Valleys and the middle Atlantic states.

CLINICAL FINDINGS

Blastomycosis is extremely rare in horses. Multiple nodules, abscesses, and draining tracts were present around the vulva, anus, and udder of a mare with blastomycosis.[233]

DIAGNOSIS

A history of travel to an endemic area should increase the clinician's index of suspicion. Cytologic examination of aspirates or direct smears is often diagnostic, revealing suppurative to pyogranulomatous to granulomatous inflammation containing round to oval yeastlike fungi (5 to 20 μm in diameter) that show broad-based budding and have a thick, refractile, double-contoured cell wall. Biopsy findings include nodular to diffuse pyogranulomatous to granulomatous dermatitis, wherein the fungus is usually found easily. Culture of cytologic specimens is not recommended for in-hospital laboratories because of the danger of infection from the mycelial form of the organisms. The value of serologic testing (agar-gel immunodiffusion, enzyme-linked immunosorbent assay) in horses is unknown.

CLINICAL MANAGEMENT

All animals with clinical blastomycosis should be treated because spontaneous remission is rare.[9,28] In humans, dogs and cats, amphotericin B, ketoconazole, or itraconazole are effective chemotherapeutic agents.

Coccidioidomycosis

CAUSE AND PATHOGENESIS

Coccidioides immitis is a dimorphic saprophytic soil fungus.[5-7,13,26,28] The ecologic niche of this fungus is characterized by sandy, alkaline soils, high environmental temperature, low rainfall, and low elevation. Geographically, this area is referred to as the Lower Sonoran Life Zone, and includes the southwestern United States, Mexico, and Central and South America. Serologic surveys indicate that most human and canine inhabitants of the endemic area become infected. Coccidioidomycosis has also been called *San Joaquin Valley Fever*.

CLINICAL FINDINGS

Coccidiomycosis is rare in horses.[25,235] There are no apparent age (6 months to 12 years) or sex predilections, but Arabians may be predisposed. Affected horses most commonly present for chronic weight loss, persistent cough, musculoskeletal pain, phasic pyrexia, and skin lesions. Cutaneous lesions occur in about 20% of the cases and may be the initial clinical sign. The lesions are abscesses, most commonly over the shoulder or pectoral region.[234,235]

DIAGNOSIS

A history of travel to an endemic area should increase the clinician's index of suspicion. Cytologic examination of aspirates or direct smears reveals suppurative to pyogranulomatous to granulomatous inflammation. Fungal elements are seldom found. Biopsy findings include nodular to diffuse, suppurative to pyogranulomatous to granulomatous dermatitis and panniculitis. Fungal elements are usually present but may be sparse. The organisms are present in spherule (20 to 200 μm in diameter) and endospore (2 to 5 μm in diameter) forms.[1-3,181]

Attempts should not be made to culture *C. immitis* in veterinary practices because of the risk of human infection.[28] Culturing of the organism should be limited to laboratories with appropriate facilities. Serologic tests (precipitin, complement fixation) are of no apparent value in the horse.[235]

CLINICAL MANAGEMENT

All animals with clinical coccidioidomycosis should be treated because spontaneous remission is unlikely.[9,28] In humans, dogs, and cats, the current drug of choice is ketoconazole.[14,181,182] Treatment of animals with disseminated disease should continue for a minimum of 1 year. Amphotericin B is used to treat animals that cannot tolerate or do not respond to ketoconazole. A few horses have been treated with ketoconazole (3 to 15 mg/kg/day) PO, or amphotericin B (0.5 mg/kg twice weekly) IV with no benefit.[235]

Cryptococcosis

Cryptococcus neoformans v. *neoformans* is a ubiquitous, saprophytic, yeast-like fungus that is most frequently associated with droppings and the accumulated filth and debris of pigeon roosts.[5-7,11,13,26] *C. neoformans* v. *gattii* has a more restricted distribution and appears to have an environmental association with the flowery eucalyptus tree.[11] Currently there are four serotypes (A, B, C, D) and two varieties of *C. neoformans*: *C. neoformans* v. *neoformans* (serotype A and D), and *C. neoformans* v. *gattii* (serotypes B and C).[28] *Cryptococcus neoformans* v. *neoformans* is most prevalent in the United States and Europe, while *C. neoformans* v. *gattii* is prevalent in Southern California, Australia, Southeast Asia, Africa, and South America. In humans, *C. n. gattii* infects immunocompetent individuals and may be more difficult to treat.[28] The establishment and spread of infection are highly dependent on host immunity; however, underlying diseases are usually not detected in horses with cryptococcosis.[25] Both experimental and natural cases of cryptococcosis in horses are accelerated or worsened by glucocorticoid therapy.[28] Cryptococcosis has also been called *European blastomycosis* and *torulosis*.

CLINICAL FINDINGS

Cryptococcosis is very rare in horses.[25,236] The most common presentations are rhinitis and/or nasal granulomas, and CNS disease (especially meningitis). Multiple cryptococcal granulomas may occur on the lips.[4,28] A 10-year-old saddlebred gelding had a subcutaneous mass on the left lateral thorax.[236] The mass enlarged from 1.5 cm to 35 cm in diameter, eventually becoming fluctuant, ruptured, and developed draining tracts which discharged thick purulent to serosanguineous material.

DIAGNOSIS

Cytologic examination of aspirates or direct smears reveals pyogranulomatous to granulomatous inflammation with numerous pleomorphic (round to elliptical, 2 to 20 μm in diameter) yeast-like organisms. These show narrow-based budding and are surrounded by a mucinous capsule of variable thickness, which forms a clear or refractile halo. Biopsy findings include a cystic degeneration or vacuolation of the dermis and subcutis that is surprisingly acellular (sometimes likened to an infusion of soap bubbles) or a nodular to diffuse pyogranulomatous to granulomatous dermatitis and panniculitis containing numerous organisms. Mayer's mucicarmine is a useful special stain because it stains the organism's capsule (carminophilic) a red color. The value of serologic testing in horses is unknown.

CLINICAL MANAGEMENT

In humans, dogs, and cats, the drugs of choice are ketoconazole, itraconazole, and fluconazole.[9,28] The combination of ketoconazole and flucytosine, with lower doses of both, may produce more rapid cures and a reduction in side effects.[28] Amphotericin B, flucytosine, and the combination of both drugs have also been successfully used to treat cryptococcosis.[28] Rarely, solitary lesions in animals with primary cutaneous cryptococcosis can be surgically excised and the animals may be cured.[28] The value of chemotherapy in horses is unknown.

Histoplasmosis Farciminosi

CAUSE AND PATHOGENESIS

Histoplasmosis farciminosi (cryptococcosis) is endemic in Africa, Asia, and Eastern Europe. It is caused by the dimorphic fungus *Histoplasma* (*Cryptococcus*, *Saccharomyces*, *Zymonema*) *farciminosum*. Except for very rare reports in humans,[25,254] infections with *H. farciminosum* appear to be limited to equines (horse, mule, donkey). The disease may be transmitted by intra-cutaneous, subcutaneous, oral, or respiratory inoculation. Trauma appears to be an essential prerequisite for infection to take place. Mosquitoes and biting and nonbiting flies may serve as vectors. Bedding, grooming, utensils, blankets, and harness can serve as fomites. The fungus survives for up to 8 to 10 weeks in soil and water at 26° C (79° F).[248] Temperature and moisture content of soil influences fungal viability. The environmental niche of *H. farciminosum* is unknown, and horses appear the major reservoir for infection.[25,238] The average incubation period for clinical infections is 35 days, with a range of 4 to 72 days.

CLINICAL FINDINGS

Equine histoplasmosis farciminosi has no apparent age (8 months to 11 years), breed, or sex predilections.[*] Most cases occur in fall and winter.[25,237] Initial lesions consist of unilateral nodules, 1.5 to 2.5 cm diameter, in the skin of the face, head, neck, and less commonly the legs (especially the cranial aspect of the front legs, and the medial aspect of the rear legs near the hocks). Initially, the nodules are firm; then they become fluctuant and rupture to discharge a light-green, blood-tinged exudate. Resultant ulcers increase in size—up to 10 cm diameter—due to the formation of bright red granulation tissue. In some horses, nodules develop in a chain along enlarged, thickened, and tortuous lymphatics, resulting in a "corded" or "knotted" appearance. Lesions are neither painful nor pruritic. Regional lymph nodes may also become enlarged and rupture. After a period of 8 to 12 weeks, infection often spreads to the other side of the body, especially the medial thigh and prepuce. General health is initially unaffected, but chronically-affected horses usually become debilitated. Affected animals remain afebrile. A small percentage of horses may develop small papules to nodules inside the nostrils, keratoconjunctivitis (usually unilateral in association with a skin lesion) or pneumonia.[†] Infections on the limbs may involve joints, producing a purulent synovitis.

H. farciminosum infections are rare in humans.[25,254] Painful, migratory, cutaneolymphatic nodules, abscesses, and pyrexia may result from the contamination of open wounds.

DIAGNOSIS

The differential diagnosis includes other mycotic and bacterial infections, especially glanders, sporotrichosis, and ulcerative lymphangitis.[8,25,27] In glanders, there is systemic illness, pyrexia, and nasal septum lesions: these are not seen in histoplasmosis. Definitive diagnosis is based on cytologic examination, biopsy, and culture. The organism is difficult to culture (positive in only 59% of the horses in one study), and may require two or three serial samplings to identify.[237-239,249] Demonstration of the organism in tissues by cytologic or histopathologic examinations is considered the most reliable means of laboratory diagnosis.[‡]

Cytologic examination reveals pyogranulomatous or granulomatous inflammation wherein many macrophages contain an average of 4 to 6 yeasts: spherical to ovoid to pear-shaped; 1 to 5 µm in diameter, double-contoured wall. Histopathologic findings include nodular to diffuse granulomatous to pyogranulomatous dermatitis with numerous fungal elements.

---

[*]References 25, 27, 237, 239, 240, 244, 246, 247, 252, 256, 257, 259.
[†]References 25, 237, 239, 241-245, 257.
[‡]References 25, 27, 237-239, 243, 247, 250, 253, 260.

Preliminary investigations indicated that serologic tests (tube and passive hemagglutination), intradermal skin testing with histoplasmin, and a fluorescent antibody technique could be useful tools.[249,250]

Many infected horses have a leukocytosis, neutrophilia, and lymphopenia.[237]

CLINICAL MANAGEMENT

Equine histoplasmosis runs a chronic, debilitating course. Although the mortality rate is only 10% to 15%, loss of function and economic impact are significant.[25,27,239,246,247] Occasional horses undergo spontaneous remission.[25,237,239] The disease is currently managed by strict hygiene, quarantine, and slaughter. There is currently no effective treatment, although the organism is susceptible to amphotericin B and nystatin *in vitro*.[251]

Geotrichum Dermatitis

CAUSE AND PATHOGENESIS

Geotrichum candidum is a ubiquitous soil saprophyte and a minor component of the normal flora of the oral cavity, gastrointestinal tract, and integument.[28] The organism is believed to produce opportunistic infections by invading mucosal or cutaneous surfaces.

CLINICAL FINDINGS

Geotrichum dermatitis appears to be extremely rare. In Brazil, *Geotrichum* was cultured from horses with a skin condition characterized by well-circumscribed areas of alopecia, scaling, and occasional exudation and crusting.[262,263] Lesions were usually multiple and occurred on the head and neck.

DIAGNOSIS

Cytologic examination of aspirates or direct smears reveals suppurative to pyogranulomatous inflammation with broad (3 to 6 μm in diameter), septate, infrequently branched hyphae, spherical yeastlike cells, and rectangular or cylindrical arthroconidia (4 to 10 μm wide) with rounded or squared ends. Biopsy findings include nodular to diffuse, suppurative to pyogranulomatous dermatitis with numerous fungal elements. *Geotrichum* grows on Sabouraud's dextrose agar, at 25° C and punch biopsies are the preferred material for culture.

CLINICAL MANAGEMENT

There is little information available on the treatment of *Geotrichum* dermatitis. One cat and its owner were cured with amphotericin B.[28] One dog was cured with the topical application of miconazole.[28]

● ANTIFUNGAL THERAPY

Topical

Topical therapy (see Table 5-1) is often curative in superficial yeast infections (*Malassezia*, *Candida*) and may be curative or adjunctive in dermatophytosis. Dermatophyte infections are difficult because the fungi are relatively protected within hair shafts and hair follicles. Many topical antifungal agents are of historical interest only and will not be discussed in this text. Examples of such products include povidone-iodine, sodium hypochlorite, captan, tolnaftate, copper naphthenate (Kopertox), thiabendazole, Whitfield's ointment (benzoic and salicylic acids), Gentian violet, potassium permanganate, and so forth.° Dermatophytosis is a difficult situation. Topical

---

°References 8, 12, 14, 22, 27, 28, 265.

antifungal agents kill unprotected hyphae and spores rapidly, but not hyphae and spores within hairs.[28]

SPOT TREATMENTS

Focal applications of topical antifungal agents are useful for the treatment of candidiasis, *Malassezia* dermatitis, and localized dermatophyte lesions.

Nystatin and *amphotericin B 3%* are polyene antibiotics that bind with ergosterol in fungal cell membranes, resulting in altered cell permeability and eventual cell death.[265] Either product may be applied q12h to treat *Candida* or *Malassezia* infections, but they are *not* effective against dermatophytes. Nystatin is also available in combination with triamcinolone for highly inflammatory lesions.

Azoles inhibit the synthesis of ergosterol, triglyceride, phospholipid, chitin, and oxidative and peroxidative enzymes.[28,265,266] The imidazoles *clotrimazole* 1% and *miconazole* 1% or 2% may be applied q12h for the treatment of dermatophytosis, candidiasis, and Malassezia dermatitis.[165] *Thiabendazole* 4% with dexamethasone 0.1% may be applied q12h for the treatment of highly inflammatory dermatophyte lesions (kerions) or highly inflammatory *Malassezia* lesions (skin or ear).

Naftifine 1% (Naftin cream or gel) and *terbinafine* 1% (Lamisil cream) are allylamines that bind to stratum corneum and penetrate into hair follicles.[166] They inhibit ergosterol biosynthesis and squalene epoxidase, and may be applied q12h for the treatment of dermatophytosis and candidiasis. Naftifine also has anti-inflammatory activity and is useful for highly inflammatory dermatophyte lesions.

Chlorhexidine 4% (ChlorhexiDerm Maximum spray) is a synthetic biguanide (see Chapter 3 for details) that may be applied q12h for the treatment of *Malassezia* and *Candida* infections and dermatophytosis.

Benzalkonium chloride 0.6% spray (TrichoBan, Vet Genix) is marketed for the spot treatment of equine dermatophytosis in the United States, but no published information confirms its clinical efficacy.

SHAMPOOS

Antifungal shampoos are very useful for the treatment of *Malassezia* dermatitis. However, due to their lack of demonstrated efficacy against dermatophytes and the danger of dispersing arthrospores into the haircoat and environment as a result of their application, shampoos are not recommended for the treatment of dermatophytosis. However, one study suggested that simultaneous treatment of dermatophytosis due to *T. equinum* in horses with environmental applications (enilconazole foggers and potassium monopersulfate sprays) and a 2% chlorhexidine/2% miconazole shampoo (Malaseb) twice weekly resulted in resolution of clinical signs within 6 weeks.[106]

Shampoos containing 2% to 4% chlorhexidine or 2% miconazole are effective for the treatment of *Malassezia* dermatitis and are the least likely to be drying or irritating. Daily application is most effective, but this frequency is more likely to be irritating and is impractical for most owners. Twice weekly (every 3 days) applications seem to be adequate in most cases.

For animals that are particularly greasy or waxy, selenium sulfide 1% is very effective. This product can be too drying and is more likely to be irritating than chlorhexidine or miconazole.

RINSES

Antifungal rinses are the most effective topical products for the treatment of widespread superficial mycoses. They have more residual activity than shampoos. The preferred products are lime sulfur 2% (see Chapter 3 for details) or enilconazole 0.2%.[28] *Enilconazole* is an imidazole that is not presently approved in the United States. Enilconazole is reported to be safe and effective.

Total body applications of enilconazole, every 3 to 4 days[50] or once weekly,[106] were reported to be effective for the treatment of dermatophytosis in horses. Many people find the odor of the product to be objectionable. *Lime sulfur* is typically applied once or twice weekly for *Malassezia* dermatitis and for dermatophytosis (see Chapter 3 for details).[27,28]

Another very useful rinse for the treatment of *Malassezia* dermatitis is *acetic acid 2.5%* (see Chapter 3 for details). The solution can be prepared by combining equal parts of vinegar (5% acetic acid) and water. The solution is well tolerated on the skin.

Natamycin is a polyene macrolide that is similar in structure and mode of action to amphotericin B and nystatin.[97] It has *in vitro* efficacy against dermatophytes, *Candida*, and other fungi. Natamycin was applied total body, every 4 days, as a 100 ppm spray solution to horses with dermatophytosis and was reported to cause resolution of lesions within 4 to 6 weeks.[97,144] Natamycin is inactivated by sunlight; hence treatments were administered inside stables or outside at night. Natamycin is not approved for use on horses in the United States.

Systemic

The most common indication for systemic antifungal therapy is dermatophytosis. Griseofulvin is still the systemic antifungal agent of choice in these cases. However, if it is ineffective, has caused complications, or is otherwise contraindicated, ketoconazole or itraconazole may be acceptable alternatives. For *Malassezia* infections, griseofulvin is not effective and ketoconazole is the drug of choice. Other regimens or treatments may be necessary for the less commonly encountered mycotic infections. Newer antifungals, particularly the triazole compounds and the allylamines are available, but in general, they still have not been shown to be preferred over griseofulvin for routine use. Neither are they approved for use in the United States. Furthermore, they are quite expensive.

GRISEOFULVIN

Griseofulvin is a fungistatic antibiotic obtained by fermentation from several species of *Penicillium*. Its antifungal activity results from the inhibition of cell wall synthesis, nucleic acid synthesis, and mitosis. This agent is primarily active against growing cells, although dormant cells may be inhibited from reproducing.[28,263a,265,269] The drug inhibits nucleic acid synthesis and cell mitosis by arresting division at metaphase, interfering with the function of spindle microtubules, morphogenetic changes in fungal cells, and possibly by antagonizing chitin synthesis in the fungal cell wall. In humans, after oral administration, the drug may be detected in the stratum corneum within 8 hours to 3 days. The highest concentrations are attained in the stratum corneum and the lowest are in the basal layers. The drug is carried to the stratum corneum by diffusion, sweating, and transepidermal fluid loss and is deposited in keratin precursor cells and remains bound during the differentiation process. Consequently, new growth of hair or nails is the first to be free from disease. Because griseofulvin is not tightly bound to keratin, tissue levels drop rapidly when therapy is stopped. Thus, it must be administered until an infected nail grows out, which takes months.

Griseofulvin is in a state of flux in the skin, and consequently, a dosage administered once or twice daily is needed to maintain constant blood levels. When therapy is stopped, stratum corneum levels are gone in 2 to 3 days. This drug is indicated for only dermatophyte infections (*Microsporum* and *Trichophyton*). It is not effective against yeasts (*Candida* and *Malassezia*).

In dogs and cats, griseofulvin is variably and incompletely absorbed from the gastrointestinal tract.[28] Therefore, not all animals respond at the lower end of the dosage scale. If a poor response is seen, the dosage may have to be increased. It should be given with a fatty meal to enhance absorption. Griseofulvin has a disagreeable taste, and nausea may be seen. Dividing daily doses increases absorption and reduces nausea. The particle size of the drug also affects absorption, and this influences the dosage.

In the United States, griseofulvin powder (Fulvicin-U/F Powder, Schering-Plough) is approved for the treatment of equine dermatophytosis. Dosage recommendations are as follows: 1 packet (2.5 g)/day for adults; $\frac{1}{2}$ to 1 packet (1.25 to 2.5 g)/day for yearlings; $\frac{1}{2}$ packet (1.25 g)/day for foals. The powder is given orally, on a small amount of feed or in a drench, daily for not less than 10 days. If cases do not respond within 3 weeks, it is recommended that the diagnosis be evaluated. The product is not for use in horses intended for food. Unfortunately, no pharmacokinetic data on griseofulvin in horses have been published.

Only two clinical trials using oral griseofulvin powder for the treatment of equine dermatophytosis have been publsihed.[66,68] In both studies, horses were given 10 mg/kg/day (higher than the doses recommended by the manufacturer) for 7 days. All treated horses were reported as "healed" (no *active* clinical signs of dermatophytosis) or "clear" (no clinical signs of dermatophytosis) within 30 days. Reinfection was reported to be "not uncommon" within 3 months after the cessation of treatment. Most authors have found no evidence that oral griseofulvin powder—at currently recommended treatment protocols—is efficacious in horses.[27]

Griseofulvin is a potent teratogen in dogs and cats;[28] therefore, it is absolutely contraindicated in pregnant animals. Because griseofulvin can cause abnormalities in spermatozoa in rodents, it is advisable to avoid using recently treated male cats and dogs for breeding.[28] The safety of griseofulvin in pregnant or breeding horses is not known. The most common problem in dogs, cats, and humans is gastrointestinal upsets that resolve when administration of the drug is discontinued.[9,28] Anemia, leukopenia, depression, ataxia, and pruritus have also been reported. Rarely reported adverse cutaneous reactions include maculopapular or exfoliative eruptions, as well as erythema multiforme or toxic epidermal necrolysis. Although produced by various species of *Penicillium*, griseofulvin, penicillins, and cephalosporins rarely exhibit cross-reactive side effects. Adverse effects of griseofulvin have not been reported in horses.

Griseofulvin does have anti-inflammatory and immunomodulatory properties and is known to suppress delayed-type hypersensitivity reactions and irritant reactions in the skin.[28] These properties can lead to important clinical misinterpretations. The authors have seen dogs and cats whose inflammatory skin diseases (e.g., bacterial pyoderma and pemphigus foliaceus) showed significant improvement while the animals were receiving large doses of griseofulvin for presumed dermatophytosis.

AZOLES

The systemically administered azoles include the imidazole, ketoconazole, and the triazoles, itraconazole and fluconazole.[28,263a,265-268] They inhibit the cytochrome P-450 enzyme, lanosterol 14-demethylase, thereby inhibiting the conversion of lanosterol to ergosterol and causing the accumulation of C14 methylated sterols. Other actions include an inhibition of intracellular triglyceride and phospholipid biosynthesis, inhibition of cell wall chitin synthesis, and inhibition of oxidative and peroxidative enzymes. The potency of each azole is related to its affinity for binding the cytochrome P-450 moiety. The relative toxicity of each azole is associated with the selectivity of its action on fungal versus mammalian enzymes. Side effects are seen in about 10% of the dogs and 25% of the cats treated with ketoconazole. Side effects are much less frequent and, in general, less severe with itraconazole and fluconazole.

Because the triazoles and allylamines are lipophilic and keratinophilic, and therapeutic levels persist in skin and nails of humans for several days to weeks after treatment is stopped, shorter durations of treatment and pulse regimens (e.g., once-a-week dosing or 1 week of treatment per month) are feasible.[264-267,270] This has not been investigated in horses.

KETOCONAZOLE

Ketoconazole (Nizoral, Janssen) is an imidazole that is active against many fungi and yeasts, including dermatophytes, *Candida*, *Malassezia*, and numerous dimorphic fungi responsible for systemic mycoses.[28,263a,265,268,269] The therapeutic effect of ketoconazole is delayed for about 5 to 10 days. Consequently, in serious cases of systemic fungal disease, amphotericin B, which acts rapidly, is often used in combination with ketoconazole to compensate for this initial delay. Alternatively, one can use itraconazole or fluconazole.

Ketoconazole is insoluble in water but soluble in dilute acid solutions, and increased gastric acidity promotes absorption. When it is given with food, absorption is enhanced. Still, ketoconazole is variably absorbed, which probably accounts for the variation of doses needed in certain patients. It should not be given with gastric antacids, H_2 blockers, or anticholinergics. The major routes of delivery of ketoconazole to the stratum corneum are via sweat, sebum, and incorporation into basal keratinocytes. Ketoconazole is not approved for use in dog, cats, or horses in the United States. In dogs and cats, a dosage of 10 mg/kg every 24 hours is effective for dermatophytosis, *Malassezia* dermatitis, and candidiasis.[28] For systemic mycoses, higher dosages (30 to 40 mg/kg/day) are more commonly needed. Because ketoconazole does not readily enter the CNS, a dosage of 40 mg/kg every 24 hours is commonly necessary for life-threatening CNS and nasal mycoses.

About 10% of the dogs treated will develop side effects, including inappetence, vomiting, pruritus, alopecia, and a reversible lightening of the haircoat.[28] Side effects are more common with doses in excess of 10 mg/kg/day. It also enhances the effects of anticoagulants and increases the blood levels of cyclosporine and antihistamines, and its concentration may be decreased if it is given concurrently with rifampin. At dosages higher than 40 mg/kg/day, anorexia, nausea, and increased liver enzyme levels occurred. Cats are more sensitive, and about 25% will have side effects, including anorexia, fever, depression, vomiting, diarrhea, elevated liver enzymes, rarely icterus or neurologic abnormalities, and even death; therefore, one rarely exceeds 10 mg/kg/24 hours or 20 mg/kg/48 hours in cats.[28] Cholangiohepatitis has also been seen in cats treated with ketoconazole. Ketoconazole is embryotoxic and teratogenic in rodents, causes mummified fetuses and stillbirths in bitches, and is not recommended in pregnant animals. In dosages of ≥10 mg/kg/day, it suppressed basal cortisol concentration and response to ACTH, suppressed serum testosterone concentrations, and increased serum progesterone concentrations in dogs.[28] When administration of the drug is halted, a sharp rebound of testosterone levels occurs. In therapeutic use, one should be aware of the possible effect on libido and breeding effectiveness in male animals, adrenal insufficiency, the possibility of inducing or exacerbating prostate disease, as well as the potential for managing prostate disease, mammary carcinoma, and spontaneous hyperadrenocorticism.[13] Ketoconazole also has various immunomodulatory and anti-inflammatory effects, including suppression of neutrophil chemotaxis and lymphocyte blastogenic responses, inhibition of 5-lipoxygenase activity, and inhibition of leukotriene production.[28]

In dogs and cats, ketoconazole is effective in the treatment of dermatophytosis, candidiasis, *Malassezia* dermatitis, blastomycosis, coccidioidomycosis, histoplasmosis, and cryptococcosis.[28] In addition, it may be effective in some cases of mycetoma, phaeohyphomycosis, zygomycosis, sporotrichosis, alternariosis, aspergillosis, and prototothecosis. Ketoconazole is often prescribed in combination with amphotericin B for systemic infections, because the antifungal activity of both seems to be enhanced.

Very little information is available on the use of oral ketoconazole in horses.[263a] Ketoconazole (3 to 15 mg/kg PO q24h) was ineffective for the treatment of equine coccidioidomycosis[235] and equine pythiosis.[201] Limited pharmacokinetic data in horses suggest that the daily dose should be 30 mg/kg.[269b] The use of ketoconazole is limited in horses due to the low absorption from the gastrointestinal tract (23% oral bioavailability), the apparent need to administer the drug intragastrically (dissolved in 0.2 N hydrochloric acid [HCl]), the cost, and the long-term treatment required for most mycoses.[263a,269b]

ITRACONAZOLE

Itraconazole (Sporonox, Janssen) is a triazole, and, compared with ketoconazole, has increased potency, decreased toxicity, and wider spectrum of action.[28,263a,268,269] Susceptible organisms include dermatophytes, *Candida* spp., *Malassezia*, those causing many intermediate and deep mycoses, *Aspergillus*, *Sporotrichum*, and the protozoans *Leishmania* and *Trypanosoma*. The drug is given orally with food; concurrent antacids, H_2 blockers, and anticholinergics are contraindicated. In cats, 10 mg/kg/day should be sufficient in most cases.[28] Some cats may require 10 mg/kg q12 hours. Occasionally, cats better tolerate 20 mg/kg q48 hours. In dogs, most authors recommend 5 to 10 mg/kg/day.[28] The major routes of delivery to the stratum corneum are sweat, sebum, and incorporation into basal keratinocytes. Itraconazole is lipophilic and keratinophilic and levels in skin and claws may be 3 to 10 times higher than those in plasma. In humans, skin and nail levels persist up to 4 weeks and 6 to 9 months, respectively, after therapy is stopped.[270] Side effects are similar to those seen with ketoconazole but occur much less frequently and with reduced severity. Because itraconazole is more specific for fungal than mammalian cytochrome P-450 enzymes, endocrinologic side effects are not produced. Like ketoconazole, itraconazole also has various immunomodulatory and anti-inflammatory properties.[28] It is not recommended during pregnancy because of teratogenic effects. In dogs and cats, anorexia, nausea, and hepatotoxicity are occasionally seen.[28] In dogs, doses of 10 mg/kg/day produce vasculitis and necroulcerative skin lesions in 7.5% of the dogs treated.[28] These lesions did not occur at doses of 5 mg/kg/day.

Very little information is available on the use of itraconazole in horses.[263a] Doses of 5 to 10 mg/kg PO q24h have been recommended.[201,218b,263a]

FLUCONAZOLE

Fluconazole (Diflucan, Roerig) is a triazole; compared with ketoconazole, it has increased potency, decreased toxicity, and wider spectrum of action. Susceptible organisms include dermatophytes, *Candida*, *Malassezia*, and those causing deep and intermediate mycoses.[28] The drug can be given with or without food. The major routes of delivery to the stratum corneum are sweat, sebum, and incorporation into basal keratinocytes. High levels are achieved in skin, claw, and even the CSF. Therapeutic levels persist in stratum corneum for 10 days after therapy is stopped. In humans, fluconazole persists in nails for 3 to 6 months posttreatment.[267] Because fluconazole is the most fungal enzyme–specific of the three systemic azoles, side effects are very infrequent. Only extremely high doses are embryotoxic and teratogenic, and endocrinologic side effects are not produced.

Based on the results of one pharmacokinetic and bioavailability study in horses,[269a] a single loading dose of 14 mg of fluconazole/kg followed by 5 mg/kg orally q24h should be effective.

IODIDES

Iodides are given orally in daily doses of saturated solutions.[265,269,271] They have a disagreeable taste and may cause nausea and iodism. The disagreeable taste and gastrointestinal irritation may be avoided by adding the solution to molasses or milk. Iodism in horses may manifest as scaling and alopecia, depression, anorexia, fever, cough, lacrimation, serous nasal discharge, salivation, nervousness, or cardiovascular abnormalities.[16,27,263a] Although iodides are widely distributed in the body, their mechanism of action is unknown because they have no efficacy against fungal organisms *in vitro*. Iodides do enhance the halide-peroxidase killing system of phagocytic cells. Iodides are anti-inflammatory agents by virtue of their ability to quench toxic oxygen metabolites and inhibit neutrophil chemotaxis.[271]

Iodides are highly effective in the treatment of cutaneous and cutaneolymphatic sporotrichosis.[16,24,27,29] Many protocols using iodides have been recommended for horses, but all are anecdotal: for instance, sodium iodide (NaI) given intravenously, twice weekly, at 1 gm/15 kg (about 67 mg/kg); or potassium iodide (KI) given orally once daily, at 1.2 gm/30 kg (40 mg/kg).[27] A supersaturated solution of KI has been administered orally, 1 to 2 mg/kg q12-24h for 1 week, then 0.5 to 1 mg/kg q24h.[228] Probably the most commonly used protocol is the following: NaI (a 20% solution) is administered slowly intravenously at 20 to 40 mg/kg q24h for 2 to 5 days, then orally at the same dose.[16,27,29] An organic iodide, ethylenediamine dihydroiodide (EDDI 20GR, Phoenix, Vedco; not labeled for use in horses in the United States), has been used orally at 20 to 40 mg/kg q24h.[27] Because the iodides have a disagreeable taste and can be gastric irritants, they are administered with sweet feed or mixed with molasses and given by syringe. Tolerance to iodides is variable and, if signs of iodism appear, treatment is stopped until the horse is normal and reinstituted at a lower dose. Systemic iodides may cause abortion in horses.[16,27,29]

Systemic iodides are also the fist-line agents for the treatment of basidiobolomycosis (see page 293) and conidiobolomycosis (see page 293), and should be combined with surgical debulking where feasible.[27,219a,271] Iodides are not effective in the treatment of other zygomycoses, such as those caused by *Absidia*, *Mucor*, and *Rhizopus*.[271] NaI was reported to be effective in the treatment of a horse with nodular cutaneous candidiasis (see page 278).

AMPHOTERICIN B

Amphotericin B (Fungizone, Squibb) is a generally fungistatic polyene antibiotic that disrupts fungal (and bacterial) cell membranes by irreversible binding with ergosterol.[28,263a,265,269] This results in altered cell permeability, leakage of intracellular constituents, and cell death. It also binds to a lesser extent to other sterols, such as cholesterol in mammalian cell membranes, and therefore is relatively toxic. Other possible mechanisms of action include oxidative membrane damage and enhanced cell-mediated immunity. Amphotericin B stimulates lymphocyte, macrophage, and neutrophil function, and induces TNF production.[28] Amphotericin B is most effective for blastomycosis, histoplasmosis, coccidioidomycosis, cryptococcosis, and candidiasis. Problems of therapy include nephrotoxicity (especially in dehydrated and hyponatremic animals), anemia, urticaria, phlebitis, depression, anorexia, pyrexia, weight loss, and hypokalemia.[27,172a,201] If urticaria becomes severe, it can be diminished by the prior administration of antihistamines.[172a] One should avoid concurrent use of nephrotoxic drugs (e.g., aminoglycosides) and potassium-depleting diuretics. Amphotericin B has been suspected of producing abortions and birth defects.[14,27] Amphotericin B may also be useful toward the treatment of *Aspergillus*, *Trichosporon*, *Zygomycetes*, *Pythium*, and disseminated *Sporotrichum* infections.

Amphotericin given systemically must be given intravenously dissolved only in 5% dextrose and water. The recommended initial daily dosage for horses is 0.3 mg/kg.* Every third day the dose is increased by 0.1 mg/kg until a maximum of 0.8 to 0.9 mg/kg/day is reached. Amphotericin B is administered at this dose daily or every other day until day 30. Water consumption, urine output, and blood urea nitrogen and creatinine concentrations should be monitored.[145a,172a,263a] Treatment with this drug is dangerous, complicated, and expensive, and clinicians are advised to consult other references for specific guidelines.[172a,263a]

FLUCYTOSINE

Flucytosine (Ancobon, Roche) is an orally administered fluorinated pyrimidine that has been useful against *Candida*, *Cryptococcus*, *Aspergillus*, and some fungi associated with phaeo-hyphomycosis.[28,263a,265,269] Fungal cells are susceptible if they contain the enzyme cytosine permease, which enables 5-fluorocytosine to be taken into the fungal cell where it is deaminated by cytosine deaminase to 5-fluoro-21-deoxyuridylic acid. These substances inhibit thymidylate

---

*References 14, 27, 172a, 184, 184a, 201.

synthetase and subsequent DNA synthesis. Resistant, mutant organisms emerge regularly and rapidly in the presence of the drug, which is why it is combined with amphotericin B. In dogs and cats, the oral dosage is 60 mg/kg every 8 hours, but it is used as a second-line treatment, when more effective drugs, such as the imidazole and thiazole derivatives, are not available or are not well tolerated. As a single agent, flucytosine rarely produces side effects. Hematologic, gastro-intestinal, and hepatic toxicities are reported. Fixed drug eruptions on the scrotum of dogs and toxic epidermal necrolysis have been seen.

Use of flucytosine has not been reported in horses.

TERBINAFINE

Terbinafine (Lamisil, Novartis) is an allylamine that is well-absorbed orally in the presence or absence of food.[266] It inhibits ergosterol biosynthesis and squalene epoxidase, resulting in fungal cell wall ergosterol deficiency and the intracellular accumulation of squalene. Terbinafine is fungistatic and fungicidal. Because it is generally not inhibitory to cytochrome P-450 systems, it is more selective than the azoles.

Terbinafine is lipophilic and keratinophilic and, in humans, achieves high concentrations in stratum corneum, hair, sebum, and subcutaneous fat. The stratum corneum/plasma ratio varies from 13:1 to 73:1. The drug is delivered to the stratum corneum primarily via the sebum, then through the basal keratinocytes, and to a lesser extent by diffusion through the dermis and epidermis. In humans, terbinafine persists in therapeutic levels in the skin for 2 to 3 weeks and in the nails for 2 to 3 months.

Terbinafine is active against dermatophytes, *Candida* spp., *Sporotrichum*, and *Aspergillus* spp. The major side effects are gastrointestinal. No embryonic or fetal toxicity or teratogenicity has been demonstrated.

There have been anecdotal reports of the use of oral terbinafine for the treatment of dogs and cats with dermatophytosis. Terbinafine was reported to be effective for dermatophytosis in cats (20 mg/kg q48h) and dogs (20 mg/kg q24h), and no toxicities were seen.[28]

No pharmacokinetic data or significant clinical trials with terbinafine in horses have been published. In one anecdotal report,[41] two horses with "dermatophytosis" were treated with 750 mg (1.5 to 3 mg/kg?) of terbinafine, powdered with a coffee grinder and spread on the grain, once daily for 10 days. This study is basically uninterpretable because no clinical description was given (weight of horses? age of horses? distribution of lesions? and so forth), the duration of disease prior to treatment was not indicated, and fungal cultures were reported as "positive" (no details).

● REFERENCES

General

1. Ainsworth GC, Austwick PKC: A survey of animal mycoses in Britain: general aspects. Vet Rec 67:88, 1955.
2. Ainsworth GC, Austwick PKC: Fungal Disease of Domestic Animals, 2nd ed. Commonwealth Agricultural Bureau, Farnham Royal, London, 1973.
3. Blackford J: Superficial and deep mycoses in horses. Vet Clin N Am Large Anim Pract 6:47, 1984.
4. Bridges CH: Mycotic diseases. In: Catcott EJ, Smithcors JF (eds): Equine Medicine and Surgery, 2nd ed. American Veterinary Publications, Santa Barbara, 1972, p 199.
5. Carter GR, Cole JR Jr: Diagnostic Procedures in Veterinary Bacteriology and Mycology, 5th ed. Academic Press, New York, 1990.
6. Carter GR, Chengappa MM: Essentials of Veterinary Bacteriology and Mycology, 4th ed. Lea & Febiger, Philadelphia, 1991.
7. Chandler FW, Watts JC: Pathologic Diagnosis of Fungal Infections. ASCP Press, Chicago, 1987.
8. Chatterjee A: Skin Infections in Domestic Animals. Moitri Publication, Calcutta, 1988.
9. Friedberg IM, et al: Fitzpatrick's Dermatology in General Medicine, 5th ed. McGraw-Hill Book Co, New York, 1999.
10. Jungerman PF, Schwartzman RM: Veterinary Medical Mycology. Lea & Febiger, Philadelphia, 1972.
11. Kowalski JJ: Mechanisms of infectious disease. In: Reed SM, Bayly WM (eds): Equine Internal Medicine. W.B. Saunders Co, Philadelphia, 1998, p 61.

12. Kral F, Schwartzman RM: Veterinary and Comparative Dermatology. J.B. Lippincott Co, Philadelphia, 1964.

13. Kwon-Chung KJ, Bennett JE: Medical Mycology. Lea & Febiger, Philadelphia, 1992.

14. McMullen WC: The skin. In: Mansmann RA, et al (eds): Equine Medicine and Surgery, 3rd ed. American Veterinary Publications, Inc, Santa Barbara, 1982, p 789.

15. Miller RI, Campbell RSF: A survey of granulomatous and neoplastic diseases of equine skin in North Queensland. Aust Vet J 59:33, 1982.

16. Moriello KA, et al: Diseases of the skin. In: Reed SM, Bayly WM (eds): Equine Internal Medicine. W.B. Saunders Co, Philadelphia, 1998, p 513.

17. Mullowney PC, Fadok VA: Dermatologic diseases of horses. Part III. Fungal skin diseases. Comp Cont Educ 6:S324, 1984.

18. Murray DR, et al: Granulomatous and neoplastic diseases of the skin of horses. Aust Vet J 54:338, 1978.

19. Page EH: Common skin diseases of the horse. Proc Am Assoc Equine Practit 18:385, 1972.

20. Panel Report: Skin conditions in horses. Mod Vet Pract 56:363, 1975.

21. Pascoe RR: The nature and treatment of skin conditions observed in horses in Queensland. Aust Vet J 49:35, 1973.

22. Pascoe RR: Equine Dermatoses. University of Sydney Post-Graduate Foundation in Veterinary Science, Veterinary Review No. 14, 1974.

23. Pascoe RR: Equine Dermatoses. University of Sydney Post-Graduate Foundation in Veterinary Science, Veterinary Review No. 22, 1981.

24. Pascoe RR, Knottenbelt DC: Manual of Equine Dermatology. W.B. Saunders Co, Philadelphia, 1999.

25. Radostits OM, et al: Veterinary Medicine. A Textbook of the Diseases of Cattle, Sheep, Pigs, Goats, and Horses, 8th ed. Baillière Tindall, Philadelphia, 1994.

26. Rippon JW: Medical Mycology, 3rd ed. W.B. Saunders Co, Philadelphia, 1988.

27. Scott DW: Large Animal Dermatology. W.B. Saunders Co, Philadelphia, 1988.

27a. Scott DW: Diagnostic des dermatoses inflammatoires équines: Analyse de la modalité de réaction histopathologique. Étude personnelle portant sur 315 cas. Point Vét 24:245, 1992.

28. Scott DW, et al: Muller & Kirk's Small Animal Dermatology, 6th ed. W.B. Saunders Co, Philadelphia, 2001.

29. Williams MA, Angarano DW: Diseases of the skin. In: Kobluk CN, et al (eds): The Horse. Diseases and Clinical Management. W.B. Saunders Co, Philadelphia, 1995, p 541.

30. Yager JA, Scott DW: The skin and appendages. In: Jubb KVF, et al (eds): Pathology of Domestic Animals, 4th ed, vol 1. Academic Press, New York, 1993, p 531.

Dermatophytosis

31. Abdel-Halim MM, Kubesy AA: Evaluation of dermatophyte test medium for diagnosis of dermatophytosis among farm animals. J Egypt Vet Med Assoc 53:207, 1993.

32. Abdel-Halim MM, Kubesy AA: The practical application of chlor-pheno-lac solution for immediate diagnosis of animal dermatophytoses. J Egypt Vet Med Assoc 54:107, 1994.

33. Adeyefa CAO: Survey of zoophilic dermatophytes from symptomatic and asymptomatic horses in Nigeria. Bull Anim Prod Afr 40:219, 1992.

34. Aho R: Studies on fungal flora in hair suspected of dermatophytosis. Acta Pathol Microbiol Scand B 88:79, 1980.

35. Aho R, Soveri T: Equine dermatophytosis caused by *Trichophyton equinum* and *Microsporum canis*. Suomen Eläinlääj 90:192, 1984.

36. Aho R: Mycological studies on zoophilic dermatophyte isolates of Finnish and Swedish origin. Mycoses 31:295, 1988.

37. Aho R, et al: Karvaäytteiden mikroskooppinen tutkimus. Suomen Eläinlääk 99:165, 1993.

37a. Al-Ani FK, et al: Ringworm infection in cattle and horses in Jordan. Acta Vet Brno 71:55, 2002.

38. Bibel DJ, Smiljanic RJ: Interactions of *Trichophyton mentagrophytes* and micrococci in skin culture. J Invest Dermatol 72:133, 1979.

39. Bohm KH, et al: Mykologische Befunde bei Pferden mit Hautveranderungen in Nordwest Deutschland-Zugleich ein Beitrag zur Frage der Entstehung equiner Dermatomykosen. Berl Much Tierärztl Wochenschr 81:397, 1968.

40. Brown GW, Donald GF: Equine ringworm due to *Trichophyton mentagrophytes var quinckeanum*. Mycopathol Mycol Appl 23:269, 1964.

41. Burkhart CG, Burkhart KM: Dermatophytosis in horses treated with terbinafine. J Equine Vet Sci 19:652, 1999.

42. Cabañes FJ, et al: Dermatophytes isolated from domestic animals in Barcelona, Spain. Mycopathologia 137:107, 1997.

43. Carman MG, et al: Dermatophytes isolated from domestic and feral animals. NZ Vet J 27:136, 1979.

44. Carter GR, et al: Ringworm of horses caused by an atypical form of *Microsporum canis*. J Am Vet Med Assoc 156:1048, 1970.

45. Carter ME: *Microsporum gypseum* isolated from ringworm lesions in a horse. NZ Vet J 14:92, 1966.

46. Chermette R: Les teignes zoonoses. Aspects épidémiologiques. Point Vét 13:63, 1981.

47. Connole MD: A review of dermatomycoses of animals in Australia. Aust Vet J 39:130, 1963.

48. Connole MD: *Microsporum gypseum* ringworm in a horse. Aust Vet J 43:118, 1967.

49. Connole MD, Pascoe RR: Recognition of *Trichophyton equinum var equinum* infection of horses. Aust Vet J 61:94, 1984.

50. Consalvi PJ: L'énilconazole: une nouvelle molécule utilisable dans le traitement par voie externe des dermatomycoses des chiens, des chevaux et des bovins. Prat Méd Chir 18:16, 1983.

51. Dahl MV: Suppression of immunity and inflammation by products produced by dermatophytes. J Am Acad Dermatol 28:S19, 1993.

52. Dekeyser J, et al: Activité thérapeutique de l'iturine et du chinosel sur la teigne du cheval à *Microsporum equinum*. Bull Epiz Dis Afr 8:279, 1960.

53. Dom P, et al: Voorkomen van pathogene bacterien en dermatophytien in huidaandoeningen bij paarden in Belgie. Vlaams Diergeneesk Tijdsch 64:15, 1995.

54. Dvorak J, Otcenasek M: Mycological Diagnosis of Animal Dermatophytes. W. Junk, The Hague, 1969.

55. English MP: An outbreak of equine ringworm due to *Trichophyton equinum*. Vet Rec 73:578, 1961.

55a. Faravelli G, et al: Dermatomicosi equine. Sci Vet Biol Anim 17:3, 1991.

56. Fischman O, et al: Ringworm infection by *Microsporum canis* in a horse. Mycopathol Mycol Appl 30:271, 1966.

57. Gabal MA, et al: Animal ringworm in upper Egypt. Sabouraudia 14:33, 1976.

58. Georg LK: Conversion of tryptophane to nicotinic acid by *Trichophyton equinum*. Proc Soc Exp Biol Med 72:653, 1949.

59. Georg LK: Epidemiology of the dermatophytoses, sources of infection, modes of transmission and epidemicity. Ann NY Acad Sci 89:69, 1960.

60. Georg L, et al: Equine ringworm with specific reference to *Trichophyton equinum*. Am J Vet Res 18:798, 1957.

61. Georg L, et al: *Trichophyton equinum*—a reevaluation of its taxonomic status. J Invest Dermatol 29:27, 1957.

62. Gupta PK, Singh RP: Effect of some therapeutics on dermatomycoses (ringworm) in animals. Indian Vet J 46:1001, 1969.

63. Gupta PK, et al: A study of dermatomycoses (ringworm) on domestic animals and fowls. Indian J Anim Hlth 9:85, 1970.

64. Gupta PK, Singh RP: A note on the effect of age on the incidence of ringworm in cattle, buffaloes, and horses. Indian J Anim Sci 39:69, 1969.

65. Haack D: Zum Nachweis von Hautpilzinfektionen des Pferdes mit dem Dermatophyten-Test Medium Fungassay. Tierärztl Prax 15:269, 1987.

66. Harding RB: Treatment of ringworm in the horse with griseofulvin. Vet Dermatol News 6:40, 1981.

67. Hasegawa A, Usui K: Isolation of *Trichophyton equinum* and *Microsporum canis* from equine dermatophytosis. Jpn J Med Mycol 16:11, 1975.

68. Hiddleston WA: The use of griseofulvin mycelium in equine animals. Vet Rec 86:75, 1970.

69. Hoerlein AB: Studies on animal dermatomycoses. Clinical studies. Cornell Vet 35:287, 1945.

70. Hoerlein AB: Studies on animal dermatomycoses. II. Cultural studies. Cornell Vet 35:299, 1945.

71. Hopes R: Ringworm in the horse—the clinical picture. Vet Dermatol News 6:33, 1981.

72. Ichijo S, et al: Equine ringworm by *Trichophyton verrucosum*. Jpn J Vet Sci 37:407, 1975.

73. Ichijo S, et al: *Trichophyton equinum* isolated from race horse dermatophytosis. Res Bull Obihiro Univ 10:803, 1978.

74. Ichijo S, et al: Dermatomycosis due to *Trichophyton verrucosum* in cows, horses, sheep, and human beings. Jpn J Vet Med Assoc 37:506, 1984.

75. Jaksch : Dermatomykosen der Equiden, Karnivoren und einiger Rodentiere in Osterreich, mit einem Beitrag zur normalen Pilzflora der Haut. Wien Tierärztl Monatschr 50:831, 1963.

76. Jillson OF, Buckley WR: Fungus disease in man acquired from cattle and horses due to *T. faviforme*. N Engl J Med 246:996, 1952.

77. Jones HE: Immune response and host resistance of humans to dermatophyte infection. J Am Acad Dermatol 28:S12, 1993.

78. Kaben U, Ritscher D: Mikrosporie bei Pferden, unter besonderer Berucksichtigung einer *Microsporum gypseum*—Infektion bei einem Fohlen. Mykosen 11:337, 1968.

79. Kane J, et al: *Microsporum equinum* in North America. J Clin Microbiol 16:943, 1982.

80. Kaplan WA, et al: Isolation of the dermatophyte, *Microsporum gypseum*, from a horse with ringworm. J Am Vet Med Assoc 129:381, 1956.

81. Kaplan W, et al: Ringworm in horses caused by the dermatophyte *Microsporum gypseum*. J Am Vet Med Assoc 131:329, 1957.

82. Knudsen EA: The areal extent of dermatophyte infection. Br J Dermatol 92:413, 1975.

83. Kosuge J, et al: Dermatomycosis in a horse caused by *Microsporum gypseum*. J Vet Med (Japan) 51:200, 1998.

84. Kostro K: Wlaściwości morfologiczne i hodowlane *Trichophyton equinum*. Polski Arch Wet 29:15, 1989.

85. Kostro K: Badania nad struktur antygenow *Trichophyton equinum*. Polskie Arch Wet 29:27, 1989.

86. Kostro K: Wlaściwości biochemiczne krajowych i wzorcowych szczepów *Trichophyton equinum*. Polskie Arch Wet 29:37, 1989.

87. Kral F: Classification, symptomatology and recent treatment of animal dermatomycoses (ringworm). J Am Vet Med Assoc 127:395, 1955.

88. Kral F: Ringworm in the horse. Mod Vet Pract 42:32, 1961.

89. Kulkarni MP, Chaudhari PG: A note on the successful treatment of unusual equine ringworm due to *Trichophyton tonsurans var sulfureum*. Indian Vet J 46:444, 1969.

90. Kulkarni VB, et al: Equine ringworm caused by *Trichophyton tonsurans var sulfureum*. Indian Vet J 46:215, 1969.

91. Londero AT, et al: An epizootic of *Trichophyton equinum* infection in horses in Brazil. Sabouraudia 3:14, 1963.

92. Mallet V, et al: Human dermatophytoses: relation to horses. In: Kwochka KW, et al (eds): Advances in Veterinary Dermatology III. Butterworth-Heinemann, Boston, 1998, p 537.

93. Maslen M, Thompson PG: Human infections due to *Trichophyton equinum var autotrophicum* in Victoria. Aust J Dermatol 25:29, 1984.

94. McPherson EA: The influence of physiological factors on dermatomycoses in domestic animals. Vet Rec 69:1010, 1957.

95. Meckenstock E: Clinical signs and treatment of dermatomycoses in domestic animals. Vet Med Rev 2:79, 1969.

96. Moretti A, et al: Epidemiological aspects of dermatophyte infection in horses and cattle. J Vet Med B 45:205, 1998.

97. Oldenkamp EP: Treatment of ringworm in horses with natamycin. Equine Vet J 11:36, 1979.

98. Onizuka S: Dermatophyte isolated from horses. Rikugun Jui Dampo 270:1471, 1934.

99. Ot enášek M, et al: Zwei Befunde der *Trichophyton equinum* in menschlichen Lasionen. Dermatol Wochenschr 149:438, 1964.

100. Otčenášek M, et al: *Microsporum equinum* als Erreger einer Dermatophytose des Pferdes. Zbl Vet Med B 22:833, 1975.

101. Pal M, Lee CW: *Microsporum canis* infection in a horse and its transmission to man. Korean J Vet Clin Med 15:196, 1998.

102. Papini R, Mancianti F: Extracellular enzymatic activity of *Microsporum canis* isolates. Mycopathologia 132:129, 1996.

103. Pascoe RR, Connole MD: Dermatomycosis due to *Microsporum gypseum* in horses. Aust Vet J 50:380, 1974.

104. Pascoe RR: Studies on the prevalence of ringworm among horses in racing and breeding stables. Aust Vet J 52:419, 1976.

105. Pascoe RR: The epidemiology of ringworm in race horses caused by *Trichophyton equinum var autotrophicum*. Aust Vet J 55:403, 1979.

106. Paterson S: Dermatophytosis in 25 horses—a protocol of treatment using topical therapy. Equine Vet Educ 9:171, 1997.

107. Paula CR, et al: *Scopulariopsis brevicaulis:* agente etiológico de dermatose em cães equinos. Rev Microbiol (São Paulo) 18:366, 1987.

108. Pepin GA, Austwick PKC: Skin diseases, mycological origin. Vet Rec 72:208, 1968.

109. Petrovich SV: Efficacy of the treatment of ringworm in horses. Veterinariiya 5:49, 1977.

110. Petrovich SV, Sarkisov AC: Specificeskaja profilaktika trichofitii lošadej. Veterinarija (Moscow) 9:40, 1981.

111. Petzold K, et al: Enzootien durch *Trichophyton equinum* bei Pferden. Dtsch Tierärztl Wochenschr 72:302, 1965.

112. Pier A, Hughes J: *Keratinomyces ajelloi* from skin lesions of a horse. J Am Vet Med Assoc 138:484, 1961.

113. Pier AC, Zancanella PJ: Immunization of horses against dermatophytosis caused by *Trichophyton equinum*. Equine Pract 15:23, 1993.

114. Polonelli L, Morace G: Antigenic characterization of *Microsporum canis, M. distortum, M. equinum, M. ferrugineum,* and *Trichophyton soudanense* cultures. Mycopathologia 92:7, 1985.

115. Rebell G, Taplin D: Dermatophytes. Their Recognition and Identification. University of Miami Press, Coral Gables, 1974.

116. Reifinger M, et al: *Trichophyton equinum* als Ursache von Pseudomyzetomen bei einem Pferd. Wien Tierärztl Monat 86:88, 1999.

117. Reith H, El Fiki AY: Dermatomykose bein Pferd durch *Keratinomyces ajelloi* Van breuseghem 1952. Bull Pharm Res Inst 21:1, 1959.

118. Ritscher D, Kaben U: Hautpilzer-krankungen bei Pferden. Monat Vet Med 26:944, 19791.

119. Rybniká A, et al: Vaccination of horses against trichophytosis. Acta Vet Brno 60:165, 1991.

120. Sarkisov AK, Petrovich S: Immunity of horses to spontaneous and experimental ringworm. Veterinariya (Moscow) 11:39, 1976.

121. Schmidt A: Diagnostic results in animal dermatophytoses. Zbl Vet Med B 43:539, 1996.

122. Scott DW, Manning TO: Equine folliculitis and furunculosis. Equine Pract 2:20, 1980.

123. Scott DW: Folliculitis and furunculosis. In: Robinson NE (ed): Current Therapy in Equine Medicine. W.B. Saunders Co, Philadelphia, 1983, p 542.

124. Scott DW: Marked acantholysis associated with dermatophytosis due to *Trichophyton equinum* in two horses. Vet Dermatol 5:105, 1994.

125. Shimozawa K, et al: Fungal and bacterial isolation from race horses with infectious dermatoses. J Equine Sci 8:89, 1997.

126. Shwayder T, et al: *Trichophyton equinum* from riding bareback: First reported US case. J Am Acad Dermatol 30(5):785, 1994.

126a. Sloet van Oldruitenborgh-Oosterbaan MM, et al: De differentiele diagnose van niet genezende "schimmel"—Plekken bij hetpaard. Tijdschr Diergeneesk 119:756, 1994.

127. Smith JMB, et al: *Trichophyton equinum var autotrophicum*: its characteristics and geographic distribution. Sabouraudia 6:296, 1968.

128. Smith JMB, et al: An unusual dermatophyte from horses in New Zealand. Sabouraudia 5:124, 1966.

129. Stannard AA: Diagnostic aids in dermatology. Mod Vet Pract 60:548, 1979.

130. Stenwig H: Isolation of dermatophytes from domestic animals in Norway. Nord Vet Med 37:161, 1985.

131. Takatori K, et al: Occurrence of equine dermatophytosis in Hokkaido. Jpn J Vet Sci 43:307, 1981.

132. Takatori K, et al: The isolation and potential occurrence of keratinophilic fungi from hairs of healthy domesticated animals. Trans Mycol Soc Jpn 21:122, 1980.

132a. Takatori K, Ichijo S: Observation on human and animal hairs invaded by *Trichophyton equinum in vitro*. Jpn J Vet Sci 41:655, 1979.

133. Takatori K, Hasegawa A: Mating experiment of *Microsporum canis* and *Microsporum equinum* isolated from animals with *Nannizzia otae*. Mycopathologia 90:59, 1985.

134. Takatori K, Ichijo S: Human dermatophytosis caused by *Trichophyton equinum*. Mycopathologia 90:15, 1985.

135. Tanner AC, Quaife RA: *Microsporum gypseum* as the cause of ringworm in a horse. Vet Rec 111:396, 1982.

136. Thomsett LR: Laboratory procedures in the diagnosis of equine ringworm. Vet Dermatol News 6:35, 1981.

137. Thorold PW: Equine dermatomycosis in Kenya caused by *Microsporum gypseum*. Vet Rec 65:280, 1953.

138. Tsuji Y, Kuchii T: Ringworm in military horses. II. Studies on *Microsporum equinum*. Rikugun Jui Dampo 417:138, 1944.

139. Vrzal V, et al: *Trichophyton equinum*—Hlavni p vodce dermatofytóz n koni. Veterinářstvi 35:119, 1985.

140. Wegmann E: Trichlorfon treatment of ringworm in horses. Mod Vet Pract 67:636, 1986.

141. Weiss R, et al: 13 Jahre veterinärmedizinische mykologische Routinediagnostik. Dermatophyten-nacheweise in den Jahren 1965 bis 1977. Sabouraudia 17:345, 1979.

142. Woloszyn S, et al: Badania nad wystepowaniem i zwalczaniem grzybic skórnych koni. Med Wet 32:14, 1976.

143. Zdovc I, et al: Primer trihofitoze pri konjih, povzročene s *Trichophyton verrucosum*. Vet Novice 24:451, 1998.

144. Zukerman I, et al: An outbreak of ringworm (trichophytosis) in horses accompanied by human infection. Israel J Vet Med 47:34, 1992.

Candidiasis

145. Barnett JA, et al: Yeasts: Characteristics and Identification. Cambridge University Press, Cambridge, 1990.

145a. Madison JB, et al: Amphotericin B treatment of *Candida* arthritis in two horses. J Am Vet Med Assoc 206:338, 1995.

146. McClure JJ, et al: Immunodeficiency manifested by oral candidiasis and bacterial septicemia in foals. J Am Vet Med Assoc 186:1195, 1985.

146a. Montes AN, et al: Vulvovaginal candidiasis in thoroughbred mares following progestogen administration. Intravaginal treatment with clotrimazole. J Equine Vet Sci 21:68, 2001.

147. Nicolet J, et al: *Candida guilliermondii* als wahrscheinliche Ursache einer disseminierten Hautgranulomatose beim Pferd. Schweiz Arch Tierheilk 107:185, 1965.

Malessezia Dermatitis

147a. Guillot J, et al: Could *Malassezia* dermatitis be diagnosed in animals other than pet carnivores? Vet Dermatol 11(suppl):38, 2000.

147b. Nell A, et al: Identification and distribution of a novel *Malassezia* species yeast on normal equine skin. Vet Rec 150:395, 2002.

147c. Senczek D, et al: Characterization of *Malassezia* species by means of phenotypic characteristics and detection of electrophoretic karyotypes by pulsed-field gel electrophoresis (PFGE). Mycoses 42:409, 1999.

Piedra

148. Fambach D: *Trichosporon equinum*. Ztschr Infektionskr 29:124, 1925.

Eumycotic Mycetoma

149. Boomker J, et al: Black-grain mycetoma (maduromycosis) in horses. Onderstepoort J Vet Res 44:249, 1977.

150. Bridges CH: Maduromycotic mycetomas in animals. *Curvularia geniculata* as an etiologic agent. Am J Pathol 33:411, 1957.

151. Keegan KG, et al: Subcutaneous mycetoma-like granuloma in a horse caused by *Aspergillus versicolor*. J Vet Diagn Invest 7:564, 1995.

152. McEntee M: Eumycotic mycetoma: Review and report of a cutaneous lesion caused by *Pseudallescheria boydii* in a horse. J Am Vet Med Assoc 191:1459, 1987.

153. Miller RI, et al: Black-grained mycetoma in two horses. Aust Vet J 50:347, 1986.

154. Schiefer VB, Mehnert B: Maduromykose beim Pferd in Deutschland. Berl Munch Tierärztl Wochenschr 78:230, 1965.

Phaeohyphomycosis

155. Abid HN, et al: Chromomycosis in a horse. J Am Vet Med Assoc 191:711, 1987.

156. Bridges CH, Beasley JN: Maduromycotic mycetomas in animals—*Brachycladium speciferum* bainier as an etiologic agent. J Am Vet Med Assoc 137:192, 1960.

157. Brown RJ, et al: Equine maduromycosis: a case report. Mod Vet Pract 53:47, 1972.

158. Cabañes FJ, et al: Phaeohyphomycosis caused by *Alternaria alternata* in a mare. J Med Vet Mycol 26:359, 1988.

158a. Genovese LM, et al: Cutaneous nodular phaeohyphomycosis in five horses associated with *Alternaria alternata* infection. Vet Rec 147:55, 2001.

159. Hall JE: Multiple maduromycotic mycetomas in a colt caused by *Helminthosporium*. Southwest Vet 18:233, 1965.

160. Kaplan W, et al: Equine phaeohyphomycosis caused by *Drechslera speciferum*. Can Vet J 16:205, 1975.

161. Pal M, Lee CW: *Exserohilum rostratum*: first isolation from equine dermatitis. Korean J Vet Clin Med 11:187, 1994.

162. Percebois G, et al: Discussion du pouvoir pathogène de certaines espèces d'*Alternaria*: propos de trois observations. Bull Soc Franç Mycol Méd 7:15, 1978.

162a. Schauffler AF: Maduromycotic mycetoma in an aged mare. J Am Vet Med Assoc 160:998, 1972.

163. Simpson JG: Chromoblastomycosis in a horse. Vet Med Small Anim Clin 61:1207, 1966.

Pythiosis

164. Alfaro AA, Mendoza L: Four cases of equine bone lesions caused by *Pythium insidiosum*. Equine Vet J 22:295, 1990.

165. Allison N, Gillis, JP: Enteric pythiosis in a horse. J Am Vet Med Assoc 196:462, 1990.

166. Austin RJ: Disseminated phycomycosis in a horse. Can Vet J 17:86, 1976.

167. Austwick PKC, Copland JW: Swamp cancer. Nature 250:84, 1974.

167a. Berrocol A, van den Ingh TSGAM: Pathology of equine phycomycosis. Vet Quart 9:180, 1987.

168. Bridges CH, Emmons CW: Phycomycosis of horses caused by *Hyphomyces destruens*. J Am Vet Med Assoc 138:579, 1961.

169. Brown CC, Roberts ED: Intestinal pythiosis in a horse. Aust Vet J 65:88, 1988.

170. Brown CC, et al: Immunohistochemical methods for diagnosis of equine pythiosis. Am J Vet Res 49:1866, 1988.

171. Campbell CK: Pythiosis. Equine Vet J 22:227, 1990.

172. Chaffin MK, et al: Multicentric cutaneous pythiosis in a foal. J Am Vet Med Assoc 201:310, 1992.

172a. Chaffin MK, et al: Cutaneous pythiosis in the horse. Vet Clin N Am Equine Pract 11:91, 1995.

173. de Cock WAW, et al: *Pythium insidiosum* sp. nov. the etiologic agent of pythiosis. J Clin Microbiol 25:344, 1987.

173a. de Haan J, Hoog Kamer R: Hyphomycosis destruens equi barsatige Schimmelkrankeit des Pferdes. Arch Wissench Prakt Tierheilk 29:395, 1903.

174. dos Santos MN, et al: Pitiose cutânea em eqüinos no Rio Grande do Sul. Pesq Vet Bras 7:57, 1987.

175. Dowling BA, et al: Cutaneous phycomycosis in two horses. Aust Vet J 77:780, 1999.

176. Eaton SA: Osseous involvement by *Pythium insidiosum*. Comp Cont Educ Pract Vet 15:485, 1993.

177. Goad MEP: Pulmonary pythiosis in a horse. Vet Pathol 21:261, 1984.

178. Gonzalez HE, Ruiz A: Espundia equina: Etiología y pathogenesis de una ficomicosis. Rev ICA Bogota 10:175, 1975.

179. Gonzalez HE, et al: Tratamiento de la ficomicosis equina subcutanea empleando yoduro de potasio. Rev ICA Bogota 14:115, 1979.

179a. Grooters AM, et al: Evaluation of microbial culture techniques for the isolation of *Pythium insidiosum* from equine tissues. J Vet Diag Invest 14:288, 2002.

180. Guedes RMC, et al: Ficomicose e habronemose cutânea. Estudo retrospectivo de casos diagnosticados no período de 1979 a 1996. Arq Bras Med Vet Zootec 50:465, 1998.

181. Habbinga R: Phycomycosis in an equine. Southwest Vet 20:237, 1967.

182. Ichitani T, Ameniya J: *Pythium gracile* isolated from the foci of granular dermatitis in the horse. Trans Mycol Soc Jpn 21:263, 1980.

183. Johnston KG, Henderson AWK: Phycomycotic granuloma in horses in the Northern territory. Aust Vet J 50:105, 1974.

184. McMullen WC, et al: Amphotericin B for the treatment of localized subcutaneous phycomycosis in the horse. J Am Vet Med Assoc 170:1293, 1977.

184a. McMullen WC: Phycomycosis. In: Robinson NE (ed): Current Therapy in Equine Medicine. W.B. Saunders Co, Philadelphia, 1983, p 550.

185. Mendoza L: ?Cual es su diagnóstico? Cien Vet 9:153, 1987.

186. Mendoza L, Alfaro AA: Equine pythiosis in Costa Rica: report of 39 cases. Mycopathologia 94:123, 1986.

187. Mendoza L, et al: Immunodiffusion test for diagnosing and monitoring pythiosis in horses. J Clin Microbiol 23:813, 1986.

187a. Mendoza L, et al: Antigenic relationship between the animal and human pathogen *Pythium insidiosum* and nonpathogenic *Pythium* species. J Clin Microbiol 25:2159, 1987.

188. Mendoza L, et al: Bone lesions caused by *Pythium insidiosum* in a horse. J Med Vet Mycol 26:5, 1988.

189. Mendoza L, Prendus J: A method to obtain rapid zoosporogenesis of *Pythium insidiosum*. Mycopathologia 104:59, 1988.

190. Mendoza L, et al: Evaluation of two vaccines for the treatment of pythiosis insidiosi in horses. Mycopathologia 119:89, 1992.

191. Mendoza L, et al: Life cycle of the human and animal oomycete pathogen *Pythium insidiosum*. J Clin Microbiol 31:2967, 1993.

192. Miller RI, Campbell RSF: Immunological studies on equine phycomycosis. Aust Vet J 58:227, 1982.

193. Miller RI, Campbell RSF: Haematology of horses with phycomycosis. Aust Vet J 60:28, 1983.

193a. Monteiro AB, et al: Pitiose eqiina no Pantanal brasilíero: aspectos clínicopatológicos de casos típicos e atípicos. Pesq Vet Bras 21:151, 2001.

194. Murray DR, et al: Metastatic phycomycosis in a horse. J Am Vet Med Assoc 172:834, 1978.

195. Neuwirth L: Radiographic appearance of lesions associated with equine pythiosis. Comp Cont Educ Pract Vet 15:489, 1993.

196. Newton JC, Ross PS: Equine pythiosis: an overview of immunotherapy. Comp Cont Educ Pract Vet 15:491, 1993.

197. Purcell KL, et al: Jejunal obstruction caused by a *Pythium insidiosum* granuloma in a mare. J Am Vet Med Assoc 205:337, 1994.

198. Sedrish SA, et al: Adjunctive use of a neodymium: yttrium-aluminum-garnet laser treatment of pythiosis granulomas in two horses. J Am Vet Med Assoc 211:464, 1997.

199. Shipton WA, et al: Cell wall, zoospore, and morphological characteristics of Australian isolates of *Pythium* causing equine phycomycosis. Trans Brit Mycol Soc 79:15, 1982.

200. Smallwood JE: A case of phycomycosis in the equine. Southwest Vet 22:150, 1969.

200a. Vivrette SL, et al: Dermatitis and pythiosis in North Carolina horses following hurricane Floyd. Vet Dermatol 11(suppl)21, 2000.

201. Worster AA, et al: Pythiosis with bone lesions in a pregnant mare. J Am Vet Med Assoc 216:1795, 2000.

201a. Znajda NR, et al: PCR-based detection of *Pythium* and *Lagenidium* DNA in frozen and ethanol-fixed animal tissues. Vet Dermatol 13:187, 2002.

Zygomycosis

Basidiobolomycosis

202. Babu KKR: *In vitro* susceptibility of *Basidiobolus haptosporus* and other Zygomycetes to ketoconazole. Mykosen 25:439, 1982.

203. Connole MD: Equine phycomycosis. Aust Vet J 49:214, 1973.

204. Mendoza L, Alfaro AA: Equine subcutaneous zygomycosis in Costa Rica. Mykosen 28:545, 1985.

205. Miller RI, Pott B: Phycomycosis of the horse caused by *Basidiobolus haptosporus*. Aust Vet J 56:224, 1980.

206. Miller RI: Treatment of equine phycomycosis by immunotherapy and surgery. Aust Vet J 57:377, 1981.

207. Miller RI, Campbell RSF: Clinical observations on phycomycosis. Aust Vet J 58:221, 1982.

208. Miller RI: Investigations into the biology of three phycomycotic fungi pathogenic for horses. Mycopathologia 81:23, 1983.

209. Miller RI: Equine phycomycosis. Comp Cont Educ 5:S472, 1983.

210. Miller RI, Campbell RSF: The comparative pathology of equine cutaneous phycomycosis. Vet Pathol 21:325, 1984.

211. Owens WR, et al: Phycomycosis caused by *Basidiobolus haptosporus* in two horses. J Am Vet Med Assoc 186:703, 1985.

212. Torres G, et al: Rinozigomicosis y zigomicosis cutánea eu equinos. I. Caracterización clinicopatológica y etiología. Rev Inst Colombiano Agro 20:176, 1985.

Conidiobolomycosis

213. Bridges CH, et al: Phycomycosis of horses caused by *Entomophthora coronata*. J Am Vet Med Assoc 140:673, 1962.

214. Chauhan HVS, et al: A fatal cutaneous granuloma due to *E. coronata* in a mare. Vet Rec 92:425, 1973.

215. Emmons CW, Bridges CH: *Entomophthora coronata*, the etiological agent of a phycomycosis of horses. Mycopathologia 53:307, 1961.

216. French DD, et al: Surgical and medical management of rhinophycomycosis (conidiobolomycosis) in a horse. J Am Vet Med Assoc 186:1105, 1985.

217. Hanselka DV: Equine nasal phycomycosis. Vet Med Small Anim Clin 72:251, 1977.

218. Hutchins DR, Johnston KG: Phycomycosis in the horse. Aust Vet J 48:269, 1972.

218a. Kaufman L, et al: Immunodiffusion test for sero-diagnosing subcutaneous zygomycosis. J Clin Microbiol 28:1187, 1990.

218b. Korenek NL, et al: Treatment of mycotic rhinitis with itraconazole in three horses. J Vet Intern Med 8:224, 1994.

219. Restrepo LF, et al: Rhinophycomycosis from *Entomophthora coronata* in horses. Information on 15 cases. Antioquia Medica 23:13, 1973.

219a. Steiger RR, Williams MA: Granulomatous tracheitis caused by *Conidiobolus coronatus* in a horse. J Vet Intern Med 14:311, 2000.

220. Zamos DT, et al: Nasopharyngeal conidiobolomycosis in a horse. J Am Vet Med Assoc 208:100, 1996.

Mucormycosis

220a. Guillot J, et al: Two cases of equine mucormycosis caused by *Absidia corymbifera*. Equine Vet J 32:453, 2000.

221. López-Sanromán J, et al: Cutaneous mucormycosis caused by *Absidia corymbifera* in a horse. Vet Dermatol 11:151, 2000.

Sporotrichosis

222. Davis HH, Worthington WE: Equine sporotrichosis. J Am Vet Med Assoc 145:692, 1964.

223. Fishburn F, Kelley DC: Sporotrichosis in a horse. J Am Vet Med Assoc 151:45, 1967.

224. Gibbons WJ: Sporotrichosis: case report. Mod Vet Pract 43:92, 1962.

225. Greydanus-van der Putten SWM, et al: Sporotrichosis bij een paard. Tijdschr Diergeneesk 119:500, 1994.

226. Jones TC, Maurer FD: Sporotrichosis in horses. Bull US Army Med Dept 74:63, 1944.

227. Kirkham WW, Moore RW: Sporotrichosis in a horse. Southwest Vet 7:354, 1954.

228. Morris P: Sporotrichosis. In: Robinson NE (ed): Current Therapy in Equine Medicine. W.B. Saunders Co, Philadelphia, 1983, p 555.

229. Thorold PW: Equine sporotrichosis. J So Afr Vet Med Assoc 22:81, 1951.

Rhinosporidiosis

230. Myers DD, et al: Rhinosporidiosis in a horse. J Am Vet Med Assoc 145:345, 1964.

231. Smith HA: Rhinosporidiosis in a Texas horse. Southwest Vet 15:22, 1961.

Alternaria Dermatitis

232. Coles BM, et al: Equine nodular dermatitis associated with *Alternaria tenuis* infection. Vet Pathol 15:779, 1978.

Blastomycosis

233. Benbrook EA, et al: A case of blastomycosis in the horse. J Am Vet Med Assoc 112:475, 1948.

Coccidioidomycosis

234. Crane CS: Equine coccidioidomycosis: case report. Vet Med 57:1073, 1962.

235. Ziemer EL, et al: Coccidioidomycosis in horses: 15 cases (1975-1984). J Am Vet Med Assoc 201:910, 1992.

Cryptococcosis

236. Chandra VK, et al: Localized subcutaneous cryptococcal granuloma in a horse. Equine Vet J 25:166, 1992.

Histoplasmosis Farciminosi

237. Al-Ani FK, et al: Epizootic lymphangitis in horses: clinical, epidemiological, and haematological studies. Pakistan Vet J 6:96, 1986.

238. Al-Ani FK, et al: Epizootic lymphangitis in horses: mice inoculation studies. Pakistan Vet J 8:5, 1988.

239. Al-Ani FK, et al: *Histoplasma farciminosum* infection of horses in Iraq. Vet Arhiv 68:101, 1998.

240. Awad FI: Studies on epizootic lymphangitis in the Sudan. J Comp Pathol 70:457, 1960.

241. Bennett SCJ: *Cryptococcus* pneumonia in equidae. J Comp Pathol 44:85, 1931.

242. Bennett SCJ: *Cryptococcus* infection in equidae. J Roy Army Vet Corps 16:108, 1944.

243. Bullen JJ: The yeast-like form of *Cryptococcus farciminosus* (Rivolta): (*Histoplasma farciminosum*). J Pathol Bacteriol 61:117, 1949.

244. Bullen JJ: Epizootic lymphangitis: clinical symptoms. J Roy Army Vet Corps 22:8, 1951.

245. Fawi MT: *Histoplasma farciminosum*, the aetiological agent of equine cryptococcal pneumonia. Sabouraudia 9:123, 1971.

246. Gabal MA, et al: Study of equine histoplasmosis "epizootic lymphangitis." Mykosen 26:145, 1983.

247. Gabal MA, et al: Study of equine histoplasmosis farciminosi and characterization of *Histoplasma farciminosum*. Sabouraudia 21:121, 1983.

248. Gabal MA, Hennager S: Study on the survival of *Histoplasma farciminosum* in the environment. Mykosen 26:481, 1983.

249. Gabal MA, Khalifa K: Study on the immune response and serological diagnosis of equine histoplasmosis "epizootic lymphangitis." Mykosen 26:89, 1983.

250. Gabal MA, et al: The fluorescent antibody technique for diagnosis of equine histoplasmosis (epizootic lymphangitis). Zentralb Vet Med B 30:283, 1983.

251. Gabal MA: The effect of amphotericin B, 5-fluorocytosine and nystatin on *Histoplasma farciminosum in vitro*. Zentralb Vet Med B 31:46, 1984.

252. Guerin C, et al: Epizootic lymphangitis in horses in Ethiopia. Med Mycol 2:1, 1992.

253. Khater AR, et al: A histomorphological study of cutaneous lesions in equine histoplasmosis (epizootic lymphangitis). J Egypt Vet Med Assoc 28:165, 1968.

254. Negre L, Bridre J: Un cas de lymphangite épizootique chez l'homme. Bull Soc Pathol Exot 4:384, 1911.

255. Plunkett JJ: Epizootic lymphangitis. J Roy Army Vet Corps 20:94, 1949.

256. Roberts GA: Epizootic lymphangitis of solipeds. J Am Vet Med Assoc 98:226, 1941.

257. Singh S: Equine cryptococcosis (epizootic lymphangitis). Indian Vet J 32:260, 1956.

258. Singh T: Studies on epizootic lymphangitis. I. Modes of infection and transmission of equine histoplasmosis (epizootic lymphangitis). Indian J Vet Sci 35:102, 1965.

259. Singh T: Studies on epizootic lymphangitis. Indian J Vet Sci 36:45, 1966.

260. Singh T, et al: Studies on epizootic lymphangitis. II. Pathogenesis and histopathology of equine histoplasmosis. Indian J Vet Sci 35:111, 1965.

261. Singh T, Varmani BML: Some observations on experimental infection with *Histoplasma farciminosum* (Rivolta) and the morphology of the organism. Indian J Vet Sci 37:471, 1967.

Geotrichosis

262. Moss EN, et al: Geotricose em eqüino puro sangue ingls. Rev Fac Med Vet Zootec Univ So Paulo 15:93, 1978.

263. Santos MRS, et al: Geotricose cutânea em eqüinos. Biológico So Paulo 49:75, 1983.

Antifungal Therapy

263a. Beard LA: Principles of antimicrobial therapy. In: Reed SM, Bayly WM (eds): Equine Internal Medicine. W.B. Saunders Co, Philadelphia, 1998, p 157.

264. deDoncker P, et al: Antifungal pulse therapy for onychomycosis. Arch Dermatol 132:34, 1996.

265. Gupta AK, et al: Antifungal agents: an overview. Part I. J Am Acad Dermatol 30:677, 1994.

266. Gupta AK, et al: Antifungal agents: an overview. Part II. J Am Acad Dermatol 30:911, 1994.

267. Faergemann J: Pharmacokinetics of fluconazole in skin and nails. J Am Acad Dermatol 40:S14, 1999.
268. Heit MC, Riviere JE: Antifungal therapy: ketoconazole and other azole derivatives. Comp Cont Educ 21.123, 1995.
269. Hill PB, et al: A review of systemic antifungal agents. Vet Dermatol 6:59, 1995.
269a. Latimer FG, et al: Pharmacokinetics of fluconazole following intravenous and oral administration and body fluid concentrations of fluconazole following repeated oral dosing of horses. Am J Vet Res 62:1606, 2001.
269b. Prades M, et al: Body fluid and endometrial concentrations of ketoconazole in mares after intravenous injection or repeated gavage. Equine Vet J 21:211, 1989.
270. Scher RK: Onychomycosis: therapeutic update. J Am Acad Dermatol 40:S21, 1999.
271. Sterling JB, Heymann WR: Potassium iodide in dermatology: a 19th century drug for the 21st century—uses, pharmacology, adverse effects, and contraindications. J Am Acad Dermatol 43:691, 2000.

Chapter 6

Parasitic Diseases

Dermatoses caused by ectoparasites are common skin disorders of large animals.[1,2,4-16,18-21] They account for 7.7% of the equine dermatoses seen at the Cornell University Clinic:

Chorioptic mange	2.67
Onchocerciasis (none since 1990)	1.67
Pediculosis	1.22
Habronemiasis (none since 1995)	1.00
Ventral midline dermatitis	0.89
Halicephalobiasis	0.11
Strawmite dermatitis	0.11

Already-diseased skin is more vulnerable to fly or mosquito parasitism and makes the diagnosis of the underlying disease more difficult. Animal suffering through annoyance, irritability, pruritus, disfigurement, secondary infections, and myiasis is often great. Many of the ectoparasites are important in the transmission of various viral, protozoal, helminthic, fungal, and bacterial diseases. The important arachnids, insects, and helminths associated with skin disease in horses are listed in Tables 6-1 through 6-3.

• THERAPEUTICS

The treatment of ectoparasitism is a complex topic.[6,12,22,27,28] Significant differences exist in the regional availability of, and regulations governing, parasiticidal agents. In general, most agents used to treat or prevent parasitic skin disorders of the horse are registered pesticides rather than drugs.[25,27,28] Pesticides are under the regulation of the Environmental Protection Agency (EPA) in the United States. Other countries have similar agencies. Because of the long lasting consequences of some chemicals, many are not available today and some can only be applied by a registered pesticide applicator. Nonrestricted pesticides must be used in accordance with their labeled directions. It is a violation of Federal law in the United States to use an EPA-registered pesticide in an extra-label fashion. Commonly accepted veterinary practice is not a legitimate excuse for extra-label use. Extra-label usage includes the treatment of a nonlabeled species, a higher frequency of application than the label allows, or usage for a disorder not listed under the indications. Since textbooks are read worldwide and not all countries have pesticide regulation as restrictive as those in the United States, the authors have included published treatments that are currently illegal in the United States. The reader should follow all pertinent regulations in his or her country.

The Food and Drug Administration (FDA) regulates drugs in the United States. Since many drugs commonly used in veterinary practice are not licensed for veterinary use, the FDA recognizes the need for extra-label drug usage. Provided that the drug does not enter the food chain, extra-label usage is allowed. However, adverse reactions that occur because a drug is used in a

Table 6-1 ARACHNIDS ASSOCIATED WITH SKIN DISEASE IN HORSES

Class: Arachnida
  Order: Acarina
    Suborder: Astigmata
      Family: Sarcoptidae
        Sarcoptes scabiei
      Family: Psoroptidae
        Psoroptes cuniculi
        P. equi
        P. matalensis
        P. ovis
        Chorioptes equi
      Family: Acaridae
        Acarus farinae
        A. siro
        Caloglyphus berlesei
    Suborder: Prostigmata
      Family: Trombiculidae
        Trombicula alfreddugési
        T. autumnalis
        T. sarcina
        T. splendens
      Family: Demodicidae
        Demodex equi
        D. caballi
    Suborder: Mesostigmata
      Family: Dermanyssidae
        Dermanyssus gallinae
    Suborder: Metastigmata
      Family: Argasidae
        Otobius megnini° (North and South America, Africa)
        Ornithodorus coriaceus° (North America)
        O. lahorensis (Asia)
        O. moubata (Africa)
        O. savignyi (Africa, Near East)
    Suborder: Metastigmata
      Family: Ixodidae
        Ixodes ricinus (Europe, Africa, Asia)
        I. hexagonus (Europe, Africa)
        I. persulcatus (Europe, Asia)
        I. canisuga (Europe)
        I. pilosus (Africa)
        I. rubicundus (Africa)

Ixodes scapularis° (North America)
I. cookei° (North America)
I. pacificus° (North America)
I. holocyclus° (Australia)
Boophilus annulatus (Central America, Africa)
B. microplus (Central and South America, Australia, Africa, Asia)
B. calcaratus (Africa)
B. decoloratus (Africa)
Margaropus winthemi (Europe, Asia, Africa)
Hyalomma plumbeum (Europe, Asia, Africa)
H. excavatum (Europe, Asia, Africa)
Rhipicephalus appendiculatus (Africa)
R. capensis (Africa)
R. neavei (Africa)
R. jeanelli (Africa)
R. ayrei (Africa)
R. pulchellus (Africa)
R. sanguineus° (cosmopolitan)
R. evertsi (Europe, Africa)
R. bursa (Europe)
R. turanicus (Europe)
Haemaphysalis cinnabarina (Africa, Asia, Europe)
H. longicornis (Asia, Australia, New Zealand)
H. bancrofti (Australia)
Dermacentor reticulatus (Europe)
D. marginatus (Africa, Asia)
D. variabilis° (North America)
D. nitens° (North, Central, and South America)
D. albipictus° (North America)
D. andersoni (North America)
D. occidentalis° (North America)
D. nigrolineatus (North America)
Amblyomma hebraeum (Africa)
A. gemma (Africa)
A. variegatum (Africa)
A. americanum° (North America)
A. cajennense° (North, Central, and South America)
A. maculatum° (North America)
Anocentor nitens (South America)
Order: Araneidea
Spiders

°Ticks recovered from large animals in the United States.

nonlabeled fashion are the responsibility of the prescribing veterinarian and may result in legal action.[24,26,30] The reader is encouraged to fully research a drug or treatment before it is used.

Topical Treatments

Topical antiparasitic therapy is primarily directed against ectoparasites that feed or live on the horse.[22,25,27,28] In treating the dermatosis, it is critical to consider the parasite; its life cycle, epidemiology, and natural behavior; and the pathogenesis of the disease the parasite is causing. Topical therapy may be just one aspect of an overall treatment plan, or it may be the sole therapy prescribed. Proper application becomes critical when it is the sole therapy.

Parasitic Diseases • 323

Table 6-2 INSECTS ASSOCIATED WITH SKIN DISEASE IN HORSES

Class: Insecta
 Subclass: Pterygota
  Division: Exopterygota
   Order: Mallophaga
    Suborder: Ischnocera
     Damalinia equi
   Order: Siphunculata
    Family: Haematopinidae
     Haematopinus asini
  Division: Endopterygota
   Order: Siphonaptera
     Ctenocephalides felis felis
     Echidnophaga gallinacea
     Pulex irritans
     Tunga penetrans
   Order: Diptera
    Suborder: Nematocera
     Family: Culicidae
      Aedes spp.
      Anopheles spp.
      Culex spp.
     Family: Ceratopogonidae
      Culicoides spp.
     Family: Simuliidae
      Simulium spp.
    Suborder: Brachycera
     Family: Tabanidae
      Tabanus spp.
      Haematopota spp.
      Chrysops spp.

Order: Diptera
 Suborder: Cyclorrhapha
  Family: Gasterophilidae
   Gasterophilus spp.
  Family: Muscidae
   Musca spp.
   Stomoxys calcitrans
   Hydrotaea spp.
   Haematobia spp.
  Family: Calliphoridae
   Calliphora spp.
   Chrysomyia spp.
   Phormia spp.
   Cochliomyia spp.
   Booponus intonsus
   Auchmeromyia luteola
  Family: Sarcophaginae
   Sarcophaga spp.
   Wohfahrtia spp.
  Family: Oestridae
   Hypoderma bovis
   H. lineatum
  Family: Cuterebridae
   Dermatobia hominis
   Cuterebra spp.
  Family: Hippoboscidae
   Hippobosca spp.
 Order: Hymenoptera
  Bees and Wasps

Table 6-3 HELMINTHS ASSOCIATED WITH SKIN DISEASE IN HORSES

Class: Nematoda
 Order: Ascaridida
  Superfamily: Oxyuroidea
   Family: Oxyuridae
    Oxyuris equi
 Order: Rhabditida
  Superfamily: Rhabditoidea
   Family: Rhabditidae
    Halicephalobus deletrix
    Pelodera strongyloides
   Family: Strongyloididae
    Strongyloides westeri
 Order: Spirurida
  Superfamily: Spiruroidea
   Family: Spiruridae
    Habronema muscae
    H. majus
    Draschia megastoma

Superfamily: Filarioidea
 Family: Filariidae
  Parafilaria multipapillosa
 Family: Onchocercidae
  Onchocerca cervicalis
  O. gutturosa
  O. reticulata
Superfamily: Dracunculoidea
 Family: Dracunculidae
  Dracunculus insignis
  D. medinensis

CHLORINATED HYDROCARBONS

Chlorinated hydrocarbons, which are dangerous insecticides, have become outdated and replaced by safer products. They persist in the environment and animal tissue for long periods of time. Several methoxychlor products are still marketed for horses, but the authors suggest the use of safer alternatives.

CHOLINESTERASE INHIBITORS

Two kinds of cholinesterase inhibitors are available: carbamates and organophosphates. They were once the mainstay of insect control. However, with the advent of safer products and better alternative treatment regimens, their use on animals is decreasing. Cholinesterase inhibitors are still valuable for environmental treatment.

Carbamates

Carbamates are typified by carbaryl. At this writing, carbaryl-containing products are not marketed for topical use in the horse.[25] Products for barn treatments are available. If those products are used in the barn, insecticides other than an organophosphate should be used on the horse to prevent profound cholinesterase depression.

Organophosphates

The most toxic insecticides in use are organophosphates. They are potent cholinesterase inhibitors, and a cumulative effect may be seen if animals are exposed to similar insecticides in another preparation or in barn applications. Currently, products containing dichlorvos (Vapona), tetra-chlorvinphos (Rabon), coumaphos (Co-Ral) are marketed for on-horse use.[25] A variety of other organophosphates are available for use in barns.

FIPRONIL

Fipronil is a relatively new insecticide and acaricide in the phenylprazole class. It acts as an antagonist at the insect γ-aminobutyric acid (GABA) receptor. Fipronil is marketed in a spray (Frontline, Merial) or spot application product (Frontline Top Spot, Merial) for flea control in dogs and cats. Its efficacy in nonfollicular mite and lice infestations has been demonstrated in horses.

FORMAMDINES

These acaricidal agents act by inhibition of monoamine oxidase. They are also prostaglandin synthesis inhibitors and α-adrenergic agonists. Amitraz (Mitaban, Upjohn and Pharmacia), the veterinary form, is available as a rinse and a collar for tick control. Amitraz is contraindicated in horses.[24,30,31] Horses sprayed with a 0.025% solution developed somnolence, depression, ataxia, weakness, and colonic impaction.

PYRETHRINS

Pyrethrin is a volatile oil extract of the chrysanthemum flower. It contains six active pyrethrins that are contact poisons and have a fast knockdown action and flushing action on insects but no residual activity. It is rapidly inactivated by moisture, air, and light. Pyrethrins, because of their low toxicity, rapid inactive, and lack of tissue residue and buildup, are relatively environmentally safe, although they are still toxic to fish and bees. For clients concerned with chemicals, the use of pyrethrins may be more acceptable, because this is an organic natural insecticide.

There is no cholinesterase suppression. Pyrethrin demonstrates a rapid kill but low toxicity, and the low concentration of 0.06% to 0.4% is effective if it is synergized with 0.1% to 2% piperonyl butoxide, which forms a stable complex with cytochrome P450, thus limiting the metabolism of pyrethrins in insects. Spray and wipe-on formulations are available.

PYRETHROIDS

These synthesized chemicals are modeled after pyrethrin and include D-trans-allethrin, bioallethrin, resmethrin, tetramethrin, deltamethrin, fenvalerate, and permethrin. A fourth-generation of potent and long-lasting pyrethroids are available for ear tag use. The LD_{50} varies with the agent selected. In action and toxicity, the pyrethroids are relatively comparable, although not identical, to pyrethrin. They produce a quick kill that is improved by the addition of a synergist and pyrethrin. Some of the early pyrethroids degrade on exposure to ultraviolet light, so there is little or no residual activity. The new pyrethroids are relatively photostable compared with pyrethrin.

The most popular pyrethroid agent in equine products is permethrin.[25] Part of permethrin's desirability is its low toxicity, relative stability on exposure to ultraviolet light, and potential for use as a repellent. As with pyrethrins, the synthetic pyrethroids are often combined with other active agents, particularly repellents.

REPELLENTS

Although these chemicals are capable of keeping insects away, they need frequent applications (often, every few hours depending on temperature, humidity, the density of insects, the movement of the animal, and the drying effect of the wind). Compounds with repellent action include pyrethrin, permethrin, citronella, diethyltoluamide (DEET), ethohexadiol, dimethyl phthalate, butoxypropylene glycol, MGK-264, and ingredients in Skin-So-Soft (Avon) bath oil (some believe that the fragrance is the effective ingredient).

SULFUR

With the emphasis on newer, more effective drugs, it is sometimes forgotten that sulfur and its derivatives are excellent and safe parasiticides. The commercial lime sulfur solution (LymDyp, DVM Pharmaceuticals) is safe for horses of all ages; is an inexpensive effective treatment of infestations of nonfollicular mites; and is fungicidal, bactericidal, keratolytic, and antipruritic. A 28% lotion (Happy Jack Mange Medicine, Happy Jack, Inc.) and 10% sulfur ointment USP are other forms of sulfur medications These high concentration products can be irritating.

Sulfur is a natural parasiticide that is relatively nontoxic and environmentally safe. Its major drawback is the foul odor. It also stains jewelry and temporarily discolors hair, especially white hair. It is drying but only rarely irritating when used at a 2% concentration. A 2% to 5% lime sulfur solution is effective against *Sarcoptes*, *Psoroptes*, *Chorioptes*, chiggers, bird and straw mites, and lice.

Systemic Antiparasitic Agents

The use of systemic agents should be approached with knowledge regarding the parasite to be treated and, most important, the biology of the parasite. For example, feeding habits of the parasite may influence efficacy. Systemic agents are particularly valuable in treating obligate parasites that feed on blood or serum, such as *Sarcoptes*, *Psoroptes*, or *Demodex* mites. Parasites such as *Chorioptes bovis* and *Damalinia equi*, which feed on tissue debris, may not be killed. Systemics can be useful adjunctive treatments when dealing with nonobligate parasites. For example, bird and straw mites will be killed when they feed on a horse recently treated with ivermectin. However, unless the source of the infestation is eliminated, new mites will continue to reach the horse and the dermatitis will continue.

SYSTEMIC ENDECTOCIDES

These parasiticides were developed from macrocyclic lactones produced by the fermentation of various actinomyces. This class of drugs includes avermectins (ivermectin, doramectin, abamectin, selamectin) and milbemycins (milbemycin, moxidectin). At present, the product used most in equine dermatology is ivermectin. Preliminary studies suggest that all of these products may have equal efficacy when administered at the appropriate dosage. All partly act by potentiating the release and effects of GABA. GABA is a peripheral neurotransmitter in susceptible nematodes, arachnids, and insects. Avermectins and milbemycins are also agonists of glutamate-gated chloride channels. In mammals, GABA is limited to the central nervous system. Because these drugs do not cross the blood-brain barrier in most adult animals, they are relatively safe and have a wide margin between efficacy and mammalian toxicity. Their use in foals less than 4 months old is contra-indicated.[26] In general, these drugs are effective for nematodes, microfilaria, lice, and mites.

IVERMECTIN

Ivermectin is a derivative of avermectin B from fermentation products of a *Streptomyces avermitilis*.[23,25a,27,29] This drug is licensed for the treatment of various intestinal parasites, including pinworms, bots, summer sores caused by *Habronema* and *Draschia* spp., and *Onchocerca* spp. It is also highly effective in the treatment of sucking lice, chiggers, *Sarcoptes*, *Psoroptes*, *Demodex*, and other serum-feeding mites. A partial response is seen when biting lice or *Chorioptes* mites are treated. Ivermectin does not affect trematodes and cestodes, because GABA is not involved in neurotransmission in those species. Parasite paralysis is the main action of ivermectin, but it also suppresses reproduction. Ticks are not killed, but their egg production and molting are suppressed.

Ivermectin is rapidly absorbed orally and has a plasma resident time of up to 5 days.[25a,29] This is important because it does not have a rapid killing effect on susceptible parasites. The dosage used to treat all nonfollicular mites is 0.2 mg/kg at 14-day intervals.

MOXIDECTIN

Moxidectin (Quest, Fort Dodge) is derived from fermentation products of *Streptomyces cyaneo-griseus* subsp. *noncyanogenus*. It is marketed for the treatment of various intestinal parasites, including pinworms and bots. It is administered at 0.4 mg/kg orally. Its plasma resident time is approximately 18 days.[25a,29] Since it is equally as effective in treating onchocerciasis as is ivermectin,[204] the two products probably can be used interchangeably.

DORAMECTIN

Doramectin (Dectomax, Pfizer) is derived from fermentation of selected strains of *Streptomyces avermitilis*. In the United States, it is marketed for the treatment and control of various nematodes, mites, and lice in cattle and swine. In horses, it has a 3-day plasma resident time.[25a]

● MITES

Of the tens of thousands of mite species, only a relatively few species are parasitic.[3,22] Adult females lay a highly variable number of eggs each day and six-legged larvae hatch from them. They molt through one to three nymphal instars before a new adult develops. The life cycle varies from species to species and ranges from 8 to 28 days.

Except for demodicosis, the most serious mite infestations are recognized during the late winter and early spring. Crowding, prolonged stabling, and suboptimal nutrition all contribute to the relatively high mite burdens seen during this period. Environmental temperature also plays a role. Mite burdens and the animal's symptomatology will decrease and may disappear during a hot summer.

Older parasitology texts list a varying number of species for each genus of mite. In separate studies on *Psoroptes* and *Sarcoptes* mites from different species located on different continents, Zahler found that "different" species within the same genus differ phenotypically but not genotypically.[47,56] Since different species of *Psoroptes* mites (*P. ovis* and *P. cuniculi*) are known to interbreed,[47] it is likely that all species of nonfollicular mites within a given genus are related and have limited host specificity.

Erythematous, crusted papules develop where the nonfollicular mites feed or burrow. The animal's level of pruritus should be in proportion to the number of mites present. When the level of pruritus far exceeds the number of mites present, hypersensitivity to the mite or its excrement must be considered. This phenomenon is well documented in humans and companion animals.[17] Hypersensitive animals are extremely pruritic and it is difficult to demonstrate a mite on their body. In many instances a mite will not be found on the horse and the confirmation or negation of the diagnosis will be determined by the response to treatment. If a positive response is noted, all contact horses should be examined carefully and probably treated. Since the nonburrowing mites can be transferred by brushes or tack, it may be prudent to treat all horses in the same barn.

Psoroptic Mange

Psoroptic mange is a pruritic dermatitis and/or otitis externa of horses.[32-47]

CAUSE AND PATHOGENESIS

Psoroptes spp. mites are large (0.4 to 0.8 mm long) (Fig. 6-1) and nonburrowing and feed on tissue fluids.[46] Their life cycle on the host is completed in approximately 10 days. Median life expectancy of an adult female is about 16 days.[22] Off-host survival time is significantly influenced by local

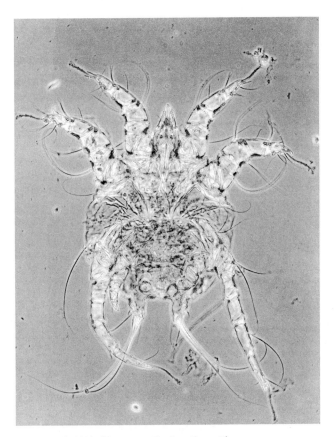

FIGURE 6-1. Psoroptes mite (×100). (*Courtesy Dr. Jay Georgi.*)

temperature and humidity.[43] Environmental conditions in the corners of stalls, organic debris and bedding, etc. can be very different from those in the rest of the barn with a prolonged off-host survival time. High temperatures and low humidity disfavor survival. In the typical barn, a 14- to 18-day off-host survival can be expected.[33] However, *P. ovis* and *P. cuniculi* maintained under various environmental conditions survived for up to 48 and 84 days, respectively.[35] The researchers suggested stable quarantine periods of 7 and 12 weeks, respectively.

As mentioned earlier, the number of distinct species with *Psoroptes* mites is probably much smaller than previously described. Presently, *P. equi*, *P. natalensis*, *P. ovis*, and *P. cuniculi* are reported to parasitize the horse.[3,22] Since *Psoroptes* mites show little-to-no host specificity and appear to be genetically homogeneous,[47] it is probably best not to assign a specific clinical presentation to any individual species (e.g., otoacariasis due to *P. cuniculi*).

Psoroptic mites from horses have not been reported to cause disease in humans. Since *Otodectes cynotis*, the ear mite of companion animals, behaves like a *Psoroptes* mite and can cause disease in humans,[17] it is likely that humans could be infested by *Psoroptes* mites from a horse if the horse had a high parasite burden and the contact time was long.

CLINICAL FEATURES

Transmission of *Psoroptes* mites is by direct or indirect contact. The incubation period varies from two to eight weeks. If the horse has been infested previously and became hypersensitive during the initial exposure, the incubation period will be shorter.

Clinical signs are quite variable. Infested horses may be asymptomatic or may show signs of ear disease, truncal dermatitis, or both. Signs of ear disease (Fig. 6-2) include head shaking, ear scratching, or head shyness, and the horse may have a lopeared appearance.[4-6,7-9,11-16,18-21] The dermatitis tends to be focused around the ears, mane, and tail. Pruritus is variable but can be intense. In mildly pruritic horses, the presentation will be of mane and tail seborrhea (see Chapter 11). In more pruritic horses, one sees nonfollicular papules, crusts, excoriation, and alopecia. In severe cases the entire topline may be involved.

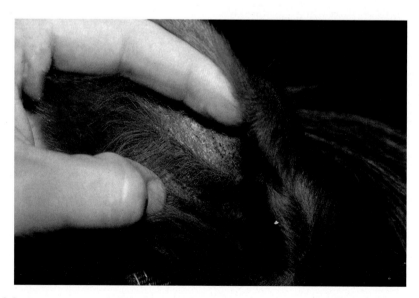

FIGURE 6-2. Psoroptic mange. Multiple crusted papules with scaling on the pinna of a headshy horse.

DIAGNOSIS

The differential diagnosis includes sarcoptic mange, chorioptic mange, lice, *Culicoides* hypersensitivity, and fly-bite dermatitis. Definitive diagnosis is based on history, physical examination, skin scrapings, and otoscopic examination. Body mites, depending on the degree of infestation, may be easily demonstrated in skin scrapings. Ear mites can be very difficult to demonstrate even with a thorough otoscopic examination (usually requires chemical restraint) and microscopic examination of material gathered from deep within the ear canal. Skin biopsy reveals varying degrees of superficial perivascular to interstitial dermatitis with numerous eosinophils.[45] Eosinophilic microabscesses and focal areas of epidermal edema, leukocytic exocytosis, and necrosis (epidermal "nibbles") may be found. Mites are rarely seen.

CLINICAL MANAGEMENT

There are various reports on the treatment of *Psoroptes* otoacariasis with numerous topical parasiticides.[34,36,38-40,42] After a thorough ear cleaning, the product is applied twice weekly for 3 weeks. If the horse is extremely head shy, owner compliance will be a problem and relapses can be expected. Since mites can survive outside the ear canal, simultaneous treatment of the body is recommended to prevent a relapse. Pyrethrin, pyrethroid, organophosphate, or lime sulfur sprays or dips can be effective when applied every 7 to 14 days for 3 to 4 weeks. Amitraz is contraindicated in horses.[24,30,31]

Ivermectin (200 µg/kg PO) is very effective in the treatment of psoroptic otoacariasis and/or dermatitis.[6,27,33] A single dosage rapidly decreases mite and egg counts with parasitologic cure 20 days after treatment. To ensure a cure, a second dose 14 days after the initial treatment is recommended. Since ivermectin and topical parasiticides do not kill eggs, the treated horse should be considered infectious for the first few weeks of treatment.

Sarcoptic Mange

Sarcoptic mange is a rare cause of pruritic dermatitis in horses.[48-56]

CAUSE AND PATHOGENESIS

Sarcoptes spp. mites (0.25 to 0.6 mm in diameter) (Fig. 6-3) tunnel through the epidermis and feed on tissue fluids and possibly epidermal cells.[3,22] The life cycle on the host is completed in 2 to 3 weeks. The mites are quite susceptible to drying and survive only a few days off the host. Transmission is by direct and indirect contact. The incubation period varies from a few hours to several weeks, depending on the method and severity of exposure and on prior sensitization of the host.

Sarcoptes scabiei mites are found on a number of different hosts. It is currently believed that all the various mites are genotypically identical.[56] Through adaptations for survival on a particular host, the mites may be phenotypically different but these phenotypic differences do not confer strict species specificity. Cross-infestation among animals and between animals and humans are not uncommon.

The primary clinical sign in sarcoptic mange of any species is pruritus, and much of this is associated with a hypersensitivity reaction to mite product(s).[11]

CLINICAL FEATURES

Once common,[91] equine sarcoptic mange is now rare throughout the world.[5,9,11,48-56] In the United States, equine sarcoptic mange has been eradicated. There are no apparent age, breed, or sex predilections. The chief clinical sign is pruritus, which usually begins on the head, ears, and neck, and spreads caudally.[10] Nonfollicular papules, crusts, excoriations, alopecia, and lichenification are usually seen.

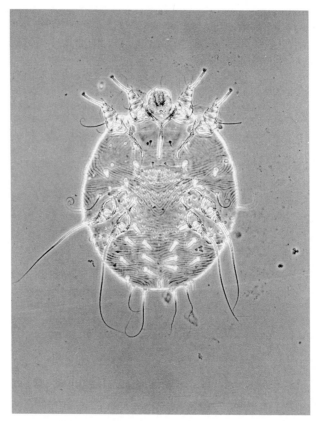

FIGURE 6-3. *Sarcoptes* mite (×100). (*Courtesy Dr. Jay Georgi.*)

DIAGNOSIS

The differential diagnosis includes psoroptic mange, lice, fly-bite dermatoses, and allergic skin disease. Definitive diagnosis is based on history, physical examination, skin scrapings, skin biopsy, and response to therapy. Mites are often very difficult to find in scrapings. If the pinnae are involved, scrapings along cranial edge should be most rewarding.

Skin biopsy reveals varying degrees of superficial perivascular to interstitial dermatitis with numerous eosinophils. Eosinophilic microabscesses and focal areas of epidermal edema, leukocytic exocytosis, and necrosis (epidermal nibbles) may be seen. Mites may be seen within parakeratotic scale crusts and in subcorneal "tunnels," but this is uncommon. Occasionally, deep perivascular dermatitis with lymphoid nodules may be seen.

Because of the frequently negative results of skin scrapings and skin biopsy, response to therapy is often employed in determining a presumptive diagnosis.[5] A positive response to treatment, especially when ivermectin was used, strongly supports the diagnosis of a nonfollicular mite infestation but does not differentiate scabies from the other mite infestations of the horse. Currently, none of the equine manges are specifically listed in the United States Department of Agriculture (USDA) list of Reportable Diseases and Conditions. Regulations in individual states may be more stringent. Since scabies would be disastrous if it entered the horse population, state or federal veterinarians should be contacted when scabies is confirmed or strongly suspected. Since quarantines might be imposed while the point source of infestation is determined, some barn owners will try to talk the veterinarian out of placing the call. If the clinical presentation is strongly suspicious of scabies, the regulatory agencies should be called.

CLINICAL MANAGEMENT

Sarcoptic mange is a severe disease. Intense, constant pruritus results in annoyance, irritability, anemia, secondary infections and myiasis, increased susceptibility to other diseases, and even death.[11] All animals that have come into contact with infected animals should be treated. Since mites can be transferred by grooming tools and other fomites, serious consideration should be given to the treatment of all horses in the barn.

In horses, sarcoptic mange may be treated with spray or dip applications of 0.5% malathion, 0.03% lindane, 0.06% coumaphos, 0.5% methoxychlor, or 2% lime sulfur.[4,11,22] At least two treatments at 14-day intervals should be administered. Ivermectin should be useful in equine sarcoptic mange.

Chorioptic Mange

Chorioptic mange (leg mange, tail mange, symbiotic scab, foot mange) is a common cause of dermatitis in horses.

CAUSE AND PATHOGENESIS

Chorioptic mites (0.3 to 0.5 mm long) (Fig. 6-4) are surface-inhabiting parasites that feed on epidermal debris.[63] The life cycle takes about 3 weeks and is completed on the host. Adult mites

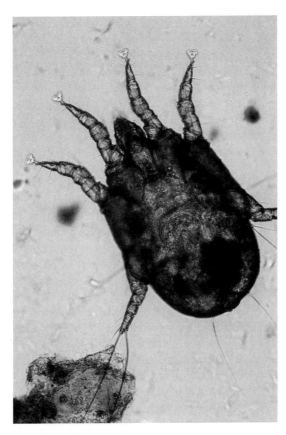

FIGURE 6-4. *Chorioptes* mite (×100).

can survive off-host for nearly 70 days depending on the presence of epidermal debris as a food source and the local environmental conditions.[35,60] Transmission is by direct and indirect contact.

Four species of mites, *Chorioptes bovis* (cattle), *C. caprae* (goats), *C. equi* (horses), and *C. ovis* (sheep) are listed in texts as individual species. However, once genotypic testing is performed, it is likely that *C. caprae*, *C. equi*, and *C. ovis* will be phenotypic variants of *C. bovis*.[22,63] Currently, interspecies transmission with chorioptic mange has not been reported and the mite has not been reported to cause human disease.

Mite populations are usually much larger during cold weather.[4,63] Thus, clinical signs are usually seen, or are more severe, in winter. This seasonality of mite populations and clinical signs is thought to be influenced by temperature, humidity, and wetting of the host. Hot and dry conditions decrease mite survival times. The signs of disease often spontaneously regress during summer when mite numbers become very small. During this clinically inapparent stage of infestation, mites may only be demonstrated around the coronet.

CLINICAL FEATURES

Chorioptic mange occurs in horses in most parts of the world.[4-6,7-9,11-16,18-21] In general, there are no apparent age, breed, or sex predilections.

In horses, *C. equi* infestations are most commonly seen in draft horses and other horses with feathered fetlocks, especially during winter.* Clinical signs are seen with the fetlocks, pasterns (Fig. 6-5), and tail being particularly affected. Pruritus may be intense or absent. Horses with widespread lesions have been seen.[11,41,57,62]

DIAGNOSIS

The differential diagnosis includes tail rubbing (insect hypersensitivity, food allergy, atopy, lice, oxyuriasis, or stable vice) and pastern dermatitis (see Chapter 15). Definitive diagnosis is based on history, physical examination, and examination of skin scrapings. During cool weather, *Chorioptes* spp. mites are usually easy to demonstrate. These mites are usually quite active and fast-moving. To prevent them from walking off the slide, the authors recommend using an insecticide-containing solution for the skin-scraping solution. Skin biopsy reveals variable degrees of superficial perivascular to interstitial dermatitis with numerous eosinophils. Eosinophilic epidermal microabscesses and focal epidermal necrosis, leukocytic exocytosis, and edema (epidermal nibbles) may be seen (Fig. 6-6).

CLINICAL MANAGEMENT

All animals that have come into contact with infected animals should be treated simultaneously. Horses stabled near the infected animal are at risk and probably should be treated.

Because of the mites' feeding habits, treatment with a conventional ivermectin regimen (e.g. 200 µg/kg PO q14d for 2 treatment) is ineffective. Treatment with higher dosages (300 µg/kg) at higher frequencies (weekly for 4 treatments) can improve the response rate, but therapeutic failures will occur.[59]

Topical treatments are labor-intensive but effective. To allow better access of agent to the mites, feathers should be clipped from draft horses. The most labor-intensive treatment involves bathing the horse with a 2% selenium sulfide shampoo.[58] The shampoo is prediluted with water (1:2), and the horse is bathed three times at 5-day intervals. After a 10-minute contact time, the lather is rinsed off and the horse is allowed to dry.

Over the years, various topical insecticides, applied at 7- to 14-day intervals, have proven to be effective. Effective agents include 0.25% crotoxyphos, 0.5% malathion, 0.5% methoxychlor,

---

*References 1, 4, 6, 9, 11, 13, 14, 21.

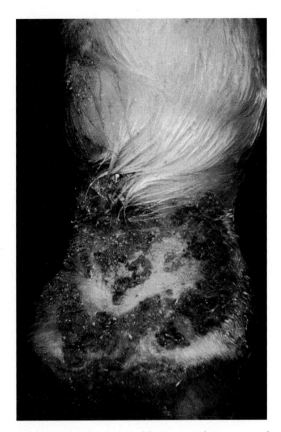

FIGURE 6-5. Chorioptic mange. Crusted, ulcerated lesions on the pastern of a draft horse. The feathers have been clipped.

0.06% coumaphos, and 2% lime sulfur.[6,12,22,27,28] Recently, a 0.25% fipronil spray has been shown to be curative in one treatment.[59] Horses to be treated are sprayed from the elbows and stifles down with 125 ml of product applied to each leg. To ensure cure, a second treatment in 3 to 4 weeks is recommended. This application constitutes an extra-label use of an EPA-registered pesticide.

Regardless of the treatment selected, the barn should be cleaned thoroughly. Grooming tools, tack, and other fomites should also be disinfected.

Demodectic Mange

Demodectic mange (follicular mange, demodicosis) is a follicular dermatosis rarely seen in horses.[64-78]

CAUSE AND PATHOGENESIS

Demodectic mites are normal residents of the skin in all large animals.[11,64,65,70,71] The mites live in hair follicles and sebaceous glands, are host-specific, and complete their entire life cycle on the host. The life cycle of most demodicids has not been carefully studied but is assumed to be completed in 20 to 35 days.

Under most environmental conditions, demodicids can survive only several minutes to a few days off the host.[73] Studies in cattle[69] and dogs[17] have shown that (1) demodectic mites are acquired during the first 2 to 3 days of life by direct contact with the dam, (2) animals delivered

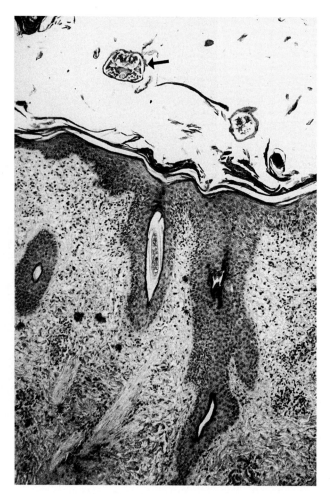

FIGURE 6-6. Chorioptic mange. Superficial perivascular to interstitial dermatitis with mite segments (*arrow*) in surface keratin.

by cesarean section and raised away from other animals did not harbor demodectic mites, and (3) confining normal adult animals with severely infested and diseased animals for several months did not produce disease in the normal animals. In addition, attempts to transmit clinical demodicosis to horses by direct contact and by applying mites to the skin were unsuccessful.[65] Thus, demodectic mange is not thought to be a contagious disease.

Because demodectic mites are normal residents of the skin, it is likely that animals manifesting clinical disease resulting from this parasite are, in some manner, immunocompromised. Demodicosis in dogs is known to occur as a result of immunosuppression (drugs or diseases) and genetic predilection (selective immunodeficiency?).[17] In large animals, many authors have suggested that clinical demodicosis probably occurs only in animals that are immunocompromised (debilitation, concurrent disease, poor nutrition, or stress).[75] In horses, demodicosis has been reported in association with chronic treatment with systemic glucocorticoids.[75]

CLINICAL FEATURES

Equine demodectic mange is recognized worldwide but is very rare in occurrence and has no apparent age, breed, or sex predilections.[9,11,21,65-67,70-78] The authors have rarely seen equine

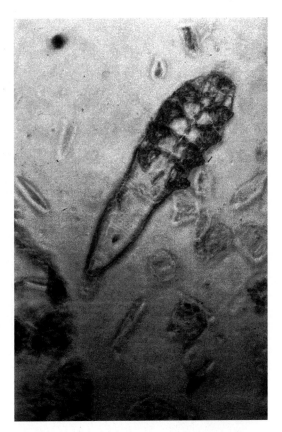

FIGURE 6-7. *Demodex equi* mite (×400).

demodicosis, and only in association with longterm glucocorticoid administration. Horses possess two species of demodicid mites: *D. caballi* (264 to 453 μm in length; eyelids and muzzle) and *D. equi* (179 to 236 μm in length; body) (Fig. 6-7). Clinical signs consist of usually asymptomatic alopecia and scaling, especially over the face (Fig. 6-8), neck, shoulders, and forelimbs. Papules and pustules may be seen.

DIAGNOSIS

The differential diagnosis includes other follicular dermatoses: staphylococcal folliculitis, dermatophytosis, and dermatophilosis. Definitive diagnosis is based on history, physical examination, skin scrapings, and skin biopsy. Alopecic, erythematous, scaling areas of skin should be squeezed firmly and scraped deeply until blood is drawn.

Skin biopsy reveals hair follicles distended to varying degrees with demodectic mites.[75] In many cases, there is minimal inflammatory response (Fig. 6-9). Alternatively, varying degrees of perifolliculitis, folliculitis, furunculosis, and foreign body granuloma formation may be seen.

CLINICAL MANAGEMENT

Because demodectic mange (1) is usually asymptomatic, (2) may spontaneously regress, and (3) has been refractory to most therapeutic agents and regimens, treatment is not usually attempted.[4,71,75] There is one report in which a horse received ivermectin for 15 days and was cured with that treatment.[77]

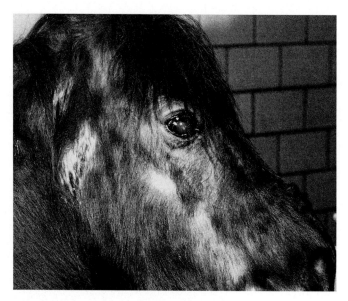

FIGURE 6-8. Demodectic mange. Patchy alopecia and scaling on the face.

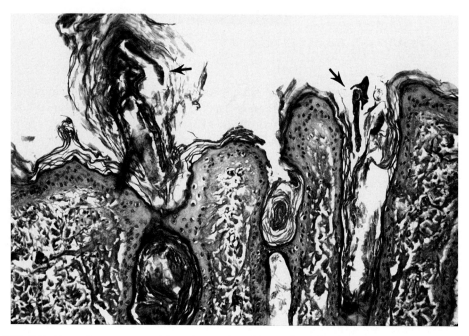

FIGURE 6-9. Demodectic mange. Mites (*arrows*) visible in the follicular keratin in a horse receiving glucocorticoids.

Trombiculidiasis

Trombiculidiasis (trombidiosis, chiggers, harvest mite, scrub itch mite, leg itch, heel bug) is a fairly common dermatosis of horses in many parts of the world.[79-81]

CAUSE AND PATHOGENESIS

Trombiculid adults and nymphs are free-living and feed on invertebrate hosts or plants.[3-5,22] Eggs are laid in the soil and hatch to larvae in approximately 1 week.[7] The larvae normally feed on tissue fluids of small rodents but are not host-specific and will attack horses and humans. Skin lesions produced by feeding larvae consist of papules and wheals. Because some animals manifest extreme pruritus, and other animals none, it is theorized that the pruritic animals may have developed a hypersensitivity reaction to larval salivary antigen(s).

Trombiculid larvae measure 0.2 to 0.4 mm in length and vary in color from red to orange to yellow. In North and South America, *Trombicula (Eutrombicula) alfreddugèsi* (Fig. 6-10) and *T. splendens* are important trombiculids that inhabit forested and swampy areas. *T. (Neotrombicula) autumnalis*—the harvest mite, or heel bug, of Europe and Australia—inhabits chalky soils, grasslands, and cornfields. *T. sarcina* is the blacksoil itch, or leg itch, mite of Australia.

Trombiculid larvae are usually active in summer and fall. After feeding (7 to 10 days), the larvae drop off the host to molt. The entire life-cycle typically takes 50 to 70 days.[3,22]

CLINICAL FEATURES

Trombiculidiasis generally occurs in the late summer and fall, when larvae are active.* The infestation is seen primarily in pastured animals, horses in infested paddocks, or horses taken on trail rides through infested fields and woods. There are no apparent age, breed, or sex predilections.

Skin lesions consist of papules and wheals at the site of larval attachment. Typical sites include the muzzle, nares, false nostril, face, ears, neck, and distal limbs. Horses pastured in tall grass may have lesions on the ventral thorax or abdomen. Close examination of an early lesion reveals a brightly colored, typically orange or red, chigger in the center of the papular lesion. Infested

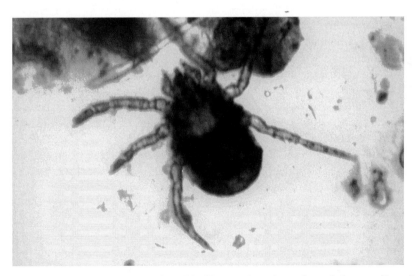

FIGURE 6-10. *Trombicula (Eutrombicula) alfreddugèsi* (×100). Six-legged larva collected in a skin scraping.

---

*References 1, 4, 5, 9, 11, 13, 14, 21, 79, 81.

horses may be asymptomatic or may be variably pruritic. With involvement of the nares, false nostril, or ears, the horse may present for sneezing or headshaking.[80] With a massive infestation or marked pruritus, cutaneous edema, exudation, crusting, and ulceration may be prominent.

DIAGNOSIS

If the larvae are still attached to the skin, the diagnosis is straightforward. Without visible larvae, the differential diagnosis includes chorioptic mange, psoroptic mange, sarcoptic mange, contact dermatitis, forage mites, biting flies, staphylococcal folliculitis, and dermatophilosis. Definitive diagnosis is based on history, physical examination, and demonstration of the trombiculids grossly or microscopically, or both, in skin scrapings. Because the larvae only feed on the animal for a short period, demonstrating the trombiculids may be impossible in chronic cases. Presumptive diagnosis is then based on the time of year, exposure to trombiculid-infested areas, physical findings, and response to therapy. Skin biopsy reveals varying degrees of superficial perivascular to interstitial dermatitis with numerous eosinophils.

CLINICAL MANAGEMENT

Treatment of trombiculidiasis may not be necessary, since the disease is self-limiting if further contact with the trombiculids is avoided. In severe cases, a single application (dip or spray) of a topical parasiticidal agent such as lime sulfur or a pyrethrin will kill any larvae still feeding.[4,22,27,28] In companion animals, monthly treatment with a 0.25% fipronil spray prevents reinfestation.[17] Severely pruritic animals may benefit from a few days' treatment with systemic glucocorticoids.

Forage Mites

Mites from the families Acaridae (Tyroglyphidae) and Pediculoididae (Pyemotidae) may cause dermatitis in animals and humans.[4,82-85] Because these free-living mites normally feed on organic matter (Acaridae) or insects in hay and grain (Pediculoididae), the dermatoses they produce are often called grain itch, straw itch, cheese itch, copra itch, and so on. The life cycle of these mites is influenced by temperature and humidity with populations typically lowest in winter.[82]

These so-called forage mites (*Pediculoides ventricosus, Pyemotes tritici; Acarus farinae*) have been reported to cause pruritic or nonpruritic papulocrustous dermatoses in horses in areas of skin that contact the contaminated foodstuff (muzzle, head, neck, limbs, ventral thorax, and abdomen).[13,14,83-85] Horses stabled under a hay loft are at risk for developing topline disease when mites fall from the loft. In humans, forage mites produce a pruritic papular to urticarial dermatosis in contact areas within 12 to 16 hours after attacking.

The differential diagnosis includes sarcoptic mange, psoroptic mange, chorioptic mange, contact dermatitis, trombiculidiasis, and fly bites. Definitive diagnosis is based on history, physical examination, and microscopic demonstration of the mites (0.3 to 0.6 mm long) in skin and forage samples. The authors find that mite recovery rates increase when a flea comb, rather than a scalpel blade, is used to collect the skin samples. The material collected in the comb can be examined directly or can be treated like feces and subjected to whatever floatation technique is used to identify internal parasites. Skin biopsy reveals varying degrees of superficial perivascular to interstitial dermatitis with numerous eosinophils.

Therapy consists of eliminating the contaminated forage. The dermatosis resolves spontaneously within a few days.[84] Severely pruritic animals may benefit from a few days of treatment with systemic glucocorticoids.

Poultry Mite

The poultry mite, *Dermanyssus gallinae* (Fig. 6-11), is known to occasionally attack horses and humans.[11,14] Adult mites live and lay eggs in cracks and crevices in the walls of poultry houses or

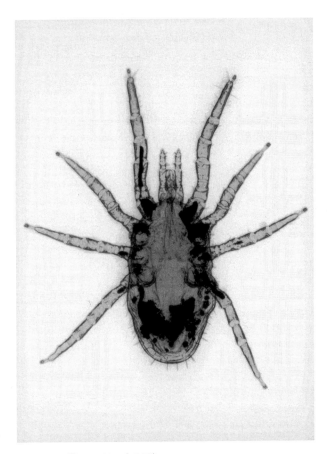

FIGURE 6-11. *Dermanyssus gallinae* mite (×100).

in bird nests. Adult mites suck blood and are 0.6 to 1 mm in length. Lesions consist of pruritic papules and crusts in contact areas (especially limbs, muzzle, and ventrum). Topline disease can be seen if birds are nesting above the horse's stall.

Diagnosis is based on history, physical examination, and demonstration of the mites in skin scrapings or the environment. Since the mite may be difficult to demonstrate on the horse, the areas it frequents (e.g., run-ins, stall, etc.) should be inspected carefully. Therapy involves eradication of the mite from the premises by removal of nests or spraying with an approved environmental pesticide. A one-time treatment of the horse with a parasiticidal spray or dip will kill the mites feeding on the horse.

Miscellaneous Mite Infestations

There is one report in which the hypopodes, a deutonymph stage of mites in the suborder Astigmata, family Glicyphagidae, caused skin disease in a horse.[85a] The horse had an acute onset of a pruritic dermatitis of her face and neck with hypotrichosis, excoriations, and crusting. Small deutonymphs, but no adults, were found on skin scraping. The horse was treated daily for 3 days with a topical 3% trichlorfon solution and was cured.

Since adult mites were not available, the mite's genus and species could not be determined. Since the hypopodes lack mouth parts, the reason for the horse's pruritus is uncertain. An allergic response to body fluids of crushed deutonymphs is possible.

● TICK INFESTATION

Ticks are an important ectoparasite of animals all around the world (Table 6-1).[86-96]

Cause and Pathogenesis

Ticks may harm their hosts by (1) injuries done by bites, which may predispose to secondary infections and myiasis, (2) sucking blood (a single adult female tick may remove 0.5 to 2.0 ml blood), (3) transmitting various viral, protozoal, rickettsial, and bacterial diseases,[10,89,90-91] and (4) causing tick paralysis.[10] Economic losses through diagnostic, therapeutic, or control programs may be sizable.

Argasid (soft) ticks, such as *Otobius megnini* and *Ornithodorus spp.*, lay their eggs in sheltered spots, such as cracks in poles, under boxes or stones, and in crevices in walls. Larvae and nymphs suck blood and lymph and drop off the host to become adults.[3,22]

Ixodid (hard) ticks, such as *Dermacentor albipictus* and *Amblyomma americanum*, lay their eggs in sheltered areas, such as wall crevices, cracks in wood near the ground, and under stones and clods of soil. Larvae (seed ticks) climb onto grass and shrubbery and wait for a suitable host to pass by.[3,22]

According to the number of hosts required during their life cycle, ticks can be classified into three groups: (1) one-host ticks (all three instars engorge on the same animal; two ecdyses take place on the host), (2) two-host ticks (larva engorges and molts on host, and nymph drops off after engorging; nymph molts on the ground, and the imago seeks a new host), and (3) three-host ticks (require a different host for every instar, drop off host each time after engorging, and molt on the ground). Most ticks found on horses in the United States are three-host ticks. Each species of tick is adapted to certain ranges of temperature and moisture. In general, ticks are not especially host-specific. Local reactions to tick bites are variable, depending on the properties of the tick in question and on the host-parasite relationship.

Clinical Features

Ticks are important ectoparasites of horses.[6,11,13,14,86-96] Tick-related dermatoses are most commonly seen in spring and summer. Although ticks may attack any portion of the body surface, favorite areas include the ears, false nostril, face, neck, mane, axillae, groin, distal limbs, and tail. Initial skin lesions consist of papules, pustules, wheals, and, occasionally, nodules centered around a tick. These primary lesions develop crusts, erosions, ulcers, and alopecia. Pain and pruritus are variable.

Otobius megnini (the spinose ear tick) induces an otitis externa, characterized by considerable irritation, inflammation, and a waxy discharge. Secondary bacterial infection is common. Affected animals may exhibit head tilting, head shaking, and ear rubbing and appear lopeared. Some infested horses develop muscle cramping and discomfort manifested by stiffness and sweating.[92]

In Australia, a hypersensitivity syndrome in horses is associated with the larvae of *Boophilus microplus*.[11,14,93] Most cases occur in late summer or early fall, and only sensitized horses are affected. The onset of clinical signs is rapid and may be evident within 30 minutes of infestation. Affected horses exhibit multiple papules and wheals, which are most numerous on the lower legs and muzzle. Close examination reveals larval ticks embedded in a serous exudate in the center of the lesions. Pruritus is intense.

Diagnosis

A definitive diagnosis of tick infestation is simply based on demonstrating the ticks. Specific identification of the ticks is of value in determining the control measures required (Figs. 6-12 and 6-13).

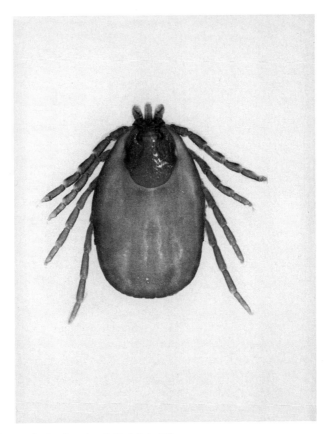

FIGURE 6-12. *Rhipicephalus* female adult tick (×20).

Skin biopsy findings vary with the duration of the lesion and the host-parasite relationship.[86] Reactions in primary infestations are characterized by varying degrees of focal epidermal necrosis and edema, with the subjacent dermis showing edema and infiltration with neutrophils, eosinophils, and mononuclear cells. Reactions in previously infested hosts are characterized by marked intra-epidermal vesiculopustular dermatitis (marked spongiosis, microabscesses containing eosinophils and basophils), marked subepidermal edema, and marked dermal infiltration with basophils, eosinophils, and mononuclear cells. Persistent nodular reactions are distinguished by diffuse dermatitis in which lymphohistiocytic cells predominate, with lesser numbers of eosinophils and plasma cells and frequent lymphoid nodules or follicles (pseudolymphomatous reaction). In all histopathologic forms of tick-bite reactions, tick mouthparts (chelicerae and hypostomes) may be found penetrating the epidermis or embedded in the dermis or both.

Clinical Management

Therapy is usually directed at temporarily reducing the tick population.[3,6,7,10,28] Total eradication is usually very difficult and is generally reserved for vectors of economically important infectious diseases. Suitable insecticides are applied to the entire body surface according to the label indications or in an as-needed fashion if application frequency is not specified. One-host ticks may require only two to three applications, whereas multiple-host ticks often require periodic applications throughout tick season. Knowledge of the insecticidal resistance of the local tick population is extremely important.

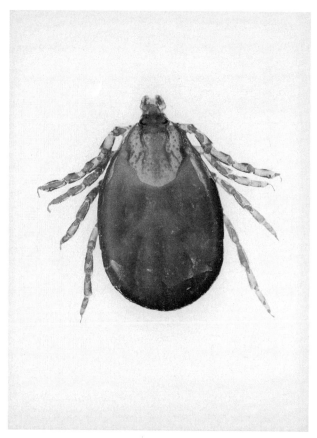

FIGURE 6-13. *Dermacentor* adult tick (×20).

Treatment of *O. megnini* ear infestations is relatively simple.[14] As many ticks as possible should be mechanically removed and the ear cleared of exudate. Xylol (two parts) with pine oil (17 parts) has been a popular, effective otic tickicide and repellent when applied every 3 to 4 weeks. In addition, many commercial otic miticides and tickicides are effective.

Other methods of tick control having variable application and efficacy include: (1) burning of pasture, (2) land cultivation, (3) repellents, and (4) sterile hybrids.[3,6,7,10,28]

● SPIDERS

Spiders have poison glands in their cephalothorax that open through pores on the tips of the chelicerae. They apparently attack large animals rarely.

In Australia, *Ixeuticus robustus* (black house spider, window spider) has been known to bite horses.[13,14] The spider (5 to 10 mm in diameter) is commonly found in unused buildings and older stables, in characteristic funnel-like webs. It is nocturnal, often being found on stable walls and floors at night. Edematous plaques are produced by spider bites, usually on the neck and body of affected horses. The condition occurs overnight. Diagnosis is based on history, physical examination, presence of spiders, and elimination of other causes. Treatment consists of local cold packs and systemic glucocorticoids and antihistamines for 2 to 3 days. Control consists of avoiding infested premises or having a commercial exterminator power-spray the premises.

• LICE INFESTATION

Infestation with lice (pediculosis) is a common cause of skin disease in horses throughout the world.

Cause and Pathogenesis

Lice are highly host-specific, obligate parasites that spend their complete life cycle (20 to 40 days) on the host.[3,4,22,97-99] Poultry lice will feed on horses.[99] Biting lice feed on exfoliated epithelium and cutaneous debris. Sucking lice feed on blood and tissue fluid. Nits 1 to 2 mm long are attached to hairs by a clear adhesive secretion by female lice (3 to 6 mm in length). Under favorable environmental conditions, lice can live 2 to 3 weeks off the host, but less than 7 days is more typical. Transmission is by direct and indirect contact.

Lice populations are much larger and, therefore, clinical signs most obvious in winter. This seasonality of pediculosis is related to lower skin and hair temperatures, longer winter coats, overcrowding, poor nutrition, and possibly other stresses associated with cold weather.

Clinical Features

In horses, lice are common ectoparasites in most parts of the world.[*] There are no apparent age, breed, or sex predilections. Biting lice (*Damalinia equi*) (Fig. 6-14) prefer the dorsolateral trunk, whereas sucking lice (*Haematopinus asini*) (Fig. 6-15) favor the mane, tail, and fetlocks.[10] Clinical signs depend on the parasite burden and site of infestation. Varying degrees of scaling, dishevelment of the coat, alopecia, and pruritus occur (Fig. 6-16, A). In most cases, the pruritus is mild to moderate.

Diagnosis

The differential diagnosis of pediculosis includes psoroptic mange, chorioptic mange, flybite dermatoses, trombiculidiasis, forage mites, seborrheic skin disease, and shedding. Definitive diagnosis is based on history, physical examination, and demonstration of lice or nits, or both. Skin biopsy reveals varying degrees of superficial perivascular to interstitial dermatitis with numerous eosinophils. Focal areas of epidermal necrosis, edema, and leukocytic exocytosis (epidermal nibbles) as well as eosinophilic intraepidermal microabscesses may be seen.

Clinical Management

Treatment of pediculosis is usually easy and effective. Treatment selection depends on the number of horses affected and the time of year. In warm weather or with heated bathing facilities in the barn, insecticidal shampoos or 1% selenium sulfide shampoo can be very effective.[58,98] Between 150 and 450 ml of shampoo is used on the horse every tenth day for a total of three baths. A 5-10-minute contact time is needed. The lice will disappear after the first bath, but the nits can persist until after the second.

With a winter infestation or the involvement of large numbers of horses, insecticides typically are used. The agent can be applied as a spray, pour-on, or powder. Most currently marketed produces for the horse contain pyrethrins or pyrethoids. Products containing Rabon, malathion, coumaphos, or sulfur are also available.[25] Label directions should be followed. In most cases, two applications at 14-day intervals is sufficient.[27] Pour-on permethrin products at or above 1% can irritate some horses.[99] Recently, a 0.25% fipronil spray has been shown to be curative with one application.[97]

---

[*]References 1, 4, 6, 9, 21, 157, 158.

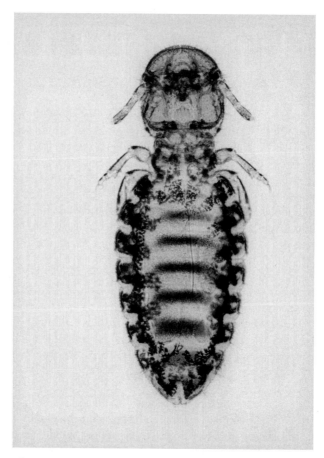

FIGURE 6-14. *Damalinia equi* adult louse (×50).

● FLEAS

Fleas are a rarely reported parasite of the horse. Since fleas show little host specificity and many barns have cats and kittens with heavy infestations, flea bites on horses may be more common than recognized. Adult fleas are blood-sucking, wingless, laterally compressed insects 2 to 4 mm long.[3,17] Eggs (about 0.5 mm long) are deposited on the host but fall to the ground for development. The viability, longevity, and length of the life cycle of the flea are highly dependent on temperature and humidity. In general, temperatures between 20° and 30° C with a relative humidity less than 70% are ideal. Dryness (less than 33% relative humidity), high heat (greater than 35° C) or extreme cold (less than 8° C) are lethal to flea larvae in a short period of time.[17] Remember that the local environmental conditions in a bedded stall or riding ring can be very different than those found in aisle ways or paddocks. Adult fleas can survive in the environment for long periods provided that they have not started to feed. A displaced adult will die quickly if it does not find a new host.

Fleas are not host-specific and have been reported to infest horses (*Ctenocephalides felis felis, Tunga penetrans, Echidnophaga gallinacea*).[10,11,100] Foals, ill animals, and those not brushed regularly will have the highest flea burden. Since approximately 70 female fleas will consume 1 ml of blood per day, heavily infested animals can become anemic. Dermatologic signs include varying

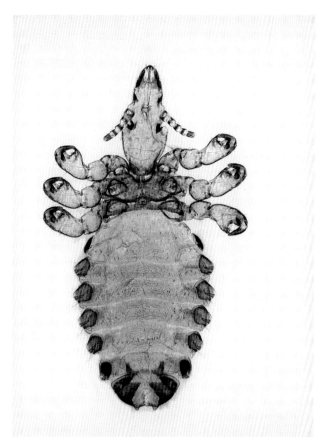

FIGURE 6-15. *Haematopinus asini* adult louse (×50).

degrees of rubbing, scratching, and chewing, as well as alopecia, excoriations, nonfollicular papules, and crusts. The face, distal limbs, and trunk are typical sites of involvement.

Environmental management is crucial in flea control. First, the point source of the barn's infestation must be identified and treated. Next, the horse's stall or run-in should be stripped of its bedding and then sprayed with an approved area product that contains both an adulticide plus a growth regulator. Products licensed for kennel use can be used in barns.

With eradication of the flea from the barn, treatment of the horses is easy. Regular brushing and combing will remove most adults. The application of most fly sprays will kill the few fleas that the grooming missed.

• FLIES

Domestic livestock are liable to almost perpetual attack from a variety of flies.[1,7,10,14,22]

Biting Flies

MOSQUITOES

Mosquitoes (*Aedes* spp., *Anopheles* spp., *Culex* spp.) are important nuisances and vectors of numerous viral and protozoal diseases to large animals throughout the world.[1,3,10,22]

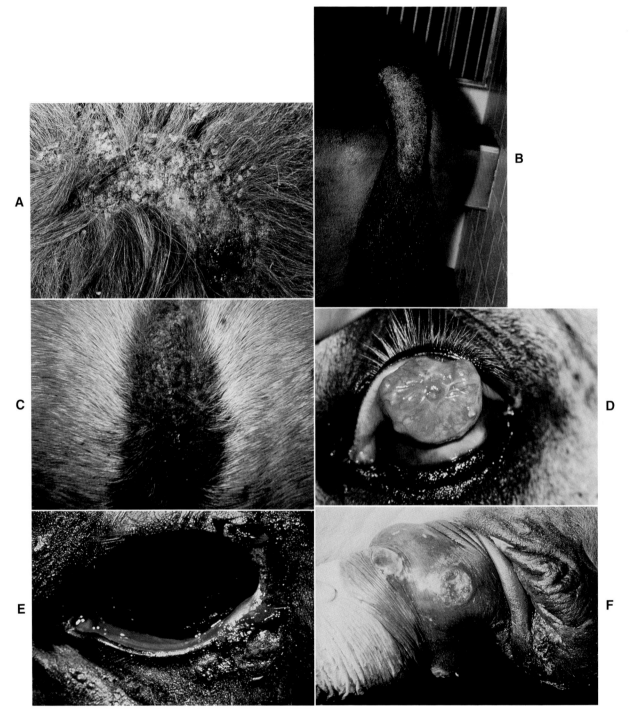

FIGURE 6-16. A, Pediculosis. Alopecia, crusting, and excoriation over the back of a horse. Note the lice. **B,** *Culicoides* hypersensitivity. Traumatic hair loss at the tail head. **C,** Ventral midline dermatitis. Linear alopecia and crusting near the umbilicus. Note punctate ulcers. (Courtesy A. A. Stannard.) **D,** Habronemiasis. Granulomatous mass on the palpebral conjunctiva. Note multiple yellow granules on surface. **E,** Habronemiasis. Multiple ulcerated, crusted papules on the eyelid and conjunctiva. (Courtesy T. J. Kern.) **F,** Halicephalobiasis. Multiple ulcerated papules and nodules on the prepuce.

Anopheles and *Culex* sp. mosquitoes lay their eggs on water and, once mature, will hatch even if the water disappears. *Aedes* spp. lay their eggs on moist vegetable material and require the presence of water for hatching to occur. The life cycle varies from 3 to 20 days. Mosquito populations are largest during warm weather and after rainfall. Adults are strong fliers and may fly distances up to several kilometers. They tend to feed (suck blood) at night.

Mosquito bites produce wheals and papules that are variably pruritic or painful.[13,14] Unlike the papules and wheals caused by the bites of many other insects, close examination of mosquito bites reveals no central crust. Individual lesions resolve spontaneously in 1 to 2 days. Large swarms of mosquitoes cause animals to be very restless at night.

Control measures are usually directed against both the larval and the adult stages.[7,10,22] Areas in which stagnant water accumulates, such as old tires, should be eliminated. Since breeding sites are on or near water, larvicidal and adulticidal products must be selected carefully. The local Department of Environmental Conservation should be contacted to see which products, if any, can be used in a particular situation. Since repellent sprays have a very short duration of action, treatment of the individual horse is unrewarding. If mosquitoes are a significant problem on a farm, the owner may want to consider using one of the newly marketed propane mosquito traps. These traps produce CO_2 and water vapor, which attract feeding females. As they approach the trap, they are pulled inside, where they die. Some traps claim coverage of 1 acre or more.

CULICOIDES GNATS

Culicoides spp. (biting midges, gnats, "punkies," sandflies, "no-see-ums") (Fig. 6-17) are important nuisances and vectors of various diseases to large animals throughout the world.[3,11,22]

There are over 1000 species of *Culicoides* gnats. Although probably not absolute, individual species of gnats have strong host preference. In the United States, *Culicoides spinosus, C. stellifer, C. variipenis,* and *C. venustus* are most problematic for horses. *Culicoides brevitarsus (robertsi), C. obsoletus, C. peregrinus, C. pulicaris, C. nubeculosus, C. circumscriptus, C. imicola, C. puncticollis* are species important in other parts of the world (see Chapter 8).[104,115,121]

The gnats are small (1 to 4 mm) in size and typically are heard but not seen, hence the name "no-see-ums." Eggs are laid in damp marshy areas, on decaying vegetation, or in manure.[3,22] The larvae of most species are aquatic and have a very variable rate of development. Most species overwinter in the larval state.

Adult gnats are blood suckers. Hosts are located not only by sight but also by body temperature, heart sound, and smell. Host odors that attract gnats include CO_2, lactic acid, and octenol.[105] Although adults are capable of flying long distances,[104] they are weak fliers and tend to feed close to their breeding grounds. Most species feed from dusk to dawn. Air that is warm (>10° C), humid, and still is ideal for feeding.

In addition to causing skin disease, *Culicoides* gnats are vectors for *Onchocerca cervicalis* and various infectious agents.

Clinical signs depend on the species of gnat involved, the gnat burden, and the degree of hypersensitivity of the host. *Culicoides* hypersensitivity (see Chapter 8) is a common and severe allergic condition of horses worldwide, as long as the local climate supports a gnat population. Because of their hypersensitivity, allergic horses react sooner, more dramatically, and longer to gnat bites.

Gnat populations start to develop from preexisting larvae in the spring and increase in numbers during the summer provided that it is not too hot or dry. Different species of gnats have preferred feeding sites on the horses' body. The two most common are the topline (ears, mane, back, and tail region) and the ventrum.[1,2,4-6,7-9,11-16,18-21] The bites are painful and pruritic and develop into papules and wheals. Nonallergic horses either show no clinical signs or only mild ones if the gnat population is exceedingly high. The number of nonrelated horses affected can be used

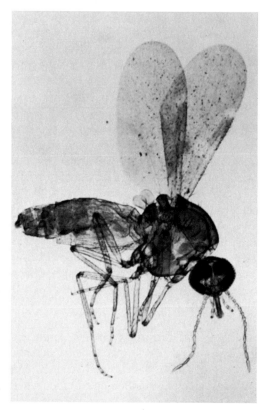

FIGURE 6-17. *Culicoides* gnat. (*Courtesy Dr. Jay Georgi.*)

to gauge the gnat burden. Because there is a genetic predisposition to develop *Culicoides* hypersensitivity,[20] it is unusual to have more than one allergic horse in a small group of unrelated horses. If multiple horses in the herd are showing clinical signs, the gnat population probably is high and control will be difficult.

If a horse is going to respond to the gnat bite, it will do so by itching. Since other mosquitoes and flies are probably also feeding on these horses, it can be difficult to attribute the nonallergic horse's summer pruritus to *Culicoides* gnats. One should be suspicious when the horse is rubbing its mane and/or tail (see Fig. 6-16, *B*).

Skin biopsy reveals a perivascular to interstitial dermatitis with eosinophils and lymphocytes.[121] The inflammation may be superficial or also involve deep vessels. Focal areas of spongiosis and eosinophilic exocytosis; eosinophilic mural and/or luminal folliculitis; or palisaded eosinophilic granulomas can also be seen (see Chapter 8).

Control of these gnats is difficult, especially when the horse is allergic to them. Although removal of manure and decaying vegetation won't eliminate the gnats, it will help reduce the local population and should be encouraged. The propane mosquito trap mentioned earlier can have octenol strips added to increase its attractiveness to mosquitoes and gnats. Other traps that are held at body temperature and contain octanol are available and specifically tout their efficacy in "no-see-um" control. No data are offered to support the claims.

When the gnats cannot be eliminated, the dermatitis can be prevented or minimized by the horse wearing a body suit, repeated application of a fly spray or pour-on, or modification of the horse's lifestyle. Body suits, although effective, are not widely used. Since many fly sprays or pour-ons have a short duration of action, especially when the horse is sweating, the best results are seen with a combination of parasiticidal application and management changes.

Since the gnats feed primarily from dusk to dawn, the horse should be stabled during those times. The stall should be in the middle of the barn since the gnats rarely enter buildings.[104] However, the gnat will enter the stall through a window. Old recommendations included screening the window with a 32-mesh screen and the installation of a time-operated insecticide spray system. Recently the authors have recommended that the owner put a 20-inch window fan in the stall window. Since the gnats are weak fliers,[7,10] a strong wind stream will keep the gnats from landing. A similar set up can be developed in a paddock when no barn is available. A large barn-sized fan is placed in the paddock to create the wind stream. Some horses quickly recognize the benefits of the wind and will voluntarily stand in the air flow.

BLACK FLIES

Simulium spp. (black flies, buffalo gnats, sandflies) are severe nuisances and vectors of various viral, protozoal, and filariid diseases to horses throughout the world.[1,3,11,14,22]

Simulid eggs are laid on stones or plants just below the surface of the water in running streams.[3,22] Eggs hatch in 6 to12 days, and they attach themselves to a stone or vegetation near fast flowing water. Typical adult life span is 2 to 3 weeks. Black fly populations are largest and most active in spring and early summer, especially in the morning and evening.

Adult black flies (1 to 5 mm long) are strong fliers and can travel over 10 km to feed. Swarms can travel over 100 km to feed provided that the air currents are correct.[22] They, like other insects, are attracted to host CO_2 and other odors. Black flies are blood suckers and vicious biters. Their saliva contain allergens and a heat-, alcohol-, and ether-stable toxin.[3,14,22] The toxin causes increased capillary permeability. With a large number of bites, significant intravascular fluid loss can occur with resultant cardiorespiratory dysfunction.

Black flies cause great annoyance and irritation and even deaths in all large animal species.[1,6,7,10,114] Simulid bites (*S. pecuarum* and *S. venustum* in the United States) cause painful papules and wheals, which often become vesicular, hemorrhagic, and necrotic. Favorite biting sites are in thinly haired areas, which included the face, ears, neck, ventrum, and legs. Localization of lesions to the intermandibular skin of horses may be seen. Simulid bites have been incriminated in the pathogenesis of equine aural plaques (see Chapter 16). Black flies may also be an important cause of insect hypersensitivity in horses (see Chapter 8). Horses caught in a swarm can be depressed and weak with tachypnea, tachycardia, and weak pulse. Without prompt treatment, shock and death can result.

Skin biopsy reveals varying degrees of superficial perivascular to interstitial dermatitis with numerous eosinophils. Focal areas of epidermal necrosis (nibbles), purpura, and subepidermal hemorrhagic bullae may be seen.

Control of simulids is difficult because the adults can fly long distances.° Stabling during the day and frequent applications of repellents to animals are helpful, whenever possible or practical. Treatment of severe cutaneous reactions is accomplished with systemic glucocorticoids.

HORSE FLIES

Tabanids (*Tabanus* spp., *Chrysops* spp., and *Haematopota* spp.), commonly called "horseflies," "deerflies," or "breeze flies," are large (up to 25 mm long) flies that cause great economic losses worldwide through their disturbing effects as nuisances and through transmission of various viral, protozoal, bacterial, and filariid diseases.[6,7,10]

°References 7, 10, 14, 22, 27, 28.

350 • Parasitic Diseases

Fed females lay their eggs on the leaves or stems of vegetation overhanging water.[10,22] After 4 to 7 days the eggs hatch and the first-stage larvae move to damp areas to complete the life cycle. Tabanids have a very protracted life cycle (10 to 42 weeks) and can hibernate if environmental conditions are unsatisfactory. Adults typically live 2 to 4 weeks. Fly populations are largest in summer and most active on hot, sultry days. Adult tabanids are blood-suckers and vicious biters. Twenty to 30 flies can take approximately 100 ml of blood in a 6-hour period of feeding.

Horseflies cause great annoyance and irritation.[6,11,14,114,125] Their loud buzzing spooks horses and will make them stop grazing. Tabanid bites produce painful, pruritic papules and wheals with a central ulcer and hemorrhagic crust. Favorite biting sites are the ventrum, legs, neck, and withers. When the fly stops feeding, rivulets of blood will appear on the skin, attracting various nonbiting flies.

Control of tabanids is very difficult.[6,7,10] Fly sheets will prevent truncal feeding, but the flies usually find some uncovered area to feed on. When possible or practical, stabling during the day and frequent applications of repellents to animals are helpful.

STABLE FLIES

Stomoxys calcitrans, the stable fly, is a cosmopolitan cause of annoyance and disease transmission (viral, protozoal, and helminthic).[3,22]

After a blood meal, the fly rests on a barn wall, fence, or other structure. Eggs are laid in wet straw, bedding, or manure. Aging manure is more attractive to stable flies.[22] The life cycle is temperature-dependent but usually is about 4 weeks in warm weather.

Stable flies cause great annoyance and irritation.[6,7,10] They are strong fliers that feed during the day. Stable fly bites cause pruritic and painful papules and wheals with a central crust. Favorite biting sites are the neck, back, chest, groin, and legs.[124] *Stomoxys calcitrans* may be one cause of insect hypersensitivity (see Chapter 8) in horses.

Control measures are directed at destroying breeding places and the use of residual environmental sprays and aerosols.[6,12,22,27,28] Regular (at least twice weekly) removal of moist bedding, hay, and manure, along with preventing the accumulation of weed heaps, grass cuttings, and vegetable refuse, is very helpful.

HORN FLIES

Haematobia (Lyperosia) spp. flies, the horn flies, are a ubiquitous cause of annoyance and disease transmission (protozoal and helminthic)[3,22] in horses.

Horn flies are small (3 to 4 mm), strong flying, blood-sucking insects that spend their entire adult life on the host. Fed females leave the host briefly to lay their eggs in fresh cow manure. Eggs laid in horse manure will not develop.[7,10,22] With a 10- to 14-day life cycle, the fly population can be very large in the summer. The preferred feeding site of the fly varies with the temperature and sun exposure. On sunny, warm (>22° C) days, the flies feed on the ventrum, whereas the topline is favored in rainy or cool weather.

Horn flies cause great annoyance and irritation.[6,7,10] Bites produce pruritic to painful papules and wheals with a central crust, which occur over the dorsum or ventrum. In horses, *H. irritans* is a cause of ventral midline dermatitis in the United States. Since each fly feeds 20 to 30 times each day, anemia can occur with a large fly burden.

Control of horn flies is much easier than that of other flies. Removal of cow manure interrupts the life cycle. Since horn flies are strong fliers, they can seek out horses from adjacent cattle farms. Because the adult fly rarely leaves its host, daily application of a fly spray should control the infestation. Since some strains have developed a resistance to pyrethroids,[106,113] spray selection must be individualized.

EQUINE VENTRAL MIDLINE DERMATITIS

Ventral midline dermatitis is a distinctive, common, fly-related dermatosis of horses.* The condition is caused by the bites of *Haematobia* (*Lyperosia*) *irritans* (the horn fly) and *Culicoides* spp. gnats. Thus, the dermatosis is quite seasonal, corresponding to fly season (spring to fall). Ventral midline dermatitis occurs most commonly in horses over 4 years of age, with no apparent breed or sex predilections.

Clinical signs consist of one to several sharply demarcated areas of punctate ulcers, hemorrhagic crusts, thickening, and alopecia on the ventral midline (see Fig. 6-16, *C*). The umbilical area is most commonly affected, but lesions may occur anywhere on the ventral midline, thorax to abdomen. Leukoderma is commonly seen. The majority of horses on the premises should be affected. Pruritus varies from intense to minimal, possibly reflecting the presence or absence of a hypersensitivity reaction to fly salivary antigen(s) in a given horse.

Diagnosis is based on history, physical examination, and the presence of the flies. Skin biopsy reveals varying degrees of superficial perivascular to interstitial dermatitis with numerous eosinophils.[4,20] Intraepidermal eosinophilic microabscesses, focal areas of epidermal necrosis (nibbles), and hypomelanosis may be seen.

Treatment consists of gentle cleansing and topical applications of antibiotic-glucocorticoid creams or ointments until healed. Severely pruritic animals may require systemic glucocorticoids for 2 to 3 days. Control is achieved by the frequent topical application of fly repellents (two to three times daily) or a thick layer of petrolatum.

MUSCA SPP. AND *HYDROTAEA* SPP. FLIES

Musca spp. and *Hydrotaea* spp. flies are cosmopolitan causes of annoyance.[14] *M. autumnalis*, *M. domestica*, *M. sorbens*, and *M. vetustissima* are the most important species.[3,22] These flies do not have biting mouth parts but feed from wounds; on secretions from the eyes, nose, and the mouth; or on blood. Eggs are laid in feces, manure, or decomposing material. The face fly, *M. autumnalis*, must lay its eggs on freshly deposited cow manure. The life cycle of the species is temperature-dependent and varies from 7 to 14 days in good conditions.

These flies are important as nuisances to production or performance and as vectors for infectious agents. *M. domestica* can carry the eggs or larvae of *Habronema* spp.

Fly masks are important in the control of face flies in horses. Fly sprays used for the biting flies will kill these flies. Cuts and wounds should be bandaged or treated with an insecticide-containing agent to prevent habronemiasis.

LOUSE FLIES

Louse flies, including *Hippobosca equina* (cosmopolitan), *H. maculata* (Africa and South America), and *H. rufipes* (Africa), parasitize horses in many parts of the world.[3,22] These flies are often called "forest flies" or "keds." Female flies (about 1 cm long) deposit larvae in sheltered spots where there is dry soil or humus. The flies are most numerous in sunny weather.

Adult louse flies suck blood and tend to cluster in the perineal and inguinal regions.[6,7,10] They remain for long periods on their hosts and are not easily disturbed. Louse flies are a source of irritation and fly-worry. Louse flies are readily killed by routinely used fly sprays.

BEES AND WASPS

Bees and wasps have been reported to attack large animals.[3,22,127,128] The venom of each species contains various peptides and proteins that cause pain and inflammation. All immunologically normal horses will develop a typical edematous wheal or plaque at the site of envenomation. Honeybees leave their stinger with attached venom sac at the sting site. All others retract the stinger and can sting multiple times. In most animals, the inflammation of a sting peaks at 48 hours.[127]

Severe reactions can be seen when the horse is allergic or is stung by a large number of insects. In an allergic horse, one sting can result in widespread urticaria, angioedema, or anaphylaxis. With massive envenomation, signs of shock and disseminated intravascular coagulation will accompany the skin changes.[128] These horses are difficult to save even with emergency treatments.

GASTEROPHILIASIS

Gasterophiliasis (bots) is a rare cause of skin disease in the horse.[11] Adult flies (botflies) are active in summer, and the females glue their eggs to the hairs of horses on the distal legs and shoulders (*G. intestinalis*), intermandibular area (*G. nasalis*), and face (*G. haemorrhoidalis*, *G. pecorum*, and *G. inermis*).[3,22] Eggs apparently hatch in response to temperature increases and licking. Larvae penetrate skin or mucosa, develop in the stomach, pass with the feces, and pupate in the ground.

Gasterophilus spp. larvae that penetrate facial skin and oral mucosa, including *G. haemorrhoidalis* (global), *G. pecorum* (Europe, Asia, and Africa), and *G. inermis* (northern hemisphere), have been reported to rarely cause dermatitis and stomatitis.[11] Cutaneous gasterophiliasis is characterized by 1- to 2-mm wide grayish-white, crooked streaks in the skin of the cheeks, neck, and shoulders (Fig. 6-18). These streaks may extend by 1.5 to 3 cm in 24 hours. The hair over these palpable, twine-like tracts may become rough and fall out, revealing a scaling skin surface. Depigmentation may be seen, but pruritus is mild or absent.

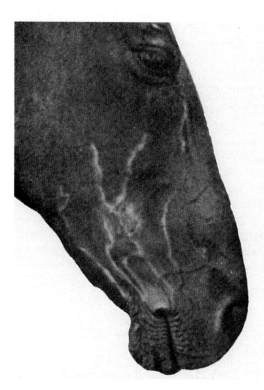

FIGURE 6-18. Gasterophiliasis. Crooked streaks in the skin caused by larval migration.

Diagnosis is based on history, physical examination, and demonstration of the migrating larvae. Skin biopsy reveals larvae in an apparently normal or mildly inflamed dermis.[11]

Therapy for cutaneous gasterophiliasis is not necessary, as the disease is self-limiting and, rarely symptomatic.

Myiasis

HYPODERMIASIS

Hypodermiasis (warbles, grubs) is a common disorder of cattle and, occasionally, horses in many parts of the world.[109]

Cause and Pathogenesis

The larval stages of *Hypoderma bovis* and *H. lineatum*, the ox warbles, are common parasites of cattle and, occasionally, horses in many countries in the northern hemisphere.[11] Adult flies (13 to 15 mm long) occur in summer and fix their eggs (1 mm long) to the hairs of horses, especially on the legs. *H. bovis* lays its eggs singly, while *H. lineatum* deposits a row of six or more on a hair. Larvae hatch in about 4 days and crawl down the hair to the skin, which they penetrate. The larvae wander in the subcutaneous tissue, apparently via the elaboration of proteolytic enzymes,[101,103] up the leg and toward the diaphragm, and they gradually increase in size. The winter resting sites of first-stage larvae are the submucosal connective tissue of the esophagus for *H. lineatum* and the region of the spinal canal and epidural fat for *H. bovis*. Larvae reach these sites weeks or months after hatching and remain in them for fall and winter, growing to 12 to 16 mm in length. During January and February, the now second-stage larvae migrate toward the dorsum of the host's body and reach the subcutaneous tissue of the back (the spring resting site), where they mature to third-stage larvae. When the parasites arrive under the skin of the back, swellings begin to form. The skin over each swelling becomes perforated (breathing pore). This is the "warble" stage of infestation, and it lasts about 30 days. In spring, the mature larvae (25 to 28 mm long) wriggle out of their cysts and fall to the ground to pupate.

In horses, *Hypoderma* larvae will migrate to the topline, especially near the withers, but usually do not mature and complete the life cycle. The nodule may or may not have a breathing hole.[4,11,20,229] In addition, aberrant migrations may cause serious effects, such as neurologic disorders.

Przhevalskiana silenus (synonyms: *Hypoderma silenus*, *H. crossi*, *P. crossi*, and *P. aegagi*) occasionally parasitizes horses in Europe and Asia. Adult flies are active from April to June and fix their eggs to hairs on the legs and chest. Larvae hatch out and crawl down to the skin, which they penetrate. The larvae migrate in the subcutaneous connective tissue up the legs to the back. All larval stages are found in the subcutaneous tissues of the back. Third-stage larvae produce subcutaneous nodules and cysts in spring, cut breathing pores, and drop on the ground to pupate.

Hypoderma diana warbles, a normal parasite of roe deer in Europe, have been identified in horses.[112] The second-stage larvae are incapable of developing further in horse skin and die within the nodule.

Clinical Features

In horses, *Hypoderma* larvae infestations are occasionally seen.° Affected horses are often in close proximity to cattle, and younger horses or those in poor condition seem to be more susceptible. Subcutaneous nodules and cysts are most commonly seen over the withers in spring and are usually few in number. Most lesions develop a breathing pore. Many lesions are painful. Rupture

---

°References 4, 5, 9, 11, 21, 102, 110, 120, 157-158, 229.

of the third-stage larvae may produce anaphylactoid reactions.[4,9] Intracranial migration of first-stage *Hypoderma* larvae with resultant neurologic disorders have been reported.[111,116]

Diagnosis

The differential diagnosis includes infectious granulomas, follicular and dermoid cysts, neoplasms, and equine eosinophilic granuloma. Definitive diagnosis is based on history, physical examination, and demonstration of the larvae. Dermatohistopathologic findings vary from a larva confined in a subcutaneous and dermal cyst (the walls of which are formed by dense connective tissue, which is often infiltrated by neutrophils and eosinophils) (Fig. 6-19) to severe suppurative, pyogranulomatous, or granulomatous reactions containing numerous eosinophils and larval segments.

Clinical Management

In horses, *Hypoderma* infestations are usually treated by gently enlarging the breathing pore with a scalpel and extracting the grub.[4,21,157,158,229] Routine wound care is rendered as needed. Alternatively, the entire nodule may be surgically excised, or the larvae may be allowed to drop out by themselves.[9] In areas of high incidence, routine worming with ivermectin or moxidectin should prevent larval migration and development.

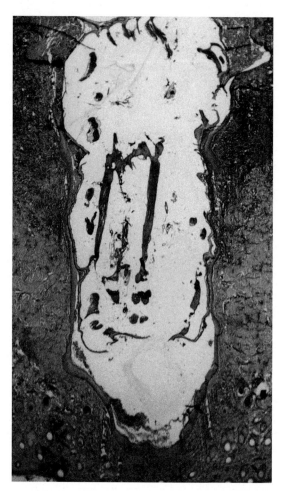

FIGURE 6-19. Hypodermiasis. Warble surrounded by fibrosis and pyogranulomatous dermatitis.

CALLIPHORINE MYIASIS

Calliphorine myiasis (blowfly strike) is a common disorder of all large animals in most areas of the world.

Cause and Pathogenesis

Calliphorine myiasis is caused by flies from the genera *Calliphora, Condylobia, Lucilia, Protophormia* and *Phormia*.[1,14,126] *L. cuprina* and *L. sericata* are the chief cause of calliphorine myiasis in Australia and Great Britain, respectively, whereas *L. caesar* and *L. illustris* are cosmopolitan in distribution. In North America, the most important blowflies are *Phormia regina* and *P. terrae-novae*.

Adult blowflies (6 to 12 mm long) lay clusters of light-yellow eggs (up to 3000 altogether) in wounds, or carcasses, being attracted by the odor of decomposing matter. Larvae hatch from eggs in 8 to 72 hours and reach full size in 2 to 19 days, depending on the temperature, amount and suitability of food, and competition with other larvae. Fullgrown larvae (10 to 14 mm long) are grayish white or pale yellow and hairy or smooth. Larvae pupate in the ground, in dry parts of a carcass, or even in the long hairs of the tail.

The factors that influence the occurrence of calliphorine myiasis can be classified into two groups: those controlling the number of flies and those determining the susceptibility of the host.

The proliferation of flies is seasonal because the adults are adapted to definite ranges of temperature and humidity. They are most abundant in late spring, early summer, and early fall. The abundance and suitability of food for the adults and larvae are of great importance.

The flies can be classified as (1) *primary flies*, which initiate a strike by laying eggs on living animals, (2) *secondary flies*, which usually lay their eggs on animals already struck, the larvae extending the injury done by the larvae of the primary flies, and (3) *tertiary flies*, which come last of all, the larvae of which do little further damage. The most important primary blowflies are *Phormia regina* (North America), *L. cuprina* (Australia), and *L. sericata* (Great Britain and New Zealand). Important secondary flies include *Chrysomyia* spp. and *Sarcophaga* spp. The ubiquitous *Musca domestica* is a common tertiary fly. The susceptibility of the host depends on inherent factors, which can be influenced by selective breeding, and on temporary factors, which can be otherwise controlled.

Clinical Features

Calliphorine myiasis is an important disorder of all large animals in most parts of the world.[122,123] The disorder is most severe in spring, early summer, and early fall.

Clinically, blowfly strike is frequently classified in terms of the anatomic site attacked. Wound strike may occur on any wounded part of the body, such as results from fighting, accidents, or surgical procedures. Any primary dermatologic condition—especially those characterized by oozing, erosion, ulceration, and draining tracts—can be struck. Blowflies will also infest the perineum if feces is trapped on the skin or tail. Lesions consist of foul smelling ulcers, often with scalloped margins. The ulcers often have a "honeycombed" appearance and are filled with larvae (maggots). Affected animals may die of toxemia and septicemia.

Diagnosis

Definitive diagnosis is based on history, physical examination, and identification of the larvae. The different larvae may be identified by means of the structure of their spiracles and the cephalopharyngeal skeleton,[126] and must be differentiated from screw-worm larvae.

Clinical Management

Treatment of individual animals includes (1) a thorough cleansing and débriding of the wound, (2) application of topical insecticide in ointment or spray form (persists long enough to prevent reinfestation), and (3) other symptomatic therapy (e.g., antibiotics) as needed.

SCREW-WORM MYIASIS

Screw-worm myiasis is a serious disease of livestock in many parts of the world.

Cause and Pathogenesis

The name "screw-worm" is given to the larvae of *Cochliomyia hominivorax* and *C. macellaria*, both of which occur in North, Central, and South America, and *Chrysomyia bezziana*, which occurs in Africa and Asia.[119,126]

Adult flies (10 to 15 mm long) deposit clusters of eggs at the edge of a wound of any size and near natural body openings, such as the nostrils and prepuce, on the host. These species have become so adapted to parasitic life that they breed only in wounds and sores on their hosts and not in carcasses. Larvae hatch within 24 hours and burrow into living tissue. They mature in 5 to 7 days, after which they leave to pupate in the ground. Mature larvae are about 15 mm long.

Wounds (accidental or surgical), rainy weather, and virtually any dermatosis predispose to screw-worm attack. The larvae (maggots) penetrate into the tissues, which they liquefy, and extend the lesion considerably.

Clinical Features

Screw-worm myiasis is a serious disease of all large animals.[1,11,14,126] The disease is most severe in spring, early summer, and early fall. There are generally no age, breed, or sex predilections.

Predisposing factors for screw-worm, and thus the areas of the body often affected, generally parallel those previously discussed for calliphorine myiasis. Common sites are wounds, wire cuts, the navel of newborn animals, and tick-bite lesions. Lesions are as described for calliphorine myiasis, but screw-worm lesions tend to be more severe and more painful and pruritic and to have a fouler smell. Severe infections are common, and death (toxemia, septicemia) from screw-worm myiasis can occur.

Diagnosis

Definitive diagnosis is based on history, physical examination, and identification of the larvae. Screw-worm myiasis is a reportable disease in the United States, and if the disease is suspected, larvae should be collected, preserved in 70% alcohol, and forwarded to an appropriate laboratory for identification.

Clinical Management

Treatment of individual animals includes (1) a thorough cleansing and débriding of the wound, (2) application of a topical insecticide in ointment or spray form, and (3) other symptomatic therapy (e.g., antibiotics) as needed.

Dermatobiasis

Dermatobiasis is an uncommon cause of subcutaneous nodules (subcutaneous furuncular myiasis) in horses in Mexico and South America.[16a,113a,114a] The third-stage larva (about 20 mm long) of *Dermatobia hominis* is an obligate parasite. The disease is most commonly seen in hills and plateaus (160 to 2000 m elevation) and forests, especially during the rainy season.

The adult female fly captures other dipteran flies (e.g., *Musca* spp., *Simulium* spp., and *Stomoxys* spp.), and glues a batch of eggs on the abdomen of these. The eggs are then carried by these vector flies to the host horse, whereupon the larvae hatch and penetrate skin or wounds. The larvae spend 4 to 18 weeks in painful subcutaneous nodules before dropping through their cutaneous breathing pores to the ground to pupate.

Treatment includes surgical excision or the use of ivermectin.

● HELMINTHS

Habronemiasis

Habronemiasis is a common cause of ulcerative cutaneous granulomas in horses around the world.[129-177]

CAUSE AND PATHOGENESIS

Three nematodes are involved in producing cutaneous habronemiasis in horses: *Habronema muscae, H. majus (H. microstoma)*, and *Draschia megastoma (H. megastoma)*.* The adults of all three nematodes inhabit the horse's stomach, *D. megastoma* residing in nodules. Eggs and larvae are passed with the feces and are ingested by the maggots of intermediate hosts: *Musca domestica*, the housefly (for *H. muscae* and *D. megastoma*), and *Stomoxys calcitrans*, the stable fly (for *H. majus*). Infectious larvae are deposited on the horse, especially in moist areas or open wounds, whereas the flies are feeding. Larvae are also capable of penetrating intact skin.[3,22,155] Larvae deposited near the mouth are swallowed and complete the parasitic life cycle in the horse's stomach. Larvae deposited on the nose migrate to the lungs, and those on other areas of the body migrate locally within the skin.

There is reason to believe that cutaneous habronemiasis is, at least in part, a hypersensitivity disorder.† First, the disease is seasonal, with spontaneous remission occurring in winter and with larvae *not* over-wintering in tissues. Second, the disease is sporadic, often affecting a single horse in a herd. Third, the disease often recurs in the same horse every summer. Fourth, systemic glucocorticoids, as the sole form of treatment, may be curative.

CLINICAL FEATURES

Habronemiasis (summer sores, bursautee, bursatti, swamp cancer, "kunkurs," "esponja," granular dermatitis) has been reported in horses from most parts of the world.‡ There are no apparent age, breed, or sex predilections. The disease usually begins in spring and summer when fly populations are active and often regresses partially or totally during the winter.

Lesions are most commonly seen on the legs (Fig. 6-20), ventrum, prepuce (Fig. 6-21), urethral process of the penis, and medial canthus of the eyes. Often, chronic wetting or wounds are predisposing factors. The onset of cutaneous habronemiasis is often characterized by the rapid development of papules or the failure of a wound to heal and the development of exuberant granulation tissue. Lesions may be solitary or multiple and are characterized by the rapid development of granulomatous inflammation, ulceration, intermittent hemorrhage, a serosanguineous exudate, and exuberant granulation. Pruritus varies from mild to severe. Small (1 mm in diameter) yellowish granules may be seen within the diseased tissue. The granules do not branch as do those (leeches) seen with pythiosis and zygomycosis. These granules represent necrotic, caseous to calcified foci surrounding nematode larvae. Habronemiasis involving the urethral process may result in dysuria and pollakiuria.[139,167,170]

Conjunctival habronemiasis is common and usually characterized by yellowish, gritty plaques on the palpebral and bulbar conjunctivae (see Fig. 6-16, *D*).[114,145,149,160,170] Eyelid granulomas and blepharitis may be seen in some cases (see Fig. 6-16, *E*). Pulmonary habronemiasis is apparently uncommon and is usually asymptomatic.§ Multiple granulomas with central caseous necrosis are found at necropsy in the interstitial and peribronchial areas of the lungs.

---

*References 5, 144, 146, 155, 164, 165, 175.
†References 4, 14, 20, 75, 114, 146.
‡References 14, 114, 134, 135, 143, 144, 146, 149, 151, 159,174, 175.
§References 114, 129, 146, 169, 173, 175.

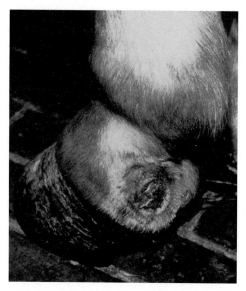

FIGURE 6-20. Habronemiasis. Ulcerated nodule on the pastern.

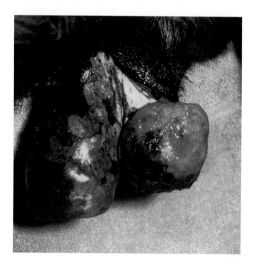

FIGURE 6-21. Habronemiasis. Large ulcerative granuloma on the prepuce.

Gastric habronemiasis is usually asymptomatic,[14,114,175] although a fatal gastric abscess attributed to *D. megastoma* has been reported.[172]

Habronema and *Draschia* larvae have been suspected of facilitating tissue invasion by *Corynebacterium pseudotuberculosis* (cutaneous abscesses) and *Rhodococcus equi* (lung abscess).[114,129,163]

DIAGNOSIS

The differential diagnosis includes bacterial and fungal granulomas, eosinophilic granuloma, equine sarcoid, squamous cell carcinoma, and exuberant granulation tissue. In some cases, the habronemiasis is superimposed on one of these other conditions.[141] Definitive diagnosis is based on history, physical examination, direct smears, and biopsy. Deep scrapings or smears from lesions, especially if the yellowish granules are retrieved, may reveal nematode larvae (40 to 50 mm long and 2 to 3 mm wide) in association with numerous eosinophils and mast cells. However, such scrapings and smears are frequently negative and *Habronema* and *Draschia* larvae may invade other ulcerative dermatoses, such as equine sarcoid, squamous cell carcinoma, and infectious granulomas.

Biopsy reveals varying degrees of nodular to diffuse dermatitis (Fig. 6-22).* The inflammatory reaction contains numerous eosinophils and mast cells. A characteristic feature of habronemiasis is multifocal areas of discrete coagulation necrosis, which consume all cutaneous structures in the area. Nematode larvae, few to many, may be found in these necrotic foci in about 50% of the specimens examined (Fig. 6-23). Palisading granulomas may develop around the necrotic foci.

CLINICAL MANAGEMENT

Habronemiasis has been managed with a plethora of therapeutic regimens.[†] However, there is little to suggest that an optimal therapeutic protocol for equine habronemiasis exists. Any therapeutic regimen will need to be individualized, with factors such as site of lesion, size of lesion, number of lesions, economics, and practicality receiving appropriate consideration.

In general, a combination of local and systemic therapy is most effective. Massive or medically refractory lesions may be eliminated surgically or, at least, debulked prior to vigorous topical and systemic therapy.[‡] Lesions of a thickness within the capability of a cryotherapy unit have been treated successfully using a double freeze-thaw cycle.[14,139,152,167,175]

Since the larvae within the lesion will die spontaneously but do not die immediately with systemic parasiticidal treatments, the need for such treatments is questionable.[161] Since ivermectin

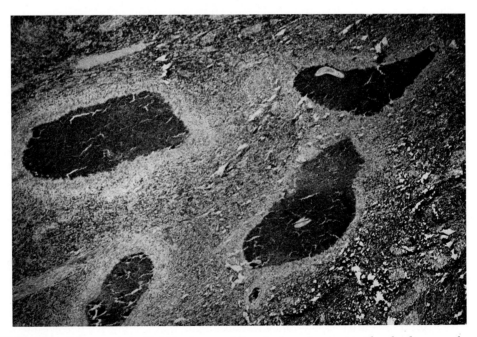

FIGURE 6-22. Habronemiasis. Multifocal areas of discrete dermal necrosis with palisading granuloma.

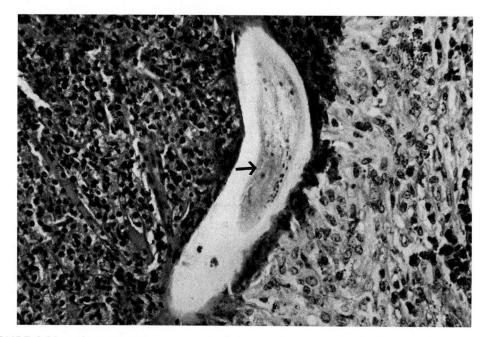

FIGURE 6-23. Habronemiasis. Larva (*arrow*) within area of necrosis and palisading granuloma.

and moxidectin, both very effective larvicides, have wide margins of safety, most investigators recommend these treatments. Two doses are given at a 21-day interval.[10]

Systemic glucocorticoids have been found to be very effective as the sole systemic agent in equine habronemiasis.[4,5,20,146,175] Prednisolone or prednisone given orally at 1 mg/kg, once daily, results in a marked resolution of most lesions within 7 to 14 days. Since high levels of glucocorticoids might induce laminitis or enterocolitis in some horses, some investigators prefer to use topical steroids.[161]

A myriad of concoctions have been used for topical therapy of habronemiasis.* Since summer sores will disappear spontaneously and most of the concoctions contain a glucocorticoid, it is difficult to determine which of these products or which of their ingredients is effective. Tresaderm, a solution containing thiabendazole, dexamethasone, and neomycin sulfate, has been effective in the authors' hands. Synotic, a solution of 0.01% fluocinolone acetonide in 60% DMSO, also can be very effective. Any topical treatment should be applied under bandage to prevent the deposition of new larvae during the healing process. When bandaging is impossible, a fly repellant ointment should be applied.

Fly control, though difficult, will reduce the incidence of habronemiasis.[6,7,10] Prompt and proper removal and disposal of manure and soiled bedding are vital. Application of residual sprays in the barn and on the horses will be beneficial.

Elimination of adult *Habronema* and *Draschia* nematodes from the stomach is another logical point of attack.[6,12,22,27,28] Since ivermectin and moxidectin have become the routine wormers for many horses, the incidence of summer sores has decreased noticeably.

---

*References 11, 14, 114, 135, 160, 175.

Onchocerciasis

Onchocerciasis was an important cause of skin disease in horses throughout the world.[178-241]

CAUSE AND PATHOGENESIS

Three species from the genus *Onchocerca* are associated with cutaneous lesions in horses in different parts of the world.[3,22,180,213] The prevalence of infection for all *Onchocerca* species is very high, ranging from 20% to 100% of a given population of animals.[109] The microfilaria numbers and location within the skin vary with the season.[194] The microfilaria are in the most superficial portion of the dermis during warm weather. Their numbers are highest in the spring and decrease to the lowest level during the winter. These variations allow easier "infection" of the intermediate hosts.

O. gutturosa infests horses in North America, Africa, Australia, and Europe.[182,191,214,215] Adult worms (up to 60 cm long) inhabit the ligamentum nuchae in horses. Microfilariae (200 to 230 μm long) are most numerous in the dermis of the face, neck, back, and ventral midline. Numerous *Simulium* spp. and *Culicoides* spp. gnats serve as intermediate hosts.

O. reticulata infests horses in Europe and Asia.[3,22,180,216,232] Adult worms (up to 50 cm long) live in the connective tissue of the flexor tendons and the suspensory ligament of the fetlock, especially in the frontlegs. Microfilariae (310 to 395 μm long) are most numerous in the dermis of the legs and ventral midline. *Culicoides* spp. gnats serve as intermediate hosts.

O. cervicalis infests horses throughout the world.[°] Adult worms (up to 30 cm long) inhabit the funicular portion of the ligamentum nuchae. They are usually encased in a necrotizing, pyogranulomatous to granulomatous reaction with marked fibrosis and dystrophic mineralization. Microfilariae (200 to 240 μm long) are most numerous on the ventral midline (especially at the umbilicus), then the face and neck. Microfilariae are not evenly distributed in the skin and tend to be present in nests or pockets. Additionally, microfilariae tend to be situated more deeply in the dermis in winter. *Culicoides* spp. gnats and, possibly, mosquitoes serve as intermediate hosts.

In infestations with *O. gutturosa* and *O. reticulata*, cutaneous nodules are produced by a granulomatous and fibrous reaction to adult worms. The exception would be *O. gutturosa* infestations in the horse, which may be nonpathogenic.[214]

In equine *O. cervicalis* infestations, the cutaneous lesions are associated with the microfilariae.[†] A unique clinical syndrome, distinctive dermatohistopathologic findings, and response to microfilaricidal chemotherapy define equine cutaneous onchocerciasis. Because most horses are infested with *O. cervicalis*, but only certain horses develop clinical signs, cutaneous onchocerciasis is thought to represent a hypersensitivity reaction to microfilarial antigen(s).[4,5,114,229,230] In horses, dead and dying microfilariae provoke the most intense inflammatory reactions.[4,20,114,229,230] In fact, an exacerbation of cutaneous signs in association with microfilaricidal therapy is well known and important to anticipate.[‡] Microfilariae are more numerous in skin with lesions than in clinically normal skin. *O. cervicalis* microfilariae may also invade ocular tissues, where they may be associated with keratitis, uveitis, peripapillary choroidal sclerosis, and vitiligo of the bulbar conjunctiva of the lateral limbus.[§] Here, again, the sudden killing of numerous microfilariae with chemotherapy may produce a severe exacerbation in ocular disease. It has been reported that horses with ocular onchocerciasis usually have more microfilariae in their skin than do horses without ocular involvement.[209,230]

°References 4, 14, 21, 179, 181, 188, 189, 199, 205, 208, 210, 213, 214, 221, 228-230, 233-235.
†References 4, 14, 114, 193, 229, 230.
‡References 4, 23, 114, 196, 199, 229, 230.
§References 114, 185, 200, 212, 225, 227, 229, 230.

In the past, *O. cervicalis* adult worms were incriminated as a cause of fistulous withers and poll evil in horses.* However, necropsy examinations in large numbers of normal horses and those with fistulous withers have failed to support this belief.[209,223,228]

It is not known how long the adults and microfilariae of the various *Onchocerca* spp. survive in the host.

CLINICAL FEATURES

Equine cutaneous onchocerciasis associated with *O. cervicalis* infestation is worldwide.† In the United States, the incidence of *O. cervicalis* infestation in clinically normal horse populations varies from 25% to 100%.‡ The incidence of infection is higher in the south. Since the commercialization of the avermectins, cutaneous onchocerciasis has become a rare disease in many areas. We have not seen a case of equine cutaneous onchocerciasis since 1990.

There are no apparent breed or sex predilections. Affected horses are usually 4 years of age or older, with horses younger than 2 years rarely showing clinical signs.

The clinical signs of equine cutaneous onchocerciasis are nonseasonal in nature, although they may be more severe during warm weather. This warm weather exacerbation of clinical signs is probably attributable to the additive effects of the insect vectors, *Culicoides* spp. gnats. Lesions may be seen exclusively on the face and neck (especially close to the mane), on the ventral chest and abdomen, or in all these areas. Lesions vary in appearance from focal annular areas of alopecia, scaling, crusting, and inflammatory plaques to widespread areas of alopecia, erythema, ulceration, oozing, crusting, and lichenification. Pruritus varies from mild to severe. An annular lesion in the center of the forehead is thought to be highly suggestive of cutaneous onchocerciasis (Fig. 6-24).[4,199] Leukoderma may be seen in combination with the lesions just described or alone and is usually irreversible. Alopecia from permanent scarring may be a sequela. Seborrhea sicca (heavy scaling) may be seen in some horses.

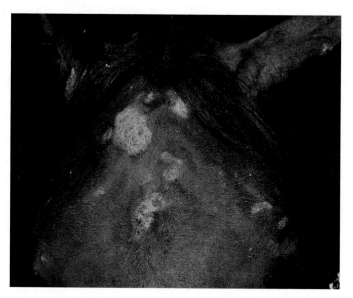

FIGURE 6-24. Onchocerciasis. Alopecic, crusted plaques on the forehead.

*References 178, 183, 197, 217, 218, 226, 231.
†References 4, 14, 21, 114, 157, 158, 181, 189, 193, 196, 199, 205, 206, 229, 232-234.
‡References 184, 186, 190, 200-202, 207, 221, 222, 228, 230.

Ocular signs may be seen in conjunction with cutaneous onchocerciasis and include variable combinations of: (1) sclerosing keratitis (originating at the temporal limbus and growing toward the center), (2) vitiligo of the bulbar conjunctiva bordering the temporal limbus, (3) white papules (0.5 to 1 mm in diameter) in the pigmented conjunctiva around the temporal limbus, (4) a round or crescent-shaped patch of depigmentation bordering the optic disc (peripapillary choroidal sclerosis), and (5) uveitis.*

O. reticulata adult worms cause subcutaneous nodules in the area of the flexor tendons and suspensory ligament of the fetlock, especially in the frontlegs, in horses in Europe and Asia.[180,192,216,232] Severely affected horses may have extensive swelling and lameness in association with the infestation.

DIAGNOSIS

The differential diagnosis for equine cutaneous onchocerciasis includes dermatophytosis, fly-bite dermatoses (seasonal), psoroptic mange, *Pelodera* dermatitis, trombiculidiasis, and food hypersensitivity. Definitive diagnosis is based on history, physical examination, and skin biopsy.

Skin scrapings and direct smears are unreliable for the demonstration of microfilariae. *Onchocerca* spp. microfilariae are rarely found in the peripheral blood. An excellent technique for demonstrating *Onchocerca* spp. microfilariae in skin involves taking a punch biopsy (4 to 6 mm in diameter), mincing the specimen with a razor or scalpel blade, placing the minced skin on a glass slide or in a Petri dish, and covering it with room temperature physiologic saline.[4,20,114,229] After allowing this preparation to incubate at room temperature for 30 minutes, examine the specimen under a microscope for the rapid motion of microfilariae in the saline. Saline containing preservatives (e.g., alcohol) should not be used, as such solutions may kill the microfilariae, not allowing their migration out of the minced skin. In addition, it must be remembered that this technique only confirms the presence of *Onchocerca* spp. microfilariae and does *not*, by itself, justify a diagnosis of cutaneous onchocerciasis.

In equine cutaneous onchocerciasis, skin biopsy reveals varying degrees of superficial and deep perivascular to interstitial dermatitis, to diffuse dermatitis with numerous eosinophils. Numerous microfilariae are usually seen in the superficial dermis, often surrounded by degranulating eosinophils (Fig. 6-25). Superficial dermal fibrosis tends to be prominent in older lesions. Occasional histopathologic findings include (1) eosinophilic infiltrative mural inflammation and necrosis of hair follicle epithelium, (2) focal small palisaded eosinophilic granulomas in the superficial dermis, where microfilariae may often be found, and (3) lymphoid nodules in the deep dermis or subcutis. Again, it must be emphasized that *Onchocerca* microfilariae may be found in the skin of normal horses as well as in lesions from potentially any equine dermatosis. Thus, the mere finding of microfilariae in a biopsy is not diagnostic of cutaneous onchocerciasis. Typical historical and physical findings must be accompanied by the indicated histopathologic changes.

CLINICAL MANAGEMENT

Equine cutaneous onchocerciasis is a cause of discomfort, irritability, and disfigurement. Permanent leukoderma and scarring alopecia are potentially devastating sequelae for valuable show horses.

Both ivermectin (0.2 mg/kg) and moxidectin (0.4 mg/kg) will kill the microfilaria within 14 days. A second treatment rarely is needed.[195,203,204,211] Regardless of which microfilaricide is used, certain ancillary procedures should be followed: (1) a thorough ocular examination prior to therapy and (2) concurrent systemic glucocorticoid administration for the first 5 days of microfilaricidal

---

*References 20, 114, 185, 225, 227, 229.

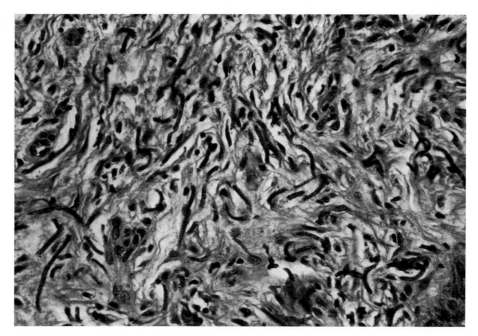

FIGURE 6-25. Onchocerciasis. Numerous microfilaria in the superficial dermis with many eosinophils.

treatment. Massive destruction of microfilariae may exacerbate both the cutaneous and ocular inflammation for the first 3 to 4 days of therapy.°

None of the microfilaricides presently in use is known to kill adult *Onchocerca* worms, and periodic flare-ups can be expected. If ivermectin or moxidectin is used regularly in the horse's worming program, flare-ups should not be seen.

Parafilariasis

Parafilariasis is a common cause of seasonal hemorrhagic nodules in horses in many parts of the world.[236-241]

CAUSE AND PATHOGENESIS

Parafilariasis (hemorrhagic filariasis, dermatorrhagie parasitaire, summer bleeding) is caused by *Parafilaria multipapillosa* in horses.[3,22] Adult worms (30 to 70 mm in length) live in the subcutaneous and intermuscular connective tissues, coiled within nodules. The subcutaneous nodules open to the surface and discharge a bloody exudate, in which embryonated eggs and larvae are found. Various flies serve as vectors or intermediate hosts: *Haematobia atripalpis* and several *Musca* spp.[236-238]

CLINICAL FEATURES

Equine parafilariasis (*P. multipapillosa*) has been reported in Eastern Europe and Great Britain.[9,11,217,236-241] The disease appears in the spring and summer. Papules and nodules arise suddenly, especially over the neck, shoulders, and trunk. The lesions, which are not usually painful or pruritic, proceed to open to the surface, discharge a bloody exudate, develop reddish-black crusts, and then heal. New lesions continue to develop as old ones heal. The disease regresses spontaneously during fall and winter. Affected horses are usually healthy otherwise.

°References 4, 20, 23, 114, 185, 196, 227, 229.

DIAGNOSIS

The differential diagnosis includes bacterial, fungal, and parasitic granulomas, and hypodermiasis. Definitive diagnosis is based on history, physical examination, direct smears, and skin biopsy. Direct smears from hemorrhagic exudate contain larvae (about 0.2 mm in length), rectangular embryonated eggs (25 μm by 50 μm), and numerous eosinophils. Skin biopsy reveals nodular to diffuse dermatitis. The centers of the lesions contain coiled adult nematodes surrounded by necrotic debris and an inflammatory infiltrate containing numerous eosinophils. Necrotic tracts lead from the central core of the lesions to the epidermal surface.

CLINICAL MANAGEMENT

Many cases of parafilariasis will recur annually for 3 to 4 years and then apparently resolve.[11,236] Avermectins are effective in the treatment of parafilariasis in cattle and should be equally as effective in the horse.

Oxyuriasis

Oxyuriasis (pin worms, thread worms) affects horses in most areas of the world.[1,3-5,22] The overall economic importance of the disease is not great. The authors have never seen this disease. *Oxyuris equi* infests the cecum and colon, and adult female worms crawl out of the anus and lay their eggs in clusters on the perineal skin. Eggs (Fig. 6-26) eventually fall off onto the ground, and infection takes place by ingestion. The activity of the female worms and, possibly, irritating substances in the material that cements the eggs to the perineal skin cause variable degrees of pruritus.

Oxyuriasis is primarily a disease of stabled horses.[1,4,14] Most infected horses show no dermatologic signs.[242] Pruritus ani results in constant rubbing of the tail base, which produces varying degrees of broken hairs and excoriation (rat-tail). Affected horses are often restless and irritable and may have a poor appetite.

The differential diagnosis includes insect hypersensitivity, pediculosis, psoroptic mange, chorioptic mange, food hypersensitivity, atopy, drug eruption, and stable vice. Definitive diagnosis

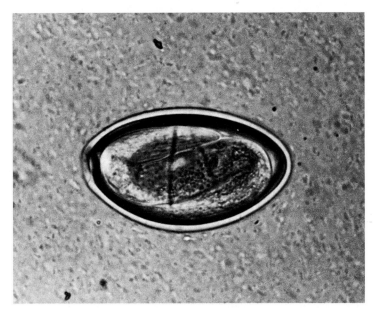

FIGURE 6-26. Oxyuriasis. *Oxyuris equi* egg. (*With permission from Bowman DD: Georgi's Parasitology for Veterinarians, 6th ed. W.B. Saunders Co, Philadelphia, 1995.*)

is based on history, physical examination, and demonstration of eggs on the perineal skin. The eggs are encased in a cream-colored, gelatinous material. Clear acetate tape applied to the area will remove the eggs. The tape is then placed on a glass slide and examined microscopically for the presence of the characteristic operculated eggs.

Therapy consists of routine worming.[243]

Strongyloidosis

Strongyloidosis has been reported in most countries throughout the world.[3,244-246] The overall economic importance of the disease is not usually very great. *Strongyloides westeri* infects the small intestine of horses.[3] Infection is acquired by ingestion or percutaneous penetration of infectious larvae. It is thought that the disruption of the skin's integrity by penetrating *S. westeri* larvae may predispose to *Rhodococcus equi* lymphangitis (see Chapter 4).[244,245]

The differential diagnosis includes contact dermatitis, *Pelodera* dermatitis, trombiculidiasis, hookworm dermatitis, chorioptic mange, and dermatophytosis. Definitive diagnosis is based on history, physical examination, and fecal flotation. Skin biopsy reveals varying degrees of superficial and deep perivascular to interstitial dermatitis with numerous eosinophils. Fortuitous sections may reveal necrotic tracts and nematode larvae surrounded by inflammatory cells.

Therapy consists of routine worming.[246]

Pelodera Dermatitis

Pelodera dermatitis (rhabditic dermatitis) is an uncommon skin condition associated with infection by the nematode *Pelodera strongyloides*.[3,247-249]

CAUSE AND PATHOGENESIS

Pelodera (*Rhabditis*) *strongyloides* is a facultative nematode parasite, 1 to 1.5 mm in length.[3,17] It usually leads a free-living existence in damp soil and decaying organic matter. Under moist, filthy environmental circumstances, the larvae can invade the skin of domestic animals, producing a parasitic folliculitis. Affected skin is that in contact with the contaminated environment. The infection is self-limited if the environmental source of the nematode is eliminated.

CLINICAL FEATURES

Pelodera dermatitis has been reported in horses.[247,248] No age, breed, or sex predilections are apparent. The disease occurs in association with moist, filthy environmental conditions.

Skin lesions are seen in areas of skin that are in close, frequent contact with the contaminated environment. The dermatitis is characterized by papules, pustules, ulcers, crusts, alopecia, scales, and erythema on the limbs, ventral thorax and abdomen, and, occasionally, the flank and neck. Pruritus is usually moderate to marked. *Pelodera* has also been identified along with a spirochete in horses with a severe pastern dermatitis.[249]

DIAGNOSIS

The differential diagnosis includes onchocerciasis, fly bites, contact dermatitis, trombiculidiasis, dermatophytosis, and various types of mange. Definitive diagnosis is based on history, physical examination, skin scrapings, and skin biopsy.

Deep skin scrapings usually reveal numerous small (about 600 μm in length), motile nematode larvae (Fig. 6-27). The adult and larval nematodes may also be detected in samples of the bedding and soil. Skin biopsy reveals varying degrees of perifolliculitis, folliculitis, and furunculosis. Nematode segments are present within hair follicles and dermal pyogranulomas. Eosinophils are numerous.

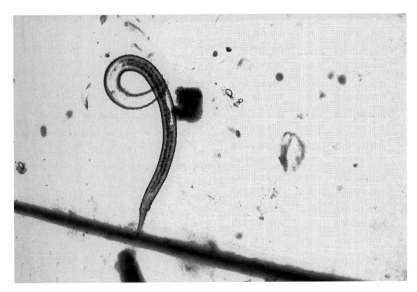

FIGURE 6-27. *Pelodera* dermatitis. *Pelodera strongyloides* larva. (*Courtesy Dr. Jay Georgi.*)

CLINICAL MANAGEMENT

Treatment is simple and effective. Complete removal and destruction of contaminated bedding and other environmental fomites is mandatory. The infected premises may be washed and sprayed with an insecticide such as malathion.

Pelodera dermatitis is a self-limited infection as long as the environmental source of the parasite is eliminated. Clinical signs regress spontaneously in one to four weeks. Severely affected animals may be treated with medicated shampoos to remove crusts and exudative debris. Secondary pyodermas may require topical antimicrobial agents or systemic antibiotics. If pruritus is severe, systemic glucocorticoids may be administered for a few days. In severe infections, recovery may be hastened by the use of topical insecticides.

Dracunculiasis

There are a few anecdotal reports of dracunculiasis in horses in the veterinary literature.[3,11] *Dracunculus medinensis* (guinea worm, dragon worm) occurs in Asia and Africa, and *D. insignis* in North America. Adult female worms (up to 100 cm in length) live in subcutaneous nodules, which ulcerate. When the lesions contact water, the uterus of the worm prolapses through its anterior end and discharges a mass of larvae (500 to 750 μm in length). Aquatic crustaceans (*Cyclops* spp.) serve as intermediate hosts, and infection occurs when contaminated water is ingested.

Lesions are usually solitary and occur most commonly on the limbs and abdomen. The subcutaneous nodules may be pruritic or painful, and just before the nodules open to the surface, the host may show urticaria, pruritus, and pyrexia.

Diagnosis is based on history, physical examination, observation of the female worm within the draining nodule, and direct smears of the exudate (larvae). Treatment classically is to gently remove the adult worm by carefully winding it up on a stick over a period of several days. Alternatively, the nodule may be surgically excised.

Control measures depend on improving contaminated water supplies.

Halicephalobiasis

CAUSE AND PATHOGENESIS

Halicephalobiasis is apparently worldwide in occurrence, but rarely recognized.[250-255] The causative agent, *Halicephalobus deletrix* (formerly *Micronema deletrix*, *Rhabditis gingivalis*), is in the order Rhabditida, where all other members are free-living saprophytic nematodes in soil and decaying organic matter. However, a free-living form of *H. deletrix* has not been found. In addition, only female nematodes, larvae, and eggs are found in tissues. Thus, details of the life cycle and mode of infection are not currently known.

CLINICAL FEATURES

No age, breed, or sex predilections are recognized. Multiple organ systems can be affected, and thus, clinical signs can be variable. Inflammation of the central nervous system is almost always present. The most commonly affected tissues are, in descending order, the brain, kidneys, oral cavity, nasal cavity, lymph nodes, lungs, spinal cord, and adrenal glands.[250,252,254,255] Cutaneous lesions appear to be uncommon. Multiple papules and nodules have been reported on the prepuce (Fig. 6-16, *F*).[251,253] Lesions were well circumscribed, firm, 0.5 to 8 cm in diameter, and tended to have surface ulceration. Other horses have had large (20 cm diameter) firm, nodular swellings with a serosanguineous discharge over the maxillary or mandibular areas in association with osteomyelitis.[250,253a,254,255]

DIAGNOSIS

At present, diagnosis can only be confirmed by biopsy. Histopathologically, a diffuse granulomatous dermatitis is seen, wherein macrophages, abundant multinucleated histiocytic giant cells, and neutrophils are present.[251-253] Eosinophils are usually few in number. Lymphoid nodules are

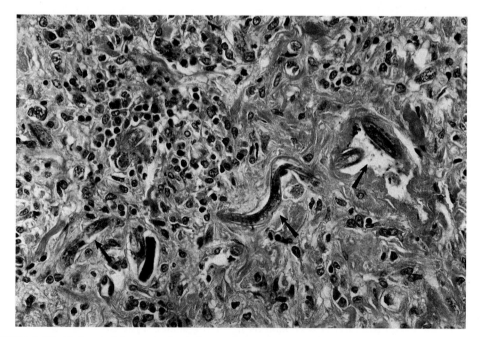

FIGURE 6-28. Halicephalobiasis. Multiple larvae (*arrows*) surrounded by a granulomatous dermatitis.

often present. Numerous adult females (235 to 445 μm length, maximum of 20 μm width), larvae, and oval ova (average 10-15 × 32-46 μm) are scattered throughout the lesion (Fig. 6-28).

Three other rhabditid parasites—*Pelodera strongyloides*, *Strongyloides westeri*, and *Cephalobus* sp.—infect equine skin, but are distinguished by their clinical syndromes and morphology in tissues. *Pelodera strongyloides* produces a parasitic folliculitis. The life cycle of *Strongyloides westeri* involves cutaneous penetration by larvae, but adults and eggs are not found in skin. *Cephalobus* sp. differs from *H. deletrix* in the shape of the stoma and esophagus and by having a blunt posterior end. Only *H. deletrix* has a pointed tail and reflexed ovary.[251]

CLINICAL MANAGEMENT

In one horse with only preputial lesions,[251] treatment with ivermectin and diethylcarbamazine was apparently curative. With surgical débridement and six treatments of ivermectin every other week, a horse with a large (6 × 10 cm) facial mass was cured.[253a] Another horse with mandibular osteomyelitis and submandibular lymphadenopathy was treated[254] with ivermectin and fenbendazole but developed progressive neurologic disease.

Cephalobiasis

A single case of necrotic, verminous mastitis in a mare was caused by *Cephalobus* sp.[256] Histopathologic findings included multifocal areas of necrosis, wherein some areas were mineralized and heavily infiltrated with plasma cells and macrophages, with focal neutrophilic microabscesses. Thousands of adult female nematodes, larvae, and eggs were present throughout the tissue.

The nematode was identified as a member of the genus *Cephalobus*, family Cephalobidae, and order Rhabditida. Members of the genus *Cephalobus* are generally saprophytic soil inhabitants.

● REFERENCES

General

1. Arundell JH: Parasites of the Horse. University of Sydney Post-Graduate Foundation in Veterinary Science, Veterinary Review 18, 1978.
2. Bordeau P: Les tiques d'importance vétérinaire et médicale 1re partie: Principales caractéristiques morphologiques et biologiques et leurs conséquences. Point Vét 25:13, 1993.
3. Bowman DD: Georgi's Parasitology for Veterinarians, 7th ed. W.B. Saunders Co, Philadelphia, 1999.
4. Fadok VA, Mullowney PC: Dermatologic diseases of horses part I. Parasitic dermatoses of the horse. Comp Cont Educ 5:S615, 1983.
5. Fadok VA: Parasitic skin diseases of large animals. Vet Clin N Am Large Anim Pract 6:3, 1984.
6. Fadok VA (ed): Dermatology. Vet Clin North Am Equine Pract 11, 1995.
7. Foil LD, et al: Arthropod pests of horses. Comp Cont Ed 12:723, 1990.
8. Hallórsdóttir S: Hudlidelser hos hest. Norsk Veterinar 102:19, 1990.
9. Hopes R: Skin diseases in horses. Vet Dermatol News 1:4, 1976.
10. Jones CJ, DiPietro JA: Biology and control of arthropod parasites of horses. Comp Cont Educ 18:551, 1996.
11. Kral F, Schwartzman RM: Veterinary and Comparative Dermatology. J.B. Lippincott Co, Philadelphia, 1964.
12. Moriello KA, et al: Diseases of the skin. In: Reed SM, et al (eds): Equine Internal Medicine. W.B. Saunders Co, Philadelphia, 1990, p 513.
13. Pascoe RR: The nature and treatment of skin conditions observed in horses in Queensland. Aust Vet J 49:35, 1973.
14. Pascoe RR: Equine Dermatoses. University of Sydney Post-Graduate Foundation in Veterinary Science, Veterinary Review No. 22, 1981.
15. Pascoe RR: A Colour Atlas of Equine Dermatology. Wolfe Publishers, Ltd, Ipswich, 1990.
16. Pascoe RR, et al: Manual of Equine Dermatology. W.B. Saunders Co, Philadelphia, 1999.
16a. Radostits OM, et al: Veterinary Medicine. A Textbook of Diseases of Cattle, Sheep, Pigs, Goats, and Horses VIII. Baillière-Tindall, Philadelphia, 1994.
17. Scott DW, et al: Muller & Kirk's Small Animal Dermatology VI. W.B. Saunders Co, Philadelphia, 2001.
18. Sloet van Oldruitenborgh-Oosterbaan MMS, et al: Parasitäre Hauterkrankungen des Pferdes. Prakt Tier 69:6, 1988.
19. Sloet van Oldruitenborgh-Oosterbaan MMS, et al: The Practitioners Guide to Equine Dermatology. Uitgeverji Libre BV, Leeuwarden, Netherlands, 2001.
20. von Tscharner C, et al: Stannard's illustrated equine dermatology notes. Vet Dermatol 11:161, 2000.
21. Thomsett LR: Skin diseases of the horse. In Pract 1:15, 1979.

22. Wall R, et al: Veterinary Ectoparasites, 2nd ed. Blackwell Scientific, Ltd, Oxford, 2001.

Therapeutics

23. Anderson RR: The use of ivermectin in horses: research and clinical observations. Comp Cont Educ 6:S516, 1984.
24. Auer DE, et al: Illness in horses following spraying with amitraz. Aust Vet J 61:257, 1984.
25. Compendium of Veterinary Products, 6th ed. North American Compendium, Inc, Port Huron, 2001.
25a. Gokbulut C, et al: Plasma pharmacokinetics and fecal excretion of ivermectin, doramectin, and moxidectin following oral administration in horses. Equine Vet J 33:494, 2001.
26. Johnson PJ, et al: Presumed moxidectin toxicosis in three foals. J Am Vet Med Assoc 214:678, 1999.
27. Littlewood J: Control of ectoparasites in horses. In Pract 21:418, 1999.
28. Lynn RC: Antiparasitic drugs. In: Georgi's Parasitology for Veterinarians, 7th ed. W.B. Saunders Co, 1999, p 235.
29. Pérez R, et al: Comparison of the pharmacokinetics of moxidectin (Equest) and ivermectin (Eqvalan) in horses. J Vet Pharmacol Therap 22:174, 1999.
30. Roberts MC, Seawright AA: Amitraz-induced large intestinal impaction in the horse. Aust Vet J 55:553, 1979.
31. Roberts MC, Argenzio A: Effects of amitraz, several opiate derivatives and anticholinergic agents on intestinal transit in ponies. Equine Vet J 18:256, 1986.

Psoroptic Mange

32. Abu-Samra MT, et al: Five cases of psoroptic mange in the domestic donkey (*Equus asinus asinus*) and treatment with ivermectin. Equine Vet J 19:143, 1987.
33. Bates PG: Inter- and intraspecific variation within the genus *Psoroptes* (Acari: Psoroptidae). Vet Parasitol 83:201, 1999.
34. Johnston LAY: A note on psoroptic otoacariasis in a horse in North Queensland. Aust Vet J 39:208, 1963.
35. Liebisch A, et al: Untersuchungen zur Uberlebensdauer von Milben der Arten *Psoroptes ovis*, *Psoroptes cuniculi* und *Chorioptes bovis* abseits des belebten Wirtes. Dtsch Tierärztl Wochenschr 92:181, 1985.
36. Lucas KM: Psoroptic otoacariasis of the horse. Aust Vet J 22:186, 1946.
37. Meleney WP: Experimentally induced bovine psoroptic acariasis in a rabbit. Am J Vet Res 28:892, 1967.
38. Montali RJ: Ear mites in a horse. J Am Vet Med Assoc 169:630, 1976.
39. Pascoe RR: Mites in "head shaker" horses. Vet Rec 107:234, 1980.
40. Patid-Kukarni VG, et al: Successful treatment of psoroptic mange in a horse with malathion emulsion. Indian Vet J 44:65, 1967.
41. Roberts RHS: Insects Affecting Livestock. Angus and Robertson, Sydney, 1952.
42. Shaw JG: Ear mange in horses. N Z Vet J 14:127, 1966.
43. Smith KE, et al: The effects of temperature and humidity on the off-host survival of *Psoroptes ovis* and *Psoroptes cuniculi*. Vet Parasitol 83:265, 1999.
44. Stickland RK, Gerrish RR: Infestivity of *Psoroptes ovis* on ivermectin-treated cattle. Am J Vet Res 48:342, 1987.
45. Stromberg PC, Fisher WF: Dermatopathology and immunity in experimental *Psoroptes ovis* (Acari: Psoroptidae) infestation of naive and previously exposed Hereford cattle. Am J Vet Res 47:1151, 1986.
46. Sweatman GK: On the life history and validity of the species in *Psoroptes*, a genus of mange mites. Can J Zool 36:905, 1958.
47. Zahler M, et al: Genetic evidence suggests that *Psoroptes* isolates of different phenotypes, hosts, and geographic origins are conspecific. Intl J Parasitol 28:1713, 1998.

Sarcoptic Mange

48. Brizard A: Le benzoate de benzyle dans le traitement des gales du cheval. Rev Méd Vét 94:267, 1943.
49. Eberhard T: Erfahrungen bei der Gasbehundlung der Pferderaude mit Schwefeldioxyd. Monat Prakt Tierheilkd 32:81, 1921.
50. Eisenblatter K: Beitrag zur Behandlung der Pferderaude. Berl Tierärztl Wochenschr 32:185, 1916.
51. Jonk M: Arsenik in der Behandlung der Raude. Berl Tierärztl Wochenschr 35:3, 1919.
52. Lepinay R: Les essais pratiques de traitement de la gale des chevaux par les gaz sulfureaux. Rec Méd Vét 93:653, 1917.
53. Richter D: Die Behundlung der Pferderaude mit Schwefigsaureanhydrid. Berl Tierärztl Wochenschr 35:1, 1919.
54. Stresow P: Raudebehandlung mit Peruol. Berl Tierärztl Wochenschr 36:607, 1920.
55. Tomašek V, et al: Lije enje Konjiske suge u Drugan sujetskrom ratie (1941-1945). Vet Archiv 60:285, 1990.
56. Zahler M, et al: Molecular analyses suggest monospecificity of the genus *Sarcoptes* (Acari: Sarcoptidae). Intl J Parasitol 29:759, 1999.

Chorioptic Mange

57. Boersema JH: De effectiviteit van coumaphos tegen *Chorioptes bovis* bij een paard met beenschurft. Tijdschr Diergeneeskd 103:377, 1978.
58. Curtis CF: Pilot study to investigate the efficacy of a 1% selenium sulphide shampoo in the treatment of equine chorioptic mange. Vet Rec 144:674, 1999.
59. Littlewood J: Chorioptic mange: successful treatment of a case with fipronil. Equine Vet Educ 12:144, 2000.
60. Littlewood JD, et al: Oral ivermectin paste for the treatment of chorioptic mange in horses. Vet Rec 137:661, 1995.
61. Mehls HJ: Eine seltene Form der *Chorioptes*—Raude beim Pferd. Berl Munch Tierärztl Wochenschr 1:9, 1952.
62. Mirck AH: Een geval van uitebreide *Chorioptes* schurft bij een paard. Tijdschr Diergeneeskd 98:580, 1973.
63. Sweatman GK: Life history, nonspecificity, and revision of the genus *Chorioptes*, a parasitic mite of herbivores. Can J Zool 35:641, 1957.

Demodicosis

64. Baker DW, Fisher WF: The incidence of demodectic mites in the eyelids of various mammalian hosts. J Econ Entomol 62:942, 1969.
65. Bennison JC: Demodicosis of horses with particular reference to equine members of the genus *Demodex*. J R Army Vet Corps 14:34, 1943.

66. Berger D: Acariasis in the horse. Vet J 67:383, 1911.
67. Besch ED, Griffiths HJ: Demonstration of *Demodex equi* (Railliet, 1895) from a horse in Minnesota. J Am Vet Met Assoc 155:82, 1956.
68. Desch CE, Nutting WB: Redescription of *Demodex caballi* (= *D. folliculorum var. equi* Railliet, 1895) from the horse, *Equus caballas*. Acarologia 20:235, 1978.
69. Fisher WF, et al: Natural transmission of *Demodex bovis stilesi* to dairy calves. Vet Parasitol 7:233, 1980.
70. Himonas CA, et al: Demodectic mites in eyelids of domestic animals in Greece. J Parasitol 61:767, 1975.
71. Koutz FR: *Demodex folliculorum* studies. IX. The prevalence of demodectic mange various animals. Speculum 17:19, 1963.
72. Linton RC: The presence of *Demodex folliculorum* in the horse. Vet J 72:79, 1916.
73. Nutting WB, et al: Hair follicle mites (*Demodex* spp.) of medical and veterinary concern. Cornell Vet 66:214, 1976.
74. Ruther D: Zur behandlung schwer heilbarer Raudeformen. Berl Tierärztl Wochenschr 27:44, 1911.
75. Scott DW, White KK: Demodicosis associated with systemic glucocorticoid therapy in two horses. Equine Pract 5:31, 1983.
76. Scott DW: Demodicosis. In: Robinson NE (ed): Current Therapy in Equine Medicine II. W.B. Saunders Co, Philadelphia, 1987, p 626.
77. Ute Brauer VEU: Klinischer Fall einer generalisierten Demodikose bei einem Pferd und deren Behandlung mit Doramectin. Tierärztl Umschau 52:131, 1997.
78. Williamson G, Oxspring GE: Demodectic scabies in the horse. Vet J 76:376, 1920.

Trombiculidiasis
79. Fraser AC: Heel-bug in the thoroughbred horse. Vet Rec 50:1455, 1938.
80. Mair TS: Headshaking associated with *Trombicula autumnalis* larval infestation in two horses. Equine Vet J 26:244, 1994.
81. Ridgway JR: An unusual skin condition in thoroughbred horses. Vet Rec 92:382, 1973.

Forage Mites
82. Berríos AM: Analisis cualitativo de las poblaciones de ácaros (*Arthropoda: Acari*) asociados a equinos estabola dos en la ciudad de concepcion, VIII region-Chile. Advances Cien Vet 9:101, 1994.
83. Hiepe T, et al: Enzootisches Auftreten von Hautveranderungen mit Wollausfall in Schafbestanden infolge Caloglyphus-berlesei-Befalls. Monat Vet Med 33:901, 1978.
84. Kunkle GA, Greiner EC: Dermatitis in horses and man caused by the straw itch mite. J Am Vet Med Assoc 181:467, 1982.
85. Norvall J, McPherson EA: Dermatitis in the horse caused by *Acarus farinae*. Vet Rec 112:385, 1983.

Miscellaneous Mite Infestations
85a. Carelle MS, et al: Dermatitis associated with "hypopodes" in a horse: The first case reported in Italy. Vet Parasitol 93:83, 2000.

Ticks
86. Bagnall BG: The Australian paralysis tick, *Ixodes holocyclus*. Aust Vet J 51:159, 1975.
87. Baker DW: Ticks found in New York State. Cornell Vet 36:84, 1946.
88. Becklund WW: Ticks of veterinary significance found on imports in the United States. J Parasitol 54:622, 1968.
89. Borges LMF, et al: Seasonal dynamics of *Anocentor nitens* on horses in Brazil. Vet Parasitol 89:165, 2000.
90. Borges LMF, Leite RC: Fauna ixodológica do pavilho auricular de eqüinos em municipios de Minas Gerais e da Bahia. Arq Bras Med Vet Zootec 50:87, 1998.
90a. Borges LMF, et al: Horse resistance to natural infestations of *Anocentor nitens* and *Amblyomma cajennense* (Acari:Ixodidae). Vet Parasitol 104:265, 2000.
91. Bordeau P: Les tiques d'importance vétérinaire et médicale 2e partie: principales espèces de tiques dures (*Ixodidae et Ambylommidae*). Point Vét 25:27, 1993.
92. Madigan JE, et al: Muscle spasms associated with ear tick (*Otobius megnini*) infestations in five horses. J Am Vet Med Assoc 207:74, 1995.
93. Riek RF: Allergic reaction in the horse to infestation with larvae of *Boophilus microplus*. Aust Vet J 30:142, 1954.
94. Strickland RK, Gerrish RR: Distribution of the tropical horse tick in the United States and notes on associated cases of equine piroplasmosis. J Am Vet Med Assoc 144:875, 1964.
95. Theiler G: Zoological survey of the Union of South Africa: tick survey. Onderstepoort J Vet Sci 24:34, 1950.
96. Tritschler LG: Allergy in a horse due to *Amblyomma americanum*. Vet Med 60:219, 1965.

Lice
97. Hugnet C, et al: Intérêt du fipronil à 0.25 pour cent en spray dans le traitement de la phtiriose à *Damalinia equi* (pou mallophage). Prat Vét Equine 31:65, 1999.
98. Paterson S, Orrell S: Treatment of biting lice (*Damalinia equi*) in 25 horses using 1% selenium sulphide. Equine Vet Educ 7:304, 1995.
99. Wright R: Lice on horses. Can Vet J 40:590, 1999.

Fleas
100. Yeruham I, et al: *Ctenocephalides felis* flea infestation in horses. Vet Parasitol 62:341, 1996.

Mosquitos, Gnats, and Flies
101. Andrews AH: Warble fly: The life cycle, distribution, economic losses, and control. Vet Rec 103:348, 1978.
102. Baker DW, Monlux WS: *Hypoderma* myiasis in the horse. J Parasitol 25:15, 1939.
103. Beesley WN: Observations on the biology of the ox warble-fly. III. Dermolytic properties of larval extracts. Ann Trop Med Parasitol 63:159, 1969.
104. Bordeau P, et al: La dermatite estivale récidivante des équidés: Données actuelles. Point Vét 27:207, 1995.
105. Braverman Y, et al: Mosquito repellent attracts *Culicoides imicola* (Diptera: Ceratopogonidae). J Med Entomol 36:113, 1999.
106. Campbell JB, Tomas GD: The history, biology, economics, and control of the horn fly, *Haematobia irritans*. Agri-Pract 13:31, 1992.
107. Depner KR: Distribution of the face fly *Musca autumnalis* in western Canada and the relation between its environment and population density. Can Entomol 101:97, 1969.

108. Dorsey CK: Face-fly control experiments on quarter horses. J Econ Entomol 59:86, 1966.

109. Foil L, Foil C: Dipteran parasites of horses. Equine Pract 10:21, 1988.

110. Girard R: Un cas d'évolution d'*Hypoderma bovis* de Geer sur le cheval. CR Acad Sci 208:306, 1939.

111. Hadlow WJ, et al: Intracranial myiasis by *Hypoderma bovis* (*Linnaeus*) in a horse. Cornell Vet 67:272, 1977.

112. Hendrikx WML, et al: A *Hypoderma diana* (Diptera: Hypodermatidae) infection in a horse. Vet Quart 11:56, 1989.

113. Kunz SE: Strategies and tactics for prevention and management of horn fly resistance. Agri-Pract 15:24, 1994.

113a. Lello E, et al: Epidemiology of myiasis in Botucatu municipality Brazil. Argu Esc Vet Univ Fed Minas Gerais 34:93, 1982.

114. McMullen WC: Equine dermatology. Proc Am Assoc Equine Pract 22:293, 1976.

114a. Murray VLE, et al: Myiasis in man and other animals in Trinidad and Tobago (1972-1973). Trop Agric 53:263, 1976.

115. Mushi EZ, et al: *Culicoides* (Diptera: Ceratopogonidae) associated with horses at Mogoditshane, Gaborone, Botswana. Vet Res Comm 22: 295, 1998.

116. Olander HJ: The migration of *Hypoderma lineatum* in the brain of a horse. Pathol Vet J 4:477, 1967.

117. Petrikowski M, et al: Etude d'une population de chevaux atteints de D.E.R.E. en Bretagne. Point Vét 27:217, 1995.

118. Potemkin VI, Vedernikov NT: On the hypodermatosis of horses. Veterinariya (Moscow) 21:23, 1944.

119. Rajamanickam C, et al: The prevalence of myiasis of domestic animals in Peninsular Medaysia. Kajian Vet 18:153, 1986.

120. Scharff DK: Control of cattle grubs in horses. Vet Med Small Anim Pract 69:791, 1973.

121. Scott DW: Histopathologie cutanée de l'hypersensibilité aux piqûres de *Culicoides* chez le cheval. Point Vét 22:583, 1990.

122. SenGupta CM, et al: Studies on myiasis and treatment. Indian Vet J 27:340, 1951.

123. Subramamian H, Mohanan KR: Incidence and etiology of cutaneous myiasis in domestic animals in Trichur. Kerala J Vet Sci 11:80, 1980.

124. Yeruham I, Braverman Y: Skin lesions in dogs, horses, and calves caused by the stable fly *Stomoxys calcitrans* (L.) (Diptera: Muscidae). Rev Elev Méd Vét Pays Trop 48:347, 1995.

125. Zumpt F: Medical and veterinary importance of horse flies. S Afr Med J 23:359, 1949.

126. Zumpt F: Myiasis in Man and Animals in the Old World. Butterworth and Co, Ltd, London, 1965.

Hymenoptera

127. Staempfli HR, Kaushik A: Clinical reactions of horses to venoms from winged stinging insects. Equine Vet Educ 5:259, 1993.

128. Staempfli HR, et al: Acute fatal reaction to bee stings in a mare. Equine Vet Educ 5:250, 1993.

Habronemiasis

129. Bain AM, et al: *Habronema megastoma* larvae associated with pulmonary abscesses in a foal. Aust Vet J 45:101, 1969.

130. Bordin EL, et al: Efficacy of ivermectin in the treatment of equine habronemiasis in Brazil. Equine Pract 9:18, 1987.

131. Boyd CL, Bullard TL: Organophosphate treatment of cutaneous habronemiasis in horses. J Am Vet Med Assoc 153:324, 1968.

132. Bridges ER: The use of ivermectin to treat genital cutaneous habronemiasis in a stallion. Comp Cont Educ 7:S94, 1985.

133. Bull LB: A granulomatous affection of the horse—habronemic granulomata (cutaneous habronemiasis of Railliet). J Comp Pathol Ther 29:187, 1916.

134. deJesus Z: Habronemiasis seriously affecting improved types of horses in Thailand. J Thai Vet Med Assoc 10:61, 1959.

135. deJesus Z: Observations on habronemiasis in horses. Philippine J Vet Med 2:133, 1963.

136. Descazeaux M, Morel R: Relations entre les habronemoses cutanées et gastriques du cheval. Bull Acad Vet Fr 6:364, 1933.

137. Descazeaux M, Morel R: Diagnostic bioloqique des habronemoses gastriques du cheval. Bull Soc Pathol Exot 26:1010, 1933.

138. Devakula S, et al: The biopsy technic as an aid in the diagnosis of equine cutaneous habronemiasis. J Thai Vet Med Assoc 13:7, 1962.

139. Finocchio EJ, Meriam JC: Surgical correction of myiasitic urethritis granulosa. Vet Med Small Anim Clin 71:1629, 1976.

140. Gibbons WJ: Summer sores. Mod Vet Pract 49:76, 1968.

141. Guedes RMC, et al: Phycomycosis and cutaneous habronemosis: Retrospective study of 30 cases diagnosed during the period, 1979-1996. Rev Med Vet Mycol 4:465, 1998.

142. Herd RP, Donham JC: Efficacy of ivermectin against cutaneous *Draschia* and Habronema infection (summer sores) in horses. Am J Vet Res 42:1953, 1981.

143. Howell CE, Hart GH: An apparent hereditary epithelial defect factor, the possible etiology of Bursattee in horses. J Am Vet Med Assoc 71:347, 1927.

144. Johnston TJ, Bancroft MJ: The life history of *Habronema* in relation to *Musca domestica* and native flies in Queensland. Proc R Soc 32:61, 1920.

145. Joyce JR, et al: Treatment of habronemiasis of the adnexa of the equine eye. Vet Med Small Anim Clin 67:1008, 1972.

146. Kirkland KC, et al: Habronemiasis in an Arabian stallion. Equine Pract 3:34, 1981.

147. Lacerda-Neto JC, et al: Tratamento da Habronemose cutânea dos eqüideos com usointravenosa de solucao di Trichlorfon à 2,5% associado à aplicacao tópica da a'cido metacreosolsufônicó com metanal. Arg Bras Vet Zoot 45:27, 1993.

148. Lewis JC: Equine granuloma in the northern territory of Australia. J Comp Pathol Ther 27:1, 1914.

149. Lewis JC, Seddon HR: Habronemic conjunctivitis. J Comp Pathol Ther 31:87, 1918.

150. Mathison PT: Eosinophilic nodular dermatoses. Vet Clin N Am Equine Pract 11:75, 1995.

151. Meyrick JJ: Bursattee. Vet J 7:318, 1878.

152. Migiola S: Cryosurgical treatment of equine cutaneous habronemiasis. Vet Med Small Anim Clin 73:1073, 1978.

153. Mohammed FHA, et al: Cutaneous habronemiasis in horses and domestic donkeys (*Equus asinus*). Rev Elev Méd Vét Pays Trop 42:535, 1989.
154. Murray DR, et al: Granulomatous and neoplastic diseases of the skin of horses. Aust Vet J 54:338, 1978.
155. Nishiyama S: Studies on habronemiasis in horses. Bull Fac Agric Kagoshima Univ 7, 1958.
156. Page EH: Common skin diseases of the horse. Proc Am Assoc Equine Pract 18:385, 1972.
157. Panel Report: Skin conditions in horses. Mod Vet Pract 56:363, 1975.
158. Panel Report: Dermatologic problems in horses. Mod Vet Pact 62:75, 1981.
159. Railliet M: Contribution a l'étude de l' "esponja" ou plaies d'été des equides du Bresil. Rec Med Vet 91:468, 1915.
160. Rebhun WC, et al: Habronemic blepharoconjunctivitis in horses. J Am Vet Med Assoc 179:469, 1981.
161. Rebhun WC: Observations on habronemiasis in horses. Equine Vet Educ 8:188, 1996.
162. Reddy AB, et al: Pathological changes due to *Habronema muscae* and *Draschia megastoma* infection in equine. Indian J Anim Sci 46:207, 1976.
163. Reid CH: Habronemiasis and *Corynebacterium* "chest" abscess in California horses. Vet Med Small Anim Clin 60:233, 1965.
164. Roubaud E, Descazeaux J: Contribution a l'histoire de la mouche domestique comme agent vecteur des habronemoses des Equidés. Bull Soc Pathol Exot 14:471, 1921.
165. Roubaud E, Descazeaux J: Evolution de l'*Habronema muscae* Carter chez la mouche domestique et de l'*Habronema microstoma* Schneider chez le Stomoxe. Bull Soc Pathol Exot 15:572, 1921.
166. Salas-Auvert R, et al: Treatment of cutaneous equine habronemiasis with a beta-glycoside, aucubigenin. Equine Pract 7:22, 1985.
167. Shideler RK, Hultine JD: Eosinophilic granuloma removed from the equine prepuce. Vet Med Small Anim Clin 68:1330, 1973.
168. Smith F: The pathology of Bursattee. Vet J 19:16, 1884.
169. Steckel RR, et al: Equine pulmonary habronemiasis with acute hemolytic anemia resulting from organophosphate treatment. Equine Pract 5:35, 1983.
170. Stick JA: Amputation of the equine urethral process affected with habronemiasis. Vet Med Small Anim Clin 74:1453, 1979.
171. Stick JA: Surgical management of genital habronemiasis in a horse. Vet Med Small Anim Clin 76:410, 1981.
172. Topacio T: Fatal suppurating abscess of the stomach caused by stomach worm (*Habronema megastoma*). Philippine J Anim Indust 1:403, 1934.
173. Torres CA: *Habronemose pulmonaire* (*Habronema muscae* Carter) expérimentalement produit chez le cobaye. Compt Rend Soc Biol 88:242, 1924.
174. Van Saceghem R: Cause étiologique et traitement de la dermite granuleuse. Bull Soc Pathol Exot 12:575, 1918.
175. Vasey JR: Equine cutaneous habronemiasis. Comp Cont Educ 3:S290, 1981.
176. Waddell AH: A survey of *Habronema* spp. and the identification of third-stage larvae of *Habronema megastoma* and *Habronema muscae* in section. Aust Vet J 45:20, 1969.
177. Wheat JD: Treatment of equine summer sores with systemic insecticide. Vet Med 56:477, 1961.

Onchocerciasis

178. Ackert JE, O'Neal WS: Parasitism and fistulous withers. J Am Vet Med Assoc 77:28, 1930.
179. Alicata JE: Microfilarial infestation of the skin of a horse. North Am Vet 17:39, 1936.
180. Bain O: Redescription de cinq espèces d'onchocerques. Ann Parasitol Hum Comp 50:763, 1975.
181. Bellocq P, Guilhem P: Guérison spectaculaire d'un cas de Dermite estivale des Equidés. Rec Méd Vét 136:663, 1960.
182. Bremmer KC: Morphologic studies on the microfilariae of *Onchocerca gibsoni* and *Onchocerca gutturosa*. Aust J Zool 3:324, 1955.
183. Chambers F: The parasitic origin of poll evil and fistulous withers. Vet Rec 45:759, 1932.
184. Caslick E: Further study of a parasite found in the ligamentum nuchae of equines. Rep NY State Vet 32:162, 1922.
185. Cello RM: Ocular onchocerciasis in the horse. Equine Vet J 13:148, 1971.
186. Collins RC: Onchocerciasis of horses in southeastern Louisiana. J Parasitol 59:1016, 1973.
187. Collobert C, et al: Prevalence of *Onchocerca* species and *Thelazia lacrimalis* in horses examined postmortem in Normandy. Vet Rec 136:463, 1995.
188. Cummings E, James ER: Prevalence of equine onchocerciasis in the southeastern and midwestern United States. J Am Vet Med Assoc 186:1202, 1985.
189. Dikmans G: Skin lesions of domestic animals in the United States due to nematode infestation. Cornell Vet 38:3, 1948.
190. Eberhard ML, Winkler WG: Onchocerciasis among ungulate animals in Georgia. J Parasitol 60:971, 1974.
191. Eichler DA, Nelson GS: Studies on *Onchocerca gutturosa* and its development in *Simulium ornatum*. J Helminthol 65:245, 1971.
192. Eisenmenger E, et al: Filarien (*Onchocerca reticulata*) als Ursache von granulomatösen Wundheilungsstörungen an den Extremitaten von Pferden. Wien Tierärztl Mschr 73:244, 1986.
193. Foil CS: Cutaneous onchocerciasis. In: Robinson NE (ed): Current Therapy in Equine Medicine II. W.B. Saunders Co, Philadelphia, 1987, p 627.
194. Foil LD, et al: Seasonal changes in density and tissue distribution of *Onchocerca cervicalis* microfilariae in ponies and related changes in *Culicoides variipennis* populations in Louisiana. J Parasitol 73:320, 1987.
195. French DD, et al: Efficacy of ivermectin in paste and injectable formulations against microfilariae of *Onchocerca cervicalis* and resolution of associated dermatitis in horses. Am J Vet Res 49:1550, 1988.
196. Herd RP, Donham JC: Efficacy of ivermectin against *Onchocerca cervicalis* microfilarial dermatitis in horses. Am J Vet Res 44:1102, 1983.
197. Hilmy N, et al: The role of *Onchocerca reticulata* as the cause of fistulous withers and ulcerative wounds of the back in solipeds, and its treatment. Cairo Fac Vet Med J 14:149, 1967.
198. Klei TR, et al: Efficacy of ivermectin (22,23-dihydroavermectin B$_1$) against adult *Setaria equina* and microfilaria of *Onchocerca cervicalis* in ponies. J Parasitol 66:859, 1980.

199. Lees MJ, et al: Cutaneous onchocerciasis in the horse: Five cases in southwestern British Columbia. Can Vet J 24:3, 1983.
200. Lloyd S, Soulsby EJL: Survey for infection with *Onchocerca cervicalis* in horses in eastern United States. Am J Vet Res 39:1962, 1979.
201. Lyons EJ, et al: Prevalence of microfilariae (*Onchocerca* spp.) in skin of Kentucky horses at necropsy. J Am Vet Med Assoc 179:899, 1981.
202. Lyons ET, et al: *Onchocerca* spp. frequency in thoroughbreds at necropsy in Kentucky. Am J Vet Res 47:880, 1986.
203. Lyons ET, et al: Verification of ineffectual activity of ivermectin against adult *Onchocerca* spp. in the ligamentum nuchae of horses. Am J Vet Res 49:983, 1988.
204. Mancebo OA, et al: Comparative efficacy of moxidectin 2% equine oral gel and ivermectin 2% equine oral paste against *Onchocerca cervicalis* (Railliet and Henry, 1910) microfilariae in horses with naturally acquired infections in Formosa (Argentina). Vet Parasitol 73:243, 1997.
205. Marcoux M, et al: Infection par *Onchocerca cervicalis* au Québec: Signes cliniques et méthode de diagnostic. Can Vet J 18:108, 1977.
206. Maurer ND, Bell PR: Evaluation of injectable trichlorfon as a treatment for onchocerciasis in horses. Southwest Vet 30:176, 1977.
207. McCullough C, et al: Onchocerciasis among ungulate animals in Maryland. J Parasitol 63:1065, 1977.
208. Mellor PS: Studies on *Onchocerca cervicalis* Railliet and Henry, 1910. I. *Onchocerca cervicalis* in British horses. J Helminthol 47:97, 1973.
209. Mellor PS: Studies on *Onchocerca cervicalis* Railliet and Henry, 1910. II. Pathology in the horse. J Helminthol 47:111, 1973.
210. Mellor PS: Studies on *Onchocerca cervicalis* Railliet and Henry, 1910. III. Morphologic and taxonomic studies on *Onchocerca cervicalis* from British horses. J Helminthol 48:145, 1974.
211. Mogg TD, et al: Efficacy of avermectin B₁ given orally against equine intestinal strongyles and *Onchocerca* microfilaria. Aust Vet J 67:399,1990.
212. Nemeseri L: Untersuchungen uber die Haufigkeit von mikrofilarien pferdeaugen und ihre pathologische bedeutung. Acta Vet Hung Acad Sci 6:109, 1956.
213. Ottley ML, Moorehouse DE: Equine onchocerciasis. Aust Vet J 54:545, 1978.
214. Ottley ML, et al: Equine onchocerciasis in Queensland and the northern territory of Australia. Aust Vet J 60:200, 1983.
215. Ottley ML, Moorehouse DE: Morphological variations in *Onchocerca* sp. from atypical hosts and sites: the validity of *O. stilesi*. Ann Parasitol Hum Comp 57:389, 1982.
216. Pader J: Filariose du ligament suspenseur du boulet chez le cheval. Arch Parasitol 4:58, 1901.
217. Pillars AW: An exhibition of worms parasitic on equines, and remarks thereon. Vet Rec 27:234, 1914.
218. Pillars AW: The parasitic origin of poll evil and fistulous withers. Vet Rec 44:1246, 1931.
219. Polley L: *Onchocerca* in horses from western Canada and the northwestern United States: an abattoir survey of the prevalence of infection. Can Vet J 24:128, 1984.
220. Pollitt CC, et al: Treatment of equine onchocerciasis with ivermectin paste. Aust Vet J 63:152, 1986.
221. Rabalais FC, et al: Survey for equine onchocerciasis in the midwestern United States. Am J Vet Res 35:125, 1974.
222. Rabalais FC, Votava CL: Cutaneous distribution of microfilariae of *Onchocerca cervicalis* in horses. Am J Vet Res 35:1369, 1974.
223. Riek RF: A note on the occurrence of *Onchocerca reticulata* (Diresing 1841) in the horse in Queensland. Aust Vet J 30:178, 1954.
224. Roberts FHS: Onchocerciasis. Aust Vet J 14:32, 1938.
225. Roberts SR: Etiology of equine periodic ophthalmia. Am J Ophthalmol 55:1049, 1963.
226. Robson J: Filariasis of the withers in the horse. Vet Rec 31:348, 1918.
227. Schmidt GM, et al: Equine ocular onchocerciasis: histopathologic study. Am J Vet Res 43:1371, 1982.
228. Schmidt GM, et al: Equine onchocerciasis: lesions in the nuchal ligament of midwestern United States horses. Vet Pathol 19:16, 1982.
229. Stannard AA: Equine dermatoses. Proc Am Assoc Equine Pract 22:273, 1976.
230. Stannard AA, Cello RM: *Onchocerca cervicalis* infection in horses from the western United States. Am J Vet Res 36:1029, 1975.
231. Steward JS: Fistulous withers and poll evil. Vet Rec 47:1563, 1935.
232. Supperer R: Filariosen der Pferde in Osterreich. Wien Tieräztl Monatsschr 40:193, 1953.
233. Thomas AD: Microfilariasis in the horse. J S Afr Vet Med Assoc 24:17, 1963.
234. Underwood JR: Equine Dhobie itch a symptom of filariasis. A report of 56 cases. Vet Bull 28:227, 1934.
235. Webster WA, Dukes TW: Bovine and equine onchocerciasis in eastern North America with a discussion on cuticular morphology of *Onchocerca* spp. in cattle. Can J Comp Med 43:330, 1979.

Parafilariasis
236. Baumann R: Beobachtungen beim parasitaren Sommerbluten der Pferde. Wien Tierärztl Monatsschr 33:52, 1946.
237. Gibson TE, et al: *Parafilaria multipapillosa* in the horse. Vet Rec 76:774, 1964.
238. Gnedina MA, Osipov AN: Contribution to the biology of the nematode *Parafilaria multipapillosa* parasite in the horse. Helminthologia 2:13, 1960.
239. Railliet M, Moussu J: La filaire des boutons hémorragiques observée chez l'ane; découverte du male. Compt Rend Seanc Soc Biol 44:545, 1892.
240. Thomsett LR: Differential diagnosis of skin diseases of the horse. Equine Vet J 2:46, 1970.
241. Williams HE: Haematidrosis in a horse. Vet Rec 65:386, 1953.

Oxyuriasis
242. Magbool A, et al: Oxyuriasis in horses and its treatment with febantel and thiabendazole. Indian Vet J 71:650, 1994.
243. Yazwinski TA, et al: Effectiveness of ivermectin in the treatment of equine *Parascaris equorum* and *Oxyuris equi* infections. Am J Vet Res 43:1095, 1982.

Strongyloidosis
244. Dewes HF: *Strongyloides westeri* and *Corynebacterium equi* in foals. N Z Vet J 20:82, 1972.

245. Etherington WG, Prescott JF: *Corynebacterium equi* cellulitis associated with *Strongyloides* penetration in a foal. J Am Vet Med Assoc 177:1025, 1980.
246. Ludwig KG, et al: Efficacy of ivermectin in controlling *Strongyloides westeri* infections in foals. Am J Vet Res 44:314, 1983.

Pelodera

247. Dozsa L: Dermatitis in large animals . . . Selected case histories. Mod Vet Pract 47:45, 1966.
248. Farrington DO, et al: *Pelodera strongyloides* dermatitis in a horse in Iowa. Vet Med Small Anim Clin 71:1199, 1976.
249. Rashmir-Raven AM, et al: Papillomatous pastern dermatitis with *Spirochetes* and *Pelodera strongyloides* in a Tennessee walking horse. J Vet Diagn Invest 12:287, 2000.

Halicephalobiasis

250. Blunden AS, et al: *Halicephalobus deletrix* infection in a horse. Equine Vet J 19:255, 1987.
251. Dunn DG, et al: Nodular granulomatous posthitis caused by *Halicephalobus* (syn. *Micronema*) sp. in a horse. Vet Pathol 30:207, 1993.
252. Kinde H, et al: *Halicephalobus gingivalis* (*H. deletrix*) infection in two horses in southern California. J Vet Diagn Invest 12:162, 2000.
253. Payan J, et al: Granulomas en el prepucio de un equino causados por *Micronema*. Rev Inst Colomb Agropecu 14:283, 1979.
253a. Pearce SG, et al: Treatment of a granuloma caused by *Halicephalobus gingivalis* in a horse. J Am Vet Med Assoc 219:1735, 2001.
254. Ruggles AJ, et al: Disseminated *Halicephalobus deletrix* infection in a horse. J Am Vet Med Assoc 203:550, 1993.
255. Spalding MG, et al: *Halicephalobus* (*Micronema*) *deletrix* infection in two half-sibling foals. J Am Vet Med Assoc 196:1127, 1990.

Cephalobiasis

256. Greiner EC, et al: Verminous mastitis in a mare caused by a free-living nematode. J Parasitol 77:320, 1991.

Chapter 7

Viral and Protozoal Skin Diseases

● VIRAL DISEASES

Cutaneous lesions may be the only feature associated with a viral infection, or they may be part of a more generalized disease.[1-5] A clinical examination of the skin often provides valuable information that assists the veterinarian in the differential diagnosis of several viral disorders.

Many of the viral diseases discussed in this chapter do not normally occur in North America. However, to omit these diseases from consideration would be unwise. The continued freedom from major viral diseases in various areas of the world is contingent, in part, on the practicing veterinarian's recognizing them when they occur and promptly informing the appropriate veterinary authorities.

When collecting samples for the diagnosis of viral disease, the clinician must remember that the suspicion that the disease is caused by a virus may be incorrect. Thus, samples should be collected for alternative diagnoses. Assuming that it is a viral disease, the following should be remembered:[21,47,49] (1) The titer of virus is usually highest at affected sites and during the early stages of the disease, (2) viruses replicate only in living cells, and their stability is adversely affected by exposure to light, desiccation, extremes of pH, and most common disinfectants, (3) secondary bacterial or mycotic infection is a common sequela of viral disease, and (4) samples taken from the later stages of disease are less likely to contain virus.

To overcome the aforementioned problems, the samples should be protected by storage at 4° C in a virus transport medium. To avoid an erroneous or incomplete diagnosis, samples should be taken from different types of lesions and from more than one animal. When collecting a skin scraping or obtaining a biopsy for viral culture, the areas should be washed with water or saline, *not* with alcohol, because alcohol inactivates most viruses. Scraping of the skin and mucous membranes should be extended to the periphery and base of the lesion.

Electron microscopy is very useful in the rapid diagnosis of viral skin diseases,[22,47,49] but isolation of the causal virus in tissue culture is still the most widely used and most sensitive technique.

An in-depth discussion of all the viral diseases—especially their extracutaneous clinical signs and pathology and their elaborate diagnostic and control schemata—is beyond the scope of this chapter. We will concentrate on the dermatologic aspects of the diseases. The reader is referred to other excellent texts for detailed information on the extracutaneous aspects of these diseases.[1-5]

Poxvirus Infections

The Poxviridae are a large family of DNA viruses that share group-specific nucleoprotein antigens.[4,47,49] The genera include Orthopoxvirus (cowpox and vaccinia), Capripoxvirus (sheeppox, goatpox, and bovine lumpy skin disease), Suipoxvirus (swinepox), Parapoxvirus (pseudocowpox, bovine papular stomatitis, and contagious viral pustular dermatitis), and Molluscipoxvirus (molluscum contagiosum).

Infection is usually acquired by cutaneous or respiratory routes. Poxviruses commonly gain access to the systemic circulation via the lymphatic system, although multiplication at the site of inoculation in the skin may lead to direct entry into the blood and a primary viremia. A secondary viremia disseminates the virus back to the skin and to other target organs.

The poxviruses replicate autonomously in the cytoplasm of cells. After uncoating, the virion produces early enzymes and early virion proteins and late virion proteins. These replication "factories" are independent of the host nucleus and are discernible on light microscopy as basophilic staining Type B inclusion bodies.

Poxviruses induce lesions by a variety of mechanisms. Degenerative changes in epithelium are caused by virus replication and lead to vesicular lesions typical of many poxvirus infections. Degenerative changes in the dermis or subcutis may result from ischemia secondary to vascular damage. Poxvirus infections also induce proliferative lesions via epithelial hyperplasia. The host-cell DNA synthesis is stimulated before the onset of cytoplasmic virus-related DNA replication.

Pox lesions in the skin have a typical clinical evolution, beginning as erythematous macules and becoming papular and then vesicular. The vesicular stage is well developed in some pox infections and transient or nonexistent in others. Vesicles evolve into umbilicated pustules with a depressed center and a raised, often erythematous border. This lesion is the so-called pock. The pustules rupture and form a crust. Healed lesions often leave a scar.

Histologically, pox lesions begin with ballooning degeneration of the stratum spinosum of the epidermis (Fig. 7-1).[62] Reticular degeneration and acantholysis result in intraepidermal microvesicles. Dermal lesions include edema and a superficial and deep perivascular dermatitis. Mononuclear cells and neutrophils are present in varying proportions. Neutrophils migrate into the epidermis and produce intraepidermal microabscesses and pustules, which may extend into the dermis. Marked irregular to pseudocarcinomatous epidermal hyperplasia is usually seen. Poxvirus lesions contain characteristic intracytoplasmic inclusion bodies, which are single or multiple and of varying size and duration. The more prominent eosinophilic inclusions (3 to 7 μm in diameter) are called Type A and are weakly positive by the Feulgen method. They begin as small eosinophilic intracytoplasmic inclusions (Borrel's bodies) and evolve into a single, large body (Bollinger's body). The smaller basophilic inclusions are called Type B.

Diagnosis of poxvirus infections is usually based on observation of the typical clinical appearance and may be supported by characteristic histologic lesions. Demonstration of the virus by electron microscopy (Fig. 7-2) will confirm a poxvirus etiology but may not differentiate between morphologically similar viruses, such as the closely related orthopoxviruses. Poxviruses are brick-shaped or oval structures measuring 200 to 400 nm. Definitive identification of specific viruses requires the isolation of the virus and its identification by serologic and immuno-fluorescence techniques.

Poxviruses of horses can produce skin lesions in humans.[30,41,55] The presumptive diagnosis is usually made on the basis of known exposure to horses. Humans having contact with horses (ranchers, veterinarians, and veterinary students) are at risk. Transmission is by direct and indirect contact, and human-to-human transmission can occur. The incubation period is 4 to 14 days. Human skin lesions average 1.6 cm in diameter and usually occur singly, most commonly on a finger. However, multiple lesions can occur. Solitary lesions may also occur on the face and legs. Regional lymphadenopathy is common, but fever, malaise, and lymphangitis are rare. Skin lesions evolve through six stages and usually heal uneventfully in about 35 days.[20] An elevated, erythematous papule evolves into a nodule with a red center, a white middle ring, and a red periphery. A red, weeping surface is present acutely. Later, a thin dry crust through which black dots may be seen covers the surface of the nodule. Finally, the lesion develops a papillomatous surface, a thick crust develops, and the lesion regresses. Pain and pruritus are variable.

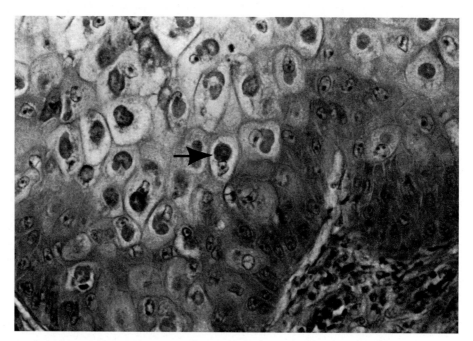

FIGURE 7-1. Poxvirus. Koilocytosis (ballooning degeneration) and intracytoplasmic inclusion bodies (*arrow*).

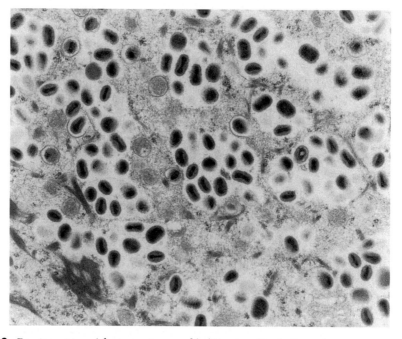

FIGURE 7-2. Poxvirus virions (electron micrograph). (*Courtesy Dr. L. Lange.*)

VACCINIA

Vaccinia is caused by an orthopoxvirus that infects horses, cattle, swine, and humans.[2,4,20,55] Vaccinia is caused by the virus propagated in laboratories and used for prophylactic vaccination against smallpox in humans. In 1979 the World Health Organization declared world-wide eradication of smallpox. Eradication was achieved by the use of a virus believed for many years to have been derived from a lesion on the udder of a cow (the very words *vaccine*, *vaccinia*, and *vaccination* are derived from the Latin word *vacca*, meaning "a cow").[55] However, from currently available information, it appears that the strain of virus used to inoculate people against smallpox may have come from a horse.[16,18,26,30,55]

"Horsepox" was a commonly described clinical disease from at least the late 18th century until the early 20th century.* However, "horsepox" is rarely described recently. Various lines of reasoning—historical, clinical, and experimental—strongly suggest that "horsepox" never existed as a separate entity and was actually vaccinia.[30,54,55] Not surprisingly, then, as smallpox was eradicated and the use of vaccinia virus immunization ceased, the disease "horsepox" literally disappeared.

In addition, from the 1940s through the 1970s, there were scattered reports on two other orthopox virus infections of the skin of horses: viral papular dermatitis[29,45] and Uasin Gishu disease.[15,34-37] Again, careful comparison of the clinical, histopathologic, and virologic features of these two syndromes with experimentally induced vaccinia in horses indicates that the three conditions are the same.[54,55]

The lesions of equine vaccinia may affect the skin of the muzzle and lips, the buccal, nasal, and genital mucosa, the skin of the caudal aspects of the pasterns or the entire body surface.[1,54] Within 4 days after inoculation of vaccinia virus, raised, discrete, 2- to 4-mm diameter papules are seen.[54] These lesions proceed through a typical pox sequence of pustules that develop dark, hemorrhagic umbilicated centers, then scabs, and then scars at about 22 days postinoculation (Fig. 7-3). In haired areas, a thin yellow exudate is produced, which dries to a fine crystalline powder-like appearance, then becomes a thick, yellow to dark brown and grease-like substance that mats the hair. Some horses manifest mild to moderate pyrexia, lameness, depression, ptyalism, and difficulties in eating and drinking.

The virus grows on chicken chorioallantoic membrane or calf kidney monolayers and has typical electron microscopic morphology.[34,35,45,54] Skin biopsy reveals typical poxvirus histopathologic changes (see above).[36,54,62]

MOLLUSCUM CONTAGIOSUM

Molluscum contagiosum is caused by a molluscipox virus.[20,23,44] The virus has not yet been grown in tissue culture or in an animal model. The disease is world-wide in distribution. Transmission occurs by intimate skin-to-skin contact, and by fomites. Immunoincompetent humans have more severe, unusual, and recalcitrant forms of the disease.

On the basis of very close homology of their viral DNA sequences, the viruses of equine and human molluscum contagiosum are either identical or very closely related.[57] It has been suggested that equine molluscum contagiosum may represent an anthropozoonosis, wherein disease is transmitted from human to animal.[57]

Molluscum contagiosum has been reported in a number of horses, from 1 to 17 years of age, many of which were in good health.† There was no evidence of contagion to contact horses. Lesions usually begin in one body region and become widespread. Most horses have hundreds of lesions (especially on the chest, shoulders, neck, and limbs). However, lesions can remain localized to areas such as the prepuce, scrotum, or muzzle. Early lesions are 1- to 8-mm diameter papules.

---

*References 1, 16, 18, 26, 30, 41, 63.
†References 7, 12, 44, 46, 47a, 50, 61.

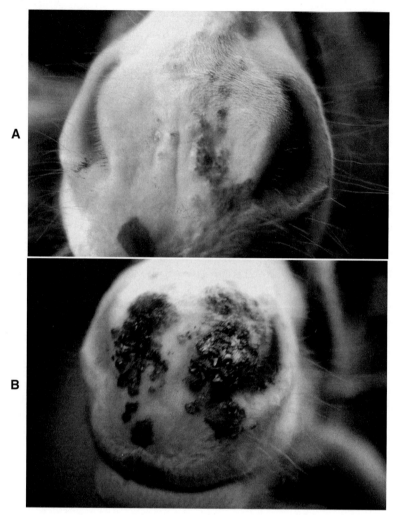

FIGURE 7-3. Vaccinia. **A,** Umbilicated papules and crusts on the muzzle. **B,** Large, thick crusts on muzzle. (*Courtesy Dr. M. Studdert.*)

In haired skin, the papules are initially tufted, but usually become alopecic and covered with a powdery crust or grayish-white scales (Fig. 7-4). Some papules have a central soft white spicule (Fig. 7-5) or firm brownish-yellow horn that projects 3 to 6 mm above the surface of the lesion. Coalescence of lesions occasionally produces 2- to 3-cm diameter cauliflower-like nodules or plaques. Some lesions bleed when traumatized. Papules in glabrous skin may be smooth, shiny, hypopigmented, and umbilicated, or hyperkeratotic and hyperpigmented (Fig. 7-6). The lesions are typically nonpruritic and nonpainful.

Biopsy reveals well-demarcated hyperplasia and papillomatosis of the epidermis and hair follicle infundibulum (Fig. 7-7).° Keratinocytes above the stratum basale become swollen and contain ovoid, eosinophilic, floccular intracytoplasmic inclusion bodies (so-called "molluscum bodies"). These inclusions increase in size and density as the keratinocytes move toward the skin surface, compressing the cell nucleus against the cytoplasmic membrane. In the stratum granu-

---

°References 12, 23, 44, 46, 47a, 50, 61.

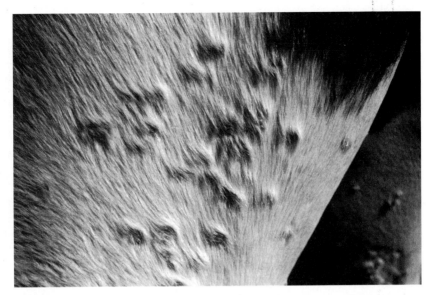

FIGURE 7-4. Molluscum contagiosum. Tufted papules that have become crusted. (*Courtesy Dr. L. Lange.*)

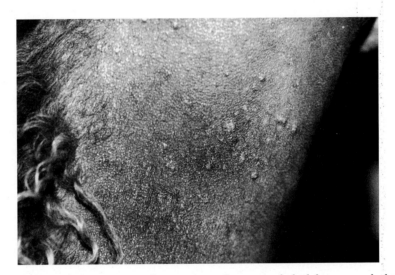

FIGURE 7-5. Molluscum contagiosum. White, waxy papules, some of which have central white spicule, on lateral neck (area has been clipped).

losum and stratum corneum, the staining reaction of the molluscum bodies changes from eosinophilic to basophilic. Molluscum bodies exfoliate through a pore that forms in the stratum corneum and enlarges into a central crater (Fig. 7-8). Usually there is no dermal inflammatory reaction, but scattered neutrophils and lymphocytes may be seen. Ultrastructural examination reveals mature virions that are brick-shaped and about 150×300 nm.*

Spontaneous regression of all lesions has not been reported, with horses remaining covered with lesions for several months to 6 years.[44,46,47a,61] Successful therapy has not been reported. An autogenous vaccine was tried in one horse, and the condition slowly worsened.[46]

---

*References 12, 23, 44, 46, 47a, 50, 61.

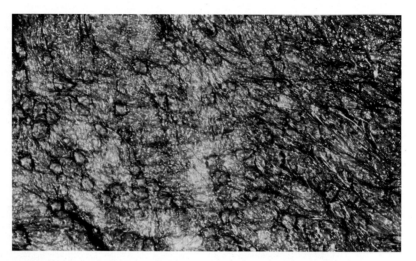

FIGURE 7-6. Molluscum contagiosum. Multiple waxy papules in the groin. (*Courtesy Dr. J. Yager.*)

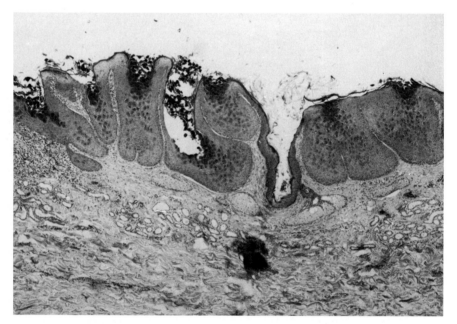

FIGURE 7-7. Molluscum contagiosum. Papillated and irregular epidermal hyperplasia with numerous inclusion bodies.

Equine Herpes Coital Exanthema

Equine herpes coital exanthema is a contagious venereal disease of horses caused by equine herpesvirus 3.[2,4-9,48,53,60] It is found in most parts of the world. In addition to transmission by coitus, transmission may also occur via insects, fomites, and inhalation. The incubation period is about 7 days.

Initial lesions include 1- to 3-mm diameter papules, vesicles, or pustules, or larger 1- to 5-cm diameter bullae on the penis and prepuce of stallions and on the vulva and perineum of mares.

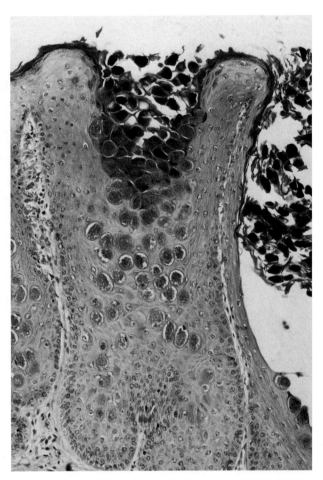

FIGURE 7-8. Molluscum contagiosum. Intracytoplasmic inclusion bodies.

These lesions are usually accompanied by edema and evolve into erosions, ulcers, and crusts (Fig. 7-9). Lesions may be pruritic but are not usually painful. Macular areas of depigmentation may persist where lesions have healed. Spontaneous healing takes place over a period of 3 to 5 weeks.

Skin biopsies are characterized by hyperplastic superficial and deep perivascular dermatitis with ballooning degeneration of keratinocytes and eosinophilic intranuclear inclusion bodies (Fig. 7-10).[2,62] Some lesions show acantholysis, necrosis, and intraepidermal vesicle formation (Figs. 7-11 and 7-12).

Treatment includes at least 3 weeks of sexual rest and the application of emollient antibiotic ointments to prevent secondary infections and preputial adhesions. Animals should not be bred while affected. Reoccurrences are seen, especially after periods of stress.

Equine Viral Arteritis

Equine viral arteritis is an infrequently encountered contagious disease of horses in many parts of the world.* Transmission occurs via coitus and inhalation. The causative virus was previously

---

*References 3, 4, 11, 16b, 19, 59.

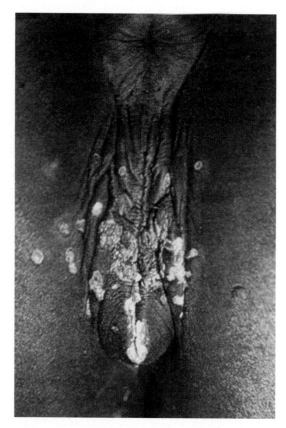

FIGURE 7-9. Herpes coital exanthema. Multiple annular areas of ulceration and depigmentation on vulva. (*Courtesy Dr. W. McMullen.*)

classified as a member of the Togaviridae family, but is currently classified as a new genus called *Arterivirus* (Arteriviridae family).[59] Equine viral arteritis is reportable in the United States.

Affected horses may develop edema of the distal limbs (especially the hind limbs), scrotum, prepuce, ventrum, and periorbital or supraorbital areas. Less frequently, edematous swelling may occur on the sternum, shoulder, mammary glands, or the intermandibular space. Rarely, affected horses may develop a papular to urticarial eruption over the dorsum and lateral thorax.[16a]

Histopathologic examination reveals lesions in the media of arteries with a well-developed muscular coat, chiefly those with a diameter of about 0.5 mm.[2,14,16a,31] Early changes include fibrinoid necrosis of the media, accompanied or followed shortly by edema and lymphocytic infiltration. Lymphocytes continue to infiltrate the media and undergo karyorrhexis, as well as accumulate in an edematous adventitia. Viral antigen can be demonstrated in affected vessels.[16a]

Vesicular Stomatitis

Vesicular stomatitis ("red nose," "sore nose," "sore mouth") is an infectious viral disease of horses, cattle, and swine, and is enzootic in North, Central, and South America.° It is caused by a vesiculovirus (lyssa virus) of the Rhabdoviridae family, and has three main serotypes (New Jersey, Indiana, and local strains). The disease is sporadic and usually seen between late spring and early

°References 1-5, 13, 17, 24, 25, 38, 56.

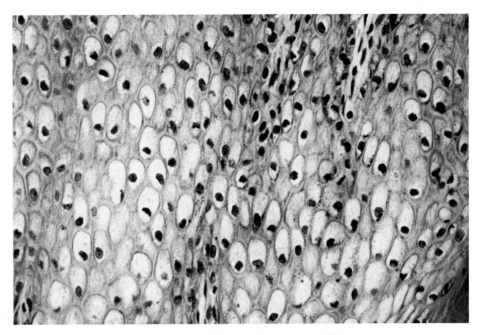

FIGURE 7-10. Herpes coital examination. Ballooning degeneration of keratinocytes.

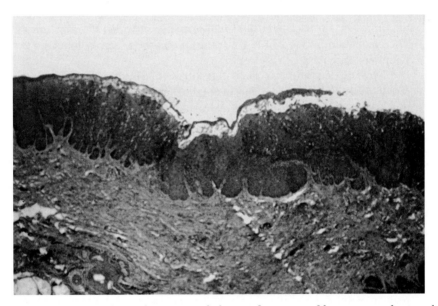

FIGURE 7-11. Herpes coital exanthema. Acantholysis and necrosis of keratinocytes has resulted in an intraepidermal vesicle.

fall. The exact mechanism of transmission is unclear, but involves biting and nonbiting insects, plants, aerosols, and secretions. Recent epidemiologic studies have indicated that: (1) horses that had access to shelter or barn had a reduced risk for developing disease, (2) the odds of developing disease are significantly greater where insect populations are greater than normal, and (3) premises with horses housed <0.25 miles from running water had significantly increased risk of disease.[28,51]

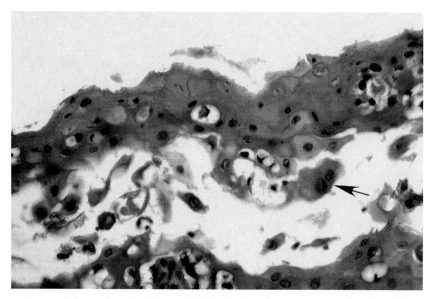

FIGURE 7-12. Herpes coital exanthema. Acantholysis (*arrow*), necrosis, and intraepidermal vesicle formation.

Hematophagous insects are probably very important in disease transmission, and vesicular stomatitis virus has been isolated from *Culicoides* spp. and *Simulium* spp. during multiple outbreaks.[28,51] The incubation period is 2 to 8 days. In humans, vesicular stomatitis virus causes influenza-like symptoms and, rarely, oral ulcers.

Excessive salivation is usually the initial clinical sign of vesicular stomatitis. Vesicles progress rapidly to painful erosions and ulcers of the oral cavity (especially the dorsal surface of the tongue), lips, and occasionally the prepuce, vulva, udder, and teats. Edema of the head is occasionally seen. Ulcers of the coronary band (Fig. 7-13) are particularly prominent in horses and may lead to severe lameness, hoof wall deformity, laminitis and, rarely, sloughed hoof. Depigmentation may persist in healed areas (Fig. 7-14). Healing usually occurs within 2 weeks. Vesicular stomatitis is reportable in the United States.

Biopsy findings include a hyperplastic superficial and deep neutrophilic perivascular dermatitis.[2,38,62] Marked intra- and intercellular edema of the epidermis may lead to reticular degeneration and spongiotic microvesicles. Epidermal necrosis follows.

Jamestown Canyon Virus Infection

Jamestown Canyon virus is a member of California encephalitis virus group (Bunyavirus, Bunyaviridae).[50a] A high prevalence of virus-specific antibody has been found in horses in various regions of the United States. The virus may be an emerging cause of encephalitis in humans. Jamestown Canyon virus was isolated from the lesions of a horse with vesicles on the coronary band and ruptured vesicles on the tongue and inner surface of the lower lip.[50a] This condition must be distinguished from vesicular stomatitis.

African Horse Sickness

African horse sickness is an acute, subacute, or mild infectious disease of horses.[4,27] The disease is caused by an orbivirus of the Reoviridae family, and is transmitted mainly by *Culicoides* spp. gnats. It occurs in Africa, the Middle East, and the Mediterranean area, and is reportable in the United

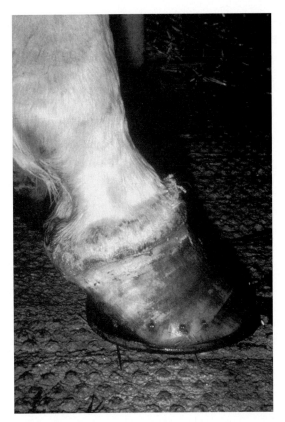

FIGURE 7-13. Vesicular stomatitis. Ulceration and crusting of coronary band. (*Courtesy Dr. N. Messer.*)

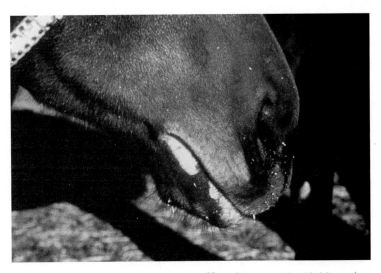

FIGURE 7-14. Vesicular stomatitis. Depigmentation of lips. (*Courtesy Dr. N. Messer.*)

● Table 7-1 **PROTOZOAN PARASITES ASSOCIATED WITH SKIN LESIONS IN HORSES**

Class: Zoomastigophorea
   Order: Kinetoplastida
      Family: Trypanosomatidae
         Genera: Trypanosoma, Leishmania
Class: Sporozoea
   Order: Eucoccidiida
      Family: Sarcocystidae
         Subfamily: Toxoplasmatinae
            Genus: Besnoitia

States. In the subacute form, affected horses may have marked edema of the eyelids and the intermandibular space.

Getah

Getah is caused by alphaviruses of the Togaviridae family, transmitted by mosquitos, and occurs in Southeast Asia.[4,43] The Getah subgroup of alphaviruses includes the Getah virus (Sakai virus) and the Sagiyama virus, both of which produce Getah disease in horses.[39,40,42]

The disease is characterized by acute pyrexia (usually 40° C) and enlarged submandibular lymph nodes followed in one to several days by a papular to urticarial eruption and/or edema of the hind limbs.* These lesions usually resolve within 1 week.

Skin biopsy reveals superficial and deep perivascular to diffuse dermatitis dominated by lymphocytes, histiocytes, and eosinophils.[33,40]

Viral Papillomatosis

DNA papovaviruses are the cause of two distinctive clinical forms of papillomatosis in horses (see Chapter 16).

Equine Sarcoid

The equine sarcoid is a fibroblastic neoplasm of viral origin (see Chapter 16).

● PROTOZOAL DISEASES

Protozoa are unicellular animals in which activities such as metabolism and locomotion are carried out by organelles of the cell.[1,4,78] Parasitic protozoa are an important cause of equine disease in many areas of the world (Table 7-1). Some of these diseases have an associated dermatosis, but the cutaneous disorders are of minimal importance compared with disorders that involve other organ systems. In this chapter, the cutaneous changes associated with various protozoal diseases of the horse will be characterized. For detailed information on other clinicopathologic, diagnostic, and therapeutic aspects of these diseases, the reader is referred to specific articles and texts within the references.[1-5] The following protozoal diseases, except giardiasis, are reportable in the United States.

Trypanosomiasis

Members of the genus Trypanosoma are found principally in the blood and tissue fluids, although a few invade tissue cells.[4,78] They are transmitted by blood-sucking arthropods and insects.

*References 32, 33, 39, 42, 43, 52.

Diagnosis is based on demonstrating the trypanosomes (elongated, central or terminal kinetoplast, flagellum, tapered ends, 12 to 35 μm in diameter) in blood or tissue fluids. Therapeutic agents include diminazene (7 mg/kg intramuscularly), suramin (10 mg/kg intravenously), or quinapyramine (3 to 5 mg/kg subcutaneously), but many horses remain inapparent carriers.

NAGANA

Nagana (also called samore, African trypanosomiasis, tsetse fly disease) is caused by *Trypanosoma congolense (T. pecorum, T. nanum)* and is transmitted mainly by the tsetse fly (*Glossina* spp.).[1,4,78] It produces edema of the distal limbs and genitalia in horses.

SURRA

Surra (Indian for "rotten") or mal de caderas is caused by *T. evansi (T. equinum)* and is transmitted mainly by blood sucking flies (especially *Tabanus* spp.) in Africa, the Middle East, Asia, and Central and South America.[1,4,78] It produces urticarial plaques that become crusted and alopecic over the neck, flanks, limbs, and genitalia.

DOURINE

Dourine (Arabic for "unclean") is caused by *T. equiperdum*, transmitted mainly by coitus, and occurs in Africa, Asia, Southeastern Europe, and Central and South America.[1,4,41,78] In stallions, initial cutaneous changes include edema of the prepuce that extends to the scrotum and surrounding skin. In mares, edema initially involves the vulva and extends to the perineum, udder, and ventral abdomen. Papules that ulcerate many occasionally be seen in both sexes, and depigmentation (leukoderma) may be a striking sequela in these areas. Later, an urticarial eruption appears, which is especially prominent over the neck, chest, flanks, and back. Urticarial plaques are 2 to 10 cm in diameter, wax and wane, and usually have a depressed center. These so-called "silver dollar spots" are alleged to be pathognomonic for dourine. Successive crops of urticarial plaques may result in skin involvement that persists for several weeks. When the lesions resolve, focal areas of hypo- or hyperhidrosis may persist.

Leishmaniasis

Members of the genus Leishmania cause disease in the horse.[*] The amastigote stages (Leishman-Donovan bodies) are found in endothelial cells and cells of the mononuclear phagocytic system. They are circular or oval in shape, 2 to 4 μm in diameter, and contain a round, basophilic nucleus and a small, rod-like kinetoplast (Fig. 7-15, *B*). The organisms are best seen with Giemsa stain. In the Old World, leishmaniasis occurs most commonly in the Mediterranean basin. In the New World, the disease is endemic in South and Central America. The disease is transmitted by blood sucking sand flies of the genus Phlebotomus in the Old World and the genus Lutzomyia in the New World. In South America, equine leishmaniasis is caused by *Leishmania braziliensis braziliensis*, which is transmitted by the sandflies *Lutzomyia cayennensis* (subspecies *viequesensis* and *puertoricensis*).[65,75,81] The disease has zoonotic potential.[65,81]

Cutaneous leishmaniasis is often diagnosed in several South American countries[†] but is extremely rarely reported elsewhere in the world.[41,68,76] No age, breed, or sex predilections are reported. Lesions are usually multiple and most commonly present on the head (especially muzzle and periocular region), pinnae, scrotum, legs, and neck. Lesions consist of papules and nodules, 5 to 10 mm in diameter, which are often crusted and ulcerated. Rarely, nonhealing ulcers with raised edges and depressed granulating centers are seen (Fig. 7-15, *A*).

---

*References 4, 64, 65, 70, 72, 74, 76, 78, 81.
†References 64, 65, 70, 72, 74, 75, 81.

Histopathologic findings include varying combinations of a multinodular to diffuse lympho-histiocytic dermatitis; a tuberculoid granulomatous dermatitis; a diffuse dermatitis containing neutrophils, macrophages, and multinucleated histiocytic giant cells.[75] The number of organisms seen is quite variable (Fig. 7-15, *C*).

One horse was treated with sodium stibogluconate (Pentostam), 600 mg intravenously daily for 10 days, repeated in 30 days.[75] Lesions had resolved after the second round of therapy, and the horse remained normal for 2 years.

Besnoitiosis

Besnoitiosis (globidiosis) appears to be a rare disease of horses in Africa and South and Central America.° The natural means of transmission of *Besnoitia bennetti* is not known, but ingestion of

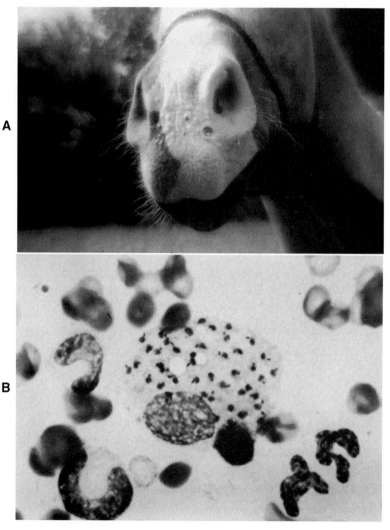

FIGURE 7-15. Leishmaniasis. **A,** Nonhealing ulcer on muzzle. (*Courtesy Dr. A. Sales.*) **B,** Macrophage containing numerous amastigotes (Leishman-Donovan bodies). (*Courtesy Dr. T. French.*)

°References 66, 67, 69, 73, 77-80.

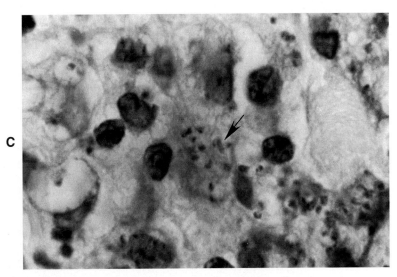

FIGURE 7-15, cont'd. C, Numerous organisms present in macrophage (*arrow*).

oocysts and mechanical transmission of bradyzoites by blood-sucking insects may be of significance. Subcutaneous injection of infected material from a diseased horse did not produce disease in rabbits nor another horse.[80]

Early cutaneous lesions appear as small, 1- to 2-mm diameter tufted papules in haired areas, or 1- to 2-mm diameter slightly raised papules in glabrous skin. These papules may become covered with a moist or gummy material within several days. Hairs overlying the papules often fall out. Hairs that regrow may be depigmented or normal in color. Severely affected horses develop widespread thickening, scaling, crusting, folding, and alopecia of the skin, especially over the legs, ventral aspect of the body, perineum, genitalia, and eyelids. Glabrous areas of skin may have multiple areas of leukoderma overlying papular lesions. Pruritus may or may not be present. Pinpoint white to glistening papules are often present on the sclera, nostrils, nasal mucosa, pharynx, larynx, and soft palate. A few of these lesions may be present in the guttural pouches. Affected horses may be febrile, depressed, weak, and show signs of upper respiratory disease (nasal and/or laryngeal stridor).

Skin biopsy reveals numerous *Besnoitia* cysts within the dermis and subcutis, which appear to develop within fibroblasts (Fig. 7-16).[67,73,80] The cysts are 300 to 600 μm in diameter, and are packed with multiple crescent- or banana-shaped bradyzoites that vary from 5 to 8 μm in length by 1.5 to 2 μm in width. The cysts are surrounded by an abundant basement membrane-like zone, and varying degrees of fibrosis and variable numbers of plasma cells. Where cyst walls have ruptured, a granulomatous or pyogranulomatous dermatitis may be present.

Successful therapy in horses has not been reported. However, trimethoprim-sulfamethoxazole (20 mg/kg q12h by mouth) was apparently effective in the treatment of cutaneous besnoitiosis in a miniature donkey.[71] The combination was given daily for 30 days, discontinued for 30 days, then readministered for an additional 45 days.

Giardiasis

Giardiasis was diagnosed in a horse with intermittent diarrhea, weight loss, poor hair coat, lethargy, inappetence, and an "exudative dermatitis" over the withers and thorax.[82] All clinical signs disappeared when the horse was treated with metronidazole orally. The relationship between the giardiasis and the "exudative dermatitis" is unclear.

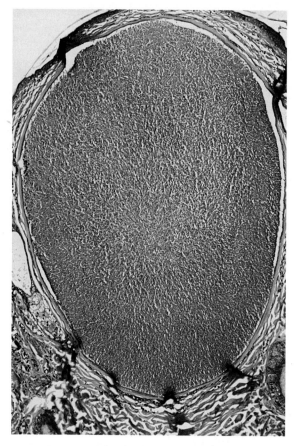

FIGURE 7-16. Besnoitiosis. *Besnoitia* cyst in skin biopsy specimen.

● REFERENCES

General

1. Chatterjee A: Skin Infection in Domestic Animals. Moitri Publication, Calcutta, 1989.
2. Jubb KVF, et al (eds): Pathology of Domestic Animals IV, vols. 1-3. Academic Press, New York, 1993.
3. Kobluk CN, et al (eds): The Horse. Diseases and Clinical Management, vols. 1-2. W.B. Saunders Co, Philadelphia, 1995.
4. Radostits OM, et al: Veterinary Medicine. A Textbook of the Diseases of Cattle, Sheep, Pigs, Goats and Horses VIII. Baillère Tindall, Philadelphia, 1994.
5. Robinson NE (ed): Current Therapy in Equine Medicine, 4th ed. W.B. Saunders Co, Philadelphia, 1997.

Viral Diseases

6. Blanchard TL, et al: Venereal disease. Vet Clin N Am Equine Pract 8:191, 1992.
7. Bourdeau P: A case of molluscum contagiosum in an immunocompromised horse. Proc Annu Congress Eur Soc Vet Dermatol Eur Coll Vet Dermatol 14:187, 1997.
8. Bowen JM: Venereal diseases of stallions. In: Robinson NE (ed): Current Therapy in Equine Medicine II. W.B. Saunders Co, Philadelphia, 1986, p 567.
9. Burki F, et al: Experimentelle genitale und nasale Infektion von Pferden mit dem Virus des equinen coital exanthems. Zbl Vet Med B21:362, 1974.
10. Burton AC: Stomatitis contagiosa in horses. Vet J 73:234, 1917.
11. Coggins L: Equine viral arteritis. In: Robinson NE (ed): Current Therapy in Equine Medicine. W.B. Saunders Co, Philadelphia, 1983, p 6.
12. Cooley AJ, et al: Molluscum contagiosum in a horse with granulomatous enteritis. J Comp Pathol 97:29, 1987.
13. Cordes T: Vesicular stomatitis strikes horse. J Am Vet Med Assoc 211:144, 1997.
14. Crawford TB, Henson JB: Viral arteritis of horses. Adv Exp Med Biol 22:175, 1972.
15. Daubney R: Uasin Gishu skin disease of horses. Kenya Dept Agric Annu Rep 3:26,1934.
16. DeJong DA: The relationship between contagious pustular stomatitis of the horse, equine variola (horse-pox of Jenner), and vaccinia (cow-pox of Jenner). J Comp Pathol Ther 30:242, 1917.

16a. Del Piero F: Diagnosis of equine arteritis virus infection in two horses by using monoclonal antibody immunoperoxidase histochemistry on skin biopsies. Vet Pathol 37:486, 2000.
16b. Del Piero F: Equine viral arteritis. Vet Pathol 37:287, 2000.
17. Donaldson AI, Ferris NP: Vesicular stomatitis. Equine Vet Educ 7:205, 1995.
18. Eby CH: A note on the history of horsepox. J Am Vet Med Assoc 132:120, 1958.
19. Elazhary Y, et al: Artérite virale équine au Québec: étude sérologique. Méd. Vét. Québec 20:23, 1990.
20. Freedberg IM, et al: Fitzpatrick's Dermatology in General Medicine, 4th ed. McGraw Hill Book Co., New York, 1999.
21. Gibbs EPJ: Collecting specimens for virus disease diagnosis. In Pract 1:21, 1979.
22. Gibbs EPJ, et al: Electron microscopy as an aid to the rapid diagnosis of virus diseases of veterinary importance. Vet Rec 106:451, 1980.
23. Gottlieb SL, Myskowski PL: Molluscum contagiosum. Int J Dermatol 33:453, 1994.
24. Green SL: Vesicular stomatitis in the horse. Vet Clin N Am Equine Pract 9:349, 1993.
25. Heiny F: Vesicular stomatitis in cattle and horses in Colorado. N Am Vet 26:726, 1945.
26. Henlick A, et al: Die Pocken II. Threme, Stuttgart, 1967.
27. House JA: African horse sickness. Vet Clin N Am Equine Pract 9:355, 1993.
28. Hurd HS, et al: Management factors affecting the risk for vesicular stomatitis in livestock operations in the western United States. J Am Vet Med Assoc 215:1263, 1999.
29. Hutchins DR: Skin diseases of cattle and horses in New South Wales. N Z Vet J 8:85, 1960.
30. Jenner E: An Inquiry into the Causes and Effects of the Variolae Vaccinae. Sampson Low, London, 1798.
31. Jones TC, et al: The lesions of equine viral arteritis. Cornell Vet 47:52, 1957.
32. Kamada M, et al: Studies on Getah virus—pathogenicity of the virus for horses. Bull Equine Res Inst 18:84, 1981.
33. Kamada M, et al: Effect of viral inoculum size on appearance of clinical signs in equine Getah virus infection. J Vet Med Sci 53:803, 1991.
34. Kaminjolo JS, et al: Vaccinia-like pox virus identified in a horse with skin disease. Zbl Vet Med B21:202, 1974.
35. Kaminjolo JS, et al: Isolation, cultivation and characterization of a poxvirus from some horses in Kenya. Zbl Vet Med B21:592, 1974.
36. Kaminjolo JS, Winquist G: Histopathology of skin lesions in Uasin Gishu skin disease of horses. J Comp Pathol 85:391, 1975.
37. Kaminjolo JS, et al: Uasin Gishu skin disease of horses in Kenya. Bull Anim Hlth Prod Afr 23:225, 1975.
38. Knight AP, Messer NT: Vesicular Stomatitis. Comp Cont Educ 5:S517, 1983.
39. Kono Y, et al: An epidemic of Getah virus infection among racehorses: Properties of the virus. Res Vet Sci 29:162, 1980.
40. Kono Y, et al: Equine Getah virus infection: pathological study of horses experimentally infected with the MI-110 strain. Jpn J Vet Sci 44:111, 1982.
41. Kral F, Schwartzman RM: Veterinary and Comparative Dermatology. JB Lippincott Co, Philadelphia, 1964.
42. Kumanomido T, et al: Pathogenicity for horses of original sagiyama virus, a member of the Getah virus group. Vet Microbiol 17:367, 1988.
43. Laegrid WW: Other exotic diseases. In: Robinson NE (ed): Current Therapy in Equine Medicine III. W.B. Saunders Co, Philadelphia, 1992, p 768.
44. Lange L, et al: Molluscum contagiosum in three horses. J So Afr Vet Assoc 62:68, 1991.
45. McIntyre RW: Virus papular dermatitis of the horse. Am J Vet Res 10:229, 1948.
46. Moens Y, Kombe AH: Molluscum contagiosum in a horse. Equine Vet J 20:143, 1988.
47. Mohanty SB, Dutta SK: Veterinary Virology. Lea & Febiger, Philadelphia, 1981.
47a. Musonda MM, et al: Molluscum contagiosum in three horses in Zambia. Bull Anim Hlth Prod Afr 44:263, 1996.
48. Pascoe RR, et al: An equine genital infection resembling coital exanthema associated with a virus. Aust Vet J 45:166, 1969.
49. Quinn PJ, et al: Clinical Veterinary Microbiology. Mosby-Year Book Europe Ltd, London, 1994.
50. Rahley RS, Mueller RE: Molluscum contagiosum in a horse. Vet Pathol 20:247, 1983.
50a. Sahu SP, et al: Isolation of Jamestown Canyon virus (California virus group) from vesicular lesions of a horse. J Vet Diagn Invest 12:80, 2000.
51. Schmidtmann ET, et al: 1995 epizootic of vesicular stomatitis (New Jersey serotype) in the western United States: An entomologic perspective. J Med Entomol 36:1, 1999.
52. Sentsui H, Kono Y: An epidemic of Getah virus infection among racehorses: Isolation of the virus. Res Vet Sci 29:157, 1980.
53. Simpson DJ: Venereal diseases of mares. In: Robinson NE (ed): Current Therapy in Equine Medicine II. W.B. Saunders Co, Philadelphia, 1986, p 513.
54. Studdert MJ: Experimental vaccinia virus infection of horses. Aust Vet J 66:157, 1989.
55. Taylor CED: Did vaccinia virus come from a horse? Equine Vet J 25:8, 1993.
56. Theiler S: Eine contagiose Stomatits des Pferdes in Sued-Afrika. Dtsch Tierärztl Wochenschr 9:131, 1901.
57. Thompson CH, et al: Close relationship between equine and human molluscum contagiosum viruses demonstrated by in situ hybridization. Res Vet Sci 64:157, 1998.
58. Timoney PJ, McCallum WH: Equine viral arteritis. Vet Clin N Am Equine Pract 9:295, 1993.
59. Timoney PJ, McCollum WH: Equine viral arteritis. Equine Vet Educ 8:97, 1996.
60. Uppal PK, et al: Equine coital exanthema (EHV-3 virus) infection in India. J Vet Med B36:786, 1989.
61. Van Rensburg IBJ, et al: Molluscum contagiosum in a horse. J So Afr Vet Assoc 62:72, 1991.
62. Yager JA, Scott DW: The skin and appendages. In: Jubb KVF, et al (eds). Pathology of Domestic Animals IV, vol. 1. Academic Press, New York, 1993, p 531.
63. Zwick W: Uber die Beziehungen der Stomatitis Pustulosa Contagiosa des Pferdes zu den Pocken der Haustiere und des Menschen. Berl Tierärztl Wochenschr 40:757, 1924.

Protozoal Diseases

64. Aguilar CM, et al: Cutaneous leishmaniasis is frequent in equines from an endemic area in Rio de Janeiro, Brazil. Mem Inst Oswaldo Cruz 81:471, 1986.

65. Aguilar CM, et al: Zoonotic cutaneous leishmaniasis due to *Leishmania braziliensis* associated with domestic animals in Venezuela and Brazil. Mem Inst Oswaldo Cruz 84:19, 1989.
66. Bennett SCJ: A peculiar equine sarcosporidium in the Anglo-Egyptian Sudan. Vet J 83:297, 1927.
67. Bennett SCJ: Globidium infections in the Sudan. J Comp Pathol Ther 46:1, 1933.
68. Bennett SCJ: Equine cutaneous leishmaniasis: Treatment with berberine sulfate. J Comp Pathol Ther 48:241, 1935.
69. Bigalke RD: Studies on equine besnoitiosis. J Parasitol 56:29, 1970.
70. Bonfante-Garrido R, et al: Enzootic equine cutaneous leishmaniasis in Venezuela. Trans Roy Soc Trop Med Hyg 75:471, 1981.
71. Davis WP, et al: Besnoitiosis in a miniature donkey. Vet Dermatol 8;139, 1997.
72. Falqueto A, et al: Cutaneous leishmaniasis in a horse (*Equus caballus*) from endemic area in the state of Espirito Santo, Brazil. Mem Inst Oswaldo Cruz 82:443, 1987.
73. Lane JG, et al: Parasitic laryngeal papillomatosis in a horse. Vet Rec 119:591, 1986.
74. Mazza S: Leishmaniosis cutánea en el caballo y neuva observación de la misma en el perro. Bol Inst Clin Quirur 3:462, 1927.
75. Ramos-Vara JA, et al: Cutaneous leishmaniasis in two horses. Vet Pathol 33:731, 1996.
76. Sales AJJ, et al: Leishmaniasis in a horse. In: Kwochka KW, et al (ed): Advances in Veterinary Dermatology III. Butterworth-Heinemann, Boston, 1998, p 458.
77. Schulz KCA, Thorburn JA: Globidiosis—a cause of dermatitis in horses. J So Afr Vet Med Assoc 26:39, 1955.
78. Soulsby EJL: Helminths, Arthropods and Protozoa of Domesticated Animals VII. Baillière Tindall, Philadelphia, 1982.
79. Terrell TG, Stookey JL: *Besnoitia bennetti* in two Mexican burros. Vet Pathol 10:177, 1973.
80. Van Heerden J, et al: Besnoitiosis in a horse. J So Afr Vet Assoc 64:92, 1993.
81. Yoshida ELA, et al: Human, canine, and equine (*Equus caballus*) leishmaniasis due to *Leishmania braziliensis* in the southwest region of São Paulo State, Brazil. Mem Inst Oswaldo Cruz 85:133, 1990.

Giardiasis

82. Kirkpatrick CE, Skand DL: Giardiasis in a horse. J Am Vet Med Assoc 187:163, 1985.

Chapter 8

Skin Immune System and Allergic Skin Diseases

• INTRODUCTION

The subject of immunodermatology has seen a tremendous emergence of new discoveries, findings, and laboratory techniques. An adequate review of this information is decidedly beyond the scope of this chapter. For the practitioner, student, and academician interested in details, numerous texts on immunology and immunodermatology are available, and a number of review articles can be recommended.* In this section, we confine ourselves to a brief overview of the concepts regarding immunology of the skin. To comprehend this discussion or to read the current scientific literature on many cutaneous diseases, the reader has to understand some newer terminology about cell surface antigens, cytokines, and adhesion molecules, which are basic components of all immunologic discussions.

Surface Antigens (Determinants) or Receptor Terminology

The understanding of current literature involving immune responses requires an understanding of cell surface determinants, which are referred to by the cluster differentiation (CD) nomenclature. This nomenclature is applied to antigens that have been detected on the surface of cells with monoclonal antibodies, and these are usually assigned a number. Initially these antigens were studied and shown to be specific to or limited to a specific group of cell types. This allowed us to identify what types of cells are present in tissues or exudates. Further studies have allowed us to recognize the function and, in many cases, the structure of these antigens. It is now known that many of the surface molecules are various immunoglobulins, carbohydrates, enzymes, adhesion molecules to bind with other cells, and receptors for the various immunoglobulins and chemicals (cytokines) secreted by cells to communicate with surrounding cells. In humans, this list of cell surface determinants has grown to well over 100 and appears to grow faster each year (Table 8-1).[10,19,20,52]

CYTOKINES

Cytokines are secreted from cells and function in communicating with surrounding cells (Table 8-2). They are soluble proteins or glycoproteins that affect the growth, differentiation, function, and activation functions of other cells. These soluble hormone-like molecules were initially discovered in association with lymphocytes and termed *lymphokines,* or in association with monocytes and termed *monokines.* As it was discovered that many other cells produced the same substances, these terms and others, such as *secretory regulins* and *peptide regulatory factors,* were

---

*References 3, 4, 7, 14, 20, 23, 30, 44, 46, 52, 55, 63, 66.

● Table 8-1 **GLOSSARY OF LEUKOCYTE ANTIGENS**

ANTIGEN FAMILY	ANTIGEN	COMMENT
CD1	CD1a CD1b CD1c	CD1 antigens are expressed in cortical thymocytes, but not on mature T cells. CD1 molecules are the best markers of dendritic/APC, although subpopulations of B cells and monocytes express CD1c.
TCR/CD3	TCR$\alpha\beta$ TCR$\gamma\delta$ CD3	The T cell receptor/CD3 complex is only expressed on the surface of mature T cells. There are two types of TCR: $\alpha\beta$ and $\gamma\delta$; each is associated with the CD3 complex, which is the signal transduction portion of both types of receptor.
CD4	CD4	Expressed by MHC class II restricted T helper cells. Macrophages and dendritic/APC can upregulate CD4 in some instances.
CD5	CD5	Expressed by almost all mature T cells; a minor subset of B cells can express CD5 (B1 cells). CD5 binds to CD72, which is expressed on B cells.
CD8	CD8α CD8β	Expressed by MHC class I restricted T cytotoxic cells. T cells usually express CD8$\alpha\beta$ heterodimers.
β_2 integrins	CD11a CD11b CD11c CD18	The β_2 integrins (CD11/CD18) are the major adhesion molecule family of leukocytes. Most leukocytes express one or more members of this family. CD18 is the β_2 subunit, which pairs with one of four α subunits to form a heterodimer. The three α subunits are CD11a (all leukocytes), CD11b (granulocytes, monocytes, dendritic antigen presenting cells). Macrophages and granulocytes express 10-fold more CD18 than do lymphocytes.
CD14	CD14	Receptor for LPS (endotoxin) and LPS-binding protein complexes. CD14 is expressed on monocytes, subsets of macrophages, subsets of B cells.
CD21	CD21	CD21 is a C3dg receptor (CR2), which complexes with components of the B cell antigen receptor complex (sIg, CD79a, CD79b), CD19, and CD35 (CR1). CD21 is expressed on mature B cells and follicular dendritic cells of the germinal center.
Link	CD44	A broadly expressed adhesion receptor (for hyaluronate) on many cell types; involved in lymphocyte trafficking and activation.
CD45	CD45 CD45RA CD45R	CD45 is the leukocyte common antigen family. CD45RA is one of these isoforms. CD45RA is expressed by all B cells and by 100% of B cell lymphomas involving lymph nodes. In skin disease, CD45RA is expressed by mast cell tumors, plasmacytomas, and rarely by T cell lymphomas.
β_1 integrins	CD49d-like	VLA family (CD49a–f) members (α subunits) occur as heterodimers with the β_1 integrin subunit. VLA-4 (CD49d) is broadly expressed on leukocytes. VLA-4 is upregulated on memory T cells.
ICAM	CD50 CD54	Intracellular adhesion molecule (ICAM) family consists of at least four members. ICAM-1 (CD54) is broadly expressed (leukocytes, endothelium) and is a major ligand of CD11a. CD54 is upregulated on endothelium, leukocytes, and even on epithelium in inflammation (by inflammatory cytokines) and is important in leukocyte transmigration. Expression of CD54 on dendritic/APC enhances T cell activation through CD11a. ICAM-3 (CD50) is expressed broadly by leukocytes, but rarely occurs on endothelium.
NCAM	CD56	Neural cell adhesion molecule isoform; marker of NK cells in humans.
Thy-1	CD90	Thy-1 expression varies considerably among different species. Dogs express Thy-1 on thymocytes and T cells (similar to mice); expression of Thy-1 in human T cells is lost at the early stages of thymocyte maturation; peripheral T cells lack Thy-1 expression. Thy-1 is highly expressed by dermal dendritic/APC and fibroblasts. It is an important marker in proliferative diseases of dendritic/APC in dogs (e.g., cutaneous and systemic histiocytosis). Thy-1 is expressed also by monocytes and eosinophils, but not by neutrophils in the dog.

Table 8-1	GLOSSARY OF LEUKOCYTE ANTIGENS—cont'd	
ANTIGEN FAMILY	ANTIGEN	COMMENT
MHCII		Major histocompatibility complex (MHC) class II molecules present oxygenously derived antigen CD4⁻ T cells. MHC class II molecules are highly expressed on dendritic/APC, B cells, resting (dog and cat!) and activated T cells (dog, cat, and human), and monocytes. Granulocytes do not express MHC class II. MHC class II can be upregulated on epithelial cells (e.g., keratinocytes) and endothelial cells by interferon γ.
BCR/CD79	CD79a	The B cell receptor complex (BCR) consists of surface Ig (sIg) complexed with two invariant molecules, which function as signal transduction molecules (CD79a, CB79b). CD79a (MB-1) is expressed throughout all stages of B cell development and persists into the plasma cell stage (despite absent or diminished sIg on plasma cells). CD79a is a useful marker for establishing the diagnosis of B cell lymphoma, since it is present in the BCR of all B cells regardless of the isotype of the sIg receptor (background associated with Ig stains in tissues is also not an issue). CD79a is useful in the diagnosis of cutaneous plasmacytoma (about 80% have focal to diffuse expression).

no longer considered appropriate. Cytokines are transiently produced and exert their biologic activities via specific cell-surface receptors of target cells, which may be expressed only after activation of the cell.* Each mediator usually has multiple overlapping activities. Numerous cytokines have been described, and typically, they may perform several different functions, depending on the tissue they interact with and the other cytokines that may be present. In different environments the same cytokine may even have opposite effects.[6,7,20,44]

Cytokines may affect the same cell in a permissive, inhibitor, additive, or suppressive manner. Cytokines are involved in virtually every facet of immunity and inflammation, including antigen presentation, bone marrow differentiation, cellular recruitment and activation, adhesion molecule expression, and acute-phase reactions (see Table 8-2).[6] The particular cytokines produced in response to an immunologic insult will determine whether an immune response develops and whether the response will be humoral, cell-mediated, or allergic. Certain cell types, particularly T lymphocytes, may secrete different patterns of cytokines, and this has been used to subclassify these cells and their associated different functions. A large group of cytokines have been identified that have as their sole or major purpose the direction of the movement of cells involved in inflammation and the immune response. These have been termed *chemokines* (Table 8-3).[1,44]

ADHESION MOLECULES

Glycoproteins critical for cell-to-cell and cell-to-matrix adhesion, contact, and communication, adhesion molecules play an integral role in cutaneous inflammation and immunology (see Chapter 1) (Table 8-4).[24,44,68] The *integrin family* includes membrane glycoproteins with α and β subunits, such as vascular cell adhesion molecule-1 (VCAM-1) on endothelial cells, which binds T lymphocytes and monocytes via vascular leukocyte adherin-4 (VLA-4), and fibronectin and laminin, which bind keratinocytes and mast cells. The *immunoglobulin gene superfamily* contains intercellular adhesion molecule-1 (ICAM-1) found on keratinocytes, Langerhans' cells, and endothelial cells, which binds leukocytes via leukocyte function-associated antigen-1 (LFA-1) or CD11a/CD18. The

*References 6 ,7 ,20, 24, 44, 46, 69, 70

● Table 8-2 **IMMUNOLOGIC PROPERTIES OF CYTOKINES**

CYTOKINE	PROPERTIES
Interleukins	
IL-1	Immunoaugmentation (promotes IL-2, IFN-α, CSF production by T cells); promotes B cell activation (promotes IL-4, IL-5, IL-6, IL-7 production and immunoglobulin synthesis); stimulates macrophages and fibroblasts; induces arachidonate metabolism
IL-2	Activates T and natural killer (NK) cells; promotes cell growth and immunoglobulin production; activates macrophages
IL-3	Promotes growth of early myeloprogenitor cells, eosinophils, mast cells, and basophils
IL-4	Promotes B cell activation and IgE switch; promotes T cell growth; synergistic with IL-3 mast cell growth
IL-5	Eosinophilic growth; B cell growth and chemotaxis; T cell growth
IL-6	Terminal differentiation factor for cells and polyclonal immunoglobulin production; enhances IL-4-induced IgE production; promotes T cell proliferation and cytotoxicity; promotes NK cell activity; activates neutrophils
IL-7	Lymphopoietin
IL-8	Chemoattractant for neutrophils, T lymphocytes, basophils, increases histamine release from basophils
IL-9	Maturation of erythroid progenitor cell tumor growth; synergistic with IL-3 for mast cell growth
IL-10	Downregulation (inhibits production of IL-1, IL-2, IL-4, IL-5, IL-5, IL-8, IL-12, TNF-α, IFN-γ, MHC class II expression)
IL-11	Megakaryocyte, lymphocyte, and plasma cell growth
IL-12	Cytotoxic lymphocyte maturation; NK cell activation and proliferation
IL-13	Similar to IL-4; enhances production of MHC class II and integrins; reduced production of IL-1 and TNF; activation of eosinophils
IL-14	Expands clones of B cells and suppresses immunoglobulin secretion
IL-15	Proliferation; increased cytotoxicity of T cells, NK cells; expression of ICAM-3; B cell growth and differentiation
IL-16	Chemoattractant, growth factor
IL-17	Autocrine proliferation and activation
IL-18	Similar to IL-12; inhibits IgE production by increasing IFN-γ
Colony-Stimulating Factors	
Granulocyte CSF	Neutrophil growth
Monocyte CSF	Monocyte growth
Granulocyte-monocyte CSF	Monomyelocytic growth
Basic fibroblast growth factor (bFGF)	Fibroblast growth and matrix production
Platelet-derived growth factor	Proliferation; chemoattractant for fibroblasts; active in wound healing
Stem cell factor	Chemoattractant; with IL-3, stimulates growth; also has histamine-releasing activity
Transforming growth factor	Inhibits IL-2–stimulated growth; acts as switch factor for IgA but inhibits IgM and IgG production; counteracts IL-4 stimulation of IgE; inhibits cytotoxicity
Interferons	
IFN-α	Antiviral; antiproliferative; immunomodulating (activation of macrophages, proliferation of B cells; stimulation of NK cells); inhibit fibroblasts
IFN-β	Antiviral; antiproliferative; immunomodulating (activation of macrophages, proliferation of B cells; stimulation of NK cells); inhibit fibroblasts
IFN-γ	Immunomodulation (activation of macrophages; proliferation of B cells; stimulation of NK cells); antiproliferative; antiviral; inhibit fibroblasts; inhibits IL-4–medicated expression of IgE–receptors and the IgE switch

● Table 8-2 **IMMUNOLOGIC PROPERTIES OF CYTOKINES—cont'd**

CYTOKINE	PROPERTIES
Tumor Necrosis Factors	
TNF-α	Inflammatory, immunoenhancing, and tumoricidal
TNF-β	Inflammatory, immunoenhancing, and tumoricidal
TNF-$\beta_{1,2,3}$	Fibroplasia and immunosuppression

● Table 8-3 **CHEMOKINES AND THEIR ACTIONS**

CHEMOKINE	TARGET CELLS	BIOLOGICAL EFFECTS
CXC (α) Family		
BCA-1 (B cell–attracting chemokine-1)	B lymphocytes	Chemotaxis
β-TG (β-thromboglobulin)	Neutrophils	Chemotaxis; activation
	Fibroblasts	Chemotaxis; proliferation; activation
CTAP-III (connective tissue–activating peptide-III)	Neutrophils	Chemotaxis; activation
	Fibroblasts	Chemotaxis; proliferation; activation
ENA-78 (epithelial cell–derived neutrophil-activating peptide-78)	Neutrophils	Chemotaxis
GCP-2 (granulocyte chemotactic protein-2)	Neutrophils	Chemotaxis; activation
GRO-α, β, δ (growth-regulated oncogene)	Neutrophils	Chemotaxis; activation
	Basophils	Chemotaxis; activation
	T lymphocytes	Chemotaxis
IL-8 (interleukin-8)	Neutrophils	Chemotaxis; activation
	Basophils	Chemotaxis; inhibition of histamine release
	T lymphocytes	Chemotaxis; inhibition of IL-4 synthesis
	B lymphs/B-CLL	Chemotaxis; inhibition of growth and IgE production
	Keratinocytes	Chemotaxis; expression of HLA-DR
IP-10 (interferon-inducible protein-10)	Activated T lymphocytes	Chemotaxis
	Monocytes	Chemotaxis
	NK cells	Chemotaxis; activation
MIG (monokine induced by γ-interferon)	Activated T lymphocytes	Chemotaxis
	NK cells	Chemotaxis
NAP-2 (neutrophil-activating peptide-2)	Neutrophils	Chemotaxis; activation
PF-4 (platelet factor-4)	Neutrophils	Chemotaxis; activation
	Monocytes	Chemotaxis
	Fibroblasts	Chemotaxis
	Basophils	Modulation of histamine release
SDF-1 (stromal cell–derived factor-1)	T lymphocytes	Chemotaxis
C-C (β) Family		
Ckβ8 (chemokine β8)	Monocytes	Chemotaxis
	Resting T lymphocytes	Chemotaxis
Eotaxin	Eosinophils	Chemotaxis
	Basophils	Chemotaxis; activation
Eotaxin-2	Eosinophils	Chemotaxis
	Basophils	Chemotaxis; activation
	Resting T lymphocytes	Chemotaxis
HCC-2	Monocytes	Chemotaxis
	T lymphocytes	Chemotaxis
	Eosinophils	Chemotaxis
	Monocytes	Chemotaxis

Continued

● Table 8-3   **CHEMOKINES AND THEIR ACTIONS—cont'd**

CHEMOKINE	TARGET CELLS	BIOLOGICAL EFFECTS
C-C (β) Family		
MCP-1 (monocyte chemoattractant protein-1)	Monocytes	Chemotaxis
	Basophils	Activation
	T lymphocytes	Chemotaxis
	NK cells	Chemotaxis; activation
	Dendritic cells	Chemotaxis
MCP-2	Monocytes	Chemotaxis
	T lymphocytes	Chemotaxis
	Eosinophils	Chemotaxis; activation
	Basophils	Chemotaxis; activation
	NK cells	Chemotaxis; activation
	Dendritic cells	Chemotaxis
MCP-3	Monocytes	Chemotaxis
	T lymphocytes	Chemotaxis
	Eosinophils	Chemotaxis
	Basophils	Chemotaxis; activation
	NK cells	Chemotaxis; activation
	Dendritic cells	Chemotaxis
MCP-4	Eosinophils	Chemotaxis; activation
	Monocytes	Chemotaxis
	T lymphocytes	Chemotaxis
	Basophils	Chemotaxis; activation
MIP-1α (macrophage inflammatory protein 1α or LD-78; also known as endogenous pyrogen)	T lymphocytes	Chemotaxis
	Monocytes/macrophages	Chemotaxis
	B lymphocytes	Increased IgE/IgG4 production
	NK cells	Chemotaxis; activation
	Basophils	Activation
	Dendritic cells	Chemotaxis
MIP-1β	NK cells	Chemotaxis; activation
	Dendritic cells	Chemotaxis
	B lymphocytes	Increased IgE/IgG4 production
NIP-3α (also known as Exodus of liver and activation-regulated chemokine [LARC])	T lymphocytes	Chemotaxis
	Dendritic cells	Chemotaxis
RANTES (regulated-upon-activation normal T cells expressed and presumably secreted)	Eosinophils	Chemotaxis
	T lymphocytes	Chemotaxis
	Monocytes	Chemotaxis
	Basophils	Chemotaxis
	NK cells	Chemotaxis; activation
	B lymphocytes	Increased IgE/IgG4 production
	Dendritic cells	Chemotaxis
SLC (secondary lymphoid tissue chemokine)	T lymphocytes	Chemotaxis
STCP-1 (stimulated T cell chemotactic protein)	Activated T lymphocytes	Chemotaxis
C (γ) Family		
Lymphotactin	Lymphocytes	Chemotaxis
	Activated NK cells	Chemotaxis; activation
CX3C Family		
Fractalkine	Monocytes	Chemotaxis
	T lymphocytes	Chemotaxis

selectin family includes lectin adhesion molecule-1 (LECAM-1 or L-selectin) on lymphocytes, which binds endothelial leukocyte adhesion molecule-1 (ELAM-1 or E-selectin), and Gmp-140 (P-selectin) as a "homing" mechanism. The *cadherin family* is important in desmosome function (see Chapter 1)

MAJOR HISTOCOMPATIBILITY COMPLEX

The major histocompatibility complex (MHC) is a cluster of genes that encodes a range of molecules of fundamental importance to the immune system.[7,23,44,52,63] MHC class I loci encode the classical histocompatibility antigens, which are expressed by all nucleated cells of the body and are target antigens in the rejection of incompatible tissue grafts. Products of the MHC class III loci include a number of factors of the complement pathways, two cytokines (TNF-α and TNF-β), and two heat-shock proteins. The MHC class II loci encode a series of transmembrane molecules with restricted expression by cells of the immune system, particularly the antigen-presenting cells: Langerhans' cells, dendrocytes, macrophages, and B lymphocytes.

● Table 8-4   **CELL ADHESION MOLECULES***

ADHESION MOLECULES	CD	FAMILY	DISTRIBUTION	FUNCTION
VLA-1	CD49a	Integrin	ECs, monocytes, activated T/B cells	Cell-matrix adhesion
VLA-2	CD49b	Integrin	ECs, EPs, activated T cells	Cell-matrix adhesion
VLA-3	CD49c	Integrin	ECs, EPs	Cell-matrix adhesion
VLA-4	CD49d	Integrin	Leukocytes	Cell-cell and cell-matrix adhesion
VLA-5	CD49e	Integrin	ECs, EPs, lymphocytes, monocytes, macrophages	Cell-matrix adhesion
VLA-6	CD49f	Integrin	ECs, EPs, T lymphocytes, mast cells	Cell-matrix adhesion
LFA-1	CD11a/CD18	Integrin	Leukocytes	Adhesion of leukocytes to ECs
MAC-1	CD11b/CD18	Integrin	Monocytes, macrophages, granulocytes, Langerhans' cells	Adhesion of leukocytes to ECs
gp150,95	CD11c/CD18	Integrin	Monocytes, macrophages, granulocytes, Langerhans' cells	Adhesion of leukocytes to ECs
ICAM-1	CD54	IgG superfamily	Monocytes, EPs, fibroblasts	Cell-cell adhesion
ICAM-2	CD102	IgG superfamily	ECs, leukocytes	Adhesion of leukocytes to ECs
ICAM-3	CD50	IgG superfamily	ECs, leukocytes, Langerhans' cells	Adhesion of leukocytes to ECs
VCAM-1	CD106	IgG superfamily	Activated ECs	Adhesion of leukocytes to ECs
PECAM-1	CD31	IgG superfamily	ECs, leukocytes	Initiation of EC-EC adhesion, platelet-monocyte/neutrophil-EC adhesion
MAdCAM-1		IgG superfamily	ECs	Adhesion of leukocytes to ECs
E-selectin	CD62E	Selectin	ECs	Adhesion of leukocytes to ECs; rolling phenomenon
P-selectin	CD62P	Selectin	Platelets, ECs	Adhesion of platelets to monocytes and neutrophils; adhesion of leukocytes to ECs; rolling phenomenon
L-selectin	CD62L	Selectin	Leukocytes	Leukocyte-EC adhesion; lymphocyte homing
Cadherins		Cadherin	EPs	EP-EP adhesion

*Abbreviations: *CD*, cluster of differentiation; *VLA*, very late activation; *ICAM*, intercellular adhesion molecule; *VCAM-1*, vascular cell adhesion molecule-1; *PECAM-1*, platelet-endothelial cell adhesion molelcule-1; *MAdCAM-1*, mucosal address in cell adhesion molecule-1; *PSGL*, P-selectin glycoprotein ligand-1; *EC*, endothelial cell; *EP*, epithelial cell.

SALT

The immune system and its inflammatory component are complex models of biologic activity and interaction. There is a tendency to dissect the immune response into its individual components and to discuss them as autonomous functional units. Immune responses are interwoven and interdependent, however, and manipulation of one component influences others. The newer studies have shown that the skin itself is a very integral and active component of the immune system. These observations led to the hypothesis that the skin, like the gastrointestinal tract, may be a functioning lymphoid organ; as such, it has been referred to as *skin-associated lymphoid tissue (SALT)*.[7,44,55] Even prior to the development of the SALT concept, it was suggested that the skin functions as a primary immunologic organ. The term *skin immune system (SIS)* has also been proposed to describe the components of the skin, excluding the regional lymph nodes, that constitute SALT.[7] In the following sections, we attempt to briefly review the specifics of the skin immune system so that the reader is familiar with the tremendous gains in knowledge and future avenues for work that will lead to further discoveries.

● SKIN IMMUNE SYSTEM

The skin immune system (SIS) contains two major components, the cellular and humoral. The cellular component comprises keratinocytes, epidermal dendritic cells (Langerhans' cells), lymphocytes, tissue macrophages, mast cells, endothelial cells, and granulocytes (see Chapter 1). The humoral components include immunoglobulins, complement components, fibrinolysins, cytokines, eicosanoids, neuropeptides, and antimicrobial peptides. Virtually all inflammatory and some noninflammatory skin diseases involve alterations of, or an interaction between, one or both parts of the SIS. As a result, it becomes inappropriate to consider immunologic disease as a category if one is to include all skin diseases that involve the immune system. Therefore, this chapter presents those diseases classically described as allergic (hypersensitive) and Chapter 9 deals with the immune-mediated skin diseases.

The epidermis is often considered the producer of the effective barrier between the outside world and the body's inside environment. In this role, the epidermis acts as a mechanical barrier, because it is often the first component of the body exposed to environmental agents such as viruses, bacteria, toxins, insects, arachnids, and allergens. The epidermis also plays an active role in the body's immunologic response to these external factors. Before the immune system can respond to these external factors, however, their presence has to be recognized. Recognition may occur at one of two levels: on the surface of the epidermis or in the dermis. If an intact epidermis is present, it would seem most likely that recognition of an environmental agent occurs in the epidermis. For many immunologic responses, including helper T cell induction, antigens must first be processed for presentation to lymphocytes. Classically, this occurs by macrophages, which express MHC class II antigens, but other cells with MHC class II antigens may be involved. Because macrophages are present in the dermis and do not normally reside in the epidermis, this function is served by another cell, the Langerhans' cell. Even before Langerhans' cells are reached, external stimuli will likely encounter keratinocytes, which we now realize do more than act as a physical barrier.

Keratinocytes

Keratinocytes do much more than produce keratin, surface lipids, and intercellular substances (see Chapter 1). They are intimately associated with Langerhans' cells and play a major role in the SIS. It is now clear that keratinocytes produce a wide variety of cytokines that have important roles in mediating cutaneous immune responses, inflammation, wound healing, and the growth and development of certain neoplasms.[20,55] Keratinocytes also produce eicosanoids, prostaglandin (PG)

E2, and neuropeptides such as proopiomelanocortin and α MSH. Though some of these are proinflammatory, some—such as PGE2 and the neuropeptides—also have anti-inflammatory effects.[20] Keratinocytes, especially when perturbed by exposure to interferon-γ (IFN-γ), express MHC II antigens.[7] This expression is required for cells to be antigen-presenting cells for T cell responses. Though keratinocytes are capable of phagocytosis, their role as antigen-processing cells is unlikely, as they do not efficiently process and present surface MHC II-bound peptide antigens, and have not been shown to be able to activate naïve T cells. However, they can induce proliferation of allogenic CD4+ T cells. There is evidence that keratinocytes expressing MHC II surface molecules may induce tolerance. Keratinocytes may also be stimulated to produce the leukocyte adhesion molecule, ICAM-1. Besides production of these immunologically important cell-surface markers, keratinocytes have been shown to be very capable producers of a variety of cytokines. They are the primary epidermal source for cytokines.[7] Probably the most immunologically important is interleukin-1 (IL-1). Keratinocytes store IL-1, which is readily released following damage to the cells. In fact, release of IL-1 from keratinocytes is essentially a primary event in skin disease.[41] Other cytokines derived from keratinocytes include IL-3, IL-6, IL-7, IL-8, IL-10, IL-12, IL-15, IL-16 and IL-18, tumor necrosis factor α (TNF-α), and a variety of growth factors and granulocyte-monocyte-macrophage stimulating and activating factors.[*] Depending on what cytokines are produced, keratinocytes may affect the type of immune response. Keratinocytes produce both IL-12 and IL-10, which may skew which type of T cells are activated or downregulate inflammation, depending on what stage T cells are exposed to them. Keratinocytes may also play a role in tissue repair by production of multiple growth factors. Therefore, it becomes apparent that keratinocytes are important in stimulating and controlling inflammation and repair of tissue. Considering the diverse functions, activities, and mediators produced by keratinocytes, it has become obvious that the epidermis plays a major role in the immune response and that keratinocytes do not function only as a mechanical barrier to environmental substances.[7,20,69,70]

Langerhans' Cells

Langerhans' cells are interdigitating dendritic cells, which appear as suprabasilar clear cells on skin sections stained routinely with hematoxylin and eosin (H & E) (see Chapter 1). They are members of a family of highly specialized antigen-presenting cells termed *dendritic cells*.[31] They are localized at the interface between organism and environment, and are important sentinels of the immune system. Langerhans' cells are the major antigen-presenting cells of the epidermis and the only epidermal cell capable of activating naïve T cells. They are bone marrow-derived monocyte/macrophage-type cells. The Langerhans' cell is characteristically identified in the epidermis by the electron-microscopic presence of Birbeck granules (see Chapter 1). Cutaneous dendritic antigen-presenting cells (APC) include both epidermal and dermal Langerhans' cells, which express abundant CD1 molecules. Recently the function of the CD1 surface receptors has been elucidated. CD1 receptors appear to be a third method of antigen presentation that is specialized and may play a more important role in cutaneous disease. A unique feature of CD1 antigen presentation is the ability to present nonpeptide antigens to T cells.[20] The epidermal Langerhans' cells do not express CD90 (Thy 1), whereas the dermal Langerhans' cells does.[55] Langerhans' cells express MHC class II antigens, as well as receptors for C3b, Fc-IgG, and Fc-IgE. The main function of Langerhans' cells is antigen-specific T cell activation. Antigenic peptides derived from endogenous protein synthesis (e.g., viral antigens, transplantation antigens, tumor-associated antigens) are generally presented in the context of MHC class I molecules, which are expressed on the surface of essentially all nucleated cells, and recognized by CD8+ antigen specific cytotoxic T cells. Exogenous antigens (not synthesized within antigen-presenting cells [e.g., extracellular

[*]References 7, 20, 36, 41, 44, 52.

bacteria, bacterial toxins, dermatophytes, vaccines, pollens, dust mites]) are presented via CD4+ helper cells that recognize antigenic peptides bound to MHC class II antigen selectively expressed by professional antigen-presenting cells (e.g., macrophages, dendritic cells, B cells).[*] Langerhans' cells bind epidermal antigens and then present the antigens along with co-stimulatory molecules, the so-called second signal to the lymphoid tissues (regional lymph node), where helper T cell lymphocytes in particular are activated. MHC II molecules are produced in the endoplasmic reticulum where they then migrate to the Golgi and endo-lysosomal compartments. The processed protein results in antigen peptides that are incorporated into the MHC II molecules at various points in this migration from endoplasmic reticulum to the cell surface. At the surface, the antigenic peptide-MHC II complex is presented to the T cell receptor (TCR) on the surface of the T cell, resulting in antigen-specific T cell activation. Effective T cell activation requires co-stimulators and cytokines that promote clonal expansion of the antigen-specific T cell. The co-stimulator or second signal is often supplied by the expression of the B7 family of cell surface molecules. These molecules may be expressed following Langerhans' cells exposure to lipopolysac-charide, TNF-α, and IL-1B as well as other signals. Langerhans' cells produce cytokines such as IL-1 and some lipid mediators that direct the T cell response.

Langerhans' cells express high levels of E-cadherin (other dendritic cells do not), which is important in selective adhesion to keratinocytes.[31] Epidermal Langerhans' cells are, thus, highly specialized cells expressing molecules that allow them to home to skin and localize in the epidermis. Tissue injury, microbial infection, and other perturbations of epidermal homeostasis provide a "danger" signal leading to local production of proinflammatory cytokines, which in turn induce mobilization and migration of Langerhans' cells to lymphoid tissue.

In humans, quantitative immunohistochemical studies demonstrated differences in Langerhans' cells in dermatitis due to internal versus external antigen sources.[51] Evaluation of skin biopsy specimens revealed significantly more Langerhans' cells and spongiosis in contact dermatitis (external antigen source) compared with drug reactions (internal antigen source).

Lymphocytes

Lymphocytes are all derived from a common stem cell in the bone marrow, and may be divided into three main types: B (bursa- or bone marrow–derived) cells, T (thymus-dependent) cells, and natural killer (NK) cells.

B cells are characterized by possessing unique surface immunoglobulins, Fc receptors, CD79 or B cell receptor complex, and C3b receptors. B cells mature into *plasma cells* following recognition of its specific antigen and activation, which produce the immunoglobulins IgG, IgM, IgA, and IgE, and they are responsible for antibody immunity. The growth and development of B cells occurs in two phases. The first is antigen-independent and yields B cells that express IgM and IgD. These initial antibodies constitute the majority of the primary antibody response to antigens, but are low affinity. The second phase or memory response is a response to a specific antigen that, with T cells, induces differentiation into IgA-, IgG-, and IgE-secreting or memory B cells.[20,44,46,52] The second phase requires T cell activation and is partly controlled by cytokines released by T cells, with IL-1, IL-2, IL-4, IL-5, and IL-10 all being shown to play roles in growth or differentiation. IL-4 and IL-13 are particularly important for B cells to switch into IgE-producing plasma cells, and this effect is enhanced by IL-5, IL-6, and TNF-α.[20,44,52] IL-4 also induces the switch to IgG4, and this precedes the switch to IgE.[44] In human beings, B lymphocytes are rarely found in normal skin and, even in dermatologic disease, are much less common than T cells.[7] Humoral immunity is described as providing primary defense against invading bacteria and neutralization activity against circulating viruses.

---

[*]References 7, 19, 20, 31, 44, 46.

NK cells are large granular lymphocytes that do not express antigen-specific receptors, but do have receptors that recognize the self MHC I molecule. When they encounter nucleated cells with self MHC I molecules, these receptors inhibit killing (killer inhibitory receptors, or KIR). Many viral or tumor cells fail to express self MHC I and will be killed. NK cells also have receptors for Fc receptor and may mediate antibody-dependent cytotoxicity.[19,20,23,52,63]

T cells are formed in the thymus, express CD3 or T cell receptor (TCR) when mature, and are divided into two major types: helper and suppressor or cytotoxic T lymphocytes.* The two major types are differentiated by their activity and their T cell receptors, which is the part of the T cell that recognizes an antigen. Classically, T cells are considered responsible for cell-mediated immunity, activation of memory B cells, and stimulation of NK cells. T cells play a central role in directing and modifying the immune response. Functions of T cells include (1) helping B cells make antibody and directing what type of antibody is made (helper T cells), (2) suppressing B cell antibody production (suppressor T cells), (3) directly damaging "target" cells, (4) mediating delayed hypersensitivity reactions, (5) suppressing delayed hypersensitivity reactions mediated by other T cells, (6) regulating macrophage function, (7) modulating the inflammatory response with chemokines and cytokines, (8) inducing graft rejection, and (9) producing graft-versus-host reactions. T cell lymphokines may amplify or dampen phagocytic activity, collagen production, vascular permeability, and coagulation phenomena. T cells can kill microorganisms and other cells, or they can recruit effector cells to perform this function. T cell function is known to be suppressed by numerous infections, cancers, and drugs.[20,32,52,55]

As T cells mature in the thymus, they develop surface receptor molecules. The receptor molecules expressed on a T cell are critical in determining the future function of the cell. CD3 represents the T cell receptor complex and marks all mature T cells. MHC II-expressing T helper cells express CD4, and MHC I-restricted CTL express CD8. CD28 is considered the major co-stimulator molecule required for the second signal from the antigen-presenting cells. CD28 is believed to react with the B7 receptor on the antigen-presenting cells. We also know that subpopulations of helper and cytotoxic T cells exist. These subpopulations have different cytokine production profiles. The initial separation and most studied are the Th1 and Th2 subpopulations of CD4+ T cells; Th2 cells produce IL-4, IL-5, and IL-10, whereas Th1 cells produce IL-2, IFN-γ, and TNF-α.[7,20,44,46] However, we now recognize that CD8 and γ-δ T cells also have type 1 and type 2 profiles.[20]

The type and diversity of T cell receptors present on lymphocytes is an area of active research and one of the most relevant markers of T cell populations. Terminology one sees regarding T cell receptors (TCR) refers to the structure of the TCR, which is usually a heterodimer consisting of two protein chains, most commonly in humans the α and β and, less commonly, γ and δ. These protein chains are divided into variable, diversity, joining, and constant regions. With polymerase chain reaction technology, T cells in tissue are now being studied by their variable region of the TCR complex, which represents a small group of antigens. These antigens are most likely representing what is initiating, or the target of, the inflammation.[20]

Tissue Macrophages

The end-stage of the mononuclear phagocyte system (MPS) is the tissue macrophage, which in the dermis has also been considered the precursor cell to the dermal dendrocyte.[7,46] In blood, lymph nodes, and other tissues, there are dendritic macrophage type cells that are also believed to be part of the MPS.[44] These cells are all bone marrow–derived and pass through the blood circulation as monocytes, which in general are CD14 positive. These cells have a wide variety of activities and morphologic appearances, especially in inflammation. Tissue macrophages, epithelioid cells, and

---

*References 7, 20, 44, 46, 52, 63.

multinucleated histiocytic giant cells are all MPS cells found in a variety of inflammatory diseases. They serve the critical function of the afferent arm of the immune system in processing and presenting antigens, especially for T cell activation, yet are also important in the efferent arm of the immune response. The MPS also plays major roles in wound healing, granulopoiesis, erythropoiesis, and antimicrobial defense (especially against intracellular pathogens). Monocytes and macrophages may secrete numerous enzymes, cytokines, inflammatory mediators, histamine-releasing factors, and inhibitors when stimulated. Some mediators upgrade inflammation, whereas others inhibit inflammatory activity in order to prevent too much tissue destruction from inflammation.

Mast Cells

Mast cells are derived from hematopoietic stem cells in the bone marrow and migrate as immature unrecognizable cells in the blood and then localize in connective or mucosal tissues (see Chapter 1). Once present in tissue they proliferate and differentiate into mature recognizable mast cells.[28] The regulation of mast cell proliferation and differentiation is the subject of much research. Cytokines from fibroblasts, stem cell growth factor, T cells, and IL-3 are particularly important.

Though mast cells were recognized many years ago, their role in preventing disease or homeostasis was unknown. Mast cells combine characteristics of both innate and acquired immune responses: they can (1) bind certain bacteria and phagocytose/kill them, (2) elaborate and secrete several biologically active products, and (3) serve as an antigen-presenting cell and promote clonal expansion of CD4+ helper T cells.[28,43,44] Their role in disease has been recognized for many years, and the importance of mast cells in immediate hypersensitivity diseases is well documented. Their role in other skin diseases, however, such as contact dermatitis and bullous pemphigoid, and in the process of fibrosis has only recently been recognized.[44] This relates to the diverse effects and interactions mast cells have with other cells and structures of the skin (Fig. 8-1). Mast cells serve as repositories for or synthesizers of numerous inflammatory mediator substances. The mediators present vary by species studied and according to the type of the mast cells (see below).[44] Some mediators are universally present, such as histamine, leukotrienes, eosinophil chemotactic factor of anaphylaxis (ECF-A), and proteolytic enzymes. There are two main categories of mediators. Preformed mediators are produced and stored in mast cell granules, which are modified lysosomes that develop from the Golgi apparatus (Table 8-5).[44] Mast cells also produce mediators that are newly synthesized at the time of activation and degranulation (Table 8-6). More recently it has been recognized that mast cells have the potential to synthesize many cytokines—IL-1, IL-2, IL-3, IL-4, IL-5, IL-6, IL-8, IL-10,IL-13, GM-CSF, TNF-α, IFN-γ—and many chemokines (e.g., MIP1α and TLA-3).[43,44] Cytokine production may result in stored cytokines or secretion independent from mediators generated from degranulation. There are differences in cytokine profiles for the different types of mast cells, further adding to the heterogeneity of mast cells.[43] Mast cells, therefore, may play many roles in the mediation of immune and inflammatory responses. Classically they are known for the recruitment of eosinophils and neutrophils, immunoglobulins, and complement from the circulation and the regulation of the immunologic response (Tables 8-5 and 8-6). In addition, mast cells can (1) produce IL-12 to drive Th1 responses; (2) produce IL-4, which is essential for the conversion of Th0 to Th2 cells; (2) produce IL-5 and IL-10 to drive Th2 responses; and (4) activate B cells without surface contact.

Mast cells may be divided in rodents morphologically and functionally into type I (atypical, mucosal) and type II (typical, connective tissue) cells.[7,44,46] *Mucosal tissue* and *connective tissue* are misleading terms, because both types of mast cells occur in mucosa and connective tissue. A more precise differentiation of mast cells has been based on the proteases, tryptase and chymase, present in the cells.[44] MC_T mast cells contain tryptase and are the predominant type found in the lung and small intestinal mucosa. MC_{TC} cells contain tryptase and chymase and are the predominant type in the skin, blood vessels, and gastrointestinal submucosa.

INFLAMMATORY CELLS

BLOOD VESSELS

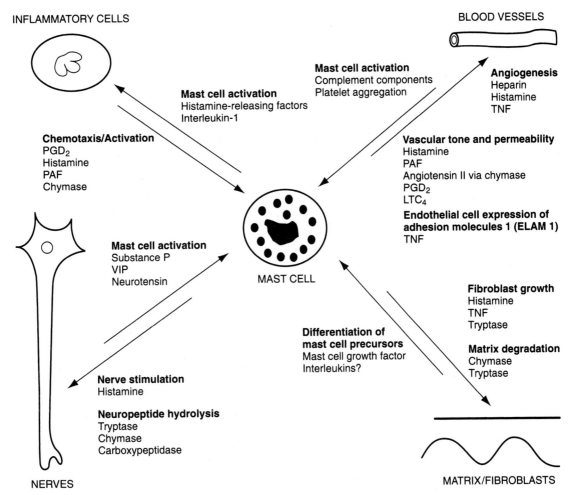

Mast cell activation
Complement components
Platelet aggregation

Angiogenesis
Heparin
Histamine
TNF

Mast cell activation
Histamine-releasing factors
Interleukin-1

Chemotaxis/Activation
PGD_2
Histamine
PAF
Chymase

Vascular tone and permeability
Histamine
PAF
Angiotensin II via chymase
PGD_2
LTC_4

Endothelial cell expression of adhesion molecules 1 (ELAM 1)
TNF

Mast cell activation
Substance P
VIP
Neurotensin

MAST CELL

Fibroblast growth
Histamine
TNF
Tryptase

Differentiation of mast cell precursors
Mast cell growth factor
Interleukins?

Matrix degradation
Chymase
Tryptase

Nerve stimulation
Histamine

Neuropeptide hydrolysis
Tryptase
Chymase
Carboxypeptidase

NERVES

MATRIX/FIBROBLASTS

FIGURE 8-1. Schematic representation of the documented interactions of human mast cells with other cells and structures in the skin. Factors identified in rodent species only are not shown. (*From Goldstein SM, Wintroub BV: The cellular and molecular biology of the human mast cell. In Fitzpatrick, TB, et al, eds: Dermatology in General Medicine V. McGraw-Hill, New York, 1993, p 365.*)

Mast cell degranulation may be initiated by a variety of substances, including allergens cross-linking two surface IgE (or IgGd) molecules, complement components C3a and C5a, eosinophil major basic protein, some hormones (estrogen, gastrin, somatostatin), substance P, and a group of cytokines referred to as *histamine-releasing factors*.[23,44,46] Other exogenous compounds known to cause mast cell degranulation include anti-IgE, compound 48/80, opiates, concanavalin A, and calcium ionophores. The different types of mast cells may be affected differently, depending on the compound that causes degranulation. Variability in degranulation, the mediators released, quantity, and time course may occur. Another secretory mechanism for histamine release has been described.[44] It has been referred to as piecemeal secretion and transfer to the cell surface by microvesicles. There is also variability in the response of different mast cells to inhibition of mast cell degranulation with the drug cromolyn. Intestinal mast cells were most affected, whereas MC_T mast cells from the lung were mildly affected, and skin MC_{TC} mast cells were not affected.[44]

The heterogeneity of mast cells has been demonstrated in dog skin, though it has not been

● Table 8-5 **PREFORMED MEDIATORS OF HUMAN MAST CELLS**

MEDIATOR	FUNCTION
Histamine	H_1 and H_2 receptor-mediated effects on smooth muscle, endothelial cells, and nerve endings
Tryptase	Cleaves C3 and C3a; degrades VIP and CGRP kallikrein-like activity;activates fibroblasts
Chymases	Function unclear; cleave neuropeptides, including substance P
Carboxypeptidase	Acts in concert with other neutral proteases
Acid hydrolase	Breaks down complex carbohydrates
Arylsulfatase	Hydrolyses aromatic sulfate esters
ECF-A	Eosinophil chemotaxis and "activation"
Neutrophil chemotactic factor	Neutrophil chemotaxis and "activation"
Heparin	Anticoagulant, anticomplementary; modifies activities of other performed mediators
Chondroitin sulfate	Function unknown
Cytokines (e.g., TNF-α, IL-4, IL-3, IL-5, and IL-6)	See Table 8-2

● Table 8-6 **PHARMACOLOGIC ACTIVITIES OF NEWLY GENERATED MAST CELL MEDIATORS**

MEDIATOR	ABBREVIATION	PHARMACOLOGIC ACTIONS
Prostaglandin D_2	PGD_2	Bronchoconstriction; peripheral vasodilation; coronary and pulmonary vasoconstriction; inhibition of platelet aggregation; neutrophil chemoattraction; augmentation of basophil histamine release
Prostaglandin F_2	9-α, 11-β–PGF_2	Bronchoconstriction; peripheral vasodilation; coronary vasoconstriction; inhibition of platelet aggregation
Thromboxane A_2	TXA_2	Vasoconstriction; platelet aggregation; bronchoconstriction
Leukotriene C_4	LTB_4	Neutrophil chemotaxis, adherence and degranulation; augmentation of vascular permeability
Leukotriene C_4	LTC_4	Bronchoconstriction; increase in vascular permeability; arteriolar constriction
Leukotriene D_4	LTD_4	Bronchoconstriction; increase in vascular permeability
Leukotriene E_4	LTE_4	Weak bronchoconstriction; enhancement of bronchial responsiveness; increase in vascular permeability
Platelet-activating factor	PAF	Platelet aggregation; chemotaxis and degranulation of eosinophils and neutrophils; increase in vascular permeability; bronchoconstriction; engenders hypotension

studied to the degree of human or rodent mast cells, and further work is warranted.[28,44] This is an important distinction, as many differences are species-specific. The skin of atopic dogs contains at least two subsets of mast cells that are distinguished in the following ways: (1) histologically, by metachromatic staining properties in different fixatives, and (2) functionally, by response to antigen *in vivo* (see discussion of Atopy). Three mast cell subtypes are distinguished in normal canine skin based on their content of the mast cell–specific proteases, chymase and tryptase: tryptase mast cells, chymase mast cells, and tryptase/chymase mast cells.[55] Whether such heterogeneity exists in equine mast cells is not known.

● Table 8-7 **CHEMOATTRACTANTS FOR NEUTROPHILS**	
Bacterial products	Lipid chemotactic factors (HETE, etc.) from mast cells
C5a (derived from complement activation; tissue, virus, and bacterial enzymes cleave C5)	Lysosomal proteases
C3a	Collagen breakdown products
C567	Fibrin breakdown products
Kallikrein	Plasminogen activator
Denatured protein	Prostaglandins
Lymphokines	Leukotrienes (especially LTB$_4$)
Monokines	Immune complexes
Neutrophil chemotactic factor (NCF) from mast cells	
ECF-A from mast cells	

Interestingly, histamine has two types of effects on hypersensitivity reactions, proinflammatory and anti-inflammatory. The proinflammatory effects of histamine are mediated through histamine 1 (H$_1$) receptors and resultant decreases in intracellular cyclic adenosine monophosphate (cAMP). Also, H$_1$ receptors mediate pruritus, and the trauma associated with pruritus may lead to further tissue and keratinocyte damage. The anti-inflammatory effects of histamine (inhibition of the release of inflammatory mediator substances from mast cells, neutrophils, lymphocytes, and monocyte-macrophages) are mediated through H$_2$ receptors and resultant increases in cAMP.

Endothelial Cells

The vascular endothelium is now known to be a very active cell type that is important in inflammation, immune responses, and tissue repair (see Chapter 1).[44,46,61] In response to various cytokines, endothelial cells express adhesion molecules (integrins, selectins, and immunoglobulin supergene family [intercellular adhesion molecules]) on their surfaces. The selectins (E-selectin and P-selectin) are expressed on endothelial cells following certain inflammatory stimuli and act to slow down and cause rolling of leukocytes along the vascular endothelium. The leukocyte activation results in integrin expression and binding to immunoglobulin supergene family molecules such as ICAM-1 and VCAM-1 on endothelial cells, resulting in adhesion. Transendothelial migration occurs following adhesion.[44] Then, in response to chemokines, the migrating lymphocytes, monocytes, and granulocytes will move towards the site of inflammation. Without this ability to home, the circulating effector cells could not respond to an immunologic or inflammatory event. In addition, activated endothelial cells can synthesize and secrete numerous substances such as cytokines (including IL-1, IL-6, and IL-8), fibronectin, collagen IV, proteoglycans, blood clotting factors, growth factors, and granulocyte-macrophage colony-stimulating factor. Defects in endothelial cell adhesion molecule expression may result in disorders that mimic immunodeficiencies owing to defective migration of lymphocytes, monocytes, or granulocytes (see Chapter 4).

GRANULOCYTES

Neutrophils have, as their major roles, the function of phagocytosis and subsequent destruction and elimination of phagocytized material. In a sense, they are the scavengers of immunologically identified debris. They are considered most important in containing infection. Owing, however, to their numerous chemoattractants (Table 8-7) and intracellular products (Table 8-8), which may be released at sites of inflammation, neutrophils are omnipresent participants in most immune and virtually all inflammatory reactions.[23,44,46,52,55]

● Table 8-8 **NEUTROPHIL PRODUCTS**

Antimicrobial Enzymes	Hydrolases
Lysozyme	Cathepsin B
Myeloperoxidase	Cathepsin D
	N-Acetyl-β-glucosaminidase
Proteases	β-Glucuronidase
	β-Glycerophosphatase
Collagenolytic proteinase	
Collagenase	**Others**
Elastase	
Cathepsin G	Lactoferrin
Leukotrienes	Eosinophil chemotactic factor
Gelatinase	Leukotrienes
	Pyrogen
	Prostaglandins
	Thromboxanes
	Platelet-activating factor

Eosinophils, effector cells in hypersensitivity reactions, also participate in the downgrading of inflammation and defense of the host against extracellular parasites.[*] They are also phagocytic (immune complexes, mast cell granules, aggregated immunoglobulins, and certain bacteria and fungi). Eosinophils have a tremendous ability to communicate with surrounding cells by the expression of surface receptors and cytokine secretion. Over 60 receptors for a variety of adhesion molecules, immunoglobulin Fc receptors, cytokines, and lipid mediators have been found on the eosinophil membrane.[39,44] Eosinophil chemotaxis has been the subject of much research. Currently a number of molecules are considered good candidates for eosinophil chemotaxis *in vivo*. These include platelet-activating factor (PAF), LTB4, LTD4, diHETEs, and the C-C subfamily of chemokines.[39,44] The C-C chemokines considered most potent and selective for eosinophil chemotaxis are eotaxin, RANTES, MCP-3 and MCP-4.[39,44] Interestingly, the response of eosinophils from normal people is less to some chemotaxins than eosinophils from allergic people. This may reflect priming of eosinophils by some cytokines such as IL-3, IL-5 and GM-CSF.[44] Eosinophils are noteworthy for their preformed mediators stored within at least two types of eosinophilic granules, but like other inflammatory cells, they also newly synthesize leukotrienes and a variety of cytokines when activated (Table 8-9). Degranulation can occur by three different mechanisms, though it appears that cytotoxic degranulation occurs commonly *in vivo*.[44]

Major basic protein (also found in basophils), eosinophil cationic protein, eosinophil-derived neurotoxin, and eosinophil peroxidase are potent toxic mediators and all have been shown to be effective at killing a variety of parasites. Eosinophil proteases may contribute to host tissue damage and wound healing as the collagenase degrades type I and type III collagen and gelatinase degrades type XVII collagen. Additionally, eosinophil degranulation results in the production of membrane-derived mediators such as leukotrienes and platelet-activating factor.

Basophils, major effector cells in some hypersensitivity reactions, may also play a role in downgrading delayed-type hypersensitivity reactions.[44] Basophils are somewhat similar to mast cells, in that they have high-affinity receptors for IgE and contain high levels of histamine, but they also are the only leukocytes to share features once thought specific for eosinophils. Basophils contain major basic protein and the Charcot-Leyden crystals (lysophospholipase).[44] Basophils express over 30 surface receptors and have preformed granule-stored mediators and newly synthesized mediators following degranulation or activation. Basophils degranulate in 4 distinct

[*]References 7, 39, 40, 44, 46, 52, 55.

● Table 8-9   **SECRETORY PRODUCTS OF EOSINOPHILS**

Granule Proteins	**Lipid Mediators**
Major basic protein	Leukotriene B_4 (small amount)
Eosinophil peroxidase	Leukotriene C_4
Eosinophil cationic protein	Leukotriene C_5
Eosinophil-derived neurotoxic	5-HETE
β-Glucuronidase	5,15- and 8,15-diHETE
Acid phosphatase	5-oxy- 15-hydroxy 6,8,11,13, HETE
Arylsulfatase	Prostaglandins E_1 and E_2
	6-Keto-prostaglandin F_1
Cytokines°	Thromboxane B_2
IL-1	PAF
IL-3	
IL-4	
IL-5	**Enzymes**
IL-6	Elastase (questionable)
IL-8	Charcot-Leyden crystal protein
IL-10	Collagenase
IL-16	92-kD Gelatinase
GM-CSF	
RANTES	
TNF-α	**Reactive Oxygen Intermediates**
TGF-β	Superoxide radical anion
TGF-β1	H_2O_2
MIP-1α	Hydroxy radicals

HETE, Hydrocyeicosatetraenoic acid; *ETE*, eicosatetraenoic acid; *diHETE*, dihydroxyeicosatetraenoic acid; *TNF*, tumor necrosis factor; *TGF*, transforming growth factor; *MIP*, macrophage inflammatory protein; *PAF*, platelet activating factor.
°Physiologic significance of these cytokines needs to be confirmed.
(From Kita H, Gleich, G J: The eosinophil: Structure and function. In: Kaplan, AP (ed). Allergy II. W.B. Saunders, Philadelphia, 1997, p 153.)

morphologic patterns, none of which are cytotoxic.[44] Basophils are important in host defense and this has been most conclusively shown in the rejection of ticks. In skin diseases, basophils are particularly important in cutaneous basophil hypersensitivity, a T cell-controlled reaction important in host responses to various ectoparasites. The late-phase allergic reaction is believed to play a major, if not *the* major, role in chronic allergic skin or respiratory disease.[44] Basophils are a key cell involved in late phase reactions.[12]

Humoral Components

The humoral components as described in the SIS include immunoglobulins, complement components, fibrinolysins, cytokines, eicosanoids, neuropeptides, and antimicrobial peptides.[7,23,44,52,63] The changes observed in inflammation are mediated, however, by numerous substances derived from the plasma, from cells of the damaged tissue, and from infiltrating monocytes, macrophages, lymphocytes, and granulocytes. The interactions among cells, neurons, expression of cell receptors, cytokines, and other soluble mediators determine the inflammatory response. Some mediators augment inflammation, and others suppress it. Some mediators antagonize or destroy other mediators, and others amplify or generate other mediators. All mediators and cells normally act together in a harmonious fashion to maintain homeostasis and to protect the host against infectious agents and other noxious substances. Many mediators may be preformed and stored with the effector cells; other mediators are produced only in response to damage or appropriate receptor activation. A complete summary of all inflammatory mediator substances is beyond the scope of this chapter; the interested reader is referred to the various references.

Complement is a group of plasma and cell membrane proteins that induce and influence immunologic and inflammatory events.[23,44,46,52,63] The critical step in the generation of biologic activities from the complement proteins is the cleavage of C3. There are two pathways for the cleavage of C3. The classic pathway requires the presence of immunoglobulin and immune complexes. The alternative (properdin) pathway does not require immunoglobulin and may be directly activated by bacteria, viruses, and some abnormal cells. There is also a pathway to amplify C3 cleavage, and an effector sequence. The final effect of this sequence is the production of a membrane attack complex, which causes cell lysis. As the effector sequence progresses, a variety of complement components are formed that have other effects. These other components play a role in neutralization of viruses, solubilization of immune complexes, and interaction with receptors on other cells. Many inflammatory cells have receptors for degradation products of C3 and C5. These activated receptors are important in phagocytosis, immune regulation, and mast cell and basophil degranulation.

Immune complexes are a heterogeneous group of immunoreactants formed by the non-covalent union of antigen and antibody.[7,23,44,46,63] Many factors influence the formation, immunochemistry, biology, and clearance of these reactants. Circulating immune complexes influence both the afferent and efferent limbs of the immune response and can mediate tissue damage in certain pathologic states. Circulating immune complexes can be measured by a number of generally unavailable techniques, including C1q-binding, solid-phase C1q, conglutinin, and Raji cell assays. Circulating immune complexes have been detected in numerous human dermatoses and probably play an important role in the pathogenesis of systemic lupus erythematosus and vasculitis.

Lipid mediators (platelet activating factor and eicosanoids) are newly synthesized unstored molecules derived from cell membranes. Cell membranes contain phospholipids, one of which is phosphatidylcholine, the parent molecule of PAF. Arachidonic acid is stored in cells as an ester in phospholipids and is the dominant fatty acid attached to the glycerol portion of PAF. Though arachidonic acid is also present in other phospholipids, this is a major source in inflammatory cells. Following specific receptor stimulation and after cellular injury, phospholipases cause the degradation of phospholipids. Phospholipase A_2 enzymes break down phosphatidylcholine into a molecule of free arachidonic acid and one of PAF. Phospholipase C activity will also result in free arachidonic acid, but it is the predominance of phospholipase A that contributes the most to the generation of inflammatory mediators. Glucocorticoids inhibit the action of phospholipases, possibly by the induction of lipocortin, at pharmacologically achieved levels. This is thought to be a major anti-inflammatory mechanism of glucocorticoid therapy.*

PAF is not an eicosanoid, but a phospholipid that also acts as an inflammatory mediator. It is produced from a variety of cells, although in humans, neutrophils and eosinophils produce the largest amounts.[7,44,46,52] PAF primes cells to have augmented responses to other stimuli and has its greatest effects on eosinophils and monocytes. It is an extremely potent eosinophil chemoattractant and stimulates their degranulation and release of leukotrienes. A chemoattractant for mononuclear cells, PAF stimulates their release of IL-1, IL-4, and TNF-α.

The metabolites of the oxidation of arachidonic acid are termed *eicosanoids* and are potent biologic mediators of a variety of physiologic or pathologic responses. Though arachidonic acid and the oxidative enzymes to degrade it are found in all human cells, only mast cells, leukocytes, endothelial cells, epithelial cells, and platelets have enough to play a major role in allergic diseases.[7,20,44,46,52] Free arachidonic acid is oxidized by one of three enzyme classes; the two most

---

*References 7, 20, 44, 46, 52, 55.

studied and important are cyclooxygenase (COX) and lipoxygenase (LO). The third is monooxygenase, and this does result in *cis/trans*–dienols (HETE) formation, which in the human epidermis leads to the formation of 12-HETE.[20]

The eicosanoids include two main types of molecules, the prostanoids and leukotrienes. Prostanoids (prostaglandins and thromboxanes) are derived by the metabolism of arachidonic acid by cyclooxygenase. Two forms of cyclooxygenase are known, COX-1 in the endoplasmic reticulum, and COX-2 in the nuclear envelope, and they serve different functions and are preferentially important in different tissues. Aspirin and the nonsteroidal anti-inflammatory drugs primarily function by blocking cyclooxygenase. Cyclooxygenase metabolism results in PGH_2 formation, which is subsequently metabolized by specific terminal enzymes that result in the formation of PGE_2, PGF_2, PGD_2, PGI_2, or thromboxane (TX) A_2. Different cell types have variations in which enzyme system is present and, therefore, in which metabolites are produced. Each final metabolite has one or more specific receptors and new therapeutic agents, such as misoprostol, are being developed as agonists or antagonists for these specific receptors.[20,44]

Leukotrienes (LTA, LTB, LTC, LTD and LTE) and their precursors—hydroperoxyeicosatetraenoic acids (HPETEs) and hydroxyeicosatetraenoic acids (HETEs)—are derived by the metabolism of arachidonic acid by the three enzymes of lipoxygenation, 5-,12-, and 15-lipoxygenase.[20,44,55] Different tissues express variable levels of the cytosolic lipoxygenases. The 5-lipoxygenase pathway predominates in neutrophils, monocytes, macrophages, and mast cells, whereas the 15-lipoxygenase pathway predominates in eosinophils and in endothelial and epithelial cells. The 12-lipoxygenase pathway predominates in platelets. The 5-lipoxygenase pathway results in the production of LTA_4, which—depending on the enzymes present in the cells—is converted to LTB_4 or LTC_4. LTD_4 or LTE_4 are produced from LTC_4. Typically, eicosanoids have autocrine and paracrine functions that are important locally for host defense, and then they are inactivated or degraded. Abnormalities in production or control mechanisms may occur, however, leading to local or systemic tissue damage and disease. The actions of eicosanoids are quite diverse and variable according to the species, tissue, cellular source, the presence of stereospecific receptors, and the generation of secondary mediators.[20,44] The understanding of how they function in disease is further complicated by the complex interactions that occur, but that are not included in many laboratory studies, and by the fact that—due to their autocrine and paracrine functions—they must be measured in the involved tissue. The effects of arachidonic acid formation and some of the activities that eicosanoids may have in skin disease are summarized in Table 8-10.[7,20,44,46,52]

● Table 8-10 **EFFECTS OF EICOSANOIDS IN SKIN DISEASE**

EICOSANOID	EFFECT
$LTC_1/D_1/E_1$	Vascular dilation and increased permeability
LTB_1	Leukocyte chemotaxis and activation; increased endothelial adherence of leukocytes; stimulates keratinocyte proliferation; enhances NK cell activity; hyperalgesia
12-HETE	Stimulates smooth muscle contraction
15-HETE	Hyperalgesia; inhibits cyclooxygenase; inhibits mixed lymphocyte reaction; stimulates suppressor T cells; inhibits NK cell activity
15-HPETE	Suppresses T lymphocyte function and Fc receptors
PGE_2	Plasma exudation; hyperalgesia; stimulates cell proliferation; suppresses lymphocyte and neutrophil function
PGF_2	Vasoconstriction; synergy with histamine and bradykinin on vascular permeability; stimulates cell proliferation
PGD_2	Smooth muscle relaxation
PGD_2/PGI_2	Suppression of leukocyte function; vasodilation and increased permeability

Aging and the Skin Immune System

With advancing age, the immune system of animals and humans undergoes characteristic changes, usually resulting in decreased immunocompetence, which is termed *immunosenescence*.[*] An age-associated decrease in immunoresponsiveness is commonly accepted for T lymphocytes but also claimed for B lymphocytes, Langerhans' cells, and other components of the immune system. Absolute cell counts of total lymphocytes, T cells, CD4+ and CD8+ T cells, and B cells were decreased in aged horses.[40a] However, immunoglobulin isotype concentrations were normal. Some studies have shown that aging humans and mice have increased susceptibility to infections or malignancies, as well as elevated titers of autoantibodies, suggestive of higher susceptibility to autoimmune diseases.

● TYPES OF HYPERSENSITIVE REACTIONS

Clinical hypersensitivity disorders were divided on an immunopathologic basis, by Gell and Coombs, into four types:[7,23,52,63]

Type I: Immediate (anaphylactic)
Type II: Cytotoxic
Type III: Immune complex
Type IV: Cell-mediated (delayed)

Subsequently, two other types of hypersensitivity reactions have been described: late-phase reactions and cutaneous basophil hypersensitivity. Clearly, these six reactions are oversimplified because of the complex interrelationships that exist among the effector cells and the numerous components of the inflammatory response. In most pathologic events, immunologically initiated responses almost certainly involve multiple components of the inflammatory process. In reality, many diseases may involve a combination of reactions, and their separation into distinct pathologic mechanisms rarely occurs. For example, IgE (classically involved in type I hypersensitivity reactions) and Langerhans' cells (classically involved in type IV hypersensitivity reactions) may interact in a previously unrecognized fashion in the development of human and canine atopic dermatitis. Even the classic type IV reaction is not as straightforward as we used to think, as evidence suggests that mast cells, eosinophils, and basophils may play a role.

Realization that this scheme has become a simplistic approach to immunopathology has provoked other investigators to modify the original scheme of Gell and Coombs, often to a seemingly hopeless degree of hairsplitting. In this section, we briefly examine the classic Gell and Coombs classification of hypersensitivity disorders, because (1) it is still somewhat applicable to discussions of cutaneous hypersensitivity diseases and (2) it is still the immunopathologic scheme used by most authors and by major immunologic and dermatologic texts.

Type I (anaphylactic, immediate) hypersensitivity reactions are classically described as those involving genetic predilection, reaginic antibody (IgE) production, and mast cell degranulation. A genetically programmed individual absorbing a complete antigen (e.g., ragweed pollen) responds by producing a unique antibody (reagin, IgE). IgE is homocytotropic and avidly binds membrane receptors on tissue mast cells and blood basophils. When the eliciting antigen comes in contact with the specific reaginic antibody, a number of inflammatory mediator substances are released and cause tissue damage. This reaction occurs within minutes and gradually disappears within an hour. It is important to note that older terms such as *reaginic antibody, homocytotropic antibody,* or *skin-sensitizing antibody* are *not* strictly synonymous with IgE, because subclasses of IgG may also mediate type I hypersensitivity reactions. The classic examples of diseases that involve type I hypersensitivity reactions in horses are urticaria, angioedema, anaphylaxis, atopy, food hypersensitivity, insect hypersensitivity, and some drug eruptions.

---

[*]References 7, 9, 23, 40a, 60, 67a.

Late-phase immediate hypersensitivity reactions have been recognized and studied.* The onset of these mast cell-dependent reactions occurs 4 to 8 hours after challenge (neutrophils, eosinophils, and basophils found histologically). They persist up to 24 hours, in contrast to classic type I reactions, which abate within 60 minutes. The initial reaction is histologically characterized by an infiltrate of neutrophils and eosinophils, which changes to a predominance of mononuclear cells. These late-phase reactions can be reproduced with intradermal injections of leukotrienes, kallikrein, or PAF. Although late-phase reactions to the intradermal injection of allergens have been recorded in horses, the clinical importance of such reactions remains to be defined. These reactions, however, are suspected to play a role in atopy and insect hypersensitivity.

Type II (cytotoxic) hypersensitivity reactions are characterized by the binding of antibody (IgG or IgM), with or without complement, to complete antigens on body tissues. This binding of antibody, with or without complement, results in cytotoxicity or cytolysis. Examples of type II hypersensitivity reactions in horses are pemphigus, pemphigoid, cold agglutinin disease, and some drug eruptions.

Type III (immune complex) hypersensitivity reactions are characterized by the deposition of circulating antigen-antibody complexes (in slight antigen excess) in blood vessel walls. These immune complexes (usually containing IgG or IgM) then fix complement, which attracts neutrophils. Proteolytic and hydrolytic enzymes released from the infiltrating neutrophils produce tissue damage. Type I hypersensitivity reactions and histamine release may be important in the initiation of immune complex deposition. Examples of type III hypersensitivity reactions in horses are systemic lupus erythematosus, leukocytoclastic vasculitis, and some drug eruptions.

Type IV (cell-mediated, delayed) hypersensitivity reactions classically do not involve antibody-mediated injury. An antigen (classically, an incomplete antigen referred to as a hapten) interacts with an antigen-presenting cell (APC). In the skin, the APC is the Langerhans' cell. The APC usually internalizes the antigen and digests it, then presents a peptide fragment bound to MHC class II immune response antigens on the cell surface. The processed antigen is then presented to T cells, leading to the production of "sensitized" T lymphocytes. These sensitized T lymphocytes respond to further antigenic challenge by releasing lymphokines that produce tissue damage. In mouse models, there is evidence that the development of type IV hypersensitivity may involve mast cells and, in some situations, small amounts of IgE.[44] It has been suggested that the term *cell-mediated* is an unfortunate misnomer for this type of immunologic reaction, which is no more or less cell-mediated than are antibody-dependent reactions, which themselves are ultimately due to the participation of a lymphocyte or plasma cell.[53] Classic examples of type IV hypersensitivity reactions in horses are contact hypersensitivity, insect hypersensitivity, and some drug eruptions.

Cutaneous basophil hypersensitivity may be mediated by T cells or homocytotropic antibody (IgE or IgG). It is characterized by a marked basophil infiltrate and fibrin deposition. These reactions occur about 12 hours after intradermal allergen injections and may peak in intensity from 24 to 72 hours.[7,23,44,46] Cutaneous basophil hypersensitivity is considered important in the development of immunity to ticks and in the pathogenesis of insect hypersensitivity.[23,52]

Type I, type II, and type III hypersensitivity reactions together form the "immediate" hypersensitivity reactions. They are all antibody-mediated; thus, there is only a short delay (from minutes to a few hours) before their tissue-damaging effects become apparent. Type IV hypersensitivity is the "delayed" hypersensitivity reaction. It is not antibody mediated, and it classically requires 24 to 72 hours before becoming detectable. This concept has also been further reevaluated so that type III, type IV, cutaneous basophil hypersensitivity, and late-phase reactions are all regarded as having delayed-in-time manifestations varying from 4 to 48 hours.[44]

---

*References 7, 12, 23, 44, 52, 55

● THERAPY FOR HYPERSENSITIVITY DISORDERS

Treatment Plans

Most horses with chronic allergies, particularly those with atopic disease, require a combination of therapeutic agents for optimal control of symptoms.[81,157a] When possible, the optimum treatment of all allergies is avoidance of the offending allergen(s). If this is not possible, most treatments are directed at blocking the effects of the allergic reaction. Prevention may also occur with allergen-specific immunotherapy (hyposensitization, desensitization) (see discussion on Atopy) and, possibly, with some immunomodulatory drugs. When allergen avoidance and/or allergen-specific immunotherapy are ineffective or partially effective, or when clients decline these approaches, other medical options will be required. Often the optimum control will require different therapeutic protocols over the life of the animal. Therefore a treatment plan will be required that takes the different problems, goals of the clients, and types of therapeutic agents into consideration. In general, these are aimed at treating the byproducts of the allergic reaction that has already occurred. The majority of therapeutic protocols are used to help alleviate pruritus (the major symptom of most allergic diseases), to treat specific problems or secondary infections, to avoid or decrease exposure to offending allergens, and to decrease inflammation. These therapeutic protocols may be specific for a problem or etiology, or they may be nonspecific. The most commonly recommended therapeutic protocols are listed in Table 8-11. These treatment options vary in their ease of administration, risks, efficacy, expense, and required monitoring. In many cases, combinations of treatments may be utilized, and an overall plan to control those aspects of the problem considered most bothersome by the client is the most effective way to manage these cases long term.

Avoidance

Avoidance requires the identification of allergens contributing to the hypersensitivity. The offending allergens may be determined by histoclinical findings, provocation testing, and "allergy testing." Avoidance frequently is effective for hypersensitivities such as insect hypersensitivity and food hypersensitivity, but it is often ineffective or impractical in atopic disease. However, even if the offending allergens cannot be completely avoided; it is helpful to eliminate exposure as much as possible. Some methods of avoidance for atopic disease will be covered in that section.

Topical Therapy

Topical therapy is often incorporated into treatment plans and is discussed in more detail in Chapter 3. The major disadvantages are the time and effort needed for administration. Expense may also be an important factor. Total body bathing and/or rinses are required for regional or generalized pruritus, and often reduce pruritus by rehydrating the stratum corneum and by removing surface debris, microbial byproducts, and allergens that may contribute to the pruritic

---

● Table 8-11   **THERAPEUTIC REGIMENS**

NONSPECIFIC THERAPY	SPECIFIC THERAPY
Soothing topical baths, rinses	Antibiotics
Moisturizers	Insect control
Topical glucocorticoids	Allergen-specific immunotherapy (hyposensitization)
Fatty acids	Novel protein diet (hypoallergenic)
Nonsteroidal anti-inflammatory agents (e.g., pentoxifylline)	Immunosuppressive therapy
Antihistamines	
Antidepressants	
Systemic glucocorticoids	

load.[82,157a] Hydrocortisone (1%) shampoo is not significantly absorbed and may help treat allergic reactions.[55] Treatment with ointments, creams, lotions, and sprays may be possible for localized areas. Topical glucocorticoids are most effective, but generally limited to localized hypersensitivity reactions. Cold water, hypoallergenic and moisturizing shampoos and creme rinses, colloidal oatmeal, and shampoos and creme rinses containing pramoxine (local anesthetic) can reduce pruritus for up to 72 hours (see Chapter 3).[82,157a] Topical therapy unfortunately is often overlooked and not presented as an option to clients. Appropriately administered topical therapy can greatly reduce the need for systemic treatment in many patients.

Fatty Acids

A large number of studies have shown that fatty acids are beneficial in the management of pruritic dogs and cats.[55] In most of these studies the pruritus was due to hypersensitivity reactions, most commonly atopic disease. Fatty acids and their role in normal skin and coat are discussed in Chapter 3. Because these agents are relatively benign, diets or supplements containing appropriate amounts and ratios could be used in most allergic horses.

The proposed mechanism, besides the inhibition of arachidonic acid metabolism, relates to metabolic byproducts of fatty acid metabolism. Supplements used for pruritus usually contain one or both of γ-linolenic acid (GLA) and eicosapentaenoic acid (EPA). GLA is found in relatively high concentrations in evening primrose, borage, and black currant oils. It is elongated to dihomo(D)GLA, which directly competes with arachidonic acid as a substrate for cyclooxygenase and 15-lipoxygenase. The result of DGLA metabolism is the formation of prostaglandin E1 and 15-hydroxy-8,11,13-eicosapentaenoic acid, both of which are believed to have anti-inflammatory effects.

EPA, which is usually supplied by using cold water marine fish oils, also competes as a substrate for cyclooxygenase and 5- and 15-lipoxygenase. The metabolism of EPA by the lipoxygenase enzymes results in the formation of leukotriene B_5 and 15-hydroxyeicosapentaenoic acid. These two products are believed to inhibit leukotriene B_4, which is a potent proinflammatory mediator. Fig. 8-2 demonstrates the interactions of GLA, EPA, and arachidonic acid.

Although the benefits of these products in dogs and cats are clear, which fatty acid, which combination of fatty acids, what ratio of omega-6 to omega-3, and what dose of these agents are most effective remains inconclusive. It appears that (1) the most anti-inflammatory ratio of omega-6:omega-3 fatty acids is 5:1 to 10:1; (2) the most important fatty acids are γ–linolenic, di-homo γ-linolenic, and eicosapentaenoic; and (3) the animal's diet (levels, ratios, and types of omega-6 and omega-3 fatty acids) has a profound effect on the efficacy of fatty acid supplementation.[55]

Little information has been published on the usefulness of these fatty acids in horses. The oral administration of linseed oil (60% α-linolenic, 17% α-linoleic) inhibited inflammation, the production of eicosanoids, and the production of TNF in a few experimental studies in horses.[75,76,78,79] Linseed oil may cause depression, anorexia, and mild colic in horses, whereas flaxseed oil (50% to 58% α-linoleic acid) does not.[74a] In two double-blinded, placebo-controlled clinical studies, no significant reduction in pruritus occurred in allergic horses treated orally with linseed oil [74] or a commercial product (evening primrose oil and cold water marine fish oil).[71] These studies are difficult to interpret because (1) it was not clear how many horses had insect hypersensitivity, atopy, or both, and (2) the horses' base diets were not analyzed. In addition, it appears that some atopic dogs have partial deficiencies in Δ-5 and Δ-6 desaturase activities, which would require supplementation with very specific omega-6 and omega-3 fatty acids in order to achieve success.[55] Whether a similar situation exists in horses is not known.

Many clinicians feel that omega-6/omega-3 fatty acid supplementation is beneficial in some allergic horses, especially those with atopy.* Although fish oils are rarely palatable to horses, a

---

*References 17, 18, 81-83, 117, 157a.

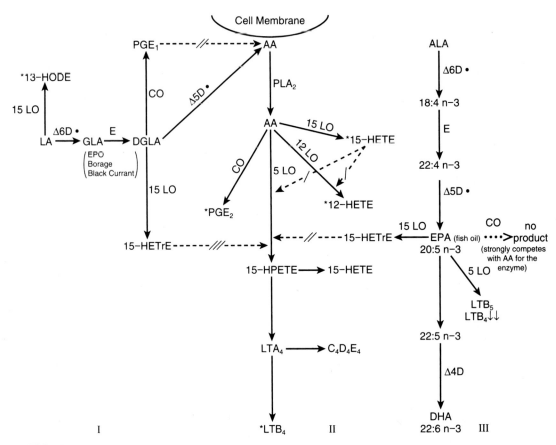

FIGURE 8-2. *I,* N-6 fatty acid metabolism with production of anti-inflammatory eicosanoids. *II,* Arachidonic acid cascade with production of proinflammatory eicosanoids. *III,* N-3 fatty acid metabolism with production of anti-inflammatory eicosanoids. *13-HODE,* 13-hydroxyoctadecadienoic acid; *PG,* prostaglandin; *E,* elongase; *Δ-6-D,* Δ-6-desaturase; *LA,* linoleic acid; *GLA,* γ-linolenic acid; *EPO,* evening primrose oil; *DGLA,* dihomo-γ-linolenic acid; *AA,* arachidonic acid; *ALA,* α-linolenic acid; *EPA,* eicosapentaenoic acid; *DHA,* docosahexaenoic acid; *DES,* desaturase; *PLA2,* phospholipase A2; *CO,* cyclooxygenase; *LO,* lipoxygenase; *HETE,* hydroxyeicosatetraenoic acid; *HPETE,* hydroperoxyeicosatetraenoic acid; *HEPE,* hydroxyeicosapentaenoic acid; *15-HETrE,* 15-hydroxy-8,11,13-eicosatriaenoic acid; *LT,* leukotriene. ★ Indicates arachidonic acid–derived eicosanoids identified in inflammatory skin disease; ? indicates inhibitory or anti-inflammatory eicosanoid (number of *slash lines* indicates degree of inhibition.) (*From White P: Essential fatty acids: Use in management of canine atopy. Comp Cont Educ 15:451, 1993.*)

commercial fatty acid supplement (DVM Derm Caps 100s), given orally at 1 capsule/50 to 100 kg q12h appears to be well tolerated and effective in some horses. These fatty acid supplements may also have synergistic effects when administered in conjunction with glucocorticoids and/or antihistamines.[55,157a] Fatty acid supplements should be given for at least 3 weeks before a judgment is made as to their benefits.[55]

Nonsteroidal Anti-Inflammatory Agents

Nonsteroidal anti-inflammatory agents are classically used to decrease pain and inflammation, but have shown little benefit for pruritus or atopic disease. A number of nonsteroidal drugs have been used to treat equine pruritus. Little or no work has been done to document the effect of these, including phenylbutazone, diethylcarbamazine, flunixin, ketoprofen, orgotein (metalloprotein, nonsteroidal anti-inflammatory), phenothiazine tranquilizers, barbiturates, and levamisole.[52,157a] Experimental studies have indicated that 5-lipoxygenase inhibitors,[72] a leukotriene synthesis inhibitor,[80] and PAF receptor antagonists[73] inhibit various aspects of the equine inflammatory response, but therapeutic trials with such agents have not been reported. Studies of nonsteroidal antipruritic agents in dogs with hypersensitivity skin disease indicated that aspirin, vitamin E, zinc methionine, vitamin C, papaverine (phosphodiesterase inhibitor), zileuton (leukotriene antagonist), doxycycline, and the combination of tetracycline and niacinamide are rarely effective.[55]

Pentoxifylline (Trental) has a variety of effects, and the benefits may result from different mechanisms, depending on the disease being treated (see Chapter 9).[55] It has been utilized for the treatment of contact hypersensitivity and atopic disease in dogs and humans. Anecdotal reports indicate that pentoxifylline may be useful in some pruritic horses (see Chapter 9).

Misoprostol acts as a PGE_1 analog. PGE_1 inhibits production of IL-1 and TNF-α in some models of inflammation, and production of LTB_4 by activated neutrophils. Of particular interest in allergic disease are its effects on decreasing histamine release, inhibiting eosinophil chemotaxis and survival, and inhibition of cutaneous late-phase allergic reactions.[44,55] Because late-phase allergic reactions may be involved in the pathogenesis of atopy, misoprostol might be useful. Misoprostol (Cytotec, Searle) is available in 100 and 200 µg tablets. Over 50% of the atopic dogs treated with misoprostol at 6 µg/kg q8h had greater than 50% reduction of pretreatment pruritus and lesion scores. The greatest risks with misoprostol are for inducing abortions (it should not be used in pregnant animals) and for causing diarrhea. No reports exist on the use of misoprostol in pruritic horses.

Antihistamines

Histamine is a potent chemical mediator that has variable actions, depending on what receptors and tissues are stimulated. The effects of histamine can be blocked in three ways: by physiologic antagonists, such as epinephrine; by agents that reduce histamine formation or release from mast cells and basophils; and by histamine receptor antagonists. We used to believe that most antihistamines worked by this latter effect. Now we have learned that most of the older first generation antihistamines also function by preventing mediator release from mast cells and basophils.[44] In veterinary dermatology, the primary indication for antihistamine therapy is the treatment of pruritus mediated by stimulation of histamine H_1 receptors, usually associated with hypersensitivity reactions.[44,55]

First-generation (classic, or traditional) antihistamines are H_1 blockers. However, not all the effects of histamine are antagonized by H_1 blockers. Because antihistamines are metabolized by the liver, they should be used with caution in patients with hepatic disease. In addition, their anticholinergic properties contraindicate their use in patients with glaucoma, gastrointestinal atony, and urinary retentive states. Some antihistamines are teratogenic in various laboratory animals. No information on teratogenicity is available for horses; however, this issue should be considered before treating pregnant mares. Finally, the efficacy of antihistamines is notoriously unpredictable and individualized in a given patient. Part of this variation may be dose-related, because antiallergic effects are concentration-dependent and some dose ranges will be antiallergic whereas others may enhance mediator release.[44] Thus, the clinician may try several antihistamines and doses before finding the one that is beneficial for a given patient.

Antihistamines block the physiologic effects of histamine. At least three different types of histamine receptors have been recognized. The role of H_3 receptors is just being uncovered, and they are primarily located in the CNS, where they affect a variety of nerve terminals and may affect neurotransmitter release.[44] Their role in dermatology has yet to be determined. The H_1-receptor antagonists are utilized in equine and small animal dermatology. This is because H_1 receptors are

● Table 8-12	**ANTIHISTAMINES FOR HORSES**	
ANTIHISTAMINE	DOSE	FREQUENCY
Amitriptyline	1 mg/kg	q12h
Chlorpheniramine	0.25 to 0.5 mg/kg	q12h
Diphenhydramine	1 to 2 mg/kg	q8-12h
Doxepin	0.5 to 0.75 mg/kg	q12h
Hydroxyzine	1 to 2 mg/kg	q8-12h

primarily responsible for pruritus, increased vascular permeability, release of inflammatory mediators, and recruitment of inflammatory cells.[44] In addition to their histamine-blocking action, some of these agents have sedative, antinausea, anticholinergic, antiserotoninergic, and local anesthetic effects. As mentioned previously, most will block mediator release if present prior to allergen challenge and if at the appropriate concentration. Most of the second generation, or nonsedating, antihistamines block mediator release to some degree.[44] However, the effects may differ with the variable or tissue being evaluated (i.e., different results may occur with various sources of mast cells, basophils, or eosinophils). Variable results may also occur depending on the method used to induce cellular responses, such as immunoglobulin E (IgE)–induced release or nonantibody inducers, though most will also decrease the response to nonimmunologic stimuli.[44] Cetirizine, a second generation antihistamine, is particularly effective in blocking the allergen-induced late-phase cutaneous reaction and in decreasing the influx of eosinophils in response to allergens.[44]

It is important to remember that antihistamines function best as *preventive* antipruritic agents.[44,55] They will *not* rapidly reduce severe ongoing pruritus and inflammation. Thus, a short course of glucocorticoids may have to be given to control the pruritus. Then the ability of an antihistamine to *prevent recurrence* of the pruritus can be assessed.

Second-generation (nonsedating) antihistamines are also H_1 blockers, but because they are poorly lipid-soluble and minimally cross the blood-brain barrier at recommended doses, they exert much less sedative action and anticholinergic effects than do first-generation antihistamines.[44] For some reason, second-generation antihistamines have not been useful in dogs to date.[55] In addition to not having any greater efficacy in dogs, second generation antihistamines are also more expensive, and some do not feel these agents are worth utilizing.[55]

There is little published information on the use of antihistamines in horses (Table 8-12). Most clinicians consider hydroxyzine (1 to 2 mg/kg q8-12h orally) to be the antihistamine of choice in the horse.* It is not known what percentage of horses respond to any given antihistamine. However, as the effects of different antihistamines vary from one horse to another,[157a] it is important to try several different ones before concluding that the pruritus is not responsive to these agents. Other antihistamines suggested for use in allergic horses include chlorpheniramine (0.25 to 0.5 mg/kg q12h orally) and diphenhydramine (1 to 2 mg/kg q8-12h orally).† "Standard" equine antihistamines—tripelennamine and pyrilamine—have not been effective. Clemastine (0.2 mg/kg PO) produced negligible inhibition of intradermal histamine reactions, suggesting poor oral bioavailability.[70a] Antihistamines should be given for at least 2 weeks before a judgment is made as to their utility. Antihistamines may act synergistically with glucocorticoids and/or fatty acids in pruritic horses.[55,157a]

*References 17, 18, 53, 81-83, 155, 157a, 167.
†References 17, 18, 81-83, 155, 157a.

Sedation and anticholinergic effects are the primary side effects from antihistamines in humans, dogs, and cats.[44,55] Antihistamine side effects are rare in the horse and include sedation, lethargy, and behavioral changes.[81,82,156,157a]

Antidepressants

A variety of the psychotropic drugs have been used to treat some hypersensitivity disorders, especially if stress or a psychogenic component may be present.[44,55] These drugs are also potent H_1 and H_2 blockers and, thus, possess many of the benefits and side effects of traditional antihistamines. In addition, these drugs lower the seizure threshold and are monoamine oxidase inhibitors. The heterocyclic (tricyclic) antidepressants—amitriptyline and doxepin—have been used with some success in humans, dogs, and cats.[44,55] Anecdotal reports indicate that doxepin (0.5 to 0.75 mg/kg q12h orally) is effective in some allergic horses.[81-83,155,157a] The authors have had success in a few allergic horses with amitriptyline (1 mg/kg q12h orally).

Systemic Glucocorticoids

Hypersensitivity diseases typically respond well to systemic glucocorticoids, and this is the treatment of choice for acute hypersensitivity diseases. It is also the treatment for many recurrent, but short-duration (under 4 months/year) disorders. It is indicated in the treatment of long-term, perennial hypersensitivity diseases only when safer options are not effective or practical. If long-term therapy is required, short-acting oral glucocorticoids (prednisone, prednisolone, or methylprednisolone) are preferred (see Chapter 3). Some human patients with atopic dermatitis cases are resistant to glucocorticoids due to altered receptor binding.[55]

Glucocorticoids are, in general, well tolerated in horses and represent the symptomatic treatment of choice for allergies.* The typical induction dose is 2 mg/kg prednisolone or prednisone q24h, in the morning, orally, until the pruritus is controlled (usually 3 to 10 days). In order to minimize side effects, long-term glucocorticoid therapy is given every other morning at the lowest possible dose (≤ 0.5 mg/kg prednisolone or prednisone q48h) (see Chapter 3). Some horses respond to prednisolone but not to prednisone (see Chapter 3). The authors recommend always beginning treatment with prednisolone.

Some horses respond best to dexamethasone (0.2 mg/kg q24h, in the morning, orally). However, dexamethasone is not as safe for long-term treatment. If dexamethasone is used for induction, prednisolone should be used for maintenance therapy (see Chapter 3).

Cyclosporine

Cyclosporine (Neoral, Novartis) is used for a wide variety of dermatologic diseases in humans, dogs, and cats.[20,44,55] This potent immunomodulatory agent has a number of actions: inhibition of IL-2, IL-3, IL-4, IL-5, TNF-α, IFN-α, and mast cell degranulation (see Chapter 3). In this way, cyclosporine inhibits T lymphocyte and macrophage function, antigen presentation, mast cell and eosinophil production, neutrophil adherence, natural killer cell activity, growth and differentiation of B cells, and histamine and eicosanoid release from mast cells. There are no reports concerning the use of cyclosporine in pruritic horses. The drug is very expensive.

Other Specific Therapies

Chronic allergic diseases, even in acute phases, predispose to secondary infections with *Malassezia* or bacteria, most often *Staphylococcus* species (see Chapters 4 and 5). When present, whether as infection or just overgrowth, they may contribute significantly to the pruritus and inflammation. It is important to recognize and treat specifically for these problems; otherwise therapies directed at

---

*References 17, 18, 81-83, 117, 157a.

the underlying hypersensitivity or pruritus will be much less effective. Parasitic diseases, besides causing a hypersensitivity reaction themselves, may aggravate other allergies by allergic or nonallergic mechanisms (see Chapter 6). These also must be identified and controlled for optimum success with antiallergy treatment protocols.

● HYPERSENSITIVITY DISORDERS

Urticaria and Angioedema

Urticaria (hives) and angioedema are variably pruritic, edematous skin disorders that are immunologic or nonimmunologic in nature. There may be multiple mechanisms involved in a given patient.[91] Urticaria is common, but angioedema is rare in the horse.

CAUSE AND PATHOGENESIS

Urticaria and angioedema result from mast cell or basophil degranulation, though the mast cell is considered the major effector cell. They may result from many stimuli, both immunologic and nonimmunologic.[°] Immunologic mechanisms include type I and III hypersensitivity reactions. Nonimmunologic factors that may precipitate or intensify urticaria and angioedema include physical forces (pressure, sunlight, heat, cold, exercise), psychologic stresses, genetic abnormalities, and various drugs and chemicals (aspirin, narcotics, foods, food additives). Chronic idiopathic urticaria in humans may be associated with autoantibodies to the high-affinity IgE receptor (Fc epsilon RI α).[20] Humans with chronic urticaria were more likely to have exposure to dogs and cats and to have positive titers to *Toxocara canis*.[103] The relationship is supported by a favorable response of many of these patients to parasiticidal therapy. Factors reported to have caused urticaria and angioedema in horses are listed in Table 8-13.

CLINICAL FEATURES

Urticaria is common, whereas angioedema is rare in horses.[†] No age, breed, or sex predilections have been reported for urticaria and angioedema in horses. Clinical signs may be acute or transient (most common) or chronic or persistent. Acute urticaria and angioedema are empirically defined as episodes lasting less than 6 to 8 weeks, whereas chronic episodes last longer. Urticarial reactions are characterized by the sudden onset of more-or-less bilaterally symmetric localized or generalized wheals, which may or may not be pruritic and usually do not exhibit serum leakage or hemorrhage. The lesions are typically flat-topped and steep-walled. Characteristically, the wheals are evanescent lesions, a few millimeters to several centimeters in diameter and a few millimeters in height, with each lesion persisting less than 24 to 48 hours. The lesions are typically of normal body temperature and pit with digital pressure. Urticarial lesions may occasionally assume bizarre patterns (serpiginous, linear, arciform, annular, papular) and coalesce to cover large areas as plaques. Hair may appear raised in these areas. Lesions can occur anywhere on the body, especially on the neck, trunk, and proximal extremities. Angioedematous reactions are characterized by localized or generalized large, edematous swellings that may or may not be pruritic and which exhibit serum leakage or hemorrhage. Angioedema most commonly involves the muzzle (Fig. 8-3), eyelids, ventrum (Fig. 8-4, A), and distal extremities. Angioedema is usually preceded or accompanied by urticaria.

The size and shape of urticarial lesions can vary considerably and these features have been used in a clinical classification:[50,67]

°References 20, 44, 55, 90, 91, 96, 100, 104.
†References 2, 8, 9, 21, 29, 32, 37, 42, 45, 47-50, 53, 56, 59, 62, 64, 65, 67, 84-102, 104

● Table 8-13 **POTENTIAL CAUSES OF URTICARIA AND ANGIOEDEMA IN HORSES**[53,91,96,100,104]

Drugs
   Penicillin, tetracyclines, sulfonamides, neomycin, ciprofloxacin, streptomycin, aspirin, phenylbutazone, flunixin, phenothiazines, guaiphensin, ivermectin, moxidectin, pethidine, iron dextrans, vitamin B complex and liver extract, hormones
Antisera, bacterins, and vaccines
   Strangles, encephalomyelitis, salmonellosis, botulinum, tetanus
Foods
   Pasture plants, hays
Plants
   Nettle, buttercup
Transfusion reactions
Hypersensitivity reactions
   Atopy, food, contact, drug
Stinging and biting insects and arachnids
   Bee, hornet, wasp, mosquito, blackfly, spider, ant
Snake bite
Infections
   Bacterial, fungal, viral, protozoal, parasitic (including intestinal parasites, onchocerciasis, hypodermiasis, *Pyomotes* straw mites)
Contactants
Vasculitis
   Many causes (e.g., drugs, purpura hemorrhagica)
Dermatographism
Cold urticaria
Exercise-induced urticaria
Stress/psychogenic factors
Idiopathy

I. *Conventional urticaria*—characterized by papules and wheals that vary from 2 mm to 5 cm in diameter (Fig. 8-5).
II. *Papular urticaria*—characterized by uniform, small, 3- to 6-mm diameter papules. This type is especially associated with stinging insects, particularly mosquitoes.
III. *Giant urticaria*—characterized by wheals that are very large, up to 40 cm in diameter.
IV. *Exudative (oozing) urticaria*—wherein severe dermal edema leads to serum oozing, matting of the hairs, and alopecia.
V. *Gyrate (polycyclic) urticaria*—wherein wheals occur in bizarre shapes: arciform, serpiginous, doughnut-like, geographic, and so forth (see Fig. 8-4, *B*). Drug reactions are a common cause of this variety.

DIAGNOSIS

It must be emphasized that urticaria and angioedema are *not* definitive diagnoses but rather cutaneous reaction patterns with many potential causes (see Table 8-13). The differential diagnosis for urticaria varies with the morphologic presentation. The major differential for conventional and giant urticaria is vasculitis. The differential for papular urticaria includes infectious and sterile folliculitides, which are particularly likely if oozing, crusts, and alopecia follow the initial appearance of papules. The major differential for gyrate urticaria is erythema multiforme. The lesions of erythema multiforme characteristically do not pit with digital pressure. Other possible differentials for urticaria include lymphoma and amyloidosis.

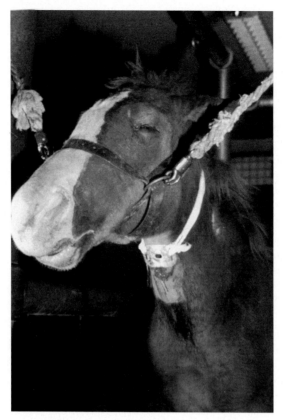

FIGURE 8-3. Penicillin-induced angioedema of face.

Because of the numerous potential causes (see Table 8-13), definitive diagnosis and treatment of urticaria can be frustrating. In humans with chronic urticaria, a definitive diagnosis is achieved in only about 25% of the cases.[20,44] This percentage may be even lower in the horse, mainly due to unwillingness on the part of owners and/or clinicians to pursue a potentially exhaustive, expensive, and time-consuming diagnostic work-up. The most commonly reported causes of equine urticaria are drugs (especially penicillin), feedstuffs (intolerance or hypersensitivity?), atopy, and infections/infestations.

Careful assessment of the patient's history and environment is key to establishing a likely differential diagnosis. In chronic cases, a daily journal of the patient's condition and exposures kept by the owner can be very instructive in sorting out the multitudinous possibilities. A seasonal recurrence of disease suggests insects, aeroallergens, seasonal food items (summer), or aeroallergens, seasonal food items, or cold (winter). Was the urticaria preceded by a drug, vaccination, deworming, or feed change? Does the urticaria occur when the horse is outdoors, indoors, or both? Do specific activities—exercise, feeding—precede the urticaria? Are there other signs—cutaneous and/or noncutaneous—of infections, ectoparasitisms, or endoparasitisms?

The localization of lesions may suggest the cause—for example, sites of contact with topical products, plants, tack, blankets, and so forth. The most commonly implicated contactants include medicated sprays, rinses, and pour-ons; tack; saddle soaps; leather conditioners; and pasture plants.[53,91,96,100,104]

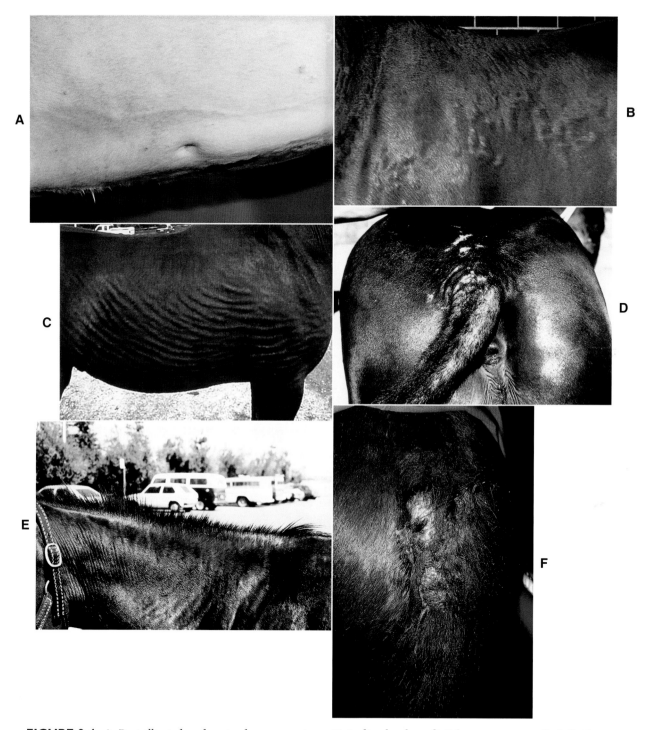

FIGURE 8-4. A, Penicillin-induced angioedema on ventrum. Note dimple where digital pressure was applied. **B,** Gyrate (polycyclic) urticaria in an atopic horse. **C,** Striped urticaria. (*Courtesy H. Schott.*) **D,** "Rat-tailed" appearance of a horse with *Culicoides* hypersensitivity. (*Courtesy A. Stannard.*) **E,** "Buzzed-off mane" appearance of a horse with *Culicoides* hypersensitivity. (*Courtesy A. Stannard.*) **F,** Secondary staphylococcal pyoderma of tail on a horse with insect hypersensitivity.

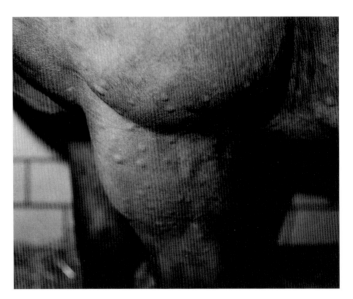

FIGURE 8-5. Conventional urticaria in an atopic horse.

Because most cases of urticaria are acute (transient), and more likely to be temporally associated with likely causes, it is often justified to treat these cases with glucocorticoids, with or without antihistamines, along with eliminating/avoiding the suspected cause(s).[100] Chronic (persistent) cases need to be investigated very thoroughly.

After the importance of drugs, biologicals, infections, and parasitisms have been determined, further specific testing could include:

- Novel protein ("hypoallergenic") diet (see Food Hypersensitivity for details).°
- Intradermal test (see Atopy for details).†
- *Dermatographism* is a specific type of pressure-induced urticaria, wherein wheals conform to a particular configuration reflecting exogenous pressure (e.g., saddle, tack).‡ Some horses manifest the dermatographism only when certain feeds have been consumed prior to the application of pressure.[91] The diagnosis is confirmed by "drawing" on the patient with a blunt tipped instrument (hemostat, tongue depressor), whereupon wheals appear in the traced areas within 15 minutes.
- *Cold urticaria* is confirmed by the application of an ice cube to the skin for about 5 minutes, which results in wheal formation at that site within 15 minutes.[67,91,100,104]
- *Exercise-induced urticaria* is only caused by exercise: passive heating does not cause wheals.[91,100,104] The diagnosis is confirmed by a 30-minute exercise period producing the urticaria.
- *Cholinergic urticaria/pruritus* is caused by a complicated interaction of exercise, passive heating, and certain feeds triggering urticaria, pruritus, or both.[91,96a,104]

Unusual cases of equine urticaria have been reported:

- Contact urticaria has occurred in horses that were clipped, scrubbed with povidone-iodine, and exposed to a contact gel for ultrasonography.[91] Neither the povidone-iodine nor the contact gel alone produced the urticaria: only the combination.

°References 18, 35, 53, 90, 91, 96, 100, 104.
†References 18, 35, 53, 89-91, 96, 100, 104.
‡References 50, 53, 67, 87, 91, 100, 104.

- Generalized gyrate urticaria was caused by garlic contained in a feed additive.[99] The affected horse had positive intradermal reactions and a precipitin line on immunodiffusion testing with garlic extracts.
- "Striped" or "zebra" urticaria has been reported.[101a,102] Affected horses have numerous parallel bands of urticaria, mostly over the trunk, and more-or-less bilaterally symmetric in distribution (Fig. 8-4, C). Lesions tended to become more severe in warm weather. The condition is mildly pruritic, and affected horses occasionally bite and/or rub the lesions. Anecdotal reports indicate that "allergy work-ups" in these horses are usually unrewarding, and that the horses respond incompletely to glucocorticoids and antihistamines. The authors have seen only one such horse. The horse had multiple positive reactions on intradermal testing and responded well to allergen specific immunotherapy.

HISTOPATHOLOGY

Skin biopsy specimens from most types of urticaria reveal a mild to moderate perivascular (superficial or superficial and deep) to interstitial dermatitis with numerous eosinophils and variable dermal edema (Fig. 8-6). [54,67,90,91] In some cases, lymphocytes are also present. The overlying epidermis is normal. Severe dermal edema can produce subepidermal vesicles through dermoepidermal separation. With exudative (oozing) urticaria, additional histopathologic features include variable degrees of intra- and extra-cellular epidermal edema, which may progress to epidermal microvesicle formation.[67] Leukocytoclastic vasculitis is rarely seen.

CLINICAL MANAGEMENT

The prognosis for urticarial reactions is favorable, because general health is not usually affected. The prognosis for angioedema varies with severity and location. Angioedematous reactions involving the nasal passages, pharynx, and larynx may be fatal. The likelihood of documenting a specific cause and, thus, rendering specific treatment in chronic equine urticaria is not great. Again, the multiplicity of causes and the owner/clinician frustration when facing a daunting diagnostic workup are important reasons for this poor performance. "Idiopathic" urticaria accounts for 2.44% of the equine dermatoses seen at the Cornell University Clinic.

Therapy consists of (1) elimination and avoidance of known etiologic factors and (2) treatment of symptoms with epinephrine (epinephrine 1:1000 at 5 to 10 ml/450 kg subcutaneously or intramuscularly) or glucocorticoids (prednisolone or prednisone at 2 mg/kg, given orally, intramuscularly, or intravenously), or both. Antihistamines have not been adequately evaluated for efficacy in treating chronic equine urticaria. They are ineffective for the treatment of acute reactions, but may be useful for the prevention of future reactions or in the management of chronic cases (see Antihistamines). Hydroxyzine may be the antihistamine of choice for chronic urticaria.[67,157a] Pentoxifylline may be helpful if vasculitis is present (see Chapter 9) Acupuncture was reported to be successful in one horse.[88]

Atopy

The term atopy, from the Greek atopo (meaning "strange"), was introduced by Coca and Cooke in 1923 in order to describe three familial human disorders with common characteristics: atopic dermatitis, allergic asthma, and hay fever.[112] It was believed that the mode of transmission was hereditary, and the antibodies implicated in the mechanism of hypersensitivity were called "reagins."[113] Today, atopy (atopic disease, atopic dermatitis) is defined as a genetically programmed disease of horses, humans, dogs, and cats in which the patient becomes sensitized to environmental antigens that in nonatopic animals create no disease.[44,52,55,157a] Additionally, atopy has been defined as a reaginic antibody-mediated disease.[22,23] Though allergen-specific IgE has been classically associated with the disease, more components of the immune system appear to be

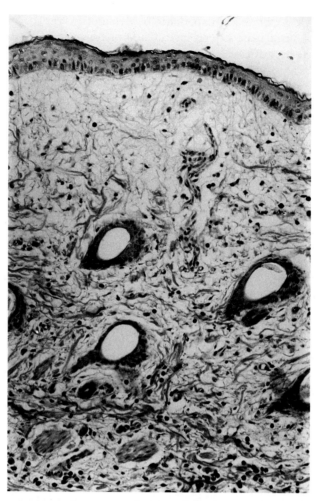

FIGURE 8-6. Biopsy specimen from conventional urticaria in an atopic horse. Note perivascular accumulation of eosinophils and pronounced superficial dermal edema.

important. Some evidence supports the importance of allergen-specific IgG.[44,52,55] The role of Langerhans' cells, T cells, and eosinophils, as well as changes in the inflammatory milieu with chronicity, are also being recognized as important components of the disease process.

CAUSE AND PATHOGENESIS

Strong breed predilections, familial involvement, and limited breeding trials have demonstrated that human and canine atopy is genetically programmed.[20,44,55] Reports[117,119,154a] of familial occurrence and breed predispositions for equine atopy could suggest a genetic programming.

In addition to genetics, other factors are important in the development of clinical atopy in dogs:[55]

- Susceptibility to sensitization during the first few months of life.
- Augmentation of the production of IgE to other environmental allergens by parasitic diseases.
- Augmentation of the production of IgE to other environmental allergens by viral infections and vaccination with modified live viral vaccines.

- The hypothesized importance of increased environmental pollutants and indoor allergens in the increase in incidence of atopic dermatitis in humans.[108a,135a,156a]

These factors could certainly explain the increased incidence of atopy, especially in young animals.

Atopenes are the environmental allergens to which atopic individuals are allergic.[157a] These depend on both the nature of the environment and the lifestyle of the animal. Young horses kept in a stable for 1 year all developed antibodies against the arachnids and molds found in the stable dust.[143] These results suggest that the repeated and/or continual exposure of young horses to antigens in stable dust could eventually lead to allergic reactions. In a study involving 448 Lippizan horses living on six different stud farms, environmental and genetic factors had a significant effect on the serum concentrations of allergen-specific IgE.[117a]

Atopy has been classified as a type I hypersensitivity reaction.[20,22,23,44,55] Genetically predisposed individuals absorb percutaneously, inhale, and possibly ingest various allergens that provoke allergen-specific IgE or IgG production. Equine IgE is (1) not precipitated in the presence of antigen, (2) inactivated at 56° C, (3) not complement-fixing, (4) antigenically similar to human IgE, and (5) capable of passively transferring atopic sensitivities to normal horses by Prausnitz-Küstner (P-K) testing.° Molecular cloning and sequencing of the low-affinity IgE receptor (CD23) has been accomplished in the horse.[168b] CD23 is expressed on the surface of B cells prior to isotype switching and is upregulated or induced by IL-4. CD23 is thought to play a central role in IgE-associated immune responses, including allergies, and these reagents will be useful in future studies of allergic diseases in horses. It has been traditional to espouse the primary importance of allergen-specific IgE, though total IgE level is not elevated in atopic dogs.[55] Numerous studies in humans and dogs show that allergen-specific IgE is associated with atopic disease.[44,55] IgE also binds to epidermal Langerhans' cells in lesional atopic skin from dogs and humans.[7,20,44,55] These findings are compelling evidence for the pathogenic role played by allergen-specific IgE in atopic disease. However, the absolute requirement for IgE is questioned because of several observations in human or canine atopics: (1) atopy has been recognized in patients with agammaglobulinemia; (2) allergen-specific IgE cannot be detected in many atopic patients and normal individuals experimentally sensitized to allergens; and (3) abnormally increased serum IgE levels generally do not fluctuate consistently during exacerbations, remissions, or treatment.[20,44,55] However, allergen-specific IgE may decrease in response to hyposensitization. Such information is not available for horses.

The advent of *in vitro* tests that measure serum allergen-specific IgE levels in humans and dogs has offered another tool to assess IgE production. These tests have shown in a number of studies that normal dogs also produce allergen-specific IgE, and that the titers do not correlate with clinical disease.[55] These observations in dogs, as well as other work in humans, have shown that heterogeneity of IgE exists, and perhaps only one type or some select types are involved in atopic disease.[7,44,55] It is hypothesized that two basic types of IgE would exist: IgE- and IgE+. Individuals with serum and tissue-bound IgE- would have minimal or no skin disease, whereas those with IgE+ would have atopic skin disease. A number of studies in dogs and cats have supported this concept of IgE heterogeneity, and this offers an explanation for the variation in serum IgE results in atopic and normal dogs, and the frequent lack of correlation between serologic and skin test results.[55] Another possibility is that the sensitivity to IgE and the ability of target cells to degranulate may constitute the underlying abnormality in atopic disease.

The classic description of the pathogenesis of atopy is that IgE (or IgGd) fixes to tissue mast cells, especially in the skin, the primary target organ of equine, canine, and feline atopy. When mast cell–fixed IgE reacts with its specific allergen or allergens, mast cell degranulation and

---

°References 120, 137, 148, 157, 163-166.

release or production of many pharmacologically active compounds ensue. This occurs following intradermal injection of allergen and is the basis of positive reactions. However, the histology and the clinical appearance of the immediate lesion (wheal) induced by intradermal allergen presentation does not mimic the clinical disease.[55] In contrast, the recognition that late-phase reactions to intradermal injections or patch test reactions produce lesions that clinically, histologically, and immmunophenotypically resemble the spontaneous disease in humans and dogs has led to newer theories regarding the pathogenesis of atopic dermatitis.

In humans and dogs it has been shown that IgE fixes to epidermal Langerhans' cells.[20,55] In atopic humans, this is mediated by the expression of high-affinity IgE receptors on Langerhans' cells, and aeroallergen-specific IgE enhances the antigen presenting capabilities of these cells. In dogs, epidermal eosinophil microaggregates and increased Langerhans' cells have been found in lesional atopic skin. Even clinically normal atopic skin has increased numbers of Langerhans' cells.[20,55] Dermal increases in eosinophils are also seen, as well as an increase in the endothelial cell expression of ICAM-1, increased numbers of T cells in lesional skin with an increase in the CD4:CD8a ratio, and increased numbers of α, ß T cells. It is likely that atopic dermatitis is caused by a combination of immediate and late-phase contact reactions to aeroallergens.[55]

In humans, the genetic abnormality in atopic dermatitis appears to be an immunologic skin dysfunction that has been induced by bone marrow transplantation.[20,44] Abnormalities of the SIS in atopic humans include (1) endothelial cells that abnormally express adhesion molecules, (2) an increase in T cells that are predominantly T helper cells (3) hyperstimulatory epidermal Langerhans' cells and increased dermal Langerhans' cells, (4) B cell overproduction of IgE, (5) IgE on Langerhans' cells, and (6) Langerhans' cells with IgE that may be able to stimulate T cells locally.[7,20,44,46] This ability could lead, in the atopic patient, to an exaggerated T lymphocyte response. Special stains of skin samples from humans with atopic dermatitis have revealed that lesional skin contains increased numbers of activated helper T cells of the subclass Th2. These helper T cells may preferentially induce IgE-producing B cells by themselves, thus resulting in the production of IL-4, IL-5, and IL-10. These interleukins stimulate mast cell and eosinophil activation and proliferation. Though eosinophils are often not seen in routine lesional skin from human atopic dermatitis patients, they do play a role in the inflammation. This assessment is based on the presence of eosinophil major basic and cationic proteins in human atopic lesional skin (confirming that eosinophils had been present) and the finding of eosinophils in early lesions at atopy patch test sites.[7,20,44,46] The T cell subclass is not a constant finding, and recent work has shown that, in chronic lesions, there is more of a mixture. Thus, early lesions are dominated by Th2 cells, but a switch to both Th1 and Th2 occurs in chronic skin lesions. It is obvious that the pathogenesis is much more complex than genetically-programmed alterations in IgE production.

Immediate intradermal test reactions do not mimic the clinical lesions seen in the atopic dog and, in many cases, they are not pruritic, suggesting that intradermally deposited antigen does not reproduce the natural disease.[55] In humans, similar changes to naturally occurring lesions can be induced at allergen patch test (the so-called "atopy patch test") sites in patients with atopic dermatitis, but not in normal patients or patients with rhinitis or asthma.[20,44,55] Though these tests are quite specific, their sensitivity is variable. When positive, the changes induced by the patch tests mimic the clinical lesion, the microscopic findings, and the cellular phenotype that occurs in the natural disease. In addition, the time course of lesion development shows initial infiltration with IL-4–containing T cells, eosinophils, and later by IFN-γ–containing T cells similar to the natural disease in human atopics.[20,44,46,55] These findings are in contrast to the late-phase reactions following intradermal injection of allergen, with resultant mast cell degranulation and subsequent neutrophilic infiltrates. These and other observations have led to the conclusion that the mast cell plays a minor role in atopic dermatitis, and that the atopy patch test is a better model to study atopic disease. Additionally, these observations strongly support the role of percutaneous absorption and the pathogenesis following helper T cell and eosinophil activation.

In atopic humans, the water-retaining capacity of even clinically normal skin is significantly decreased, and transepidermal water loss is increased.[20,55] It has been suggested that the skin of atopic humans is inherently functionally abnormal.[20]

A summary of current thought as to the possible pathogenesis of atopic skin disease might go as follows:

Percutaneously absorbed allergens (allergen penetration probably enhanced by inherent defect of epidermal barrier function) encounter allergen-specific IgE on Langerhans' cells, whereupon the allergens are trapped, processed, and presented to allergen-specific T lymphocytes. There is a subsequent preferential expansion of allergen-specific Th2 cells, which produce IL-3, IL-4, IL-5, IL-6, IL-10 and IL-13. The imbalance in allergen-specific Th2 cells (with a resultant increase in IL-4–stimulated production of allergen-specific IgE) and allergen-specific Th1 cells (with a resultant decrease in INF-γ inhibition of allergen-specific IgE production) culminates in enhanced production of allergen-specific IgE by B lymphocytes.[*] The existence of this Th1/Th2 paradigm has not been demonstrated in the horse.[157a]

An older theory focused on β-adrenergic blockade as the underlying abnormality of atopy.[44,55] Though it is not accepted as the major pathologic abnormality, it may play a role in the pathogenesis. Szentivanyi proposed the β-adrenergic theory of atopic disease in 1968. He suggested that the heightened sensitivity of atopic human beings to various pharmacologic agents could be due to a blockage of β-adrenergic receptors in the tissues. Since that time, there has been an explosion of investigative effort in the field of the cyclic nucleotides.[7,20,44,46,55] In brief, the cyclic nucleotides cyclic adenosine monophosphate (cAMP) and cyclic guanosine monophosphate (cGMP) appear to serve as the intracellular effectors of a variety of cellular events. They are viewed as exerting opposing influences in a number of systems.

A number of pharmacologic agents are known to act via various cell receptors to influence intracellular levels of cAMP and cGMP. In general, substances that elevate intracellular cAMP levels (β-adrenergic drugs, prostaglandin E, methylxanthines, histamine, and other mediator substances) or reduce intracellular cGMP levels (anticholinergic drugs) tend to stabilize the cells (lymphocytes, monocyte-macrophages, neutrophils, mast cells) and inhibit the release of various inflammatory mediators. On the other hand, substances that reduce cAMP levels (β-adrenergic drugs) or elevate cGMP levels (cholinergic drugs, ascorbic acid, estrogen, levamisole) tend to labilize the cells and promote the release of inflammatory mediators. Further studies in the area of cyclic nucleotides and biologic regulation may produce significant advances in the areas of disease pathomechanism and control of immunologic inflammation.

It has been suggested that atopic dogs have a Δ-6 desaturase deficiency and metabolize fats differently than nonatopic dogs.[55] In addition, atopic dogs have lower levels of plasma triglycerides than normal dogs after being fed corn oil, suggesting impaired fat absorption or increased plasma clearance. Recently, the existence of two subsets of atopic dogs has been proposed.[55] Atopic dogs were fed an omega-3/omega-6 fatty acid–containing diet to control their pruritus. Nonresponders had a smaller increase in plasma fatty acids, suggesting an even more pronounced abnormality in fat absorption/metabolism/clearance. Both responders and nonresponders appeared to have a Δ-5 desaturase deficiency, while nonresponders also appeared to have a Δ-6 desaturase deficiency. It was also reported that the metabolism of omega-3 fatty acids was differentially regulated among breeds of dogs.[55] All of these considerations could help explain the variable responses of atopic dogs to omega-3/omega-6 fatty acid supplementation. It is not known whether a similar situation exists in horses.

---

[*]References 7, 20, 44, 46, 55, 108a.

Atopic dogs are known to be prone to secondary bacterial pyoderma and *Malassezia* infections. A variety of abnormalities are present in atopic dogs that may explain these infections.[55] Atopic dog corneocytes have greater adherence for *S. intermedius*, and the numbers of *S. intermedius* are increased on the skin of symptomatic atopic dogs. However, the numbers of *S. intermedius* and corneocyte adhesion appear to be normal in atopic dogs that are in remission with glucocorticoids. Intradermal injection of histamine causes increased percutaneous penetration of staphylococcal antigens in normal dogs, suggesting that the inflamed skin of atopic dogs would also be more accessible to staphylococcal antigens and, perhaps, staphylococcal pyoderma. Cell-mediated immunity is depressed. A similar situation occurs in human atopic dermatitis patients.[20,44] It has been shown that, in dogs, many of these abnormalities are the result of the allergic reaction and not a primary abnormality. Atopic humans often have exaggerated responses to patch or intradermal testing with *Malassezia* antigens, and flares of their dermatitis may respond to antiyeast therapy.[20,44] A similar phenomenon is likely to occur in atopic dogs and the presence of an immunologic response has been demonstrated by intradermal testing and with *in vitro* tests for *Malassezia*-specific IgE.[55] Atopic dogs had higher serum levels of *Malassezia*-specific IgE than nonatopic dogs or dogs with *Malassezia* dermatitis without atopic disease, and the level was not related to numbers of organisms present.[55] Atopic horses certainly develop secondary staphylococcal infections,[157a] but whether or not the aforementioned abnormalities exist in atopic horses is not known.

Superantigens are a group of bacterial and viral proteins that are characterized by the capacity to stimulate large numbers of T cells.[137a,160a] They bind directly to MHC class II molecules on antigen-presenting cells and cross-link the antigen-presenting cell with T cells expressing certain receptors, leading to polyclonal T cell activation. When staphylococcal superantigens are applied to intact human skin, dermatitis is produced. Furthermore, in the presence of superantigens, keratinocytes potently activate T cells. Thus, superantigens play a role in the induction and exacerbation of inflammatory skin disease. Bacterial exotoxins also amplify allergen-specific IgE production.[140a] During exposure to allergens, IFN-γ production is decreased, leading to a predominance of Th2-like cytokines. Bacterial toxins bridge Th2 cells and B cells, inducing B cell activation. Bacterial toxins also upregulate B7.2 expression on B cells and enhance IgE synthesis. IgE binds to CD23, allowing nonspecific B cells to become potent antigen-presenting cells via the co-stimulatory molecule, B7.2. As a result, Th2-like cells may expand and induce more B cells to switch to IgE production, with subsequent overproduction of IL-4 and allergen-specific IgE. Staphylococcal superantigen-induced inflammation may explain the antibiotic-induced reduction in inflammation and pruritus seen in atopic horses that have no clinical signs of infection.

Some studies showed increased mast cell "releasability" of histamine in atopic dogs.[55] Leukocyte (basophil) histamine release was found to be significantly greater in atopic and artificially hypersensitized dogs than in normal dogs, though the total histamine content of leukocytes was not statistically significantly different between the three groups.[55] It was concluded that leukocyte releasability is a disorder of immunoregulation intrinsic to the atopic state and unrelated to the concentration of serum or tissue IgE. Whether or not a similar situation exists in horses is not known.

Histopathologic examination of cutaneous reactions produced by the intradermal injection of various allergens or inflammatory mediators in horses suggests that reactions at 15 to 30 minutes and at 4 to 6 hours represent, respectively, type I (immediate) hypersensitivity and late-phase reactions mediated by IgE.[*] IgE-mediated liberation of histamine from equine basophils has been reported.[147] The concentrations of the following substances are increased during inflammatory reactions in the horse: eicosanoids,[108a,110,121] lysosomal enzymes,[158] proteases,[149] IL-1,[149] LTB$_4$,[139] PGE$_2$,[138] histamine,[110] seratonin,[110] superoxides,[159] and TNF.[159] The most important mediator of cutaneous inflammation and pruritus in equine atopy has not yet been established.

---

*References 40, 89, 135, 136, 150, 151, 160, 164.

The eosinophil, histamine, LTB$_4$, and PAF appear to play important roles in the pathogenesis of allergic skin reactions in horses.[53,54,157a] The intradermal injection of histamine attracts numerous eosinophils and results in marked dermal edema.* Intradermal injections of histamine and bradykinin produce wheals, but those of serotonin, PGE$_1$, and PGE$_2$ do not.[108,108b,110] The migration of eosinophils is stimulated by histamine, LTB$_4$, and PAF.[150,154] The number of eosinophils is maximal 2 hours after the intradermal injection of histamine,[40,150] and 4 hours after the intradermal injection of LTB$_4$, and remains significantly elevated for up to 24 hours.[40,134,150] The intradermal injection of PAF also provokes eosinophil infiltration and edema, and the number of eosinophils is proportional to the amplitude of the edema.[114,130,157a] Eosinophils contain cytotoxic proteins,[141,144,153] and produce several mediators of inflammation: LTB$_4$, LTC$_4$, PAF, and superoxides.[106,129,132,142,144] Histamine, LTB$_4$, and IL-5 play important roles in the regulation of eosinophil adherence to various substances.[128,131,134] Eosinophils are thus capable of liberating a variety of proteins, enzymes, mediators, and oxygen radicals that are cytotoxic or proinflammatory. Eosinophils are the predominant inflammatory cell in skin biopsy specimens taken from atopic horses.[53,54,157a]

Atopy may be best described as a multifactorial disease in which genetically predisposed animals exhibit a combination of cutaneous IgE-mediated immediate and late-phase reactions to environmental antigens. Immunologic abnormalities, antigenic stimuli, altered physiologic and pharmacologic reactions, and genetic predisposition all play a role in the pathogenesis.

CLINICAL FEATURES

Reports of horses having dermatoses compatible with atopic dermatitis began to be published in the 1950s.[118] By the end of the 1980s the concept of equine atopy was well-accepted in veterinary medicine.[53,111,119] Atopy is now universally recognized.† The incidence of equine atopy is unknown. Atopy is the seventh most common equine dermatosis diagnosed at the Cornell University Clinic, accounting for 3.89% of all skin conditions. This percentage is arguably low, as 2.11% and 2.44% of our cases had a final diagnosis of "idiopathic pruritus" or "idiopathic urticaria," respectively. Because allergy testing was not performed in these horses, many of them could have been atopic.

Anecdotal reports indicate that equine atopy can have familial and breed-related predispositions.[117,119] Clinical signs most commonly begin in young horses, 1^1/$_2$ to 6 years of age.[117,119,146] No sex predilection is apparent. Some authors believe that thoroughbreds and Arabians are at risk.[117,119,146] Clinical signs may begin in any season, and they can be seasonal or nonseasonal depending on the allergens involved. Clinical signs may also progress from seasonal to nonseasonal disease.‡

The major dermatologic signs of equine atopy are pruritus and/or urticaria.§ The most common presentation is bilaterally symmetric pruritus, often in the absence of visible lesions in the beginning. The face (Fig. 8-7), pinnae, ventral thorax and abdomen, and the legs (Fig. 8-8) are the most commonly affected areas. The dorsolateral neck, mane, croup, and base of the tail are also frequently affected. Affected horses bite themselves, rub (against stalls, trees, fences, etc.), stomp their feet, flick their tail, and rarely, shake their heads. Excoriations, self-induced hypotrichosis and alopecia, secondary bacterial infections, with or without lichenification and hyperpigmentation, are commonly seen.

Urticaria, pruritic or nonpruritic, is also a common cutaneous reaction pattern in atopic horses (see Figs. 8-4, *B*, and 8-5).¶ Some atopic horses have a sterile eosinophilic folliculitis, which

---

*References 40, 105, 108, 125, 150, 152, 160.
†References 18, 50, 53, 83, 117, 123, 146, 157a.
‡References 2, 18, 22, 32, 35, 50, 52, 53, 80, 83, 90, 104, 111, 117, 123, 142a, 146, 146c, 154a, 156, 157a, 167
§References 18, 50, 53, 83, 111, 117, 123, 146, 156, 157a, 167.
¶References 18, 50, 53, 83, 111, 117, 123, 146, 156, 157a, 167.

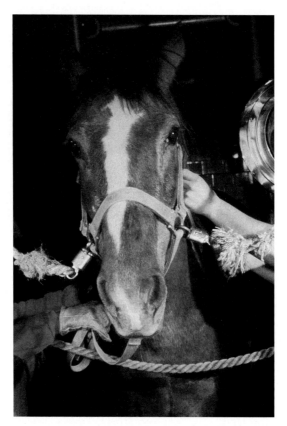

FIGURE 8-7. Atopy. Note symmetrical self-induced hypotrichosis on face.

presents with pruritic or nonpruritic tufted papules that become crusted and alopecic, and occasionally coalescent (Fig. 8-9) (see Chapter 15).[54,157a] Rarely, horses with seasonal or nonseasonal atopy will develop seasonal or nonseasonal eosinophilic granulomas (see Chapter 15). Allergic conjunctivitis and rhinitis are rarely reported in atopic horses.[111]

Chronic obstructive pulmonary disease (COPD, chronic bronchitis, heaves) is a condition affecting the respiratory tract of horses characterized by periods of acute airway obstruction followed by periods of remission.[32,52] Affected horses have decreased lung compliance, increased lung resistance, increased respiratory effort, and arterial hypoxemia. Although the cause(s) and pathogenesis of COPD is somewhat controversial, several lines of investigation suggest that COPD is an atopic disease of horses.[*] However, reports of concurrent COPD and atopic dermatitis are very rare. Most atopic horses have either skin disease or respiratory disease.

DIAGNOSIS

The differential diagnosis varies with the distribution of lesions:
- Face—food hypersensitivity, insect hypersensitivity, trombiculosis, *Dermanyssus gallinae* dermatitis, storage mites
- Pinnae—food hypersensitivity, insect hypersensitivity, psoroptic mange
- Neck—food hypersensitivity, insect hypersensitivity, storage mites

---

[*]References 89, 136, 142a, 146a-146c, 151.

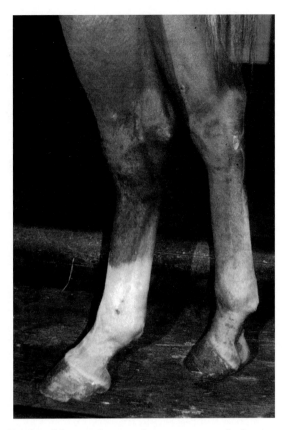

FIGURE 8-8. Atopy. Self-induced hypotrichosis and excoriations on the legs.

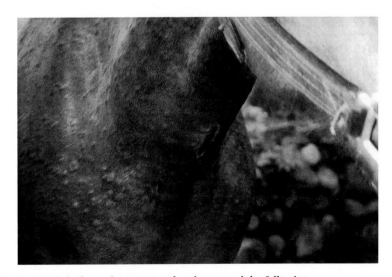

FIGURE 8-9. Atopy. Tufted papules associated with eosinophilic folliculitis.

- Mane—insect hypersensitivity, psoroptic mange, pediculosis, food hypersensitivity
- Dorsum—pediculosis, insect hypersensitivity, food hypersensitivity
- Rump—chorioptic mange, pediculosis, psoroptic mange, oxyuriasis, insect hypersensitivity, food hypersensitivity
- Legs—chorioptic mange, *D. gallinae* dermatitis, trombiculosis, strongyloidosis, contact dermatitis, insect hypersensitivity, food hypersensitivity
- Ventrum—contact dermatitis, trombiculosis, *D. gallinae* dermatitis, insect hypersensitivity, food hypersensitivity

The distribution of lesions with contact dermatitis is, in fact, extremely variable and often suggestive of the causative agent (see Contact Hypersensitivity). The possibility of an adverse cutaneous drug reaction must always be considered and excluded because these reactions can mimic almost any spontaneous skin disease (see Cutaneous Adverse Drug Reaction, Chapter 9). Horses with urticaria may have the lengthy immunologic and nonimmunologic differential diagnosis for that reaction pattern (see Urticaria and Angiodema). Horses with head shaking also have an extensive differential diagnosis (see Headshaking, Chapter 13). Rare causes of symmetrical pruritus include systemic disease (e.g., lymphoma, liver and renal neoplasia: see Chapter 16) and vertebral abnormalities (see Chapter 13).

The differential diagnosis also varies with the time of year:
- Summer—insect hypersensitivity
- Fall—trombiculosis
- Winter—pediculosis, chorioptic mange

Although food hypersensitivity is classically nonseasonal, it may be seasonal or episodic depending on the availability of the causative allergen(s) (see Food Hypersensitivity).

Some atopic horses have concurrent insect hypersensitivity and/or food hypersensitivity.[18,123,146,157a,178] The coexistence of two or three allergic conditions can greatly complicate the clinical presentation and the diagnostic work-up.

The definitive diagnosis is essentially clinical.[55,157a] Because atopy is only one of the possible causes of the clinical signs observed, it is mandatory to eliminate the other possible causes before proceeding to allergy testing. As is the case in dogs and cats,[55] allergy testing is *not* used to make a diagnosis of equine atopy, but rather to identify allergens that can be avoided or included in an allergen-specific immunotherapy protocol.[157a] It cannot be overemphasized that allergy tests are never a substitute for a meticulously gathered history, a thorough physical examination, and a careful and complete elimination of other diagnoses and concurrent problems.

Intradermal Allergy Testing

A limited number of studies have been conducted to document optimum intradermal testing procedures.* Unfortunately, different commercial allergen sources were sometimes used, making comparisons impossible, and the studies have not directly compared different commercial sources of allergens. Whichever company is used should be consulted for information regarding their testing concentrations. It is likely that some differences between studies with the same allergens reflect the animals' exposure to significant allergen levels that may induce positive but clinically insignificant reactions.[55] Preferably the allergen companies should have results of independent studies, as differences may occur. Most studies have been conducted with aqueous allergens made by Greer Laboratories. In general, the recommended aqueous test allergen concentration is 1000 PNU/ml or 1:1000 weight/volume (w/v).

●**Allergen selection.** Skin test allergen selection is an important subject. Consultations with allergen firms and national pollen charts reviewing prevalence of pollens in the practice area help

---

*References 35, 42, 53, 89, 111, 117, 122-124, 136, 142a, 146-146c, 151-156, 157a, 167.

the clinician decide what to test for. Consultations with regional veterinary dermatologists and physician allergists are also highly recommended. It is important to select allergens from a reputable allergen supply house and then not to switch suppliers, because experience with one source becomes important. Tremendous unresolved problems surround the standardization of allergenic extracts, including standards for raw material collection, methods of measuring the purity of raw materials, techniques for identifying many substances, a variety of methods of manufacturing, and determination of allergen stability and potency.[44,55] Bioactivity of commercial products varies from 10-fold to 1000-fold, and no relationship was found between bioactivity and concentrations declared in PNU or w/v.[44,55]

Testing with allergen *mixes* is not recommended.[44,55] Such mixes frequently result in false-negative reactions because individual allergens within the mix may be in concentrations too dilute for detection. More important, the patient may be allergic to only one of the allergens within the mix, making hyposensitization based on the mix result less specific. In fact, one most likely ends up hyposensitizing with allergens that the patient is not allergic to and, potentially, inducing new allergies. Skin testing with commercial "regional" allergen kits that use mixes is unsatisfactory. Instead, discussions with the supply house regarding the most important allergens for the practice area may be the most appropriate way to perform cost-effective and accurate tests for the client's budget.

Allergens commonly reported to be important in horses are mites, dusts, danders, molds, weeds, grasses, and trees.[*] It has been reported that alfalfa, grain mill dust, grain smuts, cottonseed, fireweed, yellowdock, Russian thistle, deer fly, *Rhizopus* spp., *Candida albicans*, black fly, horse fly, and black ant antigens may be irritants in the horse and that positive results must be interpreted with caution.[†]

It is essential to remember that a positive skin test reaction means only that the patient has skin-sensitizing antibody, mast cells that degranulate on antigen exposure, and target tissue that responds to the released mediators. A positive reaction does not necessarily mean that the patient has clinical allergy to the allergen(s) injected. Thus, it is essential that positive skin test reactions be interpreted in light of the patient's history. By the same token, a negative skin test reaction does not necessarily mean that the patient is not atopic. Of the otherwise classically atopic dogs, 10% to 30% may have negative skin test reactions.[55] This group probably reflects either failure (by limiting the number of test allergens used) to challenge patients with the appropriate allergens or the intervention of various factors known to produce false-negative reactions, as listed in Table 8-14.

Many factors may lead to false-positive or false-negative skin test reactions (Tables 8-14 and 8-15).[53,55] These factors must be carefully considered when skin testing is performed. The most common cause of negative skin test reactions is the recent administration of certain drugs: glucocorticoids, antihistamines, progestagens. There are no reliable withdrawal times for these drugs. Guidelines have been arbitrarily determined by clinicians. General rules of thumb for drug withdrawal times prior to skin testing are 3 weeks for oral and topical glucocorticoids, 8 weeks for injectable glucocorticoids, 10 days for antihistamines, and 10 days for products and diets containing omega-3/omega-6 fatty acids. Allergens must also be stored properly in glass and not allowed to freeze repetitively. Although it has been reported that the biologic activity of allergens stored in plastic syringes decreased faster than those stored in glass syringes,[55] no significant differences were seen in skin test reactivity.

Clearly, intradermal testing is not a procedure to be taken lightly. It requires keen attention to details and possible pitfalls, together with experience and lots of practice. Intradermal testing

---

[*]References 18, 53, 89, 90, 109, 116, 117, 122-124, 136, 142a, 146-146c, 151, 155, 156, 157a, 167.
[†]References 53, 81, 122, 123, 142a, 144a, 146c, 155, 156, 157a.

● Table 8-14 **REASONS FOR FALSE-NEGATIVE INTRADERMAL SKIN TEST REACTIONS**

Subcutaneous injections
  Too little allergen
  Testing with mixes
  Outdated allergens
  Allergens too dilute (1000 PNU/ml recommended)
  Too small volume or allergen injected
Drug interference
  Glucocorticoids
  Antihistamines
  Tranquilizers
  Progestational compounds
  Any drugs that lower blood pressure significantly
Anergy (testing during peak of hypersensitivity reaction)
Inherent host factors
  Estrus, pregnancy
  Severe stress (systemic diseases, fright, struggling)
Off-season testing (testing more than 1 to 2 months after clinical signs have disappeared)
Histamine "hyporeactivity"

● Table 8-15 **REASONS FOR FALSE-POSITIVE INTRADERMAL SKIN TEST REACTIONS**

Irritant test allergens (especially those containing glycerin; also some house dust, feather, wool, mold, and all food preparations)
Contaminated test allergens (bacteria, fungi)
Skin-sensitizing antibody only (prior clinical or present subclinical sensitivity)*
Poor technique (traumatic placement of needle; dull or burred needle; too large a volume injected; air injected)
Substances that cause nonimmunologic histamine release (narcotics)
"Irritable" skin (large reactions seen to all injected substances, including saline control)
Dermatographism
Ectoparasitism (cross-reactions with house dust mite extracts)
Mitogenic allergen

*These reactions would be more appropriately termed *clinically insignificant*.

is, however, the preferred method (the "gold standard") for identifying allergens for use in avoidance and allergen-specific immunotherapy protocols for equine atopy.* Clinicians who cannot conduct skin tests on horses on a weekly or biweekly basis will probably be unhappy with the results. In experienced hands, however, the intradermal test is a powerful tool in the diagnosis and management of equine atopy. When possible, cases should be referred to clinicians who specialize in this subject.

● **Procedure for intradermal allergy testing.** A commonly used procedure for intradermal testing is as follows:

1. Make sure the patient at least reacts to histamine. Inject 0.05 ml of 1:100,000 histamine phosphate intradermally. A wheal 15 to 30 mm in diameter should be present at 30 minutes after injection. If the histamine wheal is small (less than 10 mm) to absent, postpone intradermal skin testing, and test the animal with histamine on a weekly basis until the

*References 18, 81, 83, 89, 90, 100, 117, 123, 136, 142a, 146-146c, 151, 155, 156, 157a, 167.

expected reaction is seen. *A positive reaction does not invariably indicate that testing will be unaffected by previous drugs.* Rarely, cutaneous reactivity to histamine returns prior to cutaneous reactivity to allergen.

2. Chemical restraint is helpful and may decrease the endogenous release of glucocorticoids.

3. The horse is restrained in a standing position. Fractious animals can be sedated with xylazine. Phenothiazine tranquilizers should not be used, because they are antihistaminic. The skin over the lateral neck is the preferred test site. Because different areas of skin vary in responsiveness, the site used should be consistent from patient to patient. Gently clip the hair with a No. 40 blade, using *no* chemical preparation to clean the test site. Use a felt-tipped pen to mark each injection site. Place injection sites at least 2 cm apart, avoiding dermatitic areas.

4. Using a 26- to 27-gauge, 0.38-inch (0.9 cm) needle attached to a 1-ml disposable syringe, carefully inject, intradermally, 0.05 ml of saline or diluent control (negative control) and 0.05 ml of 1:100,000 histamine phosphate (positive control) and all the appropriately mixed test allergens. Skin testing-strength antigens should have been made fresh from concentrate within 12 weeks of use. Read the test sites at 30 minutes and 4 to 6 hours. Some information indicates that 24 hour readings may also be important. Prevent the animal from traumatizing the test area.

5. By convention, a 2-plus (2+) or greater reaction is considered to be potentially significant and must be carefully correlated with the patient's history (Fig. 8-10). With experience, positive reactions may be "guesstimated" by visual inspection. It is strongly recommended, however, that the novice measure the diameter of each wheal in millimeters. A positive skin test reaction may then be objectively defined as a wheal having a diameter that is equal to or larger than that halfway between the diameters of the wheals produced by the saline and histamine controls. In addition to the objective assessment of size, a subjective assessment of thickness and turgidity of the wheals is also utilized in determining a positive reaction.[157a] The size of positive skin test reactions does *not* necessarily correlate with their clinical importance. Some authors consider only 3+ or greater reactions in horses, indicating that 2+ reactions occur frequently in normal horses.[142a] Pruritus at some positive reaction sites occasionally

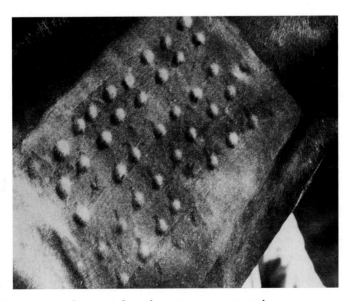

FIGURE 8-10. Positive immediate intradermal reactions in an atopic horse.

occurs and can be managed with cold compresses or topical steroids. Systemic reactions (anaphylaxis) to intradermal skin testing are extremely rare in horses.[53]

It is critical to remember that most, if not all, normal horses have one or more positive intradermal reactions.* However, atopic horses have a significantly greater number of positive reactions at all readings: immediate (30 minutes), late-phase (4 to 6 hours), and 24 hours.† It is also important to read the skin test reactions at all three time periods, because many positive late-phase reactions are not preceded by immediate reactions,[146a] and some delayed reactions are not preceded by either immediate or late-phase reactions.[146b]

Anecdotal reports indicate that (1) parasite-free horses have negative intradermal tests, (2) normal horses have increased numbers of positive intradermal test reactions (especially to insects, molds, and mites) with increasing age, (3) horses usually react to multiple insects, (4) horses in insect-free environments have negative intradermal test reactions to insect antigens, and (5) horses with chronic laminitis may have positive reactions.[81-83,143,154b,157a]

The critical "take home" message here is that reactions to individual allergens *cannot* be used to diagnose equine atopy or to determine that horses do or do not have hypersensitivity disorders. However, when overall patterns of reactivity are carefully interpreted in terms of the horse's environment, clinical signs, and previous diagnostic work-up, this information can be very valuable in establishing avoidance and allergen-specific immunotherapy protocols.[142a,146-146c]

In Vitro Testing

• **Serologic allergy tests.** The radioallergosorbent test (RAST), enzyme-linked immunosorbent assay (ELISA), and liquid-phase immunoenzymatic assay are three tests that detect relative levels of allergen-specific IgE in the serum. The RAST and ELISA attach the allergens to be tested to a solid substrate such as a paper disk or polystyrene well. The liquid-phase immunoenzymatic assay (VARL) does not use a solid phase initially, but mixes a labeled allergen with the patient's serum.[104a] The combined labeled allergen-antibody complex is subsequently bound by the label to the plastic well. This method in humans has been shown to decrease the incidence of false-positive results due to background, nonspecific, "sticky" IgE.[44,55] This liquid-phase assay also avoids the conformational distortions of antigens and resultant hiding of epitopes inherent to solid-phase techniques.

A small number of studies done with the early assays have shown problems with reproducibility of some commercial ELISA, RAST, and the liquid-phase immunoenzymatic assays.[44,55] These companies have made changes, but newer independent studies to show that these problems have been alleviated have not been presented. Although these tests are purported to be species-specific, one study revealed that the canine RAST, but not the ELISA, indicated that all horses, goats, cats, and humans tested were also allergic![55] The most recent serologic technique is the use of the Fc epsilon receptor for IgE detection[168a] With all of the technologies involving the determination of allergen-specific IgE, virtually all normal dogs and cats, all dogs and cats with any kind of skin disease, and all atopic dogs and cats have at least one, and usually multiple, positive reactions.[55] The results of serologic allergy testing correlate poorly to moderately with those of intradermal testing in dogs and cats.[55]

In part, the discrepancies between serologic and intradermal testing may be explained by numerous difficulties in technique, sensitivity, and so forth.[55] It is also important, however, to realize that they test for two different things, so complete correlations are not expected (Table 8-16). IgG anti-IgE immune complexes are present in atopic dogs, which may lead to inaccurate measurement of IgE. The differences may also indicate that two types of IgE are present, that

---

*References 18, 89, 109, 116, 117, 136, 142a, 146a-146c, 151, 156, 157a.
†References 18, 89, 109, 116, 117, 136, 142a, 146a-146c, 151, 156, 157a.

● Table 8-16   **HYPOSENSITIZATION SCHEDULE FOR AQUEOUS ALLERGENS***

INJECTION NO.	DAY NO.	VIAL 1 (100 to 200 PNU/ml)[†]	VIAL 2 (1000 to 2000 PNU/ml)	VIAL 3 (10,000 to 20,000 PNU/ml)
1	1	0.1 ml		
2	2	0.4 ml		
3	4	0.4 ml		
4	6	0.8 ml		
5	8	1.0 ml		
6	10		0.1 ml	
7	12		0.2 ml	
8	14		0.4 ml	
9	16		0.8 ml	
10	18		1.0 ml	
11	20			0.1 ml
12	22			0.2 ml
13	24			0.4 ml
14	26			0.8 ml
15	28			1.0 ml
16	38			1.0 ml
17	48[‡]			1.0 ml

*Injections are given subcutaneously.
†Protein nitrogen unit (PNU) value of each vial represents the total of all allergens used.
‡Thereafter, repeat injections (1.0 ml) every 20 to 40 days, as needed.

tissue-bound IgE does not correlate with circulating levels, that tests have different sensitivities for different allergens, or that immediate skin test reactivity and the presence of allergen-specific antibodies are no more than secondary features (epiphenomena) of atopy.[22,23,55]

The point, here, is that false- or irrelevant positive reactions are to be expected with serologic allergy testing. Hence, it is absolutely critical that (1) the candidates for testing undergo meticulous work-up, so that atopy is the only possible remaining diagnosis; and (2) the test results obtained be very carefully evaluated in light of the patient's dermatologic history. These tests are not used for the diagnosis of atopy, but to detect what allergens are important for avoidance and allergen-specific immunotherapy protocols.

Another issue has been the effects of antipruritic therapies on *in vitro* test results. In general, antihistamines, fatty acids, and other nonsteroidal drugs may be given without affecting these tests. Short-term treatment with anti-inflammatory doses of glucocorticoids probably does not influence the results of serologic allergy testing, but long-term treatment may cause false-negative reactions.[55] It is also likely that there are individual responses to clinically utilized glucocorticoid regimens. The authors presently recommend that the same withdrawal criteria used prior to intradermal testing be used prior to serologic testing.

Serologic allergy tests have numerous advantages over intradermal testing, including (1) no patient risk (no need to sedate; no risk for anaphylactic reactions); (2) convenience (no need to clip patient's haircoat, chemically restrain patient, or keep patient at clinic while preparing for, performing, and evaluating test); (3) lower likelihood that result will be influenced by prior or current drug therapy; and (4) the ability to be used in patients with widespread dermatitis or dermatographism. The disadvantages of serologic tests are that they are more expensive per item tested and that "false-positive" (clinically insignificant) results are exceedingly common. Therefore, these tests are not appropriate to use for diagnosing atopic disease, but only in selecting management protocols.

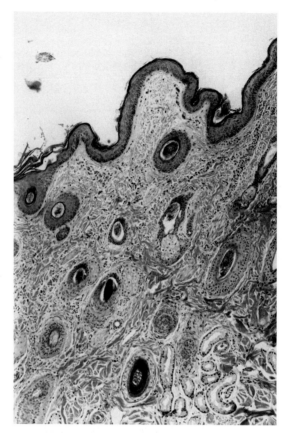

FIGURE 8-11. Superficial perivascular dermatitis with atopy.

In horses, very little information has been published on the value of serologic allergy testing. Anecdotal reports indicate that currently available serologic tests (RAST, ELISA) cannot be recommended, because (1) their reproducibility and reliability are undocumented, (2) results obtained do not correlate with intradermal test reactions or with clinical history, and (3) the vast majority of horses referred for chronic pruritus have had positive serologic tests that have either not correlated with the horses' history and/or not been successful when used to formulate avoidance and immunotherapy protocols.* One extensive study compared the results obtained with intradermal testing, RAST (Spectrum Labs, Mesa, AZ), and two ELISA (Biomedical Services, Austin, TX; Heska, Fort Collins, CO).[146c] All three serologic tests had poor sensitivity, specificity, and predictive value.

There is a great need for reliable serologic allergy tests that are available to the equine practitioner. Unfortunately, none currently exists. The authors consider the use of currently available tests to be of no diagnostic or therapeutic benefit and to be a waste of money.

HISTOPATHOLOGY

The typical histologic appearance of equine atopy is superficial and deep, perivascular to interstitial dermatitis wherein eosinophils are the dominant inflammatory cell (Fig. 8-11).[54] The epidermis is often hyperplastic, except in urticarial reactions. Eosinophilic infiltrative and/or

---

*References 17, 18, 35, 50, 81, 83, 90, 117, 123, 154a, 157a.

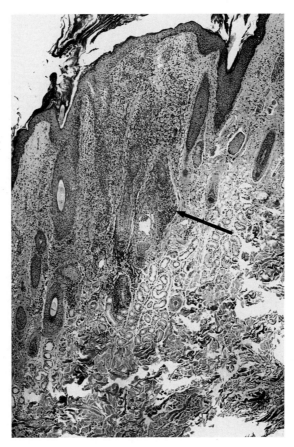

FIGURE 8-12. Skin biopsy specimen from atopic horse. Note mural folliculitis (*arrow*).

necrotizing mural folliculitides (Figs. 8-12 and 8-13) and/or eosinophilic granulomas (Fig. 8-14) are occasionally seen, but always as focal alterations.[54,157a] Some horses will have an eosinophil-rich spongiotic vesicular dermatitis.[25] Changes attributable to secondary bacterial infection (suppurative epidermitis, suppurative luminal folliculitis) may be present (Fig. 8-15). These histopathologic findings are not pathognomonic and may also be observed in insect hypersensitivity and food hypersensitivity.

CLINICAL MANAGEMENT

The client must be made aware that treatment is usually required for life and that therapeutic modifications over the life of the horse are to be expected. Before the clinician discusses the details of therapy with the client, it is imperative to mention that some allergens may be tolerated by an individual horse without any disease manifestations, but a small increase in that load (one or more allergens) may push the horse over the pruritic threshold and initiate clinical signs.[55] Equally important when considering the cause of dermatologic disorders is the concept of summation of effect; for example, a subclinical hypersensitivity in combination with an ectoparasite infestation, a mild bacterial pyoderma, or a dry environment may produce marked discomfort that would be absent if any one of the disorders existed alone.[55] Thus, it is very important to evaluate all possible contributions to the clinical signs in "allergic" horses.

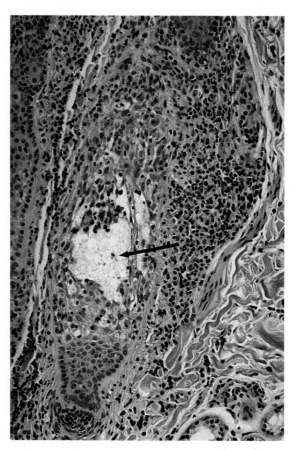

FIGURE 8-13. Close-up of Fig. 8-12. Note eosinophilic and lymphocytic mural folliculitis and follicular mucinosis (*arrow*).

The "best" therapeutic protocol varies considerably from one horse to another and depends on several factors:[157a] the severity and duration of the disease, the function and personality of the patient, the motivation and capabilities of the owner, the environment, the cost, and the existence of other concomitant dermatoses and diseases. The therapeutic options include avoidance of allergens, allergen-specific immunotherapy (hyposensitization), ectoparasite control, treatment of secondary infections, topical agents, glucocorticoids, antihistamines, omega-6/omega-3 fatty acids, and various combinations of these.

Avoidance

Avoidance of allergens is not always possible or practical. Such manipulations and their benefits are not generally possible without accurate identification of the offending allergen(s) by allergy testing. Because many patients have multiple reactivities and many allergens cannot be avoided, the effective use of this approach is not often possible as a sole therapy. It is still an important aspect of the management, however, because it will often decrease the allergen load. Some patients may greatly benefit from avoidance of confirmed allergens such as feathers (birds), danders (cats), insects, and dusts.[18,118,123.,146,157a] When changes are made in the management of the horse based on the results of intradermal testing, some animals have no further need of other medications.[146,157a]

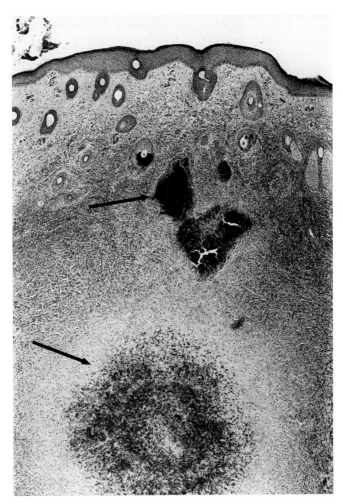

FIGURE 8-14. Skin biopsy specimen from atopic horse. Note necrotizing infiltrative mural folliculitis (*upper arrow*) and subjacent eosinophilic granuloma (*lower arrow*).

The concentrations of dusts and aeroallergens in the air are significantly higher around the nostrils of horses than in the air of their stalls.[168,170] Consequently, ventilation systems do not significantly reduce the quantity of dusts and aeroallergens at the level of the horse's nostrils when it is feeding or sniffing.[169] Controlling the sources of particulate matter, especially in forages and litters, is the only practical way to reduce the quantity of respirable dusts and aeroallergens.[168-170] In order to reduce the quantity of particles in the air, the utilization of good quality straw is preferable to wood shavings, and grass silages and alfalfa pellets are a better choice than whole grains and molassed concentrates.[168] Rolled grains are much dustier than good quality hay.[168] With other allergens, complete elimination may be impossible, but a decrease in exposure may be achievable. Cat allergen can be quite common and persistent even in environments where cats no longer live.[55]

Topical Therapy

Topical therapy is utilized in two main ways. The first is through shampoos and rinses, which remove allergens and irritants from the skin and help to eliminate dry skin. The second is through

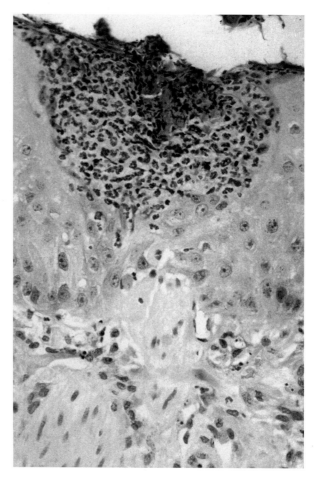

FIGURE 8-15. Neutrophilic epidermal microabscess with secondary staphylococcal dermatitis.

topical antipruritic agents (e.g., colloidal oatmeal, pramoxine, glucocorticoids), which are usually most effective for treating localized areas of pruritus. These therapies are covered in Chapter 3. In general, many atopic horses benefit from weekly baths and/or rinses where possible. Many atopic horses have sensitive, easily irritated skin. Hypoallergenic and colloidal oatmeal–containing shampoos and rinses are preferred.

Allergen-Specific Immunotherapy

Allergen-specific immunotherapy (hyposensitization, desensitization) is indicated in animals in which avoidance of antigens is impossible or ineffective, signs are present for more than 4 to 6 months of the year, and antipruritic drugs are unsatisfactory or contraindicated.[157a] This and avoidance are the only forms of therapy that stop the allergic reaction, in contrast to most medical therapies that counteract the effects of the allergic reaction. Virtually no attempts have been made to standardize immunotherapy protocols in the horse or to scientifically compare their merits. Thus, published regimens vary in the form of allergen used (aqueous, alum precipitated, propylene glycol suspended, glycerinated), the number and frequency of injections given in the induction phase, the dose of allergen administered, the potency of allergenic extract, and the route of administration (subcutaneous, intramuscular, intradermal). The vast majority of clinicians use only the subcutaneous route. Numerous authors have written about the benefits of allergen-specific immunotherapies, with most reporting a 60% to 71% rate of good to excellent responses when based on the results of intradermal testing.* It is well accepted that allergen-specific immunotherapy is an effective, valuable, relatively economical, and relatively safe treatment for atopic horses.

The mechanism of action of allergen-specific immunotherapy is complex with a variety of end organ, humoral, and cellular changes occurring in humans.[44,55] Various hypotheses were proposed in the past, such as (1) humoral desensitization (reduced levels of IgE), (2) cellular desensitization (reduced reactivity of mast cells and basophils), (3) immunization (induction of "blocking antibody"), (4) tolerization (generation of allergen-specific suppressor cells), and (5) some combination thereof. At the cellular level, an increase in allergen-induced CD25+CD8+ T lymphocytes correlates with a favorable response. Atopic humans successfully treated with IFN-γ or cyclosporine usually have no decrease, and often have an increase, in IgE levels.[55] This suggests the beneficial effect is not humoral but cellular (switch from Th2 to Th1 cytokine profile).

Aqueous allergens, which are rapidly absorbed, necessitate smaller doses and require multiple, frequent injections, constitute by far the most commonly used type today. A variety of protocols are utilized, but most of the aqueous regimens are modifications of the schedule shown in Table 8-16. Some specialists, including the authors, utilize just the two more potent concentrations.

In general, the immunotherapy prescription includes all of the positive reactions that make sense in view of the horse's history and environmental exposure. In horses with multiple sensitivities (e.g., 20 to 30 or more), the allergens should be selected on the basis of history, the probable presence of that allergen in the environment, the frequency at which the allergen is known to react in that region, and the duration of the allergen's presence. Cross-reactivity may also be utilized in the decision. In general, cross-reactivity tends to stay within families or closer relationships so that genera of the same family have some cross-allergenicity, and species of the same genus will have even greater cross-reactivity. Because grasses have fewer families, they tend to be the most cross-reactive, but the three main grass families tend to be different.[55] Bermuda grass is in the family *Eragrostoideae* and does not cross with the *Festucoideae*, the more common northern pasture grasses. Pancoideae, which includes Johnson and Bahia grass, will cross-react somewhat with the other two families. Weeds are less cross-reactive than grasses, and trees are the least cross-reactive. All this information is based on allergens that commonly are found in humans, and this may not be the same in the horse, as has been discussed for house dust mite allergens. Besides cross-reactivity, another issue is the effects allergens may have when combined. Studies have shown that molds, and to some degree insect allergens, contain proteases that may break down other allergens, especially pollens.[55] In the one veterinary study, though protease degradation was documented, the author stated that success with hyposensitization had apparently not been affected, as compared with other published studies of the mixing of mold allergens with other allergens.[55]

Depending on each individual horse's response and which form of the allergen is being utilized, a beneficial response to immunotherapy may be seen within 2 to 3 months of treatment. However, allergen-specific immunotherapy should always be continued for at least 1 year so as to appreciate the maximum benefit.[157a] "Booster" injections of allergens are administered as needed (when clinical signs first begin to reappear) and may be needed every week to every month. Experience with the patient allows the owner and the veterinarian to predict how long the patient will be asymptomatic following booster injections. Boosters are then administered shortly before clinical signs would be expected to flare up. Intervals between boosters may vary at different times of the year. It is also important to not overtreat and cause adverse reactions. Adjusting the

---

*References 18, 53, 81, 83, 111, 117, 119, 123, 124, 155, 156, 157a, 167.

immunotherapy protocol for each individual case is the most appropriate way to maximize the response, and even when adverse reactions are not seen or exacerbations prior to injections are not observed, trying different protocols may increase efficacy.[55] In general, atopic horses require lifetime administration of vaccine.

Response to immunotherapy is allergen-specific.[44,55] The response to specific types of allergens has not been well studied. Some authors have reported that the results of immunotherapy are not as good when atopic horses also have positive intradermal reactions to multiple insects.[124] However, other investigators report that results of immunotherapy are similar in atopic horses with or without positive intradermal reactions to multiple insects.[156]

Adverse reactions to allergen-specific immunotherapy are uncommon and usually benign.[156,157a,167] Adverse reactions include (1) intensification of clinical signs for a few hours to a few days, (2) local reactions (edema with or without pain or pruritus) at injection sites, and (3) urticaria. Serious reactions (anaphylaxis) are extremely rare. Adverse reactions are treated according to symptom. Intensification of pruritus and/or urticaria often indicate that the dose of the vaccine needs to be reduced.

In the severely affected, nonseasonally atopic horse, it may be necessary to control the symptoms with systemic glucocorticoids during immunotherapy. As long as oral prednisolone or prednisone doses are kept as low as possible and administered on an alternate-day basis (see Chapter 3), immunotherapy can still be successful. Avoiding glucocorticoids during at least the first few weeks of therapy will allow one to identify mild reactions and make adjustments, which is a good reason to try to avoid those drugs early on.

Systemic Antipruritic Agents

Many atopic horses require a systemic antipruritic agent, either as a sole agent or used in conjunction with other treatments for an additive effect.[157a] These agents were discussed earlier in this chapter, but some points are important to consider when treating atopic disease. Systemic glucocorticoids are usually very effective for the management of atopy. They are, however, the most dangerous of the treatments commonly utilized to treat atopy. As such, their use should be limited to cases with active seasons lasting less than 4 to 6 months, or cases for which safer options are not effective. Prednisolone or prednisone is administered orally (2.2 mg/kg q24h) in the morning until pruritus is controlled (3 to 10 days), and then on an alternate-day (morning) regimen (see Chapter 3) as needed. This schedule is relatively safe compared with long-acting corticosteroids. Many atopic horses will have more than one disease and these drugs are less effective if there is any infectious dermatitis, ectoparasitism, or other hypersensitivities present. Any animal not responding to rational treatments should be reexamined to determine whether secondary infections, ectoparasitism, or other complicating factors are present. Efficacy of treatment may change as seasons and allergen loads change, or as other complicating factors occur. Clients need to be aware of this and encouraged to treat minor flare-ups early. Combinations with topical therapy, fatty acids, and antihistamines are often more effective than single therapies.

Other Experimental and Therapeutic Agents

In humans with atopic dermatitis, studies have demonstrated therapeutic benefits of cyclosporine, leukotriene antagonists, INF-γ, injectable allergen-antibody complexes, thymopentin, extracorporeal photochemotherapy, and Chinese herbal therapy.[55] Other therapies being evaluated experimentally include peptide immunotherapy, anticytokine and cytokine receptor therapies, phosphodiesterase inhibitors, and anti-IgE therapy.[55] There is no information available on the usefulness of these modalities in the horse.

In dogs, misoprostol and pentoxifylline were reported to be of use on some patients for the partial control of pruritus.[55] Anecdotal reprints suggest that pentoxifylline may be useful in pruritic horses (see Chapter 9). Cyclosporine is useful in many atopic dogs and cats [55] but is of unknown usefulness in horses.

Contact Hypersensitivity

Contact hypersensitivity (allergic contact dermatitis) is a rare, variably pruritic, maculopapular or lichenified dermatitis affecting areas of skin coming into contact with allergens.

CAUSE AND PATHOGENESIS

Only a few reports of naturally occurring contact hypersensitivity in horses have been documented by patch testing, yet this is a common and well-studied problem in human dermatology.[20,44] Much of the veterinary literature and data on naturally occurring *allergic contact dermatitis* in horses are of dubious validity and value. In reality, there is often a huge overlap between what has been called *contact hypersensitivity* and *primary irritant contact dermatitis* in the veterinary literature.[22,23,53,55]

Classically, contact hypersensitivity represents a type IV hypersensitivity reaction wherein histologically lymphocytes are the dominant cell type.[*] Most of the work on the pathogenesis of contact hypersensitivity has been performed in laboratory animals. In contrast to irritant reactions, allergic contact reactions are characterized by a immunologic reaction to a hapten, usually a small, chemically reactive, lipid-soluble molecule that binds to a protein to become a complete antigen.[44] The hapten protein complex binds to, and most likely is pinocytosed by, epidermal Langerhans' cells, which induces an increase in Langerhans' cell size, MHC II expression, and IL-1β synthesis. The initial presentation and processing of the hapten is referred to as the *afferent phase* of allergic contact reactions. This phase is believed to require transfer of stimulated hapten-containing Langerhans' cells from the skin to regional lymph nodes. This emigration from skin to lymph may be initiated by TNF-α.[20] These T cells are stimulated to express skin homing ligands, which direct their movement to the skin. Langerhans' cell numbers are decreased in contact hypersensitivity because of their emigration to the lymph nodes, but these numbers are not decreased in primary irritant contact dermatitis.[20] The efferent phase or elicitation phase occurs in response to exposure to hapten in an already sensitized animal. Though some Langerhans' cell migration may occur, much of this reaction may occur locally. The activated memory T cells are recruited to the site of hapten exposure by expression of adhesion molecules, such as VCAM-1, E-selectin, and ICAM-1 on the vascular endothelium. ICAM-1 is also expressed on keratinocytes and may result in the diapedesis of lymphocytes. TNF-α is rapidly released from Langerhans' cells and keratinocytes following hapten exposure and stimulates the expression of E-selectin and VCAM-1 on the endothelial cells.[20,44] TNF-α is also released from cells in response to substance P, a neuropeptide that may be released as a result of the interaction between Langerhans cells and nerve fibers.[20] Other epidermal cytokines involved include IL-6 and MIP. Which cytokines are associated with allergic contact and not with irritant contact dermatitis is an area receiving extensive study. It appears the differences in IL-1β, IL-6, IL-12, and IFN-γ may be key factors.[44] The production of IL-12 may be central to the development of a Th1 cell response.[20]

Newer information blurs the distinction between immunologic and nonimmunologic events and makes differentiation problematic.[177] The clinical and histopathologic features overlap greatly. Langerhans' cells are just as actively involved in irritant reactions as allergic reactions (decreased numbers; apposition of lymphocytes). Virtually all cytokines identified in allergic reactions are also present in irritant reactions (ICAM-1, IL-2, TNF-α, LFA-1). The percentage of T cell subtypes, Langerhans' cells, macrophages, and activated antigens are not significantly different. Even patch testing produces the same cytokine profile and so forth. Some authors conclude that the difference between irritant and allergic reactions is more conceptual than demonstrable.[177]

---

[*]References 7, 20, 23, 44, 52, 55, 63, 171.

● Table 8-17 SUBSTANCES REPORTED TO CAUSE NATURALLY-OCCURRING "ALLERGIC CONTACT DERMATITIS" IN HORSES[†]
Pasture plants
Bedding
Soaps
Shampoos, rinses, and sprays (especially insecticidal/acaricidal)
Grooming aids
Blankets
Topical medicaments (e.g., antibiotics)
Tack[°]
Chrome
Cotton
Jute

[°]In most instances, these reactions are not believed to be due to leather, wool, and rubber, but rather a preservative, accelerator, or dye used in the manufacturing process.
[†]References 8, 9, 15, 17, 21, 34, 37, 45, 50, 53, 57, 58, 64, 65, 171a, 172-176, 179.

The last phase of naturally occurring contact hypersensitivity is the resolution phase. Less is known about this phase, though IL-10 may play an important role as it interferes with Th2 cell cytokine production. IL-10 is upregulated in keratinocytes in the late phase of allergic contact reactions. Basophils, which begin to migrate into late lesions, may also be involved in stimulating resolution.[44]

Spontaneous, well-documented cases of contact hypersensitivity are found rarely in the veterinary literature. The most commonly (and anecdotally) incriminated contact sensitizers in horses are listed in Table 8-17. Single instances of documented sensitivity to cotton,[172] chrome,[171a] and jute[50] have been reported. Positive reactions to patch testing with neomycin have been seen in some horses (W. Rosenkrantz, personal communication). Moisture is an important predisposing factor because it decreases the effectiveness of the normal skin barrier and increases the intimacy of contact between the agent and the skin surface. In this respect, the sweating horse is an ideal candidate for contact hypersensitivity.

CLINICAL FEATURES

Although naturally occurring contact dermatitis is reported to be common in horses,[°] true contact hypersensitivity is probably very rare. There are no reported age, breed, or sex predilections.

Although contact hypersensitivity can be produced in humans after a 3- to 5-week sensitization period, the sensitization period for patients with naturally occurring disease exceeds 2 years in over 70% of cases.[20,44,55] In horses, the culprit contactant is rarely a recent addition to the animal's environment. Substances reported to cause naturally occurring "allergic contact dermatitis" in horses are listed in Table 8-17. Again, virtually none of these substances, other than those previously listed, has been well documented with patch testing, and even less with typical histopathology of the positive patch test sites.

Clinical signs of contact hypersensitivity include varying degrees of dermatitis, from erythema, edema, and scaling, to papules, vesicles, oozing, and crusts. Pruritus varies from mild to intense. Self-mutilation and/or secondary bacterial infections may be superimposed on the contact dermatitis. Chronicity leads to alopecia, lichenification, and pigmentary disturbances of the skin and/or haircoat. The area of the body affected often suggests the nature of the contactant:

[°]References 8, 9, 15, 17, 21, 34, 37, 45, 50, 53, 57, 58, 64, 65, 172-176, 179.

- Face, neck, and ears—insecticidal/acaricidal repellents and sprays
- Muzzle and extremities—pasture plants, bedding
- Face and trunk—tack
- Area conforming to application of a topical substance

Again, because of the horse's ability to sweat, contactants have access to the skin even in heavily haired areas. Contact hypersensitivities may be seasonal or nonseasonal, depending on the allergens involved. In situations where several horses are similarly housed, involvement of a single animal would suggest hypersensitivity, whereas clinical signs in several animals would point to irritant reactions or contagious disease.

DIAGNOSIS

Depending on the distribution of lesions, the dermatitis may visually be strongly suggestive of being contact-related. The differential diagnosis could include primary irritant contact dermatitis, atopy, food hypersensitivity, sarcoptic mange, psoroptic mange, insect hypersensitivity, *Pelodera* dermatitis, and staphylococcal folliculitis. Definitive diagnosis is based on history, physical findings, and results of provocative exposure and patch testing with appropriate histopathology. Provocative exposure involves avoiding contact with suspected allergenic substances for up to 14 days. The animal is first bathed with a nonirritating, hypoallergenic shampoo to remove all possible allergenic substances from the skin and haircoat, and then placed in a "nonallergenic" environment for up to 14 days. The animal is then re-exposed to its normal environment or to suspect substances, one at a time, and is observed for an exacerbation of the dermatosis over 7 to 10 days. Provocative exposure is time-consuming, requires a patient and dedicated owner, and is frequently impossible to undertake. Additionally, without biopsy or patch testing, provocative exposure does *not* reliably distinguish between hypersensitive and irritant skin reactions. To better define the reactions, skin biopsy specimens taken from acute lesions induced by the exposure should be studied.

The patch test is the method for documenting contact hypersensitivity.[20,44,55] In the classic closed patch test, the test substance is applied to a piece of cloth or soft paper that is then placed directly on intact skin, covered with an impermeable substance, and affixed to the skin with tape. After 48 hours the patch is removed, and the condition of the underlying skin is examined. Owing to the logistical problems of applying and securing patch test substances to horses, patch testing is rarely done. The sliding of the material and irritation from tape leads to much misinterpretation of results. The use of ether to remove the tape and the adhesive (Scanpar) tends to minimize but not eliminate these problems.

For now, performing closed patch tests with suspected allergens in their natural state is probably the most sensible way to proceed. The dorsolateral thorax is gently clipped, and suspected allergens are applied to the skin (preferably with Scanpar), taped in place, and secured under a body bandage. The test materials are removed in 48 hours, and the test sites are observed for the following 3 to 5 days. Optimally, test sites should undergo biopsy, but more fulminant reactions can be considered positive. The nature of the reaction is not determined without biopsy of these acute lesions. Additionally, substances eliciting positive reactions should be tested on normal animals to make sure that they are not irritants.

HISTOPATHOLOGY

Humans and dogs with experimentally induced or naturally occurring contact hypersensitivity classically have a superficial and/or deep perivascular dermatitis wherein lymphocytes and histiocytes predominate.[20,44,55] However, some patients have numerous neutrophils and/or eosinophils present. Whether these differences represent differences in the nature of the culprit contactant and/or the immunologic reaction produced is not known. No detailed studies on the histopathologic findings in equine contact hypersensitivity have been published. Anecdotal reports,[45,174] as well as the authors' experiences, suggest that the cutaneous reaction pattern may be perivascular to interstitial (Fig. 8-16) and that lymphocytes or eosinophils may dominate. The epidermis shows variable degrees of hyperplasia, intra- and intercellular edema, and exocytosis of lymphocytes or eosinophils (Fig. 8-17). Histopathologic findings consistent with secondary bacterial pyoderma (suppurative epidermitis, suppurative luminal folliculitis) may be present.

CLINICAL MANAGEMENT

The prognosis for contact hypersensitivity depends on the offending allergen. Therapy for contact hypersensitivity in horses may include avoidance of allergens or the use of glucocorticoids. Avoidance of allergens is preferable but may be impossible, either because of the nature of the substances or because they cannot be identified. In such instances, pentoxifylline or glucocorticoids are usually very effective but will often be needed for life. Some animals can be managed with topical glucocorticoids alone (see Chapter 3). Other animals require systemic glucocorticoids. Pentoxifylline (see Chapter 9) has been effective in some humans and dogs with contact hypersensitivity.[20,44,55]

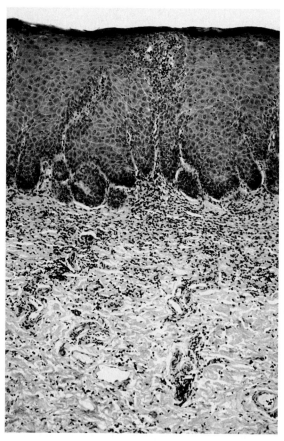

FIGURE 8-16. Skin biopsy specimen from horse with contact hypersensitivity caused by 5-fluorouracil. Note superficial interstitial dermatitis.

Food Hypersensitivity

Food hypersensitivity (adverse food reaction, food allergy, food intolerance) is a skin disorder of horses that is associated with the ingestion of a substance found in the horse's diet.[17,50,53] Presumably it is a hypersensitivity reaction to an antigenic ingredient. This may not always be the case, however. Toxic food reactions and nontoxic, nonimmunologic reactions (intolerances) may in fact be occurring, and the condition incorrectly called food hypersensitivity. Toxic reactions are usually dose-related, may occur in any individual, and are often associated with histamine or bacterial toxins in the food. Food intolerance is an individual sensitivity to a food that may occur by a variety of nonimmunologic mechanisms, including metabolic, pharmacologic, and idiosyncratic. Their clinical differentiation from allergy is rarely accomplished or necessary.[23,44,55,63] The term *food hypersensitivity* is still accepted, however, because of its common usage and because of the difficulty differentiating between hypersensitivity and intolerance in practice.

CAUSE AND PATHOGENESIS

Diet has long been recognized as a cause of hypersensitivity-like skin reactions in horses, dogs, cats, and human beings. Although the pathomechanism of food hypersensitivity is unclear, type I hypersensitivity reactions are well documented and the most common type of hypersensitivity reactions in humans, although type III and IV reactions have been suspected. Cutaneous type I reactions are associated with both immediate and late-phase reactions. Immediate (within minutes

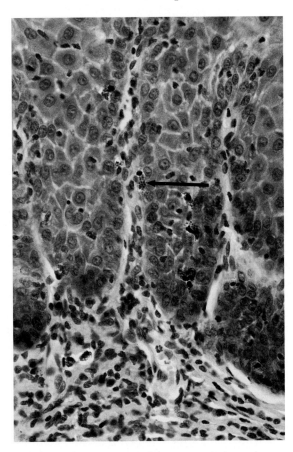

FIGURE 8-17. Close-up of Fig. 8-16. Note eosinophilic exocytosis (*arrow*).

to hours) and delayed (within several hours to days) reactions to foods have also been seen in the horse. Why the skin is a frequent target of food-induced hypersensitivity is not well known, though it has been recognized in humans that cutaneous lymphocyte antigen is induced on T cells when cutaneous disease is present, but not on T cells in food-related respiratory disease.[44] Whether sensitization occurs in the intestinal mucosa or to absorbed allergen is unknown. Normally the gut possesses several mechanisms that comprise the intestinal mucosal barrier, which blocks the absorption or the entering of foreign antigens into the body. Antigens are normally broken down by the effects of gastric acid enzymes, pancreatic and intestinal enzymes in the gut lumen, and by intestinal cell lysosomal activity. Intestinal peristalsis also acts to decrease absorption of potential antigens by removing antigens trapped in the intestinal mucous. The intestinal mucosal barrier is comprised of a protective mucous coating overlying the epithelial cells, which are sealed together by tight junctions. Together the mucous and epithelial cells block the passage of most macromolecules. This is supported by an immunologic response of secretory IgA from the plasma cells in the laminal propria. Secretory IgA binds antigens and removes them in the intestinal mucus, or for those antigens that pass through the intestinal barrier, secretory IgA binds antigen and is removed from the circulation through the liver and bile.[44,55] Antigens bypassing these protective mechanisms stimulate an immune response that, for many molecules, results in tolerance or anergy by activation of suppressor (CD8) T cells or suppressor cytokine profiles (such as IL-4, IL-10, and TGF-β) from Th2 and Th3 cells.[44] Abnormalities in the barrier or immune response may result in sensitization. Therefore, damage to the normal defense barriers along with ingestion of food molecules at the same time most likely contributes to which molecules become antigenic. The type of molecule also plays a role, as most food hypersensitivity reactions are directed against complex glycoproteins. The protection is delayed in human infants, because in the first month of life there is predominantly an IgM response, which is not as effective as secretory IgA in trapping and removing antigens.[44] Children have immature intestinal mucosal barriers that are less efficient in handling and processing food proteins.[44] Despite these defenses, an immunologic response to a variety of food antigens often occurs both in normal individuals and those with proven food hypersensitivity.[44,55] In rodents, it has been shown that antigen-presenting cells in the mononuclear phagocytic system stimulate gut CD8+ T cells that play a role in the development of immune tolerance, and if overloaded with multiple antigens, this may prevent the induction of tolerance to subsequent exposed antigens. This observation has led to the suggestion that, if a similar mechanism occurred in human infants, the observation of increased incidence of food hypersensitivity in 4-month-old human infants fed a variety of solids foods could be explained.[44] Another consideration in animals, in which gastrointestinal parasitism and viral enteritis are relatively common, is that a damaged intestinal tract allows the bypassing of the normal defense mechanisms and antigens would overload the gut mononuclear phagocytic system. The predisposition to develop IgE antibody may be enhanced by a concurrent parasitic infection.[22,55] This has been shown experimentally where endoparasites favor the development of IgE to orally administered allergens in atopy-prone dogs and in cats.[55] Poor digestion results in larger protein molecules, and because food hypersensitivity rarely occurs to small proteins and amino acids, these may be more capable of inducing a hypersensitivity reaction.[55] Additionally, because endoparasitism and various enteritides occur in young horses, and food hypersensitivity often develops in young horses, it becomes a tempting hypothesis that needs to be studied. Attention has also been focused on a heterogeneous group of cytokines called histamine-releasing factors.[23,55] After being initially generated by chronic antigenic exposures, these cytokines can cause histamine release in the absence of the provoking antigen, and this release can continue for some time after the antigen is removed. Such a mechanism could explain the long delay (10 to 13 weeks) reported between the initiation of a hypoallergenic diet and clinical improvement in some food-hypersensitive dogs. This mechanism is also believed to play a role in cutaneous hyperirritability with chronic ingestion of the offending food allergens.[44]

● Table 8-18 **DIETARY ITEMS REPORTED TO HAVE CAUSED FOOD HYPER-SENSITIVITY IN THE HORSE**

Alfalfa	"Grains"
Barley	"Grasses"
Beet pulp	"Horse cubes"
Bran	"Horse tonics"
Buckwheat	Malt
Chicory	Oats
Clover	Potatoes and their byproducts
Feed additives and supplements	St. John's wort
Glucose	Wheat

Compared with what is known in humans, little is known about the food allergens that are important in horses. Most commonly, the allergen is a water-soluble glycoprotein present in the food, and this glycoprotein may become recognizable only after digestion or heating and preparation of the food. The size of the allergenic glycoprotein in humans is generally large, with a molecular weight greater than 12,000 daltons. This has not been confirmed in the horse.

The documentation of a hypersensitive mechanism has not been confirmed in the horse. Food intolerance is also likely to occur in the horse and may mimic food hypersensitivity reactions. In humans, food intolerance is believed to account for the majority of adverse food reactions, though their importance in cutaneous diseases has not been studied in depth.

We have only skeletal information on the dietary items responsible for food hypersensitivity in horses. Good studies are difficult because few horse owners are willing to feed a novel protein diet, let alone separate a diet into its components and to feed each item individually to identify the responsible allergen. In addition, challenges are open, and in humans, the placebo effect has been shown to be very high when attempting to determine dietary allergens. Therefore, documentation is based on three positive double-blinded, placebo-controlled food challenges.[44] In dogs, *in vitro* (serologic) tests cannot be relied on to detect allergens that cause hypersensitivity, because they are positive in most normal dogs and in most dogs with other skin diseases.[55] These tests are also positive in most dogs with proven hypersensitivity to food, but not to the important allergens as determined by test meal investigations.[55] Table 8-18 lists dietary items reported to have caused food hypersensitivity in horses. The most commonly implicated (mostly anecdotal) dietary allergies are alfalfa, barley, bran, oats, wheat, concentrates, and feed supplements. Though food additives (including preservatives) are often blamed by the public (particularly by naturalists), these substances are rarely documented to cause food hypersensitivity in horses.

CLINICAL FEATURES

Food hypersensitivity is reported to be rare in horses.* This could be due, in part, to the difficulty in convincing horse owners to feed novel protein diets. Food hypersensitivity accounts for 0.44% of the equine dermatoses seen at the Cornell University Clinic. Concurrent insect hypersensitivity or atopic disease may be present.[157a,178]

No age, breed, or sex predilections have been documented for equine food hypersensitivity. Though there is no documented age predilection, it is important to note that many cases occur in young horses. The clinical signs of food hypersensitivity may be seasonal or nonseasonal, depending on the allergens involved.[17,18,157a] The most common cutaneous signs of equine food hypersensitivity are (1) multifocal or generalized pruritus, (2) pruritic or nonpruritic urticaria, or

*References 17, 18, 34, 35, 45, 48, 50, 53, 62, 64, 81, 90, 91, 100, 178, 179.

(3) a combination of these.° Commonly affected areas include the face, neck, trunk, and rump. Some affected horses exhibit predominantly or exclusively tail rubbing and perianal pruritus (Fig. 8-18). Severe pruritus may lead to self-mutilation, secondary bacterial infection, or both of these. Concurrent gastrointestinal or respiratory abnormalities have not been described in food hypersensitive horses.

DIAGNOSIS

The differential diagnosis of equine food hypersensitivity consists of atopy, drug reaction, insect hypersensitivity, pediculosis, oxyuriasis, intestinal parasite hypersensitivity, chorioptic mange, psoroptic mange, sarcoptic mange, straw mite infestation, and contact dermatitis.

At present, the definitive diagnosis of food hypersensitivity in horses is reliably made only on the basis of elimination diets and provocative exposure testing. The necessary duration of a novel protein diet is unknown. Most clinicians recommend a 4-week duration.[†]

Novel protein diets must be individualized for each patient, on the basis of careful dietary history. The objectives of the diet are (1) to feed the animals dietary substances that they are not commonly exposed to and (2) to feed the animals a diet that is free of additives, supplements, and treats. A common approach is to withhold all concentrates, additives, supplements, and treats and to feed a bulk food not previously used (e.g., alfalfa, oat, or timothy hay). If a grain must be fed, switch from sweet-mixed feeds to pure grain (e.g., oats, corn). If the dermatosis improves, all elements of the previous ration are reintroduced to see whether the dermatosis is reproduced and the diagnosis is confirmed. Reintroduction of the dietary allergen(s) usually causes clinical signs to reappear within 12 hours to 7 days. At this point, the diagnosis can be further refined by eliminating and reintroducing individual dietary items in order to pinpoint the specific substance(s) involved. Horses that have concurrent atopy or insect hypersensitivity may have a partial response to the novel protein diet (for example, a 50% reduction in pruritus).

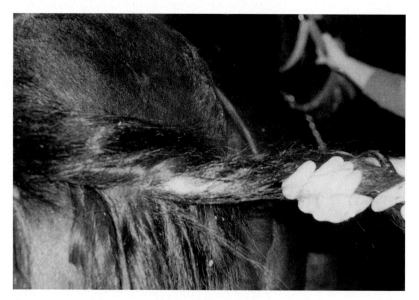

FIGURE 8-18. Tail excoriations in a butt-rubbing food-hypersensitive (oats) horse.

°References 17, 18, 34, 35, 45, 48, 50, 53, 62, 64, 81, 90, 91, 100, 179.
[†]References 17, 18, 35, 53, 90, 100.

Allergen-specific serologic allergy tests (RAST, ELISA) are available for the horse, but their reliability, reproducibility, and diagnostic merits are not documented. The authors and others[17] find that nearly all referred pruritic horses have had positive serologic reactions to foods. However, the results have either made no sense, or dietary changes implemented on the basis of the results of these tests have been of no benefit. In like fashion, the merits of intradermal testing with foods in horses are undocumented.[17,18,50,90,100] Serologic and intradermal tests for food hypersensitivity are believed to be worthless in dogs and cats.[55] The authors believe that the same is true for horses.

HISTOPATHOLOGY

Skin biopsy specimens are characterized by superficial or superficial and deep perivascular to interstitial dermatitis wherein eosinophils are the dominant inflammatory cell (Fig. 8-19).[17,50,54] The epidermis may be normal, spongiotic, or hyperplastic. Focal areas of eosinophilic infiltrative and/or necrotizing mural folliculitides and/or eosinophilic granulomas may be observed. Some horses have an eosinophil-rich spongiotic vesicular dermatitis.[25] Histopathologic findings consistent with secondary bacterial infection (suppurative epidermatitis, suppurative luminal folliculitis) may be present.

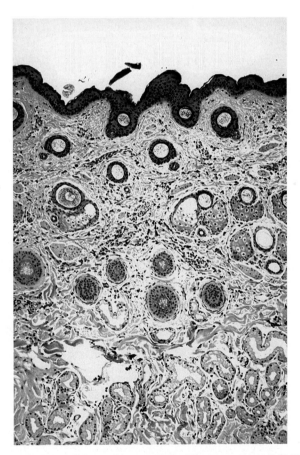

FIGURE 8-19. Skin biopsy specimen from a horse with food hypersensitivity (alfalfa). Pure superficial and deep eosinophilic dermatitis.

CLINICAL MANAGEMENT

The prognosis for food hypersensitivity is usually good. Therapy consists of avoiding offending foods or using systemic antipruritic agents. Response to glucocorticoids is variable, with some horses responding very well and others responding only partially. Antihistamines and/or omega-6/omega-3 fatty acids may also be useful, but factual information is not presently available.

Insect Hypersensitivity

Insect hypersensitivity is the most common allergic skin disease of the horse.* The disease is caused by hypersensitivity to the bites of *Culicoides* and *Simulium* species, *Stomoxys calcitrans* and, possibly, *Haematobia irritans*. It has a worldwide distribution. The incidence of the disease in the equine population varies, being 2.8% in the United Kingdom,[228] 3% in Switzerland,[208] and 4.4% in Japan,[240] to 21.8% in Israel,[191] 26% in Canada,[181] 29% in Germany,[260] and 32% in Australia.[247] Insect hypersensitivity is the third most common equine dermatosis seen at the Cornell University Clinic, accounting for 6.33% of equine skin disorders. The condition has previously been reported under a number of (often erroneous) names: Dhobie itch, Queensland itch, sweet itch, summer itch, muck itch, dermatite estivale récidivante, summer sores, summer eczema, summer dermatitis, summer mange, summer fungus, allergic dermatitis, allergic urticaria, Kasen, lichen tropicus, psoriasis, microfilarial pityriasis.

CAUSE AND PATHOGENESIS

This disorder represents type I (immediate and late-phase) and type IV (delayed) hypersensitivity to antigens (presumably salivary) from numerous *Culicoides* (gnats) and *Simulium* (black flies) species, *Stomoxys calcitrans* (stable fly), and possibly *Haematobia (Lyperosia) irritans* (horn fly).† It is possible that some horses have hypersensitivities to multiple insects. *Culicoides* gnats (biting midges, sandflies, punkies, no-see-ums) are the most important cause of equine insect hypersensitivity. There are some 800 to 1000 species of *Culicoides* worldwide.[190] Results of gnat collection techniques, intradermal testing with gnat antigens, and passive cutaneous anaphylaxis trials have incriminated numerous *Culicoides* species in various parts of the world: *C. brevitarus (robertsi)* in Australia;[47,48,249] *C. obsoletus* in Canada;[182,222] *C. pulicaris* and *C. nubeculosis* in France;[190] *C. imicola* (most), *C. obsoletus*, *C. nubeculosis*, *C. newsteadi*, *C. punctatus*, *C. puncticollis*, *C. shultzei*, and *C. circumscriptus* in Israel;[191,192,194] *C. obsoletus* and *C. peregrinus* in Japan;[257] *C. obsoletus*, *C. pulicaris*, *C. impunctactus, and C. chiopterus* in Norway;[214] *C. imicola* in South Africa and Botswana;[237] *C. pulicaris*, *C. punctatus*, and *C. nubeculosis* in the United Kingdom‡; and *C. variipenis*, *C. insignis*, *C. spinosis*, *C. niger*, *C. pusillus*, *C. alachua*, *C. scanloni*, *C. venustus*, *C. stellifer*, *C. obsoletus*, and *C. biguttatus* in the United States.§

Clinical evidence strongly suggests that this disorder has familial and genetic predispositions.Π Icelandic ponies have received the most investigation in this regard.# Icelandic ponies do not develop insect hypersensitivity in Iceland because there are no *Culicoides* gnats in Iceland.[208,216,218a,224] However, Icelandic ponies readily develop insect hypersensitivity when they are in *Culicoides*-inhabited areas. In addition, Icelandic ponies that are born in Iceland and then moved to a

---

*References 2, 8, 16-18, 21, 22, 29, 32, 37, 48-50, 52-54, 56, 62, 65, 190, 197, 207, 218a, 219, 220, 226, 229, 232, 244, 252, 262, 263.

†References 8, 16, 49, 53-55, 184-186, 191, 199, 220, 222, 231-233, 238, 240, 245, 249, 253a, 257.

‡References 186, 228, 229, 233, 245, 256.

§References 202-204, 210-213, 231, 232, 251.

ΠReferences 16, 49, 50, 181, 185, 189, 191, 195, 199, 206, 215, 216, 218a, 220-222, 224, 224a, 226, 227a, 229, 231-233, 238, 240, 244, 245, 249, 257, 260, 262.

#References 208, 216, 218a, 224, 260, 262.

Culicoides-inhabited area have a significantly higher prevalence of insect hypersensitivity (26% to 30%) and experience a more severe clinical disease than Icelandic ponies that are born in *Culicoides*-inhabited areas (2% to 8.2%).[°] This would suggest that early, repeated exposure to *Culicoides* gnats is, to some degree, protective. This susceptibility of Icelandic ponies to insect hypersensitivity has been reported to segregate with equine leukocyte antigens (ELA) Be1, Be8, W1, W7, and W23.[208,215,224a,227a,262]

German Shire horses had insect hypersensitivity with a prevalence of 11.6% in the United Kingdom and 37.7% in Germany, and a familial occurrence of disease in about 35% of the cases.[226] Other breeds reported to be possibly at increased risk include ponies, Arabians, Connemaras, and quarter horses.[†]

Intradermal injections of *Culicoides* (and occasionally *Simulium, Stomoxys*, and *Haematobia*) extracts produce immediate (30 minutes) and delayed (24 to 48 hours) reactions in over 80% and about 50%, respectively, of affected horses.[‡] Some affected horses also develop late-phase immediate (4 to 6 hours) reactions.[§] Affected horses typically react to all *Culicoides* spp. injected, suggesting shared common allergen(s).[Π] Most horses react to two or more genera of insects.[#] Whole body extracts of *Culicoides* and *Stomoxys* contain numerous fractions with allergenic activity over a range of molecular weights.[234,259] *Culicoides* antigen stimulates equine blood mononuclear cell proliferation and release of eosinophil adherence, including factor(s).[230a]

Passive cutaneous anaphylaxis studies have shown that skin test reactivity can be transferred from affected horses to normal horses and guinea pigs.[236,245,249] Intradermal injections of anti-human IgE antibodies produce an identical reaction to that seen with *Culicoides* extracts.[236] When serum from affected horses is absorbed with anti-human IgE antibodies, the ability of the serum to transfer sensitivity to normal skin is markedly reduced.[236] The skin of affected horses has increased numbers of IgE-bearing cells in the superficial dermis (predominantly mast cells) and epidermis (presumably Langerhans' cells) and increased numbers of plasma cells expressing IgE.[262,262a] These observations suggest that IgE antibodies are involved in the pathogenesis of equine insect hypersensitivity.

Eosinophils, lymphocytes, Langerhans' cells, histamine, PAF, and LTB_4 play an important role in the pathogenesis of equine insect hypersensitivity.[″] Eosinophils and lymphocytes constitute the major inflammatory cells present in naturally occurring skin lesions, those produced by intradermal injections of insect antigens, and those induced by intradermal injections of PAF and histamine.[ʃ] Horses with insect hypersensitivity have increased numbers of peripheral blood eosinophils, lymphocytes, monocytes, and elevated blood histamine levels.[¥] In particular, numbers of CD5+ and CD4+ T lymphocytes and Langerhans' cells are increased in skin lesions.[223,230] LTB_4, LTC_4, and LTD_4 concentrations are increased in affected epidermis,[255] and peripheral blood basophils produce more sulfidoleukotrienes and histamine when exposed to insect (*Culicoides* and *Simulium*) extracts.[227b] No clear correlation was found between the numbers of mast cells at lesion sites and reactivity to intradermal injections of *Culicoides* extract.[235] IgG antibodies to *Culicoides* salivary antigens are present in horses with insect bite hypersensitivity and normal horses exposed to *Culicoides* gnats, but not in native Icelandic horses (no exposure to *Culicoides* gnats).[262b] IgE

[°]References 189, 195, 208, 216, 218a, 224, 262.
[†]References 50, 62, 189, 191, 199, 229, 244.
[‡]References 122, 182, 184-186, 199, 201, 208, 214, 218, 224, 234, 235, 244, 245, 257.
[§]References 18, 89, 109, 116, 117, 136, 146a-146c, 151, 156, 200, 214, 262.
[Π]References 182a, 191, 200, 204, 214, 252, 262.
[#]References 17, 18, 66, 122, 156, 185, 190, 191, 200, 227, 244, 245.
[″]References 40, 130, 157a, 186, 200, 205, 223, 230, 247, 252, 255.
[ʃ]References 130, 157a, 204, 223, 230, 252.
[¥]References 16, 53, 130, 185, 222, 230-232, 240, 249, 250.

antibodies to *Culicoides* salivary antigens were only detected in horses with insect bite hypersensitivity.[262b] Western blots showed that horses with insect bite hypersensitivity and normal horses exposed to *Culicoides* gnats have antibodies to many different *Culicoides* antigens and that the antibody profile varies from horse to horse.[262b]

Zinc has been shown to have potent immunomodulatory capacity, particularly influencing T helper cell organization and cytokine release.[253a] However, there were no differences in plasma zinc and copper levels or plasma copper:zinc ratios among horses with insect bite hypersensitivity and normal horses.[253a]

CLINICAL FEATURES

Insect hypersensitivity is the most common hypersensitivity and pruritic skin disorder of the horse, and it is worldwide in distribution.* It may be seen in any breed, in all ages, and in either sex. However, certain breeds appear to be at increased risk: Icelandic, German Shire, ponies, Arabians, Connemaras, and quarter horses. Most horses first develop clinical signs at 3 to 4 years of age. Coat color is not a risk factor. When such information is available, familial involvement is documentable in about one-third of the cases.

Clinical signs are distinctly seasonal (spring through fall) in temperate climates, paralleling the presence of insects. In warmer, subtropical to tropical climates, the disease can be nonseasonal with seasonal exacerbations. The condition typically worsens with age. Clinical signs are often worse near dusk and dawn (the favorite feeding times for many *Culicoides* species).

Affected horses usually show one of three patterns of skin disease: (1) dorsal distribution, (2) ventral distribution, and (3) some combination thereof. These differences in lesion distribution probably reflect the different preferential feeding sites of the various insect species. *Dorsal insect hypersensitivity* is characterized by pruritus, with or without crusted papules, usually beginning at the mane, rump (croup), and base of the tail (Fig. 8-20). The condition then usually extends to involve the face, pinna, neck, shoulder, and dorsal thorax. Self-trauma and chronicity lead to excoriations (erosions, ulcers), variable hair loss (hypotrichosis, alopecia), lichenification, and pigmentary disturbances (especially melanoderma and melanotrichia [Fig. 8-21]). Severely affected horses develop a "rat tail" (Fig. 8-4, *D*) and/or a "buzzed-off mane" (Fig. 8-4, *E*). *Ventral insect hypersensitivity* is characterized by pruritus with or without crusted papules, beginning on the ventral thorax and abdomen, axillae, and groin. The legs (Figs. 8-22 and 8-23) and intermandibular space are often involved. Secondary changes may occur as described above. Horses with insect hypersensitivity rarely have involvement of the flanks. In addition, horses with insect hypersensitivity uncommonly develop urticaria, and when they do, it is typically papular (see Urticaria and Angioedema).

Affected horses scratch and chew at themselves and rub against environmental objects (stalls fences, doorways, posts, trees, and so forth). Reflex nibbling movements can often be elicited by manipulation of the skin of the mane.[62] Secondary bacterial infections (superficial folliculitis, tail pyoderma [Fig. 8-4, *F*]) are not uncommon. These infections may have typical morphologies (see Chapter 4), or they may appear as areas of severe inflammation and/or oozing, possibly as a result of staphylococcal superantigens (see Chapter 4). Affected horses may suffer behavioral changes (anxious, nervous, restless, aggressive) and be unfit for riding, showing, or working. Some horses will lose weight due to the constant irritation.

Some horses have concurrent atopy and/or food hypersensitivity, which can greatly complicate the diagnostic work-up and therapeutic management.

---

*References 2, 8, 16-18, 21, 22, 29, 32, 37, 49, 50, 52-54, 56, 62, 65, 181, 184, 187-191, 199, 200, 201, 204, 207, 213, 216, 218-220, 224, 225, 228, 231, 232, 238-240, 246, 247, 256, 258, 260, 262, 263.

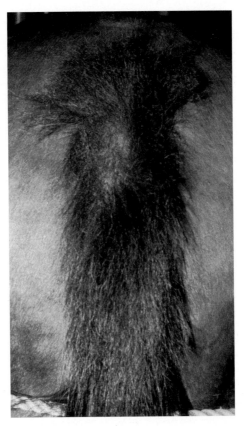

FIGURE 8-20. Self-induced tail damage in a horse with insect hypersensitivity.

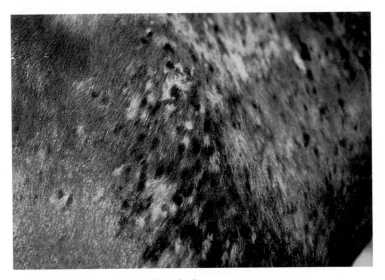

FIGURE 8-21. Melanotrichia caused by *Culicoides* hypersensitivity.

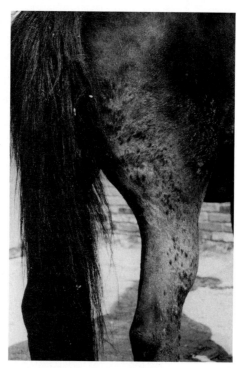

FIGURE 8-22. Traumatic hypotrichosis and melanotrichia in a horse with insect hypersensitivity.

DIAGNOSIS

The differential diagnosis will vary according to the distribution of lesions (see Atopy). The definitive diagnosis is based on history, physical examination, ruling-out other conditions, and response to insect control. Microscopic examination of affected hairs reveals fractured distal ends, which can be seen in any pruritic horse (Fig. 8-24).

Intradermal testing with insect extracts, especially *Culicoides* spp, is usually positive in horses with insect hypersensitivity.[*] Reactions may be present at 30 minutes (immediate), 4 to 6 hours (late-phase), 24 to 48 hours (delayed), or combinations of these. It must be remembered that normal horses may have positive reactions (especially at 30 minutes), and the prevalence of positive reactions in healthy horses increases with increasing age.[66,81-83,143,157a] In any case, *Culicoides* extracts for intradermal testing are not presently commercially available.

Antibodies against *Culicoides* and *Stomoxys* have been detected in the serum of affected horses by ELISA.[191] Other investigators have found no differences in ELISA scores (using *Culicoides* extract) between normal horses and horses with insect hypersensitivity.[262] The diagnostic value of ELISA results is presently undocumented.

IgG antibodies to *Culicoides* salivary antigens are present in both horses with insect bite hypersensitivity and normal horses exposed to *Culicoides* gnats.[262a] However, IgE antibodies to *Culicoides* salivary antigens were only detectable in horses with clinically active insect bite hypersensitivity.[262b] *Culicoides*-hypersensitive horses in clinical remission did *not* have detectable *Culicoides*-specific IgE.[262b]

---

[*]References 66, 122, 182, 184-186, 199, 201, 208, 214, 218, 224, 234, 235, 244, 245, 257.

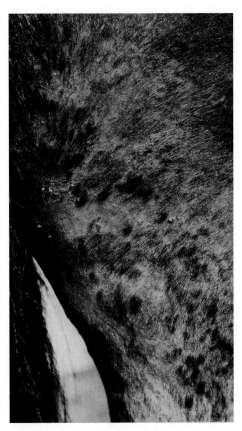

FIGURE 8-23. Close-up of horse in Fig. 8-22. Traumatic hypotrichosis, focal crusts and scales, and melanotrichia.

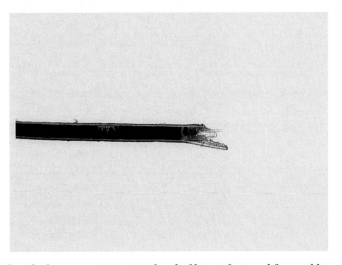

FIGURE 8-24. *Culicoides* hypersensitivity. Distal end of hair is fractured from rubbing.

Approximately 80% of the horses with insect hypersensitivity had positive basophil degranulation test results to *Culicoides* and/or *Simulium* extracts.[262] This test is not commercially available.

It was suggested that infra-red thermography was potentially useful for the early and out-of-season detection of insect hypersensitivity.[193] This has never been corroborated.

HISTOPATHOLOGY

The typical histologic appearance of insect hypersensitivity (naturally occurring lesions and those induced by intradermal injections of insect extracts) is a superficial and deep perivascular-to-interstitial dermatitis wherein eosinophils are the dominant inflammatory cell (Figs. 8-25 and 8-26).° Some horses have only a superficial perivascular-to-interstitial dermatitis. Some biopsy specimens have numerous lymphocytes, but eosinophils are usually predominant. Variable degrees of epidermal hyperplasia, hyperkeratosis (orthokeratotic and/or parakeratotic), spongiosis, eosinophilic and lymphocytic exocytosis, erosion and ulceration may be seen. Dermal edema and fibrosis are variably present. Focal areas of infiltrative-to-necrotizing eosinophilic mural folliculitis, and focal eosinophilic granulomas may be present.[252] Special stains (toluidine blue, tryptase) demonstrate increased numbers of mast cells in the superficial dermis.[262a] These histopathologic findings are not pathognomonic for insect hypersensitivity and may be seen in atopy and food hypersensitivity.

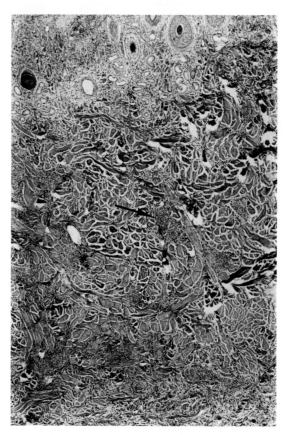

FIGURE 8-25. Deep perivascular dermatitis (*arrow*) with insect hypersensitivity.

°References 53, 185, 200, 222, 223, 230, 252, 255, 262a.

Immunohistochemical studies have shown that infiltrating lymphocytes are CD3+ and mostly CD4+ T cells and that T lymphocytes and Langerhans' cells are found in the lower layers of the epidermis and at the dermoepidermal junction.[223,230] Changes consistent with secondary bacterial infection (suppurative epidermitis, suppurative luminal folliculitis) may be seen.

CLINICAL MANAGEMENT

The management of insect hypersensitivity involves (1) insect control and (2) the use of topical and systemic antipruritic agents.* Treatment of unrugged, grazing horses is extremely difficult and frustrating.[50] Secondary infections must be recognized and treated, because they can cause the response to antipruritic agents to be poor.

When possible and practical, protective housing is effective. It may be needed from dusk to dawn or at other times, depending on the insect(s) involved. *Culicoides* gnats are able to pass through mosquito netting. A smaller mesh screen may be used. Housing and screens can be sprayed with residual insecticides as needed. Time-operated spray-mist insecticide systems are useful, but expensive. In general, *Culicoides* gnats are most active when the ambient temperature is above 50° F, when humidity is high, and when there is no breeze (see Chapter 6). Because *Culicoides* gnats are not strong fliers, powerful fans (floor, overhead) can be useful in stables. *Culicoides* gnats breed in standing water and generally fly short distances (¼ to ½ mile). Thus, avoidance or drainage of lakes, marshes, swamps, irrigation canals, and so forth can be beneficial. Rugging (using blankets and hoods on the horse) is also useful.

On-animal insect control protocols can be useful. Sprays, lotions, pour-ons, and rinses containing pyrethroids are particularly useful but must be applied daily or weekly, depending on the product and the environmental conditions and circumstances. A 4% permethrin pour-on

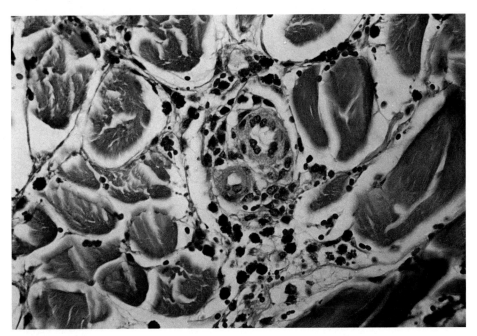

FIGURE 8-26. Skin biopsy specimen from horse with *Culicoides* hypersensitivity. Perivascular accumulation of eosinophils in deep dermis.

---

*References 2, 8, 16-18, 21, 22, 29, 32, 37, 49, 50, 52, 53, 62, 190, 194, 197-199, 220, 222, 232, 241, 244, 248, 254, 262.

(dorsal midline, once every 1 to 3 weeks) and an 0.5% fenvalerate spray (dorsal midline, every 7 days) have been recommended.[50,254] A commercial bath oil (Skin-So-Soft) diluted with equal parts of water has achieved anecdotal success as a leave-on repellent.[53,199] Cattle ear tags impregnated with various pyrethroids have been of anecdotal benefit when attached to halters and braided into manes and tails.[53,66,199] Maintaining a continuous film of liquid paraffin or mineral oil on the skin and hairs of the mane and tail has been reported to prevent *Culicoides* gnats from crawling down the hairs to the skin.[53,62,185,232]

Where protective housing and insecticidal protocols are inadequate or unfeasible, antipruritic therapy is needed. *Topical* antipruritic therapy can reduce pruritus for up to 72 hours and may help reduce the need for systemic agents (see Atopy and Chapter 3). Useful agents include cold water, hypoallergenic and moisturizing shampoos and rinses, and shampoos and rinses containing colloidal oatmeal or pramoxine.[157a,190]

Systemic antipruritic agents include glucocorticoids, antihistamines, omega-6/omega-3 fatty acids, and combinations of these (see Atopy). *Systemic glucocorticoids* are the most consistently effective agents.[*] Induction therapy may be accomplished with 2.2 mg/kg prednisolone or prednisone, or 0.22 mg/kg dexamethasone, given every morning until pruritus is controlled. Maintenance therapy is best accomplished with alternate-morning prednisolone or prednisone (see Chapter 3).

Antihistamines may be of benefit, especially for reducing needed doses of glucocorticoids and when used synergistically with omega-6/omega-3 fatty acids (see Atopy).[†] Useful antihistamines include hydroxyzine (1 to 2 mg/kg q8-12h orally), chlorpheniramine (0.25 to 0.5 mg/kg q12h orally), diphenhydramine (1 to 2 mg/kg q8-12h orally), and doxepin (0.5 to 0.75 mg/kg q12h orally). *Omega-6/omega-3 fatty acids* may be useful for reducing needed glucocorticoid doses and when used synergistically with antihistamines (see Atopy).[157a] In two double-blinded, placebo-controlled clinical studies, no significant reduction in pruritus occurred in allergic horses treated orally with linseed oil[74] or a commercial product (evening primrose oil and cold water marine fish oil).[71] These studies are difficult to interpret because (1) it was not clear how many horses had insect hypersensitivity, atopy, or both, and (2) the horses' base diets were not analyzed (see page 417). Many clinicians feel that omega-6/omega-3 fatty acid supplementation is beneficial in allergic horses.[‡] Although fish oils are rarely palatable to horses, a commercial fatty acid supplement (DVM Derm Caps 100s) given orally at 1 capsule per 50 to 100 kg q12h, appears to be well tolerated and effective in some horses (see Atopy).[157a]

The usefulness of *allergen-specific immunotherapy (hyposensitization)* in equine insect hypersensitivity is unclear. Early attempts to use immunotherapy were reported to be unsuccessful when intradermal reactions to *Culicoides* were positive.[124,155] A few horses that had positive reactions to only mosquito or black fly extracts appeared to respond well.

A small study (14 horses) was conducted in double-blinded, placebo-controlled fashion using an aqueous whole body extract of *C. variipenis*.[188] There was no difference in response to the *Culicoides* extract versus the placebo. Possible areas of concern with this study are (1) it lasted only 6 months (immunotherapy for atopy is continued for at least 1 year), and (2) injections were given every 20 days after an initial 46-day induction period.

Another small study (10 horses) was conducted in an open fashion using a whole body *C. variipenis* extract in adjuvant (mycobacterial cell wall fraction).[183] Injections were administered subcutaneously every 6 to 10 days for the first year, and every month or so for the second year. After 2 years, 8 of the 10 horses had moderate to complete control of their pruritus. This protocol should be repeated in a double-blinded, placebo-controlled fashion in a larger number of horses.

---

[*]References 2, 17, 32, 50, 52, 53, 67, 81-83, 157a, 190, 199, 200, 222, 240, 241, 244.
[†]References 17, 81-83, 157a, 205, 234, 240-242.
[‡]References 17, 18, 81-83, 117, 157a.

An aqueous whole body flea extract was administered intradermally once weekly to horses with presumptive insect hypersensitivity (intradermal testing not performed).[53] Three of 6 horses responded well.

Anecdotal reports indicate that homeopathic remedies,[253] "active biologic peptides,"[209] animal tissue preparations and autologous blood,[180] and a 10% salicylic acid topical solution[217] are useful in horses with insect hypersensitivity.

Due to the hereditary nature of insect hypersensitivity, affected horses should not be used for breeding.

PARASITE HYPERSENSITIVITIES

Although not well documented, hypersensitivity is thought to be significant in the pathogenesis of some parasite-associated equine dermatoses.[52,53] Various *intestinal parasites* have been suspected to be the cause of pruritic and variably seborrheic dermatoses, especially in foals.[34,179] *Cutaneous onchocerciasis* is believed to be a hypersensitivity reaction associated with the microfilariae of *Onchocerca cervicalis* (see Chapter 6). *Cutaneous habronemiasis* is believed to be, in part, a hypersensitivity reaction to the larval stages of *Habronema muscae, H. majus,* and *Draschia megastoma* (see Chapter 6).

● REFERENCES

General

1. Bacon KB, Schall TJ: Chemokines as mediators of allergic inflammation. Int Arch Allergy Immunol 109:97, 1996.
2. Barbet JL, et al: Diseases of the skin. In: Colahan PT, et al (eds). Equine Medicine and Surgery IV, Vol. II. American Veterinary Publications, Inc., Goleta., 1991, p 1569.
3. Benjamin E, et al: Immunology, A Short Course III. Wiley-Liss, New York, 1996.
4. Beutner EH, et al: Immunopathology of the Skin III. Churchill Livingstone, New York, 1987.
5. Bone J, et al (eds): Equine Medicine and Surgery I. American Veterinary Publications, Inc., Wheaton, 1963.
6. Borish L, Rosenwasser LJ: Update on cytokines. J Allergy Clin Immunol 97:719, 1996.
7. Bos JD: Skin Immune System. CRC Press, Boca Raton, 1990.
8. Byars DT: Allergic skin diseases in the horse. Vet Clin N Am Large Anim Pract 6:87, 1984.
9. Campbell SG: Diseases of Allergy. In: Catcott EJ, Smithcors, JF (eds). Equine Medicine & Surgery II. American Veterinary Publications, Santa Barbara, 1972, p 227.
10. Cannon AG, Affolter VK: What does 'CD' mean? Proc Annu Memb Meet Am Acad Vet Dermatol Am Coll Vet Dermatol 14:133, 1998.
11. Catcott EJ, Smithcors JF: Equine Medicine and Surgery II. American Veterinary Publications, Inc., Santa Barbara, 1972.
12. Charlesworth EN, et al: Cutaneous late phase response to allergen. Mediator release and inflammatory cell infiltration. J Clin Invest 83:1519, 1989.
13. Colahan PT, et al: Equine Medicine and Surgery IV. American Veterinary Publications, Inc., Goleta, 1991.
14. Dahl MV. Immunodermatology II. Year Book Medical Publishers, Chicago, 1988.
15. Eyre P, Hanna CJ: Equine allergies. Equine Pract 2:40, 1980.
16. Fadok VA, Mullowney PC: Dermatologic diseases of horses, part I. Parasitic dermatoses of the horse. Compend Cont Educ 5:S615, 1983.
17. Fadok VA: Dermatology. The Veterinary Clinics of North America: Equine Practice, April, 1995.
18. Fadok VA: Update on equine allergies. Vet Allergy Clin Immunol 5:68, 1997.
19. Fadok VA: Immunology can be fun! The Starwars approach to immune function. Proc Annu Memb Meet Am Acad Vet Dermatol Am Coll Vet Dermatol 15:81, 1999.
20. Freedberg IM, et al: Fitzpatrick's Dermatology in General Medicine V. McGraw-Hill, New York, 1999.
21. Halldórsdóttir S. Hudlidelser hos hest. Norsk Vet 102:19, 1990.
22. Halliwell REW. Clinical and immunological aspects of allergic skin diseases in domestic animals. In: von Tscharner C, Halliwell REW (eds). Advances in Veterinary Dermatology I. Baillière-Tindall, Philadelphia, 1990, p 91.
23. Halliwell REW, Gorman NT: Veterinary Clinical Immunology. W.B. Saunders Co., Philadelphia, 1989.
24. Hargis AM, Liggit HD: Cytokines and their role in cutaneous injury. In: Ihrke PJ, et al (eds). Advances in Veterinary Dermatology II. Pergamon Press, New York, 1993, p 325.
25. Hargis AM, et al: Spongiotic vesicular dermatitis as a cutaneous reaction pattern in seven horses. Vet Dermatol 12:291, 2001.
26. Hauser C, et al: T helper cells grown with hapten-modified cultured Langerhans' cells produce interleukin 4 and stimulate IgE production by B cells. Eur J Immunol 19:245, 1989.
27. Hauser C, et al: Superantigens and their role in immune-mediated diseases. J Invest Dermatol 101:503, 1993.

28. Hill PB, Martin RJ: A review of mast cell biology. Vet Dermatol 9:145, 1998.
29. Hopes R: Skin diseases of the horse. Vet Dermatol News 1:4, 1976.
30. Ihrke PJ, et al: Advances in Veterinary Dermatology II. Pergamon Press, New York, 1993.
31. Jakob T, Udey MC: Epidermal Langerhans' cells: From precursors to nature's adjuvants. Adv Dermatol 14:209, 1999.
32. Kobluk CN, et al: The Horse. Diseases and Clinical Management. W.B. Saunders Co., Philadelphia, 1995.
33. Kondo S, Saunder DH: Epidermal cytokines in allergic contact dermatitis. J Am Acad Dermatol 33:786, 1995.
34. Kral F, Schwartzman RM: Veterinary and Comparative Dermatology. JB Lippincott Co., Philadelphia, 1964.
35. Littlewood JD: Diagnostic procedures in equine skin disease. Equine Vet Educ 9:174, 1997.
36. Luger TA, Schwartz T: Evidence for an epidermal cytokine network. J Invest Dermatol 95:100S, 1990.
37. Manning TO, Sweeney C: Immune-mediated equine skin diseases. Compend Cont Ed 8:979, 1986.
38. Mansmann RA, et al: Equine Medicine and Surgery III. American Veterinary Publications, Inc., Santa Barbara, 1982.
39. Martin LB, et al: Eosinophils in allergy: role in disease, degranulation, and cytokines. Int Arch Allergy Immunol 109:207, 1996.
40. McEwan BJ, et al: The response of the eosinophil in acute inflammation in the horse. In: von Tscharner C, Halliwell REW (eds). Advances in Veterinary Dermatology I. Baillière-Tindall, Philadelphia, 1990, p 176.
40a. McFarlane D, et al: Age-related quantitative alterations in lymphocyte subsets and immunoglobulin isotypes in healthy horses. Am J Vet Res 62:1413, 2001.
41. McKenzie RC, Sauder DN: The role of keratinocyte cytokines in inflammation and immunity. J Invest Dermatol 95:105S, 1990.
42. McMullen WC: The skin. In: Mansmann RA, et al (eds). Equine Medicine and Surgery III. American Veterinary Publications, Santa Barbara, 1982, p 793.
43. Mecheris DB. Unraveling the mast cell dilemma: Culprit or victim of its generosity? Immunol Today 18:212, 1997.
44. Middleton E, et al: Allergy Principles and Practice V. Mosby, St. Louis, 1998.
45. Mullowney PC. Dermatologic diseases of horses part V. Allergic, immune-mediated, and miscellaneous skin diseases. Compend Cont Ed 7:S217, 1985.
46. Nickoloff BJ. Dermal Immune System. CRC Press, Boca Raton, 1993.
47. Page EH: Common skin diseases of the horse. Proc Am Assoc Equine Practit 18:385, 1972.
48. Pascoe RR: The nature and treatment of skin conditions observed in horses in Queensland. Aust Vet J 49:35, 1973.
49. Pascoe RR: Equine Dermatoses. University of Sydney Post-Graduate Foundation in Veterinary Science, Review No. 21, 1981.
50. Pascoe RRR, Knottenbelt DC: Manual of Equine Dermatology. W.B. Saunders Co., Philadelphia, 1999.
51. Prieto VG, et al: Quantitative immunohistochemical differences in Langerhans' cells in dermatitis due to internal versus external antigen sources. J Cutan Pathol 25:301, 1998.
52. Reed SM, Bagly WM: Equine Internal Medicine. W.B. Saunders Co., Philadelphia, 1998.
53. Scott DW. Large Animal Dermatology. W.B. Saunders Co., Philadelphia, 1988.
54. Scott DW: Diagnostic des dermatoses inflammatoires équines: analyse de la modalité de réaction histopathologique: étude personnelle portant sur 315 cas. Point Vét 24:245, 1992.
55. Scott DW, et al: Muller & Kirk's Small Animal Dermatology VI. W.B. Saunders Co., Philadelphia, 2001.
56. Sloet van Oldruitenborg-Oosterbaan MM: Allergisch bedingte Hauterkrankungen des Pferdes. Prakt Tier 69:9, 1988.
57. Stannard AA: Some important dermatoses in the horse. Mod Vet Pract 55:31, 1972.
58. Stannard AA: The skin. In: Catcott EJ, Smicors JR (eds). Equine Medicine & Surgery II. American Veterinary Publications, Inc., Wheaton, 1972, p 381.
59. Stannard AA: Equine dermatology. Proc Am Assoc Equine Practit 22:273, 1976.
60. Sunderkötter C, et al: Aging and the skin immune system. Arch Dermatol 133:1256, 1997.
61. Swerlick RA, Lawley TJ: Role of microvascular endothelial cells in inflammation. J Invest Dermatol 100:111S, 1993.
62. Thomsett LR. Skin diseases of the horse. In Pract 1:16, 1979.
63. Tizard IR: Veterinary Immunology: An Introduction V. W.B. Saunders Co., Philadelphia, 1997.
64. van der Haegen A, et al: Les affections cutanées allergiques 2-atopie, dermatite de contact, allergie alimentaire, urticaire, granulome éosinophilique. Prat Vét Equine 32:23, 2000.
65. von Tscharner C: Die wichtigsten Hautkrankheiten beim Pferde. Prakt Tier 69:4, 1988.
66. von Tscharner C, Halliwell REW: Advances in Veterinary Dermatology I. Baillière-Tindall, Philadelphia, 1990.
67. von Tscharner C, et al: Stannard's Illustrated Equine Dermatology Notes. Vet Dermatol 11:161, 2000.
68. Walsh LJ, Murphy GF: Role of adhesion molecules in cutaneous inflammation and neoplasia. J Cutan Pathol 19:161, 1992.
69. Yager JA: The skin as an immune organ. In: Ihrke PJ, et al (eds). Advances in Veterinary Dermatology II. Pergamon Press, New York, 1993, p 3.
70. Yager JA: The skin as an immune organ. In: Kwochka KW, et al (eds). Advances in Veterinary Dermatology III. Pergamon Press, New York, 1996, p 3.

Allergy Therapy

70a. Bergvall K, et al: Pharmacodynamics of Clemastine in healthy horses. Proc Ann Memb Meet Am Acad Vet Dermatol Am Coll Vet Dermatol 17:23, 2002.
71. Craig JM, et al: A double-blind placebo-controlled trial of an evening primrose and fish oil combination versus hydrogenated coconut oil in the management of recurrent seasonal pruritus in horses. Vet Dermatol 8:177, 1997.
72. Cunningham FM, et al: Pharmacology of the 5-lipoxygenase inhibitors BAY Y 1015 and BAY X 1005 in the horse. J Vet Pharmacol Therapy 20:296, 1997.
73. Foster AP, et al: Actions of PAF receptor antagonists in horses with the allergic skin disease sweet itch. Inflamm Res 44:412, 1995.

74. Friberg CA, Logas D: Treatment of *Culicoides* hypersensitive horses with high-dose N-3 fatty acids: a double-blinded crossover study. Vet Dermatol 10:117, 1999.

74a. Hansen RA, et al: Effects of dietary flaxseed oil supplementation on equine plasma fatty acid concentrations and whole blood platelet aggregation. J Vet Intern Med 16:457, 2002.

75. Henry MM, et al: Effect of dietary alpha-linolenic acid on equine monocyte procoagulant activity and eicosanoid synthesis. Circ Shock 32:173, 1990.

76. Henry MM, et al: Influence of an omega-3 fatty acid-enriched ration on in vivo responses of horses to endotoxin. Am J Vet Res 52:523, 1993.

77. McCann ME, Carnick JB: Potential uses of W-3 fatty acids in equine diseases. Compend Cont Educ Pract Vet 20:637, 1998.

78. Morris DD, et al: Effect of dietary linolenic acid on endotoxin-induced thromboxane and prostacyclin production by equine peritoneal macrophages. Circ Shock 29:311, 1989.

79. Morris DD, et al: Effect of dietary alpha-linolenic acid on endotoxin-induced production of tumor necrosis factor by peritoneal macrophages in horses. Am J Vet Res 52:528, 1991.

80. Olsen SC, et al: Inhibition of equine mononuclear cell proliferation and leukotriene B4 synthesis by a specific 5-lipoxygenase inhibitor, A-63162. Am J Vet Res 53:1015, 1992.

81. Rosenkrantz WS, Frank LA: Therapy of equine pruritus. In: Ihrke RJ, et al (eds). Advances in Veterinary Dermatology II. Pergamon Press, Oxford, 1993, p 433.

82. Rosenkrantz WS: Systemic/topical therapy. Vet Clin N Am Equine Pract 11:127, 1995.

83. White SD, Rosenkrantz WS: Advances in equine dermatology. In: Kwochka KW, et al (eds). Advances in Veterinary Dermatology III. Butterworth-Heinemann, Boston, 1998, p 409.

Urticaria and Angioedema

84. Anderson IL: An unusual reaction in a horse during anesthesia. NZ Vet J 31:85, 1983.

85. Anderson WI, et al: Adverse reaction to penicillin in horses. Mod Vet Pract 64:928, 1983.

86. Bhikane AU, et al: Hypersensitivity reaction in a horse following injection of Belamyl (B complex and liver extract). Indian Vet J 70:167, 1993.

87. Cornick JL, Brumbaugh GW: Dermatographism in a horse. Cornell Vet 79:109, 1989.

88. Due T: Urticarier hos hest. Dansk Veterinaer 82:540, 1999.

89. Evans AG, et al: Intradermal skin testing of horses with chronic obstructive pulmonary disease and recurrent urticaria. Am J Vet Res 53:203, 1992.

90. Evans AG: Urticaria in horses. Compend Cont Edu 15:626, 1993.

91. Fadok VA: Of horses and men: urticaria. Vet Dermatol 1:103, 1990.

92. Goldberg GP, Short CE: Challenge in equine anesthesia: a suspected allergic reaction during acetylpromazine, guaifenesin, thiamylal, and halothane anesthesia. Equine Pract 10:5, 1988.

93. Greatorex JC: Urticaria, bluenose and purpura haemorrhagica in horses. Equine Vet J 1:157, 1968.

93a. Hallebeek AJM, et al: "Haverbultjes" bij paarden. Tijd Diergeneesk 20:588, 1995.

94. Halliwell RE: Urticaria and angioedema. In: Robinson NE (ed). Current Therapy in Equine Medicine I. W.B. Saunders Co., Philadelphia, 1983, p 535.

95. Klein L: Urticaria in the horse after anesthesia. N Z Vet J 31:206, 1983.

96. Littlewood JL: Urticaria: a clinical challenge. Equine Vet Educ 3:36, 1991.

96a. Logas D, et al: Cholinergic pruritus in a horse. J Am Vet Med Assoc 201:90, 1992.

97. Matthews NS, et al: Urticaria during anesthesia in a horse. Equine Vet J 25:55, 1994.

98. McGladdery AJ: Recurrent urticaria in a Thoroughbred stallion. Equine Vet Educ 3:126, 1991.

99. Miyazawa K, et al: An equine case of urticaria associated with dry garlic feeding. J Vet Med Sci 53:747, 1991.

100. Paterson S: Investigation of skin disease and urticaria in the horse. In Pract 22:446, 2000.

101. Prickett ME: The untoward reaction of the horse to injection of antigenic substances. J Am Vet Med Assoc 155:258, 1969.

101a. Schott HC, et al: Linear "zebra" urticarial dermatosis in multiple horses. Vet Dermatol 11(suppl. 1):21, 2000.

102. Wirth D, Kyscher A: Streifenartige urtikarielle Hauterkrantung (Streifenurtikaria) bei Pferden. Wien Tierärztl Monatsschr 37:449, 1950.

103. Wolfrom E, et al: Chronic urticaria and *Toxocara canis* infection: a case-study. Ann Dermatol Venercol 123:240, 1996.

104. Yu AA: Equine urticaria: a diagnostic dilemma. Compend Cont Educ Pract Vet 22:277, 2000.

Atopy and Cutaneous Inflammation

104a. Alaba O: Allergies in dogs and cats: Allergen-specific IgE determination by VARL Liquid Gold compared with ELISA/RAST. Vet Allergy Clin Immunol 5:93, 1992.

105. Archer RK: Eosinophil leukocyte attracting effect of histamine in skin. Nature 187:155, 1960.

106. Asmis R, Jorg A: Calcium-ionophore-induced formation of platelet-activating factor and leukotrienes by horse eosinophils: A comparative study. Eur J Biochem 187:475, 1990.

107. Auer DE, et al: Superoxide production by stimulated equine polymorphonuclear leukocytes inhibition by anti-inflammatory drugs. J Vet Pharmacol Therapy 13:59, 1990.

108. Auer DE, et al: Assessment of histamine, bradykinin, prostaglandin E1 and E2 and carrageenin as vascular permeability agents in the horse. J Vet Pharmacol Therapy 14:61, 1991.

108a. Boguniewicz M, Leung DYM: Atopic dermatitis. A question of balance. Arch Dermatol 134:870, 1998.

108b. Bottoms GD, et al: Endotoxin-induced eicosanoid production by equine vascular endothelial cells and neutrophils. Circ Shock 15:155, 1985.

109. Bourdeau P, Lebis C: Common allergens in 83 horses. Proc Ann Congress Eur Soc Vet Dermatol Eur Coll Vet Dermatol 15:166, 1998.

110. Burka JF, et al: Chemical mediators of anaphylaxis (histamine, 5-HT, and SRS-A) released from horse lung and leukocytes in vitro. Res Comm Chem Pathol Pharmacol 13:379, 1976.

111. Carr SH: A practitioner report: equine allergic dermatitis. Florida Vet J 10:20, 1981.

112. Coca AF, Cooke RA: On classification of the phenomena of hypersensitiveness. J Immunol 6:163, 1923.

113. Coca AF, Grove EF: Studies in hypersensitiveness. A study of the atopic reagins. J Immunol 10:445, 1925.

114. Dawson J, et al: Eicosanoids and equine leukocyte locomotion in vitro. Equine Vet J 18:493, 1986.

115. Dawson J, et al: Platelet activating factor as a mediator of equine cell locomotion. Vet Res Commun 12:101, 1988.

116. Delger JM: Cutaneous reactivity to mold allergens in normal horses. Proc Annu Memb Meet Am Acad Vet Dermatol Am Coll Vet Dermatol 9:25, 1993.

117. Delger JM: Intradermal testing and immunotherapy in horses. Vet Med 92:635, 1997.

117a. Eder C, et al: Influence of environmental and genetic factors on allergen-specific immunoglobulin E levels in sera from Lippizan horses. Equine Vet J 33:714, 2001.

118. Elliott FA: Allergens-apparent cause of "summer itch" (equine). Calif Vet 13:29, 1970.

119. Evans AG: Recurrent urticaria due to inhaled allergens. In: Robinson NE (ed). Current Therapy in Equine Medicine II. W.B. Saunders Co., Philadelphia, 1987, 619.

120. Eyre P: Anaphylactic (skin sensitizing) antibodies in the horse. Vet Rec 90:36, 1972.

121. Eyre P: Preliminary studies on pharmacological antagonism of anaphylaxis in the horse. Can J Comp Med 40:149, 1976.

122. Fadok VA: Equine pruritus: Results of intradermal skin testing. Proc Annu Memb Meet Am Acad Vet Dermatol Am Coll Vet Dermatol 2:6, 1986.

123. Fadok VA: Overview of equine pruritus. Vet Clin N Am Equine Pract 11:1, 1995.

124. Fadok VA: Hyposensitization of equids with allergic skin/pulmonary diseases. Proc Annu Memb Meet Am Acad Vet Dermatol Am Coll Vet Dermatol 12:47, 1996.

125. Foster AP, et al: Inflammatory effects of platelet activating factor (PAF) in equine skin. Equine Vet J 24:208, 1992.

126. Foster AP, et al: Platelet activating factor is a mediator of equine neutrophil and eosinophil migration in vitro. Res Vet Sci 53:223, 1992.

127. Foster AP, et al: Inhibitory effects of the PAF receptor antagonist WEB 2086 on antigen-induced responses in equine allergic skin disease. Br J Pharmacol 108:13P, 1993.

128. Foster AP, Cunningham FM: PAF- and LTB4-induced migration of eosinophils and neutrophils isolated from horses with allergic skin disease. Agents Actions 41:C258, 1994.

129. Foster AP, Cunningham FM: Histamine induces equine eosinophil superoxide production via H1 receptor activation. Inflammation Res 44:S266, 1995.

130. Foster AP, et al: Platelet activating factor mimics antigen-induced cutaneous inflammatory responses in sweet itch horses. Vet Immunol Immunopathol 44:115, 1995.

131. Foster AP, et al: Agonist-induced adherence of equine eosinophils to fibronectin. Vet. Immunol Immunopathol 56:205, 1997.

132. Foster AP, Cunningham FM: Differential superoxide anion generation by equine eosinophils and neutrophils. Vet Immunol Immunopathol 59:222, 1997.

133. Foster AP, et al: Inhibition of antigen-induced cutaneous responses of ponies with insect hypersensitivity by the histamine-1 receptor antagonist chlorpheniramine. Vet Rec 143:189, 1998.

134. Foster AP, Cunningham FM: Histamine-induced adherence and migration of equine eosinophils. Am J Vet Res 59:1153, 1998.

135. Foster AP, Cunningham FM: The pathogenesis and immunopharmacology of equine insect hypersensitivity. In: Kwochka KW, et al (eds). Advances in Veterinary Dermatology III. Butterworth Heinemann, Boston, 1988, p 177.

135a. Graham-Brown RAC: Therapeutics in atopic dermatitis. Dermatol 13:3, 1998.

136. Halliwell REW, et al: The role of allergy in chronic pulmonary diseases of horses. J Am Vet Med Assoc 174:277, 1979.

137. Hanna CJ, et al: Equine immunology 2: immunopharmacology-biochemical basis of hypersensitivity. Equine Vet J 14:16, 1982.

137a. Hauser C, Orbea HA: Superantigens and their role in immune-mediated diseases. J Invest Dermatol 101:503, 1993.

138. Higgins AJ, Lees P: Phenylbutazone inhibition of prostaglandin E2 production in equine acute inflammatory exudate. Vet Rec 113:622, 1983.

139. Higgins AJ, Lees P: Detection of leukotriene B4 in equine inflammatory exudate. Vet Rec 115:275, 1984.

140. Higgins AJ, et al: Influence of phenylbutazone on eicosanoid levels in equine acute inflammatory exudate. Cornell Vet 74:198, 1984.

140a. Hofer MF, et al: Staphylococcal toxins augment specific IgE responses by atopic patients exposed to allergen. J Invest Dermatol 112:171, 1999.

141. Jorg A, et al: Purification of horse eosinophil peroxide. Biochem Biophys Acta 701:185, 1982.

142. Jorg A, et al: Leukotriene generation by eosinophils. J Exper Med 155:390, 1982.

142a. Jose-Cunilleras E, et al: Intradermal testing in healthy horses and horses with chronic obstructive pulmonary disease, recurrent urticaria, or allergic dermatitis. J Am Vet Med Assoc 219:1115, 2001.

143. Kamphues J: Risiken durch Mängel in der hygienischen Qualität von Futtermitteln für Pferde. Pferdeheilk 12:326, 1996.

144. Klebanoff SJ, et al: Comparative toxicity of the horse eosinophil peroxidase-H_2O_2 halide system and granule basic proteins. J Immunol 143:239, 1989.

144a. Kolm-Stark G, Wagner R: Intradermal skin testing in Icelandic horses in Austria. Equine Vet J 34:405, 2002.

145. Lees P, et al: Eicosanoids and equine leukocyte locomotion in vitro. Equine Vet J 18:493, 1986.

146. Littlewood JD, et al: Atopy-like skin disease in the horse. In: Kwochka KW, et al (eds). Advances in Veterinary Dermatology III. Butterworth-Heinemann, Boston, 1988, p 563.

146a. Lorch G et al: Results of intradermal tests in horses without atopy and horses with chronic obstructive pulmonary disease. Am J Vet Res 62:389, 2001.

146b. Lorch G, et al: Results of intradermal tests in horses without atopy and horses with atopic dermatitis or recurrent urticaria. Am J Vet Res 62:1051, 2001.

146c. Lorch G, et al: Comparison of immediate intradermal test reactivity with serum IgE quantitation by use of a radioallergosorbent test and two ELISA in horses with and without atopy. J Am Vet Med Ass 218:1314, 2001.

147. Margo AM, et al: Characterization of IgE-mediated histamine release from equine basophils. Equine Vet J 20:352, 1988.

148. Matthews AG, et al: A reagin-like antibody in horse serum: 1. Occurrence and some biological properties. Vet Res Commun 6:13:, 1983.

149. May SA et al: Late-stage mediators of the inflammatory response: identification of interleukin-1 and a casein-degrading enzyme in equine acute inflammatory exudates. Res Vet Sci 50:14, 1991.

150. McEwen BJ, et al: The effect of leukotriene B4, leukotriene C4, zymosan-activated serum, histamine, tabanid extract and n-formyl-methionyl-leucyl-phenylalanine on the in vitro migration of equine eosinophils. Can J Vet Res 54:400, 1990.

151. McPherson FA, et al: Chronic obstructive pulmonary disease (COPD) in horses: aetiological studies: responses to intradermal and inhalation antigenic challenge. Equine Vet J 11:159, 1979.

152. Morrow A, et al: Dermal reactivity to histamine, serotonin and bradykinin in relation to allergic skin reactions of the horse. J Vet Pharmacol Therapy 9:40, 1986.

152a. Navarro P, et al: The complete cDNA and deduced amino acid sequence of equine IgE. Mol Immunol 32:1, 1995.

153. Piller K, Portmann P: Isolation and characterization of four horse basic proteins from horse eosinophilic granules. Biochem Biophys Res Commun 192:373, 1993.

154. Potter KA, et al: Stimulation of equine eosinophil migration by hydroxyacid metabolites of arachidonic acid. Am J Pathol 121:361, 1985.

154a. Rees CA: Response to immunotherapy in six related horses with urticaria secondary to atopy. J Am Vet Med Assoc 218:753, 2001.

154b. Rees CA: Equine pruritic skin disease part II. Proc Ann Memb Meet Am Acad Vet Dermatol Am Coll Vet Dermatol 17:149, 2002.

155. Rosenkrantz W, Griffin C: Treatment of equine urticaria and pruritus with hyposensitization and antihistamines. Proc Annu Memb Met Am Acad Vet Dermatol Am Coll Vet Dermatol 2:33, 1986.

156. Rosenkrantz WS, et al: Responses in horses to intradermal challenge of insects and environmental allergens with specific immunotherapy. In: Kwochka KW, et al (eds). Advances in Veterinary Dermatology III. Butterworth-Heinemann, Boston, 1998, p 200.

156a. Ruzicka T: Atopic eczema: between rationality and irrationality. Arch Dermatol 134:1462, 1998.

157. Schatzmann U, et al: Active and passive cutaneous anaphylaxis in the horse following immunization with benzyl-penicilloyl-bovine gammaglobulin (BPO20-BGG). Res Vet Sci 15:347, 1973.

157a. Scott DW: La dermatite atopique du cheval. Méd Vét Québec 30:82, 2000.

158. Sedgwick AD, et al: Lysosomal enzyme release in equine nonimmune acute inflammatory exudate. Equine Vet J 18:68, 1986.

159. Seethanathan P, et al: Characterization of release of tumor necrosis factor, interleukin-1, and superoxide anion from equine white blood cells in response to endotoxin. Am J Vet Res 51:1221, 1990.

160. Shipstone M, et al: The use of compound 48/80 as a positive control in equine intradermal allergy testing. Vet Dermatol 10:291, 1999.

160a. Skov L, Baadsgaard O: Superantigens: do they have a role in skin disease? Arch Dermatol 131:829, 1995.

161. Slauson DO, et al: Complement-induced equine neutrophil adhesiveness and aggregation. Vet Pathol 24:239, 1987.

162. Sloet van Oldruitenborgh-Oosterbaan MM, et al: Intradermal allergy testing in normal horses. In: Kwochka KW, et al (eds). Advances in Veterinary Dermatology III. Butterworth-Heinemann, Boston, 1998, p 564.

163. Suter M, Fey H: Isolation and characterization of equine IgE. Zbl Vet Med B 28:414, 1981.

164. Suter M, et al: Histologische und morphologische Charakterisieurung von Pferde-Reagin (IgE) mittels Prausnitz-Küstner-Technik. Schweiz Arch Tierheilk 123:647, 1981.

165. Suter M, Fey H: Further purification and characterization of horse IgE. Vet Immunol Immunopathol 4:545, 1983.

166. Suter M, Fey H: Allergen-specific ELISA for horse IgE. Vet Immunol Immunopathol 4:555, 1983.

167. Tallarico NJ, Tallarico CM: Results of intradermal allergy testing and treatment by hyposensitization of 64 horses with chronic obstructive pulmonary disease, urticaria, head shaking, and/or reactive airway disease. Vet Allergy Clin Immunol 6:25, 1998.

168. Vanderput S, et al: Airborne dust and aeroallergen concentrations in different sources of feed and bedding for horses. Vet Quart 19:154, 1997.

168a. Wassom DL: Principles and history of the Fc epsilon receptor (FcRI) for IgE detection. Compend Cont Educ Pract Vet 19(suppl):6, 1997.

168b. Watson JL, et al: Molecular cloning and sequencing of the low-affinity IgE receptor (CD23) for horse and cattle. Vet Immunol Immunopathol 73:323, 2000.

169. Webster AJF, et al: Air hygiene in stables 1: effects of stable design, ventilation, and management on the concentration of respirable dust. Equine Vet J 19:448, 1987.

170. Woods PSA, et al: Airborne dust and aeroallergen concentration in a horse stable under two different management systems. Equine Vet J 25:208, 1993.

Contact Hypersensitivity

171. Baadsgaard O, Wang T: Immune regulation in allergic and irritant skin reactions. Int J Dermatol 30:161, 1991.

171a. Baltus V, Henschmann R: Toxische Kontaktdermatitis bei Pferden durch erhöhte Werte von 6 wertigen Chrom in Ledersattelgurten. Pferdheilk 12:839, 1996.

172. Brose E, et al: Nicht-IgE-vermittelte Allergien beim Pferd-Falldarstellung einer Typ IV—Allergie auf Baumwolle. Prakt Tierärztl 80:1072, 1999.

173. Bryce A, et al: Skin conditions – horse – following spraying for ticks. Univ Sydney Post-Grad Comm Vet Sci Control & Therapy 132:227, 1986.

174. Cordes T: Apparent contact dermatitis in hunter/jumper show horses. Mod Vet Pract 68:240, 1987.

175. Ihrke PJ: Contact dermatitis. In: Robinson NE (ed). Current Therapy in Equine Medicine I. W.B. Saunders Co., Philadelphia, 1983, p 547.

176. Reddin L, Steven DW: Allergic contact dermatitis. N Am Vet 27:561, 1946.

177. Rietschel RL: Irritant contact dermatitis. Mechanisms in irritant contact dermatitis. Clin Dermatol 15:557, 1997.

Food Hypersensitivity

178. Littlewood JL: Case report—allergic skin report in a horse. Vet Dermatol News 14:24, 1992.
179. Walton GS: Allergic responses involving the skin of domestic animals. Adv Vet Sci Comp Med 15:201, 1970.

Insect Hypersensitivity

180. Aichinger O: Aus der praxis: Summerekzem der Pferde-Erfolgreiche Behandlung mit injektionen und Eigenblut. Tierärztl Umschau 54:322, 1999.
181. Anderson GS, et al: The hypersensitivity of horses to *Culicoides* bites in British Columbia. Can Vet J 29:718, 1988.
182. Anderson GS, et al: *Culicoides* (Diptera: Ceratopogonidae) as a causal agent of *Culicoides* hypersensitivity (sweet itch) in British Columbia. J Med Entomol 28:685, 1991.
182a.Anderson GS, et al: Hypersensitivity of horses in British Columbia to extracts of native and exotic species of *Culicoides* (Diptera: Ceratopogonidae). J Med Entomol 30:657, 1993.
183. Anderson GS, et al: Immunotherapy trial for horses in British Columbia with *Culicoides* (Diptera: Ceratopogonidae) hypersensitivity. J Med Entomol 33:458, 1996.
184. Baker KP: Sweet itch in horses. Vet Rec 93:617, 1973.
185. Baker KP, Quinn PJ: A report on clinical aspects and histopathology of sweet itch. Equine Vet J 10:243, 1978.
186. Baker KP: The pathogenesis of insect hypersensitivity. Vet Dermatol News 8(2):11, 1983.
187. Baker KP, Collin EA: A disease resembling sweet itch in Hong Kong. Equine Vet J 16:467, 1984.
188. Barbet JL, et al: Specific immunotherapy of *Culicoides* hypersensitive horses: A double-blind study. Equine Vet J 22:232, 1990.
189. Becker W: Uber Vorkommen, Ursachen und Behandlung des Sogenannten "Sommerekzems" bei Ponys. Berl Munch Tierärztl Wschr 77:120, 1964.
190. Bourdeau P, Petrikowski M: La dermatite estivale récidivante des équidés: données actuelles. Point Vét 27:207, 1995.
191. Braverman Y, et al: Epidemiological and immunological studies of sweet itch in horses in Israel. Vet Rec 112:521, 1983.
192. Braverman Y: Preferred landing sites of *Culicoides* species (Diptera: Ceratopogonidae) on a horse in Israel and its relevance to summer seasonal recurrent dermatitis (sweet itch). Equine Vet J 20:426, 1988.
193. Braverman Y: Potential of infra-red thermography for the detection of summer seasonal recurrent dermatitis (sweet itch) in horses. Vet Rec 125:372, 1989.
194. Braverman Y: Control of biting midges *Culicoides* (Diptera Ceratopogonidae), vectors of bluetongue and inducers of sweet itch: A review. Isr J Vet Med 45:124, 1989.
195. Brostrom H, et al: Allergic dermatitis (sweet itch) of Icelandic horses in Sweden: an epidemiological study. Equine Vet J 19:229, 1987.
196. Datta S: Microfilarial pityriasis in equines (*Lichen tropicus*). Vet J 95:213, 1939.

197. Fadok VA, Mullowney PC: Dermatologic diseases of horse, part 1. Parasitic dermatoses of the horse. Compend Cont Ed 5:615, 1983.
198. Fadok VA: Parasitic skin diseases of large animals. Vet Clin N Am Large Anim Pract 6:3, 1984.
199. Fadok VA: *Culicoides* hypersensitivity. In: Robinson NE (ed). Current Therapy in Equine Medicine II. W.B. Saunders Co., Philadelphia, PA, 1987, p 624.
200. Fadok VA, Greiner EC: Equine insect hypersensitivity: Skin test and biopsy results correlated with clinical data. Equine Vet J 22:236, 1990.
201. Faravelli G, et al: Valore diagnostico dell' intradermoreazione con estratto di zanzara (genere Culex) in corso di "sweet itch" nel cavallo. Prax Vet Italy 7:17, 1986.
202. Foil L, Foil C: Parasitic skin diseases. Vet Clin N Am Equine Pract 2:403, 1986.
203. Foil L, Foil C: Dipteran parasites of horses. Equine Pract 10:21, 1988.
204. Foil LD, et al: Studies on *Culicoides* hypersensitivity "sweet itch" in Louisiana horses. Proc Annu Memb Meet Am Acad Vet Dermatol Am Coll Vet Dermatol 6:8, 1990.
205. Foster AP, et al: Inhibition of antigen-induced cutaneous responses of ponies with insect hypersensitivity by the histamine-1 receptor antagonist chlorpheniramine. Vet Rec 143:189, 1998.
206. Frost RDI: Sweet itch. Vet Rec 94:28, 1974.
207. Ginel PJ, et al: Dermatitis por hipersensibilidad a insectos en el caballo. Med Vet Spain 12:453, 1995.
208. Glatt PA: Contribution a l etude de la dermatite estivale; approche immuno-genetique. Schweiz Arch tierheilk 128:46, 1986.
209. Gramel T, Müller E: Einsatz von biologisch aktiven Peptiden bei Pferden mit Sommerekzem. Tierärztl Umschau 44:317, 1989.
210. Greiner EC, Fadok VA: Determination of the *Culicoides* spp. associated with hypersensitivity in horses. Proc Annu Memb Meet Am Acad Vet Dermatol Am Coll Vet Dermatol 1, 1985.
211. Greiner EC, et al: *Culicoides* hypersensitivity in Florida: biting midges collected in light traps near horses. Med Vet Entomol 2:129, 1988.
212. Greiner EC, et al: Equine Culicoides hypersensitivity in Florida: biting midges aspirated from horses. Med Vet Entomol 4:375, 1990.
213. Greiner EC: Entomologic evaluation of insect hypersensitivity in horses. Vet Clin N Am Equine Pract 11:29, 1995.
214. Halldórsdóttir S, Larsen HJ: Intradermal challenge of Icelandic horses with extracts of four species of the genus Culicoides. Res Vet Sci 47:283, 1989.
215. Halldórsdóttir S, et al: Distribution of leukocyte antigens in Icelandic horses affected with summer eczema compared to non-affected horses. Equine Vet J 23:300, 1991.
216. Halldórsdóttir S, Larsen HJ: An epidemiological study of summer eczema in Icelandic horses in Norway. Equine Vet J 23:296, 1991.
217. Hasslacher D: Sommerekzem beim Pferd. Ein Feldversuch zur Behandlungmit mit einer steroidfreien, galenisch neuen 10 prozentigen Salicylölzubereitung. Prakt Tierärztl 72:856, 1991.
218. Henry A, Bory L: Dermatose estivale récidivante du cheval. Rec Méd Vét 113:65, 1937.

218a. Hesselholt M, Agger N: "Summereksem" hos hest. Dansk Vet Tidsskrift 16:715, 1977.

219. Hutchins DR: Skin diseases of cattle and horses in New South Wales. N Z Vet J 8:85, 1960.

220. Holmes M: Culicoides hypersensitivity. Equine Vet J 22:230, 1990.

220a. Isharo T, Ueno H: Studies on summer mange ("Kasen" disease) of the horse. IV. Etiology considered from prevention and treatment. Bull Natl Inst Anim Hlth 34:105, 1958.

221. Ishihara T, Ueno H: Studies on summer mange ("Kasen" disease) of the horse in Japan. I. Genetic study on predisposition for summer mange. Bull Natl Inst Anim Hlth, Tokyo, 37:179, 1957.

222. Kleider N, Lees MJ: Culicoides hypersensitivity in the horse: 15 cases in southwestern British Columbia. Can Vet J 25:26, 1984.

223. Kurotaki T, et al: Immunopathological study on equine insect hypersensitivity ("Kasen") in Japan. J Comp Pathol 110:145, 1994.

224. Larsen HJ, et al: Intradermal challenge of Icelandic horses in Norway and Iceland with extracts of Culicoides spp. Acta Vet Scand 29:311, 1988.

224a. Lazary S, et al: ELA in horses affected by sweet itch. Anim Blood Grps Biochem Genet, Suppl:93, 1985.

225. Le Seach G: La dermatite estivale des équidés en Algérie. Rec Méd Vét 122:442, 1946.

226. Littlewood JD: Incidence of recurrent seasonal pruritus ("sweet itch") in British and German Shire horses. Vet Rec 142:66, 1998.

227. Lowe JE: Heat bumps, sweet feed bumps, sweet itch. In: Robinson NE (ed). Current Therapy in Equine Medicine I. W.B. Saunders Co., Philadelphia, 1983, p 110.

227a. Marti E, et al: On the genetic basis of equine allergic diseases: II. Insect bite dermal hypersensitivity. Equine Vet J 24:113, 1992.

227b. Marti E, et al: Sulfidoleukotriene generation from peripheral blood leukocytes of horses affected with insect bite dermal hypersensitivity. Vet Immunol Immunopathol 71:307, 1999.

228. McCaig JA: A survey to establish the incidence of sweet itch in ponies in the United Kingdom. Vet Rec 93:444, 1973.

229. McCraig J: Recent thought on sweet itch. Vet Annu 15:204, 1975.

230. McKelvie J, et al: Characterisation of lymphocyte subpopulations in the skin and circulation of horses with sweet itch (Culicoides hypersensitivity). Equine Vet J 31:466, 1999.

230a. McKelvie J, et al: Culicoides antigen extract stimulates equine blood mononuclear (BMN) cell proliferation and the release of eosinophil adherence-inducing factor(s). Res Vet Sci 70:115, 2001.

231. McMullen WC: Allergie dermatitis in the equine. Southwest Vet 24:121, 1971.

232. McMullen WC: The skin. In: Mansmann RA, et al (eds). Equine Medicine and Surgery III. American Veterinary Publications, Wheaton, Illinois, 1982, p 789.

233. Mellor PS, McCaig J: The probable cause of "sweet itch" in England. Vet Rec 95:411, 1974.

234. Morrow AN, et al: Allergic skin reactions in the horse: response to intradermal challenge with fractionated Culicoides. J Vet Med B 33:508, 1986.

235. Morrow AN, et al: Skin lesions of sweet itch and the distribution of dermal mast cells in the horse. J Vet Med B 34:347, 1987.

236. Morrow AN, et al: Some characteristics of the antibodies involved in allergic skin reactions of the horse to biting insects. Br Vet J 143:59, 1987.

237. Mushi EZ, et al: Culicoides (Diptera: Ceratopogonidae) associated with horses at Mogoditshane, Gaborone, Botswana. Vet Res Commun 22:295, 1998.

238. Nakamura R, et al: Studies on "Kasen" of horses in Hokkaido. I. Results obtained in 1953. Jpn J Vet Res 2:109, 1954.

239. Nakamura R, et al: Studies on "Kasen" of horses in Hokkaido. II. Results obtained in 1954. Jpn J Vet Res 3:73, 1955.

240. Nakamura R, et al: Studies on "Kasen" of horses in Hokkaido. III. Research on the actual state of the disease. Jpn J Vet Res 4:81, 1956.

241. Nakamura R, et al: Studies on "Kasen" of horses in Hokkaido. V. Preliminary experiments concerning the effects of anti-allergic drugs applied to horses with the disease. Jpn J Vet Res 5:97, 1957.

242. Nakamura R, et al: Studies on "Kasen" of horses in Hokkaido. VI. Therapeutic significance of antihistamine preparations for horses affected with the disease. Jpn J Vet Res 6:123, 1958.

243. Nakamura R, et al: Studies on "Kasen" of horses in Hokkaido. VII. Applications of repellents against "Kasen" in 1958 and 1959. Jpn J Vet Res 8:53, 1960.

244. Petrikowski M, Bourdeau P: Etude d'une population de chevaux atteints de D.E.R.E. en Bretagne. Point Vét 27:217, 1995.

245. Quinn PJ, et al: Sweet itch: Responses of clinically normal and affected horses to intradermal challenge with extracts of biting insects. Equine Vet J 15:266, 1983.

246. Ralbag ED: Allergic urticaria in horses. Refuah Vet 11:166, 1954.

247. Riek RF: Studies on allergic dermatitis ("Queensland Itch") of the horse. I. Description, distribution, symptoms, and pathology. Aust Vet J 29:177, 1953.

248. Riek RF: Studies on allergic dermatitis ("Queensland Itch") of the horse. II. Treatment and control. Aust Vet J 29:185, 1953.

249. Riek RF: Studies on allergic dermatitis ("Queensland Itch") of the horse: the aetiology disease. Aust J Agric Res 5:109, 1954.

250. Riek RF: Studies on allergic dermatitis ("Queensland Itch") of the horse: the origin and significance of histamine in the blood and its distribution in the tissues. Aust J Agric Res 6:161, 1955.

251. Schmidtmann ET, et al: Comparative host seeking activity of Culicoides species (Diptera: Ceratopogonidae) attracted to pastured livestock in central New York State, USA. J Med Entomol 17:221, 1980.

252. Scott DW: Histopathologie cutanée de l'hypersensibilité aux piqures de Culicoides chez le cheval. Point Vét 22:583, 1990.

253. Sommer H: Präventive und Therapie des Sommerekzems beim Pferd mit homöopathischen Mitteln. Tierärztl Umschau 52:271, 1997.

253a. Stark G, et al: Zinc and copper plasma levels in Icelandic horses with Culicoides hypersensitivity. Equine Vet J 33:506, 2001.

254. Stevens DP, et al: High-cis permethrin for the control of sweet itch in horses. Vet Rec 122:308, 1988.

255. Strothmann-Lüerssen A, et al: Das Sommerekzem beim Islandpferd: Epidermale Eicosanoidkonzentration, Proliferationsparameter un histologische Veränderungen in betroffenen Hautpartien. Pferdheilk 8:385, 1992.

256. Townley P, et al: Preferential landing and engorging sites of *Culicoides* species landing on a horse in Ireland. Equine Vet J 16:117, 1984.

257. Ueno H, Ishihara T: Studies on summer mange ("Kasen" disease) of the horse in Japan. III. Skin test sensitivity tests with insect allergens. Bull Natl Inst Anim Hlth Tokyo 32:217, 1957.

258. Underwood JR: Equine dhobie itch a symptom of filariasis. Vet Bull US Army, 28:227, 1934.

259. Ungar-Waron H, et al: Immunogenicity and allergenicity of *Culicoides imicola* (Diptera: Ceratopogonidae) extracts. J Vet Med B 37:64, 1990.

260. Unkel M: Epidemiologische Erhebung zum Sogenannten Sommerekzem bei Islandpferden. Prakt Tierärztl 8:656, 1984.

261. Vallis J: Microfilaires et dermatose estivale récidivante du cheval. Rev Méd Vét 97:65, 1946.

262. van der Haegen A, et al: Les affections cutanées allergiques 1- la dermatite estivale récidivante. Prat Vét Equine 32:15, 2000.

262a. van der Haegen A, et al: Immunoglobulin E–bearing cells in skin biopsies of horses with insect bite hypersensitivity. Equine Vet J 33:699, 2001.

262b. Wilson AD, et al: Detection of IgG and IgE serum antibodies to *Culicoides* salivary gland antigens in horses with insect dermal hypersensitivity (sweet itch). Equine Vet J 33:707, 2001.

263. Wisniewski E, et al: Lip owka-sezonowe alergiczme zapalenie skóry koni. Med Wet 48:294, 1992.

264. Yamashita J, et al: Studies on "Kasen" of horses in Hokkaido. IV. Research on the punkies in Hokkaido with description of a new species. Jpn J Vet Res 5:89, 1957.

Chapter 9

Immune-Mediated Disorders

Immune-mediated dermatoses are well recognized but uncommon skin diseases in the horse.[6,8,10-14] These dermatoses have been reported to account for 2% of all equine dermatoses examined by the dermatology service at a university practice.[11] They have been subdivided into primary or autoimmune, and secondary or immune-mediated disorders, the latter believed to be primarily diseases wherein tissue destruction results from an immunologic event that is not directed against self-antigens.[4,18]

In autoimmune disease, antibodies or activated lymphocytes develop against normal body constituents and will induce the lesions of the disease by passive transfer. A major level of control of the autoreactive clones of lymphocytes is suppression by suppressor T cells that are specific for those clones.[4,18] The development of autoimmune diseases is a reflection of a lack of control or a bypass of the normal control mechanisms. Over the years, a variety of possible defects have been described, but the exact abnormal mechanism and what induces these diseases still remains unknown. Some of the possibilities include (1) suppressor T cell bypass, (2) suppressor T cell dysfunction, (3) abnormal MHCII expression or interaction, (4) cytokine and receptor ligand abnormalities, (5) autoantigen modification, (6) cross-reacting antigens, (7) inappropriate IL-2 production, (8) idiotype-antiidiotype imbalance, (9) mutations in receptor affinity, and (10) failure of clonal deletion of low affinity autoreactive lymphocytes.[2-4,15,16,18] In addition, there is sexual dimorphism in the immune response, with female sex hormones tending to accelerate immune responses and male sex hormones tending to suppress responses.[2,15]

In secondary immune-mediated diseases, the antigen is foreign to the body. Most commonly, the inciting antigens are drugs, bacteria, and viruses that stimulate an immunologic reaction that results in host tissue damage.[2,4,18] Superantigens are gene products that are recognized by a large fraction of T cells and have the potential to interfere with the recognition and elimination of conventional antigens.[5] These gene products may play a role in the genesis of immune-mediated diseases. So-called "epitope spreading" may also be important in autoimmune diseases.[15,21] In this situation, an autoimmune or inflammatory disease process can cause tissue damage such that certain protein tissue components originally hidden from autoreactive T or B cells become exposed and evoke a secondary or primary autoimmune response, respectively.

• DIAGNOSIS OF IMMUNE-MEDIATED SKIN DISEASE

The diagnosis of these dermatoses requires demonstration of characteristic dermatopathologic changes and, optimally, the autoantibodies, immune complexes, or mediators (e.g., cytotoxic T cells) involved in the immunologic injury. Establishing the presence of characteristic dermatopathology requires skin biopsy (see Chapter 2). In general, the following guidelines should be observed:[1,12,15]

1. Multiple biopsy specimens should always be taken, because diagnostic changes may be focal.
2. Samples should be selected from the most representative lesions of the suspected immune-mediated diseases.
3. Punch biopsy specimens should be taken in as gentle a fashion as possible; wedge biopsy by scalpel excision may be necessary.
4. Whenever possible, biopsy specimens should be taken when the horse is not under the effects of any glucocorticoid or immunosuppressive therapy.
5. Dermatopathologic examination should be performed by a veterinary pathologist who has a special interest in dermatopathology or by a veterinary dermatologist trained in dermatopathology.

Establishing the mediator of the immunologic damage may require biopsy and/or analysis of the patient's serum for auto- or abnormal antibodies. The biopsies for immunopathologic examination often must be processed in special ways that may require fresh tissue, frozen tissue, or specially fixed samples, depending on the test that will be performed. The veterinary immunopathology laboratory will be able to tell you what is required. Tests used to detect the presence of autoantibodies or various immunoreactants (e.g., immunoglobulins, complement components, microbial antigens) in skin lesions include immunofluorescence and immunohistochemical (e.g., immunoperoxidase) methods.[1,7,15,49]

Biopsy specimens for direct antibody testing should be selected from areas not secondarily infected and generally representing the earliest lesion typical for that disease; a possible exception is discoid lupus erythematosus, wherein older lesions may be preferred. Vasculitis lesions under 24 hours old are best. For bullous diseases, the blister itself is not sampled, but the adjacent normal skin or erythematous skin. Samples for direct immunofluorescence testing need to be fixed and mailed in Michel's fixative. Samples for direct immunoperoxidase testing may be formalin-fixed. The results of studies of tissues processed by quick-freezing and of those kept in Michel's fixative for up to 2 weeks are comparable.[11,15] Studies in horses suggest that specimens may be reliably preserved in Michel's fixative for at least 7 to 14 days,[11,12,49] and in some instances, specimens have been successfully preserved for 4 to 8 years.[49] The pH of Michel's fixative must be carefully maintained at 7.0 to 7.2 to ensure accurate results.[11,12,15] Samples for direct antibody detection should be sent to a veterinary immunopathology laboratory.

Testing for abnormal antibody or immune complex deposition is considered highly valuable in human medicine and for many of the immune-mediated dermatoses. For the similar equine diseases, however, their value has been considerably less. Techniques and results appear to be improving based on reports from veterinary immunopathology research laboratories.[15] These tests are fraught with numerous procedural and interpretational pitfalls, including method of specimen handling, choice of substrates used, method of substrate handling, specificity of conjugates, fluorescein-protein-antibody concentrations, and unitage of conjugates. An in-depth discussion of these factors is beyond the scope of this chapter; the reader is referred to Beutner and colleagues[1] for details. The incidence of positive results in the equine disorders typically varies from about 25% to 90% for direct immunofluorescence testing.[10-12] Positive results are much more commonly achieved with the immunoperoxidase method. However, with this technique the incidence of false-positive results is also much higher.[15] In fact, the intercellular and basement membrane zone deposition of immunoglobulins or complement components can be detected from time to time in a wide variety of inflammatory dermatoses.[10-12,15,57] The authors and others[7,15] do not believe that these tests need to be routinely done in the work-up of a suspected case of immune-mediated skin disease in a horse. Results of immunopathologic testing can *never* be appropriately interpreted in the absence of histopathologic findings.[7,15] On the other hand, histopathologic findings are sufficiently characteristic to be diagnostic in the majority of cases.[19] The clinician's time and the owner's money are better spent in the careful selection and procuring of representative skin specimens and their forwarding to a knowledgeable dermatopathologist.

Autoimmune dermatoses are classified on the basis of the specific autoallergen being targeted.[15,17] This cannot be determined on the basis of routine immunofluorescence or immuno-histochemical testing. Specific identification requires techniques such as immunoprecipitation, immunoblotting, and antigen-specific ELISA.[28] This is rarely done in routine veterinary diagnostic laboratories and is limited to certain veterinary immunologic research laboratories. As a result, we may still be lumping together different diseases or variants that share clinical, histopathologic, and routine immunopathologic features.

Indirect immunofluorescence testing (testing serum for the presence of circulating auto-antibody) has been positive in less than 50% of affected horses, and is not recommended as a cost-effective test.[11,12,49,57] In addition, these tests can be positive in normal horses and horses with dermatoses of nonimmune-mediated origin.[10-13,57] Now that better technology is available,[15] we should be sending tissue and serum samples to researchers that are performing these tests correctly and frequently. Only then will we be able to identify whether or not the variants described in humans also exist in horses and whether their differentiation leads to prognostic or therapeutic value.

• THERAPY OF IMMUNE-MEDIATED SKIN DISEASES

As a group, all of these immune-mediated dermatoses are characterized by an inappropriate immune response that, to be adequately controlled, may require the use of potent immunosuppressive and immunomodulating drugs. The diseases are not all optimally treated in the same way, however, nor do they have the same prognosis. Therefore, it is important that the clinician make as specific a diagnosis as possible. Although much work is occurring in human medicine regarding new approaches to the management of these diseases, very little of this information is being applied in veterinary medicine.

The drugs used to treat immune-mediated skin diseases are generally referred to as *immunosuppressive agents*. However, for some of these drugs, their exact mechanism is unknown. They may act in methods different from those of the more classic immune-suppressive agents. They are considered together because, whatever their mechanism of action, they share the features of being beneficial in managing the immune-mediated skin diseases. Glucocorticoids are the most common class of drugs used as immunosuppressive agents. They are discussed in Chapter 3. The following immunomodulating drugs are used in the horse, but very little specific data are available. Hence, the discussions are primarily based on information available for humans, dogs, and cats.[3,15]

Azathioprine

Azathioprine (Imuran, Glaxo Wellcome) is a synthetic modification of 6-mercaptopurine that can be given orally or by injection.[15] However, for skin diseases, the oral route is usually used. It is metabolized in the liver to 6-mercaptopurine and other active metabolites; 6-mercaptopurine is then metabolized by three enzyme systems. Xanthine oxidase and thiopurine methyltransferase (TPMT) produce inactive metabolites. Humans and possibly dogs that have absent (homozygous) or low (heterozygous) TPMT activity are more likely to develop myelosuppression. The drug antagonizes purine metabolism, thereby interfering with DNA and RNA synthesis. Azathioprine primarily affects rapidly proliferating cells, with its greatest effects on cell-mediated immunity and T lymphocyte-dependent antibody synthesis. Primary antibody synthesis is affected more than secondary antibody synthesis. Azathioprine is preferred over 6-mercaptopurine because it has a more favorable therapeutic index.

Even so, azathioprine is a potent drug with potential toxicities, which include anemia, leukopenia, thrombocytopenia, vomiting, hypersensitivity reactions (especially of the liver), pancreatitis, elevated serum alkaline phosphatase concentrations, skin rashes, and alopecia. The most common significant side effect is diarrhea, which may be hemorrhagic. This often responds to dose reductions or temporary discontinuation of the drug. More than 90% of the cases experience anemia and lymphopenia, but usually not to the degree that treatment needs to be discontinued. It has also been suggested that patients that are not responding to therapy, that are not lymphopenic, and are otherwise tolerating the drug very well, should have their dose of azathioprine increased. The authors have not seen, or heard of, adverse reactions to azathioprine in horses.[57]

Patients should be monitored initially every 2 weeks with complete blood counts and platelet counts. After the patient's condition is stable, monitoring can be tapered to once every 4 months. If other symptoms occur, or at least yearly, a chemistry panel should also be run. Hepatitis and pancreatitis are the major conditions to monitor with chemistry panels.

In horses, azathioprine may be beneficial for pemphigus complex, bullous pemphigoid, and both types of lupus erythematosus, as well as other autoimmune and immune-mediated disorders.[57] It is most commonly used in cases of equine pemphigus foliaceus and vasculitis that do not respond to glucocorticoids.[57] Azathioprine is usually not used alone, but is combined with systemic glucocorticoids. There is often a lag phase, with clinical improvement occurring in 3 to 6 weeks. After remission is achieved, the dosages of both drugs are tapered, but initially, unless side-effects are a problem, the glucocorticoid dosage is tapered to levels approaching 1 mg/kg q48h (prednisolone equivalents). The oral dosage of azathioprine for horses is 2.5 mg/kg q24h until clinical response is achieved, and then it is continued every other day for a month or longer. Slow tapering to the lowest dose possible decreases side effects and the expense of therapy. Glucocorticoids can be given on the alternate days when azathioprine is not given.

Chrysotherapy

Chrysotherapy is the use of gold as a therapeutic agent. Gold compounds are capable of modulating many phases of immune and inflammatory responses, but the exact mechanisms of this effect are unknown.[12,15] Gold is available in two dosage forms, which have dissimilar pharmacokinetics: the oral compound auranofin (Ridaura, SmithKline Beecham) contains 29% gold, and the parenteral compound aurothioglucose (Solganal, Schering) contains 50% gold. Neither form is approved for use in horses, but their distribution, metabolism, and actions have been established in humans and laboratory animals. Studies in humans show that the oral forms are 25% absorbed and attain blood levels with a 21-day half-life, but only small amounts can be detected in tissues and skin. In a few clinical trials in dogs with immune-mediated dermatoses, the results with oral gold were equivocal, but no adverse side-effects were observed. The parenteral form is 100% absorbed, but has only a 6-day half-life in blood. It is 95% protein-bound and is well distributed to cells of the mononuclear phagocytic system, liver, spleen, bone marrow, kidneys, and adrenal glands. Much lower levels are detected in skin. In humans, serum concentrations reach a plateau after 1 to 2 months of weekly aurothioglucose injections, and urinary excretion can be detected for as long as 1 year after chronic therapy is stopped.

Gold may act at several levels of the inflammatory and immune response.[15] Auranofin appears to have an additional immunomodulating action, while gold sodium thiomalate inhibits interleukin-5-mediated eosinophil survival, but both oral and parenteral golds inhibit bacteria, the first component of complement, and the epidermal enzymes that may be responsible for blister formation in pemphigus. Gold inhibits phagocytosis by macrophages. Gold also reduces the release of inflammatory mediators, such as lysosomal enzymes, histamine, and prostaglandin, inactivates complement components, interferes with immunoglobulin-synthesizing cells, inhibits antigen and mitogen induced T cell proliferation, and suppresses interleukin-2 and interleukin-2 receptor synthesis.

Toxic effects are worrisome in humans, because 33% of patients have some adverse reaction, although 80% of these are minor.[3,15] Most common are skin eruptions, oral reactions, proteinuria, and bone marrow depression. During the induction phase, a hemogram and urinalysis should be checked weekly, and monthly thereafter. In over 100 dogs treated with injectable gold salts, the most common side effect was pain at the injection site. In addition, two dogs developed reversible thrombocytopenia, and four dogs developed fatal toxic epidermal necrolysis when switched immediately from azathioprine to aurothioglucose therapy for pemphigus foliaceus. This may be enhanced by previous or concurrent administration of azathioprine. Aurothioglucose-related erythema multiforme has been seen in both dogs and cats. Side effects have not been reported in horses.[12,44,57] In laboratory rodents, gold is known to cross the placenta, be secreted in milk, and to be teratogenic.

Aurothioglucose has been reported to be effective for the treatment of cases of equine pemphigus foliaceus, including those that were unresponsive to glucocorticoids.[12,44,57] Auranofin has not been used. Most adverse reactions (in humans, dogs, and cats) develop late in therapy. Horses are given 1 mg/kg intramuscularly weekly until remission occurs. If no response is seen after 16 weeks of therapy, the aurothioglucose is unlikely to be of benefit. After remission, one dose is given every 2 weeks for a month, and then once monthly for several months. It is advisable to halt medication administration eventually for observation, because some patients go into complete remission, whereas other animals can be maintained on a reduced dosage. Two points of caution: (1) the treatment takes up to 16 weeks for beneficial effects to occur, so other medication—typically glucocorticoids—should be maintained, if needed, at full dosage until this lag period is passed; and (2) gold compounds should not be administered simultaneously with other cytotoxic drugs (such as azathioprine), because toxicity is thereby enhanced.

Gold is seldom the first-choice drug for pemphigus. Patients are usually started on a glucocorticoid regimen, with azathioprine added to reduce the steroid dosage. In cases with excessive side effects, or when azathioprine and glucocorticoids are ineffective, gold is a logical choice. Gold injections should be delayed for 4 weeks following the discontinuation of azathioprine.

Gold compounds should not be used in pregnant animals, and in animals with blood dyscrasias, hepatic disease, or renal disease. As of this writing, aurothioglucose is unavailable in the United States, and its availability in the future is unknown. Gold sodium thiomalate (Myochrysine, Taylor-Acorn) can be used in the identical fashion. Anecdotal reports indicate that gold sodium thiomalate is also effective.

Pentoxifylline

Pentoxifylline (Trental, Hoechst-Roussel or generic) is a methylxanthine derivative that produces a variety of physiologic changes at the cellular level.[15] Immunomodulatory and rheologic effects include increased leukocyte deformability and chemotaxis, decreased platelet aggregation, decreased leukocyte responsiveness to interleukin-1 (IL-1) and tumor necrosis factor (TNF)-α, decreased production of TNF-α from macrophages, decreased production of IL-1, IL-4, and IL-12, inhibition of T- and B-lymphocyte activation, and decreased natural killer cell activity. It also has been shown to inhibit T cell adherence to keratinocytes. In humans, these effects are beneficial in the treatment of peripheral vascular disease, vasculitis, and contact hypersensitivity.

Pentoxifylline also has been used for a variety of inflammatory diseases such as necrobiosis lipoidica, granuloma annulare, and brown recluse spider bites. The drug also affects wound healing and connective tissue disorders through increased production of collagenase and decreased production of collagen, fibronectin, and glycosaminoglycans. In humans, the drug has been used to treat scleroderma. Anecdotal reports indicate that pentoxifylline has been used in equine medicine for the treatment of atopy, vasculitis, erythema multiforme, pemphigus foliaceus, and sarcoidosis. Pentoxifylline improved the respiratory function of horses with chronic obstructive pulmonary disease ("heaves") maintained in an unfavorable environment.[5a]

Pentoxifylline is available in a 400-mg coated tablet. It is usually crushed and dosed at 8 to 10 mg/kg q12h.[2a] Anecdotal reports indicate that an oral pentoxifylline powder (Navicon, J. Webster Laboratories) is also effective.

Side effects are minimal and may include transient sweating, behavioral change, and conjunctivitis.

● AUTOIMMUNE DISEASES

Pemphigus Complex

The pemphigus complex is a group of uncommon autoimmune diseases described in horses that is comparable to the human, canine, and feline diseases.[3,15] These disorders are vesiculobullous to pustular disorders of the skin or mucous membranes characterized by acantholysis (loss of cohesion between keratinocytes). In humans, there are at least eight varieties of pemphigus, while horses have at least three varieties.[3,15,17,30]

CAUSE AND PATHOGENESIS

In humans, the pemphigus complex is characterized histologically by intraepithelial acantholysis leading to vesicle formation, and immunologically by the presence of autoantibodies to components of the keratinocyte desmosome, both bound in the skin and circulating in the serum.[3,21,22,30] The clinical lesions, both in severity and in body location, appear to relate to which components of the desmosome the autoantibodies are targeting.[15,21,22,25,30] For instance, humans with mucosal-dominant pemphigus vulgaris have antibodies against desmoglein III, those with pemphigus foliaceus produce antibodies against desmoglein I, and patients with mucocutaneous pemphigus vulgaris produce both.[21,22] Using a neonatal mouse model, the injection of antidesmoglein III IgG alone is not efficient at inducing gross skin lesions, whereas combining both antidesmoglein III and antidesmoglein I does produce lesions.[21,22] As pemphigus vulgaris progresses to cutaneous involvement, antidesmoglein I antibodies are produced, possibly as a result of epitope spreading.

Pemphigus antigens are heterogeneous (85 to 260 kd), present in all mammalian and avian skin, and those identified specifically are associated with desmosomal components.* In humans, regional variation exists in the expression of both pemphigus foliaceus and pemphigus vulgaris antigens, which also differ from each other.[25] This regional difference and the specific profile of the patient's autoantibodies correlates with, and helps to explain, the distribution of lesions seen in clinical disease.[15,21,22,25,30] The pemphigus vulgaris and pemphigus foliaceus antibodies from human patients reproduce their respective clinical, histopathologic, and immunopathologic syndromes when injected into neonatal mice. Antibodies to some of these antigens are not, however, associated with pathology.

The pathomechanism of blister formation in pemphigus is unknown, though it has been proposed to be as follows: (1) the binding of pemphigus antibody on the antigen, (2) internalization of the pemphigus antibody and fusion of the antibody with intracellular lysosomes, and (3) resultant activation and release of a keratinocyte proteolytic enzyme (plasminogen activator or another factor), which diffuses into the extracellular space and converts plasminogen into plasmin, which hydrolyzes the adhesion molecules.[3,15,17] The resultant loss of intercellular cohesion leads to acantholysis and blister formation within the epidermis. The pemphigus antibody-induced acantholysis is not dependent on complement or inflammatory cells. Experimentally, however, complement potentiates the acantholysis. Urokinase-type plasminogen activator receptors were shown to have increased expression in the skin lesions of humans with pemphigus vulgaris and

---

*References 1, 3, 15-17, 21 23, 30.

pemphigus foliaceus.[32] Other studies have shown that plasminogen activator activity does not correlate with lesion development, and studies conducted in genetically engineered mouse models also have suggested that direct interference with the antibody targets creates similar lesions.[3]

In desmoglein III[null] mice, treatment with human pemphigus vulgaris serum induces extensive acantholysis and blistering, suggesting that autoantibodies against cell surface molecules other than desmoglein I and desmoglein III can induce pemphigus vulgaris.[29] Patients with pemphigus vulgaris and pemphigus foliaceus have IgG antibodies that precipitate cholinergic receptors.[29] Because cholinergic receptors control keratinocyte adhesion and motility, their inactivation by autoantibodies may elicit cell signals that cause desmosomal disassembly. Although keratinocyte desmosomal cadherins (desmoglein I and III) hold the cells together, desmoglein III[null] mice do *not* develop spontaneous acantholysis and blisters. In addition, activation of cholinergic receptors can prevent, stop, and reverse the acantholysis elicited by pemphigus antibodies *in vitro*. Thus, the acantholysis in pemphigus may be mediated by at least two complementary pathogenic pathways: (1) anticholinergic receptor autoantibodies that weaken intercellular adhesion between keratinocytes via inactivation of the cholinergic receptor-mediated physiologic control of cadherin (desmoglein) expression and/or function, which causes dyshesion, cell detachment, and rounding up (acantholysis); and (2) autoantibodies to other adherence molecules (e.g., desmoglein) that prevent the formation of new desmosomes.

Syndecan-1 is a membrane heparin sulfate proteoglycan expressed over the entire surface of keratinocytes and at points of cell-cell contact. It acts as an extracellular matrix receptor and binds to interstitial collagens, fibronectin, and tenascin. In humans, lesions of pemphigus vulgaris and pemphigus foliaceus have a marked loss of syndecan-1 expression in areas of acantholysis.[22a] It has been proposed that syndecan-1 and E-cadherin are co-expressed, and that pemphigus vulgaris and pemphigus foliaceus autoantibodies impair syndecan-1 function too.

What initiates the autoantibody formation is still unknown, though a virus spread by an insect vector is suspected in an endemic form of pemphigus foliaceus (fogo selvagem) seen in South America.[3,24] It has been suggested that the black fly may play the role of vector. This hypothesis has been supported by an epidemiologic study correlating exposure to black flies as a risk factor for the development of endemic pemphigus foliaceus.

Genetic factors in humans and dogs also appear to be important.[3,15] In humans, both pemphigus foliaceus and pemphigus vulgaris have HLA associations and some populations may be susceptible to pemphigus vulgaris due to differences in their immune response genes.[3] Breed predispositions and familial cases are recognized in dogs.[15] Other factors thought to be involved in the pathogenesis of some cases of pemphigus are drug provocation (especially penicillamine and phenylbutazone), ultraviolet light, and emotional upset.[3,15] One horse developed pemphigus foliaceus after a third course of penicillin, and spontaneously resolved after penicillin administration was stopped.[20]

Diet has been implicated as a cause of pemphigus in humans.[15,31] The molecular structure of many food ingredients is similar to that of known pemphigus-inducing drugs. For instance: *thiols* contained in garlic, onion, leek, and chive; *isothiocyanates* in mustard, horseradish, turnip, radish, cabbage, cauliflower, and Brussel sprouts; *phenols* in mango, cashews, and many food additives; *tannins* in tea, coffee, ginseng, certain berries, banana, pear, apple, and avocado. Interestingly, most humans with fogo selvagem live in close proximity to rivers, many of which contain high levels of tannins due to decomposing leaves and other vegetable matter.[31] Heat and humidity cause tannin decomposition. Perhaps consumption of such substances is more important than black flies!

Owing to the thinness, or other characteristics, of equine epidermis, intraepidermal vesicles, bullae, and pustules are fragile and transient. Thus, clinical lesions usually include erosions and ulcers bordered by epidermal collarettes.

DIAGNOSIS OF PEMPHIGUS: GENERAL COMMENTS

The pemphigus complex is uncommon in horses, accounting for about 1.6% of all equine skin disorders seen at one university clinic.[11] In general, the various forms of pemphigus have relatively distinct clinical differences. Certain diagnostic features, however, can be applied to the whole group. The most important diagnostic aspects are the history, physical examination, and histopathologic findings. Detection of pemphigus antibody by direct immunofluorescence or immunohistochemical testing may also be helpful, but owing to costs, technical problems, and relatively poor diagnostic sensitivity and specificity, those tests are not routinely recommended. If they are performed, however, all the pemphigus variants should show an intercellular deposition of IgG or complement components (Fig. 9-1).[10,15,54] Occasionally, immunoglobulins of other classes may be found. Indirect immunofluorescence testing is frequently negative. Microscopic examination of direct smears from intact vesicles or pustules or from recent erosions often reveals numerous nondegenerate neutrophils and/or eosinophils, and numerous acantholytic keratinocytes.[10,12,54,57] One or two acantholytic keratinocytes may be seen in an occasional high-power microscopic field during the microscopic examination of any suppurative condition, but

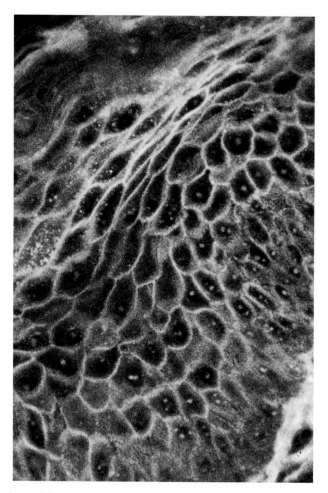

FIGURE 9-1. Pemphigus foliaceus. IgG is present in the intercellular spaces on direct immunofluorescence testing.

when these cells are present in clusters or large numbers in several microscopic fields, they are strongly suggestive of pemphigus. Marked acantholysis has rarely been observed cytologically in cases of equine dermatophytosis.[56]

Skin biopsy findings may be diagnostic or strongly supportive in pemphigus.[10,12,13,53-55] Intact vesicles, bullae, or pustules are preferred. Because these fluid-filled lesions are so fragile and transient, it may be necessary to hospitalize the animal so that it can be scrutinized every 2 to 4 hours for the presence of primary lesions. In some cases, the diagnosis may be made by selecting recently exudative, crusted areas of skin, wherein the acantholytic keratinocytes are found within the crusts and exudate. Multiple biopsy specimens and serial sections will greatly increase the chances of demonstrating diagnostic histopathologic changes.

Electron microscopic examination of pemphigus lesions suggests that dissolution of the intercellular cement substance is the initial pathologic change, followed by the retraction of tonofilaments, disappearance of desmosomes, and acantholysis.[54]

Results of routine laboratory determinations (hemogram, serum chemistries, urinalysis, serum protein electrophoresis) are nondiagnostic, often revealing mild to moderate leukocytosis and neutrophilia, mild nonregenerative anemia, mild to moderate hypoalbuminemia, and mild to moderate elevations of α_2, β, and γ globulins.[10,54]

CLINICAL MANAGEMENT OF PEMPHIGUS: GENERAL COMMENTS

Therapy of equine pemphigus is often difficult, requiring large doses of systemic glucocorticoids with or without other potent immunomodulating drugs.[10,13,54,57] Close physical and hematologic monitoring of the patient is critical. Therapy usually must be maintained for prolonged periods, if not for life. Thus, the therapeutic regimen must be individualized for each patient, and owner education is essential.

Large doses of glucocorticoids (2 to 4 mg/kg prednisolone or prednisone, or 0.2 to 0.4 mg/kg dexamethasone orally q24h in the morning) will induce remission in most horses. Marked clinical improvement should be seen within 10 to 14 days. When glucocorticoids are ineffective or undesirable, other immunomodulating drugs can be used in an attempt to reduce the dosage or eliminate the need for the former. Chrysotherapy (gold salts) or azathioprine are most commonly used (see Therapy of Immune-Mediated Skin Diseases).[10,12,13,54,57] Omega-3/omega-6 fatty acid-containing products may also be useful.[57]

Exposure to ultraviolet light can exacerbate or even precipitate pemphigus.[3,12,13,15,57] Thus, photoprotection is an important therapeutic adjunct. Avoidance of sunlight between 8 AM and 5 PM is helpful.

PEMPHIGUS FOLIACEUS

Pemphigus foliaceus is the most common form of pemphigus and the most common autoimmune dermatosis in the horse.* It is, however, an uncommon disease, accounting for only 1.89% of the equine skin diseases seen at the Cornell University Clinic. In humans and dogs, the major pemphigus foliaceus antigen is desmoglein I, a 150-kd glycoprotein from the cadherin group of adhesion molecules.[3,15,17,21,22] The exact antigen in the horse has not been specifically identified.[17] There are no apparent sex or age predilections, and the disease has been reported in horses 2 months to 20 years of age. In one study of nine horses,[10] Appaloosas accounted for 33.3% of the cases, but only 6.8% of the general equine hospital population. However, other authors have found no breed predilection.

In dogs, one form of pemphigus foliaceus is seen in animals with a history of chronic skin disease, especially chronic pruritic or allergic skin disease.[15] Similarly, pemphigus foliaceus has

---

*References 10, 12, 13, 16a, 17, 20, 33-50, 52-55, 57-60.

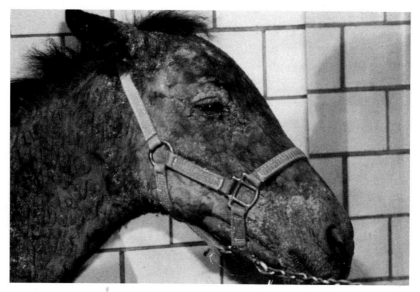

FIGURE 9-2. Pemphigus foliaceus. Severe crusting, scaling, and alopecia on the face and neck.

been reported to occur in a group of horses that had *Culicoides* hypersensitivity for 1 to 3 years.[61] However, in a retrospective study of 10 horses with pemphigus foliaceus, no seasonality or environmental risk factors were detected.[46]

Anecdotal reports indicate that, in many cases, a triggering event (drug administration, variety of systemic diseases, "stressful situations") precedes the onset of disease.[16a]

Skin lesions commonly begin on the face (Fig. 9-2) and/or the legs (Fig. 9-3, *A*), and frequently become generalized within 1 to 3 months (Figs. 9-3, *B*, and 9-4). In some cases, lesions are localized to the face or coronary bands (Fig. 9-5) for long periods of time. Preputial and mammary areas may be targeted in some cases. The primary skin lesions are vesicles, bullae, or pustules (Fig. 9-3, *C*). However, due to the fragile and transient nature of these lesions, the clinician typically sees annular erosions with or without epidermal collarettes, annular thick crusts, annular areas of alopecia, and variable degrees of oozing and scaling. In some horses, early lesions are tufted papules and crusts over the withers, saddle area (Fig. 9-6), or brisket (Fig. 9-7). Nikolsky's sign may be present. Some cases present with extensive exfoliative dermatitis without distinct annular primary or secondary lesions. It has been reported that transient, persistent, or recurrent urticaria can precede the development of typical pemphigus lesions for days to weeks.[16a]

Over 50% of the cases have varying degrees of edema of the distal limbs (Fig. 9-8) and ventral abdomen.[13,44,61] The degree of edema may be out of proportion to, or occur in the absence of, surface lesions. Pruritus and pain may or may not be present. Skin lesions may be exacerbated in warm, humid, sunny weather.[13,61] Some animals experience spontaneous waxing and waning of their skin disease.[13,61] Over 50% of the horses manifest variable systemic signs, including depression, lethargy, poor appetite, weight loss, and fever.[13,44,61] One horse with pemphigus foliaceus was found to have erosions in the esophagus and esophageal zone of the stomach.[60]

Diagnosis

The differential diagnosis of pemphigus foliaceus includes dermatophytosis, dermatophilosis, bacterial folliculitis, sarcoidosis, multisystemic eosinophilic epitheliotropic disease, seborrhea, drug reaction, and epitheliotropic lymphoma.

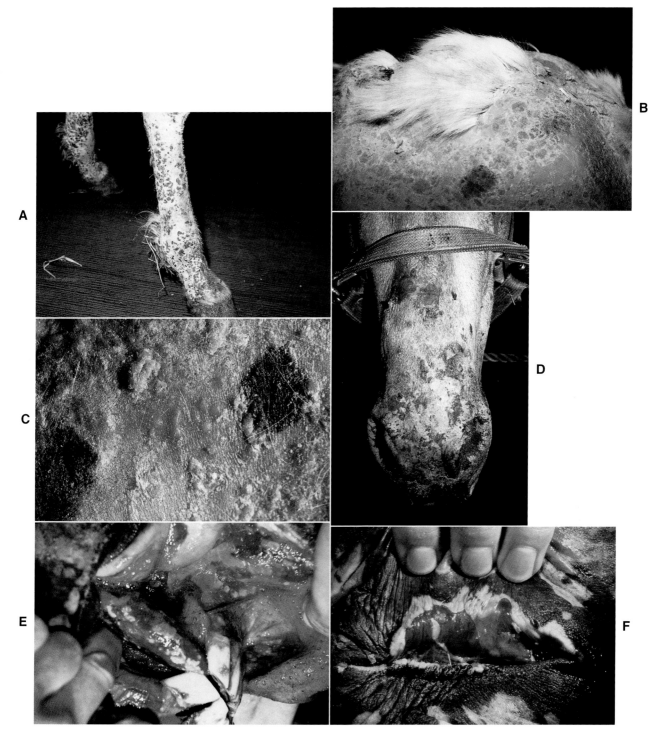

FIGURE 9-3. A, Pemphigus foliaceus. Annular crusts and erosions and alopecia on the leg. **B,** Pemphigus foliaceus. Annular crusts, erythema, and alopecia over the rump. **C,** Pemphigus foliaceus. Intact vesicles on erythematous, alopecic thoracic skin. **D,** Bullous pemphigoid. Annular ulcers, crusts, and erythema on the face. **E,** Bullous pemphigoid. Ulcerative stomatitis. **F,** Bullous pemphigoid. Ulcers bordered by epithelial collarettes on the vulva.

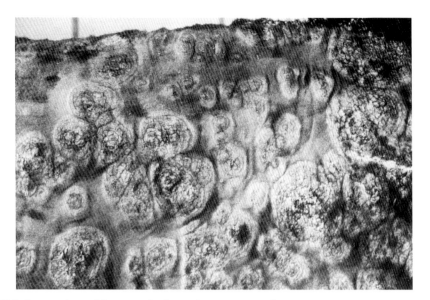

FIGURE 9-4. Pemphigus foliaceus. Thick annular crusts over thorax.

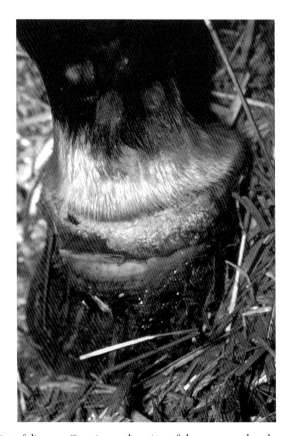

FIGURE 9-5. Pemphigus foliaceus. Crusting and oozing of the coronary band.

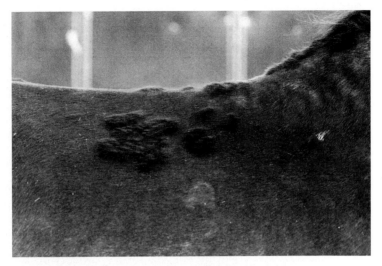

FIGURE 9-6. Pemphigus foliaceus. Tufted papules and crusts on saddle area.

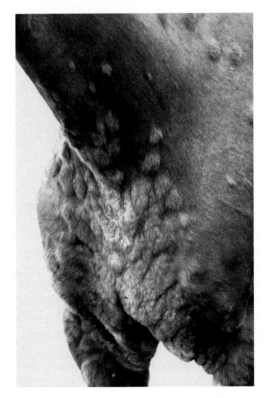

FIGURE 9-7. Pemphigus foliaceus. Tufted papules and crusts on brisket.

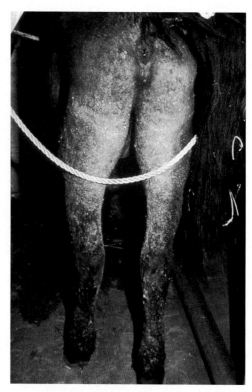

FIGURE 9-8. Pemphigus foliaceus. Exfoliative dermatitis and edema of hind legs.

The definitive diagnosis is based on history, physical examination, direct smears (Fig. 9-9), skin biopsy, immunofluorescence or immunohistochemical testing, and demonstration of the antigen being targeted (desmoglein I). Pemphigus foliaceus is characterized by intragranular or subcorneal acantholysis with resultant cleft and vesicle or pustule formation (Figs. 9-10 and 9-11).[12,13,16a,19] Within the vesicle or pustule, cells from the stratum granulosum may be seen attached to the overlying stratum corneum (granular cell "cling-ons") (Fig. 9-12, A). Either neutrophils or eosinophils may predominate. Other helpful histopathologic findings that may be seen include (1) eosinophilic exocytosis and microabscess formation within the epidermis or follicular outer root sheath or both, (2) frequent involvement of the follicular outer root sheath in the acantholytic and pustular process (pustular mural folliculitis), (3) acantholytic, dyskeratotic granular epidermal cells ("grains") at the surface of erosions, and (4) surface crusts containing numerous acantholytic keratinocytes singly or in clusters (Fig. 9-12, B). It must be emphasized, here, that cases of acantholytic dermatophytosis can be histologically indistinguishable from pemphigus foliaceus (see Chapter 5). Hence, sections must be scrutinized for the presence of fungal elements, and special stains and fungal cultures may be indicated.

In some cases of equine pemphigus foliaceus, the remarkable ventral or limb edema is *not* explained by hypoalbuminemia.[42] Skin biopsies taken from some of these animals has revealed a vasculitis.[42]

Management

Rarely, equine pemphigus foliaceus will resolve spontaneously.[16a,20,54,55,61] However, the vast majority of horses require aggressive treatment. The age at onset appears to be of prognostic

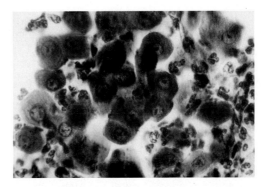

FIGURE 9-9. Pemphigus foliaceus. Nondegenerate neutrophils and acantholytic keratinocytes.

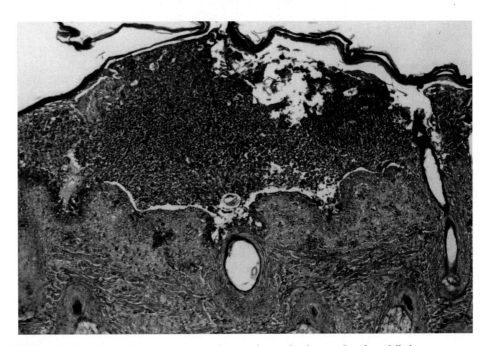

FIGURE 9-10. Pemphigus foliaceus. Large subcorneal pustule also involves hair follicles.

significance.[16a,57] In general, younger horses (≤1 year) may have less severe disease, may respond better to treatment, and may eventually remain in remission when treatment is withdrawn.

In most cases, the initial treatment of choice is oral prednisolone or prednisone (2 to 4 mg/kg orally q24h [see Chapter 3]).[10,13,57,61] The induction dose should be maintained until the disease is inactive (usually 10 to 14 days). Following induction, the dosage is tapered to an alternate-morning regimen (see Chapter 3). Patients failing to respond to prednisolone or prednisone may respond to dexamethasone (0.2 to 0.4 mg/kg orally q24h).[13,44,57,61] Dexamethasone is not as safe as prednisolone or prednisone for chronic alternate-morning maintenance therapy (see Chapter 3). Hence, if dexamethasone was used to achieve remission, one should attempt to substitute prednisolone or prednisone for maintenance.

In horses that do not respond to glucocorticoids or when glucocorticoids are undesirable, azathioprine (2.5 mg/kg orally q24h for induction, then q48h for maintenance) or aurothioglucose

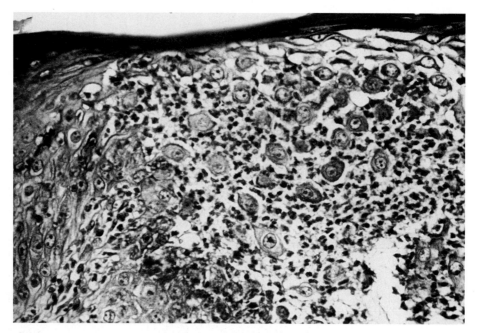

FIGURE 9-11. Pemphigus foliaceus. Numerous acantholytic keratinocytes and neutrophils within a sub-corneal pustule.

(1 mg/kg intramuscularly every week for induction, then every 1 to 2 months for maintenance) may be useful (see Therapy of Immune-Mediated Skin Diseases).* Both of these agents, or an omega-3/omega-6 fatty acid–containing product may be useful for reducing required dosages of glucocorticoids.[57] Anecdotal reports indicate that pentoxifylline may be useful for the treatment of pemphigus foliaceus.

Some horses respond to therapy and remain in prolonged remission without further treatment.[13,57,61] However, about 50% of these cases relapse within 2 to 30 months. In general, rapid relapses and multiple recurrences often become progressively less responsive to previous treatment regimens.[57,61] Some mares requiring low-dose alternate-morning prednisone to control their pemphigus foliaceus have been successfully bred.[61]

Pemphigus foliaceus is often worse and more difficult to control in sunny, hot, humid weather.[13,57,61] Sun avoidance is very important. Gentle cleansing is often useful for decreasing the increased pruritus often associated with sweating.[57,61]

PEMPHIGUS VULGARIS

In humans, the major pemphigus vulgaris antigen is desmoglein III, a 130-kd glycoprotein from the cadherin group of adhesion molecules.[15,21,22] In more severe cases that also have cutaneous involvement, antibodies to desmoglein I are also present.[21,22] The exact antigen in the horse has not been specifically identified.[17]

Pemphigus vulgaris is extremely rare in the horse.[16a,61] Vesicles, bullae, and resultant painful ulcers were present in the mouth and on the head and neck. Skin biopsy specimens revealed suprabasilar acantholysis, cleft, and vesicle formation. Direct immunofluorescence testing revealed the intercellular deposition of immunoglobulin within affected epidermis.

Prognosis appears to be grave. Systemic glucocorticoid therapy has not been effective.[16a]

---

*References 12, 13, 44, 48, 57, 61.

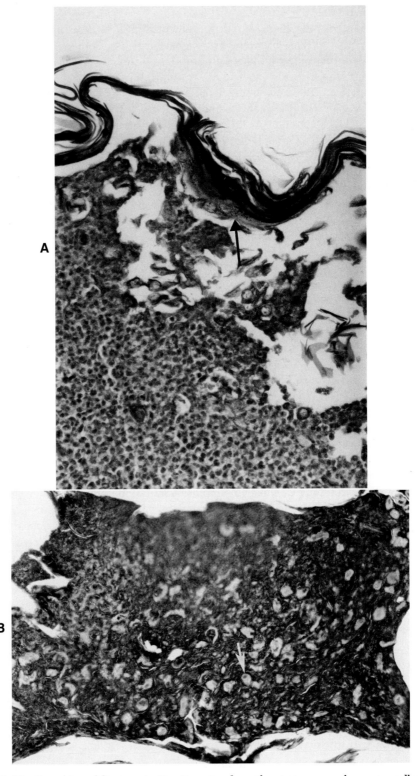

FIGURE 9-12. Pemphigus foliaceus. **A,** Keratinocytes from the stratum granulosum are adhered to the overlying stratum corneum ("cling-ons") (*arrow*). **B,** Numerous acantholytic keratinocytes (*arrow*) in crust with pemphigus foliaceus.

PARANEOPLASTIC PEMPHIGUS

This form of pemphigus was first characterized in humans in 1990 and recently described in horses.[3,15,30,62,63] The diagnostic criteria established in humans include the following: severe oral ulceration with polymorphous skin eruptions; histology that includes intraepithelial acantholysis, keratinocyte apoptosis, and vacuolar interface changes; direct immunofluorescence testing findings that include the intercellular deposition of IgG with the epithelium, and C3 in a granular pattern along the basement membrane zone; and indirect immunofluorescence findings that include IgG deposition in the intercellular spaces on monkey esophagus and rodent urinary bladder.[30,62] The immunofluorescence findings on rodent urinary bladder have a specificity of 83% and a sensitivity of 75%; thus, false-positive and false-negative results occur.[30,62] Immuno-precipitation studies are needed to confirm the diagnosis by identifying the characteristic antigen complex: plakins (desmoplakins I [250 kd] and II [210 kd], bullous pemphigoid antigen I [230 kd], envoplakin [210 kd], periplakin [190 kd]), desmoglein III (130 kd), and an unidentified (170 kd) transmembrane antigen.[30,62] Antibodies from human patients reproduce the cutaneous lesions when injected into newborn mice.

The pathogenesis of paraneoplastic pemphigus is unknown. It has been hypothesized that antitumor immune responses cross-react with normal epithelial proteins, perhaps associated with anomalous expression of desmosomes and/or desmoplakins by the neoplasms, and/or dysregulated cytokine production (e.g., IL-6) by neoplastic cells.[30,62] Autoantibodies against desmoglein III and the 170-kd protein probably initiate acantholysis and cell membrane damage, resulting in auto-antibody formation against desmoplakins. The antidesmoplakin antibodies then enter keratinocytes and bind target autoantigens by an epitope-spreading phenomenon.

A 6-year-old Tennessee walking horse gelding had a history of painful bullae and ulcers of the tongue, gingiva, and lips, along with progressive lethargy, inappetence, and weight loss.[63] These signs were accompanied by a slowly enlarging firm, round, intramuscular mass on the neck. Biopsy specimens from the oral mucosa revealed subepidermal clefts and vesicles in association with a perivascular accumulation of lymphocytes, plasma cells, and neutrophils. Direct immunofluo-rescence testing revealed the intercellular deposition of IgG in the epithelium. Treatment with prednisone, 2.2 mg/kg q12h orally, was of no benefit.

Eight weeks later the horse returned for progressive disease, and the cervical mass was excised and reported to be a hemangiosarcoma. A later publication indicated that the mass was probably a reticulum cell sarcoma.[62] Within 1 week following surgery, the horse began to improve and went on to totally recover. Serum from the horse that had been frozen since the initial visit reacted with the keratinocytes in monkey esophagus and the transitional cells of murine urinary bladder. Immunoprecipitation studies demonstrated that the horse's antibodies reacted with polypeptides at 250 kd and 210 kd (desmoplakin I and II), 230 kd (bullous pemphigoid antigen 1), 210 kd (envoplakin), 190 kd (periplakin), and 170 kd (uncharacterized).[62]

The clinical, immunopathologic, and immunoprecipitation findings in this horse fulfilled four of the five criteria used to diagnose paraneoplastic pemphigus in humans.[3,30,62] Only the histopathology was inconsistent: no acantholysis indicative of pemphigus, rather subepidermal vesiculation more indicative of bullous pemphigoid. At the least, this most interesting case appears to be a good example of a paraneoplastic syndrome.

In humans, paraneoplastic pemphigus is usually associated with malignancies, especially lymphomas.[3,30,62] Unless the associated neoplasm can be cured, immunosuppressive therapy is not very effective.[3,30,62]

Autoimmune Subepidermal Bullous Dermatoses

The classification of autoimmune blistering diseases is based on the antigen(s) targeted by pathogenic autoantibodies. The autoimmune subepidermal bullous diseases represent different nosologic entities.[3,15] Recent studies conducted by Olivry and colleagues have demonstrated that canine subepidermal bullous diseases include bullous pemphigoid (autoantibodies against bullous pemphigoid antigen 2 [type XVII collagen]), epidermolysis bullosa acquisita (autoantibodies against type VII collagen), bullous systemic lupus erythematosus (IgG autoantibodies against the noncollagenous aminoterminus of type VII collagen), linear IgA bullous dermatosis (IgA and IgG autoantibodies against the extracellular portion of bullous pemphigoid antigen 2, from which the intracellular, transmembrane, and NC16A domains have been removed by proteolysis), and mucous membrane pemphigoid (autoantibodies against a 97-kd antigen—possibly the C-terminus of bullous pemphigoid antigen 2—in the lower lamina lucida).[15] These entities are similar clinically, histopathologically, and with routine immunofluorescence or immunohistochemical testing. However, they are different diseases and studies of larger numbers of cases may reveal important prognostic and therapeutic differences. A similar situation may exist with equine subepidermal bullous diseases.

The use of salt-split skin as a substrate for indirect immunofluorescence testing is a practical contribution to the study of autoimmune subepidermal bullous diseases.[3,15] A 1-molar solution of NaCl splits skin through the lamina lucida, allowing the recognition of autoantibodies that bind to the roof (epidermal), floor (dermal), or combined both sides of the split.

BULLOUS PEMPHIGOID

Bullous pemphigoid is a very rare autoimmune, vesiculobullous, ulcerative disorder of skin or oral mucosa or both.*

Cause and Pathogenesis

Bullous pemphigoid is characterized histologically by subepidermal vesicle formation and immunologically by the presence of one or two autoantibodies against antigens at the basal cell hemidesmosomes of skin and mucosa.[3,15,71] The bullous pemphigoid antigens are present in all mammalian and avian skin and are associated with hemidesmosomes and the lamina lucida of the basement membrane.

The first antigen is bullous pemphigoid antigen 1 (BPAg 1, BP230) which is a 230-kd intracellular antigen that is a homolog to desmoplakin I.[3] Serum antibodies to this antigen have not yet been described in horses. The second bullous pemphigoid antigen (BPAg 2, BP180), also called *collagen XVII*, is a 180-kd hemidesmosomal transmembranous molecule.[3] Equine cases of bullous pemphigoid exhibit antibodies to this latter molecule.[70] The cause of antibody production is still unknown, but genetic factors have been determined in humans and dogs. In humans, the expression of BPAG is greatest in skin where lesions commonly occur.[67] Pemphigoid antibodies from affected humans produce locally the clinical, histologic, and immunopathologic features of bullous pemphigoid when injected into rabbit cornea, guinea pig skin, or neonatal mice.[1,3,70]

The proposed pathomechanism of blister formation in bullous pemphigoid is as follows: (1) the binding of complement-fixing pemphigoid antibody to the antigen of the hemidesmosomes, (2) complement fixation and activation, (3) activation of mast cells and release of chemotactic cytokines, (4) chemoattraction of neutrophils and eosinophils, and (5) release of proteolytic enzymes from the infiltrating leukocytes, which disrupt dermoepidermal cohesion, resulting in dermoepidermal separation and vesicle formation.[3,15] In humans, elevated concentrations of eosinophil cationic protein, major basic protein, and neutrophil-derived myeloperoxidase and elastase were detected in blister fluid and serum of patients with bullous pemphigoid, suggesting that the release of these substances from activated granulocytes may be important in the

References 10, 13, 16a, 57, 61, 66, 68-70, 72.

pathogenesis of blister formation.[65] An eosinophil-derived enzyme, gelatinase, may be involved in cleaving the type XVII collagen.[64]

Other factors thought to be involved in the pathogenesis of some cases of bullous pemphigoid are drug provocation (especially sulfonamides, penicillins, and furosemide) and ultraviolet light.[3,15]

Clinical Features

Bullous pemphigoid is very rare, accounting for only 0.22% of the equine skin diseases seen at the Cornell University Clinic. It is a severe, rapidly progressive, mucocutaneous disorder.[16a,57,70,72] No breed or sex predilections are apparent, and affected horses have varied from 5 to 14 years. The oral cavity, mucocutaneous junctions (lips, vulva, anus, eyelids), and intertriginous areas (axilla, groin) are ulcerated, oozing, and crusted (Fig. 9-3, *D* through *F*). Epidermal collarettes are prominent, but intact vesicles and bullae are transient and not commonly seen. Lesions are painful. One horse had corneal ulcers and edema of the distal limbs and ventrum.[69] Another horse had immune deposits in the kidneys.[61] All horses have been severely ill (depression, anorexia, weight loss, pyrexia).

Diagnosis

The differential diagnosis of bullous pemphigoid includes pemphigus vulgaris, systemic lupus erythematosus, erythema multiforme, drug reaction, vesicular stomatitis, herpes coital exanthema, stachybotryotoxicosis, paraneoplastic stomatitis, and candidiasis.

The definitive diagnosis is based on history, physical examination, skin or mucosal biopsy, immunofluorescence or immunohistochemical testing, and demonstration of the antigen targeted (BPAG2). Histopathologically, bullous pemphigoid is characterized by subepidermal cleft and vesicle formation (Fig. 9-13, *A*).[10,12,69,70,72] Acantholysis is not seen. Inflammatory infiltrates vary from mild and perivascular to moderate and interstitial. Neutrophils and mononuclear cells usually predominate. Tissue eosinophilia is uncommon. Subepidermal vacuolar alteration is the earliest prevesicular histopathologic finding (Fig. 9-13, *B*).

Electron microscopic examination reveals the following features: smudging, thickening, and interruption of the basement membrane zone; fragmentation and disappearance of the anchoring fibrils, anchoring filaments, and hemidesmosomes; basal cell degeneration; and separation occurring within the lamina lucida.[72]

Direct immunofluorescence testing or immunohistochemical testing reveals a linear deposition of immunoglobulin, and usually complement, at the basement membrane zone of skin or mucosa.[10,61,69,70,72] Indirect immunofluorescence testing is usually positive (IgG autoantibodies directed at the basement membrane) (Fig. 9-14).

Clinical Management

All reported cases have had severe, progressive disease, and have died prior to or in spite of glucocorticoid therapy. It would appear that early diagnosis and institution of aggressive immuno-suppressive treatment (e.g., glucocorticoids and azathioprine) will be needed to successfully manage equine bullous pemphigoid. Because cutaneous lesions of bullous pemphigoid in humans can be induced by exposure to ultraviolet light, it would be prudent to avoid direct exposure to sunlight between 8 AM and 5 PM.[3,15]

Lupus Erythematosus

Lupus erythematosus is a term that encompasses a group of diseases with different clinical syndromes that share a similar underlying autoimmune process.[3,15,79] The appropriate terminology and classification of the syndromes and cases with these disorders have led to, and still create, differing views and controversy. The terminology and a classification system used in humans,

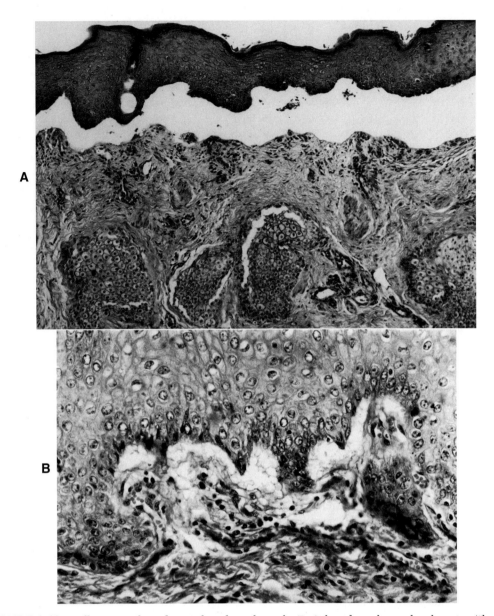

FIGURE 9-13. Bullous pemphigoid. **A,** Subepidermal vesicle. **B,** Subepidermal vacuolar alteration ("bubbles") with bullous pemphigoid.

described by Sontheimer, is beginning to be utilized in veterinary medicine.[15,79] In Sontheimer's system the basis is that there is lupus erythematosus, which may be systemic or cutaneous. The systemic form of lupus erythematosus may be associated with any of the lupus-related skin diseases, or many nonspecific cutaneous lesions. The lupus erythematosus–related skin disease might be nonspecific, or it may be one of the forms of cutaneous lupus erythematosus that are specific skin syndromes, characterized by certain clinical and histopathologic findings. The different forms of cutaneous lupus erythematosus vary as concerns the probability of associated systemic disease. In the horse, we have classically recognized two main forms of cutaneous lupus erythematosus.

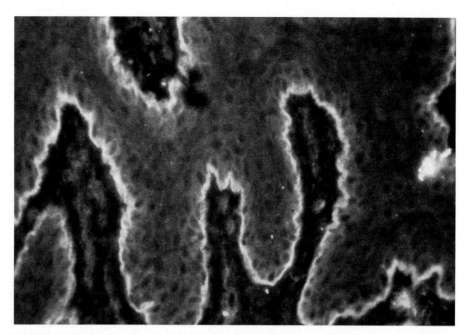

FIGURE 9-14. Bullous pemphigoid. IgG deposited on basement membrane zone on indirect immunofluorescence testing.

Lupus erythematosus is a rare autoimmune disorder that has polyclonal lymphocytic involvement. The exact etiology is unknown, but in humans, all forms are characterized by a variety of autoantibodies to nuclear antigens and/or immune complex deposition. Genetic associations have been described in humans and dogs. In humans, the different forms of cutaneous lupus erythematosus have different genetic markers. Other precipitating factors include viral infections, drugs, hormones, chemical exposure, and cigarette smoking.[3,15]

The pathogenesis of skin lesions in lupus erythematosus is unclear. All three forms of cutaneous lupus erythematosus in humans, as well as canine cutaneous lupus erythematosus, are often exacerbated by exposure to ultraviolet radiation.[3,15] In humans, it has been demonstrated that the lymphocytes infiltrating skin lesions of discoid and systemic lupus erythematosus are predominantly T cells, and that helper T cells predominate in discoid lupus, whereas suppressor T cells predominate in the systemic variety.[3]

Five characteristics of cutaneous lupus erythematosus are (1) photosensitivity (lesions may be produced by sunlight in both the UVB and UVA spectra), (2) keratinocyte damage (associated with contiguous T lymphocytes and macrophages), (3) lymphohistiocytic infiltration, (4) autoantibody production, and (5) immune complex deposition.* Skin lesions may be induced or exacerbated with ultraviolet light exposure. Infusion of antinuclear antibodies does not produce skin lesions, however, and immune complexes appear at the basement membrane zone after dermatohistopathologic changes appear (up to 6 weeks *after* inflammatory changes appear).

A current hypothesis for the pathogenesis of skin lesions in genetically susceptible individuals is as follows:
1. Ultraviolet light (both UVB and UVA) penetrating to the level of epidermal basal cells induces, on the keratinocyte surface, the enhanced expression of ICAM-1 and of autoantigens (e.g., Ro) previously found only in the nucleus or cytoplasm (e.g., native and denatured DNA).

---

*References 3, 15, 73, 75, 77, 78, 80.

2. Specific autoantibodies to these antigens that are present in plasma and in tissue fluid bathing the epidermis attach to keratinocytes and induce antibody-dependent cytotoxicity of keratinocytes.

3. Injured keratinocytes release IL-2 and other lymphocyte attractants, accounting for the resultant lymphohistiocytic infiltrate.

4. Injured keratinocytes release increased amounts of TNF-α, IL-1, and IL-6, which are associated with elevations of antinuclear antibodies (ANA), increased B cell activity, and higher production of IgM.[3,15]

In one study of cutaneous lupus erythematosus in humans,[73] there was a marked increase in Ki-67 (a protein essential for cell proliferation) and p53 (a protein that can regulate cell proliferation and down-regulate bcl-2), and a marked decrease in bcl-2 (a protein that promotes cell survival and inhibits apoptosis). It was hypothesized that basal keratinocytes, damaged by antibody-dependent cellular cytotoxicity, become hyperproliferative (thus expressing Ki-67), which includes the expression of p53, which in turn, down-regulates bcl-2 and activates an apoptotic pathway in the epidermis.

SYSTEMIC LUPUS ERYTHEMATOSUS

Systemic lupus erythematosus is a very rare multisystemic autoimmune disorder of horses, accounting for only 0.22% of the equine skin diseases seen at the Cornell University Clinic.

Cause and Pathogenesis

The etiology of systemic lupus erythematosus appears to be multifactorial, with genetic predilection, immunologic disorder (suppressor T cell deficiency; B cell hyperactivity; deficiencies of complement components), viral infection, and hormonal and ultraviolet light modulation all playing a role.[1-4,15] B cell hyperactivity results in a plethora of autoantibodies formed against numerous body constituents. In humans and dogs, a number of drugs (especially procainamide, hydralazine, isoniazid, sulfonamides, penicillamine, several anticonvulsants, and contraceptives), as well as modified live virus vaccines are thought to precipitate or exacerbate systemic lupus erythematosus.[3,15]

Clinical Features

The clinical signs associated with systemic lupus erythematosus are varied and changeable. Because of this phenomenal clinical variability and ability to mimic numerous diseases, systemic lupus erythematosus has been called the "great imitator."

Systemic lupus erythematosus is a rare, multisystemic autoimmune disorder of the horse.[12,13,74,81] No age, breed, or sex predilections are currently recognized. Cutaneous changes reported in association with equine systemic lupus erythematosus include (1) lymphedema of the distal limbs (Fig. 9-15), (2) panniculitis, (3) mucocutaneous ulceration, (4) patchy alopecia, scaling, and leukoderma of the face, neck, and trunk (Fig. 9-16), and (5) generalized exfoliative dermatitis. Skin lesions may be exacerbated in warm, sunny weather. Extracutaneous abnormalities may include various combinations of polyarthritis, anemia, purpura, peripheral lymphadenopathy, fever, depression, poor appetite, and weight loss.

Diagnosis

The differential diagnosis is lengthy due to the varied and changeable disease manifestations. When cutaneous lesions are present, the differential includes sarcoidosis, multisystemic eosinophilic epitheliotropic disease, pemphigus foliaceus, bullous pemphigoid, pemphigus vulgaris, stachybotryotoxicosis, vasculitis, erythema multiforme, drug reaction, seborrhea, and epitheliotropic lymphoma.

The definitive diagnosis of systemic lupus erythematosus is often one of the most challenging tasks in medicine. The clinicopathologic abnormalities that are demonstrated depend on the organ systems involved and may include anemia (nonregenerative or hemolytic, with or without a positive direct Coombs' test result); thrombocytopenia with or without a positive platelet factor-3 test result; leukopenia or leukocytosis; proteinuria (glomerulonephritis); hypergammaglobulinemia (polyclonal); and sterile synovial exudate obtained by arthrocentesis. The lupus

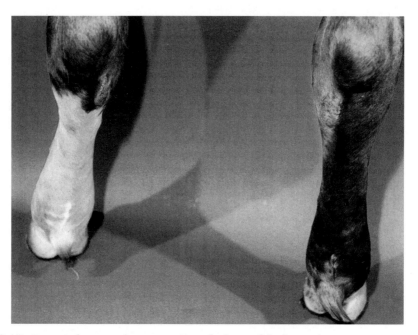

FIGURE 9-15. Systemic lupus erythematosus. Lymphedema of the legs.

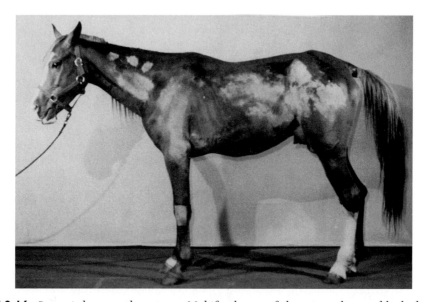

FIGURE 9-16. Systemic lupus erythematosus. Multifocal areas of alopecia, scaling, and leukoderma.

erythematosus (LE) cell test may have a positive result, but it is variable from day to day, is steroid-labile, and lacks sensitivity and specificity.[15,74] The antinuclear antibody (ANA) test is currently considered the most specific and sensitive serologic test for systemic lupus erythematosus. It must be remembered that ANA can be detected from time to time with probably *any* disease, as well as in healthy animals.[13,15,74] Thus a positive ANA titer must always be interpreted in light of other critical historical, physical, and laboratory data.

The most characteristic dermatohistopathologic finding is an interface dermatitis (hydropic or lichenoid or both), which may involve hair follicle outer root sheaths (Figs. 9-17 and 9-18).[13,15,19,74] Other helpful findings include subepidermal vacuolar alteration, focal thickening of the basement membrane zone, and dermal mucinosis.

Direct immunofluorescence or immunohistochemical testing reveals the deposition of immunoglobulin or complement or both at the basement membrane zone, often known as a positive "lupus band."[1,3,15,74]

In humans, the American Rheumatism Association developed criteria for the diagnosis of systemic lupus erythematosus, and these were modified in 1982. These have also been applied to dogs with minor modifications, primarily those reflecting the humoral immunologic responses of the canine (Table 9-1).[15] Dogs that develop four or more of the modified criteria during any given observation period have systemic lupus erythematosus. It has also been suggested that a probable diagnosis of systemic lupus erythematosus is appropriate if three criteria are present or if polyarthritis with ANAs is present. Though these criteria are helpful guidelines, they must be utilized cautiously. In humans, numerous situations that may lead to a false diagnosis based on the American Rheumatism Association criteria have been described. The presence of skin disease and subsequent diagnosis of systemic lupus erythematosus is particularly problematic, and other multipart classification schemes have been proposed.[3] The usefulness of such criteria in horses is undetermined.

Because no single laboratory test is diagnostic for systemic lupus erythematosus, the veterinarian must rely on the recognition of multisystemic disease (especially joint, skin, kidney, oral mucosa, and hematopoietic system), positive ANA result, and confirmatory histopathologic and immunopathologic findings in involved skin or oral mucosa or both.

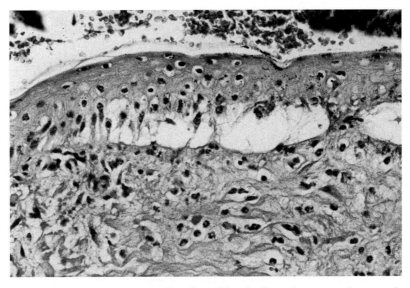

FIGURE 9-17. Hydropic degeneration of epidermal basal cells, with systemic lupus erythematosus.

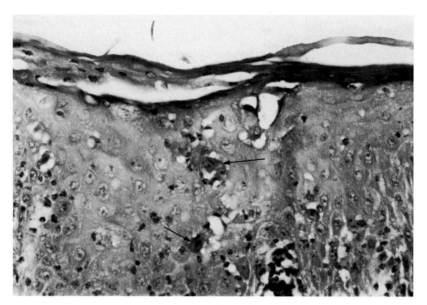

FIGURE 9-18. Apoptotic keratinocytes (*arrows*) in systemic lupus erythematosus.

● Table 9-1   **CRITERIA FOR THE DIAGNOSIS OF CANINE SYSTEMIC LUPUS ERYTHEMATOSUS***

CRITERION	DEFINITION
Erythema	Redness in areas of skin that are thin or poorly protected by the haircoat (particularly the face)
Discoid rash	Depigmentation, erythema, erosions, ulcerations, crusts, and keratotic scaling that selectively affect the face (e.g., nasal planum, forehead, lips, and periocular region)
Photosensitivity	Skin rash resulting from an unusual reaction to sunlight
Oral ulcers	Oral or nasopharyngeal ulceration, usually painless
Arthritis	Nonerosive arthritis involving two or more peripheral joints characterized mainly by pain during movement (progressive forced flexion-extension); swelling or effusion – often not very marked
Serositis	Presence of a nonseptic inflammatory cavity effusion (pleuritis or pericarditis)
Renal disorders	Persistent proteinuria (>0.5 g/L or >3+ if quantification is not performed) or cellular casts (red cell, hemoglobin, or mixed)
Neurological disorders	Seizures or psychosis in the absence of offending drugs or known metabolic disorders (e.g., uremia, ketoacidosis, or electrolyte imbalances)
Hematologic disorders	Hemolytic anemia (with reticulocytosis) or leukopenia (<3000/mm^3 total on two or more occasions) or lymphopenia (<1000/mm^3 total on two or more occasions) or thrombocytopenia (<100,000/mm^3 in the absence of offending drugs)
Immunologic disorders	Antihistone (antibody to histone at an abnormal titer) or anti-Sm (antibody to the Sm nuclear antigen) or anti-type 1 (antibody to a 43-kd nuclear antigen) or T-cell subsets (a striking decrease in the CD8+ population [<200/mm^3] or a CD4+:CD8+ ratio higher than 4.0)
Antinuclear antibodies (ANAs)	An abnormal titer of ANAs as shown by immunofluorescence or an equivalent assay in the absence of drugs known to be associated with their formation

*Adapted from the 1982 revised American Rheumatism Association Criteria.[3]
From Chabanne L, et al: Canine systemic lupus erythematosus. Part II. Diagnosis and treatment. Comp Cont Ed 21:402, 1999.

Clinical Management

The prognosis in systemic lupus erythematosus is generally unpredictable and depends on the organs involved.[3,15] In general, the earlier the diagnosis is made, the better the prognosis.

Therapy must be individualized. The initial agent of choice is probably large doses of systemic glucocorticoids (2 to 4 mg/kg prednisolone or prednisone orally q24h, or 0.2 to 0.4 mg/kg dexamethasone orally q24h). In one case[81] glucocorticoid therapy was stopped after several months, and the horse remained in remission for another 12 months. When systemic glucocorticoids are unsatisfactory, other immunomodulating drugs may be useful, such as azathioprine and omega-3/omega-6 fatty acids. Patients with systemic lupus erythematosus are prone to infections.[3,12,15] Thus, infections must be identified quickly and treated aggressively.

DISCOID LUPUS ERYTHEMATOSUS

Discoid lupus erythematosus is a rare immune-mediated dermatitis of the horse, accounting for only 0.33% of the equine skin disease seen at the Cornell University Clinic.

Cause and Pathogenesis

Equine discoid lupus erythematosus is a relatively benign cutaneous disease with no systemic involvement.[13,16a,82] Sun exposure often aggravates the disease, suggesting that photosensitivity plays a role in the pathogenesis. Anecdotal reports indicate that, in many cases, there appears to be a triggering of disease onset by various incidents, including excessive sun exposure, extremes in environmental temperature (hot or cold), drug administration, or "stressful situations."[16a] In humans, it has been demonstrated that the lymphocytes infiltrating skin lesions are predominantly T cells, especially helper T cells.[3,15] A current hypothesis concerning the pathogenesis of lesion formation is presented in the discussion on systemic lupus erythematosus.

Clinical Features

Equine discoid lupus erythematosus is a rare dermatosis in which there is no systemic involvement.[13,16a,82] No breed or sex predilections are apparent, and affected horses range from 1 to 14 years. The onset of lesions may be gradual or rapid. Skin lesions begin on the face—especially the lips, nostrils, and periocular region—and include more or less symmetric areas of erythema, scaling, and alopecia (Fig. 9-19). These lesions are annular to oval, variably well circumscribed, and manifest variable degrees of leukoderma (Fig. 9-20). Crusts, erosions, and leukotrichia (Fig. 9-21) are occasionally present. Pruritus and pain are typically mild to absent. Some horses develop lesions on the pinnae, neck, and shoulders and on the perianal, perineal, and genital areas. The disease is often exacerbated in warm, sunny weather.

DIAGNOSIS

The differential diagnosis includes photodermatitis, dermatophytosis, demodicosis, onchocerciasis, and in the absence of gross signs of inflammation, vitiligo. The definitive diagnosis is based on history, physical examination, skin biopsy, and immunofluorescence or immunohistochemical testing. Skin biopsy reveals an interface dermatitis (hydropic, lichenoid, or both) (Fig. 9-22).[16a,82] Focal hydropic degeneration and apoptosis of basal epidermal and follicular outer root sheath cells (Fig. 9-23), pigmentary incontinence (Fig. 9-24), focal thickening of the basement membrane zone (Fig. 9-24), subepidermal vacuolar alteration (Fig. 9-25), marked accumulations of lymphocytes, plasma cells, and histiocytes around dermal vessels and appendages, and variable degrees of dermal mucinosis are common features. In one horse, occasional multinucleated histiocytic giant cells were present (Fig. 9-26).[82] "Fibrinoid material" may be seen in the superficial dermis, near the basement membrane zone and/or perivascularly.[16a]

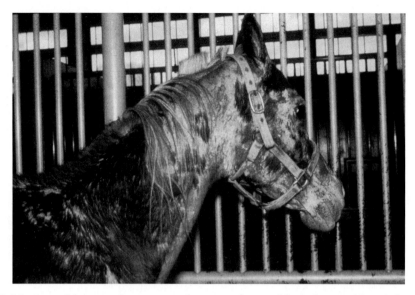

FIGURE 9-19. Discoid lupus erythematosus. Alopecia, scaling, and leukoderma of face and neck.

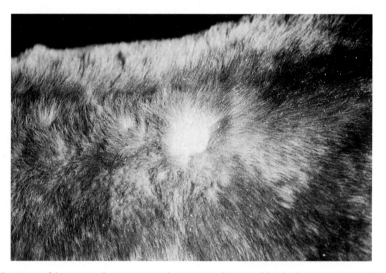

FIGURE 9-20. Discoid lupus erythematosus. Alopecia, scaling, and leukoderma over neck.

It must be emphasized, here, that the basement membrane zone in normal horse skin is thick and prominent (see Chapter 1), and caution is warranted in assessing *pathologic* thickening.[16a] It has also been suggested that hydropic degeneration of basal cells is encountered in a variety of superficial inflammatory processes in horse skin, and that this pathologic change seems to lack the specificity it has in other species.[16a] The authors do not agree.[57]

Immunopathologic tests reveal immunoglobulin or complement or both at the basement membrane zone of affected skin (Fig. 9-27). Indirect immunofluorescence testing, ANA tests, and LE cell tests are negative.

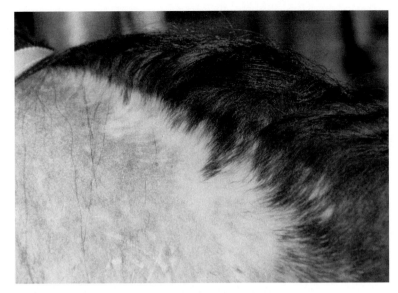

FIGURE 9-21. Discoid lupus erythematosus. Leukoderma and leukotrichia.

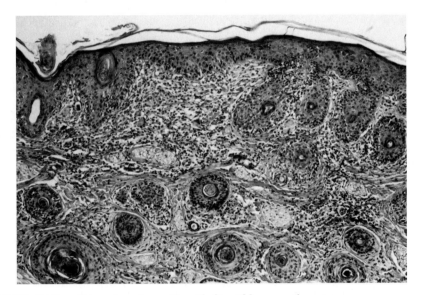

FIGURE 9-22. Lichenoid interface dermatitis with discoid lupus erythematosus.

Clinical Management

The prognosis for discoid lupus erythematosus is usually good. Therapy will probably need to be continued for life, and marked depigmentation predisposes to sunburn.

Therapy of discoid lupus erythematosus must be appropriate to the individual. Mild cases may be controlled by, and all cases benefit from, avoidance of exposure to intense sunlight (from 8 AM to 5 PM), the use of topical sunscreens, and the use of topical glucocorticoids (see Chapter 3). Initially, topical glucocorticoid therapy is most successful when potent agents, such as betamethasone or fluocinolone in DMSO (Synotic), are applied q12h. After the dermatosis is in

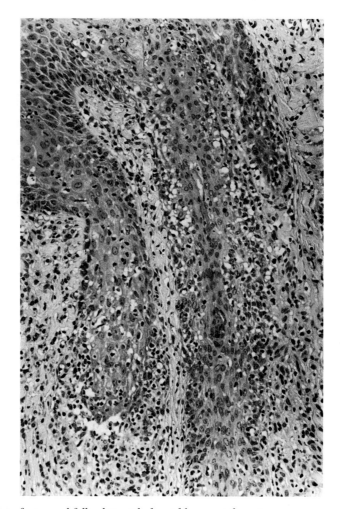

FIGURE 9-23. Interface mural folliculitis with discoid lupus erythematosus.

remission, topical glucocorticoids are applied as needed (once daily, q48h, and so forth), and less potent agents (e.g., 1% to 2% hydrocortisone) may be sufficient for maintenance. In some cases, a 1-month course of systemic prednisolone or prednisone (2.2 mg/kg orally q24h until remission is achieved, then q48h) is helpful. The topical agents may then be sufficient to maintain the remission.

Omega-3/omega-6 fatty acid–containing products (DVM Derm Caps) have been used in dogs and cats in order to reduce glucocorticoid dose requirements[15] and may be useful in horses as well.[57]

Cryoglobulinemia and Cryofibrinogenemia

Cryoglobulinemia and cryofibrinogenemia are very rare causes of ischemic skin disease in horses.

CAUSES AND PATHOGENESIS

Cryoglobulins and *cryofibrinogens* are proteins that can be precipitated from serum and plasma, respectively, by cooling and redissolve on warming.[3,15] Cryoglobulins have been classified into three types according to their characteristics. Type I cryoglobulins are composed solely of mono-

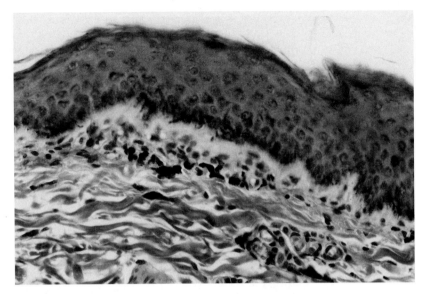

FIGURE 9-24. Thickened basement membrane zone and subjacent pigmentary incontinence with discoid lupus erythematosus.

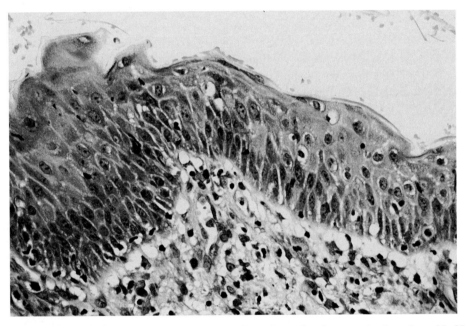

FIGURE 9-25. Discoid lupus erythematosus. Subepidermal vascular alteration ("subepidermal bubbles").

clonal immunoglobulins or free light chains (Bence Jones proteins) and are most commonly associated with lymphoproliferative disorders. Type II cryoglobulins are composed of monoclonal and polyclonal immunoglobulins and are most commonly associated with autoimmune and connective tissue diseases. Type III cryoglobulins are composed of polyclonal immunoglobulins and are seen with infections, autoimmune disorders, and connective tissue diseases. Essential forms

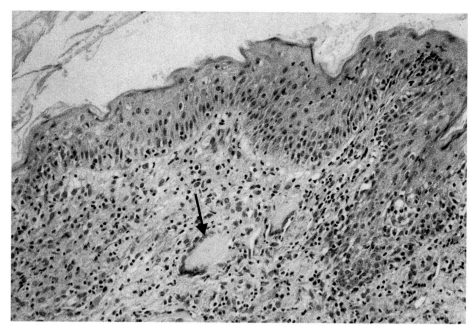

FIGURE 9-26. Discoid lupus erythematosus. Multinucleated histiocytic giant cells (*arrow*).

also may occur where no underlying cause is identifiable. Cutaneous signs associated with cryoglobulins and cryofibrinogens are due to vascular insufficiency (obstruction, stasis, spasm, thrombosis) that occur from microthrombi and vasculitis.

CLINICAL FEATURES

Cold agglutinin disease and cryoglobulinemia are rarely reported in the horse.[83-85] Cold-reacting autoantibodies (usually IgM) may be directed against erythrocytes (cold agglutinin disease, cold hemagglutinin disease, cryopathic hemolytic anemia). The cryopathic autoantibody is most active at colder temperatures (0° to 4° C), but has a wide range of thermal activity. Cold agglutinin disease was reported in a horse affected with wheals and edema of the legs.[83] The condition had occurred with the onset of cold, winter weather for 2 consecutive years. Monoclonal cryo-globulinemia was diagnosed in association with lymphoma in a horse with necrosis and sloughing of the tips of both pinnae.[85] In humans, the most common cutaneous manifestations of cold agglutinin disease are purpura, acrocyanosis, distal necrosis, urticaria, and leg ulcers.[3]

DIAGNOSIS

The differential diagnosis includes vasculitis, systemic lupus erythematosus, drug reaction, frostbite, and the numerous causes of urticaria. The definitive diagnosis of cold agglutinin disease is made by history, physical examination, and demonstration of significant titers of cold agglutinins. *In vitro* autohemagglutination of blood at room temperature can be diagnostic for cold-reacting autoantibodies. Blood in heparin or ethylenediamine-tetra-acetic acid (EDTA) is allowed to cool on a slide, thus permitting the autoagglutination to be readily visible macroscopically. The reaction can be accentuated by cooling the blood to O° C, or reversed by warming the blood to 37° C. Doubtful cases can be confirmed via Coombs' test if the complete test is performed at 4° C and the Coombs reagent has activity against IgM. Caution in the interpretation of the cold Coombs'

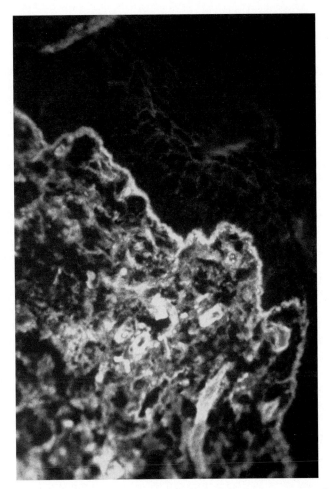

FIGURE 9-27. Discoid lupus erythematosus. IgG deposited at the basement membrane zone on direct immunofluorescence testing.

test is warranted because normal horses can have titers up to 1:100. Cryoprecipitate levels may be crudely determined by allowing venous blood collected in a warm syringe to clot at 37° C for 30 minutes; then the serum and citrated plasma are cooled to 4° C and a gel-like precipitate is formed, which will redissolve upon rewarming to 37° C.

Skin biopsy usually reveals necrosis, ulceration, and often secondary suppurative changes. Fortuitously sampled sections may show vasculitis, thrombotic to necrotic blood vessels, or blood vessels containing an amorphous eosinophilic substance consisting largely of precipitated cryoprotein. Diffuse edema, extravasation of erythrocytes, and homogenization of dermal collagen may also be seen.

CLINICAL MANAGEMENT

The prognosis for cold agglutinin disease varies with the underlying cause. Therapy of cold agglutinin disease includes (1) correction of the underlying cause, if possible, (2) avoidance of cold, and (3) immunosuppressive drug regimens. One reported equine case was treated with systemic glucocorticoids, resulting in clinical recovery and a negative cold Coombs' test.[83]

Graft-Versus-Host Disease

Graft-versus-host disease occurs whenever lymphoid cells from an immunocompetent donor are introduced into a histoincompatible recipient that is incapable of rejecting them.[3] The disease results from donor T cell responses to recipient transplantation antigens. Certain cytokines play an important role in the pathogenesis of graft-versus-host disease, as antibodies to TNF-α and IL-2 can block or ameliorate the condition in animal models.[3] Epidermal and follicular ICAM-1 expression may play a key role in tethering CD8+ T cells (cytotoxic), enabling subsequent interactions between T cells and keratinocytes.[86,88] Activated T cells produce a storm of cytokines, including IL-2, IL-3, IL-4, IFN-α, and TNF-α. These mediators recruit and activate effector cells, including additional lymphocytes, macrophages, and NK cells that attack both host and donor tissue through contact-dependent mechanisms (such as perforin) or soluble mediators (such as TNF-α). In humans, graft-versus-host disease is seen most commonly as a sequela of allogeneic bone marrow transplantation, but may also occur after syngeneic bone marrow transplantation, reinfusion of autologous marrow, blood transfusions, maternal-fetal transplacental transfer of leukocytes, and solid organ transplantation.[3] Graft-versus-host disease has occurred in horses given hepatic and thymic cells from fetuses or peripheral blood lymphocytes from unrelated horses.[87,89]

In humans and dogs, a bone marrow graft from a donor genetically identical for major histocompatibility complex antigens is followed by significant graft-versus-host disease in about 50% of recipients, despite postgraft immunosuppressive therapy.[3,15] Hence, minor histocompatibility antigens are important in the development of disease. The principal target organs in graft-versus-host disease are the skin, liver, and alimentary tract. Affected horses develop an exfoliative to ulcerative dermatitis, ulcerative stomatitis, and diarrhea.

Diagnosis is based on history, physical examination, and skin biopsy. Histopathologic findings in acute graft-versus-host disease include varying degrees of interface dermatitis (hydropic or lichenoid or both) with keratinocyte apoptosis and satellitosis. The lymphocytic exocytosis and apoptosis also target follicular epithelium. In chronic graft-versus-host disease, findings include variable sclerodermoid or poikilodermatous changes.

Therapy of graft-versus-host disease with various combinations of immunomodulatory agents has been only partially and unpredictably effective.[3,15] Leflunomide, when combined with prednisone and cyclosporine, has been reported to virtually eliminate allograft rejection responses in dogs.[15]

Cutaneous Adverse Drug Reaction

Cutaneous adverse drug reactions (drug eruption, drug allergy, dermatitis medicamentosa) in horses are uncommon, variably pruritic, and pleomorphic cutaneous or mucocutaneous reactions to a drug.[12,16a,98]

CAUSE AND PATHOGENESIS

Adverse reactions to drugs are common, and in humans, cutaneous reactions are one of the most common.[3] Drugs responsible for skin eruptions may be administered orally, topically, or by injection or inhalation. Cutaneous adverse drug reactions accounted for 4.11% of the equine skin diseases seen at the Cornell University Clinic. It is likely that this percentage is unusually high due to the referral nature of our practice. In humans, it is reported to be 2.2% of all hospitalized patients and 3 per 1000 courses of drug therapy.[3] Even these numbers are suspect, as few mechanisms exist that would accurately record the incidence of drug reactions.

Adverse drug reactions may be divided into two major groups: (1) predictable, which are usually dose-dependent and are related to the pharmacologic actions of the drugs, and (2) unpredictable or idiosyncratic, which are often dose-independent and are related to the individual's immunologic response or to genetic differences in susceptibility of patients (idiosyncrasy or intolerance), which are often related to metabolic or enzymatic deficiencies. Drug metabolites are generated by cytochrome-P-450-mixed function oxidases (phase I enzymes), but also by other oxidative metabolizing enzymes, some of which are present in skin.[99] Reactive drug metabolites then need to be detoxified by phase II enzymes, such as epoxide hydrolase or glutathione-S-transferase to prevent toxicity. Thus, there are two places for inappropriate generation and/or accumulation of toxic reactants more toxic than the parent compounds. In humans, slow acetylation contributes to sulfonamide drug reactions, and familial anticonvulsant drug reactions are linked to inherited detoxification defects.[99] A hypothesis for the drug reactions associated with sulfonamides and anticonvulsants includes (1) oxidation by cytochrome-P-450 into chemically reactive metabolites (either in liver by hepatic cytochrome-P-450 with secondary transfer to skin, or in keratinocytes by epidermal cytochrome-P-450), and (2) decreased detoxification of these reactive metabolites, which bind to proteins and induce an immunologic response.

Many cutaneous effects of certain drugs are predictable. For instance, many of the anticancer or immunosuppressive drugs can cause alopecia, purpura, poor wound healing, and increased susceptibility to infection through their effects on cellular biology.[3,15] Immunologic reactions involved in cutaneous drug reactions include types I, II, III, and IV hypersensitivity reactions. Newer techniques may help to determine the underlying immune response in some types of drug reactions.[5] Human patients with systemic lupus erythematosus and atopy are thought to be predisposed to cutaneous drug reactions,[3] but no such observations have been made for the horse.

Any drug may cause an eruption, though certain drugs are more frequently associated with the development of cutaneous adverse drug reaction. The most common drugs recognized to produce idiosyncratic cutaneous adverse drug reactions in horses are topical agents, sulfonamides (especially those that are trimethoprim potentiated, such as Tribrissen), penicillins, phenylbutazone, ivermectin, diuretics, antipyretics, and phenothiazine tranquilizers.[16a,98]

CLINICAL FEATURES

Cutaneous adverse drug reactions can mimic virtually any dermatosis (Figs. 9-28 and 9-29) (Table 9-2).* In humans the most common morphologic patterns are exanthematous, urticaria or angioedema, and fixed drug eruption.[3] In horses, the most common reactions were contact der-

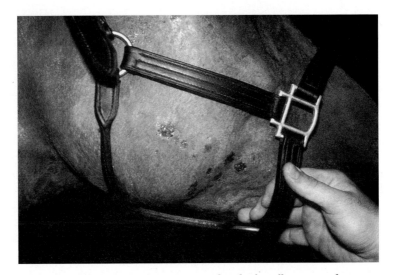

FIGURE 9-28. Vasculitis. Punched-out ulcers associated with phenylbutazone administration.

---

*References 3, 15, 90-95, 97, 98.

● Table 9-2 **CUTANEOUS ADVERSE DRUG REACTIONS IN HORSES**

REACTION PATTERN	FREQUENCY*	DRUGS
Urticaria-angioedema	C	Penicillin, tetracyclines, phenylbutazone, ciprofloxacin, streptomycin, sulfonamides, neomycin, aspirin, various contactants (shampoos, sprays, pour-ons, dips), hormones, vaccines, antisera, guaifenesin, vitamin B complex and liver extract, flunixin, iron dextrans, acepromazine
Exfoliative dermatitis-erythroderma	C	Trimethoprim-sulfonamides, various contactants (shampoos, sprays, dips, pour-ons)
Maculopapular	VR	Phenylbutazone
Erythema multiforme	C	Trimethoprim-sulfonamides, vaccines, ceftiofur
Contact dermatitis	C	Various contactants (shampoos, sprays, dips, pour-ons, ointments, creams, gels, lotions, pastes, etc.)
Injection site panniculitis/vasculitis	R	Vaccines, other injectables
Pemphigus foliaceus	VR	Penicillin
Miscellaneous		
Sterile pyogranuloma		Ivermectin
Vasculitis		Phenylbutazone
Trichorrhexis and hypotrichosis		Ivermectin
Tail dermatitis		Moxidectin
Epitheliotropic lymphoma-like		Drug combinations

*C, Common; R, rare; VR, very rare.

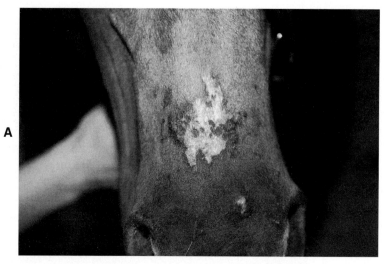

FIGURE 9-29. Trimethoprim-sulfadiazine drug eruption. **A,** Alopecia, depigmentation, and crusts on bridge of nose.

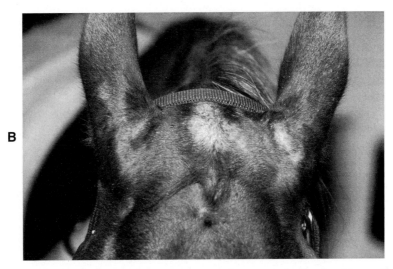

FIGURE 9-29, cont'd. B, Alopecia, depigmentation, and crusts on forehead and base of pinnae.

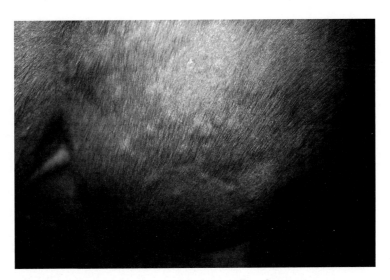

FIGURE 9-30. Urticaria over shoulder associated with penicillin administration.

matitis, exfoliative dermatitis, erythema multiforme, and urticaria.[98] No age or sex predilections have been reported for equine cutaneous drug reactions.[98]

Although no specific type of reaction is related to only one drug, certain reactions are more commonly seen with certain drugs. Urticaria is most commonly caused by penicillin (Fig. 9-30).[98] Erythema multiforme and exfoliative dermatitis (Fig. 9-31) have been most commonly seen with administration of sulfonamides.[98]

Unusual drug eruptions have been reported. One horse developed a painful, sterile pyogranulomatous dermatitis over the neck, ventrum, and limbs (Fig. 9-32, A) following the administration of ivermectin (Fig. 9-33).[98] Another horse developed multifocal trichorrhexis and hypotrichosis following the administration of ivermectin.[98] Severe pruritus over the rump and flanks occurred

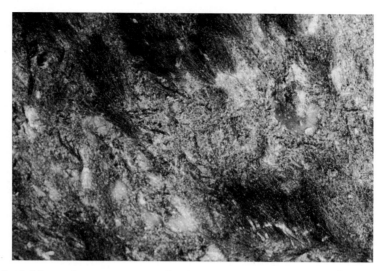

FIGURE 9-31. Exfoliative dermatitis associated with topical therapy.

during the epidural administration of morphine and detomidine.[93a] The authors have seen focal vasculitis and panniculitis in horses following subcutaneous injections. The authors have also received several anecdotal reports of rump and tail head pruritus following the administration of moxidectin.[57] Skin biopsy specimens revealed a cell-poor necrotizing folliculitis. The authors have also seen horses with well-circumscribed, often linear, hyperkeratotic to crusted plaques over the limbs in horses receiving multiple systemic and/or topical medicaments.[57] Histologically, these lesions were characterized by granulomatous mural folliculitis, which is a rare cutaneous reaction pattern apparently associated with drug administration in dogs.[15] A vesicular and ulcerative eruption of the oral, anal, and genital mucosae and the skin of the muzzle and eyelids was reported in a neonatal foal.[92a] Histological findings included subepidermal vesicles, dermal papillary neutrophilic microabscesses, and perifollicular accumulations of neutrophils. The foal recovered spontaneously, and the eruption was attributed to the topical application of iodine (iododerma).

Because drug reaction can mimic so many different dermatoses, it is imperative to have an accurate knowledge of the medications given to any patient with an obscure dermatosis. Drug eruption may occur after a drug has been given for days or years, or a few days after drug therapy is stopped. Eruptions most commonly occur within 1 to 3 weeks after initiating therapy.[98] Some reactions (vasculitis, nodules, vaccine reactions) may occur weeks to months after the drug is administered.[3,15,98] At present, the only reliable test for the diagnosis of drug eruption is to withdraw the drug and watch for disappearance of the eruption (usually in 1 to 2 weeks). Occasionally, however, drug eruptions may persist for weeks to months after the offending drug is stopped (e.g., reactions to vaccines and other injectables).[3,15,98] Purposeful readministration of the offending drug to determine whether the eruption will be reproduced is undesirable and may be dangerous.

DIAGNOSIS

The differential diagnosis is complex, because cutaneous adverse drug reaction may mimic virtually any dermatosis. In general, no specific or characteristic laboratory findings indicate drug eruption. Results of *in vivo* and *in vitro* immunologic tests have usually been disappointing. The basophil degranulation test has been reported to be a valuable test for detecting some

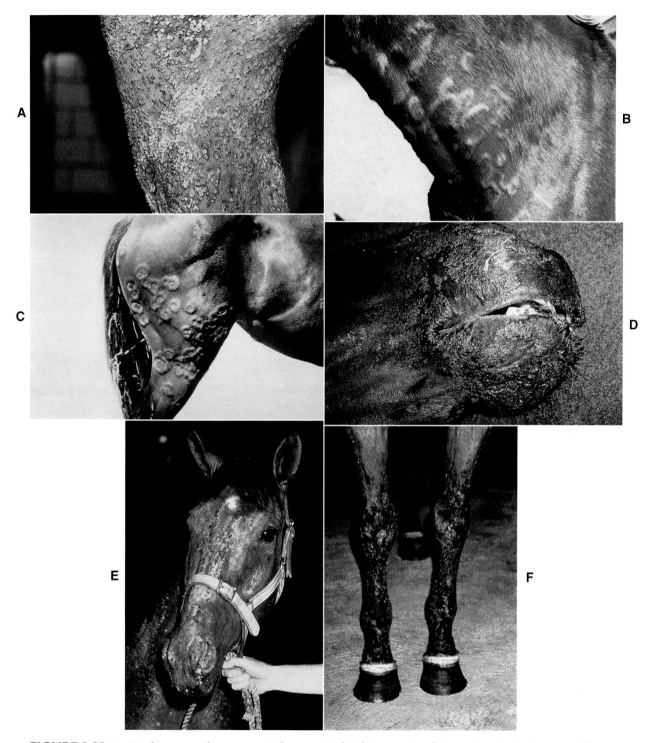

FIGURE 9-32. A, Sterile pyogranulomatous pustules associated with ivermectin administration. **B,** Erythema multiforme. Annular and serpiginous lesion over neck. (*Courtesy Dr. A. Stannard.*) **C,** Erythema multiforme. Annular, donut-like lesions with central scale-crust on thigh. (*Courtesy Dr. A. Stannard.*) **D,** Erythema multiforme due to trimethoprim-sulfadiazine administration. Well-circumscribed ulcers on muzzle. **E,** Erythema multiforme. Well-circumscribed ulcers on face and pinnae. **F,** Erythema multiforme. Well-circumscribed ulcers on legs.

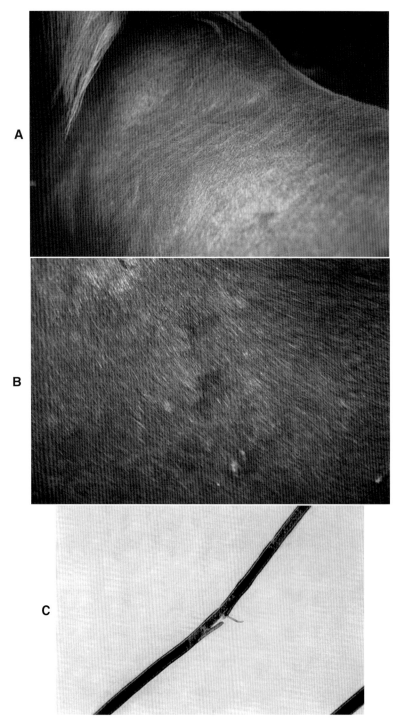

FIGURE 9-33. Drug reaction to ivermectin. **A,** Linear areas of trichorrhexis and hypotrichosis. **B,** Trichorrhexis and irregular lengths of hairs. **C,** Drug reaction (ivermectin). Anatomy of hair shaft is focally obscured, and shaft is weakened resulting in breakage.

hypersensitivity-induced cutaneous adverse drug reactions,[15] but this test is technically demanding and generally unavailable.

Helpful criteria for determining whether a drug eruption is likely are as follows:[3,15,98]

1. Hypersensitivity or reactions occur in a minority of patients receiving the drug.
2. Observed manifestations do not resemble known pharmacologic actions for the drugs.
3. Previous experience that the suspect drug is known for causing this type of cutaneous reaction.
4. Lack of alternative etiologies that could explain the cutaneous reaction that occurred while taking the suspect drug.
5. Appropriate timing—cutaneous adverse drug reactions generally will occur within the first 1 to 3 weeks of the initiation of therapy with the offending drug and while the drug is still being taken or is still present in the body. Prior exposure to the drug may have been tolerated without adverse effects, and if the reaction is a hypersensitivity, prior exposure should have occurred so that sensitization could occur. If an animal has been previously sensitized, cutaneous reactions may be seen within hours to days of drug readministration.
6. Dechallenge. Resolution begins to occur within 1 to 2 weeks after drug is discontinued. For some reactions—such as fixed drug, lichenoid, and local injection reactions—resolution may require several weeks.
7. Rechallenge. Reaction is reproduced by administration of small doses of the drugs or of cross-reacting drugs. Though this is the most definitive way to document the drug reaction, it is generally not recommended because more serious reactions may occur. In one study, 10.5% of cases of cutaneous adverse drug reaction in horses were confirmed by rechallenge.[98]

Identifying the specific cause of a cutaneous drug eruption can be difficult, because many patients are receiving several drugs at the same time.[3,15,98] In some cases the reactions only occur with drug combinations, and one drug will be tolerated.

Recently, possible causal drug exposure in dogs has been assessed by adaptation of drug implication criteria adopted by the French committee for pharmacologic surveillance in humans (Table 9-3).[15,96] The usefulness of such criteria in horses is unknown.

Just as the clinical morphology of drug reactions varies greatly, so do the histologic findings (Figs. 9-34 through 9-38). Histologic patterns recognized with cutaneous adverse drug reactions include perivascular dermatitis (pure, spongiotic, hyperplastic), interface dermatitis (hydropic, lichenoid), vasculitis/vasculopathy, intraepidermal vesiculopustular dermatitis, subepidermal vesicular dermatitis, cell-poor follicular necrosis, interstitial dermatitis, and panniculitis. Eosinophils may be absent or numerous. Some syndromes—such as erythema multiforme—have their own characteristic histopathology. Granulomatous mural folliculitis is characterized by infiltration and eventual replacement of follicular epithelium, and occasionally sebaceous glands, by granulomatous inflammation.

CLINICAL MANAGEMENT

The prognosis for drug reactions is usually good unless other organ systems are involved or there is extensive epidermal necrosis. Therapy of drug reaction consists of (1) discontinuing the offending drug, (2) treating symptoms with topical and systemic medications as indicated, and (3) avoiding chemically related drugs.[3,15,98] Drug reactions may be poorly responsive to glucocorticoids.[12,16a] Hence, a lack of response to glucocorticoids in a disorder that should respond is one indication that the clinician should consider drug reaction.[16a]

Erythema Multiforme

Erythema multiforme is an uncommon, acute, often self-limited eruption of the skin, mucous membranes, or both, characterized by distinctive gross lesions and a diagnostic sequence of pathologic changes.[3,15,105]

● Table 9-3 **PROPOSED CRITERIA FOR THE IMPLICATION OF DRUGS AS CAUSES OF CUTANEOUS ERUPTIONS**[262,292]

Drugs are given a numerical score of −3 to +3 based on the added values obtained from the following three criteria.

Delay in Appearance of Lesions as Related to Drug Administration

Drug attributed a score of:
a. +1 (suggestive) if lesions began over 7 days after the first administration of the drug *or* less than 1 day after reexposure to a culprit medication.
b. 0 (inconclusive) if a specific assessment could not be made.
c. −1 (not suggestive) if criteria for "suggestive" (+1) are not met.

Effect of Drug Interruption on Cutaneous Lesions

Drug attributed a score of:
a. +1 (suggestive) if lesions resolve solely with removal of suspect drug.
b. 0 (inconclusive)
c. −1 (incompatible) if patient does *not* improve upon drug elimination or if improvement occurs *without* removal of suspect drug.

Drug Rechallenge

Drug attributed a score of:
a. +1 (suggestive) if lesions recur with readministration of the suspect drug.
b. 0 (inconclusive) if no rechallenge performed.
c. −1 (incompatible) if rechallenge does not reproduce the lesions.

A positive total drug score (e.g., +1, +2, +3) is considered suggestive of drug causation.
A zero score is considered inconclusive.
A negative score (e.g. −1, −2, −3) is considered doubtful for drug causation.

CAUSE AND PATHOGENESIS

Despite recognition of multiple etiologic and triggering causes, the pathogenesis of erythema multiforme is not fully understood. It is currently thought to present a host-specific cell-mediated hypersensitivity reaction directed toward various antigens, including infections, drugs, neoplasia, various chemical contactants, foods, and connective tissue disease.[3,15,105] Cell-mediated immune mechanisms likely explain the main pathologic events of erythema multiforme.[3,15,86] The keratinocyte (antigenically altered by drugs, infectious agents, toxins) appears to be the primary target (apoptosis, necrosis), the dermal inflammatory infiltrate is composed of T lymphocytes (T helper > T suppressor), the exocytosing lymphocytes are T cells (T suppressor > T helper), and neighboring keratinocytes are invariably positive for ICAM-1 and class II MHC antigen. In humans, direct immunofluorescence testing reveals immunoreactants (especially C3 and IgM) at the basement membrane zone and in the walls of superficial dermal blood vessels in about 50% of the cases.[1,3] In addition, circulating immune complexes are often present.

In the horse, erythema multiforme has most commonly been associated with drug administration (especially potentiated sulfonamides, penicillin, and ivermectin), infections (especially herpesvirus), vaccinations, neoplasia (especially lymphoma), and topical agents.[16a,57,100,105] Reactions to food have occasionally been suspected.[57] Many cases have been idiopathic.[11,16a,102,103,105]

The confusion on pathogenesis and classification of erythema multiforme has been frustrating for human and veterinary medicine for years.[3,15] In humans, erythema multiforme is usually divided into two subsets.[3] An important distinction, in humans, is that the more common, mild,

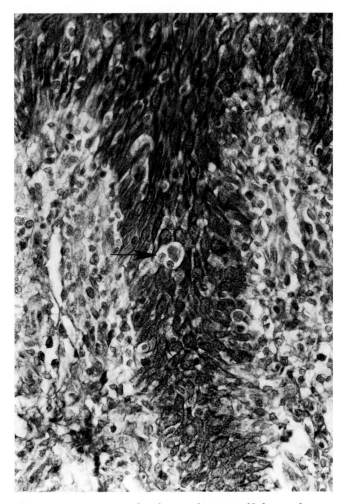

FIGURE 9-34. Satellitosis (*arrow*) associated with trimethoprim-sulfadiazine drug reaction.

relapsing cutaneous disease of erythema multiforme (erythema multiforme "minor") is most often associated with viral infections, whereas the more severe forms involving mucosa and having more widespread cutaneous disease (erythema multiforme "major") are most often associated with drug eruptions.

In addition, much confusion has existed over the relationship of erythema multiforme to the Stevens-Johnson syndrome (also referred to as *erythema multiforme major* by some authors), toxic epidermal necrolysis (Lyell's syndrome), and "overlaps" of the latter two entities. Much of the confusion in classification has stemmed from the terminology that is applied to the various syndromes in humans, and the lack of agreement on a clinical definition.[3,15] Recently, an international consensus clinical classification for the diagnosis of erythema multiforme and the Stevens-Johnson syndrome-toxic epidermal necrolysis in humans was published, and the classification system was evaluated in dogs.[15] It is unknown whether such a system would be useful in horses.

CLINICAL SIGNS

Erythema multiforme accounted for 1.89% of the equine dermatology cases seen at the Cornell University Clinic. There are no reported age, breed, or sex predilections. Prodromal or concurrent clinical signs may reflect the underlying cause. As the term *multiforme* applies, the skin lesions are variable, but they are usually characterized by an acute, rather symmetric onset of (1) urticarial papules and plaques, (2) vesicles and bullae, or (3) some combination thereof. The lesions and

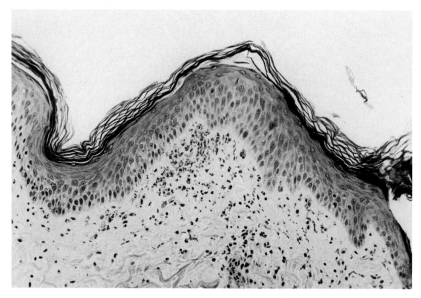

FIGURE 9-35. Papillary microabscess with trimethoprim-sulfadiazine drug reaction.

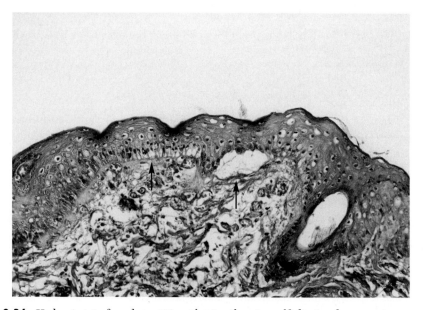

FIGURE 9-36. Hydropic interface dermatitis with trimethoprim-sulfadiazine drug reaction.

patients with urticarial lesions (0.5-cm diameter papules to 10-cm diameter plaques) are usually asymptomatic (erythema multiforme minor). These lesions often exhibit fairly rapid peripheral expansion and central resolution, resulting in annular, arciform, serpiginous, "donut," and polycyclic shapes (Figs. 9-32, *B*, 9-39, and 9-40). The overlying skin and hair coat are usually normal. The urticarial lesions of erythema multiforme do *not* pit with digital pressure, unlike the wheals of true urticaria (hives). Some urticarial lesions are painful when touched and may develop central areas of necrosis, ulceration, and yellowish-brown crusting (Fig. 9-32, *C*). Although any area of the body can be affected, the neck and dorsum are the most common sites for lesions. Occasionally, horses become systemically ill (fever, depression, anorexia) and have rather extensive, painful, vesiculobullous, necrotizing, and ulcerative lesions of the mucocutaneous areas, oral mucosa, conjunctiva, intertriginous areas (axilla, groin), and other cutaneous sites (erythema multiforme major, Stevens-Johnson syndrome) (Fig. 9-32, *D* through *F*).

It has been suggested that two characteristic equine dermatoses—reticulated leukotrichia and hyperesthetic leukotrichia—may be forms of erythema multiforme (see Chapter 12).[16a,101] Many of these cases are associated with herpesvirus infection or vaccination, and will recur with subsequent vaccination.

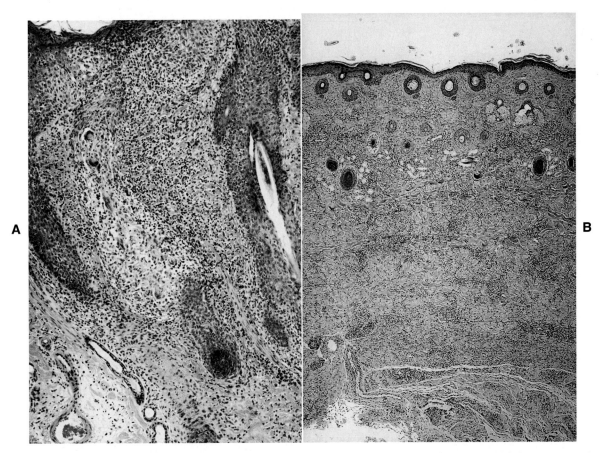

FIGURE 9-37. A, Infiltrative and granulomatous mural folliculitis in linear alopecia. **B,** Superficial and deep interstitial dermatitis due to drug eruption.

Continued

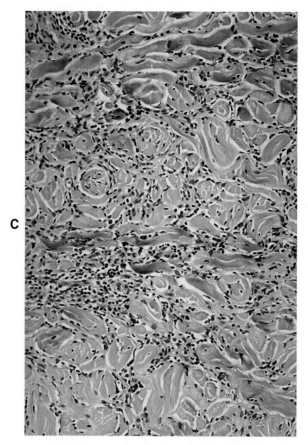

FIGURE 9-37, cont'd. C, Close-up of *B*. Interstitial infiltrate of lymphocytes.

DIAGNOSIS

The differential diagnosis of the urticarial form includes urticaria, vasculitis, drug reaction, lymphoma, amyloidosis, and mast cell tumor. Unlike the individual wheals of urticaria, which are evanescent and disappear within hours, the individual wheals of erythema multiforme persist for days to weeks. The differential diagnosis of the vesiculobullous form includes bullous pemphigoid, pemphigus vulgaris, systemic lupus erythematosus, stachybotryotoxicosis, viral vesicular diseases, and epitheliotropic lymphoma. Definitive diagnosis is made on the basis of history, physical examination, and skin biopsy. *Urticarial* lesions are characterized histologically by hydropic interface dermatitis, prominent apoptosis of keratinocytes, satellitosis of lymphocytes and macrophages, focal pigmentary incontinence, dermal edema, and variable purpura (Figs. 9-41 and 9-42).[102-105] Dermal collagen fibers may become vertically oriented and attenuated, presenting a web-like appearance ("gossamer" collagen). *Vesiculobullous* lesions are characterized by hydropic interface dermatitis, marked apoptosis of keratinocytes, and segmental, full-thickness coagulation necrosis of epithelium. Coalescent hydropic degeneration may produce intrabasal cleft and vesicle formation and even dermoepidermal separation (Fig. 9-43). Full-thickness necrosis of the epithelium (necrolysis) may also result in dermoepidermal separation. In all forms of erythema multiforme, hair follicle outer root sheath may be affected. Chronic lesions may have marked surface parakeratotic hyperkeratosis.[16a]

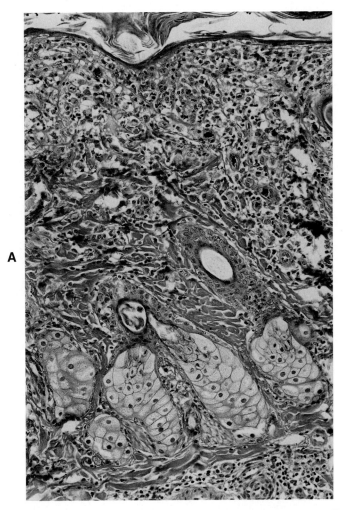

FIGURE 9-38. A, Epitheliotropic lymphoma-like drug reaction. Epitheliotropic infiltrate of pleomorphic lymphohistiocytic cells. *Continued*

CLINICAL MANAGEMENT

Erythema multiforme may run a mild course, spontaneously regressing within weeks to months.[11,102,103] An underlying cause should be sought and corrected, whenever possible, a procedure that will also result in spontaneous resolution of the erythema multiforme. Severe vesiculobullous cases of erythema multiforme require supportive care and an exhaustive search for underlying causes. The usefulness of systemic glucocorticoids and other immunomodulating drugs in erythema multiforme is controversial, and severe vesiculobullous eruptions may respond only partially or not at all to these drugs.[3] In the absence of concurrent conditions that would contraindicate their use (e.g., infections), the early, short-term use of high doses of glucocorticoids would make sense in horses with painful, vesiculobullous, or necrotizing disease.[105] If used, glucocorticoids should be given in high, immunosuppressive doses (prednisolone or prednisone 2.2 to 4.4 mg/kg orally q24h; dexamethasone 0.2 to 0.4 mg/kg orally q24h). Anecdotal reports indicate that pentoxifylline may be useful for the treatment of erythema multiforme.

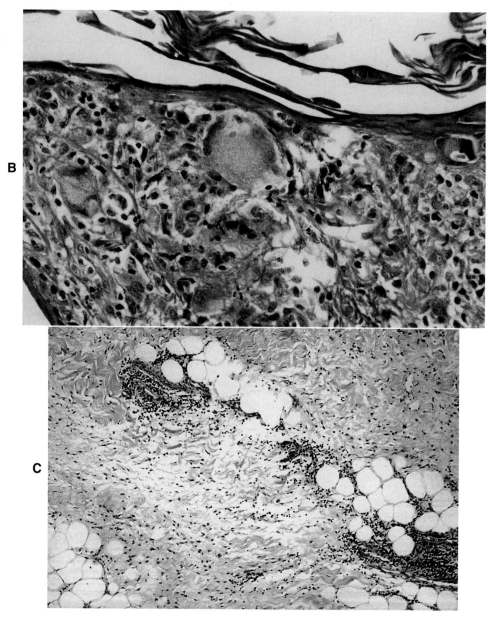

FIGURE 9-38, cont'd. B, Close-up of *A.* Intraepidermal multinucleated histiocytic giant cells. **C,** Injection reaction. Panniculitis.

Vasculitis

Cutaneous vasculitis is an uncommon disorder in horses that is characterized by purpura (often palpable), wheals, edema, papules, plaques, nodules, necrosis, and ulceration often involving the distal limbs and head.

CAUSE AND PATHOGENESIS

Vasculitis can occur via immune and nonimmune mechanisms.[1,3,5,9,15] Cutaneous vasculitis most commonly is believed to be immunologically mediated. The pathomechanism of most cutaneous

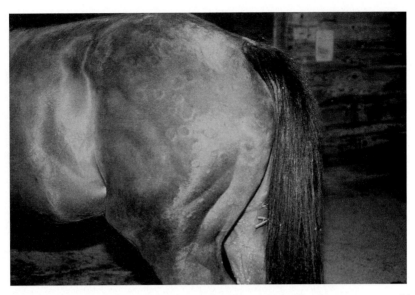

FIGURE 9-39. Erythema multiforme. Multiple annular, donut-shaped lesions over rump and lateral thigh.

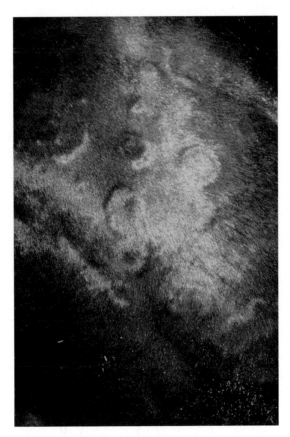

FIGURE 9-40. Multiple annular, donut-shaped lesions on neck.

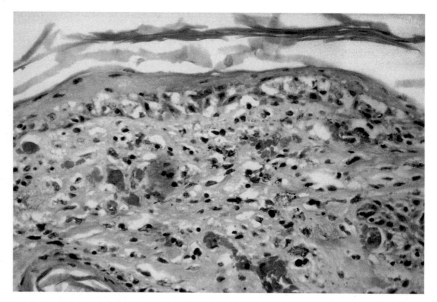

FIGURE 9-41. Erythema multiforme. Hydropic interface dermatitis.

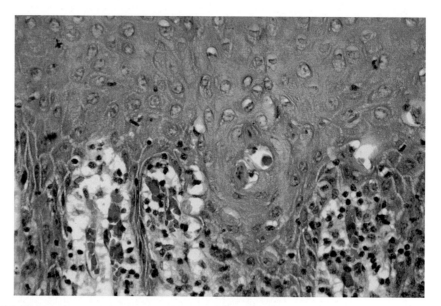

FIGURE 9-42. Erythema multiforme. Hydropic degeneration of basal cells and apoptotic keratinocytes.

vasculitides is assumed to involve type III (immune complex) hypersensitivity reactions. Type I hypersensitivity reactions may be important in the initiation of immune complex deposition in blood vessel walls. However, it appears to be more complex, and multiple mechanisms likely play a role. It has been postulated that differences in membrane receptors (probably, adhesion molecules and cytokines) for immunoglobulin and complement on leukocytes may account for the different histologic appearances of neutrophilic and lymphocytic vasculitides.[1-3] Additionally, initial neutrophil-induced damage to endothelial cells could result in the expression of "not self"

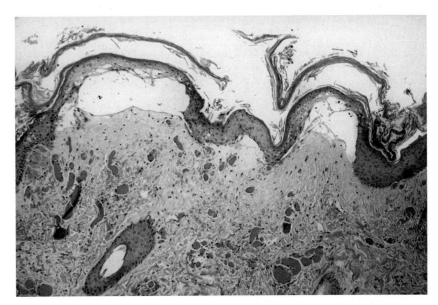

FIGURE 9-43. Erythema multiforme. Subepidermal vesicles with necrotic epidermis.

antigens, whereupon dendritic cells and T cells could initiate a secondary cell-mediated immune response, thus perpetuating the vascular disease and producing a lymphocyte-dominated infiltrate.[3,115] In cutaneous necrotizing vasculitis, endothelial cells show increased expression of ICAM-1 and E-selectin.[3,115] E-selectin is an adhesion molecule for neutrophils. In some cases and forms of vasculitis there has been an association with the presence of autoantibodies that react with neutrophil cytoplasmic structures (e.g., proteinase-3, myeloperoxidase) or endothelial cells.[3,115]

The most common cutaneous vasculitis in the horse may be that seen in purpura hemorrhagica.[11,12,108,118,120] In this disorder, the most common inciting cause is *Streptococcus equi* infection (strangles). Immune complexes in the sera of horses with poststrangles purpura hemorrhagica contain predominantly IgA with specificity for *S. equi*–specific antigen (M protein).[111] Only 1% to 5% of horses with strangles develop purpura hemorrhagica, and the predisposing factors are not known.[12,123] Purpura hemorrhagica is similar to Henoch-Schönlein purpura in humans.[3,12,111] Other forms of cutaneous vasculitis may be associated with other infectious agents (bacteria, viruses), drug administration, connective tissue disorders, other diseases (immune-mediated enterocolitis; omphalitis; bronchopneumonia; necrotic colitis; cholangiohepatitis), or neoplasia.[*] Some cases of cutaneous vasculitis are idiopathic.[†] Focal cutaneous vasculitis reactions may rarely be seen at the site of injections.[57] In some instances, vasculopathies are restricted to white-skinned, white-haired areas of the distal limbs and muzzle, even when large areas of the skin may be nonpigmented, suggesting that some environmental substances (pasture plants, and so forth) are acting as photoactivated allergens (photoactivated contact dermatitis).[11,12,16a,121a,122] Large doses of phenylbutazone were reported to cause a degenerative vasculopathy in horses.[116]

Anecdotal reports indicate that pastern dermatitis in Shires and Clydesdales is a cutaneous vasculitis.[110a] It has been hypothesized that this vasculitis probably has many triggering factors (infections, infestations, contactants, etc.) and that genetically determined immunodysregulation plays an important role in the pathogenesis.

---

*References 3, 11, 12, 14, 57, 112, 113, 116, 118, 120.
†References 3, 11, 12, 15, 57, 117, 118, 120, 126.

CLINICAL FEATURES

Skin is often the only organ system involved. However, other organ systems may be affected, wherein the skin lesions may represent the initial sign of a systemic disease. Skin lesions are typically seen in dependent areas of the body, in skin over areas of pressure and normal "wear and tear," and in skin covering extremities (pinnae, tip of tail, and so forth) that are more susceptible to cold environmental influences.

Cutaneous vasculitis is uncommon, accounting for 3.33% of the equine dermatoses seen at the Cornell University Clinic. There are no apparent age, breed, or sex predilections, but most horses are over 2 years old.[*] Severe necrotizing cutaneous vasculitis has been seen in foals secondary to omphalitis and salmonellosis (Figs. 9-44 and 9-45).[57,124] Cutaneous lesions occur most commonly on the distal limbs, pinnae, lips, and periocular area (Figs. 9-46, *A* through *C*, and 9-47). Lesions consist of purpura, wheals, edema, erythema, nodules, necrosis, punched-out (crateriform) ulcers, and crusts, and may obviously follow vascular structures (Fig. 9-46, *D*). The coronary bands may be severely affected (Fig. 9-46, *E*). Lesions may be painful. Oral purpura, vesicles, bullae, and ulcers may be present.[†] Diascopy may be useful for confirming the purpuric nature (nonblanching) of suspicious erythematous lesions. Affected horses may show signs of systemic illness, including fever, depression, decreased appetite, and weight loss.

Purpura hemorrhagica may be the most common cause of cutaneous vasculitis in the horse.[‡] It is an acute disease that typically occurs two days to several weeks following an infectious disease or vaccination.[§] The most common causative infectious disorder is strangles (*S. equi*), but other associated infectious processes include equine influenza, equine viral arteritis, equine infectious anemia, glanders, ehrlichiosis, *Corynebacterium pseudotuberculosis* infection, and *Streptococcus zooepidemicus* infection.[¶] The most commonly incriminated vaccines are those against strangles

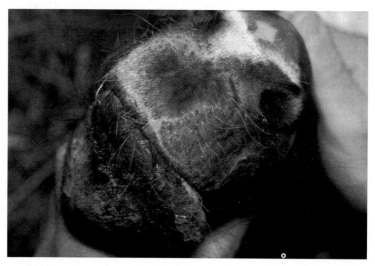

FIGURE 9-44. Vasculitis associated with salmonellosis. Well-circumscribed areas of necrosis on muzzle.

[*]References 11, 14, 117, 118, 120, 125, 126.
[†]References 11, 14, 107, 114, 118, 120.
[‡]References 12, 14, 108, 110, 112, 120.
[§]References 12, 14, 107, 108, 110, 119, 120, 123.
[¶]References 12, 14, 108, 110, 120.

and influenza, as well as tetanus antitoxin.* There may be substantial variation in severity and clinical course of the disease. Typically there is an acute onset of extensive subcutaneous edema of the face, muzzle, distal limbs, and ventral abdomen. The edema is usually symmetrical, but may begin in just one leg or area. In general the swellings are warm and painful. Petechiae and ecchymoses may be seen in visible mucous membranes. Affected horses are often depressed, stiff, and reluctant to move, but body temperatures are usually normal. Severely edematous areas may ooze serum and progress to necrosis, slough, and ulceration.

Photoactivated vasculopathies are a poorly understood, but relative common entity in the horse.[12,16a,121a,122] Mature animals are typically affected, but there are no apparent breed or sex predilections. The syndrome is most commonly seen in summer with exposure to abundant sunlight. Most animals are at pasture. Typically, only one animal on a premise is affected, even though others also have nonpigmented limbs. Oddly, affected horses often have only one leg affected, even though other legs may also be nonpigmented.[16a] Other affected animals will have lesions on all nonpigmented distal limbs and even the muzzle. The medial and lateral aspects of the pasterns and fetlocks are the preferred sites of disease. Early lesions include erythema, necrosis, oozing, crusting, and disproportionate edema (Fig. 9-48, *C*). Chronic lesions may be firm, proliferative, lichenified, and "warty" in appearance. Affected animals are not usually pruritic, but variable degrees of pain are often present.

The authors have seen a syndrome of *nodular eosinophilic vasculitis and arteritis*. Affected horses typically present with lesions on one or more legs (Fig. 9-48, *A* and *B*). Lesions begin as

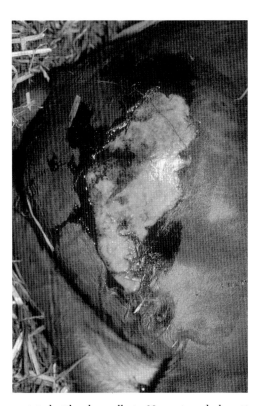

FIGURE 9-45. Vasculitis associated with salmonellosis. Necrosis and ulceration over hip.

---

*References 12, 14, 108, 110, 119, 120.

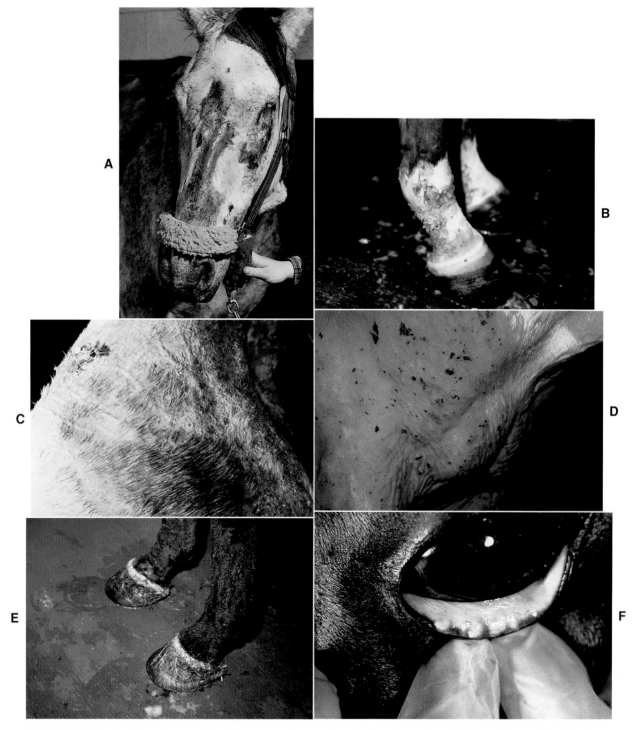

FIGURE 9-46. A, Idiopathic vasculitis. Linear areas of necrosis and ulceration on face. **B,** Idiopathic vasculitis. Erythema and necrosis of distal leg. **C,** Vasculitis associated with internal lymphoma. Alopecia, erythema, and punctate ulcers. **D,** Idiopathic vasculitis. Punctate ulcers and crusts involving vessels. **E,** Idiopathic vasculitis. Linear ulcers on distal legs and ulcerative coronitis. **F,** Amyloidosis. Yellow papules on mucocutaneous junction of lower eyelid. (*Courtesy Dr. J. King.*)

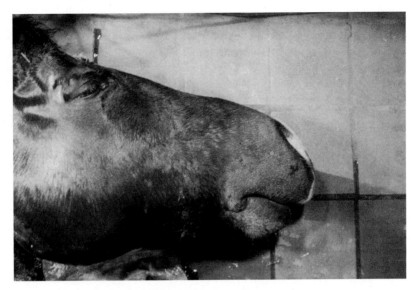

FIGURE 9-47. Swollen face due to vasculitis.

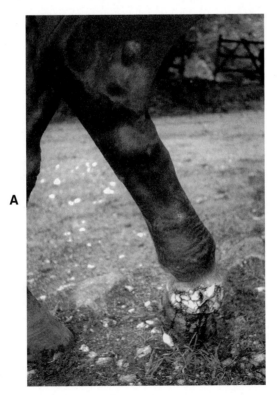

FIGURE 9-48. A, Nodular eosinophilic vasculitis. Firm to fluctuant nodules, some of which have necrosed and ulcerated on hind leg.

Continued

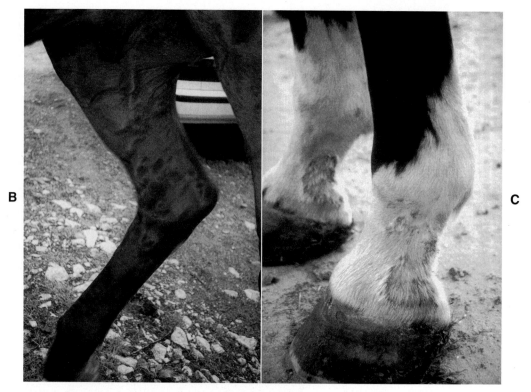

FIGURE 9-48, cont'd. B, Nodular eosinophilic vasculitis. Annular and linear lesions on hind leg. **C,** Pastern vasculitis. Edema and linear areas of necrosis and crust. (*Courtesy Dr. M. Sloet.*)

firm, usually painful nodules that may necrose, ulcerate, bleed, and crust. Lesions are sometimes linear. Affected horses are usually healthy otherwise.

Pastern vasculitis in Shires and Clydesdales begins as small, discrete ulcers on one or all pasterns.[110a] These lesions often bleed, especially during exercise and work. Initial lesions enlarge and coalesce, become infected, and discharge copious amounts of foul-smelling exudate. Chronically, lesions may spread up the leg as far as the carpi and tarsi. In severe cases the limbs show generalized swelling. Some animals develop permanent thickening, lichenification, and nodules ("grapes") the size of a golf ball or baseball. These chronic changes cause mechanical problems during movement and work, and can be easily damaged.

DIAGNOSIS

The differential diagnosis includes coagulopathy, severe erythema multiforme, bullous pemphigoid, pemphigus vulgaris, systemic lupus erythematosus, cryoglobulinemia, frostbite, drug reaction, equine viral arteritis, and stachybotryotoxicosis. The differential diagnosis for urticarial lesions includes hypersensitivity disorders (atopy, food hypersensitivity), drug reactions, erythema multiforme, amyloidosis, and lymphoma. Definitive diagnosis is based on history, physical examination, and results of skin biopsy. Varying degrees of vasculitis are seen. Most commonly, the vasculitis is neutrophilic (leukocytoclastic) (Fig. 9-49, *A*), but eosinophilic (Fig. 9-49, *B*), lymphocytic, and mixed forms may be seen.* Lesions most likely to show diagnostic changes are those less

---

*References 11, 12, 14, 16a, 19, 114, 117, 118, 122, 125, 126.

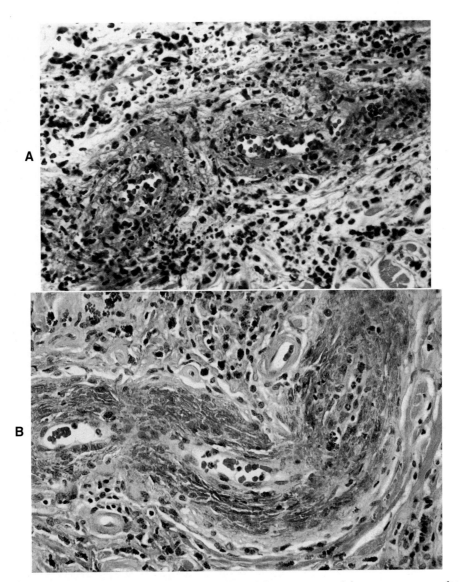

FIGURE 9-49. Vasculitis. **A,** Idiopathic necrotizing vasculitis. **B,** Eosinophilic necrotizing vasculitis.

Continued

than 24 hours old. Fibrinoid necrosis may be seen. Involvement of deep dermal vessels may suggest systemic disease. When deeper vessels are involved, necrosis of appendages and subcutaneous fat may be seen. In some biopsies, the diagnosis of vasculitis or vasculopathy is suspected on the basis of a cell-poor hydropic interface dermatitis and mural folliculitis, segmental epidermal necrosis, and the loss of definition and staining intensity and ultimate atrophy or necrosis of hair follicles ("fading follicles"). Sebaceous and sweat glands may be similarly, but less frequently affected. Subepidermal vesicles may be seen.

Early in the disease, photoactivated vasculitides are often characterized by a leukocytoclastic, necrotizing vasculitis of superficial dermal blood vessels.[16a,57] Varying degrees of thrombosis and purpura are usually seen, and the overlying epidermis is often edematous or necrotic (Fig. 9-49, *C*

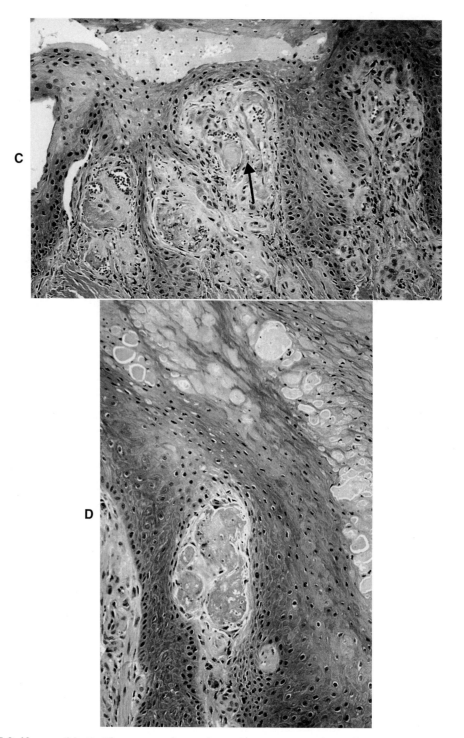

FIGURE 9-49, cont'd. C, Photoactivated vasculitis. Necrotizing vasculitis affecting several papillary dermal vessels (*arrow*). **D,** Photoactivated vasculitis. Necrosis and thrombosis of papillary dermal vessel.

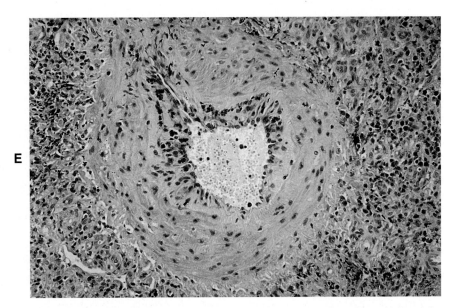

FIGURE 9-49, cont'd. E, Nodular eosinophilic vasculitis. Deep dermal arteriole with intramural eosinophils, many of which are karyorrhectic.

and *D*). In chronic lesions, superficial dermal vessel walls are usually thickened and hyalinized, the vessels may be thrombosed, and only occasional karyorrhectic nuclei are found in vessel walls.

The vascular lesions seen with photoactivated vasculopathies and phenylbutazone intoxication are often best described as degenerative and necrotic ("vasculopathic").[116,122] A true vasculitis may not be seen. Degeneration and necrosis of endothelial cells and vessel walls are seen and may be accompanied by thrombosis and purpura.

Nodular eosinophilic vasculitis and arteritis is characterized by eosinophilic inflammation that involves deep dermal arteries (Fig. 9-49, *E*).

Direct immunofluorescence and immunohistochemical testing may reveal immunoglobulin and/or complement in vessel walls (Fig. 9-50), and occasionally at the basement membrane zone.[*] However, such testing is not usually needed, is not particularly useful for the diagnosis, and if performed, must be done within the first 4 to 12 hours after lesion formation.[†]

Severely affected horses often show neutrophilia, mild anemia, hyperfibrinogenemia, and hyperglobulinemia.[‡] Rarely, affected horses will have positive antinuclear antibody tests.[11,118,120,125]

CLINICAL MANAGEMENT

Once the diagnosis of cutaneous vasculitis has been established, it is imperative that underlying etiologic factors be sought and eliminated. It is difficult to predict the course of cutaneous vasculitis in any individual case.[12,14,57,118,120] There may be only a single episode lasting a few weeks, or the disorder may be chronic or recurrent. The ultimate outcome is often dependent on the etiology, the severity of the skin disease, and the extent of internal organ involvement.[§]

---

[*]References 11, 12, 14, 16a, 117, 118, 125, 126.
[†]References 1, 3, 11, 12, 14, 15.
[‡]References 11, 12, 14, 109, 117, 118, 120, 121, 125.
[§]References 11, 12, 14, 57, 114, 118, 120, 121.

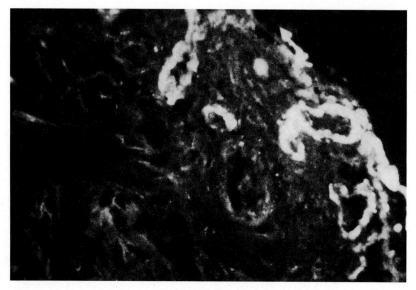

FIGURE 9-50. Vasculitis. Deposition of IgG in vessel walls (direct immunofluorescence testing).

Treatment of vasculitis consists of correction of the underlying cause and immunomodulatory drug treatment.[3,15] Systemic glucocorticoid therapy (2 to 4 mg/kg prednisolone or prednisone q24h, or 0.2 to 0.4 mg/kg dexamethasone q24h) is often successful.* Daily induction doses are maintained until remission is achieved (7 to 21 days), at which time alternate-morning therapy is established and slowly tapered. Some horses will remain in remission when therapy is terminated,[57,118,120,125] while others continue to relapse.[57,118,.120] In one series of 19 cases, the overall survival rate with glucocorticoid therapy was 63%.[118] Animals failing to respond to glucocorticoids may benefit from the concurrent administration of azathioprine or pentoxifylline.[15,57]

Concurrent administration of bactericidal antibiotics may be appropriate in some cases. Supportive care, including hydrotherapy, hand walking, and support bandages are often helpful. Some horses die of their underlying disease, from secondary bacterial infection (especially pneumonia, cellulitis), or from respiratory distress (severe edema); some are euthanized due to extensive skin necrosis and economic considerations.[11,57,118,120] In one series of 19 cases, the only abnormality that was significantly predictive of a poor response to glucocorticoid and supportive therapy was the presence of fever.[118]

In photoactivated vasculitides, therapeutic principles include sun avoidance (keep indoors during the day; use leg wraps) and large doses of systemic glucocorticoids.[16a,57,121a,122] Occasionally, lesions recur when treatment is stopped or recur in subsequent years.[16a] In these instances, an attempt should be made to identify and eliminate the antigen(s) in cause. In one report,[121a] animals confined to a sand paddock developed no lesions, while 85% of the animals at pasture had lesions.

Alopecia Areata

Alopecia areata is an uncommon disorder of horses characterized by patches of well-circumscribed, nonscarring alopecia that grossly is noninflammatory. It accounted for 1.33% of the equine dermatoses seen at the Cornell University Clinic.

---

*References 12, 14, 117, 118, 120, 125, 126.

CAUSE AND PATHOGENESIS

Alopecia areata is of complex pathogenesis with immunologic targeting of anagen hair follicles and the relatively consistent finding of antifollicular autoantibodies (IgG class), as well as CD4+ and CD8+ cells in the affected follicles in humans and rodents.[127,128,131] Antifollicular antibodies have also been documented to occur in the horse.[127,132] In horses, IgG autoantibodies are directed against trichohyalin, inner root sheath, outer root sheath, and precortex of the hair follicle.[127,132] These antibodies reacted with a 200- to 222-kd doublet, antigens of 40 to 50 kd, and particularly trichohyalin. When the IgG fractions of serum from a horse with alopecia areata were injected into murine skin, hair growth was inhibited.[132] Most intrabulbar lymphocytes are $\alpha \beta$ CD8+ T cells, and perifollicular cells include CD4+ and CD8+ T lymphocytes and CD1+ dendritic antigen-presenting cells.[127] Expression of some hair follicle antigens is increased in many human patients with alopecia. Taken together, these observations suggest that the development and/or manifestations of alopecia areata may be related to the level of certain hair follicle antigens, which may be genetically determined, and a resultant autoimmune response to these antigens.

Other observations in humans supporting the immunologic basis are (1) accumulations of lymphoid cells (helper T cells) around hair bulbs during the active phase of the disease, (2) occasional association of alopecia areata with other immune-mediated diseases, (3) increased incidence of various autoantibodies in alopecia areata, (4) decreased numbers of circulating T cells, (5) abnormal presence of Langerhans cells in the follicular bulb, (6) increased expression of class I and II MHC antigens, (7) the deposition of C3 or IgG and IgM or both at the basement membrane zone of the hair follicles in lesional and normal scalp as revealed by direct immuno-fluorescence testing, and (8) the therapeutic benefit of inducing delayed-type hypersensitivity and immunosuppressive therapies.[3] In addition, genetic, endocrine, and psychologic factors have been thought to play a role in humans with alopecia areata.[3] Morphologic abnormalities of melanocytes in follicular bulbs have been described in humans with alopecia areata.

CLINICAL FEATURES

Anecdotal reports indicate that Appaloosas and Palominos are at risk,[126b] but published cases do not corroborate this. No age or sex predilections are apparent. Alopecia areata is characterized by the insidious or sudden appearance of one or multiple well-circumscribed, more-or-less annular areas of noninflammatory alopecia.[12,16a,126a,127,129,132] Lesions vary from 2 to 25 cm in diameter, and the exposed skin appears normal (Figs. 9-51 and 9-52). Lesions are commonly seen on the face, neck, and trunk (Figs. 9-53 and 9-54). Widespread alopecia areata has been called *alopecia universalis*. Mane and tail hairs may be lost. Pruritus and pain are absent, and affected horses are otherwise normal. Exposed skin may become hyperpigmented and/or scaly.

It has been reported that at least one form of so-called "mane and tail dysplasia" is a form of alopecia areata.[16a,101] In this syndrome, focal areas of alopecia and/or short, brittle, dull hairs are present in the mane and/or tail. Because this syndrome is particularly common in Appaloosas, genetic predilection may be important in the etiopathogenesis.

Some cases of so-called "spotted leukotrichia" (see Chapter 12) with hair loss in the leukotrichic areas may be alopecia areata.[16a]

DIAGNOSIS

The differential diagnosis includes infectious folliculitides (*Staphylococcus* spp., *Dermatophilus congolensis*, dermatophytes, *Demodex* mites), occult sarcoid, injection reaction, anagen or telogen defluxion, and follicular dysplasia. The surface changes of scaling and crusting, which typically accompany the infectious folliculitides and occult sarcoid, are *not* a feature of alopecia areata.

Definitive diagnosis is based on history, physical examination, trichogram, and skin biopsy. Microscopic examination of hairs plucked from the margin of enlarging lesions may reveal

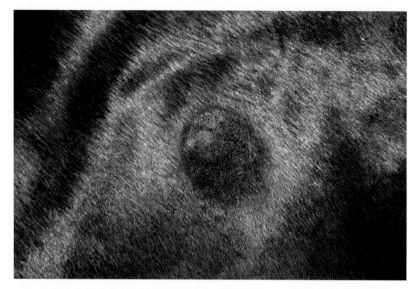

FIGURE 9-51. Alopecia areata. Annular alopecia on shoulder.

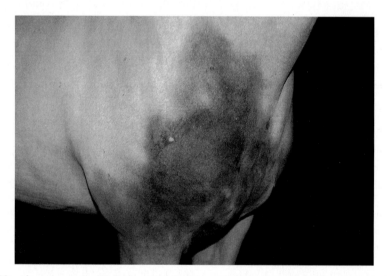

FIGURE 9-52. Alopecia areata. Well-circumscribed area of noninflammatory alopecia over brisket.

dysplastic and "exclamation point" hairs—short, stubby hairs with frayed, fractured, pigmented distal ends whose shafts undulate or taper toward the proximal end. The characteristic early histopathologic findings include a peribulbar accumulation of lymphocytes which has been described as looking like "a swarm of bees" (Fig. 9-55).[*] Lymphocytes infiltrate the hair bulb, as well as the root sheaths of the inferior segment of the hair follicle, and apoptotic keratinocytes may be seen. These early changes may be quite focal and difficult to demonstrate, requiring multiple biopsies from the advancing edge of early lesions and serial sections of these. Later, the histopathologic findings consist of a predominance of telogen and catagen hair follicles, peribulbar

---

[*]References 12, 16a, 57, 126a, 127, 129, 130, 132.

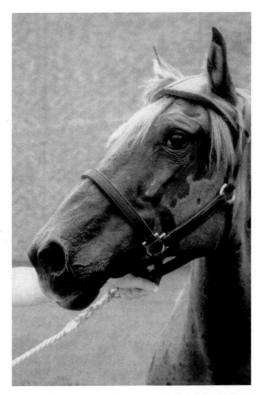

FIGURE 9-53. Alopecia areata. Well-circumscribed noninflammatory alopecia on the face. (*Courtesy Dr. J. Baird.*)

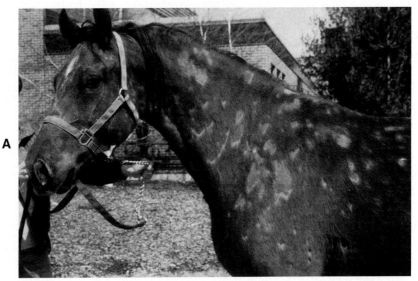

FIGURE 9-54. Alopecia areata. **A,** Widespread areas of well-circumscribed noninflammatory alopecia. (*Courtesy Dr. J. Baird.*)

Continued

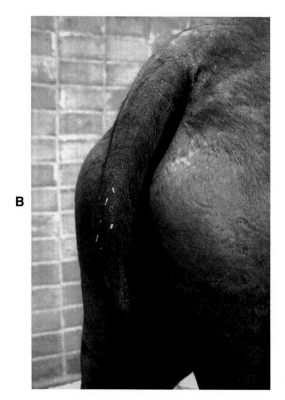

B

FIGURE 9-54, cont'd. **B,** Hypotrichosis and alopecia of the tail. (*Courtesy Dr. M. Sloet.*)

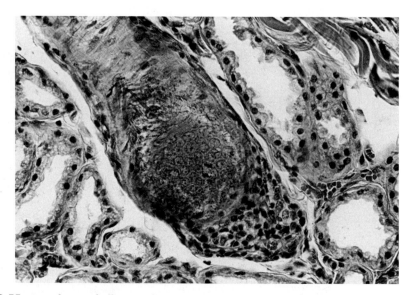

FIGURE 9-55. Lymphocytic bulbitis in alopecia areata.

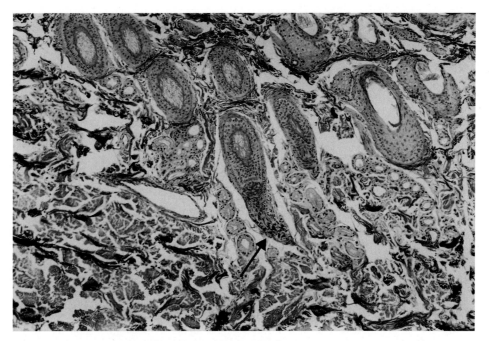

FIGURE 9-56. Alopecia areata. Peribulbar melanosis (*arrow*).

melanosis (Fig. 9-56), follicular atrophy, changes consistent with follicular dysplasia (dysplastic hair shafts, distorted hair follicle contours), and orphaned sebaceous and epitrichial sweat glands. Miniaturized hair follicles and hairs may be seen.[16a,57] Inflammation may be subtle or absent. In chronic lesions, where inflammation is gone, follicular dysplasia (mane and tail or otherwise) is a potential misdiagnosis.[16a,57]

CLINICAL MANAGEMENT

The prognosis for equine alopecia areata appears to vary with the distribution of the lesions. Solitary lesions or multiple lesions restricted to one anatomic site often undergo spontaneous remission within several months to 2 years. When hair grows back, it may be finer and lighter in color than normal. Usually these hairs gradually regain a normal diameter and color. Widespread lesions appear to persist.[12,127,129] However, one horse that had been almost totally alopecic after 12 months of disease made a complete, spontaneous recovery.[130] In one horse, hair loss occurred 3 times—and spontaneously regrew twice—over a period of 3 years.[132]

No curative treatment is currently available for alopecia areata. In humans, a number of treatment modalities are available that have resulted in varying degrees of hair regrowth, including glucocorticoids (systemic or topical), inducing contact hypersensitivity at the site of lesions (dinitrochlorobenzene, squaric acid dibutyl ester), cyclosporine, and topical minoxidil.[3,127] However, hair loss usually recurs after treatment is discontinued.

In the horse, anecdotal reports indicate that systemic glucocorticoids had no effect in one patient and seemed to be effective in one other.[127] One horse was treated with oral prednisone for 12 weeks, and slow hair growth was seen over the period of one year, suggesting that the hair regrowth was spontaneous and not associated with treatment.[126a] Topical triamcinolone was of no benefit in one horse.[130] Minoxidil is a vasodilator that possesses hair growth stimulant properties that are useful for the treatment of patchy alopecia areata in humans. Anecdotal reports indicate that the twice daily topical application of a 2% minoxidil solution (Rogaine Hair Regrowth, Pharmacia and Upjohn) may be effective in patchy alopecia areata in horses.

Amyloidosis

Amyloidosis is a rare cause of cutaneous and upper respiratory disease in horses. It accounted for 0.33% of the equine dermatoses seen at the Cornell University Clinic.

CAUSE AND PATHOGENESIS

Amyloidosis is a generic term that signifies the abnormal extracellular deposition of one of a family of unrelated proteins that share certain characteristics, staining properties, and ultrastructural findings.[3,15,153] Amyloidosis is not a single disease entity, and amyloid may accumulate as a result of a variety of different pathogenetic mechanisms.

Different amino acid compositions of amyloid may be seen.[153] Amyloid deposits contain a nonfibrillar protein called *amyloid P*, which is identical to a normal circulating plasma globulin known as *serum amyloid P* (an elastase inhibitor that may help protect amyloid deposits from degradation and phagocytosis). Primary and myeloma-associated systemic amyloidosis have immunoglobulin light chains (mostly the lambda type) as precursors to the amyloid fibril protein, which is termed *amyloid L*. In secondary systemic amyloidosis (associated with chronic inflammation), a serum precursor protein, serum amyloid A (a high density lipoprotein and acute-phase reactant), forms the fibrils in the amyloid deposits. Serum amyloid A is thought to be cleaved proteolytically by macrophages to amyloid and excreted extracellularly.

Although the pathogenesis of amyloidosis is unclear, it is morphologically related to cells of the mononuclear phagocytic system, plasma cells, and keratinocytes. Functional studies suggest that such cells play at least a partial role in the genesis of amyloid. Ultimately, amyloid deposits lead to changes in tissue architecture and function.

In the horse, two forms of amyloidosis—systemic and organ-limited—are most commonly reported.[14,154] Systemic amyloidosis, which rarely produces skin lesions, is usually associated with chronic infections (e.g., tuberculosis, coccidioidomycosis, glanders, strangles, osteomyelitis, chronic purulent inflammations) and chronic antigenic stimulus (immune sera production),* and is also referred to as *secondary* or *reactive amyloidosis*. The amyloid fibrils (termed *AA amyloid*) in this form are produced from a serum α-globulin (the hepatic acute phase protein, serum amyloid A protein or protein SAA) by macrophages. Recently, a systemic amyloidosis with multiple skin lesions with an AL amyloid was reported in a horse.[135]

Organ-limited amyloidosis usually affects the skin and/or upper respiratory tract, is usually not associated with known triggering factors, and is also referred to as *primary* or *immunocytic amyloidosis*.† The amyloid fibrils (termed *AL amyloid*) in these forms are produced from monoclonal immunoglobulin light chains. Amyloid has also been reported within the skin and lymph node lesions of histiolymphocytic lymphoma[134] and plasmacytoma.[133] Inhaled allergens or toxins have been suggested as possible etiologic factors in upper respiratory tract amyloidosis.[143] The hereditary forms of amyloidosis in humans associated with prealbumin-derived AH amyloid have not been described in horses.[3]

CLINICAL FEATURES

Organ-limited amyloidosis is rare in the horse, accounting for about 0.04% of the cases seen by two university large animal clinics.[143,154] Cutaneous and upper respiratory tract amyloidosis occurs without breed or age (3 to 19 years) predilections; it occurs in males twice as frequently as

---

*References 12, 135-137, 140-142, 148, 149, 154.
†References 133, 138-140, 143-145, 147, 150-152, 154.

females.[12,14,151] Cutaneous lesions are characterized by multiple papules, nodules, or plaques, which are most commonly present in the head, neck, shoulders, and pectoral region (Figs. 9-46, *F*, and 9-57).° Lesions are firm, well circumscribed, 0.5 to 10 cm in diameter, nonpainful, and nonpruritic. The overlying skin and hair coat are usually normal in appearance. Regional lymph nodes may be enlarged. In some horses, the lesions have an initial rapid onset and urticarial appearance. Such lesions may regress spontaneously or in conjunction with systemic glucocorticoid therapy, only to recur and assume a chronic, progressive course.

Rarely, cutaneous lesions may be preceded, accompanied, or followed by upper respiratory tract lesions (nasopharyngeal amyloidosis).[†] Such horses are presented for epistaxis, difficult breathing (rhinodyspnea), or deteriorating athletic performance. Lesions may be unilateral or bilateral, papular to nodular to plaque-like, and solitary or multiple. They are often confluent and are often ulcerated or bleed easily when palpated. Lesions most commonly occur on the rostral portion of the nasal septum or on the rostral floor of the nasal cavity. Occasionally, lesions may involve the entire nasal septum, entire nasal cavity, pharynx, larynx, guttural pouch, trachea, bronchi, and conjunctiva.

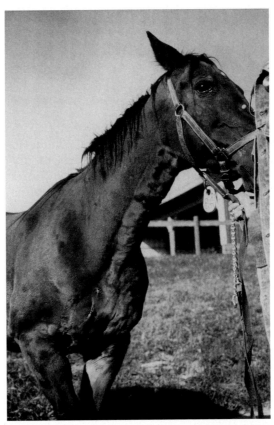

FIGURE 9-57. Cutaneous amyloidosis. Multiple firm nodules on neck and chest.

°References 12, 14, 133, 140, 147, 151, 152, 154.
[†]References 12, 14, 138-140, 143, 145-147, 150, 151, 154.

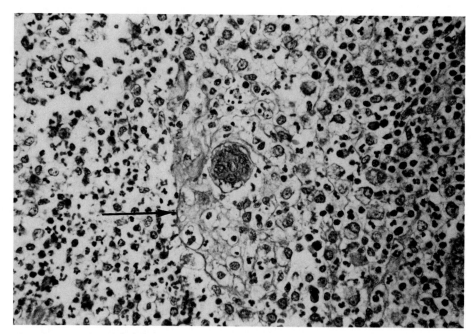

FIGURE 9-58. Cutaneous amyloidosis. Pyogranulomatous dermatitis and small amount of extracellular amyloid (*arrow*).

DIAGNOSIS

The differential diagnosis includes other asymptomatic papulonodular skin diseases, especially eosinophilic granuloma, lymphoma, and mast cell tumor. The definitive diagnosis is based on history, physical examination, and results of skin biopsy. Cytologic examination of needle aspirates may reveal granulomatous inflammation with multinucleated histiocytic giant cells and irregular sheets of amorphous eosinophilic material.[135] If the cut surface of lesions is painted with Lugol's iodine solution and rinsed with 1% sulfuric acid, amyloid deposits stain purple-brown.[140,142,143,147,148] Histopathologic findings include nodular to diffuse areas of granulomatous dermatitis and panniculitis with numerous multinucleated histiocytic giant cells, associated with variable-sized areas of amorphous, homogeneous, hyaline, eosinophilic amyloid within the dermis and subcutis (Figs. 9-58 and 9-59). Large extracellular amyloid deposits often contain clefts or fractures. Amyloid may also be deposited in and around vessel walls, and be seen intracellularly within macrophages and multinucleated histiocytic giant cells. Amyloid typically shows congophilia and apple-green birefringence with polarized light microscopic examination of Congo red-stained sections. If sections are treated with potassium permanganate prior to Congo red staining, AA amyloid loses its congophilia, whereas AL amyloid retains its congophilia.*

Electron microscopic examination shows a characteristic pattern of randomly intermingled, nonbranching, 7.5 to 10 nm wide, linear, tubular fibrils. Each fibril is composed of several filaments with a twisted β-pleated sheet configuration.[140,153,154]

CLINICAL MANAGEMENT

The prognosis varies with presence and severity of any upper respiratory tract or systemic amyloid deposits. As most horses with cutaneous amyloidosis do not have involvement of other organ

---

*References 135, 140, 143, 146, 153, 154.

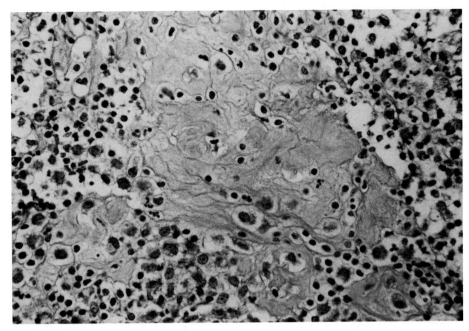

FIGURE 9-59. Cutaneous amyloidosis. Pyogranulomatous dermatitis and large extracellular amyloid deposit.

systems, the prognosis for life is good. Presently, no effective treatment is available for horses with multiple cutaneous lesions. In horses with nasopharyngeal amyloidosis, surgical excision of large nodules and/or the alar folds have allowed some animals to return to their former uses for over 1 year.[143,146,150] In humans, skin lesions of both primary and myeloma-associated amyloidosis have responded to DMSO, which may inhibit amyloid synthesis or act to promote amyloid degradation.[153]

● REFERENCES

General References

1. Beutner EH, et al: Immunopathology of the Skin III. Churchill Livingstone, New York, 1987.
2. Bos JD: Skin Immune System (SIS). CRC Press, Boca Raton, 1990.
2a. Crisman MV, et al: Pharmacokinetic disposition of intravenous and oral pentoxifylline in horses. J Vet Pharmacol Ther 16:23, 1993.
3. Freedberg IM, et al (eds): Dermatology in General Medicine V. McGraw-Hill, New York, 1999.
4. Halliwell REW, Gorman NT: Veterinary Clinical Immunology. W.B. Saunders Co, Philadelphia, 1989.
5. Hauser C, Orbea HA: Superantigens and their role in immune-mediated diseases. J Invest Dermatol 101:503, 1993.
5a. Léguillette R, et al: Effects of pentoxifylline on pulonary function and results of cytologic examination of bronchoalveolar lavage fluid in horses with recurrent airway obstruction. Am J Vet Res 63:459, 2002.
6. Manning TO, Sweeney C: Immune-mediated equine skin diseases. Comp Cont Educ 8:979, 1986.
7. Mottier S, von Tscharner C: Immunohistochemistry in skin disease. Diagnostic value? In: von Tscharner C, Halliwell REW (eds): Advances in Veterinary Dermatology I. Baillière-Tindall, 1990, p 479.
8. Mullowney PC: Dermatologic diseases of horses, part V: Allergic, immune-mediated, and miscellaneous skin diseases. Comp Cont Educ 7:S217, 1985.
9. Nickoloff BJ: Dermal Immune System. CRC Press, Boca Raton, 1993.
10. Scott DW, et al: Immune-mediated dermatoses in domestic animals: ten years after—Part I. Comp Cont Educ 9:423, 1987.
11. Scott DW, et al: Immune-mediated dermatoses in domestic animals: ten years after—Part II. Comp Cont Educ 9:539, 1987.
12. Scott DW: Large Animal Dermatology. W.B. Saunders Co, Philadelphia, 1988.
13. Scott DW: Autoimmune skin diseases in the horse. Equine Pract 11(10):20, 1989.
14. Scott DW: Unusual immune-mediated skin diseases in the horse. Equine Pract 13(2):10, 1991.

15. Scott DW, et al: Muller & Kirk's Small Animal Dermatology VI. W.B. Saunders Co, Philadelphia, 2000.

16. Soter N, Baden HA: Pathophysiology of Dermatologic Disease II. McGraw-Hill, New York, 1991.

16a. von Tscharner C, et al: Stannard's illustrated equine dermatology notes. Vet Dermatol 11:161, 2000.

17. Suter MM, et al: Autoimmune diseases of domestic animals: an update. In: Kwochka KW, et al (eds): Advances in Veterinary Dermatology III. Butterworth-Heinemann, Boston, 1998, p 321.

18. Tizard IR: Veterinary Immunology: An Introduction IV. W.B. Saunders Co, Philadelphia, 1992.

19. Yager JA, Scott DW: The skin and appendages. In: Jubb KVF, et al (eds): Pathology of Domestic Animals IV, Vol I. Academic Press, New York, 1993, p 531.

Pemphigus Complex

20. Amory H, et al: Pemphigus foliacé dans l'espèce équine: synthèse et description de 2 cas. Ann Méd Vét 141:139, 1997.

21. Amagai M, et al: The clinical phenotype of pemphigus is defined by the antidesmoglein autoantibody profile. J Am Acad Dermatol 40:167, 1999.

22. Anhalt GJ: Making sense of antigens and antibodies in pemphigus. J Am Acad Dermatol 40:763, 1999.

22a. Bayer-Garner IB, et al: Acantholysis and spongiosis are associated with loss of syndecan-1 expression. J Cutan Pathol 28:135, 2001.

23. Buxton RS, et al: Nomenclature of the desmosomal cadherins. J Cell Biol 121:481, 1993.

24. Dmochowski M, et al: Desmocollins I and II are recognized by certain antisera from patients with various types of pemphigus, particularly Brazilian pemphigus foliaceus. J Invest Dermatol 100:380, 1993.

25. Ioannides D, et al: Regional variation in the expression of pemphigus foliaceus, pemphigus erythematosus, and pemphigus vulgaris antigens in human skin. J Invest Dermatol 96:15, 1991.

26. Iwatsuki K, et al: Ultrastructural binding site of pemphigus foliaceus antibodies: comparison with pemphigus vulgaris. J Cutan Pathol 18:160, 1991.

27. Lombardi C, et al: Environmental risk factors in endemic pemphigus foliaceus (fogo selvagem). J Invest Dermatol 98:847, 1992.

28. Nishikawa T: Desmoglein ELISAs. Arch Dermatol 135:195, 1999.

29. Nguyen T, et al: The pathophysiological significance of nondesmoglein targets of pemphigus autoimmunity. Arch Dermatol 134:971, 1998.

30. Robinson ND, et al: The new pemphigus variants. J Am Acad Dermatol 40:649, 1999.

31. Tur E, Brenner S: Diet and pemphigus. Arch Dermatol 134:1406, 1998.

32. Xue W, et al: Functional involvement of urokinase-type plasminogen activator receptor in pemphigus acantholysis. J Cutan Pathol 25:469, 1998.

Pemphigus Foliaceus

33. Anderson FE, Findlay VS: Pemphigus foliaceus, or bullous exfoliative dermatitis in the horse. Ann Vet Rev 26:334, 1902.

34. Barnick W, Gutzeit R: Ein Fall von acuten Pemphigus beim pferde. Zschr Vet Kd 3:241, 1891.

35. Day MJ, Penhale WJ: Immunodiagnosis of autoimmune skin disease in the dog, cat, and horse. Aust Vet J 63:65, 1986.

36. Edmond RJ, Frevert C: Pemphigus foliaceus in a horse. Mod Vet Pract 67:527, 1986.

37. Grabnickel W: Über je einen Fall von Pemphigus und Pemphigusähnlicher Erkrankung des Pferdes. Monat Vet Med 15:735, 1901.

38. Graffunder H: Allgemeiner acuter Pemphigus bei einem Pferde. Berl Tierärztl Wschr 6:153, 1980.

39. Griffith G: Pemphigus foliaceus in a Welch Pony. Comp Cont Educ 9:347, 1987.

40. Holubar K: Pemphigus: A disease of man and animal. Historical and other perspectives. Int J Dermatol 27:516, 1988.

41. Johnson ME, et al: Pemphigus foliaceus in the horse. Equine Pract 3(2):40, 1981.

42. Johnson PJ: Pemphigus foliaceus in a horse. Vet Allergy Clin Immunol 5:131, 1997.

43. Laing JA, et al: Pemphigus foliaceus in a 2-month-old foal. Equine Vet J 24:490, 1992.

44. Manning TO: Pemphigus foliaceus. In: Robinson NE (ed): Current Therapy in Equine Medicine. Philadelphia, W.B. Saunders Co, 1983, p 541.

45. Messer NT, Knight AP: Pemphigus foliaceus in a horse. J Am Vet Med Assoc 180:938, 1982.

46. Pascal A, et al: Seasonality and environmental risk factors for pemphigus foliaceus in animals: a retrospective study of 83 cases presented to the Veterinary Medical Teaching Hospital, University of California, Davis from 1978 to 1994. Proc Am Acad Vet Dermatol Am Coll Vet Dermatol 11:24, 1995.

47. Peter JE, et al: Pemphigus in a Thoroughbred. Vet Med Small Anim Clin 76:1203, 1981.

48. Power HT, et al: Use of a gold compound for the treatment of pemphigus foliaceus in a foal. J Am Vet Med Assoc 180:400, 1982.

49. Rosser EJ, et al: The duration and quality of positive direct immunofluorescence testing in skin biopsies using Michel's fixative on a case of equine pemphigus foliaceus. J Equine Vet Sci 3:14, 1983.

50. Rothwell TLW, et al: Possible pemphigus foliaceus in a horse. Aust Vet J 62:429, 1985.

51. Ruocco V, Sacerdoti G: Pemphigus and bullous pemphigoid due to drugs. Int J Dermatol 30:307, 1991.

52. Schulte A, et al: Pemphigus foliaceus beim Pferd. Pferdeheilk 5:23, 1989.

53. Scott DW, et al: The comparative pathology of non-viral bullous skin diseases in domestic animals. Vet Pathol 17:257, 1980.

54. Scott DW: Pemphigus in domestic animals. Clin Dermatol 1:141, 1983.

55. Scott DW, et al: Pemphigus and pemphigoid in dogs, cats, and horses. Ann N Y Acad Sci 420:353, 1983.

56. Scott DW: Marked acantholysis associated with dermatophytosis due to *Trichophyton equinum* in two horses. Vet Dermatol 5:105, 1994.

57. Scott DW, Miller WH Jr: Unpublished observations.

58. Wessendorf W: Pemphigus acutus beim pferde. Arch Wiss Prakt Tierheilk 19:321, 1893.

59. Wohlsein P, et al: Pemphigus foliaceus bei einem Fohlen. Ein kasuistischer Beitrag. Tierärztl Prax 22:151, 1994.

60. Wohlsein P, et al: Pemphigus foliaceus in a horse. Vet Dermatol 4:27, 1993.

Pemphigus Vulgaris

61. White SL: Bullous autoimmune skin diseases: diagnosis, therapy, prognosis. Proc Am Assoc Equine Practit 38:507, 1992.

Paraneoplastic Pemphigus

62. Anhalt GJ: Paraneoplastic pemphigus. Adv Dermatol 12:77, 1997.
63. Williams MA, et al: Paraneoplastic bullous stomatitis in a horse. J Am Vet Med Assoc 207:331, 1995.

Bullous Pemphigoid

64. Borreyo L, et al: Deposition of eosinophil granule proteins preceding blister formation in bullous pemphigoid: comparison with neutrophil and mast cell granule proteins. Am J Pathol 148:897, 1996.
65. Czech W, et al: Granulocyte activation in bullous diseases: release of granular proteins in bullous pemphigoid and pemphigus vulgaris. J Am Acad Dermatol 29:210, 1993.
66. George LW, White SL: Autoimmune skin diseases of large animals. Vet Clin N Am Large Anim Pract 6:79, 1984.
67. Goldberg DJ, et al: Regional variation in the expression of bullous pemphigoid antigen and location of lesions in bullous pemphigoid. J Invest Dermatol 82:326, 1984.
68. Halliwell REW: Autoimmune diseases in domestic animals. J Am Vet Med Assoc 181:1088, 1982.
69. Manning TO, et al: Pemphigus-pemphigoid in a horse. Equine Pract 3(5):38, 1981.
70. Olivry T, et al: Equine bullous pemphigoid IgG autoantibodies target linear epitopes in the NC16A ectodomain of collagen XVII (BP180, BPAG2). Vet Immunol Immunopathol 73:45, 2000.
71. Onodera Y, et al: Difference in binding sites of autoantibodies against 230- and 170-kD bullous pemphigoid antigens on salt-split skin. J Invest Dermatol 102:686, 1994.
72. Scott DW: Pemphigoid in domestic animals. Clin Dermatol 5:155, 1987.

Systemic Lupus Erythematosus

73. Chung JH, et al: Apoptosis in the pathogenesis of cutaneous lupus erythematosus. Am J Dermatopathol 20:233, 1998.
74. Geor RJ, et al: Systemic lupus erythematosus in a filly. J Am Vet Med Assoc 197:1489, 1990.
75. Lehmann P, et al: Experimental reproduction of skin lesions in lupus erythematosus by UVA and UVB radiation. J Am Acad Dermatol 22:181, 1990.
76. Mooney E, et al: Characterization of the changes in matrix molecules at the dermoepidermal junction in lupus erythematosus. J Cutan Pathol 18:417, 1991.
77. Norris DA: Pathomechanisms of photosensitive lupus erythematosus. J Invest Dermatol 100:58S, 1993.
78. Sauder DN, et al: Epidermal cytokines in murine lupus. J Invest Dermatol 100:42S, 1993.
79. Sontheimer RD: The lexicon of cutaneous lupus erythematosus: a review and personal perspective on the nomenclature and classification of the cutaneous manifestations of lupus erythematosus. Lupus 6:84, 1997.
80. Velthuis PJ, et al: Immunohistopathology of light-induced skin lesions in lupus erythematosus. Acta Dermatol Venereol (Stockh) 70:93, 1990.
81. Vrins A, Feldman BF: Lupus erythematosus-like syndrome in a horse. Equine Pract 5(6):18, 1983.

Discoid Lupus Erythematosus

82. Scott DW: Le lupus discoïde équin: description de trois cas. Point Vét 22:7, 1990.

Cryoglobulinemia and Cryofibrinogenemia

83. Coffman J: Immunity: autoimmunity, isoimmunity, and immunodeficiency in the foal. Vet Med Small Anim Clin 74:1430, 1979.
84. Maede Y, et al: Cryoglobulinemia in a horse. Jap J Vet Med Sci 53:379, 1991.
85. Traub-Dargatz J, et al: Monoclonal aggregating immunoglobulin cryoglobulinemia in a horse with malignant lymphoma. Equine Vet J 17:470, 1985.

Graft-Versus-Host Disease

86. Affolter VK, et al: Immunohistochemical characterization of canine acute graft-versus host disease and erythema multiforme. In: Kwochka KW, et al (eds): Advances in Veterinary Dermatology III. Butterworth-Heinemann, Boston, 1998, p 103.
87. Ardans AA, et al: Immunotherapy in two foals with combined immunodeficiency, resulting in graft-versus-host reaction. J Am Vet Med Assoc 167:1970, 1977.
88. Johnson ML, Farmer ER: Graft-versus-host reactions in dermatology. J Am Acad Dermatol 38:369, 1998.
89. Perryman LE, Liu IKM: Graft-versus-host reactions in foals with combined immunodeficiency. Am J Vet Res 41:187, 1980.

Cutaneous Adverse Drug Reaction

90. Anderson WI, et al: Adverse reaction to penicillin in horses. Mod Vet Pract 64:928, 1983.
91. Bhikane AU, et al: Hypersensitivity reaction in a horse following injection of Belamyl (B complex and liver extract). Indian Vet J 70:167, 1993.
92. Byars DT: Allergic skin diseases in the horse. Vet Clin N Am Large Anim Pract 6:87, 1984.
92a. Ginn PE, et al: Self-limiting subepidermal bullous disease in a neonatal foal. Vet Dermatol 9:249, 1998.
93. Goldberg GP, Short CE: Challenge in equine anesthesia: a suspected allergic reaction during acetylpromazine, guaifenesin, thiamylal, and halothane anesthesia. Equine Pract 10:5, 1988.
93a. Haitjema H, Gibson KT: Severe pruritus associated with epidural morphine and detomidine in a horse. Aust Vet J 79:248, 2001.
94. Matthews NS, et al: Urticarial response during anesthesia in a horse. Equine Vet J 25:55, 1994.
95. MVP Staff Report: Adverse drug reactions. Mod Vet Pract 59:689, 1978.
96. Perez T, et al: Hypersensitivity reactions to drugs: correlation between clinical probability score and laboratory diagnostic procedure. J Invest Clin Immunol 5:276, 1995.
97. Pricke HME: The untoward reaction of the horse to injection of antigenic substances. J Am Vet Med Assoc 155:258, 1969.
98. Scott DW, Miller WH Jr: Idiosyncratic cutaneous adverse drug reactions in the horse: literature review and report of 19 cases (1990-1996). Equine Pract 19:12, 1997.
99. Wolkensstien P, et al: Metabolic predisposition to cutaneous adverse drug reactions. Arch Dermatol 131:544, 1995.

Erythema Multiforme

100. Affolter VK, Shaw SE: Cutaneous drug eruptions. In: Ihrke PJ, et al (eds): Advances in Veterinary Dermatology II. Pergamon Press, New York, 1993, p 447.
101. Fadok VA: Update on four unusual equine dermatoses. Vet Clin N Am Equine Pract 11:105, 1995.

102. Marshall C: Erythema multiforme in two horses. J S Afr Vet Assoc 62:133, 1991.

103. Scott DW, et al: Erythema multiforme in a horse. Equine Pract 6(8):26, 1984.

104. Scott DW: Diagnostic des dermatoses inflammatoires équines: analyse de la modalité de réaction histopathologique; étude personelle portant sur 315 cas. Point Vét 24:245, 1992.

105. Scott DW, Miller WH Jr: Erythema multiforme in the horse: literature review and report of 9 cases (1988-1996). Equine Pract 20(6):6, 1998.

106. Stannard AA: Personal communication, 1990.

Vasculitis

107. Bennett PM, King AS: Studies on equine purpura haemorrhagica. 2. Symptomatology. Br Vet J 104:414, 1948.

108. Biggers JD, Ingraham PL: Studies on equine purpura haemorrhagica. Review of the literature. Br Vet J 104:214, 1948.

109. Biggers JD, et al: Studies on equine purpura haemorrhagica. 4. Haematology. Br Vet J 105:191, 1949.

110. Byars TD, Divers TJ: Equine purpura haemorrhagica. Georgia Vet 32:14, 1980.

110a. Ferraro SL: Pastern dermatitis in Shires and Clydesdales. J Equine Vet Sci 21:524, 2001.

111. Galan JE, Timoney JF: Immune complexes in purpura hemorrhagica of the horse containing IgA and M antigen of *Streptococcus equi.* J Immunol 135:3134, 1985.

112. Greatorex JC: Urticaria, blue nose and purpura haemorrhagica in horses. Equine Vet J 1:157, 1969.

113. Gunson DE, Rooney JR: Anaphylactoid purpura in a horse. Vet Pathol 14:325, 1977.

114. King AS: Studies on equine purpura haemorrhagica. 3. Morbid anatomy and histology. Br Vet J 105:35, 1949.

115. Lotti T, et al: Cutaneous small-vessel vasculitis. J Am Acad Dermatol 39:667, 1998.

116. Meschter CL, et al: Vascular pathology in phenylbutazone intoxicated horses. Cornell Vet 74:282, 1984.

117. Morris DD, et al: Chronic necrotizing vasculitis in a horse. J Am Vet Med Assoc 183:579, 1983.

118. Morris DD: Cutaneous vasculitis in horses: 19 cases (1978-1985). J Am Vet Med Assoc 191:460, 1987.

119. O'Dea JC: Comments on vaccination against strangles. J Am Vet Med Assoc 155:427, 1969.

120. Reef VB: Vasculitis. In: Robinson NE (ed): Current Therapy in Equine Medicine II. Philadelphia, W.B. Saunders Co, 1987, 312.

121. Roberts MC, Kelly WR: Renal dysfunction in a case of purpura haemorrhagica in a horse. Vet Rec 110:144, 1982.

121a. Sloet van Oldruitenborgh-Oosterbaan MM, et al: Pasture dermatosis in the nonpigmented lower limb in the horse. Vet Dermatol 11(suppl):21, 2000.

122. Stannard AA: Photoactivated vasculitis. In: Robinson NE (ed): Current Therapy in Equine Medicine II. Philadelphia, W.B. Saunders Co, 1987, p 646.

123. Sweeney CR, et al: Complications associated with *Streptococcus equi* infection on a horse farm. J Am Vet Med Assoc 191:1446, 1987.

124. Van Huffel X, et al: Successful treatment of an unusual case of extensive skin necrosis on the limbs of a foal. Vlaams Diergeneesk Tijdschr 56:400, 1987.

125. Werner LL, et al: Acute necrotizing vasculitis and thrombocytopenia in a horse. J Am Vet Med Assoc 185:87, 1984.

126. Woods PR, et al: Granulomatous enteritis and cutaneous arteritis in a horse. J Am Vet Med Assoc 203:1573, 1993.

Alopecia Areata

126a. Black SS, et al: Clinical snapshot #4. Comp Cont Educ 23:758, 2001.

126b. Conroy TD: Alopecia areata. In: Andrews EJ, et al (eds). Spontaneous Animal Models of Human Disease. New York, Academic Press, 1979, p 30.

127. McElwee KJ, et al: Comparison of alopecia areata in human and nonhuman mammalian species. Pathobiol 66:90, 1998.

128. Michie HJ, et al: The DEBR rat: an animal model of human alopecia areata. Br J Dermatol 125:94, 1991.

129. Middleton DJ, Church S: Alopecia universalis in a horse. Vet Dermatol 5:123, 1994.

130. Schott HC, et al: Spontaneous recovery from equine alopecia areata/universalis: case report and comparison of the disorder in other species. In: Kwochka KW, et al (eds): Advances in Veterinary Dermatology III. Butterworth-Heinemann, Boston, 1998, p 469.

131. Sundberg JP, et al: Alopecia areata in aging C3H/HeJ mice. J Invest Dermatol 102:847, 1994.

132. Tobin DJ, et al: Equine alopecia areata autoantibodies target multiple hair follicle antigens and may alter hair growth. A preliminary study. Exp Dermatol 7:289, 1998.

Amyloidosis

133. Geisel O, et al: Kutane Amyloidose vom Immunglobulin-Ursprung bei einem Pferd. Pferdeheilk 5:299, 1989.

134. Gliatto JM, Alroy J: Cutaneous amyloidosis in a horse with lymphoma. Vet Rec 137:68, 1995.

135. Hawthorne TB, et al: Systemic amyloidosis in a mare. J Am Vet Med Assoc 196:323, 1990.

136. Hayden DW, et al: Amyloid-associated gastroenteropathy in a horse. J Comp Pathol 98:195, 1988.

137. Hjärre A: Uber der Amyloiddegeneration bei Tieren. Acta Pathol Microbiol Scand 16 (suppl.):132, 1933.

138. Hjärre A, Nordlund I: Om atypisk amyloidos hos djuren. Skand Vet Tidskr 32:385, 1942.

139. Hjärre A: Uber Amyloidose bei Tieren mit Besonderer Berücksichtigung atypischer Formen. Berl Münch Tierärztl Wschr 93:331, 1942.

140. Husby G: Equine amyloidosis. Equine Vet J 20:277, 1988.

141. Husebekk A, et al: Characterization of amyloid protein AA and its serum precursor SAA in the horse. Scand J Immunol 23:703, 1986.

142. Jakob W: Spontaneous amyloidosis of mammals. Vet Pathol 8:292, 1971.

143. Kasper CA, et al: Nasal amyloidosis: a case report and review. Equine Pract 16(3):25, 1994.

144. Linke RP, Trautwein G: Immunoglobulin lambda-light-chain-derived amyloidosis in two horses. Blut 58:129, 1989.

145. Mould JRB, et al: Conjunctival and nasal amyloidosis in a horse. Equine Vet J 10 (suppl):8, 1990.

146. Nappert G, et al: Nasal amyloidosis in two quarter horses. Can Vet J 29:834, 1988.

147. Nieberle K: Pathologisch-anatomische mitterlungen. 2. Lokale, tumorförmige Amyloidosis der Nasenscheidewand eines Pferdes. Tierärztl Umsch 31:404, 1925.

148. Nieberle K, Cohrs P: Lehrbuch der Speziellen Pathologischen Anatomie der Haustiere. Gustav-Fischer, Jena, 1961.

149. Schützler H, Beyer J: Klinische und histologische Untersuchungen an Serumpferden unter besonderer Berücksichtigung der Leberruptur. Arch Exp Vet Med 18:1119, 1964.

150. Shaw DP, et al: Nasal amyloidosis in four horses. Vet Pathol 24:183, 1987.

151. Stannard AA: Equine dermatology. Proc Am Assoc Equine Practit 22:273, 1976.

152. Stünzi H, et al: Systemische Haut-und Unterhautamyloidose beim Pferd. Vet Pathol 12:405, 1975.

153. Touart DM, Sau P: Cutaneous deposition diseases. Part I. J Am Acad Dermatol 39:149, 1998.

154. van Andel ACJ, et al: Amyloid in the horse: a report of nine cases. Equine Vet J 20:277, 1988.

Chapter 10

Endocrine, Nutritional, and Miscellaneous Haircoat Disorders

● ENDOCRINE DISORDERS

Glucocorticoids

Hyperadrenocorticism is the most common endocrinopathy affecting the skin of the horse.

GLUCOCORTICOIDS AND THE SKIN

In many species, the protein catabolic, antienzymatic, and antimitotic effects of glucocorticoids are manifested in the following ways: (1) the epidermis becomes thin and hyperkeratotic, (2) hair follicles and sebaceous glands become atrophic, (3) the dermis becomes thin, (4) dermal vasculature becomes fragile, (5) wound healing is delayed, and (6) cutaneous infections are more common.[1,11,11a] Histologic correlates of these abnormalities include diffuse orthokeratotic hyperkeratosis, epidermal and follicular atrophy, telogenization of hair follicles, excessive trichilemmal keratinization of hair follicles ("flame follicles"), sebaceous gland atrophy, thin dermis, and telangiectasia.[1,11,11a]

In horses, the findings are quite different. Instead of easy epilation, alopecia, thin skin, and hypotonic skin, the cushingoid horse becomes hypertrichotic. Calcinosis cutis has not been reported in cushingoid horses. As is the case in other species, cushingoid horses do appear to be more susceptible than normal horses to skin infections.

ADRENAL FUNCTION TESTS

Adrenal function tests are basically of two types: those that are single measurements of basal glucocorticoid levels in blood or urine and those that are provocative, dynamic response tests. Single measurements of basal glucocorticoid levels, while cheaper and easier to perform, are unreliable.[2,8,9,11]

Blood Cortisol

Baseline blood cortisol concentrations in normal horses approximate 1 to 13 µg/dl.[*] Baseline blood cortisol concentrations are not affected by breed, age, gender, or pregnancy. However, important considerations to keep in mind when interpreting blood cortisol levels include the following: (1) different laboratories may differ in their normal and abnormal values, (2) stress (exercise, hypoglycemia, anesthesia, surgery, severe disease, transport, hospitalization, blood taking, unaccustomed to environment or routine) can markedly elevate blood cortisol levels, (3) episodic daily secretion of cortisol occurs, and (4) single measurements of blood cortisol are of limited value in the diagnosis of hyperglucocorticoidism.[†] In the horse, blood cortisol levels are highest in the morning and

---

[*]References 11, 13a-16a, 18-21, 23-26, 29, 35, 36, 38, 42, 44, 50-52, 54, 73.
[†]References 2, 8, 9, 11a, 12a, 13a, 16a-21a, 23-27, 34a-36, 38, 53, 62, 66, 68, 85, 87.

lowest at night.* Because of the endogenous rhythmic and episodic fluctuations, and the exogenously provoked fluctuations in baseline cortisol concentrations, as well as the overlap with baseline concentrations found in horses with hyperadrenocorticism, this test is highly unreliable for the diagnosis of equine hyperadrenocorticism. Basal cortisol concentrations in cushingoid horses may be low, normal, or high.

Cortisol Response Tests

To overcome unreliability of basal blood cortisol levels, various provocative tests have been developed.[†] Two commonly used ACTH response test procedures for the horse are as follows: (1) plasma or serum cortisol determinations are made before and 8 hours after the intramuscular injection of 1 IU/kg of ACTH gel or (2) plasma or serum cortisol determinations are made before and 2 hours after the intravenous injection of 100 IU synthetic aqueous ACTH. By either procedure, normal horses will double to triple their basal cortisol levels, whereas horses with pituitary-dependent hyperadrenocorticism will have exaggerated responses. The sensitivity of the ACTH stimulation test in the diagnosis of equine hyperadrenocorticism varies from 70% to 79%.[62,85,86] Thus, it does not consistently discriminate between normal and cushingoid horses. If the ACTH stimulation test results are combined with the measurement of plasma ACTH concentrations, sensitivity is reported to be 100%.[85]

Older literature indicated that the dexamethasone suppression test was not a sensitive indicator of adrenocortical function in horses.[‡] In horses, dexamethasone does *not* have the suppressive effect seen in dogs and humans, presumably because the hypersecretion of ACTH is from the pars intermedia (rather than the pars distalis) and is relatively insensitive to glucocorticoid negative feedback. These observations were based on dexamethasone suppression tests performed by measuring plasma or serum cortisol before and 6 hours after the intramuscular administration of 20 mg dexamethasone.

More recently an overnight dexamethasone suppression test has been reported to be 100% sensitive and 100% specific for the diagnosis of equine hyperadrenocorticism.[48,52,53,56,66] Basal blood cortisol concentrations are measured prior and 19 to 24 hours following the administration of 40 μg (0.04 mg)/kg dexamethasone intramuscularly. Dexamethasone suppression tests have occasionally been avoided or discouraged in horses with hyperadrenocorticism because of the hypothetical risk of causing laminitis.[85] However, no side effects were reported with the overnight protocol. It has been reported that starting a dexamethasone suppression test at 9 AM or 9 PM gave the same results.[33] After an overnight dexamethasone suppression test, normal horses will have post-dexamethasone cortisol concentrations of <1 μg/dl while cushingoid horses will have concentrations of >1 μg/dl.

Plasma ACTH

Plasma ACTH levels are measured by radioimmunoassay.[§] Basal plasma ACTH concentrations in normal horses approximate 5 to 37 pg/ml. Blood for ACTH assays is typically drawn in EDTA tubes, the plasma is separated within 3 hours and frozen at -20°C in a plastic tube. Once frozen, the plasma can be kept for up to 1 month before being assayed. Samples of frozen plasma should be shipped to the appropriate laboratory on dry ice overnight to ensure that they do not thaw during shipment.

---

*References 14, 16a, 18, 20-21a, 23, 24, 35, 36.

[†]References 8, 9, 11, 13a, 45, 48, 52, 53, 62, 66, 76, 85-87.

[‡]References 11, 42, 44, 50, 62, 71, 73, 74, 90.

[§]References 8, 9, 13a, 28, 42, 48, 49, 71, 73, 74, 85, 90.

Plasma ACTH concentrations were reported to be sensitive and specific for the diagnosis of hyperadrenocorticism in horses and ponies.[48,49] Plasma ACTH concentrations >27 pg/ml (ponies) and >50 pg/ml (horses) are "strongly supportive" of the diagnosis of hyperadrenocorticism. It has been reported that the simultaneous performance of an ACTH stimulation test and basal plasma ACTH concentrations was 100% accurate for the diagnosis of equine hyperadrenocorticism.[55]

Other Tests

The *TRH stimulation* test resulted in a significant increase in plasma cortisol concentrations in cushingoid horses compared with normal horses.[*] However, the sensitivity and specificity of this test in equine hyperadrenocorticism are unknown.

The *combined dexamethasone suppression/ACTH stimulation test* often yields ambiguous results.[†]

The *combined dexamethasone suppression/TRH stimulation test* is of unproven sensitivity and specificity in equine hyperadrenocorticism.[8,54,66]

Although the mean *urinary corticoid:creatinine ratio* is significantly higher in cushingoid than in normal horses, there is much overlap in test results, resulting in both false-negative and false-positive test results.[8,46a,66,83]

Basal plasma insulin concentrations, the *glucose tolerance test*, and the *insulin response test* have good sensitivity, but are only applicable to horses with hyperglycemia.[8,48,58,86] Although insulin-resistant hyperglycemia is commonly seen in cushingoid horses, stress-induced hyperglycemia in normal horses may result in glucose concentrations of the same order of magnitude.[8,48,66] In addition, hyperglycemia with normal basal insulin concentrations has been reported.[48,64] Furthermore, ponies often have a relative insensitivity to insulin compared with horses.[43,48,76a]

In a very small number of horses, *salivary concentrations of cortisol* in cushingoid horses were higher than those in normal horses.[88a]

HYPERADRENOCORTICISM

Hyperadrenocorticism (Cushing's disease, Cushing's syndrome, equine hirsutism), an uncommon disorder of the horse, is caused by excessive endogenous glucocorticoid production, usually in association with a functional lesion of the pars intermedia of the pituitary gland. Classically, equine hyperadrenocorticism has been associated with the presence of a functional chromophobe adenoma of the pars intermedia (intermediate lobe) of the pituitary gland (hypophysis).[‡] It is currently believed that the condition actually results from loss of normal inhibitory control,[52,53,87] eventuating in the classic endocrine processes of hypertrophy, hyperplasia, and, rarely, adenoma formation. For reasons that are currently unknown, there is a decrease or loss of the neurotransmitter dopamine in the innervation of the pars intermedia. The function of melanotropes in the pars intermedia is normally inhibited when dopamine and, perhaps, serotonin are released from nerve endings extending from the hypothalamus. Loss of inhibition is followed by increased synthesis and secretion of various peptides. Over time there is hypertrophy and hyperplasia of the pars intermedia. In most cases of equine hyperadrenocorticism, the pars intermedia is enlarged because of hypertrophy and hyperplasia, with progression to true adenoma being a late and uncommon event. The cells of pituitary tumors are sometimes difficult to distinguish, but most closely resemble hyperplastic melanotrophs.[§]

---

*References 8, 13a, 43, 44, 66, 87.
†References 8, 13a, 15a, 48, 49, 52, 53, 62, 66, 68, 86.
‡References 2, 4, 5, 7, 8, 9, 11, 13a, 37, 39, 40, 42, 44-46, 50, 51, 55-57, 59, 61-68, 71, 75-82, 89.
§References 8, 62, 68, 70, 76, 82.

The normal equine pituitary gland produces a variety of closely related peptides by cleavage of a common precursor protein known as *pro-opiomelanocortin (POMC)*.[*] The pars distalis processes POMC to adrenocorticotropin (ACTH), β-lipotropin (βLPH) and α-lipotropin (αLPH), whereas in the pars intermedia the main POMC-derived peptides are α-melanocyte stimulating hormone (αMSH), β-melanocyte stimulating hormone (βMSH), corticotropin-like intermediate lobe peptide (CL1P), and β-endorphin (βEND).[†] In normal horses, the pars intermedia produces only about 2% of the ACTH. Cushingoid horses have elevated levels of these POMC-derived peptides in pituitary tissue and blood, and a loss of the diurnal (circadian) rhythm of cortisol secretion. ACTH release from the pars distalis is under neuroendocrine control from the hypothalamus, mediated via corticotropin-releasing hormone (CRH) and arginine vasopressin and is subject to negative feedback by cortisol. In contrast, pars intermedia POMC-peptide secretion is under dopaminergic control and does not appear to be influenced by plasma cortisol.[‡]

The alteration in POMC-derived hormones contributes to adrenocortical dysfunction by at least two mechanisms.[52] Release of ACTH in horses with hyperadrenocorticism is much greater than that observed in clinically normal horses and, although it is not as pronounced as the release of other POMC-derived peptides, it is sufficient to stimulate adrenocortical steroidogenesis. Also, other POMC-derived peptides can potentiate the actions of ACTH. Thus, a small increase in ACTH concentration, coupled with a large increase in potentiating peptides (e.g., MSH and βEND), can contribute to melanotrope-mediated adrenocortical dysfunction.

The pituitary lesion grows by expansion, has a low mitotic index, and does not metastasize. The enlarged pituitary gland can weigh up to 11.4 g (normal <3.5 g).[87] The size of the pituitary lesion does not correlate with the severity of clinical signs. Adrenocortical hyperplasia is typically, but not always, present, and may be diffuse, nodular, or both.[§]

Other causes of equine hyperadrenocorticism are extremely rare. Single cases caused by a pituitary meningioma[64a] and an adrenocortical adenoma[88] are reported. Classical hyperadrenocorticism due to exogenous steroids (iatrogenic disease) has not been reported.

The pathogenesis of the clinical signs seen in equine hyperadrenocorticism are complex and, in many instances, undocumented.[¶] Weight loss and muscle weakness and atrophy are presumably due to the catabolic effects of glucocorticoids. The occurrence of fat pads is thought to be due to fat redistribution under the influence of glucocorticoids. Increased susceptibility to bacterial and fungal infections and poor wound healing are due to the immunosuppressive and anti-inflammatory effects of glucocorticoids. Laminitis is hypothesized to be associated with the enhancement of the vasoconstrictor potency of endogenous biogenic amines by glucocorticoids. Glucocorticoid excess is also believed to be the cause of frequent low blood concentrations of thyroid hormones, abnormal estrus cycles, and rarely, fractures.

Behavioral changes could be due to high levels of βEND in blood and cerebrospinal fluid or pressure of the pituitary lesion on the hypothalamus.[Π] The pressure of an enlarging pituitary mass can also cause central blindness, thermoregulatory disturbances, and seizures.

Polydipsia and polyuria are thought to be due to glucocorticoid antagonism of antidiuretic hormone (ADH) resulting in diabetes insipidus and/or the antagonism of insulin resulting in diabetes mellitus.

The most puzzling clinical abnormality is the hypertrichosis, which has been postulated to be due to (1) increased adrenocortical production of androgens, (2) increased secretion of MSH, or

---

[*]References 8, 9, 11, 48, 52, 53, 61, 66, 68, 73, 74, 87, 90.

[†]References 8, 9, 13, 28, 30, 34, 48, 52, 53, 61, 64, 70, 73, 74, 87, 90.

[‡]References 8, 11, 48, 53, 66, 71.

[§]References 8, 9, 11, 42, 44, 50, 59, 61, 68, 71, 73, 74, 78, 82, 87.

[¶]References 8, 9, 11, 37, 44, 53, 61, 62, 66, 68, 70, 76, 78, 85, 87.

[Π]References 8, 53, 61, 66, 68, 70, 87.

(3) pressure of the pituitary lesion on thermoregulatory areas of the hypothalamus.[*] Although the haircoat abnormality has classically been referred to as *hirsutism*, this is inappropriate. Hirsutism refers to hair growth in women in areas of the body where hair growth is under androgen control and in which normally only postpubescent males have terminal hair growth (e.g., mustache, beard, chest).[1] The haircoat abnormality in equine hyperadrenocorticism is properly called *hypertrichosis*, which specifically refers to hair density or length beyond the accepted limits of normal for a particular age, race, or sex.[1]

Hyperhidrosis may be caused by pressure of the pituitary lesion on thermoregulatory areas of the hypothalamus, or the dramatic haircoat change.[†]

Clinical Features

Equine hyperadrenocorticism (Cushing's disease, Cushing's syndrome, hirsutism) is an uncommon to rare disorder, accounting for 0.44% of all the equine dermatoses examined at the Cornell University Clinic.

Horses that present with many or most of the classical historical and physical features of hyperadrenocorticism make for a straightforward clinical diagnosis.[‡] However, the clinical signs often develop sequentially and in random order over a variable period of time (months to years). Signs may wax and wane. The presenting complaint for horses with hyperadrenocorticism is frequently not directly related to the pituitary dysfunction, and evidence to suggest pituitary dysfunction is often revealed by a carefully developed history and thorough physical examination.

Hyperadrenocorticism is generally a disease of elderly horses (average 20 years, range 7 to 42 years). There are no breed predilections, but ponies seem to be at increased risk.[53,62,66] There is controversy in the literature over any sex predilection, with some authors indicating female,[44,50,59,61] others male,[62,73] and still others no predilection.[48,53,82,87]

One of the most striking clinical abnormalities in equine hyperadrenocorticism is hypertrichosis (Fig. 10-1), which is present in 85% to 100% of the cases. The haircoat is typically long, thick, shaggy, and curly, often most noticeably on the limbs. The mane and tail are typically unaffected. Early signs may be delayed shedding in spring, often followed by early regrowth of winter coat in fall. Some horses exhibit incomplete shedding, with long hairs persisting in the jugular groove, under the shins, the belly, and the legs, or in a few round patchy areas over the entire body. Some horses with early hyperadrenocorticism develop transient alopecia with shedding, commonly confined to the head. In exceptional cases, there may be a coat color change.[87] The skin may be normal, dry and scaly, or greasy.

Cushingoid horses are increasingly susceptible to skin infections (especially dermatophilosis, staphylococcal folliculitis, abscesses, and draining tracts). Hyperhidrosis—usually episodic but occasionally persistent—is seen in up to 60% of the cases. This can lead to matting of the haircoat into thick tufts. Rarely, papular and nodular xanthomas are present over the thorax.[11]

Weight loss, muscular weakness, and muscular atrophy are present in up to 88% of the cases. The epaxial, lumbar, and abdominal muscles are particularly affected, often leading to a pot-bellied and sway-backed appearance. Muscle wasting can also result in an increased prominence of the croup, tuber coxae, and tuber sacrale regions. Fat pads may develop on the body, especially in the supraorbital, tailhead, lumbar, and scapular regions.

Polydipsia and polyuria are seen in 39% to 76% of the cases, and are usually associated with diabetes mellitus and/or diabetes insipidus. Changes in behavior and attitude (lethargy, docility,

---

[*]References 8, 11, 63, 67, 68, 82, 87, 89.
[†]References 8, 11, 67, 68, 87, 89.
[‡]References 2, 5-9, 11, 37, 39, 40, 42-46, 48-50, 53, 56, 57, 59, 61-64, 65-68, 73-82, 85-87, 89.

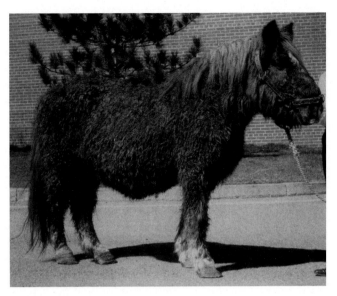

FIGURE 10-1. Hyperadrenocorticism. Note hypertrichosis, pot-belly, and sway back.

dullness, drowsiness, somnolence, decreased responsiveness to painful stimuli) are common (15% to 82% of cases).

Laminitis is seen in 24% to 82% of affected horses. Often all four feet are affected, and horses suffer repeated bouts of laminitis that is refractory to conventional therapy. Intractable pain is probably the most common reason for euthanasia.

Other signs that may be seen in cushingoid horses include polyphagia or anorexia, buccal ulcers, episodic tachypnea and tachycardia, bacterial or mycotic infections (conjunctivitis; sinusitis; pneumonia; joint or tendon sheath infections; abscesses in teeth, pharynx, mandible, and lung), neurologic abnormalities (blindness, ataxia, seizures), infertility, abnormal estrus cycles, delayed wound healing, skeletal problems (fractures, hypertrophic osteopathy), and colic.

Diagnosis

When many of the classical abnormalities are present, a presumptive diagnosis of hyperadreno-corticism is justified on the basis of history and physical examination. However, in early cases, wherein only one or two of the clinical signs (e.g., weight loss, behavioral change, neurologic disturbance, laminitis, infection) are present, the differential diagnosis can be quite lengthy.[2,7-9] Retention of a long winter haircoat can be seen in horses with chronic illnesses and dietary deficiencies.[11]

Results of routine laboratory testing are variable, often reflective of disease chronicity, and never used to confirm or refute the diagnosis.* Typical, fully developed cases frequently have insulin-resistant hyperglycemia; glucosuria; varying combinations of relative or absolute neutrophilia, lymphopenia, and eosinopenia; elevated plasma insulin concentrations; and low serum T_4 and T_3 concentrations. Urine specific gravity may be normal or low. Horses with chronic infections may have leukocytosis and nonregenerative anemia. Occasional horses have elevated serum liver enzyme concentrations, others have lipemia and hypercholesterolemia.

Basal plasma cortisol concentrations are of no diagnostic benefit, because they may be low, normal, or elevated in cushingoid and normal horses (see Adrenal Function Tests). Definitive

---

*References 2, 7-9, 11, 32, 44, 50, 53, 56, 59, 61, 62, 66, 68, 78, 82, 87.

diagnosis is most consistently and practically confirmed by means of the overnight dexamethasone suppression test (see Adrenal Function Tests).

Computed tomography and ventrodorsal radiography with contrast venography have been shown to be useful for demonstrating an enlarged pituitary gland.[38,56,66,87] However, both techniques require general anesthesia and the availability of specialized equipment. In addition, the rate of false-negative studies (masses less than 2 mm in diameter) and false-positive studies (nonfunctional pituitary lesion) is unknown.

To the authors' knowledge, no studies have been published concerning the histologic appearance of the skin from horses with hyperadrenocorticism. Papular and nodular xanthomas are characterized by xanthogranulomatous inflammation, which may be nodular and/or diffuse in pattern (Figs. 10-2 and 10-3).[11]

Clinical Management

Appropriate management of equine hyperadrenocorticism is dependent on many considerations: severity of the disease, rate of progression of the disease, what the horse is used for, economics, and owner dedication. In all cases, excellent husbandry practices are essential: excellent quality feed, access to sufficient drinking water, regular deworming (every 8 weeks if horse at pasture or in a group), routine dental care (every 6 months or as needed), routine vaccination program, hoof care, early and aggressive treatment of infections, and routine clipping of the haircoat (decreases heat stress, matting associated with hyperhidrosis, and risk of infections).[*]

Medical management involves the use of one of two types of drugs: dopamine agonists or serotonin antagonists.[†] The goal of medical treatment is to help reestablish a balance between the neurotransmitters dopamine and serotonin.

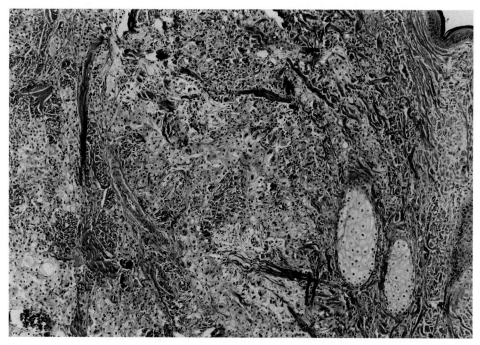

FIGURE 10-2. Hyperadrenocorticism and cutaneous xanthoma. Skin biopsy specimen reveals xanthogranuloma.

---

[*]References 2, 7-9, 42, 44, 45, 53, 60a, 66, 87.
[†]References 2, 8, 9, 42, 44, 45, 53, 66, 87.

Pergolide (dopamine agonist) is the current drug of choice.[*] In general, treatment is begun at 0.5 mg/day per os. Response to treatment is evaluated after 4 to 8 weeks and, if no improvement is seen, the dose is increased by 0.25 mg. The dose is increased by 0.25 mg increments every 4 to 8 weeks until improvement is observed. Most horses require 0.75 to 1.25 mg/day, though doses as high as 5 mg/day have been reported.[42,44] When the appropriate dose is achieved, clinical and biochemical improvement is typically seen within 1 month. The first clinical signs to improve are usually polydipsia and polyuria (if these are present). Side effects are uncommon and include anorexia, diarrhea, depression, dizziness, dry mouth, sweating, and colic.

Cyproheptadine (serotonin antagonist) is erratic as concerns its therapeutic efficacy.[†] In general, treatment is begun at 0.25 mg/kg q24h per os. The horse is reevaluated in 4 weeks and, if no improvement is observed, the dose is increased to 0.25 mg/kg q12h PO. Occasional horses require up to 0.36 mg/kg q12h PO. Pergolide is usually effective in horses that fail to respond to cyproheptadine.

Bromocriptine (dopamine agonist) has been used in very few horses, either orally at 15 mg/horse q12h (it is poorly absorbed) or subcutaneously/intramuscularly at 5 mg/horse q12h).[‡] This drug is expensive, has no apparent advantage over pergolide and cyproheptadine, and requires more investigation before its use can be recommended.

Trilostane (3β-hydroxysteroid dehydrogenase inhibitor) was given (0.4 to 1 mg/kg orally for 30 days) to Cushingoid horses.[69a] Improvements in polyuria, polydipsia, and demeanor were seen, but adrenal function tests were not significantly different at the end of therapy.

Mitotane (op-DDD) is ineffective in equine hyperadrenocorticism.[§] Anecdotal reports indicate the benefits of "glandulars," "antioxidants," free-choice minerals, low-sugar feeds (corn,

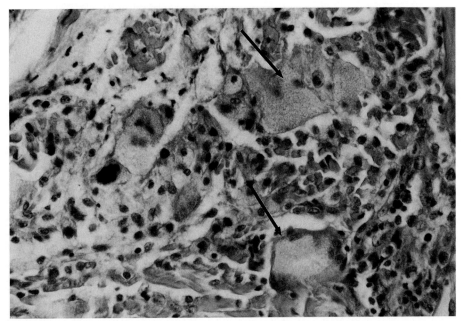

FIGURE 10-3. Close-up of Fig. 10-2. Xanthogranuloma with multinucleated histiocytic giant cells (*arrows*).

[*]References 2, 8, 9, 45, 53, 66, 72, 87.
[†]References 2, 8, 9, 42, 44, 45, 53, 66, 69, 87.
[‡]References 8, 9, 41, 45, 53, 66, 73, 87.
[§]References 8, 9, 44, 53, 59, 66, 87.

oats, barley), constitutional homeopathy, and Chinese herbs.[60] No details or science were presented.

The prognosis for equine hyperadrenocorticism is very dependent on the clinical stage of the disease and any complications (e.g., laminitis). However, mildly affected animals can sometimes be maintained for years with the husbandry practices mentioned above, and animals responsive to husbandry practices and medical management can be kept in satisfactory to near-normal health for up to 10 years.

Thyroid Hormones

Naturally occurring hypothyroidism is extremely rare, if it exists at all, in adult horses.

THYROID HORMONES AND THE SKIN

Thyroid hormones play a dominant role in controlling metabolism and are essential for normal growth and development.[1,11,11a] The primary mechanisms of action of thyroid hormones are stimulation of cytoplasmic protein synthesis and increasing tissue oxygen consumption. These effects are thought to be initiated by the binding of thyroid hormones to nuclear chromatin and the augmentation of the transcription of genetic information. Available data suggest that thyroid hormones play a pivotal role in differentiation and maturation of mammalian skin, as well as in the maintenance of normal cutaneous function.

Hypothyroidism results in epidermal atrophy and abnormal keratinization as a result of decreased protein synthesis, mitotic activity, and oxygen consumption.[11,11a] The thyroid hormone-deficient epidermis is characterized by both abnormal lipogenesis and decreased sterol synthesis by keratinocytes. Epidermal melanosis may be seen, but the pathologic mechanism is unclear. Sebaceous gland atrophy occurs, and sebum excretion rates are reduced. Thyroid hormones are necessary for the initiation of the anagen phase of the hair follicle cycle. In hypothyroid individuals, anagen is not initiated, resulting in the hair follicles being retained in telogen and leading to failure of hair growth and alopecia.

Hypothyroidism results in the accumulation of glycosaminoglycans in the dermis, leading to an increase in the interstitial ground substance and a thick, myxedematous dermis.[1,11,11a] The exact cause of this tissue myxedema is unknown, although evidence suggests that (1) elevated levels of TSH in primary hypothyroidism result in an increased synthesis of ground substance and (2) the transcapillary albumin escape rate is increased while lymphatic drainage is inadequate in myxedema.

Thyroid hormone has been reported to heal the ulcers and reduce the scarring associated with chronic radiodermatitis in humans and to improve the healing of deep dermal burns in rats.[11] These effects were thought to be due to thyroid hormone actions on the proliferation and metabolism of fibroblasts and collagen synthesis. Not surprisingly, the skin of hypothyroid dogs and humans exhibits poor wound healing and easy bruising.[1,11a]

THYROID FUNCTION TESTS

No single area of veterinary diagnostics is more misunderstood, confused, and abused than thyroid function testing. For the most part, this situation is referable to the failure to recognize the significance of (1) the euthyroid sick syndrome and (2) the unreliability of basal serum thyroid hormone levels.

Thyroid function tests (e.g., basal metabolic rate; radioactive iodine uptake; protein-bound iodine; butanol-extractable iodine; thyroxine (T_4) by competitive protein-binding or column chromatography; triiodothyronine (T_3 resin uptake; and free thyroxine index, T_7 test) are either inaccurate, impractical, or inferior to modern techniques and will not be discussed here.*

---

*References 11, 105-108, 117, 121, 129, 135.

Serum T_4 and T_3

Radioimmunoassay (RIA) and enzyme-linked immunosorbent assay (ELISA) methods are used for determining serum levels of total T_4 and total T_3.[*] Serum samples may be held at room temperature for at least 1 week with no significant deterioration. Reported basal levels of thyroid hormones in horses approximate 1 to 3 µg/dl T_4 and 30 to 170 ng/dl T_3. However, because not all laboratories may use the same assay kit or technique to determine their results, normal ranges can vary from laboratory to laboratory.

Other factors to consider when assessing basal serum T_4 and T_3 levels include the following: (1) T_4 and T_3 levels are lower in euthyroid patients with the euthyroid sick syndrome (discussed later), (2) T_4 and T_3 levels are lower in euthyroid patients associated with recent drug therapy (e.g., glucocorticoids, anabolic steroids, phenylbutazone),[†] (3) normal T_4 and T_3 levels may be lower during warm weather and, conversely, higher in cold weather,[8,9,11] (4) normal T_4 and T_3 levels tend to be lower in horses in training,[‡] (5) normal T_4 and T_3 levels are higher in neonates (as much as 10 times greater than those of adults),[§] (6) T_4 levels are lower in fasted animals,[8,9,100,114,130] (7) T_4 and T_3 levels are lower in horses fed endophyte (*Acremonium* sp.)–infected fescue,[8,9,137] (8) there is diurnal variation in T_4 and T_3 levels, and (9) thyroid hormone values change in a given horse over time.[¶]

A number of conditions (chronic illness, acute illnesses, surgical trauma, fasting, starvation, and fever) can produce moderate to marked reductions in serum T_3 and T_4 levels. Under these circumstances, the patients are euthyroid and in no need of thyroid medication. This situation is referred to as the *euthyroid sick syndrome* and is a common source of misdiagnosis regarding basal serum T_4 and T_3 levels.[Π] It is thought that this metabolic switch in the sick patient is protective by counteracting the excessive calorigenic effects of T_3 in catabolic states.

In summary, basal serum levels of T_4 and T_3 are significantly influenced by numerous conditions that have nothing to do with thyroidal disease and hypothyroidism. In the absence of classic historical, clinical, and clinicopathologic evidence of thyroid hormone deficiency, low basal serum T_4 and T_3 levels are unreliable for a diagnosis of hypothyroidism.

Thyroid Function Testing

Because of the numerous factors that influence T_4 and T_3 concentrations, it is very risky to make a diagnosis of hypothyroidism using baseline values as the sole criteria. Function testing using thyroid-stimulating hormone (TSH) or thyroid-releasing hormone (TRH) is often necessary. To avoid confounding factors, function testing should be performed in horses that have been free of medication for at least 30 days.

TSH Stimulation Test

All published studies in horses involve the use of bovine TSH. Methodology of the TSH response test in horses varies considerably from one report to another, and there are no data suggesting that one method is superior to another.[**] Morris and Garcia[115] reported that equine serum T_4 and T_3 responses to 5, 10, or 20 IU of TSH were similar. A dose of 2.5 IU of TSH also provokes an increase in thyroid hormone concentrations. The recommended procedure for the TSH stimulation test in horses is as follows: (1) serum T_4 levels measured before and 4 to 6 hours after the

---

[*]References 89, 96, 97, 101, 120, 122, 124-128, 132, 134.
[†]References 8, 9, 11, 95, 115, 116, 119.
[‡]References 8, 9, 91, 106, 107, 131, 147.
[§]References 8, 9, 11, 92, 104, 107, 108, 119, 147.
[¶]References 8, 9, 98, 109, 112, 134, 146.
[Π]References 8, 9, 11, 99, 134, 146.
[**]References 8, 9, 11, 101, 102, 107, 115, 122, 123, 127, 138, 140, 144, 147, 148, 152, 158, 163.

intravenous administration of 2.5 to 5 IU of TSH and (2) serum T_3 concentrations measured before and 2 hours after the intravenous administration of 2.5 to 5 IU of TSH. In normal horses, basal T_4 levels should at least double at 4 to 6 hours, and T_3 concentrations should at least double at 2 hours. It has been reported that the TSH response is normal in horses with low basal serum T_4 and T_3 levels associated with phenylbutazone administration.[115,116]

In most parts of the world today, bovine TSH is not available. Recombinant human TSH is available and might be useful. However, it is very expensive and no information is available on the use of this product in horses.

TRH Stimulation Test

The TRH stimulation is reported to be a valuable indicator of equine thyroid function. TRH given intravenously at a dose of 0.5 to 1 mg causes at least a doubling of serum T_4 and T_3 concentrations at 4 and 2 hours, respectively, after injection.[°] TRH, when available, is very expensive. Recombinant human TRH is also available, but it is very expensive and untested in horses.

HYPOTHYROIDISM

Cause and Pathogenesis

A clinical syndrome of hypothyroidism and dysmaturity in foals has been well described.[†] Musculoskeletal abnormalities predominate, and foals are typically affected at birth. The cause of this congenital hypothyroidism is not known, and dams of affected foals are normal and have normal thyroid function. Because this syndrome is not associated with notable cutaneous abnormalities, it will not be discussed here. The interested reader is referred to other excellent sources.[7-9]

Hypothyroidism may occur if horses are fed diets that contain abnormal amounts of iodine.[8,9,11] Mares that receive iodine-deficient diets have dead or weak foals with goiters and no haircoats.[7-9] Goiters and hypothyroidism may develop in horses fed low-iodine feeds exclusively.[7-9] Outbreaks of goiter, weakness, fetal death, and limb abnormalities have been reported when excessive amounts of iodine have been fed to mares.[7-9] The interested reader is referred to other excellent sources for details on these diet-related thyroid abnormalities.[7-9]

Naturally occurring idiopathic hypothyroidism in adult horses is difficult to characterize and quite controversial.[8,9,11] Some authors believe the condition to be common, while others consider it to be rare. "Many" horses diagnosed as hypothyroid are obese and have laminitis and thickened necks. Anecdotal or poorly documented reports suggest that naturally occurring hypothyroidism in adult horses may be responsible for such conditions as laminitis, infertility, anhidrosis, irregular or absent estrus cycles, myopathy, decreased libido in stallions, alopecia, anemia, exercise intolerance, poor growth and agalactia in mares.[†] None of these "associations" have been corroborated.

The only documented clinical signs of hypothyroidism in adult horses were produced experimentally via surgical thyroidectomy.[140a,147,148,160] The horses exhibited retarded growth, lethargy, sensitivity to cold (shivering), decreased rectal temperature, decreased heart rate, decreased respiratory rate, decreased cardiac output, decreased feed consumption and weight gain (*not* obesity!). Dermatologic abnormalities included a dull, rough haircoat, delayed shedding of winter haircoat; and "edema" (myxedema?) of the face and distal limbs. Hematologic abnormalities included normochromic, nonregenerative anemia, increased serum cholesterol, increased serum triglyceride, and increased serum very low-density lipoproteins.[140a,148,160] These abnormalities were reversed when the horses were treated with thyroid hormone.

°References 93, 101, 111, 138, 140, 152, 158.
†References 2, 7-9, 136, 139, 140, 142, 143, 145, 149-151, 154, 156.
‡References 1, 7-9, 11, 127, 128, 133, 138, 147, 153, 155, 158, 161-163.

Clinical Reports

Only three reports of putative naturally occurring equine hypothyroidism with dermatologic abnormalities were found. Two horses had normal haircoats at birth, and began to lose hair at 5 months of age.[141,159] Both horses had bilaterally symmetric alopecia over a large part of the body, including the tail in one horse. One of the horses was lethargic and shivered frequently,[159] while the other horse was otherwise normal.[141] A third horse, 11 years old, developed bilaterally symmetric alopecia over the neck, head, and flanks.[157]

Diagnosis

The diagnosis is based on history, physical examination, and thyroid function testing. Stimulation tests, using either TSH or TRH, are used infrequently in horses because of the expense and limited availability of the stimulating hormones. However, these tests are much more reliable than measurement of baseline thyroid hormone concentration (see Thyroid Function Tests).

The three horses with putative hypothyroidism and alopecia did have thyroid tests performed. One horse had low baseline serum concentrations of T_4 and T_3.[157] A second horse had suppressed responses of T_4 and T_3 to TSH.[141] The third horse had normal baseline serum concentration of T_4, but low baseline concentration of T_3.[159] The authors hypothesized that there was inadequate conversion of T_4 to T_3 in this horse.

Skin biopsies were performed on two of the horses. In one horse, histopathologic findings included "collagenization" of the dermis and small hair follicles that contained disorganized keratin material.[159] Histopathologic findings in the other horse included an increased number of hair follicles, many of which were filled with "irregular keratin material."[141]

Clinical Management

If a horse has clinical signs suggestive of hypothyroidism and low baseline serum concentrations of thyroid hormones, and if known nonthyroidal factors affecting thyroid function have been ruled out, thyroid hormone supplementation should be considered. Thyroid hormone supplementation consists of administering either l-thyroxine at 20 µg/kg orally q24h, or iodinated casein at 5 g (contains approximately 50 mg T_4 and 30 mg T_3)/horse orally q24h.* Clinical abnormalities resulting from surgical thyroidectomy resolved with T_4 (2.5 µg/kg, q12h) or T_3 (0.6 µg/kg q12h).[160] Response to therapy is evaluated by clinical response as well as by monitored serum concentrations of T_4 and T_3. It must be emphasized that many conditions associated with low levels of thyroid hormones have multifactorial causes, and what appears to be a favorable response to thyroid hormone supplementation may actually be spontaneous resolution of another disorder. It is also critical to remember that thyroid hormone supplementation can cause varying degrees of hair growth in normal dogs, as well as in dogs and cats with various nonthyroidal causes of hair loss.[11a] This is likely to occur in horses.

The three horses with putative hypothyroidism and alopecia were treated with thyroid hormones. The horse with "inadequate conversion" of T_4 to T_3 was treated with T_3 for 10 days, and its hair began to regrow in 1 week![159] Six weeks after supplementation was stopped, the horse's hair began to fall out again. The horse was subsequently lost to follow-up.

A second horse was treated with T_3 for 10 days and also regrew hair.[141] However, this horse was also reported to be regrowing hair prior to treatment! This horse was also subsequently lost to follow-up. The third horse was reported to respond to T_4, but further details were not available.[157]

---

*References 8, 9, 94, 148, 152, 158.

• NUTRITIONAL SKIN DISEASES

The nutritional factors that influence the health of the skin are exceedingly complex.[7-9,11,164-170] Dermatoses may result from numerous nutritional deficiencies, excesses, or imbalances, but the skin responds with only a few types of clinical reaction patterns and lesions. These include fairly widespread scaling, crusting, alopecia, and a dry, dull, brittle haircoat. Consequently, physical examinations alone can seldom reveal a specific nutritional cause.

Twenty years ago, nutritional imbalances were thought to be a common cause of skin disease, especially poor haircoats and "seborrhea," in horses.[171] Even today, horses are routinely administered various nutritional supplements and "cocktails" for everything from poor haircoat, to scaly skin (see Chapter 11), to pigmentary abnormalities of skin and haircoat (see Chapter 12), to pruritus. In North America, horses are increasingly fed good to excellent quality diets, making disorders caused by nutritional deficiencies and/or imbalances increasingly uncommon.[9] It is the authors' opinion that inappropriate nutrition is a rare cause of skin disease in horses.

General malnutrition (protein and calorie deficiency), whether strictly dietary in origin or secondary to debilitating diseases, causes the skin to become dry, scaly, thin, and inelastic.[6,11] The skin may become more susceptible to infections and may show hemorrhagic tendencies and pigmentary disturbances. The haircoat becomes dry, dull, brittle, thinned, and perhaps faded in color. Normal hair shedding and regrowth can be impaired, resulting in long coats or patchy shedding. Malnutrition can develop via interference with intake, absorption, or utilization of nutrients; via increased requirements or excretion of nutrients; or via inhibition.

An inappropriate supply of almost any essential nutrient can cause undesirable skin conditions in the horse. Some of the nutrients most likely to be involved in skin disorders are discussed below.

Protein Deficiency

Protein deficiency may be produced by starvation, inanition, or diets very low in protein.[6,11,168] Hair is 95% protein, with a high percentage of sulfur-containing amino acids. The normal growth of hair and the keratinization of skin require 25% to 30% of the animal's daily protein requirements. Animals with protein deficiency may have hyperkeratosis, cutaneous atrophy, and pigmentary disturbances of skin and haircoat. The haircoat may be dry, dull, brittle, thin, faded, and easily epilated. Hair growth is retarded, and shedding may be prolonged. Animals suffering from protein deficiency also manifest decreased growth or weight loss, decreased packed cell volume (PCV), and decreased serum concentrations of protein and albumin.[169] Severe hypoproteinemia results in cutaneous edema. The National Research Council (NRC) requirement for dietary protein in horses is 13%.[170]

Fatty Acid Deficiency

Fatty acid deficiency has not been convincingly described in the horse. However, the use of unsaturated fat supplements has long been thought to improve coat appearance.[6,168] As early as 1917, it was reported that 0.45 kg (1 pound) of linseed meal per day was a helpful conditioner for run-down horses with rough haircoats and was excellent in the spring to hasten shedding of the hair and to give bloom and finish to show or sale horses.[165] Coats that fail to shed and lack luster may improve within 40 to 60 days by adding 60 ml (2 ounces) of vegetable oil to the grain ration daily.[168] It has also been reported that late winter coats are often improved by dietary supplementation of a vegetable oil over 20 to 60 days.[6]

Most horses readily accept fat-supplemented grain mixes up to 10% added fat.[172] In general, high-quality vegetable oils are best accepted. For best acceptability, the fat supplements are introduced into the diet in small amounts (2 to 3 oz/meal), then gradually increased to the desired concentration.

Mineral Deficiencies

COPPER

Copper is an essential component of many oxidative enzymes, such as tyrosinase, ascorbic acid oxidase, lysyl oxidase, and cytochrome oxidase.[7,11,174] Copper deficiency (hypocuprosis) may occur because of a dietary deficiency or as a result of interference with absorption of copper by zinc or cadmium. A deficiency in copper may cause haircoat fading or leukotrichia (hypochromotrichia, achromotrichia) because copper is needed for the enzymatic conversion of tyrosine to melanin.[168] Affected horses may develop hair loss and faded haircoat color around the eyes, giving the horse a "spectacled" appearance.[6] The NRC suggests that the ration of horses contain at least 10 mg of copper per kg of feed (90% dry matter basis).[170]

IODINE

Iodine is required for the proper development and function of the thyroid gland and is an indispensable component of thyroid hormones, which control metabolism.[7,11,173,174] Dietary iodine deficiency in the mare resulting in goitrous neonates has been reported.[7,11,175-178] Certain soils and pastures are known to be iodine-deficient, such as those in the Great Lakes, Northern Plains, and Pacific Northwest regions of the United States. In addition, goitrogens such as thiocyanates, perchlorates, rubidium salts, and arsenic are known to interfere with thyroidal iodine uptake.[7,174] Clinical signs include weak foals with variable hair loss and thickened, puffy (myxedematous) skin. Goiter may or may not be visible externally. The NRC recommends an iodine content of 0.1 mg/kg of diet.[170] Free choice feeding of iodized or trace mineralized salt should supply the needed iodine.[168]

ZINC

Zinc has many functions in body metabolism.[7,11,174] It is needed for muscle and bone growth, feed utilization, normal reproductive function, taste and smell acuity, normal leukocyte function, normal keratogenesis, and wound healing, and is a component of over 70 metalloenzymes.

Naturally occurring zinc deficiency has not been reported in the horse. However, foals fed experimental diets containing 5 mg of zinc per kg of diet developed skin lesions.[179] Early changes included alopecia and scaling of the legs, which progressed to the ventrolateral abdomen and thorax. Chronically deficient foals developed severe crusting in the same areas. Wound healing was poor, and serum alkaline phosphatase concentrations were decreased.

The authors have received skin biopsy specimens from a few horses that were presented to their veterinarians for erythema, scaling, and crusting around the lips, eyes, coronets, and pressure points. Histologic findings included a hyperplastic superficial perivascular dermatitis with marked parakeratotic hyperkeratosis. Variable degrees of intra- and intercellular epidermal edema were present. The dominant inflammatory cells were lymphocytes, then eosinophils. The horses responded to oral zinc supplementation. Dietary details were not available.

The NRC recommends that the diet contain at least 40 mg of zinc/kg of dry matter.[170] Thus, a 500-kg horse needs about 400 to 600 mg of zinc daily. Zinc sulfate contains 40.5% zinc and 1 to 1.5 gm/day will supply the total requirement.[168] Zinc oxide contains 80.3% zinc, so 500 to 600 mg daily will supply the total requirement.[168]

Vitamin Deficiencies

VITAMIN A

Vitamin A maintains the structure and functional integrity of epithelial tissues.[7,11,174] In the horse, either vitamin deficiency or excess can cause a rough, dull haircoat, which progresses to alopecia, scaling, and hyperkeratosis.[6,168,180,181] Vitamin A deficiency is also associated with night blindness, excessive lacrimation, reproductive problems (failure to conceive and abortions in mares; decreased libido and testicular atrophy in stallions), and neurologic disorders. Some horses develop coronitis, and hooves may become dry, scaly, and develop multiple vertical cracks.[6,9,11] Vitamin A–deficient horses also had decreased serum concentrations of iron, albumin, and cholesterol.[180]

The NRC suggests that the diets of horses contain 2,000 IU of vitamin A activity per kg of dry matter.[170] This is equivalent to about 20,000 to 50,000 IU of vitamin A per day for a mature horse.[168] According to the NRC, the maximum tolerance level is 16,000 IU per day of dry matter, or about 160,000 to 240,000 IU per day for a mature horse. Horses fed high-quality roughage or commercial grains containing supplemental vitamin A are not likely to develop vitamin A deficiency. A likely candidate for deficiency would be a growing horse fed poor-quality forage, particularly a forage that has been stored for a prolonged period, and grains such as barley or oats, which contain low levels of vitamin A activity.[168] Vitamin A is rapidly destroyed by exposure to oxygen and light.[173]

● MISCELLANEOUS HAIRCOAT DISORDERS

Abnormal Shedding

Normal shedding in the horse is basically controlled by photoperiod and, to a lesser extent, factors such as ambient temperature and nutrition (see Chapter 1). In some horses, abnormal excessive spring shedding may result in visible hair loss.[3,4,11] Areas of more-or-less symmetrical hypotrichosis or alopecia are seen, especially on the face, shoulders, and rump. The skin in affected areas is normal and the horses are otherwise healthy. The pathogenesis of the abnormal shedding is not known. Affected animals recover spontaneously and completely within 1 to 3 months.

Anagen and Telogen Defluxion

In *anagen defluxion*, a special circumstance (e.g., infectious diseases, metabolic diseases, fever) interferes with the anagen phase of the hair cycle, resulting in abnormalities of the hair follicle and hair shaft.[1,11,11a,182] Hair loss occurs suddenly, within days of the insult, as the growth phase continues. Anagen defluxion accounts for 1% of the equine dermatology cases seen at the Cornell University Clinic.

In *telogen defluxion*, a stressful circumstance (e.g., high fever, pregnancy, shock, severe illness, surgery, anesthesia) causes the abrupt, premature cessation of growth of many anagen hair follicles and the synchronization of these hair follicles in catagen, then in telogen.[1,4,5,11-12] Within 1 to 3 months of the insult, a large number of telogen hairs are shed as a new wave of hair follicle activity begins. Telogen defluxion accounts for 1.11% of the equine dermatology cases seen at the Cornell University Clinic.

Hair loss in anagen and telogen defluxion may be regional, multifocal, or fairly generalized, and is more-or-less bilaterally symmetric (Fig. 10-4). The haircoat in affected areas may be thin and easily epilated, or completely absent. Alopecic areas may be roughly annular and up to 5 cm in diameter or may be coalescent and produce large areas of well-circumscribed hair loss. Skin in the affected areas is normal.

Diagnosis is based on history, physical examination, and direct hair examination. Telogen hairs are characterized by a uniform shaft diameter and a slightly clubbed, nonpigmented root end that lacks root sheaths (Fig. 10-5). Anagen defluxion hairs are characterized by irregularities and dysplastic changes. The diameter of the shaft may be irregularly narrowed and deformed, and breaking occurs at such structurally weakened sites. Skin biopsy is only rarely helpful. When the alopecia due to telogen defluxion begins, histologic examination reveals normal skin and hair follicle activity. In anagen defluxion, the characteristic changes are usually most evident in the

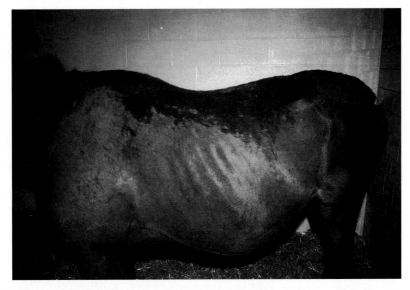

FIGURE 10-4. Telogen defluxion postmetritis. Note alopecia of shoulder, lateral thorax and abdomen, and hip.

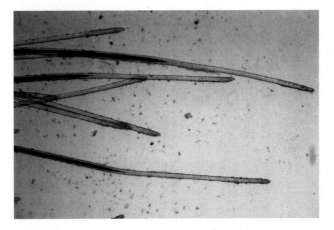

FIGURE 10-5. Telogen defluxion. All epilated hairs are in telogen phase.

affected hairs, and these are usually lost when the skin is clipped for biopsy. Typical histopathologic findings in anagen defluxion include apoptosis and fragmented cell nuclei in the keratinocytes of the hair matrix of anagen hair follicles, as well as eosinophilic dysplastic hair shafts within the pilar canal.

Both telogen and anagen defluxion spontaneously resolve when the inciting factor is eliminated.

Trichorrhexis Nodosa

Trichorrhexis nodosa appears along the hair shaft as small, beaded swellings. The "nodes" are composed of frayed cortical fibers through which the hair shaft fractures. The basic cause is trauma, and a contributing factor may be inherent weakness of the hair shaft.[1,3,10-11a] Examples of

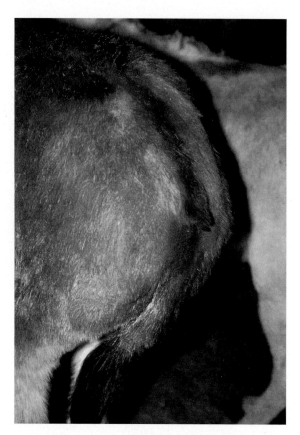

FIGURE 10-6. Trichorrhexis nodosa due to insecticidal rinse. Hairs over rump are broken off at varying lengths.

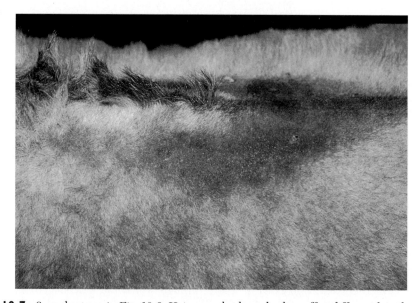

FIGURE 10-7. Same horse as in Fig. 10-6. Hairs over back are broken off at different lengths.

physical trauma include excessive grooming and prolonged ultraviolet light exposure. Sources of chemical trauma include shampoos, rinses, and sprays. Trichorrhexis nodosa accounts for 0.67% of the equine dermatology cases seen at the Cornell University Clinic.

The characteristic lesions are small nodules along the hair shafts, which may be visible with the naked eye. Hair shaft breakage occurs through these nodes, resulting in multifocal or generalized hypotrichosis (Fig. 10-6). Affected areas contain hairs that are broken off at varying lengths (Fig. 10-7).

The differential diagnosis includes piedra (see Chapter 5). Diagnosis is based on history, physical examination, and microscopic examination of hairs. Microscopically, the hair shaft swellings are focal areas of cortical splitting that have the appearance of two brooms pushed together. The ends of broken hairs have longitudinal splits.

Therapy requires eliminating the source(s) of physical and/or chemical trauma.

Hypertrichosis

Hypertrichosis implies a greater than normal amount of hair.[11] It may be seen as a multifocal or generalized abnormality in horses with hyperadrenocorticism and numerous chronic diseases.[11] Hypertrichosis may also be seen focally as a result of local injury or irritation, such as with wounds from ill-fitting tack.[3,11] The hair in these focal areas may become excessive, thicker, stiffer, and darker than normal.

● REFERENCES

General

1. Freedberg IM, et al (eds): Fitzpatrick's Dermatology in General Medicine IV. McGraw Hill, New York, 1999.
2. Kobluk CN, et al (eds): The Horse. Diseases and Clinical Management. W.B. Saunders Co, Philadelphia, 1995.
3. Kral F, Schwartzman RM: Veterinary and Comparative Dermatology. J.B. Lippincott Co, Philadelphia, 1964.
4. McMullen WC: The Skin. In: Mansmann RA, et al (eds): Equine Medicine and Surgery III. American Veterinary Publications Inc, Santa Barbara, 1982, p 789.
5. Pascoe RR: Equine Dermatoses. University of Sydney Post-Graduate Foundation in Veterinary Science, Review No. 22, 1981.
6. Pascoe RRR, Knottenbelt C: Manual of Equine Dermatology, W.B. Saunders Co, Philadelphia, 1999.
7. Radostits OM, et al: Veterinary Medicine. A Textbook of the Diseases of Cattle, Sheep, Pigs, Goats, and Horses. VIII. Ballière-Tindall, Philadelphia, 1994.
8. Reed SM, Bayly WM (eds): Equine Internal Medicine. W.B. Saunders Co, Philadelphia, 1998.
9. Robinson NE (ed). Current Therapy in Equine Medicine. IV. W.B. Saunders Co, Philadelphia, 1997.
10. Schindelka H: Hautkrankheiten bei Haustieren II, Braumuller, Vienna, 1908.
11. Scott DW: Large Animal Dermatology. W.B. Saunders Co, Philadelphia, 1988.
11a. Scott DW, et al: Muller & Kirk's Small Animal Dermatology VI. W.B. Saunders, Co, Philadelphia, 2001.

12. Stannard AA: The Skin. In: Mansmann RA, et al (eds): Equine Medicine and Surgery II, American Veterinary Publications, Inc, Santa Barbara, 1972, p 381.

Adrenal Function

12a. Alexander SL, et al: The effect of acute exercise on the secretion of corticotropin releasing factor, arginine vasopressin, and adrenocorticotropin as measured in pituitary venous blood from the horse. Endocrinol 128:65, 1991.
13. Beech J: Evaluation of thyroid, adrenal, and pituitary function. Vet Clin N Am Equine Pract 3:649, 1987.
14. Bottoms GD, et al: Circadian variation in plasma cortisol and corticosterone in pigs and mares. Am J Vet Res 33:785, 1972.
15. Eiler H, et al: Adrenal gland function in the horse: Effect of dexamethasone on hydrocortisone secretion and blood cellularity and plasma electrolyte concentrations. Am J Vet Res 40:727, 1979.
15a. Eiler H, et al: Combined dexamethasone-suppression cosyntropin (synthetic ACTH) stimulation test in the horse: A new approach to testing of adrenal gland function. Am J Vet Res 41:430, 1980.
16. Eiler H, et al: Adrenal gland function in the horse: Effects of cosyntropin (synthetic) and corticotropin (natural) stimulation. Am J Vet Res 40:724, 1979.
16a. Evans JW, et al: Rhythmic cortisol secretion in the equine: analysis and physiological mechanisms. J Interdiscipl Cycle Res 8:11, 1977.
17. Ganjam V: Episodic nature of the -ENE and -ENE steroidogenic pathways and the relationship to the adrenogonadal axis in stallions. J Reprod Fertil 27:67, 1979.

18. Hoffsis GF, et al: Plasma concentration of cortisol and corticosterone in the normal horse. Am J Vet Res 31:1379, 1970.

19. Hoffsis GF, Murdick PW: The plasma concentrations of corticosteroids in normal and diseased horses. J Am Vet Med Assoc 157:1590, 1970.

20. Irvine CHG, Alexander SL: Factors affecting the circadian rhythm in plasma cortisol concentrations in the horse. Dom Anim Endocrinol 11:227, 1994.

21. James VHT, et al: Adrenocortical function in the horse. J Endocrinol 48:319, 1970.

21a. Johnson AL, Malinowski K: Daily rhythm of cortisol, and evidence for a photo-inducible phase for prolactin secretion in nonpregnant mares housed under non-interrupted and skeleton photoperiods. J Anim Sci 63:169, 1986.

22. Klein HJ, et al: Funktionstest der equinen Nebennierenrinde. Pferdeheilk 5:225, 1989.

23. Kumar MSA, et al: Diurnal variation in serum cortisol in ponies. J Anim Sci 42:1360, 1976.

24. Larsson M, et al: Plasma cortisol in the horse, diurnal rhythm and effects of exogenous ACTH. Acta Vet Scand 20:16, 1979.

25. Linden A, et al: Comparison of the adrenocortical response to both pharmacological and physiological stresses in sport horses. J Vet Med A 37:601, 1990.

26. Lindner A, et al: Cortisol, T_4, T_3, und T-uptake-Bestimmung in Serum and Plasma von Pferden. J Vet Med A 37:455, 1990.

27. Luna SP, et al: Pituitary-adrenal activity and opioid release in ponies during thiopentone/halothane anesthesia. Res Vet Sci 58:35, 1995.

28. MacFarlane D, et al: Hematologic and serum biochemical variables and plasma corticotropin concentration in healthy aged horses. Am J Vet Res 59:1247, 1998.

29. MacHarg MA, et al: Effects of multiple intramuscular injections and doses of dexamethasone in plasma cortisol concentrations and adrenal responses to ACTH in horses. Am J Vet Res 46:2285, 1985.

30. Okada T, et al: Immunocytochemical localization of adrenocorticotropic hormone immunoreactive cells of the pars intermedia in Thoroughbreds. Am J Vet Res 58:920, 1997.

31. Redekopp C, et al: Spontaneous and stimulated adrenocorticotropin and vasopressin pulsatile secretion in the pituitary effluent of the horse. Endocrinol 118:1410, 1986.

32. Rossdale PD, et al: Changes in blood neutrophil/lymphocyte ratio related to adrenocortical function in the horse. Equine Vet J 14:293, 1982.

33. Sojka JE, et al: The effect of starting time on dexamethasone suppression test results in horses. Dom Anim Endocrinol 10:1, 1993.

34. Tan JH, et al: Immunocytochemical differences in adenohypophyseal cells among adult Mongolian pony mares, stallions, and geldings. Am J Vet Res 59:262, 1998.

34a. Taylor PM: Equine stress responses to anaesthesia. Br J Anaesth 63:702, 1989.

35. Toutain PL, et al: Diurnal and episodic variations of plasma hydrocortisone concentrations in horses. Dom Anim Endocrinol 5:55, 1988.

36. Zokolovick A, et al: Diurnal variation in plasma glucocorticosteroid levels in the horse (*Equus caballus*). J Endocrinol 35:249, 1966.

Hyperadrenocorticism

37. Allen JR, et al: Diagnosis of equine pituitary tumors by computed tomography—Part I. Compend Cont Edu 10:1103, 1988.

38. Allen JR, et al: Diagnosis of equine pituitary tumors by computed tomography—Part II. Compend Cont Edu 10:1196, 1988.

39. Andreasen M, et al: Hypofysetumor hos hest. Dansk Veterinaer 77:97, 1994.

40. Backstrom G: Hirsutism associated with pituitary tumors in horses. Nord Vet Med 15:778, 1963.

41. Beck DJ: Effective long-term treatment of a suspected pituitary adenoma with bromocriptine mesylate in a pony. Equine Vet Edu 4:119, 1992.

42. Beech J: Tumors of the pituitary gland (pars intermedia). In: Robinson NE (ed): Current Therapy in Equine Medicine. W.B. Saunders Co, Philadelphia, 1983, p 164.

43. Beech J, Garcia M: Hormonal response to thyrotropin-releasing hormone in healthy horses and in horses with pituitary adenoma. Am J Vet Res 46:1941, 1985.

44. Beech J: Tumors of the pituitary gland (pars intermedia). In: Robinson NE (ed). Current Therapy in Equine Medicine II. W.B. Saunders Co, Philadelphia, 1987, p 182.

45. Beech J: Treatment of hypophysial adenomas. Compend Cont Edu 16:921, 1994.

46. Brandt AJ: Uber Hypophysenadenome bei Hund und Pferd. Skand Vet Tidskrift 30:875, 1940.

46a. Chandler KJ, Dixon RM: Urinary cortisol: creatinine ratios in healthy horses and horses with hyperadrenocorticism and non-adrenal disease. Vet Rec 150:773, 2002.

47. Cohen ND, Carter GK: Steroid hepatopathy in a horse with glucocorticoid-induced hyperadrenocorticism. J Am Vet Med Assoc 200:1682, 1992.

48. Couëtil L: New developments in equine Cushing's disease. Equine Pract 18:28, 1996.

49. Couëtil L, et al: Plasma adrenocorticotropin concentration in healthy horses and in horses with clinical signs of hyperadrenocorticism. J Vet Intern Med 10:1, 1996.

50. Deem DA, Whitlock RH: The pituitary gland. In: Mansmann RA, et al (eds): Equine Medicine and Surgery II, American Veterinary Publications Inc, Santa Barbara, 1982, p 885.

51. Douglas R: Circadian cortisol rhythmicity and equine Cushing's-like disease. J Equine Vet Sci 19:684, 1999.

52. Dybdal NO, et al. Diagnostic testing for pituitary pars intermedia dysfunction in horses. J Am Vet Med Assoc 204:627, 1994.

53. Dybdal NO: Pituitary pars intermedia dysfunction (equine Cushing's-like disease). In: Robinson NE (ed): Current Therapy in Equine Medicine IV, W.B. Saunders Co, Philadelphia, 1997, p 499.

54. Eiler H, et al: Results of a combined dexamethasone suppression/thyrotropin-releasing hormone stimulation test in healthy horses and horses suspected to have a pars intermedia pituitary adenoma. J Am Vet Med Assoc 211:79, 1997.

55. Ericksson K, et al: A case of hirsutism in connection with hypophyseal tumor in a horse. Nord Vet Med 8:87, 1956.

56. Feige K, et al: Klinische Symptomatik und diagnotische Moylichkeiten des Hypophysenadenoms beim Pferd. Schweiz Arch Tierheilk 142:49, 2000.
57. Field JR, Wolf C: Cushing's syndrome in a horse. Equine Vet J 20:301, 1988.
58. Garcia MC, Beech J: Equine intravenous glucose tolerance test: glucose and insulin responses of healthy horses fed grain or hay and of horses with pituitary adenoma. Am J Vet Res 47:570, 1986.
59. Gribble DH: The endocrine system. In: Mansmann RA, et al (eds): Equine Medicine and Surgery II. American Veterinary Publications Inc, Santa Barbara, 1972, p 433.
60. Harman JC: Natural medicine for Cushing's syndrome. J Equine Vet Sci 20:84, 2000.
60a. Harman JC, Ward M: The role of nutritional therapy in the treatment of equine Cushing's syndrome and laminitis. Altern Med Rev 6(suppl.):S4, 2001.
61. Heinrichs M, et al: Immunocytochemical demonstration of proopiomelanocortin-derived peptides in pituitary adenomas of the pars intermedia on horses. Vet Pathol 27:419, 1990.
62. Hillyer MH, et al: Diagnosis of hyperadrenocorticism in the horse. Equine Vet Edu 4:131, 1992.
63. Holscher MA, et al: Adenoma of the pars intermedia and hirsutism in a pony. Vet Med Small Anim Clin 73:1197, 1978.
64. Horvath CJ, et al: Adenocorticotropin-containing neoplastic cells in a pars intermedia adenoma in a horse. J Am Vet Med Assoc 192:367, 1988.
64a. Johansson B, Segall T: Meningiomen ovanlig tumörform hos häst. Svensk Veterinär Tidning 46:123, 1994.
65. King JM, et al: Diabetes mellitus with pituitary neoplasm in a horse and a dog. Cornell Vet 52:133, 1962.
66. Levy M, et al: Diagnosis and treatment of equine Cushing's disease. Compend Cont Edu 21:766, 1999.
67. Loeb WF, et al: Adenoma of the pars intermedia associated with hyperglycemia and glycosuria in two horses. Cornell Vet 56:623, 1966.
68. Love S: Equine Cushing's disease. Brit Vet J 149:139, 1993.
69. Mazan MR: Medical management of a full-thickness tear of the retroperitoneal portion of the rectum in a horse with hyperadrenocorticism. J Am Vet Med Assoc 210:665, 1997.
69a. McGowan CM, Neiger R: Efficacy of trilostane in the management of equine Cushing's disease. J Vet Intern Med 15:322, 2001.
70. Millington WR, et al: Equine Cushing's disease: differential regulation of β-endorphin processing in tumors of the intermediate pituitary. Endocrinol 123:1598, 1988.
71. Moore J, et al: A case of pituitary adrenocorticotropin-dependent Cushing's syndrome in the horse. Endocrinol 104:576, 1979.
72. Muñoz MC, et al: Pergolide treatment for Cushing's syndrome in a horse. Vet Rec 139:41, 1996.
73. Orth DN, et al: Equine Cushing's disease: plasma immunoreactive proopiolipomelanocortin peptide and cortisol levels basally and response to diagnostic tests. Endocrinol 110:1430, 1982.
74. Orth DN, Nicholson WE: Bioactive and immunoreactive adrenocorticotropin in normal equine pituitary and in pituitary tumors of horses with Cushing's disease. Endocrinol 111:559, 1982.
75. Pauli BU, et al: Swischenzelladenom der Hypophyse mit "Cushing-ahnlicher": Symptomatologie beim Pferd. Vet Pathol 11:417, 1974.
76. Reed SM: Pituitary adenomas: Equine Cushing's disease. In: Reed SM, Bayly WM (eds): Equine Internal Medicine. W.B. Saunders Co, Philadelphia, 1998, p 912.
76a. Reeves HJ, et al: Measurement of basal serum insulin concentration in the diagnosis of Cushing's disease in ponies. Vet Rec 149:449, 2001.
77. Richard S, Ribot Y: Quel est votre diagnostic? Point Vét 26:382, 1994.
78. Roarty G: Cushing's syndrome in the horse: A review. Irish Vet J 43:118, 1990.
79. Urman HK, et al: Pituitary neoplasms in two horses. Zbl Vet Med 10:257, 1963.
80. van der Kolk JH, et al: Een paard met de ziekte van Cushing. Tijdschr Diergeneeskd 116:670, 1991.
81. van der Kolk JH, et al: Anorexie bij een pony met de ziekte van Cushing. Tijdschr Diergeneeskd 118:298, 1993.
82. van der Kolk JH, et al: Equine pituitary neoplasia: a clinical report of 21 cases (1990-1992). Vet Rec 133:594, 1993.
83. van der Kolk JH, et al: Urinary concentration of corticoids in normal horses and horses with hyperadrenocorticism. Res Vet Sci 56:127, 1994.
84. van der Kolk JH, et al: Lipid metabolism in horses with hyperadrenocorticism. J Am Vet Med Assoc 206:1010, 1995.
85. van der Kolk JH, et al: Diagnosis of equine hyperadrenocorticism. Equine Pract 17:24, 1995.
86. van der Kolk JH, et al: Laboratory diagnosis of equine pituitary pars intermedia adenoma. Dom Anim Endocrinol 12:35, 1995.
87. van der Kolk JH, et al: Equine Cushing's disease. Equine Vet Edu 9:209, 1997.
88. van der Kolk JH, et al: Pituitary-independent Cushing's syndrome in a horse. Equine Vet J 33:110, 2000.
88a. van der Kolk JH, et al: Salivary and plasma concentration of cortisol in normal horses and horses with Cushing's disease. Equine Vet J 33:211, 2001.
89. Wallace MA, et al: Central blindness associated with a pituitary adenoma in a horse. Equine Pract 18:8, 1996.
90. Wilson MG, et al: Proopiolipomelanocortin peptides in normal pituitary, pituitary tumor, and plasma of normal and Cushing's horses. Endocrinol 110:941, 1982.

Thyroid Function

91. Blackmore DJ, et al: Observations on thyroid hormones in the blood of thoroughbreds. Res Vet Sci 25:284, 1978.
92. Chen CL, Riley AM: Serum thyroxine and tri-iodothyronine concentrations in neonatal foals and mature horses. Am J Vet Res 42:1415, 1981.
93. Chen CL, Li WI: Effect of thyrotropin releasing hormone (TRH) on serum levels of thyroid hormones in thoroughbred mares. J Equine Vet Sci 6:58, 1986.

94. Chen CL, et al: Serum levels of thyroxine and triiodothyronine in mature horses following oral administration of synthetic thyroxine (Synthroid). J Equine Vet Sci 4:5, 1984.

95. DeGroot LJ, Hoye K: Dexamethasone suppression of serum T_3 and T_4. J Clin Endocrinol Metab 42:976, 1976.

96. deMartin BW: Study on the thyroid function of thoroughbred horses by means of "in vitro" ^{125}I-T_3 modified and ^{125}I-T_4 tests. Rev Fac Met Vet Zootec Univ Sao Paulo 12:107, 1975.

97. deMartin BW: Study on the thyroid function of thoroughbred females in varying stages of pregnancy using "in vitro" tests ^{125}I-T_3 and ^{125}I-T_4 tests. Rev Fac Met Vet Zootec Univ Sao Paulo 12:121, 1975.

98. Duckett WM, et al: Thyroid hormone periodicity in healthy adult geldings. Equine Vet J 21:123, 1989.

99. Furr MO, et al: The effects of stress on gastric ulceration, T_3, T_4, reverse T_3, and cortisol in neonatal foals. Equine Vet J 24:37, 1992.

100. Glade MJ, Reimers TJ: Effects of dietary energy supply on serum thyroxine, triiodothyronine and insulin concentration in young horses. J Endocrinol 104:93, 1985.

101. Harris P, et al: Equine thyroid function tests: a preliminary investigation. Br Vet J 148:70, 1992.

102. Held JP, Oliver JW: A sampling protocol for the thyrotropin-stimulation test in the horse. J Am Vet Med Assoc 184:326, 1984.

103. Hightower D, et al: Comparison of serum and plasma thyroxine determinations in horses. J Am Vet Med Assoc 159:449, 1971.

104. Irvine CHG, Evans MJ: Post-natal changes in total and free thyroxine and triiodothyronine in foal serum. J Reprod Fertil 23:709, 1975.

105. Irvine CHG: Protein bound iodine in the horse. Am J Vet Res 28:1687, 1967.

106. Irvine CHG: Thyroxine secretion rate in the horse in various physiological states. J Endocrinol 39:313, 1967.

107. Kallfelz FA, Lowe JE: Some normal values of thyroid function in horses. J Am Vet Med Assoc 156:1888, 1970.

108. Kallfelz FA, Erali RP: Thyroid tests in domesticated animals: free thyroxine index. Am J Vet Res 34:1449, 1973.

109. Kelley ST, et al: Measurement of thyroid gland function during the estrous cycle of nine mares. Am J Vet Res 35:657, 1974.

110. Larsson M, et al: Thyroid hormone binding in serum from 15 vertebrate species: isolation of thyroxine-binding globulin and prealbumin analogs. Gen Compar Endocrinol 58:360, 1985.

111. Lothrop CD, Nolan HL: Equine thyroid function assessment with the thyrotropin-releasing hormone response test. Am J Vet Res 47:942, 1986.

112. Malinowski K, et al: Age and breed differences in thyroid hormones, insulin-like growth factor (IGF)-1 and IGF binding proteins in female horses. J Anim Sci 74:1936, 1996.

113. Messer NT, et al: Effect of dexamethasone administration on serum thyroid hormone concentrations in clinically normal horses. J Am Vet Med Assoc 206:63, 1995.

114. Messer NT, et al: Effect of food deprivation on baseline iodothyronine and cortisol concentrations in healthy adult horses. Am J Vet Res 56:116, 1995.

115. Morris DD, Garcia M: Thyroid-stimulating hormone: response test in healthy horses, and effect of phenylbutazone on equine thyroid hormones. Am J Vet Res 44:503, 1983.

116. Morris DD, Garcia M: Effects of phenylbutazone and anabolic steroids on adrenal and thyroid gland function tests in healthy horses. Am J Vet Res 46:359, 1985.

117. Motley JS: Use of radioactive triiodothyronine in the study of thyroid function in normal horses. Vet Med Small Anim Clin 67:1225, 1972.

118. Murray MJ, Luba NK: Plasma gastrin and somatostatin, and serum thyroxine (T_4), triiodothyronine (T_3), reverse triiodothyronine (r T_3) and cortisol concentrations in foals from birth to 28 days of age. Equine Vet J 25:237, 1993.

119. Ramirez S, et al: Duration of effects of phenylbutazone on serum total thyroxine and free thyroxine concentrations in horses. J Vet Intern Med 11:371, 1997.

120. Reap M, et al: Thyroxine and triiodothyronine levels in 10 species of animals. Southwest Vet 31:31, 1978.

121. Refetoff S, et al: Parameters of thyroid function in the serum of 16 selected vertebrate species: a study of PBI, serum T_4, free T_4, and the pattern of T_4 and T_3 binding to serum proteins. Endocrinol 86:793, 1970.

122. Reimers TJ, et al: Validation of radioimmunoassays for triiodothyronine, thyroxine, and hydrocortisone (cortisol) in canine, feline, and equine sera. Am J Vet Res 42:2016, 1981.

123. Shaftoe S, et al: Thyroid-stimulating response tests in one-day-old foals. Equine Vet Sci 8:310, 1988.

124. Singh AK, et al: Validation of nonradioactive chemiluminescent immunoassay methods for the analysis of thyroxine and cortisol in blood samples obtained from dogs, cats, and horses. J Vet Diagn Invest 9:261, 1997.

125. Sojka JE, et al: Serum triiodothyronine, thyroxine, and free thyroxine concentrations in horses. Am J Vet Res 54:52, 1993.

126. Sojka JE: Factors which affect serum T_3 and T_4 levels in the horse. Equine Pract 15:15, 1993.

127. Sojka JE: Hypothyroidism in horses. Compend Cont Edu 17:845, 1995.

128. Solter PF, Farner S: Correlation of two nonradioactive immunoassays to a radioimmunoassay technique for thyroxine measurement in equine serum. J Vet Diagn Invest 12:51, 2000.

129. Sutherland RL, Irvine CHG: Total plasma thyroxine concentrations in horses, pigs, cattle, and sheep. Anion exchange resin chromatography and ceriarsenite colorimetry. Am J Vet Res 34:1261, 1973.

130. Swinkler AM, et al: Effects of dietary excesses on equine serum thyroid hormone levels. J Anim Sci 65:255, 1989.

131. Takayi S, et al: Effects of training on plasma fibrinogen concentration and thyroid hormone level in young racehorses. Exp Res Equine Hlth 11:94, 1974.

132. Thomas CL, Adams JC: Radioimmunoassay of equine serum for thyroxine: reference values. Am J Vet Res 39:1239, 1978.

133. Thompson FN, et al: Thyroidal and prolactin secretion in agalactic mares. Theriogenol 25:575, 1986.

134. Thompson JC, et al: Serum thyroid hormone concentrations in New Zealand horses. N Z Vet J 45:11, 1997.
135. Tram BF, Wasserman RH: Studies on the depression of radioiodine uptake by the thyroid after phenothiazine administration II. Effect of phenothiazine on the horse thyroid. Am J Vet Res 17:271, 1956.

Hypothyroidism
136. Allen AL, et al: A case-control study of the congenital hypothyroidism and dysmaturity syndrome of foals. Can Vet J 37:349, 1996.
137. Boosinger TR, et al: Prolonged gestation, decreased triiodothyronine concentration, and thyroid gland histomorphologic features in newborn foals of mares grazing *Acremonion coenophialum*-infected fescue. Am J Vet Res 56:66, 1995.
138. Chen CL, Li OWI: Hypothyroidism. In: Robinson NE (ed): Current Therapy in Equine Medicine II. W.B. Saunders Co, Philadelphia, 1987, p 185.
139. Doige CE, McLaughlin BG: Hyperplastic goitre in newborn foals in western Canada. Can Vet J 22:42, 1981.
140. Ducket WM: Thyroid gland. In: Reed SM, Bayly WM (eds): Equine Internal Medicine, W.B. Saunders Co, Philadelphia, 1998, p 916.
140a. Frank N, et al: Effect of hypothyroidism on blood lipid concentrations in horses. Am J Vet Res 60:730, 1999.
141. Hillyer MH, Taylor FGR: Cutaneous manifestations of suspected hypothyroidism in a horse. Equine Vet Educ 4:116, 1992.
142. Irvine CHG, Evans MJ: Hypothyroidism in foals. N Z Vet J 25:354, 1977.
143. Irvine CHG: Hypothyroidism in the foal. Equine Vet J 16:302, 1984.
144. Kallfelz FA: The thyroid gland. In: Mansmann RA, et al (eds): Equine Medicine and Surgery II. American Veterinary Publications Inc, Santa Barbara, 1982, p 891.
145. Kreplin C, Allen A: Congenital hypothyroidism in foals in Alberta. Can Vet J 32:751, 1991.
146. Lori DN, MacLeary JM: Hypothyroidism in the horse. J Equine Vet Sci 21:9, 2001.
147. Lowe JE: Thyroid diseases. In: Robinson NE (ed): Current Therapy in Equine Medicine. W.B. Saunders Co, Philadelphia, 1983, p 159.
148. Lowe JE, et al: Equine hypothyroidism: the long-term effects of thyroidectomy on metabolism and growth in mares and stallions. Cornell Vet 64:276, 1974.
149. McLaughlin BG, Doige CE: A study of ossification of carpal and tarsal bones in normal and hypothyroid foals. Can Vet J 23:164, 1982.
150. McLaughlin BG, Doige CE: Congenital musculoskeletal lesions and hyperplastic goitre in foals. Can Vet J 22:130, 1981.
151. McLaughlin BG, et al: Thyroid hormone levels in foals with congenital musculoskeletal lesions. Can Vet J 27:264, 1986.
152. Messer, NT: Thyroid disease (dysfunction). In: Robinson NE (ed): Current Therapy in Equine Medicine IV. W.B. Saunders Co, Philadelphia, 1997, p 502.
153. Mooney CT, Murphy D: Equine hypothyroidism: the difficulties of diagnosis. Equine Vet Edu 7:242, 1995.
154. Murray MJ: Hypothyroidism and respiratory insufficiency in a neonatal foal. J Am Vet Med Assoc 197:1635, 1990.
155. Schlotthauer CF: The incidence and types of disease of the thyroid gland of adult horses. J Am Vet Med Assoc 78:211, 1931.
156. Shaver JR, et al: Skeletal manifestations of suspected hypothyroidism in two foals. J Equine Med Surg 3:269, 1979.
157. Shearer D. Bilateral alopecia in a Welsh pony associated with hypothyroidism. Proc Annu Cong Eur Soc Vet Dermatol 5:25, 1988.
158. Sojka JE: Hypothyroidism in horses. Compend Cont Edu 17:845, 1995.
159. Stanley O, Hillidge CJ. Alopecia associated with hypothyroidism in a horse. Equine Vet J 14:165, 1982.
160. Vischer CM, et al: Hemodynamic effects of thyroidectomy in sedentary horses. Am J Vet Res 60:14, 1999.
161. Vischer CM, et al: Hypothyroidism and exercise intolerance in horses. J Vet Intern Med 10:151, 1996.
162. Vivrette SL, et al: Skeletal disease in a hypothyroid foal. Cornell Vet 74:373, 1984.
163. Waldron-Mease E: Hypothyroidism and myopathy in racing thoroughbreds and standardbreds. J Equine Med Surg 3:124, 1999.

Nutritional Skin Diseases
164. Galligan DT: Principles of nutrition. In: Colahan PT, et al (ed). Equine Medicine and Surgery IV, Vol I. American Veterinary Publications, Inc., Goleta, 1991, p 152.
165. Henry WA, Morrison FB: Feed and Feeding XVII. Henry Morrison Co, Madison, 1917.
166. Hintz HF: Nutrition. In: Mansmann RA, et al (eds): Equine Medicine and Surgery III, Vol I. American Veterinary Publications, Santa Barbara, 1982, p 87.
167. Hintz HF: Nutrition. In: Robinson NE (ed): Current Therapy in Equine Medicine II. W.B. Saunders Co, Philadelphia, 1987, p 387.
168. Hintz HF: Nutrition and skin diseases. In: Current Therapy in Equine Medicine III. W.B. Saunders Co, Philadelphia, 1992, p 687.
169. Lawrence LM, Raub RH: Nutritional management. In: Kobluk CN, et al (eds): The Horse. Diseases and Clinical Management, Vol 1. W.B. Saunders Co, Philadelphia, 1995, p 93.
170. National Research Council (NRC). Nutritional Requirements of Horses V. National Academy Press, Washington, DC, 1989.
171. Panel Report: Dermatologic problems in horses. Mod Vet Pract 62:75, 1981.
172. Potter GD: Fat-supplemented diets for horses. J Equine Vet Sci 19:614, 1999.
173. Tyznik WJ: Nutrition and diseases. In: Catcott EJ, Smithcors JF (eds): Equine Medicine and Surgery II. American Veterinary Publications, Wheaton, 1972, p 239.
174. Underwood EJ: Trace Elements in Human and Veterinary Nutrition IV. Academic Press, New York, 1977.

Iodine Deficiency
175. Evvard JM: Iodine deficiency symptoms and their significance in animal nutrition and pathology. Endocrinol 12:539, 1928.

176. Irvine CHG, Evans MJ: Hypothyroidism in foals. N Z Vet J 25:354, 1977.
177. Jovanovic M, et al: Goiter in domestic animals in Serbia. Acta Vet (Belgr.) 3:31, 1953.
178. Welch H: Hairlessness and goiter in newborn domestic animals. Bull 119, Agric Exp Stat, Univ Montana, 1917.

Zinc Deficiency

179. Harrington DD, et al: Clinical and pathological findings on horses fed zinc-deficient diets. Proc Symp Equine Nutrit Physiol 3:51, 1973.

Vitamin A Deficiency

180. Donoghue S, et al: Vitamin A nutrition of the equine: growth, serum biochemistry, and hematology. J Nutr 111:365, 1981.
181. Howell CE, et al: Vitamin A deficiency in horses. Am J Vet Res 2:60, 1941.

Anagen Defluxion

182. Milne EM, Rowland AC: Anagen defluxion in two horses. Vet Dermatol 3:139, 1993.

Chapter *11*

Keratinization Defects

Keratinization defects are those that alter the surface appearance of the skin. The epidermis of animals is being replaced constantly by new cells. The epidermal cell renewal time in normal horses is approximately 17 days.[1] Despite this high turnover rate, the epidermis maintains its normal thickness, has a barely perceptible surface keratin layer, and loses its dead cells invisibly into the environment. If the delicate balance between cell death and renewal is altered, the epidermal thickness changes, the stratum corneum becomes noticeable, and the normally invisible sloughed cells of the stratum corneum become obvious. The causes of keratinization defects are numerous; they produce clinical signs by altering proliferation, differentiation, desquamation, or some combination of these.[10,19] Alterations in epidermal lipid formation and deposition can accompany these other changes.[11]

A characteristic of healthy skin is that the relationship between transepidermal water loss and hydration remains directly proportional.[3] Following skin damage or a decrease in efficiency of the water barrier, a dissociation between hydration (water-holding capacity) and transepidermal water loss occurs. In pathologic skin, the correlation between transepidermal water loss and stratum corneum water content shows an inverse relationship due to a damaged skin barrier or alterations in keratinization, or both. Hence, there is increased transepidermal water loss and decreased hydration.

Dryness (xerosis) of the skin is caused by decreased water content, which must be more than 10% for skin to appear and feel normal.[4] Moisture loss occurs through evaporation to the environment under low humidity conditions and must be replenished by water from lower epidermal and dermal layers. In xerotic skin, the stratum corneum is thickened, disorganized, and fissured. An important part of the stratum corneum barrier is the presence of three intercellular lipids: sphingolipids, free sterols, and free fatty acids. Lamellar bodies are an essential part of this barrier both to trap and to prevent excess water loss. The optimal stratum corneum water concentration to promote softness and pliability is 20% to 35%.

• ANTISEBORRHEIC TREATMENTS

Antiseborrheic agents are available as ointments, creams, gels, lotions, and shampoos. In veterinary medicine, seborrheic lesions are usually widespread in nature and occur in haired skin, thus making shampoo the most appropriate vehicle. For the most part, veterinary shampoo formulations are not patented, and "identical" products can be marketed by one or more generic manufacturers. The reader is advised to approach these products carefully. Although the active ingredients may be identical in name and concentration, the purity, stability, and irritability of the active and inert ingredients may be very different and the shampoo may perform poorly. If a change from one brand of the "same" shampoo to another is contemplated, it is best to give the new product to the clients who have been using the shampoo to be replaced. If they believe that the new product is equally as good or better than the old one, the change can be made.

Antiseborrheics are commercially available in various combinations.[12] The clinician must decide which combination of drugs to use and needs to know each drug's actions and concentrations. Ideal therapeutic response depends on the correct choice, but variations among individual patients do occur. For dry and scaly seborrhea (seborrhea sicca), a different preparation is needed than for oily and greasy seborrhea (seborrhea oleosa). Sulfur, for instance, is useful in dry seborrhea, but it is not a good degreaser. Benzoyl peroxide, on the other hand, degreases well but can be too keratolytic and drying for dry, brittle skin. The following discussion may help the clinician understand the differences and uses and help distinguish the correct medication from among the myriad of commercially available pharmaceuticals.

Antiseborrheic drugs include keratolytic and keratoplastic ingredients. Keratolytic agents facilitate decreased cohesion among corneocytes, desquamation, and shedding, resulting in a softening of the stratum corneum with easy removal of scale. They do not dissolve keratin. Keratoplastic agents attempt to renormalize the keratinization and abnormal epithelialization that is present in keratinization disorders. The complete mechanism of these effects is not known, although some keratoplastic agents (particularly tar) are believed to normalize epidermal proliferation by decreasing deoxyribonucleic acid (DNA) production with a resultant decrease in the mitotic index of the epidermal basal cells. *Follicular flushing* is a term used to describe agents that help remove follicular secretions, remove bacteria, and decrease follicular hyperkeratosis. The most common major ingredients in antiseborrheic shampoos include tars, sulfur, salicylic acid, benzoyl peroxide, and selenium sulfide. Other commonly included active agents are urea, glycerine, and lactic acid.

Sulfur is both keratoplastic and keratolytic, probably through the interaction of sulfur with cysteine in keratinocytes. It is a mild follicular flushing agent, but not a good degreaser. Sulfur is also antibacterial, antifungal, and antiparasitic, and these actions are attributed to the formation of pentathionic acid and hydrogen sulfide. The smaller the sulfur particles (colloidal are smaller than precipitated), the greater the efficacy. The best keratolytic action occurs when sulfur is incorporated in petrolatum. This is in sharp contrast to the findings with salicylic acid, which produces its effect faster when employed in an emulsion base. The keratolytic effect of sulfur results from its superficial effect on the horny layer and the formation of hydrogen sulfide. The keratoplastic effect is caused by the deeper action of the sulfur on the basal layer of the epidermis and by the formation of cystine.

In the shampoos marketed in North America by the well-recognized manufacturers of dermatologicals, a pure sulfur product cannot be purchased. Because of the synergistic activity between sulfur and salicylic acid, all "sulfur" shampoos contain both ingredients. Popular sulfur shampoos include SebaLyt (DVM Pharmaceuticals), SeboRx (DVM Pharmaceuticals), Micro Pearls Advantage Seba-Moist shampoo (EVSCO), Micro Pearls Advantage Seba-Hex shampoo (EVSCO), and Sebolux (Virbac).

Salicylic acid (0.1% to 2%) is keratoplastic and exerts a favorable influence on the new formation of the keratinous layer. It is also mildly antipruritic and bacteriostatic. In stronger concentrations (3% to 6%), it solubilizes the intercellular "cement," thus acting as a keratolytic agent, causing shedding and softening of the stratum corneum. When salicylic acid is combined with sulfur, it is believed that a synergistic effect occurs. A common combination is a 2% to 6% concentration of each drug. In human dermatologic practice, a 40% salicylic acid plaster is used to treat calluses and warts.

Tar preparations are derived from destructive distillation of bituminous coal or wood. Birch tar, juniper tar, and coal tar are crude products listed in order of increasing capacity to irritate. Coal tar solution (5%, 10%, or 20%) produces a milder, more readily managed effect. Coal tar solution contains only 20% of the coal tar present in coal tar extract or refined tar. Most pharmaceutical preparations for dermatologic use have been highly refined to decrease the staining effect and the strong odor. In this refining process, some of the beneficial effects of tar are lost, and its potential carcinogenic danger is also decreased. Unadulterated tar products have no place in equine practice because of their toxicity and tendency to cause local irritation. All tars are odiferous, potentially irritating and photosensitizing, and carcinogenic. Some tars may stain light-colored coats. In one of the author's (DWS) experience, tars are the most irritating topical antiseborrheic medications in veterinary dermatology, and this author does not use tar-containing topical preparations.

Tar shampoos are widely used, however, and seem to be helpful in managing seborrhea. They are keratolytic, keratoplastic, and mildly degreasing. As with sulfur shampoos, tar products usually contain other ingredients, usually sulfur and salicylic acid. Micro Pearls Advantage EVSCO-tar shampoo (EVSCO) is a pure tar product. Popular combination products include LyTar (DVM Pharmaceuticals), NuSal-T (DVM Pharmaceuticals), Allerseb-T (Virbac), and T-Lux (Virbac).

Benzoyl peroxide (2.5% to 5%) is keratolytic, antibacterial, degreasing, antipruritic, and follicular-flushing. It is metabolized in the skin to benzoic acid, which lyses intercellular substance in the horny layer to account for its keratolytic effect. It is not a stable ingredient and should not be repackaged, diluted, or mixed with other products. Benzoyl peroxide is drying, can induce a contact dermatitis (in less than 10% of patients), and bleaches hair, clothing, and furniture. Skin tumor–promoting activity has been documented in laboratory rodents, but no such activity has been documented in any other species.

Benzoyl peroxide is available as a 5% gel (OxyDex, DVM Pharmaceuticals; and Pyoben, Virbac) and as a 2.5% to 3% shampoo (OxyDex, DVM Pharmaceuticals; Micro Pearls Advantage Benzoyl-plus shampoo, EVSCO; and Pyoben, Virbac). One product is available that also contains sulfur (Sulf OxyDex, DVM Pharmaceuticals). Only reputable benzoyl peroxide products should be used, because poor products have short shelf lives, little activity, or increased irritation potential. Because of its potent degreasing action, benzoyl peroxide excessively dries out normal skin with prolonged use, and it is generally contraindicated in the presence of dry skin or significant irritation, or both. A study in dogs showed that benzoyl peroxide combined with a liposome-based (Novasome microvesicles) humectant (Micro Pearls Advantage Benzoyl Plus shampoo) eliminates or minimizes this drying effect.[18]

Selenium sulfide alters the epidermal turnover rate and interferes with the hydrogen bond formation in keratin. It is keratolytic, keratoplastic, and very degreasing. At this writing, there are no selenium sulfide shampoos marketed specifically for veterinary use in North America. The human product that contains 1% selenium sulfide (Selsun Blue, Abbot Laboratories) is effective in horses and usually is not too irritating.

In human medicine, there are dozens of keratolytic and keratoplastic agents marketed in the cream, gel, or ointment formulation. Very few are marketed in veterinary medicine, and most are generic products (e.g., 10% sulfur ointment, ichthammol ointment, zinc oxide, and thuja) or products marketed for other purposes (e.g., petroleum jelly, udder balm). KeraSolv Gel (DVM Pharmaceuticals) contains 6.6% salicylic acid, 5% sodium lactate, and 5% urea in a propylene glycol gel and is an effective local treatment for hyperkeratotic lesions; for example, cannon keratosis.

In the process of removing the excessive scale or grease, antiseborrheic products can damage the stratum corneum and alter the hydration of the epidermis.[16] Excessively low humidity can cause similar alterations. Emollients and moisturizers are used to counteract these effects.

Emollients are agents that soften or soothe the skin, whereas moisturizers increase the water content of the stratum corneum. Both types of drugs are useful in hydrating and softening the skin. Many of the occlusive emollients are actually oils (safflower, sesame, and mineral oil) or contain lanolin. These emollients decrease transepidermal water loss and cause moisturization. These agents work best if they are applied immediately after saturation of the stratum corneum with water. For maximal softening, the skin should be hydrated in wet dressings, dried, and covered with an occlusive hydrophobic oil. The barrier to water loss can be further strengthened by covering the local lesion with plastic wrap under a bandage. Nonocclusive emollients are relatively ineffective in retaining moisture. Examples of emollients include vegetable oils (olive, cottonseed, corn, and peanut oil), animal oils (lard, whale oil, anhydrous lanolin, and lanolin with 25% to 30% water), silicones, hydrocarbons (paraffin and petrolatum [mineral oil]), and waxes (white wax [bleached beeswax], yellow wax [beeswax], and spermaceti). Hygroscopic (humectant) agents are moisturizers that work by being incorporated into the stratum corneum and attracting water. These agents draw water from the deep epidermis and dermis, and from the environment if the relative humidity is greater than 70%.[4] These agents, such as propylene glycol, glycerin, colloidal oatmeal, urea, sodium lactate, and lactic acid, may also be applied between baths. Both occlusive and hygroscopic agents are found in a variety of veterinary spray and cream rinse formulations, which are matched to a corresponding shampoo—for example, HyLyt°efa cream rinse and shampoo (DVM Pharmaceuticals).

The addition of novasomes or spherulites to veterinary antiseborrheics has increased the efficacy of the products while decreasing the labor intensity of the treatments. As discussed in Chapter 3, these are tiny capsules incorporated into shampoos that adhere to the skin and hair and remain there after rinsing. In a time-dependent fashion, some of the capsules disintegrate and release either water and lipids (novasomes) or active ingredients with or without moisturizers (spherulites). Because of the newness of these products, the number of studies documenting their efficacy is limited. In one study, Micro Pearls Advantage Hydra-Pearls Cream Rinse (EVSCO) was shown to be superior to a traditional humectant emollient (Humilac, Virbac) for the treatment of dry skin in dogs.[17]

Systemic antiseborrheic agents are used primarily in the treatment of the congenitohereditary seborrheic disorders (e.g., primary seborrhea, ichthyosis).[6,16] Because most of the generalized secondary seborrheas are due to altered environmental conditions, dietary deficiency, metabolic abnormalities, or other correctable disorders, systemic treatments are rarely considered and probably would be of little value. These agents might be of some value in those idiopathic conditions in which the defect appears to be due to altered keratinization; for example, primary seborrhea and cannon keratosis.

Retinoids are the most commonly used systemic antiseborrheic agents in veterinary medicine. *Retinoids* refer to all the chemicals, natural or synthetic, that have vitamin A activity. Synthetic retinoids are primarily retinol, retinoic acid, or retinal derivatives or analogs. They have been developed with the intent of amplifying certain biologic effects while being less toxic than their natural precursors. More than 1500 synthetic retinoids have been developed and evaluated.[6,16] Different synthetic drugs, all classed as synthetic retinoids, may have profoundly different pharmacologic effects, side effects, and disease indications.

Naturally occurring vitamin A is an alcohol, all-*trans* retinol. It is oxidized in the body to retinal and retinoic acid. Each of these compounds has variable metabolic and biologic activities, although both are important in the induction and maintenance of normal growth and differentiation of keratinocytes. Only retinol has all of the known functions of vitamin A. The two most widely used retinoids in veterinary dermatology were isotretinoin (11-*cis*-retinoic acid; Accutane, Roche), synthesized as a natural metabolite of retinol, and etretinate (Tegison, Roche), a synthetic retinoid. Etretinate is no longer available because tissue residues in humans can persist for years after drug withdrawal and might result in fetal defects. It was replaced with acitretin (Soriatane, Roche), a free-acid metabolite of etretinate. Acitretin appears to be comparable to etretinate in efficacy and acute toxicity, but because it has a much shorter terminal elimination half-life (2 days versus etretinate's 100 days), its long-term safety should be better.

The biologic effects of retinoids are numerous and diverse, but their ability to regulate proliferation, growth, and differentiation of epithelial tissues is their major benefit in dermatology. They also affect proteases, prostaglandins, humoral and cellular immunity, and cellular adhesion and communication.[6,16] In dogs and cats, isotretinoin is usually given in a dose of 1 to 3 mg/kg q12-24h hours and appears to be indicated in diseases that require alteration or normalization of adnexal structures, although some epidermal diseases may respond.[6,16] Etretinate or acitretin is indicated in disorders of epithelial or follicular development or keratinization.[6,16] In dogs and cats, etretinate or acitretin is given at 0.5 to 1 mg/kg every 24 hours.

Numerous toxicities can be seen with the systemic use of retinoids. All retinoids are potent teratogens. There are no reports of the use of systemic retinoids in the horse, and these agents would be prohibitively expensive to use in this species.

● EQUINE SEBORRHEA

Seborrhea is a chronic skin reaction pattern in the skin of horses that is characterized by a defect in keratinization with increased scale formation, excessive greasiness of the skin and haircoat, and sometimes by secondary inflammation.[14,15] Some patients are both flaky and greasy, depending on the region of the body involved. Ingrained in the veterinary literature are the terms *seborrhea sicca*, *seborrhea oleosa*, and *seborrheic dermatitis*. *Seborrhea sicca* denotes dryness of the skin and coat. There is focal or diffuse scaling of the skin with the accumulation of white to gray nonadherent scales, and the coat is dull and dry. *Seborrhea oleosa* is the opposite; the skin and hairs are greasy. The greasy keratosebaceous debris is best appreciated by touch and smell. *Seborrheic dermatitis* is characterized by scaling and greasiness, with gross evidence of local or diffuse inflammation. It may be associated with folliculitis. Animals with seborrhea oleosa or seborrheic dermatitis should be examined carefully for *Staphylococcus* bacteria and *Malassezia* yeast. The initial seborrheic condition encourages bacteria and yeast overgrowth, and then the bacteria and yeast continue to stimulate seborrheic change.

These three terms appropriately describe the horse's clinical appearance and aid in initial shampoo selection, but they cannot be used to direct the diagnostic effort to find the cause of the seborrhea. Individuals respond to the same seborrheic insult in different manners. Regardless of the nature of the seborrhea, all causes of seborrhea should be considered and excluded only by the appropriate testing.

Etiologically, seborrhea is classified into primary and secondary types. *Primary seborrhea* in dogs is an inherited disorder of epidermal hyperproliferation.[16] The etiology of equine primary seborrhea is unknown. A veterinarian does the owner and animal a great injustice if seborrheic signs in a horse are immediately classified as primary seborrhea. The diagnosis of primary seborrhea is tenable only if the signs started early in life and if appropriate diagnostic tests have failed to reveal a cause for the keratinization defect.

Secondary seborrheas are those caused by some external or internal insult that alters the proliferation, differentiation, or desquamation of the surface and follicular epithelium (Table 11-1).[14-16] Secondary seborrheas are common in the horse.° Virtually any disorder discussed in this textbook can result in seborrheic signs during the acute or healing phase of the disease.

Cause and Pathogenesis

Any disorder that alters cellular proliferation, differentiation, or desquamation produces seborrheic signs. In most instances, the mechanisms by which the following seborrhea-inducing factors cause their changes are incompletely understood.

°References 2, 3, 7-9, 11-15, 20, 25, 26.

● Table 11-1   THE DIFFERENTIAL DIAGNOSIS OF EQUINE SEBORRHEA

Primary
    Mane and tail seborrhea
    Generalized seborrhea (dry and/or greasy)

Secondary
    Infectious agents (dermatophytes, *D. congolensis*, staphylococci)
    Ectoparasites (lice, *Onchocerca*)
    Endoparasites
    Nutritional imbalances
    Maldigestion/malabsorption (intestinal, pancreatic, hepatic)
    Contactants (shampoos, rinses, sprays)
    Warm, dry environment
    Chronic catabolic states
    Immunologic disorders (pemphigus foliaceus, systemic lupus erythematosus, sarcoidosis,
        multisystemic eosinophilic epitheliotropic disease)
    Drug reaction (e.g., iodism, potentiated sulfonamides)
    Neoplasia (epitheliotropic lymphoma, internal malignancy)

INFLAMMATION

Inflammatory skin diseases are typically characterized by epidermal hyperplasia, which probably results from the release or production of dermal eicosanoids, histamine, and cytokines. Leukotriene B_4 (LTB_4) concentrations have been reported to be increased in the skin lesions of dogs with seborrhea.[16] Both LTB_4 and prostaglandin E_2 increase DNA synthesis in the basal layer and stimulate epidermal proliferation.[16] If the inflammation is mild, seborrheic signs can develop in the absence of pruritus. Examples include grooming that is too vigorous, bacterial folliculitis, dermatophilosis, dermatophytosis, lice, low-grade contact dermatitis, and early epitheliotropic lymphoma.

NUTRITIONAL FACTORS

Glucose, protein, essential fatty acids, and various vitamins and trace minerals are necessary for normal cellular proliferation and differentiation. Deficiency, excess, or imbalance in one or more of these nutrients can produce seborrhea (see Chapter 10). Because the vast majority of horses in developed countries eat high-quality, balanced diets, nutritional seborrheas are very uncommon. When they do occur, they usually are secondary to malabsorption, maldigestion, or metabolic disease.

ENVIRONMENTAL FACTORS

The water and lipid content of the skin is important to maintain normal invisible desquamation.[3,4,10,16] If transepidermal water loss increases, desquamation changes and the squames (packets of dead cells) become visible. Low environmental humidity, excessive bathing (especially with harsh products), and fatty acid deficiency can produce this change.

As can be seen from the above-mentioned factors, virtually any disease can cause seborrhea and can do so by many different mechanisms.

Clinical Features

The clinical signs of *secondary seborrhea* include flakiness, greasiness, seborrheic dermatitis, or some combination of these (Figs. 11-1 through 11-3). The nature, distribution, and severity of the signs depend on the cause of the seborrhea and the individual patient. In general, systemic causes

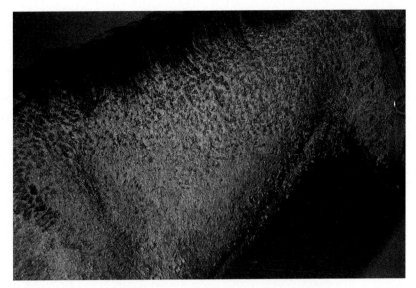

FIGURE 11-1. Severe scaling and alopecia in a horse with sarcoidosis (generalized granulomatous disease).

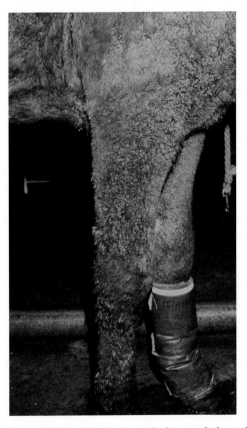

FIGURE 11-2. Severe secondary seborrhea in a horse with chronic cholangiohepatitis.

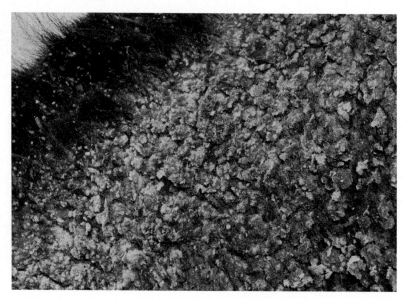

FIGURE 11-3. Same horse as in Fig. 11-2. Severe scaling, crusting, and alopecia over lateral neck.

(e.g., metabolic disease, dietary deficiency, hepatic or gastrointestinal disease, and primary or secondary lipid abnormalities) result in generalized signs that are not pruritic at their onset. These animals can become pruritic, however, as the seborrhea worsens or if there is a secondary staphylococcal or *Malassezia* overgrowth. They often have more pronounced seborrheic changes on the neck and trunk and in intertriginous areas.

Except for low environmental humidity and overzealous or inappropriate topical treatments (e.g., excessive bathing, dipping, or powdering; contact dermatitis to a shampoo), external causes (e.g., pediculosis, dermatophilosis, dermatophytosis) result in focal, multifocal, or regionalized signs of secondary seborrhea. At examination, these horses have areas of normal skin.

Primary seborrhea is uncommon in the horse.* The most common form of primary seborrhea in the horse is **mane and tail seborrhea**,[2,5,8,11-15,20] which accounts for 0.33% of the equine dermatology cases seen at the Cornell University Clinic. No age, breed, or sex predilections have been reported. Moderate to severe scaling is seen in the mane or tail regions or both (Fig. 11-4). Crusts may be present. Both dry and oily forms of the disorder are seen. There is little or no inflammation, pruritus, or alopecia. **Generalized primary seborrhea** is rare, accounting for 1.22% of the equine dermatology cases seen at the Cornell University Clinic (Fig. 11-5).[2,5,11-15,20-27] The dermatosis is more-or-less symmetric, tending to spare the extremities. Both dry and oily forms are seen. With oily forms, a rancid odor is usually present. Pruritus is rare unless secondary bacterial or yeast infections arise.

Diagnosis

The diagnosis of seborrhea is straightforward and is based on the characteristic lesions. Determining the cause of the seborrhea is far more difficult. A thorough history, dietary review, and physical examination will often direct further diagnostic testing (see Table 11-1).[2,5,11-15,20] Primary seborrhea is a diagnosis made by exclusion.

---

*References 2, 5, 8, 11-15, 20-27.

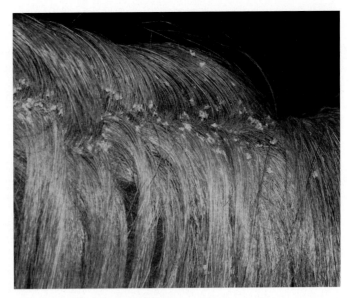

FIGURE 11-4. Mane and tail seborrhea. Multiple waxy, adherent scales in mane.

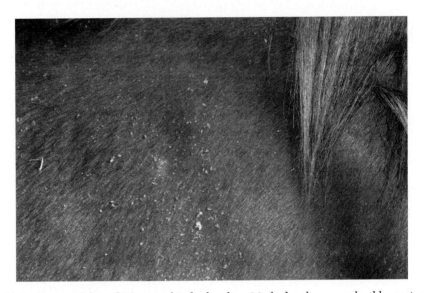

FIGURE 11-5. Primary (idiopathic) generalized seborrhea. Marked scaling over shoulder region.

The histopathologic findings in mane and tail seborrhea have not been described. Histopathologic findings reported in generalized primary seborrhea include a hyperplastic superficial perivascular dermatitis with prominent orthokeratotic and/or parakeratotic hyperkeratosis (Fig. 11-6, *A*).[14,15] The parakeratotic hyperkeratosis is usually present multifocally (in "caps" at the shoulder of hair follicle infundibula), often overlying edematous ("squirting") dermal papillae (Fig. 11-6, *B*). The inflammatory infiltrate is predominantly composed of lymphocytes, histiocytes, and a few neutrophils. Changes consistent with secondary infection (suppurative epidermitis, suppurative luminal folliculitis) may be present.

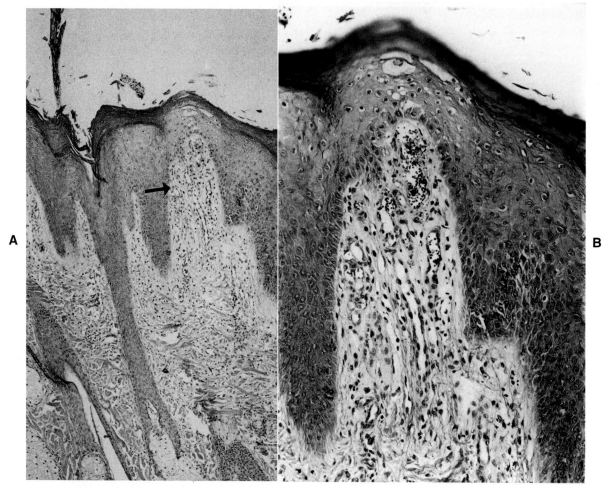

FIGURE 11-6. Primary generalized seborrhea. **A,** Hyperplastic superficial perivascular dermatitis with focal parakeratotic hyperkeratosis and "squirting" dermal papilla (*arrow*). **B,** Close-up of A. Classic papillary squirting.

Clinical Management

Secondary seborrhea is best managed by treating the underlying cause, whereupon the seborrheic signs resolve spontaneously within 1 to 2 months. Primary seborrhea is incurable.[14,15] It is important for the owner to understand that, similar to the case with dandruff in humans, control rather than cure is the goal of therapy. Because mane and tail seborrhea is often essentially a cosmetic problem, many owners elect not to treat affected horses.

Topical therapy is the mainstay for seborrheic skin disease.[2,14-16] Clipping the haircoat may be indicated in order to facilitate delivering topical agents to the skin surface. In addition, bathing the horse initially with an inexpensive detergent (e.g., Ivory or Joy dishwashing detergent) to remove surface debris will facilitate the access of antiseborrheic agents to the skin surface, as well as reduce the amount needed of the more expensive therapeutic agents. Topical antiseborrheic therapy is used temporarily to improve skin and coat condition in secondary seborrhea, and for the lifetime of the individual to control primary seborrhea. There are a large number of grooming or antiseborrheic shampoos and rinses, and product selection depends on the nature of the seborrhea

Table 11-2 ANTISEBORRHEIC TOPICAL PRODUCTS USED IN HORSES

BRAND NAME (MANUFACTURER)	INGREDIENTS
Allergroom shampoo (Virbac)	Moisturizers
Allerseb-T shampoo (Virbac)	Coal tar, sulfur, salicyclic acid
Epi-Soothe shampoo (Virbac)	Colloidal oatmeal
Epi-Soothe cream rinse (Virbac)	Colloidal oatmeal
°Humilac spray (Virbac)	Moisturizers
°HyLyt°efa hypoallergenic shampoo (DVM)	Moisturizers
†HyLyt°efa creme rinse (DVM)	Moisturizers
LyTar shampoo (DVM)	Coal tar, sulfur, salicyclic acid
Micro Pearls Advantage Benzoyl-Plus Shampoo (EVSCO)	Benzoyl peroxide
†Micro Pearls Advantage Hydra-Pearls Cream Rinse (EVSCO)	Moisturizers
†Micro Pearls Advantage Hydra-Pearls Shampoo (EVSCO)	Moisturizers
†Micro Pearls Advantage EVSCO-Tar shampoo (EVSCO)	Moisturizers, coal tar
†Micro Pearls Advantage Seba-Hex shampoo (EVSCO)	Chlorhexidine, sulfur, salicylic acid
Micro Pearls Advantage Seba-Moist shampoo (EVSCO)	Sulfur, salicylic acid
NuSal-T shampoo (DVM)	Coal tar, salicylic acid, methol
OxyDex shampoo (DVM)	Benzoyl peroxide
Pyoben shampoo (Virbac)	Benzoyl peroxide
SebaLyt shampoo (DVM)	Sulfur, salicylic acid, triclosan
Sebolux shampoo (Virbac)	Sulfur, salicylic acid
SeboRx shampoo (DVM)	Sulfur, salicylic acid, triclosan
Selsun Blue (Abbott)	Selenium sulfide
Sulf/OxyDex shampoo (DVM)	Benzoyl peroxide, sulfur
T-Lux shampoo (Virbac)	Coal tar, sulfur, salicylic acid

°Labeled for "animals."
†Labeled for horses.

(e.g., dry or greasy), veterinary and client preference, and individual responses and idiosyncrasies of affected horses (see Chapter 3). A partial listing of some of the antiseborrheic shampoos used for horses is in Table 11-2.

For mildly dry and flaky horses, moisturizing hypoallergenic shampoos (Micro Pearls Advantage, Hydra-Pearls shampoo, HyLyt°efa hypoallergenic shampoo, Allergroom shampoo) or colloidal oatmeal shampoos (Epi-Soothe shampoo) are commonly used. For more severe flaking, sulfur salicylic acid products (Micro Pearls Advantage Seba-Moist shampoo, Sebolux shampoo, SebaLyt shampoo) are appropriate. If the horse becomes flaky again soon after the bath, the application of an afterbath rinse (Micro Pearls Advantage Hydra-Pearls cream rinse, Humilac spray, HyLyt°efa creme rinse) is indicated.

For horses with greasy skin and coat, the shampoos need to be stronger degreasing agents. Horses that are mildly to moderately greasy can be treated with sulfur-salicylic acid or mild tar products (Micro Pearls Advantage EVSCO-Tar shampoo, T-Lux shampoo). Very greasy horses are bathed with benzoyl peroxide (Micro Pearls Advantage, Benzoyl-Plus shampoo, Pyoben shampoo, OxyDex shampoo), selenium sulfide (Selsun Blue dandruff shampoo), or stronger tars (LyTar shampoo, Allerseb-T shampoo). All strong shampoos can remove too much surface lipid, disrupt the epidermal barrier, and increase transepidermal water loss; these are thus contraindicated in horses with dry, flaky skin (see Chapter 3).

Whichever shampoo is chosen, it should be lathered well, allowed to stand for 15 minutes, then rinsed thoroughly. In general, shampooing is recommended twice weekly until control is achieved, followed by weekly or biweekly administration (see Chapter 3). Some horses may initially require daily shampooing.[14]

● LINEAR KERATOSIS

Linear keratosis is a rare, possibly inherited dermatosis of the horse.[*] It accounts for 0.67% of equine dermatology cases seen at the Cornell University Clinic.

Cause and Pathogenesis

The etiopathogenesis is unknown. The lesions do not follow blood or lymphatic vessels, nerves, or dermatomes. Because of the early (sometimes congenital) onset of lesions and the occurrence in related quarter horses, it has been suggested that the disorder may be hereditary.[5,11-15,28-30] Clinico-pathologically, equine linear keratosis resembles a linear epidermal nevus (see Chapter 16).[15]

Clinical Features

Linear keratosis is most commonly seen, and may be inherited in, quarter horses, thoroughbreds, and standardbreds.[†] The condition is seen in a wide variety of breeds. Lesions may be present at birth, noticed shortly after birth, or noticed within the first 5 years of life. Linear keratosis is characterized by the gradual, asymptomatic occurrence of one or more unilateral, linear, usually vertically oriented bands of alopecia and hyperkeratosis, occurring most commonly over the neck, shoulder, and lateral thorax (Figs. 11-7 and 11-8). They vary from 0.25 to 3.5 cm in width and 5 to 70 cm in length. Lesions have also occurred on the legs, hip, and pectoral region. Often lesions begin as multiple hyperkeratotic papules that coalesce into vertical bands. Pruritus and pain are absent, and affected horses are otherwise healthy.

Diagnosis

Linear keratosis is visually distinctive. External linear trauma—such as scratches, whip marks, dripping caustic substances—might be considered as differential diagnoses. Histopathologic findings include irregular to papillated epidermal hyperplasia and marked compact orthokeratotic hyper-keratosis (Fig. 11-9). A mild superficial perivascular accumulation of lymphocytes and histiocytes may be present.

Clinical Management

Linear keratosis persists for life. Because the lesions are asymptomatic, treatment is not necessary. If desired, the regular application of antiseborrheic shampoos and keratolytic ointments, creams, or gels can be used (see Chapter 3). Linear keratosis responds poorly to treatment. Perhaps the most reasonable palliative treatment is the topical application of equal parts propylene glycol and water as needed. In dogs with epidermal nevi, the oral administration of retinoids (etretinate, isotretinoin) has been effective in some cases.[16] Whether or not these agents would be effective in equine linear keratosis is unknown. The owner must be warned about the possible hereditary nature of this condition.

● CANNON KERATOSIS

Cannon keratosis is rare idiopathic dermatosis of the horse.[8,11-15] It accounts for 0.78% of the equine dermatology cases seen at the Cornell University Clinic.

Cause and Pathogenesis

The etiopathogenesis of cannon keratosis is unknown. The condition is *not* caused by stallions urinating on their own legs.

---

[*]References 2, 5, 8, 11-15, 20, 28-30.
[†]References 2, 5, 8, 11-15, 20, 28-30.

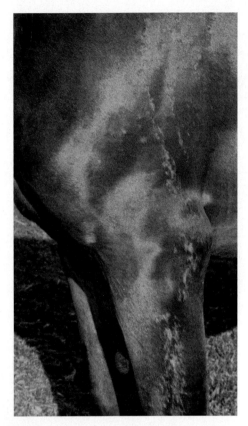

FIGURE 11-7. Linear keratosis. Linear, vertically oriented hyperkeratotic papules and alopecia on shoulder and leg.

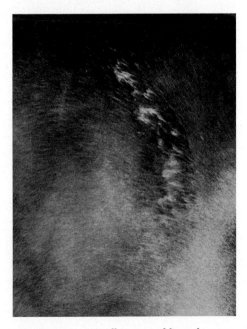

FIGURE 11-8. Linear keratosis. Linear, vertically oriented hyperkeratotic plaque on hip.

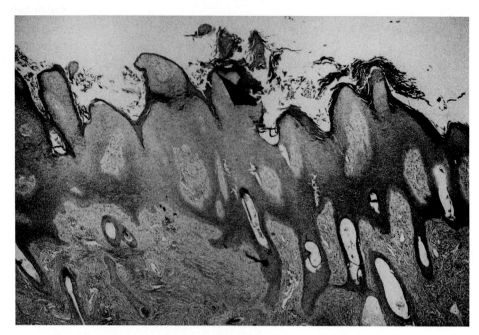

FIGURE 11-9. Linear keratosis. Papillated epidermal hyperplasia, hyperkeratosis, and papillomatosis.

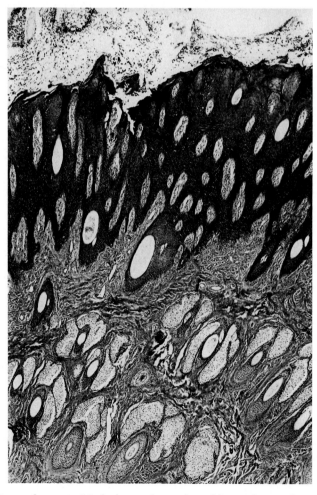

FIGURE 11-10. Cannon keratosis. Marked irregular epidermal hyperplasia and compact hyperkeratosis.

Clinical Features

Cannon keratosis ("stud crud") has no reported age, breed, or sex predilections.[5,8,11-15] Moderately well-circumscribed plaques of scaling, crusting, hyperkeratosis, and alopecia are seen bilaterally over the cranial surface of the rear cannon bone areas. Pruritus and pain are absent, and affected horses are otherwise healthy. Occasionally, lesions become fissured, inflamed or secondarily infected.

Diagnosis

The differential diagnosis includes dermatophilosis, dermatophytosis, and staphylococcal dermatitis. Histopathologic findings include marked irregular epidermal hyperplasia, marked compact ortho-keratotic and parakeratotic hyperkeratosis, and occasionally a mild perivascular accumulation of lymphocytes, histiocytes, and fewer neutrophils (Fig. 11-10).[15]

Clinical Management

Cannon keratosis persists for life. Since the condition is asymptomatic, no treatment is necessary. If desired, regular applications of antiseborrheic shampoos or keratolytic ointments, creams, or gels are beneficial (see Chapter 3). A mixture of equal parts of propylene glycol and water is the authors' preferred topical for focal hyperkeratoses. It is applied every 12 hours until maximum improvement is obtained, then as needed to prevent worsening of the lesions. Other authors[14] have suggested the use of a topical retinoid, 0.1% tretinoin cream (Retin-A, Ortho Pharmaceutical).

● REFERENCES

General References

1. Baker BB, et al: Epidermal cell renewal in the horse. Am J Vet Res 49:520, 1988.
2. Barbet JL, et al: Diseases of the skin. In: Colahan PT, et al. (eds): Equine Medicine and Surgery IV, Vol II. American Veterinary Publications, Goleta, 1991, p 1569.
3. Berardesca E, Borroni G: Instrumental evaluation of cutaneous hydration. Clin Dermatol 13:323, 1995.
4. Draelos ZD: New developments in cosmetics and skin care products. Adv Dermatol 12:3, 1997.
5. Fadok VA: An overview of equine dermatoses characterized by scaling and crusting. Vet Clin N Am Equine Pract 11:43, 1995.
6. Freedberg IM, et al (eds): Fitzpatrick's Dermatology in General Medicine, IV. McGraw-Hill Book Co, New York, 1999.
7. Hutyra F, Marek J: Special Pathology and Therapeutics of the Diseases of Domestic Animals III. Alexander Eger Publisher, Chicago, 1926.
8. Ihrke PJ: Diseases of abnormal keratinization (seborrhea). In: Robinson NE (ed): Current Therapy in Equine Medicine. W.B. Saunders Co, Philadelphia, 1983, p 546.
9. Kral R, Schwartzman RM: Veterinary and Comparative Dermatology. J.B. Lippincott, Philadelphia, 1964.
10. Kwochka KW: Keratinization abnormalities: Understanding the mechanism of scale formation. In: Ihrke PJ, et al (eds): Advances in Veterinary Dermatology II. Pergamon Press, Oxford, 1993, p 91.
11. Kwochka KW: The structure and function of epidermal lipids. Vet Dermatol 4:151, 1993.
12. Kwochka KW: Shampoos and moisturizing rinses in veterinary dermatology. In: Bonagura JD (ed): Kirk's Current Veterinary Therapy XII. W.B. Saunders Co, Philadelphia, 1995, p 590.
13. McMullen WC: The skin. In: Mansmann RA et al (eds). Equine Medicine and Surgery III. American Veterinary Publications, Santa Barbara, 1982, p 798.
14. Moriello KA, et al: Diseases of the skin. In: Reed SM, Bayley WM (eds): Equine Internal Medicine. W.B. Saunders Co, Philadelphia, 1998.
14a. Rosenkrantz WS: Systemic/topical therapy. Vet Clin N Am Equine Pract 11:127, 1995.
15. Scott DW: Large Animal Dermatology. W.B. Saunders Co, Philadelphia, 1988.
16. Scott DW, et al (ed): Muller & Kirk's Small Animal Dermatology VI. W.B. Saunders Co, Philadelphia, 2001.
17. Scott DW, et al: A Clinical study on the efficacy of two commercial veterinary emollients (Micro Pearls and Humilac) in the management of wintertime dry skin in dogs. Cornell Vet 81:419, 1991.
18. Scott DW, et al: A clinical study on the effect of two commercial veterinary benzoyl peroxide shampoos in dogs. Canine Pract 19:7, 1994.
19. Suter MM, et al: Keratinocyte biology and pathology. Vet Dermatol 8:67, 1997.
20. Williams MA, Angarano DW: Diseases of the skin. In: Kobluk CN, et al (eds): The Horse. Diseases and Clinical Management. W.B. Saunders Co, Philadelphia, 1995, p 541.

Seborrhea
21. Opperman T: Ueber das Eczema seborrhoeicum siccum beim Pferde. Dtsch Tierärztl Wschr 44:435, 1936.

22. Page EH: Common skin diseases of the horse. Proc Am Assoc Equine Pract 18:385, 1972.
23. Panel Report: Skin conditions in horses. Mod Vet Pract 56:363, 1975.
24. Panel Report: Dermatologic problems in horses. Mod Vet Pract 62:75, 1981.
25. Stannard AA: The skin. In: Mansmann RA, et al (eds): Equine Medicine and Surgery II. American Veterinary Publications, Santa Barbara, 1972, p 381.
26. Stannard AA: Some important dermatoses in the horse. Mod Vet Pract 53:31, 1972.
27. Thomsett LR: Skin diseases of the horse. In Pract 1:15, 1979.

Linear Keratosis

28. Scott DW: Equine linear keratosis. Equine Pract 7:39, 1985.
29. Stannard AA: Equine dermatology. Proc Am Assoc Pract 22:273, 1976.
30. von Tscharner C, et al.: Stannard's illustrated equine dermatology notes. Vet Dermatol 11:161, 2000.

Chapter 12

Pigmentary Abnormalities

● TERMINOLOGY AND INTRODUCTION

The color of normal skin depends primarily on the amount of melanin, carotene, and oxyhemoglobin or reduced hemoglobin that it contains and the location of the pigments within the subcutis, vessels, dermis, epidermis, and hair.[7] Epidermal and hair pigmentation results primarily from melanin, which has two forms and imparts four basic colors. Black and brown pigments are derived from eumelanins. The phaeomelanins are yellow and red pigments and contain cysteine thiol groups that react to form 5-S-cysteinyl dopa. Intermediate melanins are a blend of eumelanin and pheomelanin. A lack of melanin results in white hair or skin. See Chapter 1 for a complete discussion of the process of melanization and its control. Some aspects of the local regulation of melanization are mentioned below.

In lower animals, melatonin is believed to play a major regulatory role in cutaneous pigmentation. In humans, cats, and dogs, adrenocorticotropic hormone (ACTH) and pituitary lipotrophins regulate melanization to some degree. The interaction between keratinocytes and melanocytes is also important. In humans, keratinocytes are known to produce multiple factors that influence the growth, differentiation, tyrosinase activity, dendritic growth, pigmentation, and morphology of melanocytes.[7,23] Basic fibroblast growth factor and endothelin-1 are produced by cultured human keratinocytes.[24] Both of these factors are melanocyte mitogens, and endothelin-1 also increases tyrosinase activity in vitro. Tumor necrosis factor-α (TNF-α) and interleukin-1 (IL-1) stimulate intercellular adhesion molecule 1 (ICAM-1) expression on human melanocytes. A variety of cytokines and leukotrienes influence melanocyte function, with leukotriene B$_4$ (LTB$_4$) locally stimulating and IL-1, IL-6, and IL-7 inhibiting melanogenesis in humans. These local factors would better explain the patterns and localized control of the pigment changes seen in animals.

Hair pigmentation is separate from that of the skin, and a follicular melanin unit has also been described. In the hair, melanocytes are found in the hair bulb. In contrast to epidermal melanocytes, which are always active, hair melanocytes are active only during anagen. The controlling mechanism for hair pigmentation is still unknown.[10] Follicular melanocytes produce larger melanin granules. Variations in hair coloration reflect the melanosome size, type, shape, and dispersion. The color of these hair melanosomes may be modulated in vivo by hydrogen peroxide. Visible pigmentation depends on which stage of melanosomes is transferred, the size of the melanosomes, and how the melanosomes are dispersed within the keratinocyte. Melanosomes larger than 0.5 to 0.7 μm are dispersed individually within keratinocytes, and smaller melanosomes are grouped into melanosome complexes. As keratinocytes migrate to the surface of the skin, melanosomes may be degraded at different rates. Lighter skin has higher levels of melanosome degradation than darker skin. If one considers all of the factors involved in normal pigmentation, it becomes apparent that defects may occur at many different levels of this complex process.

● HYPERPIGMENTATION

Hyperpigmentation (*hypermelanosis*), or *melanoderma*, is associated primarily with increased melanin in the epidermis and corneocytes. Histologically, there may also be dermal pigment, but when the majority of the pigment is in the dermis, a slate or steel blue coloration is present. Hyperpigmentation is frequently encountered as an acquired condition, usually associated with chronic inflammation and irritation.[16,20] Hyperpigmentation may affect only the skin (melanoderma), only the hair (melanotrichia), or both of these. Melanoderma is often difficult to appreciate in dark-skinned horses and is most commonly seen with chronic hypersensitivity disorders. Melanotrichia is a common response when hair regrows following inflammatory insults (Fig. 12-1). The epidermis overlying numerous neoplasms and granulomas can become hyperpigmented.

Lentigo (plural, *lentigines*) is an idiopathic macular melanosis of horses. Annular, nonpalpable, dark black spots appear, usually with age, especially on the muzzle, on mucocutaneous junctions, and in the inguinal areas. The lesions are asymptomatic and of only cosmetic significance. Lentigo can be seen in association with melanocytic neoplasia in horses (see Chapter 16).

● HYPOPIGMENTATION

Hypopigmentation (*hypomelanosis*) refers to a decrease of pigment in the skin of hair coat in areas that should normally be pigmented. *Amelanosis* (achromoderma, achromotrichia) indicates a total lack of melanin. *Depigmentation* means a loss of preexisting melanin. *Leukoderma* and *leukotrichia* are clinical terms used to indicate acquired depigmentation of skin and hair, respectively.[4,7,16,20] Hereditary hypomelanoses have been divided into *melanocytopenic* (absence of melanocytes) and *melanopenic* (decreased melanin) forms.[1] Pigment loss may occur from melanocyte destruction, dysfunction, or abnormal dispersion of melanosomes as a result of abnormal melanosome transfer or from inflammation. Lack of or decrease in melanosome production may also be a cause. The disorder may be congenital or acquired.

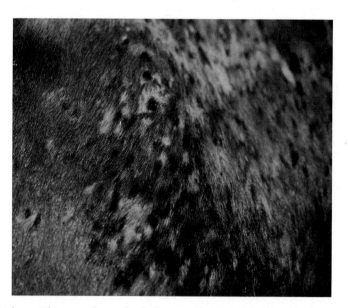

FIGURE 12-1. Melanotrichia over the neck of a horse with insect hypersensitivity.

Genetic

ALBINISM

Albinism is a hereditary lack of pigment that is transmitted as an autosomal recessive trait.[*] Albino individuals have a normal complement of melanocytes, but they lack tyrosinase for melanin synthesis and thus have a biochemical inability to produce melanin. Therefore, histopathologic studies reveal a normal epidermis with no pigment, but clear basal cells representing melanocytes are still seen. Skin, hair, and mucous membranes are amelanotic. Animals may also have unpigmented (pink) irides and photophobia.

WAARDENBURG-KLEIN SYNDROME

Waardenburg-Klein syndrome has been described in American paints.[1] In addition to blue eyes and amelanotic skin and hair, the affected animals are deaf and have blue or heterochromic irides.[1,12] The defect is in the migration and differentiation of melanoblasts. Therefore, the affected skin has no melanocytes present. The syndrome is transmitted as an autosomal dominant trait with incomplete penetrance, so these animals should not be used for breeding.

LETHAL WHITE FOAL SYNDROME

Lethal white foal syndrome (overo lethal white foal syndrome, ileocolonic aganglionosis, myenteric aganglionosis, congenital intestinal aganglionosis) is an autosomal recessive disorder resulting from the breeding of two overo spotted paint horses.[25-42]

Embryologically, the neural crest gives rise to both the myenteric plexuses and cutaneous melanoblasts. Thus, a developmental disorder of the neural crest would explain the association between lack of cutaneous pigment and absence of myenteric plexuses in the ileum, colon, and cecum. Affected foals have a mutation in the endothelin receptor B.[35,37,38,42] The endothelin signaling pathway is critical for proper development and migration of neural crest cells that ultimately form melanocytes and enteric neurons. Lethal white foal syndrome has been proposed as a model for Hirschsprung disease in humans.[34,35,37,38,42]

Affected foals are born white and apparently normal, but within a variable period of time, they show signs of colic due to an inability to pass feces. The foals do not have myenteric plexuses, and the involved gut is contracted and atretic. Affected foals typically die between 1 and 5 days of age. There is no effective treatment, and euthanasia is indicated.

LETHAL LAVENDER FOAL SYNDROME

Lethal lavender foal syndrome is a rare hereditary condition of Arabian horses.[14] The foals have a "lavender" (bluish, purplish) hair coat at birth in addition to various neurologic abnormalities (seizures, opisthotonus, paddling, blindness, no suckling reflex). The condition is fatal.

The authors have examined skin biopsy specimens from one affected foal. The histopathologic abnormalities were characterized by follicular dysplasia and abnormal clumping of melanin, similar to what is seen in dogs with color dilution alopecia.

VITILIGO

Vitiligo is an acquired, presumably genetically programmed depigmentation.[†] It accounts for 0.67% of the equine dermatoses examined at the Cornell University Clinic.

Although the exact cause of vitiligo is unknown, several theories have been proposed.[44] The *autoimmune theory* is a favored one, and antimelanocyte antibodies have been demonstrated in

---

[*]References 1, 6, 8a, 14, 21a, 22.
[†]References 3, 7, 16, 17, 22, 45-48, 50.

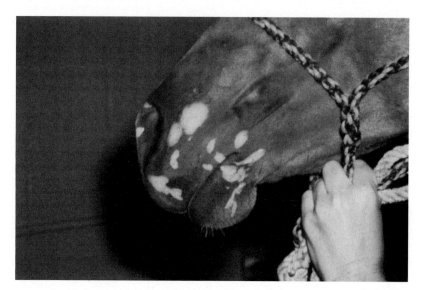

FIGURE 12-2. Early case of vitiligo on the muzzle and lips.

the serum of Arabian horses with active vitiligo.[49] The *autotoxicity theory* proposes an increased melanocyte susceptibility to melanin precursor molecules (such as dopachrome) or an inhibition of thioredoxin reductase, a free-radical scavenger located on the melanocyte membrane. The *neural theory* proposes nerve injury to explain dermatomally distributed vitiligo. A viral association has been suggested.[43] It is important to consider that multiple mechanisms could be responsible for the same phenotype.

Vitiligo is most commonly seen in Arabians (Arabian fading syndrome, pinky syndrome).* Although all colors in the breed can be affected, the disease is most common in grays. Affected animals vary in age from weanlings to 23 years old, but most are young (1 to 2 years old). Anecdotal reports indicate that vitiligo is more common in mares that are pregnant or that have recently foaled, suggesting a hormonal influence.[9,20]

Annular areas of macular depigmentation typically develop more-or-less symmetrically on the skin of the lips, muzzle (Fig. 12-2) and eyelids (Fig. 12-4, *A*), and occasionally involve the anus, vulva (Fig. 12-4, *B*), sheath, hooves, and general body areas. Occasionally larger macules coalesce to form patches (Fig. 12-3). There is no preexisting or concurrent dermatitis.

Diagnosis is based on history, physical examination, and histopathologic evaluation. Late lesions of vitiligo are characterized by a relatively normal epidermis and dermis, except that no melanocytes are seen (Fig. 12-5). In some cases (possibly early lesions), a mild lymphocytic interface dermatitis and occasional lymphocyte exocytosis may be seen.[7,44] Electron microscopy studies of melanocytes at the periphery of lesions demonstrate degenerative changes (cytoplasmic vacuolization, aggregation of melanosomes, autophagic vacuoles, fatty degeneration, and pyknosis).

The depigmentation may wax and wane in intensity but is usually permanent. Occasional horses will repigment within a year. Anecdotal reports indicate that vitamin and mineral supplements (especially vitamin A and copper) are occasionally beneficial.[9,20] Because of the waxing and waning nature of some cases of equine vitiligo, and the occasional spontaneous repigmentation, response to treatment can be difficult to interpret. Other authors report no benefit from dietary or any other

---

*References 3, 9, 11-14, 16, 17, 20, 21a, 22, 49, 50.

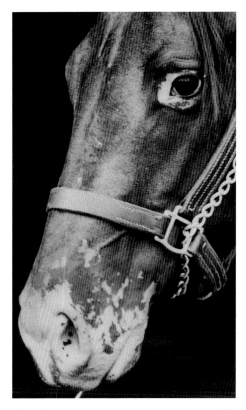

FIGURE 12-3. Chronic case of vitiligo with extensive depigmentation of the muzzle, lips, and eyelid.

form of therapy.[12,16,17] Because of the probable hereditary nature of vitiligo, affected animals should not be used for breeding.

Acquired

Acquired hypopigmentation of previously normal skin and hair can result from many factors that destroy melanocytes or inhibit melanocyte function.[4,7,15,21a] Trauma, burns, infections, and ionizing irradiation may have potent local effects. It may also be idiopathic.

Leukoderma

Leukoderma is common in horses.* It may be localized or multifocal, and temporary or permanent, depending on the cause. Leukoderma is often seen as a complication of onchocerciasis (Fig. 12-6), dourine, herpes coital exanthema, lupus erythematosus, pressure sores, ear papillomas, ventral midline dermatitis, regressing viral papillomatosis (Fig. 12-7), or freezing and burns (chemical, thermal, radiation). Leukoderma has been reported to follow contact with phenols and rubber bit guards, crupper straps, and feed buckets (Fig. 12-8).[8a,9,16,17,20] Many rubbers contain monobenzyl ether of hydroquinone (antioxidant), which inhibits melanogenesis. Leukoderma has also been associated with administration of excessive amounts of thyroprotein.[9a]

---

*References 8a, 9, 11, 13, 16, 17, 20, 21a.

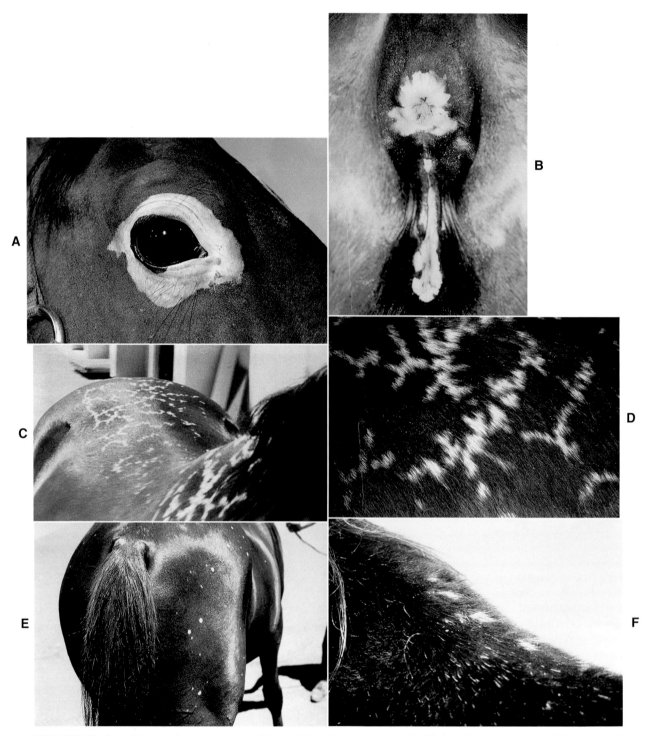

FIGURE 12-4. **A,** Vitiligo, Depigmentation of the eyelid and periocular skin. **B,** Vitiligo. Depigmentation of the anus and vulva. **C,** Reticulated leukotrichia. Cross-hatched leukotrichia over the entire dorsum—withers to rump. (*Courtesy W. McMullen.*) **D,** Reticulated leukotrichia. Close-up of cross-hatched leukotrichia. (*Courtesy A. Evans.*) **E,** Spotted leukotrichia. Multiple annular areas of leukotrichia. (*Courtesy A. Stannard.*) **F,** Hyperesthetic leukotrichia. Focal areas of leukotrichia over the withers. (*Courtesy A. Stannard.*)

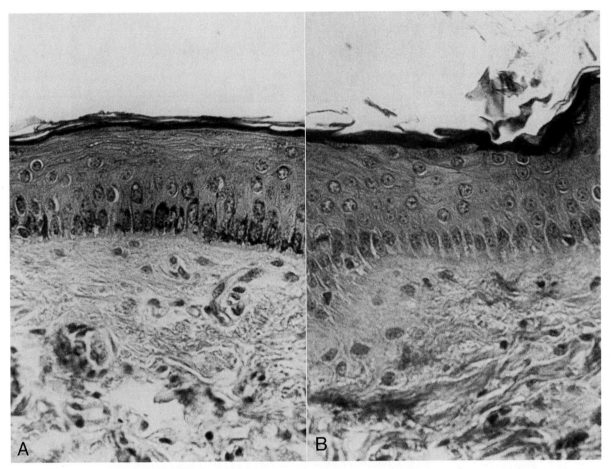

FIGURE 12-5. Equine vitiligo. **A,** Normal skin. Note heavy melanization of epidermal basal cells. **B,** Depigmented skin. Note absence of epidermal melanin.

Leukotrichia

Leukotrichia occurs commonly in horses following various traumatic and inflammatory injuries (Fig. 12-9).* Leukotrichia has also been reported in horses at the site of nerve blocks with epinephrine-containing local anesthetics.[9,20]

In the presence of the dominant allele W, a horse will, from birth, typically lack pigment in the skin and hair but have blue or brown eyes.[5,21] Such horses are often termed *albino*, *blanco*, or *cremello*. A similar appearance is produced by the C^{cr} allele of the C gene, which causes pigment dilution.[21]

A horse with the G allele is fully colored at birth but subsequently acquires an increasing number of white hairs with age.[2,5,19,20] The earliest graying begins around the eyes, at 2 to 4 years of age, and by 10 years of age such horses are practically all white. Skin and eyes remain pigmented. Examples include the Arabian, Camarque, Lippizaner, and Percheron breeds. The degree of coat pigmentation in white Camarque horses correlates directly with plasma α-MSH levels.[2]

---

*References 8a, 9, 11, 13, 16, 17, 20, 21a.

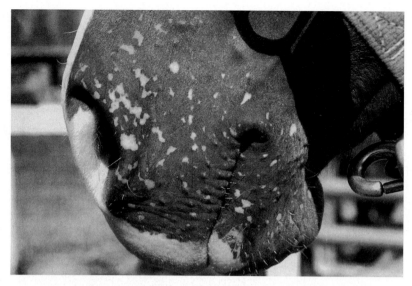

FIGURE 12-6. Equine onchocerciasis. Multiple macular areas of depigmentation on muzzle. (*Courtesy A. Evans.*)

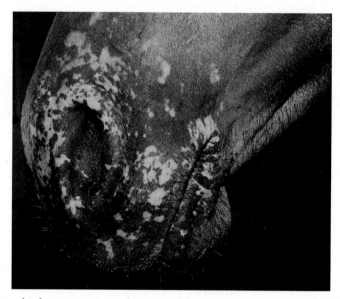

FIGURE 12-7. Macular depigmentation on the muzzle following spontaneous regression of viral papillomatosis.

Reticulated Leukotrichia

Reticulated leukotrichia (variegated leukotrichia, "tiger stripe") is an apparently uncommon dermatosis of the horse.* The cause and pathogenesis of the disorder are unknown, but apparent breed predispositions suggest that genetic factors are involved. It has been suggested the reticulated leukotrichia may be an unusual form of erythema multiforme (see Chapter 9), as some cases are temporally associated with herpesvirus infection or vaccination, and will recur with subsequent vaccination.[21a]

---

*References 3, 9, 13, 14, 16, 18, 20, 21a, 22, 51.

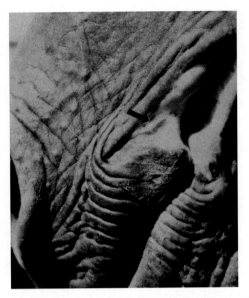

FIGURE 12-8. Depigmentation of the lips (*arrow*) due to a rubber bit.

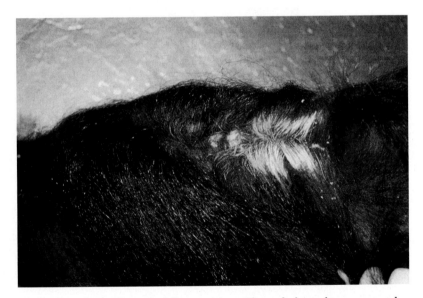

FIGURE 12-9. Leukotrichia in the mane following injury. The underlying skin was normal.

Reticulated leukotrichia is most commonly seen in quarter horses, thoroughbreds, and standardbreds, but it is occasionally recognized in other breeds.[16,18,51] There is no apparent sex predilection. Most horses develop clinical signs as yearlings. Linear crusts develop in a cross-hatched or net-like, more-or-less symmetrical pattern over the back between the withers and the base of the tail (Figs. 12-4, *C* and *D*, and 12-10). The eruption is usually asymptomatic, though some authors describe initial painful vesicles and crusts.[14] When the crusts are shed, a temporary alopecia is followed by the regrowth of white hair (leukotrichia). The underlying skin is normal. The leukotrichia is permanent.

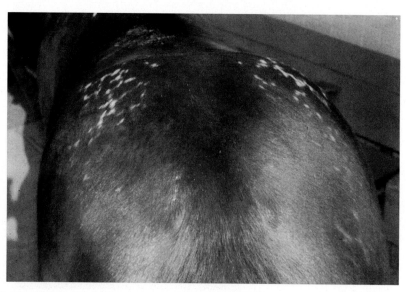

FIGURE 12-10. Reticulated leukotrichia. Linear, cross-hatched areas of leukotrichia over the rump. (*Courtesy W. McMullen.*)

Diagnosis is based on history and physical examination. Skin biopsy specimens taken at the early crusted stage are characterized by a lichenoid interface dermatitis, apoptotic keratinocytes and satellite cell apoptosis, and superficial dermal edema and pigmentary incontinence.[21a] Intra- and subepidermal vesicles may be present.

There is no known effective treatment. Due to the possible involvement of hereditary factors in this disease, affected animals should not be used for breeding.

Spotted Leukotrichia

Spotted leukotrichia is an idiopathic disorder affecting many breeds of horses, especially Arabians.[°] It accounts for 0.33% of the equine dermatoses examined at the Cornell University Clinic. Several well-circumscribed, 1- to 3-cm diameter white spots develop symmetrically or asymmetrically in the coat, especially over the sides and rump (Figs. 12-4, *E*, 12-11, and 12-12). In most cases the condition is not preceded by known skin lesions, and is asymptomatic. Leukoderma is usually absent, but when it is present, the prognosis for recovery is worse.[21a]

Diagnosis is based on history and physical examination. Detailed results of histologic examinations have not been reported. One case was reported to have melanin in the epidermis but not in the hair papillae.[52]

Individual lesions may come and go. Most horses have the condition for life, though some may undergo spontaneous remission. There is no known effective treatment.

Hyperesthetic Leukotrichia

Hyperesthetic leukotrichia is an apparently rare dermatosis of the horse.[†] The cause and pathogenesis are unknown. It has been suggested that hyperesthetic leukotrichia may be an unusual form of erythema multiforme (see Chapter 9) since some cases are temporally associated with herpesvirus infection or vaccination and will recur with subsequent vaccinations.[5a]

°References 3, 9, 13, 14, 16, 18, 20, 21a, 52.
†References 3, 5a, 9, 14, 16, 22, 53.

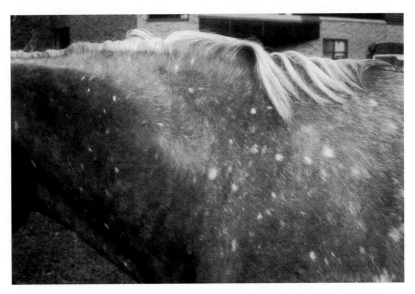

FIGURE 12-11. Spotted leukotrichia. Multiple areas of leukotrichia over the lateral thorax, shoulder, and lateral neck. The underlying skin was normal. (*Courtesy J. Baird.*)

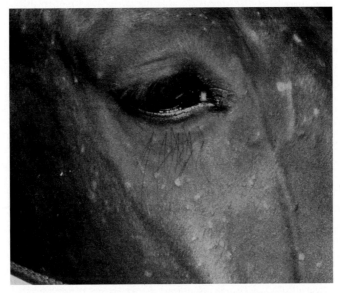

FIGURE 12-12. Spotted leukotrichia. Multiple areas of leukotrichia on the face. The underlying skin was normal.

Hyperesthetic leukotrichia usually affects mature horses with no apparent sex or breed predilections. It has apparently only been described in California. The condition is characterized by single or multiple extremely painful crusts, 1 to 4 mm in diameter, along the dorsal midline from the withers to the base of the tail. In some cases, the pain may precede the development of overt lesions. Affected horses react violently if the lesions are handled. Within a few weeks, white hairs appear in the area(s) of crusting (Fig. 12-4, *F*). The disorder runs a 1- to 3-month course, at which time the crusts and pain disappear. The leukotrichia usually persists.

Diagnosis is based on history and physical examination. Anecdotal reports indicate that biopsy specimens taken from early lesions resemble erythema multiforme (see Chapter 9).[5a,14]

There is no reported effective treatment. Some horses suffer recurrences.

• MISCELLANEOUS PIGMENT CHANGES

Some horses grow a darker coat in summer, whereas others develop a faded coat in winter.[21] Sun exposure can also bleach coats, as is seen in black horses around the muzzle and flanks.[16,21] Faded hair coats have also been attributed to various metabolic and nutritional disturbances (e.g., copper deficiency).[9,20,21] Some of these coat abnormalities are anecdotally said to respond to diet changes and/or mineral supplementation.[9,20,21]

• REFERENCES

General References

1. Alhaidari Z, et al: Melanocytogenesis and melanogenesis: genetic regulation and comparative clinical diseases. Vet Dermatol 10:3, 1999.
2. Altmeyer D, et al: The relationship between α-MSH level and coat color in white Camarque horses. J Invest Dermatol 82:199, 1984.
3. Barbet JL, et al: Diseases of the skin. In: Colohan PT, et al (eds): Equine Medicine and Surgery IV, Vol II. American Veterinary Publications, Inc, Goleta, 1991, p 1569.
4. Bologna JL, Pawelek JM: Biology of hypopigmentation. J Am Acad Dermatol 19:217, 1988.
5. Castle WE: Coat color inheritance in horses and in other mammals. Genetics 49:35, 1954.
5a. Fadok VA: Update on four unusual equine dermatoses. Vet Clin N Am Equine Pract 11:105, 1995.
6. Foil C: Comparative genodermatoses. Clin Dermatol 3:175, 1985.
7. Freedberg IM, et al (Eds): Fitzpatrick's Dermatology in General Medicine V. McGraw-Hill, New York, 1999.
8. Guaguère E, Alhaidari Z: Pigmentary disturbances. In: von Tscharner C, et al (eds): Advances in Veterinary Dermatology I. Baillière-Tindall, Philadelphia, 1990, p 395.
8a. Kral F, Schwartzman RM: Veterinary and Comparative Dermatology. J.B. Lippincott, Philadelphia, 1964.
9. McMullen WC: The skin. In: Mansmann RA, et al (eds): Equine Medicine and Surgery III. American Veterinary Publications, Inc, Santa Barbara, 1982, p 789.
9a. Mozos E, et al: Focal hypopigmentation in horses resembling Arabian fading syndrome. Equine Vet Educ 3:122, 1991.
10. Ortonne JP, Prota G: Hair melanins and hair color: ultrastructural and biochemical aspects. J Invest Dermatol 101:82S, 1993.
11. Page EH: Common skin diseases of the horse. Proc Am Assoc Equine Practit 18:385, 1972.
12. Panel Report: Skin conditions in horses. Mod Vet Pract 56:363, 1975.
13. Pascoe RR: Equine dermatoses. University of Sydney Post-Graduate Foundation in Veterinary Science, Review No. 22, 1981.
14. Pascoe RR, Knottenbelt DC: Manual of Equine Dermatology. W.B. Saunders Co, Philadelphia, 1999.
15. Pawelek J, et al: New regulations of melanin biosynthesis and the autodestruction of melanin cells. Nature 286:617, 1980.
16. Scott DW: Large Animal Dermatology. W.B. Saunders Co, Philadelphia, 1988.
17. Stannard AA: The skin. In: Mansmann RA, et al (eds): Equine Medicine and Surgery II. American Veterinary Publications, Inc, Santa Barbara, 1972, p 381.
18. Stannard AA: Equine dermatology. Proc Am Assoc Equine Practit 22:273, 1976.
19. Sturtevant AH: A critical examination of recent studies on colour inheritance in horses. J Genet 2:41, 1912.
20. Thomsett LR: Pigmentation and pigmentary disorders of the equine skin. Equine Vet Educ 3:130, 1991.
21. Trommershausen-Smith A: Positive horse identification part 3: coat color genetics. Equine Pract 1:24, 1979.
21a. von Tscharner C, et al: Stannard's illustrated equine dermatology notes. Vet Dermatol 11:161, 2000.
22. Williams MA, Angarano DW: Diseases of the skin. In: Kobluk CN, et al (eds): The Horse. Diseases and Clinical Management. W.B. Saunders Co, Philadelphia, 1995, p 541.
23. Yaar M, Gilchrest BA: Human melanocyte growth and differentiation: a decade of new data. J Invest Dermatol 97:611, 1991.
24. Yohn JJ, et al: Cultured human keratinocytes synthesize and secrete endothelin-1. J Invest Dermatol 100:23, 1993.

Lethal White Foal Syndrome

25. Blendinger C, et al: Das »Lethal-white-foal« - Syndrom. Tierärztl Prax 22:252, 1994.
26. Crowell WA: Lethal white foal syndrome. Vet Med 83:982, 1988.

27. Deeg C, Koeppel P: Lethal-white-foal syndrome - ein Fallbericht. Pferdenheilk 10:321, 1994.

28. Furugnen B: Lethal white foal syndrome hos häst. Svensk Veterinär 50:609, 1998.

29. Hultgren BD: Ileocolonic aganglionosis in white progeny of overo spotted horses. J Am Vet Med Assoc 180:289, 1982.

30. Huston R, et al: Congenital defects in foals. J Equine Med Surg 1:146, 1977.

31. Jones WE, Bogart R: Genetics of the Horse. Caballus Publications, East Lansing, 1971.

32. Jones WE: The overo white foal syndrome. J Equine Med Surg 3:54, 1979.

32a. Lightbody T: Foal with overo lethal white syndrome born to a registered quarter horse mare. Can Vet J 43:715, 2002.

33. Loeven K: Overo crosses and aganglionosis. J Equine Vet Sci 7:249, 1987.

34. McCabe L, et al: Overo lethal white foal syndrome: equine model of aganglionic megacolon (Hirschsprung disease). Am J Med Genetics 36:336, 1990.

35. Metallinos DL, et al: A missense mutation in the endothelin-B receptor-gene is associated with lethal white foal syndrome: an equine version of Hirschsprung disease. Mamm Genome 9:426, 1998.

36. Pulos WL, Hutt FB: Lethal dominant white horses. J Hered 60:59, 1969.

37. Santschi EM, et al: Endothelin receptor B polymorphism associated with lethal white foal syndrome in horses. Mamm Genome 9:306, 1998.

38. Santschi EM, et al: Incidence of the endothelin receptor B mutation that causes lethal white foal syndrome in white-patterned horses. Am J Vet Res 62:97, 2001.

39. Schneider JE, Leipold HW: Recessive lethal white in two foals. J Equine Med Surg 2:479, 1978.

40. Trommershausen-Smith A: Lethal white foals in matings of overo spotted horses. Theriogenol 8:303, 1977.

41. Vanderfecht SL, et al: Congenital intestinal aganglionosis in white foals. Vet Pathol 20:65, 1983.

42. Yang GC, et al: A dinucleotide mutation in the endothelin-B receptor gene is associated with lethal white foal syndrome: a horse variant of Hirschsprung disease. Hum Mol Genet 7:1097, 1998.

Vitiligo

43. Grimes PE, et al: Cytomegalovirus DNA identified in skin biopsy specimens of patients with vitiligo. J Am Acad Dermatol 35:21, 1996.

44. Kovacs SO: Vitiligo. J Am Acad Dermatol 38:647, 1998.

45. Meijer WCP, Eijk W: Vitiligo bij paarden en ruderen. Tijdschr Diergeneeskd 87:411, 1962.

46. Meijer WCP: Vitiligo bij het paard. Tijdschr Diergeneeskd 86:1021, 1961.

47. Meijer WCP: Dermatological diagnosis in horse and cattle judging. Vet Rec 77:1046, 1965.

48. Meijer WCP: Pigment verlust des Integumentes und die dermatologische Diagnose bei der Beurteilung von Pferden and Rindern. Dtsch Tierärztl Wochenschr 73:85, 1966.

49. Naughton GK, et al: Antibodies to surface antigens of pigmented cells in animals with vitiligo. Proc Soc Exp Biol Med 181:423, 1986.

50. Sen S, Ansari AI: Depigmentation (vitiligo) in animals and its treatment with "Meladinine." Indian J Anim Hlth 10:249, 1979.

Reticulated Leukotrichia

51. Kohli RN, Naddaf H: Reticulated leukotrichia in an Arabian horse in Iran. Indian Vet J 74:786, 1997.

Spotted Leukotrichia

52. Baker KP, Zieg H: Spotted leukotrichia in a thoroughbred three-year-old race horse. Vet Dermatol News 14:58, 1992.

Hyperesthetic Leukotrichia

53. Stannard AA: Hyperesthetic leukotrichia. In: Robinson NE (ed): Current Therapy in Equine Medicine II. W.B. Saunders Co, Philadelphia, 1987, p 647.

Chapter *13*

Environmental Skin Diseases

Environmental disorders are common and often a cause of substantial economic loss in equine medicine. In many instances—chemical toxicoses, mycotoxicoses, and hepatotoxic plant toxicoses—the dermatologic abnormalities are clinically spectacular and of important diagnostic significance, but are of less importance prognostically, therapeutically, and financially compared with abnormalities in other organ systems. An in-depth discussion of many of these diseases is beyond the scope of this chapter; therefore, we have emphasized the dermatologic feature of each condition. For detailed clinicopathologic information on many of these disorders, the reader is referred to other textbooks.[1-4,5,11,11a,14a]

• MECHANICAL INJURIES

Intertrigo

Intertrigo is a superficial inflammatory dermatosis that occurs in places where skin is in apposition and is thus subject to the friction of movement, increased local heat, maceration from retained moisture, and irritation from accumulation of debris.[4a,15] When these factors are present to a sufficient degree, dissolution of stratum corneum, exudation, and secondary bacterial infection are inevitable.

Intertrigo is occasionally seen in mares.[11,15] Congestion of the udder at parturition is physiologic, but may be sufficiently severe to cause edema of the belly, udder, and teats. In most cases, the edema disappears within 2 to 3 days after parturition. However, if extensive and persistent, the edema can lead to intertrigo in the intramammary sulcus and where the skin of the udder contacts the skin of the medial thighs. Lesions include oozing, crusting, secondary bacterial infection, and in severe cases, necrosis. A foul odor may be present. The affected areas may or may not be painful.

Diagnosis is based on history and physical examination. Treatment includes the daily applications of gentle antiseptic soaps, astringent rinses, and dusting with powders to reduce friction. Healing is usually complete within 3 to 4 weeks.

Hematoma

A hematoma is a circumscribed area of hemorrhage into the tissues.[15] It arises from vascular damage associated with sudden, severe, blunt external trauma (e.g., a fall). The lesions are usually acute in onset, subcutaneous, fluctuant, and may or may not be painful. Hematomas are most commonly seen subsequent to fractures, on the vulva subsequent to difficult deliveries, and on the brisket of foals (Fig. 13-1).[9-11,15]

Diagnosis is based on history, physical examination, and needle aspiration of the lesion that reveals blood. Most hematomas are simply allowed to organize and partially resolve. If surgical incision, evacuation, and repair are indicated, the hematoma should be allowed to organize first.

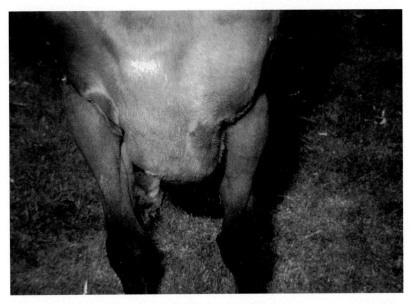

FIGURE 13-1. Hematoma on the brisket of a foal. (*Courtesy R. Pascoe.*)

Hygroma

Hygromas are cutaneous swellings associated with an underlying bursitis.[5,10a,16a,16b] Bursitis may occur after acute or chronic trauma to an existing bursa (e.g., bicipital, cunean, supraspinous, trochanteric) or after the development of an acquired bursa (e.g., capped hock, capped elbow, carpal hygroma). A local, fluctuant swelling develops over the site of injury, with variable edema and pathology of the overlying skin. Therapeutic principles include removing the cause and bandaging. Systemic anti-inflammatory agents and/or local injections of glucocorticoids may be indicated. Surgical intervention is usually a last resort.

Pressure Sore

Pressure sores (*decubital ulcers*) usually occur as a result of prolonged application of pressure concentrated in a relatively small area of the body and sufficient to compress the capillary circulation, causing tissue damage or frank necrosis.[4a,15] Tissue anoxia and full-thickness skin loss rapidly progress from a small localized area to produce ulceration, which almost invariably becomes infected with a variety of pathogenic bacteria. Within a matter of 24 to 48 hours, the edges of the ulcerated area become undermined. The ulceration may later extend to underlying bone. Because of the area of capillary and venous congestion in the base of the ulcer and at the tissue margins, systemic antibiotic therapy is virtually useless, except in the case of bacteremia.

Pressure sores (bedsores, saddle sores, saddle galls, girth galls, sit fasts) are caused by prolonged, continuous pressure—often relatively mild—leading to ischemic necrosis.[4-5,7-9,12-16] They are commonly seen in horses, especially in association with ill-fitting tack, prolonged anesthetic/surgical procedures, and prolonged recumbency. Animals that are emaciated (decreased fat and muscle layers) are at increased risk.

Lesions are initially characterized by an erythematous to reddish-purple discoloration. This progresses to oozing, necrosis, and ulceration (Fig. 13-2). The resultant ulcers tend to be deep, undermined at the edges, secondarily infected, and very slow to heal. Scarring and leukotrichia after healing are common.

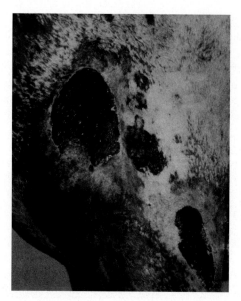

FIGURE 13-2. Pressure sore over the shoulder following anesthesia and surgery.

Diagnosis is based on history and physical examination. The most important aspect of therapy is to identify and correct the cause. Routine wound care includes daily cleansing and drying agents, and topical antiseptics or systemic antibiotics if indicated. Surgical débridement, surgical excision, or skin grafting may be necessary. Prevention is vastly superior to any kind of therapy.

Foreign Bodies

Foreign bodies occasionally cause skin lesions in horses.[11,15,18]

CAUSE AND PATHOGENESIS

Most commonly, the foreign material is of plant origin, especially wood slivers and the seeds and awns of cheatgrass, needlegrass, poverty grass, crimson clover, and foxtail.[22a] Other foreign bodies associated with skin lesions in horses include fragments of wire,[17] darts,[20] cactus spines,[19] material from gunshot injuries,[22] and suture material.[21]

Because most bullets are pointed, little material is taken in at the entry site, but large amounts of material are sucked in at the exit site, producing widespread contamination.[22] Suture sinus reactions have been associated with nonabsorbable polyamide, polyester, and polypropylene suture.[21] Suture sinuses can be associated with any suture material, but the prevalence is higher following the use of multifilament or braided suture materials.

CLINICAL FEATURES

Lesions typically produced by foreign bodies include various combinations of papules, nodules, abscesses, and draining tracts. Secondary bacterial infection is common and incompletely responsive to surgical drainage and antibiotic therapy until the foreign material is removed. The affected area may or may not be hot, painful, and edematous. Lesions occur most commonly on the legs, hips, muzzle, and ventral abdomen. Lesions may occur days to months postpenetration. Suture sinuses often appear 6 to 28 months postsurgery.[21]

DIAGNOSIS

The differential diagnosis includes infectious and sterile granulomas and abscesses, as well as neoplasia. The definitive diagnosis is based on history (exposure?), physical examination (object palpable?), radiography, ultrasonography, and surgical exploration. Ultrasonography is an excellent imaging technique for detecting various foreign bodies in the skin and muscle of horses.[19,21] Histopathologic findings include granulomatous to pyogranulomatous dermatitis and panniculitis, wherein evidence of the foreign material may or may not be found.

CLINICAL MANAGEMENT

The only successful treatment is removal of the foreign material. Systemic antibiotic therapy is often needed for secondary bacterial infection. All gunshot wounds must be treated by débridement and wound excision, and healing is by secondary intention or delayed primary closure 4 to 5 days after the primary surgery.[22]

Myospherulosis

Myospherulosis is an extremely rare granulomatous reaction thought to be due to the interaction of ointments, antibiotics, or endogenous fat with erythrocytes.[23,24] It is associated with small sac-like structures (parent bodies) filled with endobodies (spherules). Myospherulosis is most commonly reported after injection of oily medicaments or after the topical application of oily products to open wounds. Because muscle is not always involved, it has been suggested that *spherulocytosis* or *spherulocytic disease* might be a better designation for this entity.[23]

Patients are usually presented for solitary subcutaneous or dermal nodules, which may or may not have draining tracts. Histologic examination reveals several solid and cystic areas.[23,24] The walls of the cystic areas and most of the solid areas are composed of histiocytes with abundant vacuolated cytoplasm. Histiocytes surround parent bodies (20 to 350 µm in diameter) composed of thin eosinophilic walls and filled with homogeneous eosinophilic 3- to 7-µm diameter spherules. Parent bodies and spherules do not stain with PAS, GMS, or acid-fast stains, but are positive for endogenous peroxidase (diaminobenzidine reaction) and hemoglobin, indicating that the spherules are erythrocytes. The only effective treatment is surgical excision.

Arteriovenous Fistula

An *arteriovenous fistula* is a vascular abnormality, defined as a direct communication between an adjacent artery and a vein that bypasses the capillary circulation.[25] Arteriovenous fistulae may be congenital or acquired, and they are extremely rare in horses.[26] Congenital fistulae result from abnormal maturation of embryonic vasculature, whereas acquired fistulae usually result from trauma (especially penetrating wounds).

Affected areas may show persistent or recurrent edema, fluctuant swelling, and occasionally pain or secondary infection. Superficial blood vessels proximal to the fistula may be distinct and tortuous. Arteriovenous fistulae are generally characterized by pulsating vessels, palpable thrills, and continuous machinery murmurs.

Diagnosis is based on history, physical examination, and demonstration of the fistula by contrast radiography or color-flow Doppler ultrasonography.[25,26] Therapy includes surgical extirpation of the fistula.

Gangrene

Gangrene is a clinical term used to describe severe tissue necrosis and sloughing.[11,15] The necrosis may be moist or dry. The pathologic mechanism of gangrene is an occlusion of either arterial or venous blood supply. *Moist gangrene* is produced by impairment of lymphatic and venous drainage plus infection (putrefaction) and is a complication of pressure sores associated with bony prominences and pressure points in recumbent animals. Moist gangrene presents as swollen, discolored areas with a foul odor and progressive tissue decomposition. *Dry gangrene* occurs when arterial blood supply is occluded, but venous and lymphatic drainage remain intact and infection is absent (mummification). Dry gangrene assumes a dry, discolored, leathery appearance.

The causes of gangrene include (1) external pressure—pressure sores, rope galls, constricting bands, ill-fitting tack, (2) internal pressure (severe edema), (3) burns (thermal, chemical, friction, radiation, electrical), (4) frostbite, (5) envenomation (snake bite), (6) vasculitis, (7) ergotism, and (8) various infections (clostridial, staphylococcal) (Fig. 13-3). Gangrene and sloughing of the distal limbs has been described in foals and is thought to be due to hypoxia and dehydration.[26a] For diagnosis and management of these conditions, the reader is referred to appropriate sections of this book.

Subcutaneous Emphysema

Subcutaneous emphysema is characterized by free gas in the subcutis.[11,15]

CAUSE AND PATHOGENESIS

It has been described as a sequela to tracheal perforation,[28,30] esophageal rupture,[29] penetrating wounds (especially in the axillary region),[31,31a] and clostridial cellulitis/myositis.[27] Massive subcutaneous emphysema is a sequela to pneumomediastinum, which may also be caused by vigorous abdominal, diaphragmatic, and thoracic muscular contraction against a closed glottis.[32] Air from ruptured pulmonary alveoli then gains access to the perivascular spaces, migrates along the adventitia of blood vessels, reaching the mediastinum. From these, the air reaches the soft tissues of the neck and face, torso and extremities via fascial planes, producing subcutaneous emphysema.

CLINICAL FEATURES

Subcutaneous emphysema is characterized by soft, fluctuant, crepitant subcutaneous swellings. The lesions are usually nonpainful, and the animals are not acutely ill, except in the case of gas gangrene (clostridial infections).

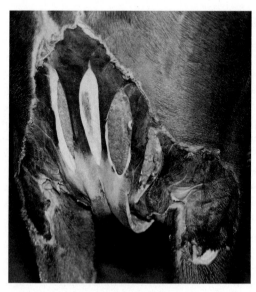

FIGURE 13-3. Clostridial infection of pectoral and proximal front leg regions. Note well-delineated area of black, leathery, sloughing, necrotic skin.

DIAGNOSIS

Diagnosis is based on history, physical examination, and possibly thoracic and abdominal radiography. Sterile subcutaneous emphysema usually requires no treatment unless extensive and incapacitating. Most cases are benign and resolve spontaneously over a course of about 1 to 2 weeks. Rarely, severe subcutaneous emphysema can lead to fatal complications, including acute thoracic restriction and respiratory acidosis, thoracic wall compression and respiratory failure, retropharyngeal emphysema and acute respiratory distress, and intracranial hypertension.[32]

CLINICAL MANAGEMENT

Treatment is directed at the underlying cause. Massive subcutaneous emphysema may require surgical decompression of the soft tissues of the thoracic wall by tracheostomy, intercostal tube placement, or multiple skin incisions.[11,32]

Draining Tracts

A *fistula* is an abnormal passage or communication, usually between two internal organs or leading from an internal organ to the surface of the body. A *sinus* is an abnormal cavity or channel or fistula that permits the escape of pus to the surface of the body.

Draining tracts are commonly encountered and are usually associated with penetrating wounds that have left infectious agents and/or foreign bodies behind.[15] Draining tracts may also result from infections of underlying tissues (e.g., bone, joint, lymph node) and previous injections. Pectoral draining tracts have rarely been caused by rib sequestration[32b] or thoracic abscess.[32a]

● THERMAL INJURIES

Burns

CAUSE AND PATHOGENESIS

Burns are occasionally seen in horses and may be thermal (barn, forest, and brush fires; accidental spillage of hot solutions), electrical (electrocution; lightning strike), frictional (rope burns; abrasions from falling), chemical (blisters; improperly used topical medicaments; maliciously applied caustic agents), or radiational (radiotherapy).*

The cause of the burn and the percentage of body involvement have great impact on the patient's survival. Patients burned by fire are at great risk for damage to the respiratory tract. Patients with large burns experience fluid and electrolyte imbalances and may die rapidly if not treated appropriately. If 25% of the body is burned, there are usually systemic manifestations (septicemia, shock, renal failure, anemia). Animals with burns over 50% or more of their body usually die. The reader is referred to other sources for in-depth discussions of the pathophysiology of burns and the management of severely burned patients with extracutaneous complications.[11a,33-36]

Loss of the skin as a protective barrier exposes the underlying tissue to invasive infection. Although microcirculation is restored within 48 hours to areas of partial-thickness injury, the full-thickness burn is characterized by complete occlusion of local vascular supply. This avascular, necrotic tissue, with impaired delivery of humoral and cellular defense mechanisms, provides an excellent medium for bacterial proliferation, with the ever-present potential for life threatening sepsis.

CLINICAL FINDINGS

Burns are most commonly seen over the dorsum and face (Fig. 13-4, *A*). They have been classified according to severity.[9,11a,33-36] *First-degree* burns involve the superficial epidermis; are character-

---

*References 4, 5-9, 11, 11a, 15, 16, 33-36.

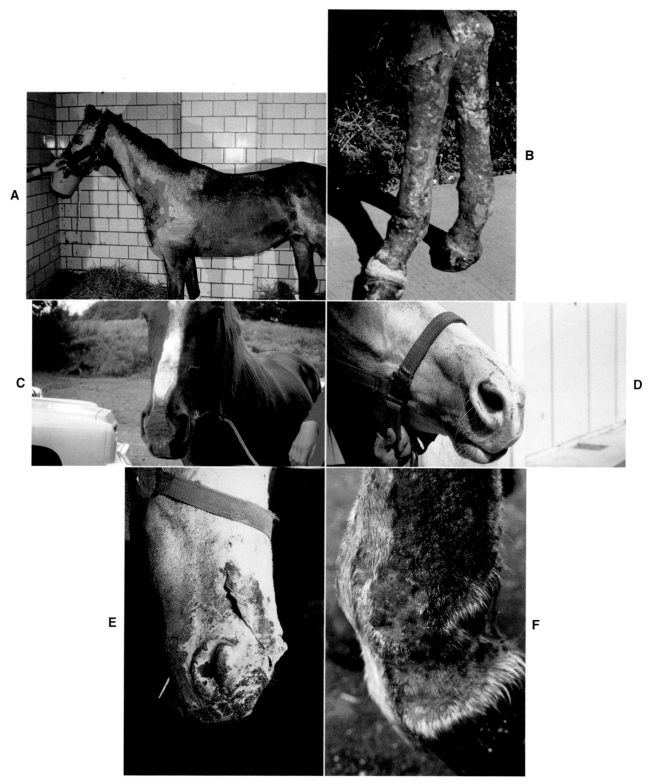

FIGURE 13-4. A, Thermal burns (barn fire). Extensive alopecia. The face, neck, and shoulder are depigmented and focally ulcerated. The pinnae have been partially burned off. **B,** Immersion foot. Note ulceration from coronets to water line. (*Courtesy F. Blacken.*) **C,** Hepatogenous photosensitization. Note marked erythema of light-skinned area of muzzle. **D,** Hepatogenous photosensitization. Erythema and scaling of muzzle. (*Courtesy A. Stannard.*) **E,** Hepatogenous photosensitization. Erythema, alopecia, ulcers, crusts, and focal sloughing of skin on muzzle. **F,** Hepatogenous photosensitization. Ulceration of distal leg. Note skin dorsal to ulcer is black, leathery, and necrotic. (*Courtesy W. McMullen.*)

ized by erythema, edema, heat, and pain; and generally heal without complication. *Second-degree* burns affect the entire epidermis; are characterized by erythema, edema, heat, pain, and vesicles; and usually reepithelialize with proper wound care. *Third-degree* burns affect the entire epidermis, dermis, and appendages; they are characterized by necrosis, ulceration, anesthesia, and scarring. Diligent therapy and possibly skin grafting are indicated. *Fourth-degree* burns involve the entire skin, subcutis, and underlying fascia, muscle, and tendon.

DIAGNOSIS

The diagnosis is usually straightforward and is based on history and physical examination. Histopathologic findings of a gradually tapering coagulation necrosis of the epidermis and deeper tissues are typical of a burn.[4a] Electrical burns may show a diagnostic histologic feature of a fringe of elongated, degenerated cytoplasmic processes that protrude from the lower end of the detached basal epidermal cells into the space separating the epidermis and the dermis. The nuclei of the basal cells and often of the higher-lying keratinocytes appear stretched in the same direction as the fringe of cytoplasmic processes. This gives the image of keratinocytes that are "standing at attention."

CLINICAL MANAGEMENT

Care of burn wounds usually includes one or more of the following: (1) thorough cleansing (povidone-iodine or chlorhexidine), (2) surgical débridement, (3) daily hydrotherapy, and (4) topical antibiotics.[11a,33-36] Occlusive dressings are avoided because of their tendency to produce a closed wound with bacterial proliferation and to delay healing. The wound should be cleaned two or three times daily, and the topical antibiotic reapplied. The most commonly used topical antibiotic is silver sulfadiazine, a painless, nonstaining, broad-spectrum antibacterial agent with the ability to penetrate eschar.[4a,15,33-36] Systemic antibiotics are not effective in preventing local burn wound infections and may permit the growth of resistant organisms. Many burned equine patients are pruritic, and measures must be taken to prevent self-mutilation (drugs, cross-tying, and so forth).[33]

Burns heal slowly and many weeks may be required to allow the wound to close by granulation. Because scarred skin is hairless and often depigmented, solar exposure should be limited. Burn scar neoplasms—squamous cell carcinoma, fibrosarcoma, fibroma, sarcoid—have been reported in horses (see Chapter 16),[33] so the areas should be examined periodically.

Frostbite

Frostbite is an injury to the skin resulting from excessive exposure to cold.[11,11a,15] It is rare in healthy animals who have been acclimatized to the cold. Frostbite is more likely to occur in neonates; animals that are sick, debilitated, or dehydrated; animals having preexisting vascular insufficiency; and animals that have recently moved from a warm climate to a cold one. The lower the temperature, the greater the risk. Lack of shelter, blowing wind, and wetting decrease the amount of exposure time necessary for frostbite to develop.

Frostbite typically affects the tips of the ears, tail tip, teats, scrotum, and feet.[6,11,15,16] These areas are often not well insulated by hair and the blood vessels are not as well protected. While frozen, the skin appears pale, is hypoesthetic, and is cool to the touch. After thawing, mild cases present with erythema, edema, scaling, and alopecia. Severe cases present with necrosis, dry gangrene, and sloughing.

Therapy varies with the severity of the frostbite. In mild cases, treatment may not be needed. Frozen tissues should be rapidly thawed by the *gentle* application of warm water (41° to 44° C). Thawing must be delayed until it is known that refreezing can be prevented, or the resultant damage may be even worse. Rewarming may be followed by the application of bland, protective ointments or creams. In severe cases with necrosis and sloughing, systemic antibiotics are also indicated. Surgical débridement or amputation is postponed until an obvious boundary between viable and nonviable tissue is present. Once-frozen tissue may be increasingly susceptible to cold injury.

• PRIMARY IRRITANT CONTACT DERMATITIS

Contact dermatitis is an inflammatory skin reaction caused by direct contact with an offending substance.[4a,11a,15,41]

Cause and Pathogenesis

Primary irritants have one thing in common: they invariably produce dermatitis if they come into direct contact with the skin in sufficient concentration for a long enough period of time.[4a,7,15,41] No sensitization is required. Moisture is an important predisposing factor, since it decreases the effectiveness of normal skin barriers and increases the intimacy of contact between the contactant and the skin surface. In this regard, the sweating horse is an ideal candidate for contact dermatitis over any area of the body. The rapidity of onset and the intensity of the reaction depend on the nature of the contactant, its concentration, the duration of the contact, and the preexisting health of the skin. Although most primary irritants are chemicals, similar skin lesions can be produced by thermal injuries, solar damage, and contact with living organisms.

Substances reported to cause primary irritant contact dermatitis include body excretions (feces and urine), wound secretions, caustic substances (acids and alkalis), crude oil, diesel fuel, turpentine, leather preservatives, mercurials, various blisters, leg sweats, improperly used topical parasiticides (sprays, dips, pour-ons, and wipes), irritating plants (*Helenium microcephalum* [small-head sneezeweed], *Cleome gynandra* [prickly spider flower], *Urtica ureus* and *U. dioica* [stinging nettle], and *Euphorbia* spp. [spurge]), wood preservatives, bedding, and a filthy environment.[4,5-9,15,16,37-43]

Clinical Features

Primary irritant contact dermatitis is common in the horse, and far more common than contact hypersensitivity (see Chapter 8).[7,15,41] Age, breed, and sex are not factors in the incidence of the condition, except as they relate to frequency of encounter with the offending contactant. Because direct contact is required, the face, distal extremities, ventrum, and areas under tack are most commonly affected. The dermatitis varies in severity from erythema, edema, papules, and scaling, to vesicles, erosions, ulcers, necrosis, and crusts (Figs. 13-5 through 13-7). Pruritus and pain are variable. Severe irritants, self-trauma, or secondary bacterial infection can result in alopecia, lichenification, and scarring. Leukotrichia and leukoderma can be transient or permanent sequelae.

In most instances the nature of the contactant can be inferred from the distribution of the dermatitis: muzzle and distal legs (plants and environmental substances, such as sprays and fertilizers); a single limb (blisters and sweats); face and dorsum (sprays, dips, wipes); perineum and rear legs (urine and feces); tack-associated areas (preservatives, dyes, and polishes); and ventrum (bedding and a filthy environment). Pentachlorophenol (a component of waste motor oil, fungicides, wood preservatives, and moth-proofers) was reported to produce severe contact dermatitis and loss of the mane and tail hairs.[38]

Immersion foot is a term that was first used to describe injuries from water immersion after shipwreck or time on a wet life raft. *Trench foot* described injuries due to soaked feet in soldiers, hunters, and outdoorsmen. *Immersion foot* is now the common name used for both scenarios. The condition is a vasoneuropathy associated with prolonged exposure to moisture, cold temperatures, and impaired blood flow to extremities.

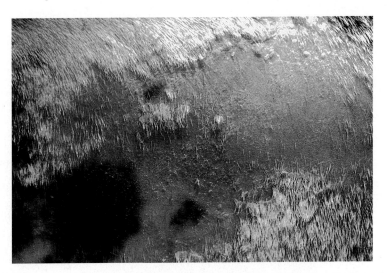

FIGURE 13-5. Primary irritant contact dermatitis due to application of motor oil. Alopecia, scaling, and erythema over thorax.

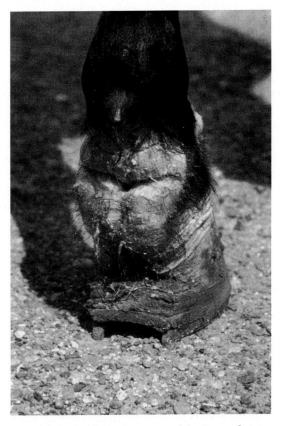

FIGURE 13-6. Primary irritant contact dermatitis on caudal pastern due to application of mustard oil. (*Courtesy W. McMullen.*)

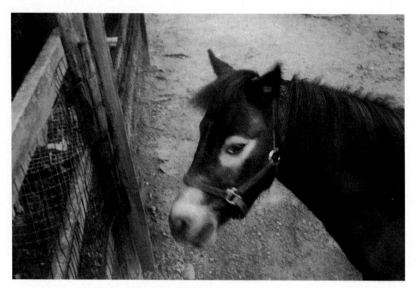

FIGURE 13-7. Primary irritant contact dermatitis due to application of fly wipe. Note alopecia and depigmentation around eye.

A condition analogous to immersion foot in humans has been reported in horses.[36a] All animals had been standing in cool water for at least 2 to 3 days. Clinical signs included early pain, stiffness, reluctance to move, and edema and erythema of the submerged areas of skin. Dermatitis progressed to necrosis and slough (Figs. 13-4, *B*, and 13-8).

Vesiculobullous lesions were seen in 24% of the horses at a Midwestern horse show.[37] Horses first acted sensitive when touched around the head and muzzle, then began developing vesicles and bullae within 2 days of arriving. The nose was affected in all horses, and the periocular region, perianal region, lips, and pinnae were also involved in 22%, 14%, 12%, and 5%, respectively, of the horses. Poor appetite was present in 26% of the horses. The dermatitis was associated with exposure to wood shavings from trees of the *Quassia* genus (family Simaronbaceae). *Quassia* spp. contain bitter elements such as quassin and neoquassin, which have cytotoxic activity *in vitro*. The dermatitis began a median of 52 hours after contact with the shavings and resolved a median of 5 days (range 2 to 21 days) after exposure to the shavings was terminated.

Diagnosis

The differential diagnosis typically includes contact hypersensitivity, *Pelodera* dermatitis, and trombiculosis. The definitive diagnosis is based on history, physical examination, and recovery when the offending contactant is removed. The cause is usually obvious, but occasionally may require considerable detective work, especially when owners are unwilling to admit to using home remedies that have produced the dermatitis. Histopathologic findings include variable degrees of superficial perivascular dermatitis wherein neutrophils or lymphocytes are the predominant inflammatory cell types. Epidermal necrosis and ulceration, as well as signs of secondary bacterial infection, may be seen.

Clinical Management

The contactant must be identified and eliminated. Residual contactant and other surface debris should be removed with copious amounts of cool water and gentle cleansing soaps. Other symptomatic treatments may include topical and/or systemic antibiotics and glucocorticoids. In

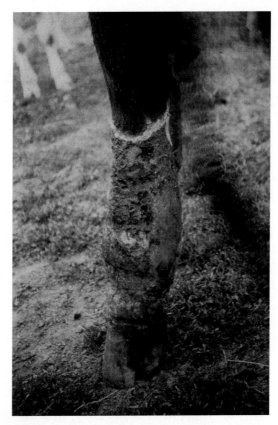

FIGURE 13-8. Immersion foot. Note ulceration, crusting, swelling, and alopecia from coronet to water line. (*Courtesy J. Servantie.*)

most cases, the dermatitis will resolve within 7 to 14 days after the contactant is removed. For *immersion foot*, therapy includes warming, symptomatic topical medicaments, and surgical intervention as required.

• CHEMICAL TOXICOSES

Selenosis

Chronic selenium poisoning causes lameness, hoof changes, emaciation, and loss of the long hairs of the mane, tail, and fetlocks.[11,11a,15]

CAUSE AND PATHOGENESIS

Selenosis is seen in the Great Plains and Rocky Mountain belt areas of the United States and in certain regions of Australia, Canada, China, South America, Mexico, Israel, and the United Kingdom.[11,15,44-52] The condition is associated with high levels of selenium in the soil (generally >5 ppm) or the presence of selenium-concentrating plants. Selenium levels are highest in low-rainfall areas with alkaline soils. On seleniferous soils, "converter" or "indicator" plants such as *Astragalus* spp., *Xylorrhiza* spp., *Gutierrezia* spp., *Grindelia* spp., *Sideranthus* spp., *Greyia* spp., *Aster* spp., *Atriplex* spp., *Penstemon* spp., *Castilleja* spp., *Oonopsis* spp., and *Stanleya* spp. accumulate selenium to a much higher level than do other plants on the same soil. In addition, these plants grow preferentially in seleniferous soil and have some value as indicators of possible toxicosis. Chronic selenosis can also be seen when drinking water contains as little as 0.1 to 2 ppm selenium. Selenium concentrations in feed should not exceed 5 ppm. Clinical signs usually appear after 3 weeks to 3 months of consuming the seleniferous plants.

The pathologic mechanism of chronic selenosis is unclear.[11,15,52] Selenium probably interferes with oxidative enzyme systems that possess sulfur-containing amino acids. The defective hoof and hair keratinization characteristic of chronic selenosis probably results from the substitution of sulfur with selenium in the sulfur-containing amino acids.

CLINICAL FEATURES

Chronic selenosis (alkali disease, bob-tailed disease) occurs in horses with no age, breed, or sex predilections.[11,15,44-52] Horses typically develop sore feet and lameness, which begins in the hind feet and progresses to involve all four feet. The coronary band area becomes tender, and various hoof wall deformities appear: hoof rings, corrugations, or horizontal cracks. In severe cases, the hooves may become necrotic and slough. The hair coat is rough, and there is easy breakage and progressive loss of the long hairs of the mane, tail (Fig. 13-9), and fetlocks. Generalized alopecia may be seen.

DIAGNOSIS

The differential diagnosis includes arsenic toxicosis, mercurialism, mimosine toxicosis, and malnutrition. The definitive diagnosis is based on history, physical examination, selenium levels in tissues, and selenium levels in soil, water, and feed.[11,15,44-52] Chronic selenosis is characterized by the following tissue levels of selenium: >2 ppm (blood), >10 ppm (hair), and 8 to 20 ppm (hoof).

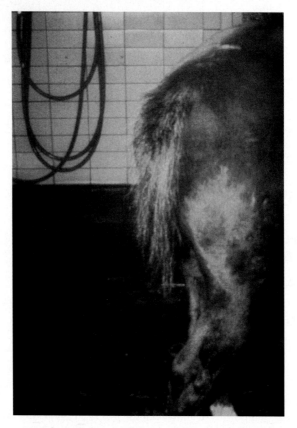

FIGURE 13-9. Selenosis. Note hypotrichotic tail. (*Courtesy W. McMullen.*)

CLINICAL MANAGEMENT

Fatalities are rare in chronic selenosis, but affected horses are often destroyed or sold because owners become impatient or discouraged with the chronic, prolonged recovery period, which usually takes several months.[11,15,44-52] The source of selenium must be identified and eliminated. Addition of inorganic arsenic, such as sodium arsenate, to drinking water (5 ppm) or salt supplements (30 to 40 ppm) is reported to be beneficial.[15] Naphthalene, given orally at a dosage of 4 to 5 gm for an adult horse, q24h for 5 days is reported to be effective.[15] The naphthalene is stopped for 5 days, then readministered for a second 5-day course. Other measures reported to be of some benefit include a high-protein diet (high in sulfur-containing amino acids) and the daily oral administration of 2 to 3 gm of DL-methionine.[15] Pretreatment with copper is reported to be an effective preventive measure.[15]

Arsenic Toxicosis

Chronic arsenic poisoning causes gastroenteritis, emaciation, and exfoliative dermatitis.[9,11,11a,15]

CAUSE AND PATHOGENESIS

Sources of arsenic include parasiticide dips and sprays, weed and orchard sprays, insect baits, and arsenical medicaments.[1-3,6,9,12-15] Arsenic is a general tissue poison and combines with and inactivates sulfhydryl groups in tissue enzymes.

CLINICAL FEATURES

Clinical signs include gastroenteritis, emaciation, variable appetite, and a dry, dull, rough, easily epilated haircoat, progressing to alopecia and exfoliative dermatitis.[1-3,6,9,12-15] Occasionally focal areas of skin necrosis and slow-healing ulcers may be seen. Some horses develop a long haircoat along with severe exfoliation.

DIAGNOSIS

The differential diagnosis includes selenosis, mercurialism, mimosine toxicosis, malnutrition, and hyperadrenocorticism. The definitive diagnosis is based on history, physical examination, and arsenic levels in the liver or kidneys greater than 10 to 15 mg/kg wet matter.[1-3,8,11-14]

CLINICAL MANAGEMENT

The source of arsenic must be identified and eliminated. More-or-less anecdotal treatment recommendations have included (1) D-penicillamine at 11 mg/kg orally q6h for 7 to 10 days,[12,13,15] or (2) sodium thiosulfate (10% to 20% aqueous solution) at 10 to 30 gm intravenously, followed by 20 to 60 gm orally q6h for 3 to 4 days,[3,7,8,11-15] or (3) dimercaprol (BAL) at 3 to 5 mg/kg intramuscularly q6h for 2 days, then q12h for 8 more days,[3,7,8,11-15] or (4) thioctic acid (with or without BAL) at 50 mg/kg intramuscularly q8h.[7,8,11-15] The relative success rate achieved with any of these protocols is not reported.

Mercurialism

Chronic mercury poisoning causes gastroenteritis, nephrosis, lameness, oral ulceration, emaciation, and progressive generalized alopecia.[9,11-15]

CAUSE AND PATHOGENESIS

Mercurialism is usually caused by the accidental feeding of grain that has been treated with organic mercurials used as antifungals.* It may also occur from the accidental overdosage of

---

*References 1-3, 11, 15, 53, 53a, 54.

mercury-containing medicaments, the licking-off of mercury-containing skin dressings, or from the percutaneous absorption of mercury-containing skin dressings. In addition, mercury-containing topical medicaments (e.g., mercurial "blisters") may produce severe primary irritant contact dermatitis.* The pathologic mechanism of mercurialism is not known.

CLINICAL FEATURES

Clinical signs with accidental feeding include gastroenteritis, oral ulceration, depression, anorexia, emaciation, nephrosis, a generalized loss of body hair, and then the loss of the long hairs of the mane, tail, and fetlocks. With topical application, the clinical signs vary from contact dermatitis to ulcers. Oral ulcers may be seen as a result of licking affected skin. Rarely, enough mercury is absorbed transcutaneously and/or orally to produce systemic illness.

DIAGNOSIS

The differential diagnosis includes selenosis, arsenic toxicosis, mimosine toxicosis, and malnutrition. The definitive diagnosis is based on history, physical examination, and mercury levels in the kidneys equal to or greater than 100 ppm.[1-3,11]

CLINICAL MANAGEMENT

The source of mercury must be identified and eliminated. Sodium thiosulfate as well as dimercaprol has been recommended for treatment (see Arsenic Toxicosis).[3,11,13,15] In addition, 4 gm of potassium iodide given orally q24h for 10 to 14 days has been reported to be beneficial.[9]

Iodism

Excessive intake of iodine is usually due to therapeutic overdosage or oversupplemented feeds.† Clinical signs include seromucoid nasal discharge, lacrimation, cough, variable appetite, and joint pain. Cutaneous changes are characterized by severe scaling (seborrhea sicca), with or without partial alopecia, which is most commonly seen over the dorsum, neck, head, and shoulders. Because iodine is rapidly metabolized and excreted from the body, removal of the source results in rapid recovery.

● PLANT TOXICOSES

Mimosine Toxicosis

Mimosine poisoning is characterized by alopecia.[7a,11,15,16]

CAUSE AND PATHOGENESIS

The toxic amino acid, mimosine, is a potent depilatory agent and occurs in *Mimosa pudica* (sensitive plant) and *Leucaena leucocephala* (jumbey tree). These plants are best suited to humid and subhumid tropical lowlands, and there is a great deal of variation in the effects of poisoning depending on the variety of the plant, the amount of other fodder available, and the selection of the feed by the horse. Mimosine toxicosis has been reported in Australia, New Zealand, New Guinea, the West Indies, Africa, Hawaii, and Florida.

CLINICAL FEATURES

Mimosine toxicosis is characterized by a gradual loss of the long hairs of the mane, tail (Fig. 13-10), and fetlocks. Hoof dystrophies and laminitis may be seen.

---

*References 6, 8, 9, 11, 15, 53a, 55.
†References 1-3, 6, 8, 9, 11, 11a, 15, 56.

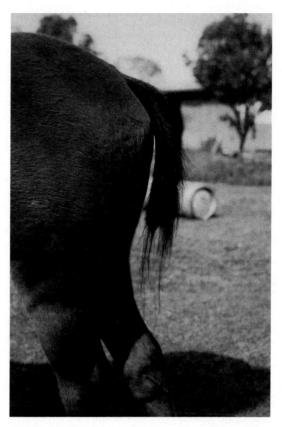

FIGURE 13-10. Mimosine toxicosis. Note hypotrichotic tail. (*Courtesy R. Pascoe.*)

DIAGNOSIS

The differential diagnosis includes selenosis, mercurialism, alopecia areata, and mane and tail dysplasias.

CLINICAL MANAGEMENT

All toxic effects are quickly reversible by removing horses from access to the plants. The addition of 1% $FeSO_4$ to the feed has been reported to reduce the severity of the toxicosis.[9,11,15]

Hairy Vetch Toxicosis

Hairy vetch (*Vicia villosa*) has been reported to be the possible cause of a rare generalized granulomatous disease in horses.[57,58] Clinical signs included severe generalized exfoliative dermatitis, weight loss, fever, and enlargement of palpable lymph nodes. At necropsy, multiple organ systems were affected. Histopathologic findings included sarcoidal granulomatous inflammation with numerous multinucleated histiocytic giant cells. This condition was likened to hairy vetch toxicosis in cattle. However, major differences in the bovine disease include marked pruritus, diarrhea, and large numbers of eosinophils involved in the granulomatous inflammatory process.[15]

The equine syndrome bears a striking resemblance to equine sarcoidosis (see Chapter 15). Either hairy vetch toxicosis is clinically and pathologically a little different in horses than in cattle and is, indeed, the cause of the described generalized granulomatous disease, or the two horses actually had sarcoidosis and the presence of hairy vetch in pasture was just coincidental.

Sorghum Toxicosis

Plants from the genus *Sorghum* (Johnson, milo, and Sudan grasses) were hypothesized to produce ataxia, cystitis, and urinary incontinence, which result in urine scalding (primary irritant contact dermatitis) in the perineal region,[11,11a,15,16,59-59c] medial thighs, and cranial, medial, and distal pelvic limbs. The toxin is presently speculative, and candidates included hurrin, a cyanogenic glycoside, and lathyrogens.[59-59c] It has been hypothesized that exposure to sublethal doses of hydrocyanic acid produces axonal degeneration and demyelination. Successful therapy has not been reported.

Hoary Alyssum Toxicosis

Hoary alyssum (*Berteroa incana*) toxicosis is characterized by edema of the legs, laminitis and fever.[60] Clinical signs begin 18 to 36 hours after the plant is eaten, and disappear 2 to 4 days after the plant source is removed. The plant, a member of the *Cruciferae* family (mustards), is widespread in the United States. Not all exposed horses become affected. Under experimental conditions,[60] edema of one or more legs was the most consistent clinical sign, and this occurred with or without laminitis, and with or without fever in 56% of the horses.

● MYCOTOXICOSES

Ergotism

Ergotism is an extremely rare mycotoxicosis of horses caused by alkaloids produced by *Claviceps purpurea*, and is characterized by dry gangrene and sloughing of distal extremities.[11,11a,15,61,62]

CAUSE AND PATHOGENESIS

Ergotism is caused by a series of active alkaloids (ergotamine, ergotoxine, ergonovine, ergocryptine, and so forth) contained in grains infected with the fungus *Claviceps purpurea*.[1-3,11,15] Ergot is the common name given to the sclerotium formed by *C. purpurea*. The sclerotium is the fungal mass that replaces the seed or kernel of the infected plant. *C. purpurea* infects over 200 grasses and cultivated cereals, especially wheat, barley, rye, and oats. Infection develops abundantly during wet seasons. The fungal alkaloids cause persistent spasm of arterioles, resulting in congestion proximal to the spasm and ischemia distal to the spasm. The vasospasm is exaggerated by cold.

CLINICAL FEATURES

Clinical signs may occur as soon as 7 days after exposure to contaminated feed. Typically, lameness of the hind limbs is noted first, followed by swelling at the coronary band, which progresses to the fetlocks. The feet become necrotic, cold, and insensitive, and a distinct line separates viable from dead tissue. The front feet, ears, and tail may be similarly affected and, in severe cases, may slough.

DIAGNOSIS

The differential diagnosis includes frostbite, traumatic or chemical gangrene, vasculitis, and septicemia. The definitive diagnosis is based on history, physical examination, and feed analysis.[11,15] The purple to black ergot sclerotia can be visualized in unmilled grain. Histopathologic findings include degeneration and necrosis of vascular endothelium, thrombosis, and necrosis of surrounding tissues.[15]

CLINICAL MANAGEMENT

The source of ergot must be identified and eliminated. Symptomatic treatment may include warm packs and gentle cleansing to increase circulation, and antibiotics. Suggested preventive measures include using ergot-free seed, crop rotation, plowing deeply, and mowing down surrounding grasses.[61]

Stachybotryotoxicosis

Stachybotryotoxicosis is characterized by ulceronecrotic lesions of the mucous membranes and skin, bone marrow suppression, and hemorrhage.[11,15]

CAUSE AND PATHOGENESIS

Stachybotrys atra is a saprophytic fungus that grows on hay and straw and produces toxins referred to as *macrocytic trichothecenes (satratoxins)*.[3,11,15,66,67] These toxins cause bone marrow suppression, resulting in profound thrombocytopenia, neutropenia, and hemorrhage. In addition, ulceronecrotic lesions are produced in skin and mucous membranes.

CLINICAL FEATURES

Stachybotryotoxicosis has mainly been reported in Europe. Clinical signs are usually seen within 1 to 2 days of beginning to eat toxin-containing feed, and the severity is dependent on the amount of toxins ingested. Initial lesions consist of painful necrotic ulcers in the mouth, nasal region, and lips.[63-65,67,68] Large scales, crusts, and fissures then appear. These mucocutaneous lesions are accompanied by conjunctivitis, rhinitis, and mandibular lymphadenopathy. Within 2 weeks, systemic signs are seen: fever, depression, anorexia, bleeding diathesis, colic, diarrhea, weakness, lameness, and hyperexcitability. Endoscopic examinations may reveal ulcers in the nasal passages, pharynx, and larynx. Electrocardiographic examination often reveals second-degree heart block. Death frequently occurs when systemic signs are present.

DIAGNOSIS

The differential diagnosis includes pemphigus vulgaris, bullous pemphigoid, systemic lupus erythematosus, vasculitis and drug reaction. The definitive diagnosis is based on history, physical examination, and the isolation of *S. atra* and its toxins (dermonecrotoxic in 3 days after applied topically to the skin of young rats) from contaminated feed.[63,67] Systemically ill horses are neutropenic and thrombocytopenic. Histopathologic findings include purpura and necrosis.

CLINICAL MANAGEMENT

There is no specific treatment for the disease, other than to remove the source of toxins. If further intoxication is prevented, spontaneous remission may occur within a few days (early, mild cases) to 2 weeks.

● ZOOTOXICOSES

Snake Bite

Two families of snakes in the United States contain venomous species: the *Elapidae* and the *Viperidae*.[11a,71,78b] The *Elapidae* include the coral snakes, whose venom is highly neurotoxic but which are regarded as a minor danger to horses. The *Viperidae* are commonly referred to as "pit vipers" and account for most reported snake bites. Three genera of pit vipers are present in the United States: *Agkistrodon* (copperheads and cottonmouths), *Crotalus,* and *Sistrusus* (rattlesnakes). The pit vipers can deliver venom efficiently and rapidly. Rattlesnakes are the most numerous: the Mojave, the western diamondback, the western, the timber, the Massasauga, and the eastern diamondback. Each species has a defined ecologic niche.

Snake venoms include varying amounts of hemotoxic and neurotoxic constituents (Table 13-1). These substances can produce a variety of systemic abnormalities.[71-76]

Snake bites occur most commonly during spring and summer and are seen most commonly on the nose, head, neck, and legs.[11-13,15,69-73a,77,78b] Cutaneous reaction to venom is characterized by rapid, progressive edema, which usually obliterates fang marks, pain, and occasionally local

● Table 13-1	COMMON SNAKE VENOM CONSTITUENTS[71-75]	
PROINFLAMMATORY EFFECTS	BLOOD DYSCRASIAS AND ALTERED HEMOSTATIC EFFECTS	DESTRUCTION OF CONNECTIVE TISSUE AND MYONECROTIC EFFECTS
Kininogenases	Phospholipases	Collagenase
Bradykinin-potentiating factor	Crotalase	Hyaluronidase
Direct lytic factor	Proteases	Elastase
Crotamine	Platelet adhesion factor	Phospholipase A_2
		Ribonuclease
Amine-liberating factor	Hemorrhagic toxins a, b, c	Deoxyribonuclease
	Thrombin-like enzyme	5′ Nucleotidase
	Factor X activator	
	Prothrombin activator	

hemorrhage. Pain is variable. Bites around the face are potentially serious because of rapid swelling and respiratory involvement. Ecchymoses and discoloration become apparent several hours later and may progress to necrosis and sloughing. Various systemic signs, including profuse sweating, may be present or develop with time.[70-76] In one study of horses bitten by prairie rattlesnakes,[70a] the most commonly observed clinical signs were swelling associated with the bite wound (100% of cases), fever (63%), tachycardia (56%), dyspnea (56%), tachypnea (33%), and epistaxis (45%). Commonly observed hematologic and biochemical abnormalities included anemia, leukocytosis, hyperfibrinogenemia, and elevated levels of creatine kinase, aspartate transaminase, and L-iditol dehydrogenase.

The management of snake bites is often complicated, arduous, and controversial.[70a,71,74-76] During the general acute phase (the first 24 hours after envenomation), first aid includes calming and immobilization to help decrease venom absorption and distribution. Tourniquets are useful only in the first 30 minutes after the bite and are only applicable to legs. Incision and suction of bites is ineffective, destructive to underlying tissues, and dangerous to the caregiver.

The goals of therapy are to prevent or control shock, neutralize the venom, minimize tissue necrosis, and prevent secondary bacterial infection.[70a,71,74-76,78b] Minimal tissue reaction in the area of the fang marks indicates that the horse was bitten by a nonvenomous snake, or a venomous snake that liberated little or no venom. In this case, therapy includes routine wound care, tetanus prophylaxis, and antibiotics. When moderate to marked local tissue reaction is present, with or without concurrent systemic signs, treatment may also include the use of antivenin, glucocorticoids, nonsteroidal anti-inflammatory agents, sedatives and painkillers, intravenous fluids, surgical débridement, and other forms of supportive care. The reader is referred to recent publications on the intricacies, possible complications, and controversy attending the various modes of therapy.[11a,70a,71,73-76,78b] Some authors believe that antivenin is unnecessary in adult horses because of their great body weight, relatively low mortality rates, and the cost of the antivenin. Antivenin may be considered in small horses, ponies, or foals with moderate to severe bites, but is most effective if administered within 4 hours after envenomation.[71] Antivenin therapy can be accompanied by anaphylactic and serum sickness reactions.[71]

Several factors influence the horse's prognosis, including the delay between envenomation and the initiation of therapy; the amount of physical activity postbite; the size of the snake; the size of the horse; the location of the bite; the time of year; the age of the snake; and when the snake last liberated venom.[71] Many bites do not result in envenomation.[71] In one report of horses bitten by prairie rattlesnakes,[70a] 25% of the horses died.

● PHOTODERMATITIS

Electromagnetic radiation comprises a continuous spectrum of wavelengths varying from fractions of angstroms to thousands of meters. The ultraviolet (UV) spectrum is of particular importance in dermatology.[4a] UVC (less than 290 nm) is damaging to cells but does not typically reach the earth's surface because of the ozone layer. UVB (290 to 320 nm) is often referred to as the *sunburn* or *erythema spectrum* and is about 1000 times more erythemogenic than UVA. UVA (320 to 400 nm) penetrates deeper into the skin than UVB and is the spectrum associated with photosensitivity reactions.

Ultraviolet light (UVL) is partially reflected, absorbed, and transmitted inward. Absorbed light raises the energy level of light-absorbing molecules (chromophores), resulting in various biochemical processes that can damage virtually any component of a cell. This damage can result in cellular hyperproliferation, mutagenesis, alteration of cell surface markers, and toxicity. Chromophores in the skin include keratin proteins, blood, hemoglobin, porphyrin, carotene, nucleic acids, melanin, lipoproteins, peptide bonds, and aromatic amino acids such as tyrosine, tryptophan, and histidine.[86a] Natural barriers to UVL damage include the stratum corneum, melanin, blood, and carotenes. Melanins absorb UVL and scavenge free radicals produced during the burning, but release other free radicals that can be equally or more damaging. These barriers can easily be overcome by prolonged, repeated exposure to sunlight.

Photodermatology is an ever-expanding field in human medicine and includes photodynamic mechanisms and various specific diseases not recognized in veterinary medicine.[4a,86a,86b] Phototoxicity and photosensitivity are of primary concern to veterinary clinicians. *Phototoxicity* is the classic sunburn reaction and is a dose-related response to light exposure. *Photosensitivity* occurs when the skin has increased susceptibility to the damaging effects of UVL because of the production, ingestion, and injection of or contact with a photodynamic agent. *Photoallergy* is a reaction to a chemical (systemic or contact) and UVL in which an immune mechanism can be demonstrated. *Photocontact dermatitis* occurs when contactants cause photosensitivity or photoallergy. *Phytophotodermatitis* is caused by contact with certain plants.

Phototoxicity

Phototoxicity (solar dermatitis, actinic dermatitis, sunburn) occurs from an actinic reaction on white skin, light skin, or damaged skin (e.g., depigmented or scarred areas) that is not sufficiently covered by hair.* The condition occurs when such skin is exposed to direct or reflected sunshine. The rapidity of onset and the severity of the reaction depend on various factors related to the animal, the duration of sun exposure, and the intensity of the sunlight. The sun's rays are most intense during summer months from 9 AM to 3 PM. Altitude influences solar intensity. For every 300-m (1000-ft) increase in elevation, the sun's intensity increases by 4%.[4a] The pathogenesis of phototoxicity is incompletely understood, but it involves the epidermis and blood vessels of the superficial and deep plexuses. Exposure to UVB and UVC results in the formation of clusters of vacuolated keratinocytes in the superficial epidermis (so-called "sunburn cells"), as well as apoptotic keratinocytes, vascular dilatation and leakage, depletion of Langerhans' cells and mast cells, and an increase in the tissue levels of histamine, prostaglandins, leukotrienes, other vasoactive compounds, inflammatory cytokines, adhesion molecules, and reactive oxygen species.[4a,84a]

Oxygen intermediates—superoxide radical (O_2^-), hydrogen peroxide (H_2O_2), and hydroxyl radical (HO·)—may be particularly important in the pathogenesis of solar damage.[81a] These substances deplete antioxidants, recruit neutrophils, and can destroy and degrade all components of connective tissue. Natural defenses (antioxidants) include superoxide dismutase, catalase, glutathione peroxidase, vitamin E, vitamin C, and ubiquinones.

---

*References 4a, 6, 8, 9, 11, 15.

Photosensitization

There are three features basic to all types of photosensitization: (1) the presence of a photodynamic agent within the skin, (2) the concomitant exposure to a sufficient amount of certain wavelengths of UVL, and (3) the cutaneous absorption of this UVL, which is greatly facilitated by lack of pigment and hair coat. Regardless of the type of photodynamic agent involved or how it reaches the skin, all inflammatory reactions are assumed to involve the same basic pathogenesis and to produce similar clinical signs. Factors that influence the severity of the reaction include the amount of reactive pigment within the skin and the degree of exposure to sunlight.

Photosensitization is classified according to the source of the photodynamic agent[4,5,7-16,79-93]: (1) primary photosensitization (a preformed or metabolically derived photodynamic agent reaches the skin by ingestion, injection, or contact), (2) hepatogenous photosensitization (blood phylloerythrin levels are elevated in association with liver abnormalities), (3) photosensitization due to aberrant pigment synthesis (porphyria), and (4) idiopathic photosensitization (Table 13-2).

There are instances of apparent photosensitization in horses in which the pathologic mechanism is not known. In some instances, various lush pastures have been incriminated. The photosensitization occurring in association with ingestion of clover, alfalfa, lucerne, vetch, and oats

● Table 13-2 **CAUSES OF PHOTOSENSITIZATION IN THE HORSE**

Primary Photosensitization	Photodynamic Agent
Hypericum perforatum (St. Johns' Wort, Klamath weed)	Hypericin
Fagopyrum sagittatum, Polygonum fagopyrum (buck wheat)	Fagopyrin, photofagopyrin
Lolium perenne (perennial rye grass)	Perloline
Medicago denticulata (burr trefoil)	Aphids
Phenothiazine	Phenothiazine sulfoxide
Thiazides	?
Acariflavines	?
Rose bengal	?
Methylene blue	?
Sulfonamides	?
Tetracyclines	?

Hepatogenous Photosensitization	Hepatotoxin
Kochia scoparia (burning bush, fireweed)	?
Myoporum laetum (ngaio tree)	Ngaione
Brassica spp. (rape, kale)	?
Heliotropium europaeum (heliotrope)	Pyrrolizidine alkaloids (lasiocarpine, heliotrine)
Senecio spp. (ragworts)	Pyrrolizidine alkaloids (retrorsine)
Amsinckia spp. (tarweed, fiddle-neck)	Pyrrolizidine alkaloids
Crotalaria spp. (crotalaria, rattleweed)	Pyrrolizidine alkaloids (monocrotaline, fulvine, crispatine)
Microcystis spp. (blue-green algae in water)	Cyclic peptide
Phomopsis leptostromiforms (on lupins)	Phomopsin A
Liver abscess	Bacteria/toxins
Lymphosarcoma	Malignant lymphocytes
Hepatic carcinoma	Malignant hepatocytes
Copper	
Phosphorus	
Carbon tetrachloride	
Phenanthridium	
Serum, antiserum	? (Viral? immunologic?)

(*Trifolium* spp., *Vicia* spp., and *Avena* spp.) has in some instances been thought to be primary, and in others hepatogenous. Photodermatitis has been seen in association with *Dermatophilus congolensis* infections of light-skinned areas of horses (see Chapter 4). The condition disappears when the dermatophilosis is cured. Photodermatitis has also been recognized in association with some cases of metritis in mares.

Cutaneous lesions are usually restricted to light-skinned, sparsely haired areas but, in severe cases, may extend into the surrounding dark-skinned areas as well. Restlessness and discomfort often precede visible skin lesions. Erythema and edema may be followed by vesicles and bullae, ulcers, oozing, crusting, scaling, and hair loss. Secondary bacterial infections are frequent. In severe cases, necrosis and sloughing may occur. Variable degrees of pruritus and/or pain are present. The muzzle (Fig. 13-4, *C* through *E*), eyelids, lips, face, pinnae, back, perineum, distal legs (Fig. 13-4, *F*), and coronets are most commonly affected. Conjunctivitis, keratitis, and corneal edema may be seen in some cases.[80,91] Horses often attempt to protect themselves from sunlight.

Diagnosis of photosensitization is based on history, physical examination, investigation of the premises, and laboratory evaluation. Liver function tests should always be performed, whether the horse is showing clinical signs of liver disease or not.[15] Primary photodynamic agents can be identified with several biologic assay systems. The number of animals at risk compared with the number of animals affected helps determine whether the photodermatitis is photosensitive (many animals affected) or photoallergic (one animal affected). Photodermatitis confined to the distal limbs and/or muzzle is suggestive of photocontact reactions (pasture plants, environmental sprays, topical medicaments) and photoactivated vasculopathies (see Chapter 9). The histopathology of photodermatitis in horses has not been the subject of detailed reports. By the time most cases are biopsied, the condition is somewhat chronic and histologic findings include diffuse necrotizing or fibrosing dermatitis (Fig. 13-11). Rarely, when specimens from more acute lesions are taken, changes include epidermal and dermal edema and the intramural and perivascular deposition of amorphous eosinophilic material in superficial dermal blood vessels (Fig. 13-12).

In general, the prognosis is favorable for primary photosensitization, but poor for hepatogenous photosensitization. The general principles of therapy include (1) identification and elimination of the photodynamic agent, (2) avoidance of sunlight, and (3) symptomatic treatment for hepatic disease and other extracutaneous disorders. The photodermatitis may be ameliorated with systemic glucocorticoids, nonsteroidal anti-inflammatory agents (aspirin, phenylbutazone), and cool, soothing topical applications. Systemic antibiotics may be required for secondary bacterial infections, and surgical débridement may be required for areas of necrosis and sloughing.

Actinic Keratosis

Actinic (solar) keratoses are seen in horses and are premalignant epithelial dysplasias (see Chapter 16).

• MISCELLANEOUS EFFECTS OF SOLAR EXPOSURE

Exposure to UVL is an important factor in precipitating or potentiating a number of skin lesions and may also exacerbate generalized systemic disease activity.[86a,86b] Although the role of UVL is clearly defined in some conditions, its pathogenic role in other disorders is less well understood. For example, UVL exposure may induce or exacerbate the lesions of discoid lupus erythematosus, systemic lupus erythematosus, pemphigus, and pemphigoid (see Chapter 9).

In addition, UVL exposure of skin has important local and systemic immunologic consequences (photoimmunologic changes).[86a] For example, exposure to UVB or UVA changes Langerhans' cell morphologic features and function and influences cutaneous cytokine production. Impaired antigen recognition and processing and impaired immune responses may influence susceptibility

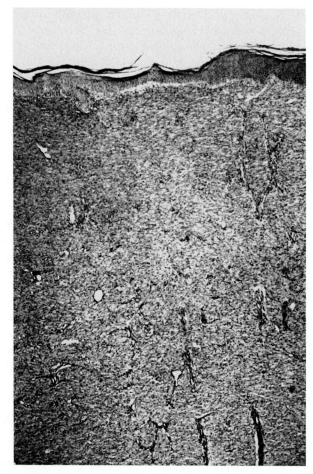

FIGURE 13-11. Photodermatitis due to hepatogenous photosensitization. Biopsy specimens from chronic lesions are typified by diffuse fibrosing dermatitis.

to cutaneous neoplasms and infections. The damaging effects on cutaneous immunity of low-dose UVB are genetically determined in mice.[92a] This UVB susceptibility is mediated almost exclusively by TNF-α, and the trait appears to be a risk factor for the development of squamous cell carcinoma and basal cell carcinoma.

● HEAD SHAKING

Head shaking is an abnormal condition wherein the horse flicks, nods, or shakes its head in the absence of obvious extraneous stimuli and with such frequency and violence that the horse becomes difficult or dangerous to use or appears to be distressed.[94-99] Although widely recognized, head shaking remains a poorly understood entity. Potential causes in horses are legion (Table 13-3).

In most instances, the clinical signs are seasonal (spring through fall). Clinical signs are usually worse when the animals are exposed to sunlight and are often first observed when the horses are exercised. Most horses shake their heads in a vertical plane and exhibit variable degrees of snorting and rubbing the muzzle on objects.

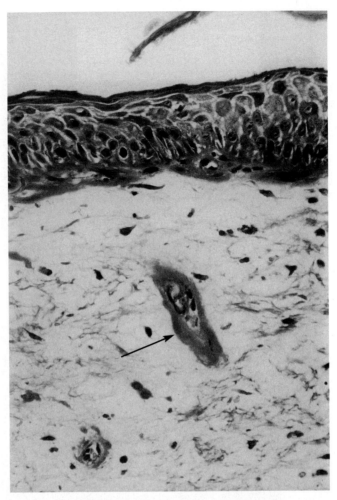

FIGURE 13-12. Photodermatitis due to hepatogenous photosensitization. Biopsy specimens from earlier lesions show epidermal and dermal edema and the intramural and perivascular deposition of amorphous eosinophilic material in superficial dermal blood vessels (*arrow*).

● Table 13-3 **CAUSES OF HEAD SHAKING IN THE HORSE**

Ear mites	Dental periapical osteitis
Trombiculosis	Periodontal disease
Protozoal myeloencephalitis	Buccal lesions
Guttural pouch mycosis	Trigeminal or infraorbital neuritis
Otitis externa/media/interna	Uveal or retinal lesions
Otic foreign body	Vasomotor rhinitis
Traumatic cranial/cervical injuries	Allergic rhinitis
Exostoses of the occipital protuberance	Stereotypic behaviour
Cerebral encephalopathy (hepatic, togavirus encephalitis)	Optic-trigeminal nerve summation (photic)
Cervical myositis	Bit/bridle problems
Osteoma of paranasal sinuses	Idiopathy

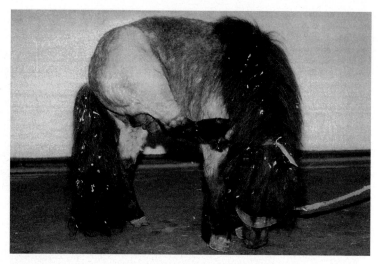

FIGURE 13-13. Constant scratching of neck associated with fracture of axis. (*Courtesy M. Sloet.*)

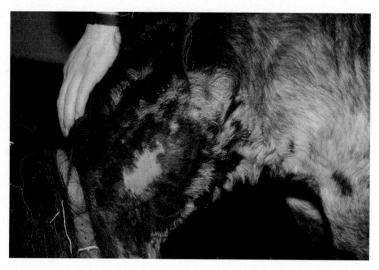

FIGURE 13-14. Close-up of horse in Fig. 13-13. Note traumatic hypotrichosis, alopecia, and excoriation of lateral neck. (*Courtesy M. Sloet.*)

Many horses are better or asymptomatic when accommodated indoors during daylight hours or when their eyes are covered to block sunlight. Many of these horses improve greatly when treated with cyproheptadine (0.3 to 0.6 mg/kg, q12h, orally).[95,96,99] It has been postulated that these horses have optic-trigeminal nerve summation similar to "photic sneezing" in humans (sunlight stimulates the facial sensory branches of the trigeminal nerve).

● PRURITUS AND NEUROLOGIC DISEASES

In humans, lesions of the central nervous system can be associated with focal pruritus.[100] Examples include brain abscess, brain neoplasm, aneurysm, and syringomyelia with dermatomal pruritus.

Localized pruritus has been recognized in a horse with a fracture of the axis.[100] The horse constantly scratched at the cranial neck area bilaterally (Figs. 13-13 and 13-14) and had some ataxia and hypermetria of the hind legs. Radiography revealed a fracture of the axis, and a CT-scan revealed compression of the local cervical nerve. The horse was euthanized.

● REFERENCES

General References

1. Buck WB, et al: Clinical and Diagnostic Veterinary Toxicology II. Kendall/Hunt, Dubuque, 1976.
2. Casarett LJ, Doull J: Toxicology. MacMillan Publishing, New York, 1975.
3. Clarke ML, et al: Veterinary Toxicology II. Baillière-Tindall, London, 1981.
4. Colahan PN, et al (eds): Equine Medicine and Surgery IV. American Veterinary Publications, Santa Barbara, 1991.
4a. Freedberg IM, et al (eds): Fitzpatrick's Dermatology in General Medicine V. McGraw-Hill Book Co, New York, 1999.
5. Kobluk CN, et al (eds): The Horse. Diseases and Management. W.B. Saunders Co, Philadelphia, 1995.
6. Kral F, Schwartzman RM: Veterinary and Comparative Dermatology. J.B. Lippincott, Philadelphia, 1964.
7. Mansmann RA, et al (eds): Equine Medicine & Surgery II. American Veterinary Publications, Wheaton, 1972.
8. Mansmann RA, et al (eds): Equine Medicine & Surgery III. American Veterinary Publications, Santa Barbara, 1982.
9. Pascoe RR: Equine Dermatoses. University of Sydney Post-Graduate Foundation in Veterinary Science, Vet Rev No 22, 1981.
10. Pascoe RRR, Knottenbelt DC: Manual of Equine Dermatology. W.B. Saunders Co, Philadelphia, 1999.
11. Radostits OM, et al: Veterinary Medicine. A Textbook of the Diseases of Cattle, Sheep, Pigs, Goats, and Horses VIII. Baillière Tindall, Philadelphia, 1994.
11a. Reed SM, Bayly WM (eds): Equine Internal Medicine. W.B. Saunders Co, Philadelphia, 1998.
12. Robinson NE (ed): Current Therapy in Equine Medicine. W.B. Saunders Co, Philadelphia, 1983.
13. Robinson NE (ed): Current Therapy in Equine Medicine II. W.B. Saunders Co, Philadelphia, 1987.
14. Robinson NE (ed): Current Therapy in Equine Medicine III. W.B. Saunders Co, Philadelphia, 1992.
14a. Robinson NE (ed): Current Therapy in Equine Medicine IV. W.B. Saunders Co, Philadelphia, 1997.
15. Scott DW: Large Animal Dermatology. W.B. Saunders Co, Philadelphia, 1988.
15a. Stannard AA: The skin. In: Catcott EJ, Smithcors JF (eds): Equine Medicine and Surgery II. American Veterinary Publications, Inc, Santa Barbara, 1972, p 381.
16. Thomsett LR: Noninfectious skin diseases of horses. Vet Clin N Am Large Anim Pract 6:59, 1984.

Hygroma

16a. Jann H, et al: Treatment of acquired bursitis (hygroma) by en-bloc resection. Equine Pract 12:8, 1990.
16b. van Veenendaal JC, et al: Treatment of hygromata in horses. Aust Vet J 57:513, 1981.

Foreign Bodies

17. Kiper ML, et al: Foreign body and abscess in the flank of a horse. Mod Vet Pract 69:97, 1988.
18. Pascoe RR: Equine nodular and erosive skin conditions: The common and not so common. Equine Vet Educ 3:153, 1991.
19. Rollins JB, et al: Ultrasonographic identification of cactus spines in the distal extremity of three horses. Equine Pract 17(10):31, 1995.
20. Spurlock GH, Spurlock SL: Projectile dart foreign body in a horse. J Am Vet Med Assoc 193:565, 1988.
21. Trostle SS, Hendrickson DA: Suture sinus formation following closure of ventral midline incisions with polypropylene in three horses. J Am Vet Med Assoc 207:742, 1995.
22. Vatistas NJ, et al: Gunshot injuries in horses: 22 cases (1971-1993). J Am Vet Med Assoc 207:1198, 1995.
22a. Williams PD: Lumps, bumps, and swellings—a clinical approach to diagnosis. Equine Vet Educ 7:300, 1995.

Myospherulosis

23. Lazaron A, et al: Dermal spherulosis (myospherulosis) after topical treatment for psoriasis. J Am Acad Dermatol J Am Acad Dermatol 30 (part 1):265, 1994.
24. Liggett AD, et al: Myospherulosis in the subcutis of a pony. Can J Vet Res 51:150, 1987.

Arteriovenous Fistula

25. Hosgood G: Arteriovenous fistulas: pathophysiology, diagnosis, and treatment. Comp Cont Educ 11:625, 1989.
26. Welch RD, et al: Pulsed spectral Doppler evaluation of a peripheral arteriovenous fistula in a horse. J Am Vet Med Assoc 200:1360, 1992.

Gangrene

26a. Steinman A, et al: Gangrene in the distal extremity of all four limbs of a 2-week-old foal. Can Vet J 41:861, 2000.

Subcutaneous Emphysema

27. Brown CM, et al: Intramuscular injection techniques and the development of clostridial myositis or cellulitis in horses. J Am Vet Med Assoc 193:668, 1988.
28. Caron JP, Townsend HGG: Tracheal perforation and widespread subcutaneous emphysema in a horse. Can Vet J 25:339, 1984.
29. DeBowes RM, Gavin P: What is your diagnosis? J Am Vet Med Assoc 180:781, 1982.
30. Fubini SL, et al: Tracheal rupture in two horses. J Am Vet Med Assoc 187:69, 1985.
31. Hance SR, Robertson JT: Subcutaneous emphysema from an axillary wound that resulted in pneumomediastinum and bilateral pneumothorax in a horse. J Am Vet Med Assoc 200:1107, 1992.

31a. Laverty S, et al: Penetrating wounds of the thorax in 15 horses. Equine Vet J 28:220, 1996.
32. Marble SL, et al: Subcutaneous emphysema in a neonatal foal. J Am Vet Med Assoc 208:97, 1996.

Draining Tracts

32a. Ferguson HR, et al: Surgical correction of a thoracic abscess in a colt. J Am Vet Med Assoc 156:868, 1970.
32b. Spoormakers TJP, Klein WR: An unusual cause of a pectoral fistula: sequestration of the first rib in the horse. Equine Vet Educ 13:83, 2001.

Burns

33. Fox SM, et al: Management of a large thermal burn in a horse. Comp Cont Educ 10:88, 1988.
34. Fubini SL: Burns. In: Robinson, NE (ed.): Current Therapy in Equine Medicine II. W.B. Saunders Co, Philadelphia, 1986, p 639.
35. Geiser DR, Walker RD: Management of large animal thermal injuries. Comp Cont Educ 7:S69, 1985.
36. Scarratt WK, et al: Cutaneous thermal injury in a horse. Equine Pract 6:13, 1984.

Primary Irritant Contact Dermatitis

36a. Bracken FK, et al: A condition akin to immersion foot. Vet Med 81:562, 1986.
37. Campagnolo, E. R. et al: Outbreak of vesicular dermatitis among horses at a midwestern horse show. J Am Vet Med Assoc 207:211, 1995.
38. Case AA, Coffmann JR: Waste oil: toxic for horses. Vet Clin N Am 3:273, 1973.
39. Cordes T: Apparent contact dermatitis in hunter/jumper show horses. Mod Vet Pract 68:240, 1987.
40. Edwards WC, Manin T: Malicious mutilation of a horse with sulfuric acid. Vet Med Small Anim Clin 77:90, 1982.
41. Ihrke PJ: Contact dermatitis. In: Robinson, N. E. (ed.): Current Therapy in Equine Medicine. W.B. Saunders Co, Philadelphia, 1983, p 547.
42. Rebhun WC: Chemical keratitis in a horse. Vet Med Small Anim Clin 75:1537, 1980.
43. Salsbury DL: Pine tar irritation in a horse. Vet Med Small Anim Clin 65:60, 1970.

Selenosis

44. Crinion RA, O'Connor JP: Selenium intoxication in horses. Irish Vet J 32:81, 1978.
45. Dewes HF, Lowe MD: Suspected selenium poisoning in a horse. N J Vet J 35:53, 1987.
46. Hultine JD, et al: Selenium toxicosis in the horse. Equine Pract 1:57, 1979.
47. Knott SG, et al: Selenium poisoning in horses in North Queensland. Queensl J Agric Sci 15:43, 1958.
48. Knott SG, McCray CWR: Two naturally occurring outbreaks of selenosis in Queensland. Aust Vet J 35:161, 1959.
49. McLaughlin JG, Cullen J: Clinical cases of chronic selenosis in horses. Irish Vet J 40:136, 1986.
50. Muth OH, Binns W: Selenium toxicity in domestic animals. Ann N Y Acad Sci 111:583, 1964.
51. Traub-Dargatz JL, et al: Selenium toxicity in horses. Comp Cont Educ 8:771, 1986.
52. Witte ST, et al: Chronic selenosis in horses fed locally produced alfalfa hay. J Am Vet Med Assoc 202:406, 1993.

Mercurialism

53. Frohner E: Case of mercurial poisoning in the horse. Vet J 14:448, 1907.
53a. Leuthold A: Mercury poisoning in the horse. Schweiz Arch Tierheilk 105:668, 1963.
54. Markel MD, et al: Acute renal failure associated with application of a mercuric blister in a horse. J Am Vet Med Assoc 185:91, 1984.
55. Schuh JCL, et al: Concurrent mercuric blister and dimethyl sulphoxide (DMSO) application as a cause of mercury toxicosis in two horses. Equine Vet J 20:68, 1988.

Iodism

56. Fadok VA, Wild S: Suspected cutaneous iodism in a horse. J Am Vet Med Assoc 183:1104, 1983.

Hairy Vetch Toxicosis

57. Anderson CA, Divers TJ: Systemic granulomatous inflammation in a horse grazing hairy vetch. J Am Vet Med Assoc 183:569, 1983.
58. Woods LW, et al: Systemic granulomatous disease in a horse grazing pasture containing vetch (Vicia sp.). J Vet Diagn Invest 4:356, 1992.

Sorghum Toxicosis

59. Adams LG: Cystitis and ataxia associated with sorghum ingestion by horses. J Am Vet Med Assoc 155:518, 1969.
59a. Knight PR: Equine cystitis and ataxia associated with grazing of pastures dominated by sorghum species. Aust Vet J 44:257, 1968.
59b. Morgan SE, et al: Sorghum cystitis ataxia syndrome in horses. Vet Hum Toxicol 32:582, 1990.
59c. Van Kampen KR: Sudan grass and sorghum poisoning of horses: a possible lathyrogenic disease. J Am Vet Med Assoc 156:629, 1970.

Hoary Alyssum Toxicosis

60. Geor RJ, et al: Toxicosis of horses after ingestion of hoary alyssum. J Am Vet Med Assoc 201:63, 1992.

Ergotism

61. Hintz HF: Ergotism. Equine Pract 10(5):6, 1988.
62. Wilcox EV: Ergotism in horses. Montana Agric Ext Sta Bull 22:49, 1899.

Stachybotryotoxicosis

63. Forgacs J, Carll WT: Mycotoxicoses. Adv Vet Sci 7:273, 1962.
64. Launer P, et al: Stachybotryotoxikose in einem Pferdebestand. Mh Vet Med 42:593, 1987.
65. LeBars J: La Stachybotryotoxicose: une mycotoxicose fatale due à Stachybotrys atra Corda. Revue Rev Méd Vét 128:51, 1977.
66. LeBars J, LeBars P: Toxinogenesis and development conditions of Stachybotrys atra in France. Acta Vet Scand 87 (suppl.): 349, 1991.
67. Lefebvre HP, et al: Three cases of equine stachybotryotoxicosis. Rev Méd Vét 145:267, 1994.
68. Servantie J, et al: Stachybotryotoxicose équine: première description en France. Rev Méd Vét 136:687, 1985.

Snake Bite

69. Arbuckle J, Theakston R: Facial swelling in a pony attributable to an adder bite. Vet Rec 131:75, 1992.
70. Clarke EGC, Clarke MZ: Snakes and snake bite. Vet Ann 10:27, 1969.
70a. Dickinson CE, et al: Rattlesnake venom poisoning in horses: 32 cases (1973-1993). J Am Vet Med Assoc 208:1866, 1996.
71. Driggers T: Venomous snakebites in horses. Comp Cont Educ 17:235, 1995.

72. Gevrey J: Les morsures de vipères. Point Vét 25:193, 1993.
73. Gonzalez D: Snake bites in domestic animals. Toxicon 28:149, 1990.
73a. Hoffman A, et al: Myocarditis following envenoming with Vipera palestinae in two horses. Toxicon 31:1623, 1993.
74. Hudelson S, Hudelson P: Pathophysiology of snake envenomization and evaluation of treatments—Part I. Comp Cont Educ 17:889, 1995.
75. Hudelson S, Hudelson P: Pathophysiology of snake envenomization and evaluation of treatments—Part II. Comp Cont Educ 17:1035, 1995.
76. Hudelson S, Hudelson P: Pathophysiology of snake envenomization and evaluation of treatments—Part III. Comp Cont Educ 17:1385, 1995.
77. Mason JH: The treatment of snake bite in animals. J So Afr Vet Med Assoc 33:583, 1962.
78. Shein M: Delayed death of a mare bitten by a snake. Isr J Vet Med 44:268, 1988.
78a. Swanson TD: Treatment of rattlesnake bite in the horse. Proc Am Assoc Equine Practit 22:267, 1976.
78b. Yathirai S, Ramachandran CTVM: Snakebite in equine—a review. Centaur 8:53, 1992.

Photodermatitis

79. Berry JM, Merriam J: Phototoxic dermatitis in a horse. Vet Med Small Anim Clin 65:251, 1970.
80. Chabchoub A, et al: Photosensibilisation et atteinte oculaire chez le pur-sang arabe: cas clinique et revue bibliographique. Rev Méd Vét 150:617, 1999.
81. Clare NT: Photosensitization in animals. Adv Vet Sci 2:182, 1955.
81a. Darr D, Fridovich I: Free radicals in cutaneous biology. J Invest Dermatol 102:671, 1994.
82. Ford EJH: Hepatogenous light sensitization in animals. In: Rook AJ, Walton GS (eds): Comparative Physiology and Pathology of the Skin. Blackwell Scientific Publ, Oxford, 1965, p 351.
83. Fowler ME: Clinical manifestations of primary hepatic insufficiency in the horse. J Am Vet Med Assoc 147:55, 1965.
84. Galitzer SJ, Oehme FW: Photosensitization: a literature review. Vet Sci Comm 2:217, 1978.
84a. Hruza LL, Pentland AP: Mechanisms of UV-induced inflammation. J Invest Dermatol 100:35S, 1993.
85. Kellerman TS, Coetzer JAW: Hepatogenous photosensitivity diseases in South Africa. Onderstepoort J Vet Res 52:157, 1985.
86. Kownacki AA, Tobin T: Plant toxicities. In: Robinson NE (ed): Current Therapy in Equine Medicine I. W.B. Saunders Co, Philadelphia, 1983, p 595.
86a. Ledo E: Photodermatoses. Part I. Photobiology, photoimmunology, and idiopathic photodermatoses. Int J Dermatol 32:387, 1993.
86b. Ledo E: Photodermatoses. Part II. Chemical photodermatoses and dermatoses that can be exacerbated, precipitated, or provoked by light. Int J Dermatol 32:480, 1993.
87. Leinonen M, et al: Valoyliberkkyys varsala-tapausse-lostus ja kirjallisuuskatsaus. Suomen Eläin 105:377, 1999.
88. Mohammed FHA, et al: Hepatogenous photosensitization in horses due to Aphis craccivora on lucerne. Bull Anim Health Prod Afr 25:184, 1977.
89. Oehme FW: Phenothiazine. In: Robinson NE (ed): Current Therapy in Equine Medicine I. W.B. Saunders Co, Philadelphia, 1983, p 590.
90. Panciera RJ: Serum hepatitis in the horse. J Am Vet Med Assoc 155:408, 1969.
91. Renner JE, et al: Fotodermatitis y queratitis en equinos por contacto con chirira (Pastinaca sativa). Vet Arq 8:450, 1991.
92. Seaman JT: Pyrrolizidine alkaloid poisoning of horses. Aust Vet J 54:150, 1978.
92a. Streilein JW: Sunlight and skin-associated lymphoid tissues (SALT). J Invest Dermatol 100:475, 1993.
93. White SD: Photosensitivity. In: Robinson NE (ed): Current Therapy in Equine Medicine II. W.B. Saunders Co, Philadelphia, 1987, p 632.

Head Shaking

94. Hassel DM, et al: Endoscopy of the auditory tube diverticula in four horses with otitis media/interna. J Am Vet Med Assoc 207:1081, 1995.
95. Madigan JE, et al: Photic headshaking in the horse: 7 cases. Equine Vet J 27:306, 1995.
96. Madigan JE, Bell SA: Owner survey of headshaking in horses. J Am Vet Med Assoc 219:334, 2001.
97. Mair TS: Assessment of bilateral infraorbital nerve blockade and bilateral infraorbital neurectomy in the investigation and treatment of idiopathic headshaking. Equine Vet J 31:262, 1999.
98. Moore LA, et al: Management of headshaking in three horses by treatment for protozoal myeloencephalitis. Vet Rec 141, 264, 1997.
99. Willis PA: Cyproheptadine: medical treatment for photic headshakers. Comp Cont Educ 17:98, 1997.

Pruritus and Neurologic Disease

100. Johnson RE, et al: Localized pruritus: a presenting symptom of a spinal cord tumor in a child with features of neurofibromatosis. J Am Acad Dermatol 43:958, 2000.
101. Sloet van Oldruitenborgh-Oosterbaan MM: Personal communication, 2000.

Chapter *14*

Congenital and Hereditary Skin Diseases

Congenital and hereditary defects of the skin are rarely reported and usually untreatable.[1,3-8,10] Many of the disorders have an unproven mode of inheritance or are transmitted as recessive traits. Breeding of apparently normal parents or siblings of an affected horse distributes the gene more widely. Breeders of animals with suspected or proven genodermatoses should be instructed to avoid breeding of all close relatives of the affected animal.

● DISORDERS OF THE SKIN AND FOLLICULAR EPITHELIUM

Aplasia Cutis Congenita

Aplasia cutis congenita (epitheliogenesis imperfecta) is a very rare congenital and, perhaps, inherited failure to form certain layers of skin.[2,8] The condition is a developmental failure of skin fusion. Dermis, epidermis, and fat may all be missing, or single layers may be absent.

Aplasia cutis congenita has been reported several times in the horse.[11-18] However, careful evaluation of the clinical findings and the histopathology (when reported and illustrated) suggests that the majority of these foals had epidermolysis bullosa. A few animals had solitary or regionalized lesions of the distal leg[12] or face[17] consistent with aplasia cutis congenita. The lesions were characterized by round, to oval, to linear areas of well-circumscribed ulcerations (Fig. 14-1). Secondary infection is a possible complication. The major differential diagnosis is obstetric trauma. Small lesions may, with supportive therapy, heal by scar formation. Alternatively, lesions may be treated by surgical excision or skin grafting techniques.

Epidermolysis Bullosa

The term *epidermolysis bullosa* refers to a group of hereditary mechanobullous diseases whose common primary feature is the formation of blisters following trivial trauma.[2,9] In humans, classification is by mode of inheritance and histopathologic and ultrastructural features (Table 14-1).[2,9]

CAUSE AND PATHOGENESIS

Although wide variation exists in clinical severity and inheritance, epidermolysis bullosa is currently divided into three groups based on histopathologic and ultrastructural findings: *epidermolysis bullosa simplex* (blister cleavage occurs within the stratum basale); *junctional epidermolysis bullosa* (blister cleavage occurs within the lamina lucida); and *dystrophic epidermolysis bullosa* (blister cleavage occurs within the superficial dermis).[2,9] The well-documented cases of equine epidermolysis bullosa fall into the junctional group. The pathogenesis of the various forms of epidermolysis bullosa is not completely described but focuses on abnormal keratin intermediate filament and keratin network formation and abnormal anchoring mechanisms (types VII and XVII collagen, laminin, plectin, integrins) (Table 14-1).[2,9]

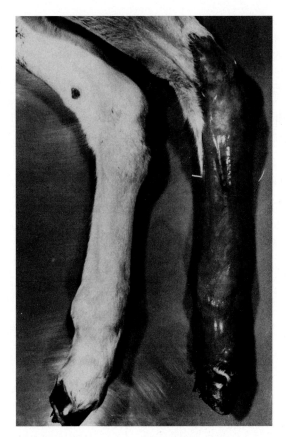

FIGURE 14-1. Aplasia cutis congenita. Extensive ulceration on leg of foal. (*Courtesy Dr. J. King.*)

● Table 14-1 **TYPES OF EPIDERMOLYSIS BULLOSA (EB)**

TYPE OF EB	STRUCTURE AFFECTED	DEFICIENT PROTEIN
EB Simplex		
Dowling-Meara, Weber-Cockayne, Koebner	Intermediate filaments	Keratin 5 or 14
With muscular dystrophy	Hemidesmosomes	Plectin
Junctional EB		
With pyloric atresia	Hemidesmosomes	Integrins α_6 or β_4
Nonlethal	Anchoring filaments/lamina densa	Type XVIII collagen or laminin 5
Lethal	Anchoring filaments/lamina densa	Laminin 5
Dystrophy EB		
Dominant	Anchoring fibrils	Type VII collagen
Recessive	Anchoring fibrils	Type VII collagen

Although epidermolysis bullosa was first described in horses in 1988,[19,22] it is very likely that most reported cases of so-called "epitheliogenesis imperfecta"[11,13,15-18] were, in fact, foals with epidermolysis bullosa. Most cases of well-documented equine epidermolysis bullosa have involved draft horses, especially Belgians and American Saddlebreds.[13,19-25] Although the mode of inheritance has not been proven, an autosomal recessive transmission is likely.[13,20,21,24,24b] In Belgians and American Saddlebreds, ultrastructural studies have demonstrated separation through the lamina lucida with severe attenuation of hemidesmosomes.[19-22,24a,24b] There is decreased immunoreactivity to laminin-5.[24a] Immunoblot analysis confirmed decreased expression of the γ-2 subunit chain of laminin-5.[24a] Results suggest a mutation in either the LAMC2 or the LAMB3 subunit gene, which would make junctional epidermolysis bullosa in Belgians most similar to the Herlitz-type junctional epidermolysis bullosa in humans.

CLINICAL FEATURES

Epidermolysis bullosa has been predominantly reported in draft horses, especially Belgians,[13,19-25] and reports indicate a similar disease has been seen in American saddlebreds.[19a,24b] However, cases of what was very likely epidermolysis bullosa have also been described in a quarter horse[18] and a saddlebred.[15] There is no sex predilection.

Foals may be born with lesions or develop lesions within the first 2 days of life. Primary skin lesions are vesicles and bullae, but these are transient, easily ruptured, and usually absent when the foals are initially examined. The predominant clinical lesions are well-demarcated ulcers, often with peripheral epidermal and mucosal collarettes. Exudation and crusting is often pronounced. Lesions are typically present on the coronets (Fig. 14-2); the mucocutaneous junctions of the lips, anus, vulva, eyelids, and nostrils; over areas of bony prominences (Figs. 14-3 and 14-4), such as the fetlocks, hocks, carpi, stifles, hips, and rump; and in the oral cavity (Figs. 14-5 and 14-6). Hoof wall separation usually progresses to complete sloughing of hooves. Lesions may also be observed on the cornea and in the esophagus. Dental dysplasia may be present.[15,19a,24b] Affected foals become progressively depressed, cachectic, and are euthanized or die of septicemia.

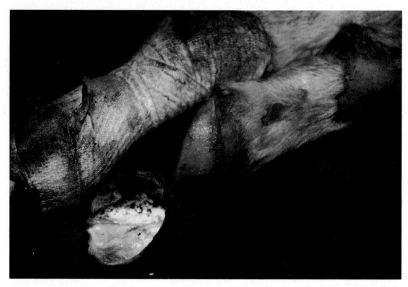

FIGURE 14-2. Junctional epidermolysis bullosa. Ulceration of the coronary band and sloughing of the hoof.

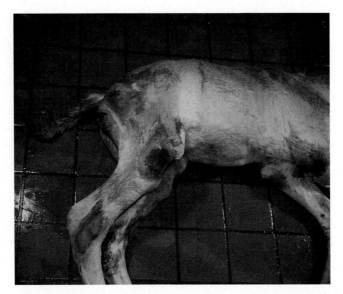

FIGURE 14-3. Junctional epidermolysis bullosa. Ulcers over hocks, stifles, elbows, and hip.

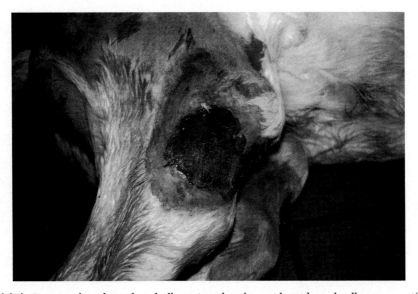

FIGURE 14-4. Junctional epidermolysis bullosa. Annular ulcer with epidermal collarette on stifle.

DIAGNOSIS

The clinical presentation is highly suggestive. Similar clinical signs could be seen with pemphigus vulgaris, bullous pemphigoid, systemic lupus erythematosus, and drug reaction, but these are most unlikely to occur as congenital or neonatal disorders.

Skin biopsy reveals subepidermal cleft and vesicle formation (Fig. 14-7).[19-23,24b] Inflammation is minimal except where ulceration, infection, or both of these have occurred. Biopsy specimens stained with PAS usually show the PAS-positive basement membrane zone attached to the dermal floor of the clefts and vesicles (Fig. 14-8).[23] Ultrastructural studies reveal that dermoepidermal

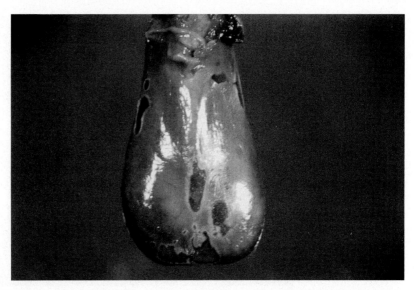

FIGURE 14-5. Junctional epidermolysis bullosa. Multiple annular ulcers and collarettes where vesicles and bullae have ruptured on the tongue. (*Courtesy Dr. J. King.*)

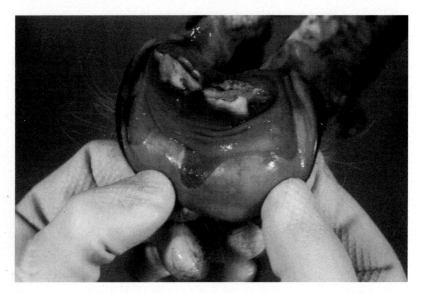

FIGURE 14-6. Junctional epidermolysis bullosa. Buccal surface of lower lip with well-circumscribed ulcers and collarettes. (*Courtesy Dr. J. King.*)

separation occurs in the lamina lucida of the basement membrane zone and that hemidesmosomes are small, abnormal, and reduced in number.[19-22,24b] Direct immunofluorescence testing is negative.[19,23,24]

CLINICAL MANAGEMENT

There is presently no effective treatment for equine epidermolysis bullosa. The clinician should inform the owner of the nature and heritability of the disorder, and the stallion and mare should not be used for further breeding.

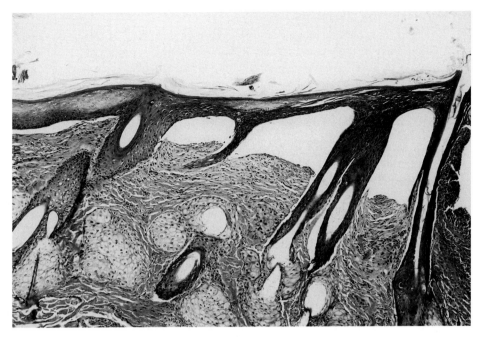

FIGURE 14-7. Junctional epidermolysis bullosa. Subepidermal vesicles.

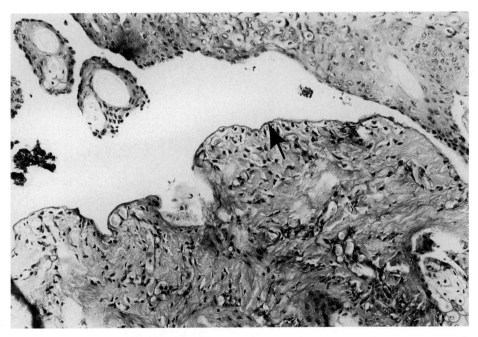

FIGURE 14-8. Junctional epidermolysis bullosa. PAS-positive basement membrane zone is at floor of vesicle (*arrow*).

Erythrokeratoderma Variabilis

The palmoplantar keratodermas are a heterogenous group of disorders characterized by abnormal thickening of the palms and soles in humans.[2] The disorders may be hereditary or acquired.

A disorder resembling erythrokeratoderma variabilis was reported in a female warmblood.[25a] The horse was born with "crumbly" hooves and symmetrical lesions over bony prominences of the limbs. The lesions were hyperkeratotic plaques. Histologic examination revealed marked hyperkeratosis and epidermal hyperplasia. The animal was euthanized at 9 weeks of age and no necropsy was performed.

In humans, erythrokeratoderma variabilis is inherited as an autosomal-dominant trait and responds well to the oral administration of retinoids.[2]

Hypotrichosis

Hypotrichosis implies a less-than-normal amount of hair and a congenital, possibly hereditary, basis for the condition.[8,9] Hypotrichosis may be regional or multifocal in distribution, but is usually generalized. Reports of hypotrichosis in the horse are extremely rare, anecdotal, and sketchy.[26] Anecdotal reports indicate that a hereditary hypotrichosis occurs in certain lines of Arabians.[5] Hair loss is symmetrical and restricted to the face, especially the periocular area (Fig. 14-9). Skin in affected areas may be scaly and feel thinner than normal.

Congenital hypotrichosis was reported in a blue roan Percheron.[27] The horse was born with poorly circumscribed patchy alopecia of the trunk and legs. Teeth and hooves were normal. Alopecia was progressive, becoming almost complete by 1 year of age (Fig. 14-10). Histopathologic findings included follicular hypoplasia and hyperkeratosis, as well as a predominance of catagen and telogen hair follicles (Figs. 14-11 and 14-12). Melanotic debris was present in the lumina of many hair follicles and sebaceous glands. The horse was in good health at 5 years of age, but was susceptible to sunburn.

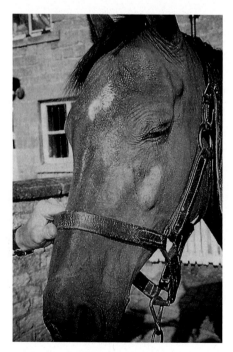

FIGURE 14-9. Hypotrichosis—poor hair density and quality. (*From Pascoe RR, Knottenbelt DC: Manual of Equine Dermatology. W.B. Saunders Co., Philadelphia, 1999.*)

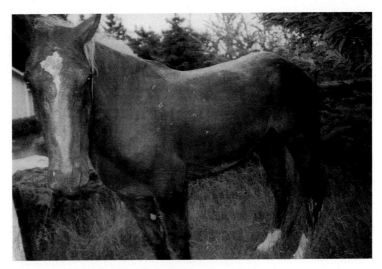

FIGURE 14-10. Congenital hypotrichosis in a Percheron.

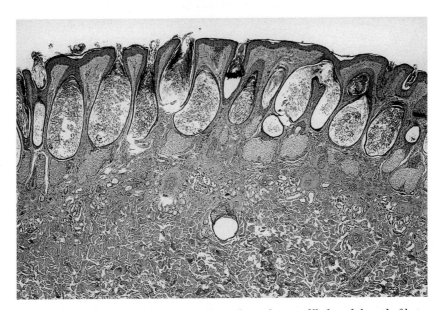

FIGURE 14-11. Hypotrichosis. Hair follicles are hypoplastic, keratin-filled, and devoid of hairs.

There is currently no effective treatment for equine hypotrichosis. Affected horses may be more susceptible to sunburn and hypothermia. Affected animals and their parents should not be used for breeding.

Trichorrhexis Nodosa

Trichorrhexis nodosa is a hair shaft defect that may be hereditary or acquired (see Chapter 10).[2,8,9]

Follicular Dysplasia

Follicular dysplasia (e.g., "mane and tail dystrophy," "black and white hair follicle dystrophies") has been recognized in horses, and is probably genetic in origin[1,7-10] *Mane and tail follicular dysplasia*

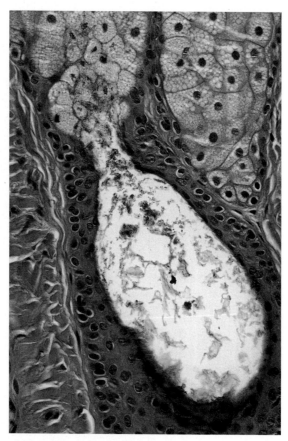

FIGURE 14-12. Hypotrichosis. Sebaceous gland melanosis.

is recognized at birth or at a few weeks of age. It is particularly common in Appaloosas.[5] Affected animals have short, brittle, dull hairs and variable alopecia in the mane and tail (Fig. 14-13). *Black or white hair follicular dysplasias* are also recognized at birth or in juvenile animals. Patches of hair coat in either black- or white-haired areas are short, brittle, and dull. Affected areas usually become hypotrichotic. The authors have received biopsies with limited clinical and follow-up information on a few horses with more widespread (trunk and neck), non-color–related follicular dysplasias. These animals had brittle, dull, hypotrichotic hair coats with irregular hair lengths (Fig. 14-14) (breakage) and a tendency toward dry, scaly skin in affected areas. Curly coat horses with hypotrichotic manes and tails may have forms of follicular dysplasia (see Curly Coat).

A major differential diagnosis is alopecia areata, which is an acquired autoimmune condition with diagnostic histopathologic findings (see Chapter 9).

Histologically, follicular dysplasias are characterized by abnormal development (shape, size, and so forth) of hair follicles, and the production of dysplastic hair shafts (abnormally shaped; abnormally stained; melanin deposition abnormalities; loss of normal hair shaft microanatomy) (Figs. 14-15 and 14-16).

There is currently no effective treatment for equine follicular dysplasia. Affected horses and their parents should not be used for breeding.

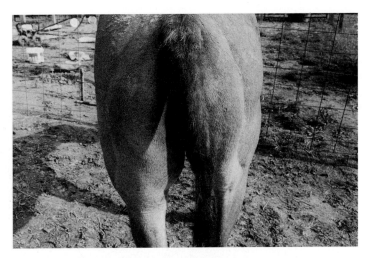

FIGURE 14-13. Follicular dysplasia involving the tail.

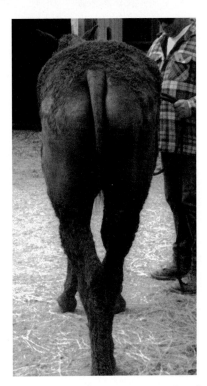

FIGURE 14-14. Follicular dysplasia. Note alopecia over rump, tail, and caudal thighs.

Curly Coat

The curly coat phenotype in most North American horses is a dominant trait.[27a] Curly coat is occasionally seen as a recessive trait in quarter horses, Percherons, Arabians, Appaloosas, Missouri fox trotters, Tennessee walking horses, paints, Morgans, and Paso Finos.[8,27a] Curly horses come in varying degrees of curliness (Fig. 14-7).

Curly horses can shed in the spring to the point of patchy alopecia. Some curlies have varying

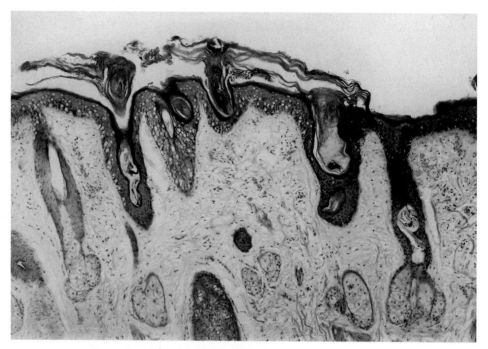

FIGURE 14-15. Follicular dysplasia. Misshapen telogen follicles, follicular keratosis, and dysplastic hair shafts.

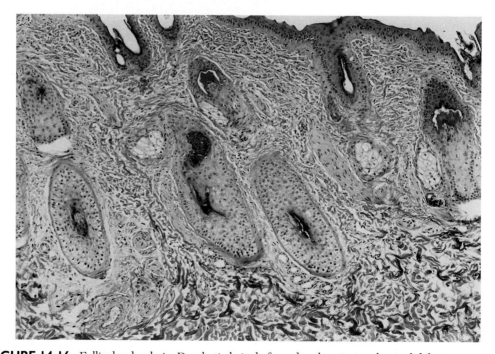

FIGURE 14-16. Follicular dysplasia. Dysplastic hair shafts and melanotic intraluminal debris.

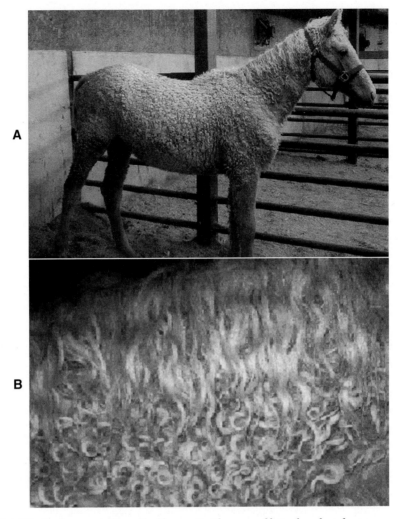

FIGURE 14-17. Curly coat. **A,** Overall of horse. **B,** Close-up of lateral neck and mane.

degrees of tail hypotrichosis, referred to as "scanty tail" or "string tail," and these same horses typically have hypotrichotic manes as well. Curly horses can also shed mane and tail hairs in the spring to the point of hypotrichosis or alopecia.

The histoanatomy of the general body skin of normal curly coat horses is similar to that of noncurly horses (hair follicles *not* curved!).[27a] However, biopsy specimens from the mane and tail of horses with scanty or string tail often show follicular keratosis, dysplastic hair shafts, and sebaceous melanosis. Either curly horses with abnormal manes and tails have forms of follicular dysplasia, or the pathological diagnosis of follicular dysplasia needs to be rendered with great caution in these individuals.

● DISORDERS OF PIGMENTATION

Albinism

Congenital, hereditary albinism has been reported in the horse (see Chapter 12).[8,10]

Lethal White Foal Syndrome

Lethal white foal syndrome is characterized by hereditary abnormalities in pigmentation and intestinal tract development (see Chapter 12).[7,8,10]

Lavender Foal Syndrome

Lavender foal syndrome is a hereditary disorder of Arabian foals wherein pigmentary abnormalities occur in conjunction with multiple extracutaneous defects (see Chapter 12).[5]

Vitiligo

Vitiligo (Arabian fading syndrome) is an idiopathic, noninflammatory, probably hereditary condition in Arabian horses (see Chapter 12).[1,7,8,10]

Reticulated Leukotrichia

Reticulated leukotrichia is a disorder of quarter horses, thoroughbreds, and standardbreds, and is probably a genodermatosis (see Chapter 12).[1,7,8]

Spotted Leukotrichia

Spotted leukotrichia is predominantly a disorder, probably genetic in origin, of Arabian horses (see Chapter 12).[1,7,8]

● DISORDERS OF COLLAGEN

Cutaneous Asthenia

Cutaneous asthenia (Ehlers-Danlos syndrome, dermatosparaxis, hyperelastosis cutis) is a group of inherited, congenital connective tissue diseases characterized by loose, hyperextensible, and abnormally fragile skin that is easily torn by minor trauma.[2,8,9]

CAUSE AND PATHOGENESIS

This disease complex resembles the Ehlers-Danlos syndromes of humans, which consists of at least 11 different disorders that are distinguishable clinically, biochemically, and genetically (Table 14-2).[2,9] Equine cutaneous asthenia has been reported almost exclusively in quarter horses, some of which were related, suggesting a hereditary basis.[19a,28a,30,31] The mode of inheritance has not been determined, but autosomal recessive transmission has been suspected.[28,30] The nature of the collagen abnormality is unknown, although the collagen fibril packing defect and elevated proportion of acid-soluble extractable collagen found in two quarter horses prompted the authors to postulate a defect at the level of assembly or stabilization of collagen fibrils.[30]

CLINICAL FEATURES

Cutaneous asthenia has been reported in several quarter horses[28,28a,30-32] and one Arabian-cross horse.[29] The authors have seen one Hafflinger with the disorder. No sex predilection is evident, and affected horses develop "loose skin" and other dermatologic problems at a very early age, always before six months of age. Most commonly, affected horses have three or more areas of abnormal skin over the dorsolateral thoracic, lumbar, and sacral areas (Fig. 14-18). Lesions may enlarge, and new lesions may appear over time. Typically, these areas are well circumscribed, round to oval, 4 to 30 cm in diameter, nonpainful, and nonpruritic. The skin in these areas is hyperextensible (Fig. 14-19), may be stretched 5 to 10 cm above the skin surface, and may return normally or quite slowly to its normal position (Fig. 14-20). Traction at the edge of lesions may cause pain. Affected skin may be thin, velvety, and depressed 1 to 2 mm below the surface of the normal skin. Affected skin is often quite fragile, being easily torn (Fig. 14-21) when the horse is

● Table 14-2   **TYPES OF EHLERS-DANLOS SYNDROME**

TYPE	TISSUE AFFECTED	ABNORMALITY
I	Skin, joints	?
II	Skin, joints	Collagen V
III	Skin, joints	?
IV	Skin, blood vessels, intestine	Collagen III
V	Skin, joints, heart	Procollagen (lysyl oxidase deficiency)
VI	Skin, joints, bone, eyes	Procollagen (lysyl hydroxylase deficiency)
VIIa, b	Skin, joints	Procollagen
VIIc	Skin, joints	Procollagen (precollagen peptidase deficiency)
VIII	Skin, joints, teeth	?
IX	Skin, bones	Copper deficiency (lysyl oxidase deficiency)
X	Skin, joints, platelets	Fibronectin
IX	Joints	?

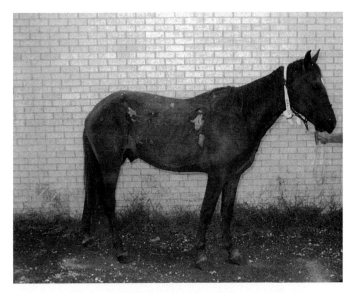

FIGURE 14-18. Cutaneous asthenia. Multiple ulcers over trunk. (*Courtesy Dr. W. McMullen.*)

ridden and so forth. Torn skin may be slow to heal, may hold sutures poorly, and may heal with large, white, cigarette paper–like scars. Some horses develop frequent leg wounds[28a,30] or tear off large sheets of skin when they rub against things.[29] Subcutaneous hematomas and abscesses can occur.[5,19a]

DIAGNOSIS

The clinical syndromes of hyperextensible, easily torn skin in a foal are highly suggestive of cutaneous asthenia. Complete documentation requires biopsies for histopathologic, ultrastructural, and perhaps, biochemical studies.

Skin biopsy may reveal striking dermal abnormalities or near-normal skin. The deep[30] or superficial and deep[29,31] dermis may be thinner than normal. Collagen fibers may appear fragmented,[30] more sparsely distributed,[29-31] separated by wide spaces,[29,30] or lacking their normal parallel

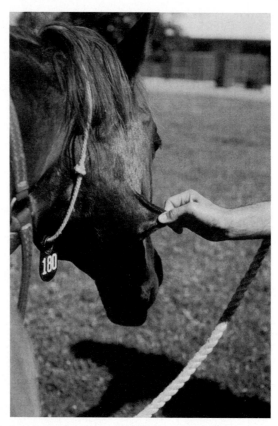

FIGURE 14-19. Cutaneous asthenia. Hyperextensibility of skin on cheek. (*Courtesy Dr. A. Evans.*)

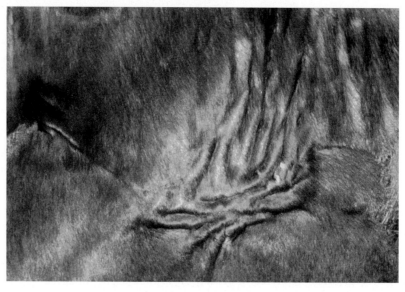

FIGURE 14-20. Cutaneous asthenia. Skin maintains wrinkled appearance after being twisted and tented. (*Courtesy Dr. W. McMullen.*)

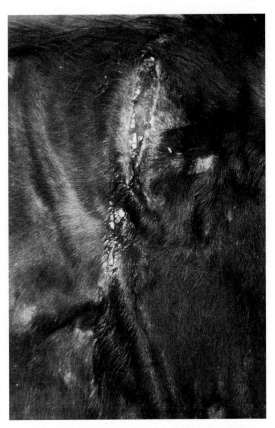

FIGURE 14-21. Cutaneous asthenia. Spontaneous tear in wrinkled skin. (*Courtesy Dr. W. McMullen.*)

arrangement (Fig. 14-22).[30] Collagen fibers may be thin, fragmented, and disorganized.[19a] Masson's trichrome–stained specimens reveal that some collagen fibers have a central red core (Fig. 14-23).[29,30] Special stains show elastic fibers to be normal. Biopsy specimens from one horse revealed a horizontal linear zone of loose collagen bundles and cleft formation through the middle of the deep dermis.[28a] These authors suggested that incisional full-thickness skin biopsies should be taken, because punch biopsies may not obtain deep dermis.

Electron microscopic examination may reveal collagen fibrils that are fragmented,[29] loosely packed,[28a,30] curved, nonparallel, disorganized,[29,30] and of an abnormal range of diameters.[28a,30]

CLINICAL MANAGEMENT

The clinician should inform the owner of the nature, heritability, and chronic incurable course of the disease. The horse, as well as its sire and dam, should not be used for breeding. The only useful management procedure is to minimize trauma to affected skin.

● ENDOCRINE AND NUTRITIONAL DISORDERS

Congenital Hypothyroidism

Congenital hypothyroidism may be a cause of congenital hypotrichosis and alopecia (see Chapter 10).[8]

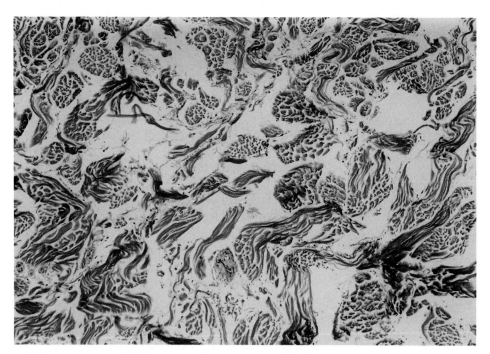

FIGURE 14-22. Cutaneous asthenia. Deep dermal collagen bundles are widely separated and lack their normal parallel arrangement.

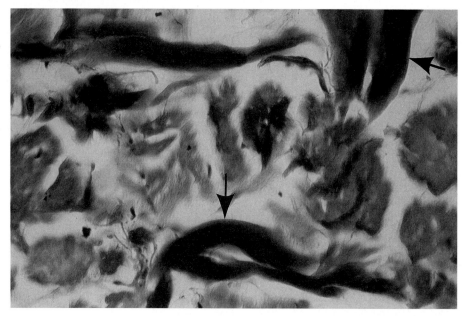

FIGURE 14-23. Cutaneous asthenia. Masson's trichrome stain reveals abnormal staining of some collagen fibers (*arrows*).

Iodine Deficiency

Maternal iodine deficiency may be a cause of congenital hypotrichosis and alopecia in foals (see Chapter 10).[8]

• MISCELLANEOUS DISORDERS

Neoplasms

Congenital skin neoplasms have been reported in horses. These include papilloma, hemangioma, melanoma, and mast cell tumor (see Chapter 16).[8]

Keratinous Cysts

Congenital cutaneous cysts have been reported in horses. These include dermoid cysts and heterotopic polyodontia (conchal sinus, temporal teratoma, dentigerous cyst) (see Chapter 16).[8] Dermoid cysts have been seen in related Paso Fino horses.[1]

Linear Keratosis

Linear keratosis (linear epidermal nevus) is a characteristic focal keratinization defect of the skin of the horse. The predilection for quarter horses and Belgians and occurrence in closely related animals suggest an inherited basis (see Chapters 11 and 16).[1,6,7]

Linear Alopecia

Linear alopecia is a characteristic focal alopecia, most commonly seen in quarter horses and of presumed genetic origin (see Chapter 15).[33]

Neonatal Vasculitis

The authors and others[34] have seen a few foals <4 days old with oral and mucocutaneous ulcerative disease. Owners originally recognized annular, well-circumscribed areas of "bruised" and ulcerated tissue. Clinical signs progressed over a period of 10 to 14 days, involving most of the oral mucosa and lips and occasionally the eyelids, nostrils, pinnae, anus, and distal limbs. All foals were thrombocytopenic and neutropenic. Lesions oozed, crusted, and healed with supportive care over a period of 3 to 4 weeks. Histopathologic findings in skin biopsy specimens included subepidermal clefting, dermal hemorrhage, leukocytoclastic vasculitis, and necrotizing dermatitis.

The etiopathogenesis of this apparently rare syndrome is unknown. It is speculated that undiagnosed infections in, or vaccines, antibiotics, or other drugs administered to the mares during, pregnancy may have produced transient immune complex disease in the foals. Some mares had more than one affected foal, but had healthy foals in subsequent pregnancies when an alternate source of colostrum was given.

• REFERENCES

General

1. Barbet JL, et al: Diseases of the Skin. In: Colahan PT, et al. (eds): Equine Medicine and Surgery IV, Vol. II. American Veterinary Publications, Inc, Goleta, 1991, p 1569.
2. Freedberg IM, et al: Fitzpatrick's Dermatology in General Medicine V. McGraw-Hill, Inc. New York, 1999.
3. Huston R, et al: Congenital defects in foals. Equine J Med Surg 1:146,1977.
4. Jayasekara MU, Leipold HW: Congenital defects of the skin. Vet Med Small Anim Clin 77:1461, 1982.
5. Pascoe RR, Knottenbelt DC: Manual of Equine Dermatology. W.B. Saunders Co, Philadelphia, 1999.
6. Radostits OM, et al: Veterinary Medicine. A Textbook of the Diseases of Cattle, Sheep, Pigs, Goats, and Horses VIII. Baillière Tindall, London, 1994.
7. Reed SM, Bayly WM: Equine Internal Medicine. W.B. Saunders Co, Philadelphia, 1998.
8. Scott DW: Large Animal Dermatology. W.B. Saunders Co, Philadelphia, 1988.
9. Scott DW, et al: Muller & Kirk's Small Animal Dermatology VI. W.B. Saunders Co, Philadelphia, 2001.

10. Williams MA, Angarano DW: Diseases of the Skin. In: Kobluk CN, et al (eds): The Horse. Diseases and Clinical Management. W.B. Saunders Co, Philadelphia, 1995, p 541.

Disorders of the Skin and Follicular Epithelium

Aplasia Cutis Congenita

11. Berthelsen H, Eriksson K: Epitheliogenesis imperfecta neonatorum in a foal possibly of hereditary nature. J Comp Pathol Ther 48:285, 1935.
12. Butz H: Todbringende Erbanlagen. Dtsch Tierärztl Wschr 47:305, 1939.
13. Butz H, Meyer H: Epitheliogenesis imperfecta neonatorum equi. Dtsch Tierärztl Wschr 64:555, 1957.
14. Crowell WA, et al: Epitheliogenesis imperfecta in a foal. J Am Vet Med Assoc 168:56,1976.
15. Dubielzig RR, et al: Dental dysplasia and epitheliogenesis imperfecta in a foal. Vet Pathol 23:325, 1986.
16. Grunth P: Klinische Mitteilungen. Monat Prakt Tierheilk 24:259, 1913.
17. Stoss A: Eine seltene Pferdemissbildung. Monat Prakt Tierheilk 7:456, 1896.
18. Wright BG: Epitheliogenesis imperfecta: understanding this rare skin anomaly. Vet Med 81:246, 1986.

Epidermolysis Bullosa

19. Frame SR, et al: Hereditary junctional mechanobullous disease in a foal. J Am Vet Med Assoc 193:1420, 1988.
20. Gourreau JM, et al: Epidermolyse bulleuse junctionnelle léthale chez le cheval de trait en France. Bull Acad Vét France 62:345, 1989.
21. Gourreau JM, et al: Epidermolyse bulleuse junctionnelle léthale chez le cheval de trait. Point Vét 22:209, 1990.
22. Johnson GC, et al: Ultrastructure of junctional epidermolysis bullosa in Belgian foals. J Comp Pathol 98:329, 1988.
23. Kohn CW, et al: Mechanobullous disease in two Belgian foals. Equine Vet J 21:297, 1989.
24. Kohn CW: Junctional mechanobullous disease in Belgian foals. In: Robinson NE (ed): Current Therapy in Equine Medicine III. W.B. Saunders Co, Philadelphia, 1992, p 705.
24a. Linder KE, et al: Mechanobullous disease of Belgian foals resembles lethal (Herlitz) junctional epidermolysis bullosa of humans and is associated with failure of laminin-5 assembly. Vet Dermatol 11(suppl):24, 2000.
24b. Lieto LD, et al: Equine epitheliogenesis imperfecta in two American Saddlebred foals is a lamina lucida defect. Vet Pathol 39:576, 2002.

25. Shapiro J, McEwen B: Mechanobullous disease in a Belgian foal in eastern Ontario. Can Vet J 36:572, 1995.

Erythrokeratoderma Variabilis

25a. Wehrend A, et al: Fallbericht: (Erythro)keratodermia variabilis bei einem neugeborenen Warmblutfohlen. Berl Münch Tierärztl Wschr 114:40, 2001.

Disorders of Hair and Hair Growth

Hypotrichosis

26. Pascoe RR: Equine Dermatoses. University of Sydney Post-Graduate Foundation in Veterinary Science, Veterinary Review No 22, 1981.
27. Valentine BA, et al: Congenital hypotrichosis in a Percheron draft horse. Vet Dermatol 12:215, 2001.

Curly Coat

27a. Scott DW: The histology of normal curly horse skin. (Submitted for publication, 2002.)

Disorders of Collagen

Cutaneous Asthenia

28. Bridges CH, McMullen WC: Dermatosparaxis in quarter horses. Proc Annu Meet Am Coll Vet Pathol 35:12, 1984.
28a. Brounts SH, et al: Zonal dermal separation: a distinctive histopathological lesion associated with hyperelastosis cutis in a quarter horse. Vet Dermatol 12:219, 2001
29. Gunson DE, et al: Dermal collagen degradation and phagocytosis. Occurrence in a horse with hyperextensible fragile skin. Arch Dermatol 120:599, 1984.
30. Hardy MH, et al: An inherited connective tissue disease in the horse. Lab Invest 59:253, 1988.
31. Lerner DJ, McCraken MD: Hyperelastosis cutis in 2 horses. J Equine Med Surg 2:350, 1978.
32. McMullen WC: The Skin. In: Mansmann RA, et al (eds): Equine Medicine and Surgery III. American Veterinary Publications, Inc, Santa Barbara, 1982, p 789.

Miscellaneous Disorders

Linear Alopecia

33. Fadok VA: Update on four unusual equine dermatoses. Vet Clin N Am Equine Pract 11:105, 1995.

Neonatal Vasculitis

34. Perkins GA, et al: Ulcerative dermatitis, thrombocytopenia, and neutropenia in neonatal foals. Proc Am Coll Vet Intern Med 20:38, 2002.

Chapter 15

Miscellaneous Skin Diseases

● EOSINOPHILIC GRANULOMA

The eosinophilic granuloma is a common equine dermatosis and the most common nonneoplastic nodular skin disease of the horse.* It accounts for 3.89% of the equine skin disorders seen at the Cornell University Clinic.

Cause and Pathogenesis

The etiopathogenesis is unknown, and probably multifactorial. Because the lesions most commonly begin in spring and summer, insect hypersensitivity has been suspected.[6,7,13] However, in the northeastern United States, about one-third of the cases appear to begin in winter. Thus, unless the insect hypersensitivity is a delayed immunologic reaction, there must be other etiologic factors.[13]

Additional evidence that hypersensitivity reactions are involved is the knowledge that histopathologically identical lesions are seen in cats (mosquito bite hypersensitivity, flea-bite hypersensitivity, atopy, food hypersensitivity) and horses (*Culicoides* hypersensitivity, atopy, onchocerciasis) with various hypersensitivity disorders.[6,7,15-17]

Because lesions commonly occur in the saddle region, some authors have suggested that trauma may be an inciting cause.[7,23,28,30]

Some horses develop eosinophilic granulomas at injection sites when standard silicone-coated needles are used.[27a] This may represent a hypersensitivity reaction to silicone, because the same horses do *not* develop reactions when noncoated stainless steel needles are used.

Classically, a characteristic histopathologic feature of the equine eosinophilic granuloma has been called "collagen degeneration," "collagenolysis," or "necrobiotic collagen" by various authors.[22] However, a recent study indicated that there is no collagen degeneration in these lesions, and that these characteristic histopathologic lesions are more appropriately called *collagen flame figures*.[22]

In some biopsy specimens, free hair shafts may be seen.[19a] In these cases, there is often a history of body clipping prior to the onset of lesions, thus suggesting a causal relationship.

Clinical Features

Eosinophilic granuloma (eosinophilic granuloma with collagen degeneration, nodular collagenolytic granuloma, acute collagen necrosis, nodular necrobiosis) is seen most commonly in spring and summer and has no apparent age, breed, or sex predilections.† Single or multiple lesions most commonly occur on the back, withers, and neck (Figs. 15-1 through 15-3). They are round, elevated, firm, well-circumscribed, 0.5 to 10 cm in diameter, and the overlying skin and hair coat

---

*References 1, 2, 7-10, 12, 13, 19a, 20, 21.
†References 1, 7-9, 13, 19, 20, 24-30.

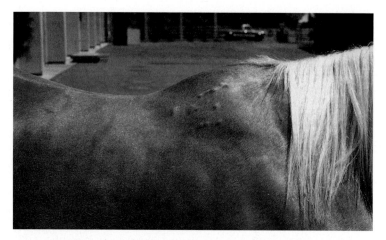

FIGURE 15-1. Eosinophilic granuloma. Multiple nodules over withers. (*Courtesy Dr. A. Stannard.*)

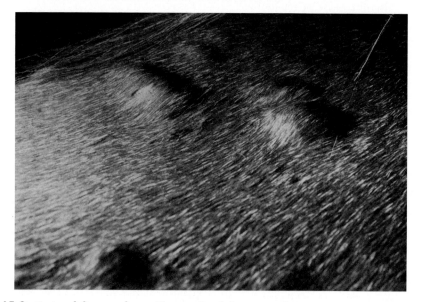

FIGURE 15-2. Eosinophilic granuloma. Cluster of nodules over withers.

are typically normal. The lesions are neither painful nor pruritic. Cystic or plaque-like lesions are occasionally seen and may discharge a central, grayish-white caseous core ("necrotic plug"). Lesions can occur anywhere on the body, and an occasional horse can have hundreds of widely disseminated papular lesions (3 to 5 mm in diameter). Horses who have concurrent *Culicoides* hypersensitivity or atopy will often have clinical signs of those entities, as well (see Chapter 8).

Diagnosis

The differential diagnosis includes the nodular skin diseases in Table 15-1.

Definitive diagnosis is based on history, physical examination, and skin biopsy. Cytologic examination reveals eosinophils, histiocytes, lymphocytes, and no microorganisms (Fig. 15-4). Peripheral blood eosinophilia is rare. Histopathologic findings include nodular-to-diffuse areas of

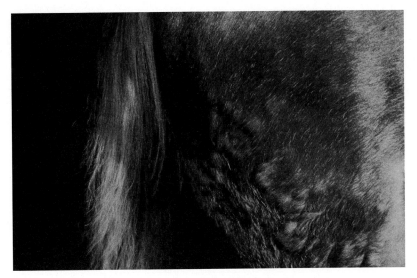

FIGURE 15-3. Eosinophilic granuloma. Clusters of nodules on thigh.

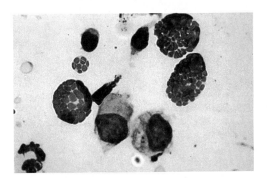

FIGURE 15-4. Eosinophilic granuloma. Eosinophils and macrophages.

eosinophilic, granulomatous inflammation of the dermis, and often the panniculus (Fig. 15-5).[3,13,15] Multifocal areas of collagen flame figures are a characteristic finding (Fig. 15-6), and small foci of eosinophilic folliculitis or furunculosis may be seen (Fig. 15-7).[3,15,22] Lymphoid nodules may be prominent. True collagen degeneration is rare (Fig. 15-8). Older lesions exhibit marked dystrophic mineralization (Fig. 15-9) and may be misdiagnosed as calcinosis circumscripta or mast cell tumors. Special stains and cultures are negative. In silicone-coated needle injection reactions, the granulomatous process is often fairly linear in shape (Fig. 15-10), suggesting reaction along the needle tract.

Clinical Management

Horses with solitary lesions, or a few lesions, may be treated by surgical excision or sublesional injections of glucocorticoids (triamcinolone acetonide, 3 to 5 mg/lesion; methylprednisolone acetate, 5 to 10 mg/lesion).* Sublesional injections are typically repeated at 2-week intervals. Lesions still present after three injections will probably require surgical removal. Alternatively, as the

*References 1, 7, 13, 18, 20, 24, 27.

● Table 15-1   **DIFFERENTIAL DIAGNOSIS OF NODULAR SKIN DISEASE IN THE HORSE***

DISEASE	COMMON SITE(S)
Bacterial	
Furunculosis (especially coagulase-positive staphylococci)	Saddle or tack areas
Ulcerative lymphangitis (especially *Corynebacterium pseudotuberculosis*)	Legs
Actinomycosis	Mandible and maxilla
Nocardiosis	?[†]
Abscess (especially *C. pseudotuberculosis*)	Chest and abdomen
Bacterial pseudomycetoma (especially coagulase-positive staphylococci)	Lips, legs, and scrotum
Tuberculosis	Ventral thorax and abdomen; medial thighs, legs
Glanders	Medial hocks
Fungal	
Dermatophytosis	Saddle or tack areas
Eumycotic mycetoma (*Curvularia geniculata*, black-grain; *Pseudoallescheria boydii*, white-grain)	Lips and legs
Phaehyphomycosis	?
Sporotrichosis	Legs
Zygomycosis	
Basidiobolus haptosporus	Chest, trunk
Conidiobolus coronatus	Nostrils
Rhinosporidiosis	Nostrils
Alternariosis (*Alternaria tenuis*)	?
Blastomycosis	?
Coccidioidomycosis	Chest, shoulder
Cryptococcosis	?
Histoplasmosis farciminosi (*Histoplasma farciminosum*)	Face, neck, and legs
Pythiosis (*Pythium* sp.)	Legs, ventral chest, and abdomen
Parasitic	
Hypodermiasis (*Hypoderma bovis, H. lineatum*)	Withers
Habronemiasis (*Habronema muscae, H. majus, Draschia megastoma*)	Legs, ventrum, prepuce, and medial canthus
Parafilariasis (*Parafilaria multipapillosa*)	Neck, shoulders, and trunk
Halicephalobiasis	Prepuce, jaw
Tick bite granuloma	Face, neck, trunk, legs
Viral	
Vaccinia	Muzzle and caudal pasterns
Immunologic	
Urticaria	Neck, trunk, proximal legs
Erythema multiforme	Neck, dorsum
Amyloidosis	Head, neck, chest, and shoulders
Neoplastic	
Papilloma	Nose and lips
Ear papilloma (aural plaque)	Pinnae

● Table 15-1 **DIFFERENTIAL DIAGNOSIS OF NODULAR SKIN DISEASE IN THE HORSE*—cont'd**

DISEASE	COMMON SITE(S)
Squamous cell carcinoma	Eyelid, prepuce, and vulva
Basal cell tumor	Legs, face, neck, and trunk
Sarcoid	Head, neck, ventrum, and legs
Epitrichial sweatgland adenoma	Pinnae and vulva
Fibroma	Periocular, neck, and legs
Fibrosarcoma	Eyelid, trunk, and legs
Hemangioma	Distal legs
Hemangiosarcoma	Neck, trunk, and proximal legs
Lymphangioma	Axilla and groin
Lipoma	Trunk and proximal legs
Schwannoma	Eyelids and periorbital region
Mast cell tumor	Head, neck, and legs
Melanocytoma	Legs and trunk
Melanoma	Perineum, perianal area, ventral tail, and genitalia
Lymphoma	Head, neck, trunk, and proximal legs
Malignant fibrous histiocytoma	Neck, thigh, and stifle
Miscellaneous	
Dermoid cysts	Dorsal midline
Heterotopic polydontia	Base of ear
Follicular cyst	Head and distal legs
Eosinophilic granuloma	Neck, withers, and back
Axillary nodular necrosis	Near axilla and girth
Unilateral papular dermatosis	Trunk
Exuberant granulation tissue	Legs
Panniculitis	Trunk, neck, proximal legs
Hematoma	Chest
Myospherulosis	?
Foreign body granuloma	Legs and ventrum
Pseudolymphoma	Head and trunk
Calcinosis circumscripta[‡]	Lateral stifle

*References 2, 10, 12, 14, 19, 21.
[†]No apparent site(s) of predilection.
[‡]Calcinosis circumscripta (tumoral calcinosis) may, in some cases, be the end stage of eosinophilic granuloma or mastocytoma.

lesions are usually asymptomatic, observation without treatment may be the preferred approach. Horses with multiple lesions may be treated with systemic glucocorticoids (prednisolone or prednisone at 2 mg/kg orally q24h; dexamethasone 0.2 mg/kg orally q24h) given for 2 to 3 weeks.[13] Some horses may suffer relapses, and retreatment is successful.[6,7,13,22] Some lesions undergo spontaneous remission in 3 to 6 months.[13,22,23] Older or larger lesions are often severely mineralized, do not respond to glucocorticoid therapy, and must be surgically excised.[1,7,13,20,27]

● UNILATERAL PAPULAR DERMATOSIS

Unilateral papular dermatosis is a relatively rare equine dermatosis characterized by multiple asymptomatic papules on only one side of the body.* It accounts for 1.22% of all the equine dermatoses seen at the Cornell University Clinic.

*References 1, 7, 8, 13, 18, 20, 21.

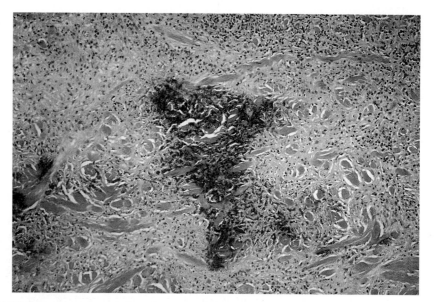

FIGURE 15-5. Eosinophilic granuloma with collagen flame figure.

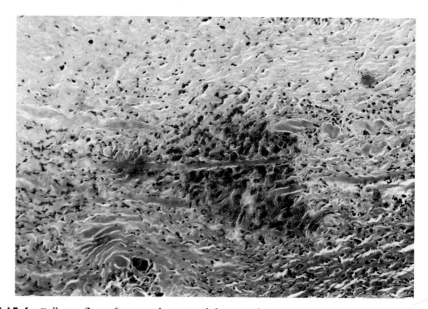

FIGURE 15-6. Collagen flame figure with eosinophilic granuloma.

Cause and Pathogenesis

The etiopathogenesis of this disorder is unknown.[1,7,13,20] Initial descriptions of the condition[18] suggested that quarter horses had a genetic predilection. However, the disorder has been seen in several breeds of horses.[13,31,32] Because many cases are seasonal (spring and summer), and the histopathologic findings of eosinophilic folliculitis and furunculosis are seen in some cats (mosquito bite hypersensitivity, flea bite hypersensitivity, atopy) and horses (*Culicoides* hypersensitivity, onchocerciasis, atopy) with various hypersensitivity disorders,[15,16] it has been hypo-

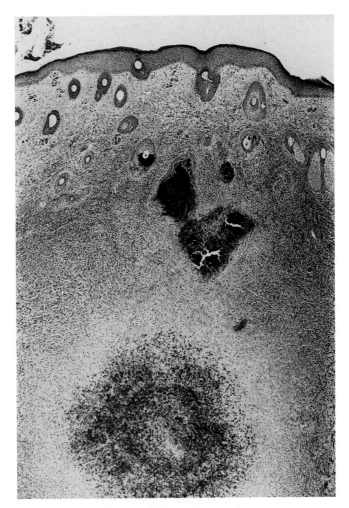

FIGURE 15-7. Foci of necrotizing eosinophilic mural folliculitis overlying eosinophilic granuloma.

thesized that unilateral papular dermatosis may represent an insect hypersensitivity.[6,21] The suspected hypersensitivity would occur on only one side of the body because of the insect's preference to feed on the leeward side of the horse in windy conditions. If this were true, one wonders why the horse always stands in the same direction, and why most horses do not have repeated seasonal recurrences of the dermatosis. Perhaps the damage is caused by an ectoparasite inhabiting bedding and direct contact is involved.[19a]

Clinical Features

There are no apparent age, breed, or sex predilections. Most horses develop lesions in spring and summer. The outstanding clinical feature of the condition is the occurrence of multiple (30 to 300) papules and occasionally nodules limited to one side of the body (Figs. 15-11 and 15-12). The lateral thorax is most commonly affected, but lesions may also be seen on the neck, shoulder, and abdomen. The early lesions are firm, rounded, elevated, well-circumscribed, tufted papules. Pruritus and pain are absent. Some lesions become crusted and alopecic. Affected horses are otherwise healthy.

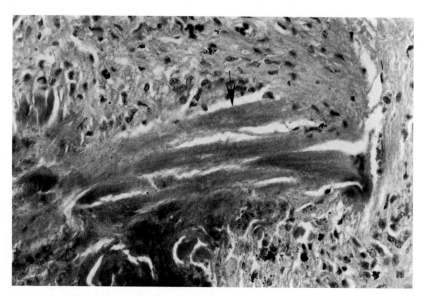

FIGURE 15-8. Collagen degeneration (*arrow*) with eosinophilic granuloma.

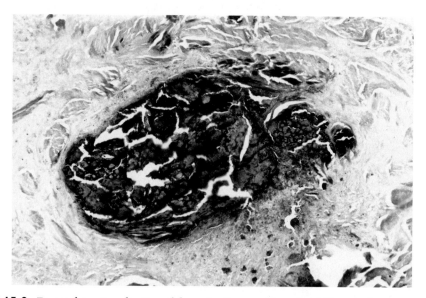

FIGURE 15-9. Dystrophic mineralization of dermal collagen with eosinophilic granuloma.

Diagnosis

Unilateral papular dermatosis is visually distinctive. Cytologic examination reveals predominantly eosinophils and no microorganisms. Skin biopsy often reveals eosinophilic folliculitis and furunculosis (Figs. 15-13 and 15-14).[13,15,31,32] Collagen flame figures may be seen in the surrounding dermis. In some cases, wedge-shaped areas of necrosis or superficial-to-mild dermal eosinophilic granulomas and necrosis, not clearly involving hair follicles, are found.[19a] Special stains and cultures are negative.

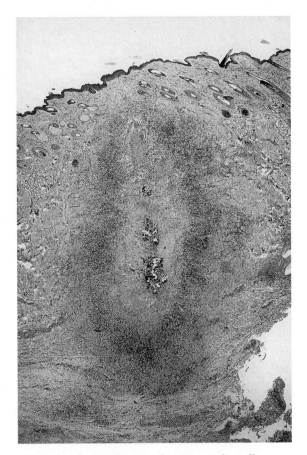

FIGURE 15-10. Eosinophilic granuloma following silicone-coated needle injection. Note linear shape of the reaction.

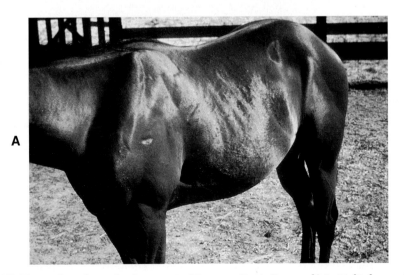

FIGURE 15-11. Unilateral papular dermatosis. (*Courtesy Dr. A. Stannard.*) **A,** Multiple papules on the left side. *Continued*

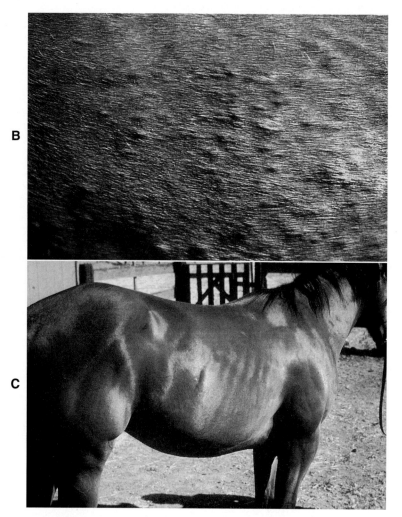

FIGURE 15-11, cont'd. B, Close-up of crusted papules. **C,** Right side of horse is normal.

Clinical Management

Unilateral papular dermatosis typically undergoes spontaneous remission within several weeks to 6 months.* Because of this and the asymptomatic nature of the disease, treatment is not usually attempted. Systemic glucocorticoids (2 mg/kg prednisolone or prednisone orally q24h; 0.2 mg/kg dexamethasone orally q24h) cause rapid resolution (2 to 3 weeks) of the dermatosis. Occasional horses suffer recurrences—on the same side or the opposite side of the body—in subsequent years.[7,13]

● AXILLARY NODULAR NECROSIS

Axillary nodular necrosis is a very rare dermatosis of the horse.[7,13,18,33] The authors' only experiences with this entity are through our telephone consultations and biopsy services.

---

*References 1, 7, 13, 18, 20, 21, 32.

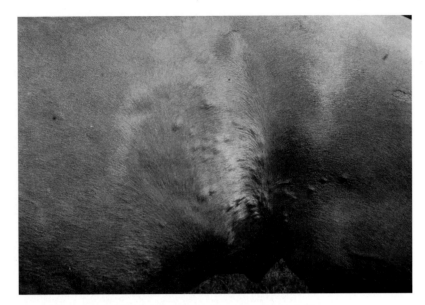

FIGURE 15-12. Unilateral papular dermatosis. Multiple papules in flank.

Cause and Pathogenesis

The etiopathogenesis is unknown. The disorder occurs at all times of the year. Vasculopathic changes have recently been described.[19a,33] It has been suggested that a more precise description for this dermatosis might be *focal nodular eosinophilic granuloma and arteritis.*[33]

Owners often erroneously call the condition "girth galls" and attribute it to overworking or ill-fitting tack.[19a] However, the condition occurs in working and nonworking horses.

Clinical Features

There are no apparent age, breed, or sex predilections. Most horses have three or less (occasionally up to 10) nodules, 1 to 10 cm in diameter, typically present in the girth area behind the elbow (Fig. 15-15).* However, lesions may be seen caudal to the shoulder and on the proximal, medial aspect of the forearm.[33] The lesions are unilateral, rounded, well-circumscribed, and firm, and the overlying skin and hair coat appear normal. Some lesions may develop crateriform ulcers. They are neither pruritic nor painful. Multiple lesions may be arranged in chains and may be connected by a thin cord of palpable tissue (diseased artery?).[19a] Affected horses are otherwise normal.

Diagnosis

The differential diagnosis includes granulomatous disorders (infectious or sterile), neoplasia, or cyst. Definitive diagnosis is based on history, physical examination, skin biopsy, and culture. Cytologic examination reveals eosinophilic to eosinophilic granulomatous inflammation, no microorganisms, and often numerous neutrophils. Histopathologic findings include interstitial-to-nodular-to-diffuse eosinophilic granulomatous dermatitis and panniculitis with focal necrosis (Fig. 15-16).[33] Foci of collagen flame figures, dystrophic mineralization of collagen, palisaded granulomas, and lymphoid nodules are present.[33] Vasculopathic changes include eosinophils associated with vacuolar changes in the tunica media and endothelium of deep dermal and subcutan-

---

*References 1, 7, 13, 18, 19a, 20, 33.

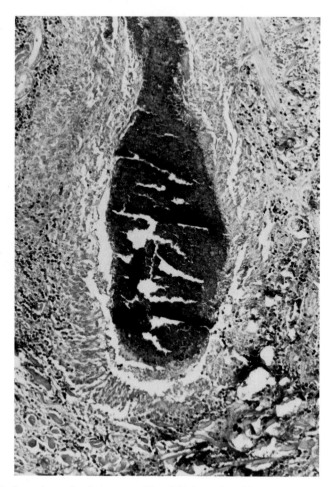

FIGURE 15-13. Unilateral papular dermatosis. Hair follicle replaced by necrotic eosinophils and follicular epithelium ("eosinophilic mush").

eous arteries, small amounts of karyorrhectic nuclear material in the tunica media, endothelial cell hypertrophy and vessel occlusion, and intimal mucinosis (Figs. 15-17 and 15-18).[33] Necrotizing arteritis is occasionally seen. Multiple specimens and multiple sections may be required in order to identify the vascular lesion.[19a] Special stains and cultures are negative.

Clinical Management

If desired, treatment may include surgical excision or sublesional glucocorticoids.[13,33] Triamcinolone acetonide (3 to 5 mg/lesion) or methylprednisolone acetate (5 to 10 mg/lesion) is effective. Some lesions spontaneously regress. Recurrences are rare but may be seen.[7]

● STERILE EOSINOPHILIC FOLLICULITIS AND FURUNCULOSIS

Sterile eosinophilic folliculitis and furunculitis is a rare cutaneous reaction pattern in the horse.[15] It accounts for 0.56% of the equine dermatoses seen at the Cornell University Clinic. Multiple lesions are present in a more-or-less symmetric distribution and may be present anywhere on the body, although the neck, shoulder, brisket, and dorsolateral thorax are most commonly affected

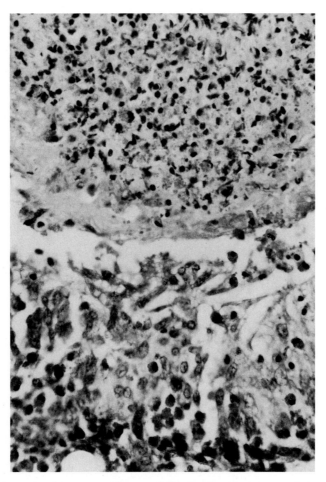

FIGURE 15-14. Unilateral papular dermatosis. Pilary canal filled with necrotic eosinophils.

(Fig. 15-19). Tufted papules become crusted and alopecic. Pruritus is usually moderate to marked, but occasionally is mild. This cutaneous reaction pattern has been seen in horses with atopy, *Culicoides* hypersensitivity, and onchocerciasis.[11] Other cases were idiopathic, but allergy testing was not done. Rarely, solitary areas of furunculosis are seen (Fig. 15-20). Solitary lesions may be reactions to insect or arachnid damage.

Cytologic examination reveals numerous eosinophils. Histopathologic findings include infiltrative-to-necrotizing eosinophilic mural folliculitis and furunculosis (Fig. 15-21) and, occasionally, focal collagen flame figures.[15] Focal areas of eosinophilic mural folliculitis and furunculosis may be seen in biopsy specimens from horses with insect hypersensitivity, atopy, and food hypersensitivity in the corresponding clinical lesions (tufted papules). Special stains and cultures are negative. The diagnostic work-up could include drug withdrawal, ectoparasite control, hypoallergenic diet, and intradermal skin testing to pursue underlying hypersensitivity disorders.

Systemic glucocorticoids (2 mg/kg prednisolone or prednisone orally q24h, 0.2 mg/kg dexamethasone orally q24h) are effective, but relapses are the rule. Long-term management is best achieved by appropriate control of the associated allergy.

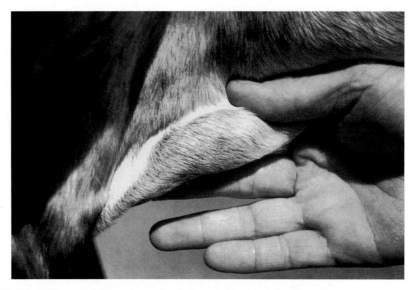

FIGURE 15-15. Axillary nodular necrosis. Nodule in axillary region. (*Courtesy Dr. A. Stannard.*)

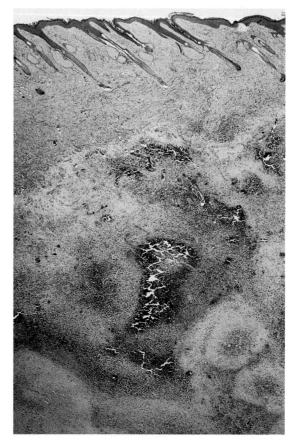

FIGURE 15-16. Axillary nodular necrosis. Eosinophilic granulomatous inflammation of deep dermis and panniculus.

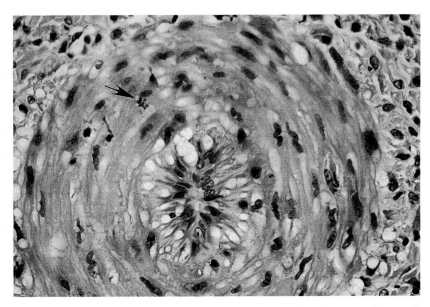

FIGURE 15-17. Axillary nodular necrosis. Subendothelial mucinosis and occasional karyorrhectic leukocyte in vessel wall (*arrow*).

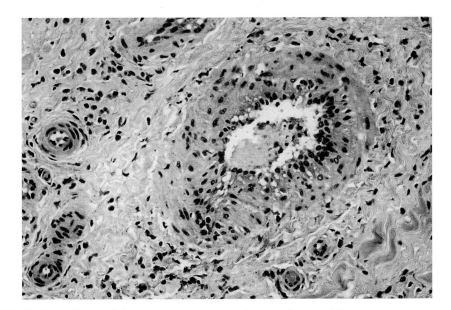

FIGURE 15-18. Axillary nodular necrosis. Intramural edema and eosinophils.

● MULTISYSTEMIC EOSINOPHILIC EPITHELIOTROPIC DISEASE

This is a rare, sporadic disorder characterized by exfoliative dermatitis, ulcerative stomatitis, wasting, and infiltration of epithelial tissues by eosinophils and lymphocytes. It accounts for 0.22% of the equine dermatoses seen at the Cornell University Clinic.

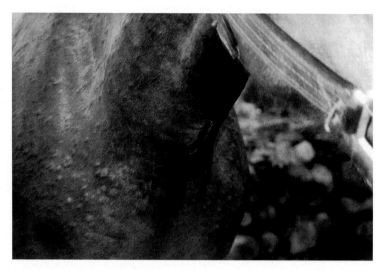

FIGURE 15-19. Sterile eosinophilic folliculitis and furunculosis. Multiple tufted papules on brisket of atopic horse.

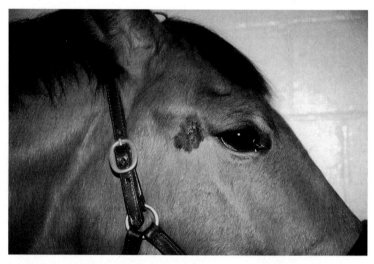

FIGURE 15-20. Sterile eosinophilic folliculitis and furunculosis. Solitary area of papules and annular alopecia near eye.

Cause and Pathogenesis

The etiopathogenesis of this condition is unknown. Various authors have suggested hypersensitivity reactions to *Strongylus equinus* larvae,[34] food allergens,[35] or an epitheliotropic cell–associated virus.[40] Swedish investigators have suggested a genetic basis for the syndrome in standardbreds.[38]

Clinical Features

Although horses can be affected at any age, most are young (mean age 3 to 4 years).[38,40] Standardbreds and thoroughbreds account for about 70% and 20%, respectively, of all reported cases.[35,36a-39] There is no sex predilection.

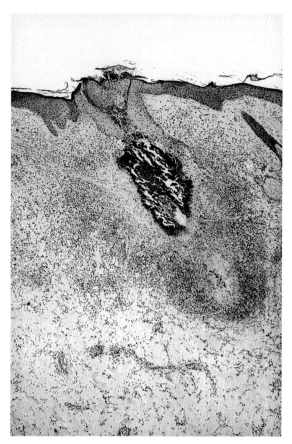

FIGURE 15-21. Sterile eosinophilic folliculitis and furunculosis. Infiltrative, necrotizing, mural folliculitis and furunculosis.

The dermatitis usually begins insidiously with scaling, crusting, oozing, alopecia, and fissures on the coronets and/or the face (Figs. 15-22, *A* through *C*). Oral ulceration is often an early finding. Some horses initially develop well-demarcated ulcers on the coronets, muzzle, and mucocutaneous junctions.[36] Rarely, vesicles and bullae are seen in these areas,[37] or urticarial eruptions may be seen in the early phase of the disease.[38] The dermatosis then develops into a more-or-less generalized exfoliative dermatitis with scaling, crusting, easy epilation, alopecia, and focal areas of ulceration (Fig. 15-22, *D*). Pruritus is variable. Peripheral lymph nodes may be enlarged.

Affected horses develop progressive weight loss with a variable appetite (poor, normal, ravenous). Pitting edema of the ventral chest and abdomen and of the distal limbs is commonly seen. Fever (38° to 40° C) or recalcitrant diarrhea may be seen in up to 50% of the cases.

Diagnosis

The differential diagnosis includes pemphigus foliaceus, systemic lupus erythematosus, sarcoidosis, bullous pemphigoid, pemphigus vulgaris, vasculitis, erythema multiforme, epitheliotropic lymphoma, drug reaction, and various toxicoses (vetch, stachybotryotoxicosis). The definitive diagnosis is based on history, physical examination, and biopsy results. The most common laboratory abnormalities are hypoalbuminemia (0.8 to 2.4 g/dl) in most horses, mild-to-moderate leukocytosis and neutrophilia (50% of the cases), and mild nonregenerative anemia (25%). Blood eosinophilia

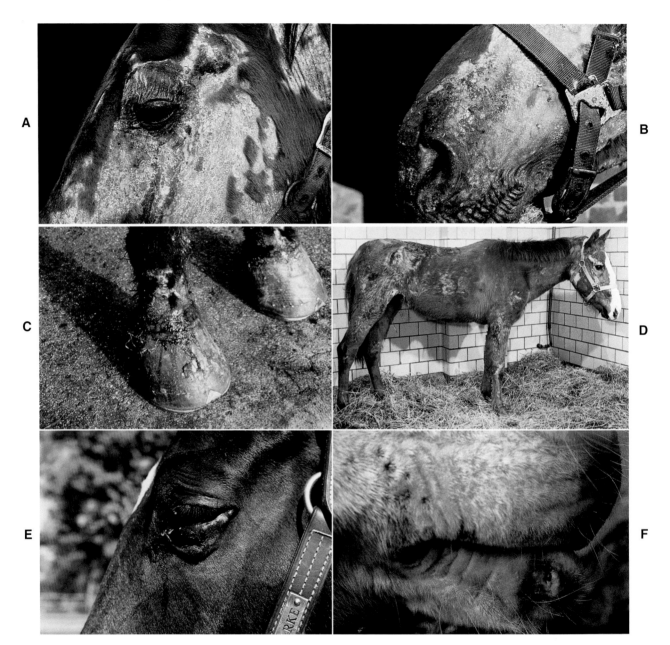

FIGURE 15-22. **A,** Multisystemic eosinophilic epitheliotropic disease. Alopecia, scaling, and ulceration on face. (*Courtesy Dr. E. Guaguère.*) **B,** Same horse as in *A.* Alopecia, scaling, and ulceration on muzzle. (*Courtesy Dr. E. Guaguère.*) **C,** Same horse as in *A* and *B.* Alopecia, ulceration, and oozing of distal leg and coronet. (*Courtesy Dr. E. Guaguère.*) **D,** Multisystemic eosinophilic epitheliotropic disease. Widespread exfoliative dermatitis. **E,** Sterile pyogranuloma. Erythematous, ulcerated nodule on lower lip. **F,** Sterile pyogranuloma. Ulcerated nodule on lower eyelid.

is rarely seen. Radiolabeled (^{51}Cr) albumin studies reveal extensive gastrointestinal protein loss, and oral glucose tolerance tests demonstrated intestinal malabsorption.[37,38] Attempts to isolate pathogenic microorganisms have not been successful.

Dermatohistopathologic findings include an intermingling of inflammatory reaction patterns: superficial and deep perivascular, lichenoid interface, interstitial, diffuse, and granulomatous (Fig. 15-23).[14,40] Eosinophils, lymphocytes, and plasma cells are the dominant inflammatory cells. Epidermal hyperplasia is marked and irregular. Hyperkeratosis is prominent and mixed (ortho-keratotic and parakeratotic). An epitheliotropic infiltration of eosinophils and lymphocytes is typical, and apoptotic keratinocytes may be prominent (Figs. 15-24 and 15-25). Eosinophilic microabscesses and eosinophilic folliculitis and furunculosis may be seen. Foci of collagen flame figures or lymphoid nodule formation are occasionally seen. Neutrophilic microabscesses and suppurative folliculitis and furunculosis may be seen; these presumably reflect secondary bacterial infection. Direct immunofluorescence testing is negative.[34,36,40]

Rectal, liver, and lymph node biopsies are frequently performed to demonstrate the multisystemic nature of the disorder. Necropsy examination reveals involvement of multiple epithelial organs, especially pancreas, salivary glands, gastrointestinal tract, esophagus, liver, and bronchi. Lymph nodes, kidneys, spleen, and adrenal glands are also commonly affected.

Clinical Management

The prognosis varies with the chronicity and severity of the disease. Most horses suffer a progressive dermatitis and wasting over the course of several months (1 to 10) and are eventually euthanized or die. Large doses of glucocorticoids (2.2 to 4.4 mg/kg prednisolone or prednisone q24h, or 0.2 to 0.4 mg/kg dexamethasone q24h) may be effective if administered early in the course of the disease.[14,35] Horses that do respond to glucocorticoids relapse when these drugs are discontinued.

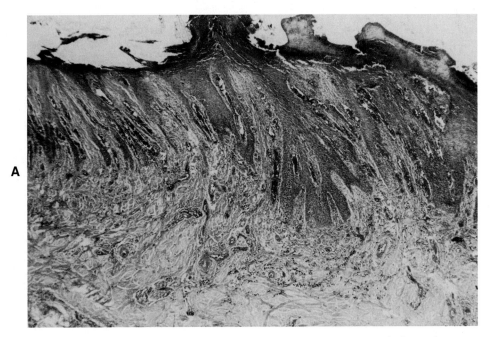

FIGURE 15-23. Multisystemic eosinophilic epitheliotropic disease. **A,** Severely hyperplastic interstitial dermatitis. *Continued*

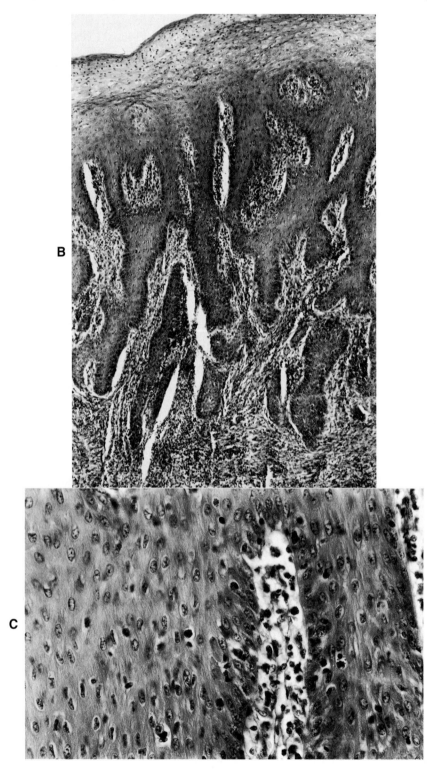

FIGURE 15-23, cont'd. B, Pseudocarcinomatous epidermal hyperplasia with multisystemic epithelio-tropic eosinophilic disease. **C**, Exocytosis of eosinophils associated with multisystemic epitheliotropic eosinophilic disease.

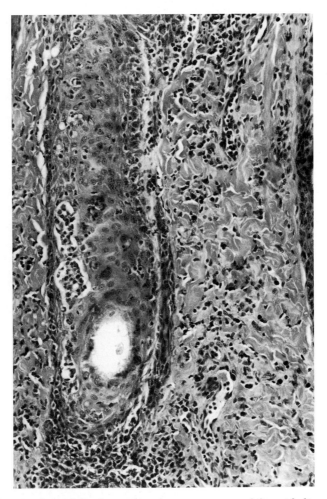

FIGURE 15-24. Pustular mural folliculitis with multisystemic eosinophilic epitheliotropic disease.

The combination of dexamethasone and hydroxyurea (20 mg/kg orally q24h) was ineffective in one horse.[37] Horses with the wasting syndrome usually do not respond.

Because of the hypersensitivity-like inflammatory reaction that characterizes this disorder, the striking involvement of skin and gastrointestinal tract, and the poor response to glucocorticoids, food hypersensitivity is an attractive etiologic hypothesis. The authors suggest that hypoallergenic diets should be evaluated in these horses (see Chapter 8).

● LINEAR ALOPECIA

Linear alopecia is a rare linear dermatosis of the horse.[19a,41] The authors' only experiences with this disorder are through telephone consultations and skin biopsy services.

Cause and Pathogenesis

The etiopathogenesis is unknown. Although the disorder has been seen in many breeds, the frequent occurrence in quarter horses would suggest genetic predisposition. It has been speculated that there may be some local dysregulation of keratinocyte function, which would allow the keratinocyte to secrete cytokines chemotactic for inflammatory cells.[41]

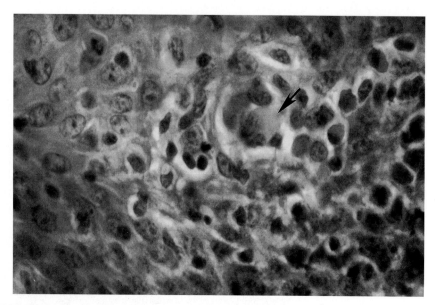

FIGURE 15-25. Multisystemic eosinophilic epitheliotropic disease. Exocytosis of lymphocytes and eosinophils and apoptotic keratinocytes (*arrow*).

Clinical Features

Circular areas of alopecia, usually in a linear vertically oriented configuration, are seen on the neck, shoulder, and/or lateral thorax areas (Fig. 15-26). One or more linear areas may be present. The lesions are usually 2 to 10 mm wide by a few centimeters to 1 meter in length. Mild surface scale and/or crust may be present. The lesions are neither painful nor pruritic. Affected horses are otherwise healthy. In some cases, linear alopecia has coexisted with so-called "linear keratosis" (see Chapter 16).

Diagnosis

The differential diagnosis includes infectious folliculitides (dermatophytosis, dermatophilosis, demodicosis, staphylococcosis), alopecia areata, and follicular dysplasia. The linearity is suggestive of trauma (e.g., scratch, whipmark) or epidermal nevus (see Chapter 16). Definitive diagnosis is based on history, physical examination, and skin biopsy. Histopathologic findings include an early infiltrative lymphocytic mural folliculitis with variable outer root sheath edema, to a later lymphohistiocytic mural folliculitis (Figs. 15-27 and 15-28). Epithelioid cells and multinucleated histiocytic giant cells are prominent in chronic lesions (Fig. 15-29), and apoptotic keratinocytes may be found in the wall of the hair follicle.[19a,41] Complete follicular destruction and permanent alopecia may occur. Sebaceous glands may be involved in some cases, and erythema multiforme-like epidermal changes may occasionally be present.[19a] Special stains and cultures are negative.

Clinical Management

Spontaneous remission is not reported. Topical or systemic glucocorticoid therapy may slow the progression or resolve the lesions, but recurrence is likely.

● PANNICULITIS

Panniculitis is a multifunctional inflammatory condition of the subcutaneous fat, characterized by deep-seated nodules that may become cystic and ulcerated and develop draining tracts. The

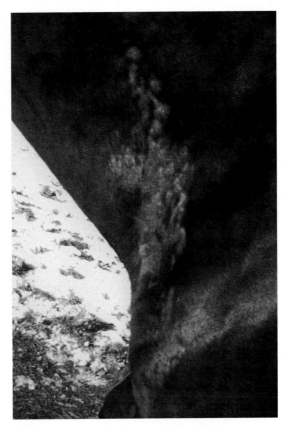

FIGURE 15-26. Linear alopecia. Annular areas of alopecia on lateral neck, cranial to shoulder.

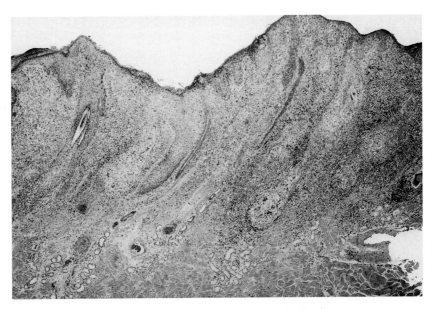

FIGURE 15-27. Linear alopecia. Granulomatous infiltrative mural folliculitis.

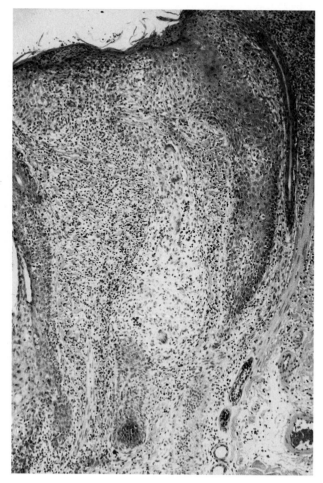

FIGURE 15-28. Linear alopecia. Central hair follicle is nearly replaced by granulomatous inflammation.

disorder is rare in horses[13,47] and accounts for 0.44% of the equine skin disorders seen at the Cornell University Clinic.

Cause and Pathogenesis

The lipocyte is particularly vulnerable to trauma, ischemia, and neighboring inflammatory disease. In addition, damage to lipocytes results in the liberation of lipid, which undergoes hydrolysis into glycerol and fatty acids. Fatty acids are potent inflammatory agents, and they incite further inflammatory and granulomatous tissue reactions.

Multiple etiologic factors are involved in the genesis of panniculitis in human beings, dogs, and cats (Table 15-2).[4,17] Most of these factors have yet to be recognized in horses. Serum α1-proteinase inhibitor concentrations were normal in two quarter horse foals with idiopathic nodular panniculitis.[42a] Infectious causes of equine panniculitis are discussed elsewhere (see Chapters 4 and 5) and are not addressed here. This section concentrates on sterile forms of panniculitis. The occurrence of idiopathic nodular panniculitis in two quarter horse foals from the same mare suggests that genetic factors could be involved in some cases.[42a]

Nodular panniculitis refers to sterile subcutaneous inflammatory nodules and is *not* a specific disease. It is a purely descriptive term, clinically representing the end result of several known and

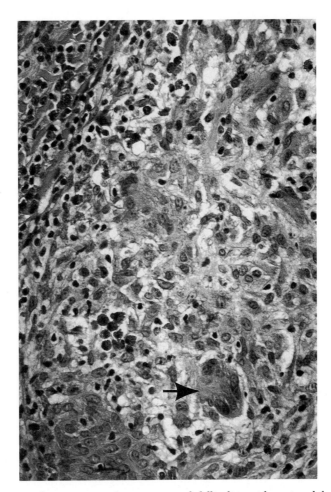

FIGURE 15-29. Linear alopecia. Granulomatous mural folliculitis with eosinophils and multinucleated giant cells (*arrow*).

unknown etiologic factors. *Weber-Christian panniculitis* has been a frequently misused term and does *not* exist as a specific disease. In horses, the majority of cases of sterile nodular panniculitis are of idiopathic origin.

One form of generalized steatitis in foals has been hypothesized to be associated with deficiencies of selenium and/or vitamin E, but this relationship is not at all clear.[11] One of the authors (DWS) has rarely encountered horses with solitary panniculitis lesions that appeared to be postinjectional.

Clinical Features

One sporadic form of equine panniculitis (steatitis, yellow fat disease) has been reported in suckling or recently weaned foals, especially in spring and early summer.* The foals develop firm, indurated, often painful, poorly demarcated, extensive plaque-like areas. The lesions are especially prominent over the dorsolateral surfaces of the body and along the nuchal crest. Affected foals often manifest signs of systemic illness: fever (up to 40.5° C), inappetence, depression, weight loss,

---

*References 45, 46, 48, 50, 52-54.

● Table 15-2   **DIFFERENTIAL DIAGNOSIS OF PANNICULITIS**

Infectious
　　Bacterial,° mycobacterial, actinomycetic,° fungal,° chlamydial, viral
Immunologic
　　Lupus erythematosus, rheumatoid arthritis, drug reaction, erythema nodosum, arthropod bite
Physiochemical (factitial)
　　Trauma, pressure, cold, foreign body° (e.g., postsubcutaneous injections of vaccines or bulky, oily, or
　　insoluble liquids)
Pancreatic disease
　　Inflammation, neoplasia
Postglucocorticoid therapy
Vasculitis
　　Leukocytoclastic, thrombophlebitis, embolism
Nutritional
　　Vitamin E deficiency
Enteropathies
Hereditary
　　α_1-Antitrypsin deficiency
Idiopathic°

°Recognized in horses.

and increased cardiorespiratory rates. Some animals develop skeletal muscle degeneration, resulting in lameness or stiff gaits. Affected fat is firm, yellowish-brown, and often contains scattered hemorrhages.

A second, rare form of equine panniculitis occurs as individual nodules.[13,47,51] No age (2 months to 15 years), breed, or sex predilections are recognized. Lesions occur singly[49] or in crops,[42-44,47,51] either localized to specific areas (rump, neck, chest, thigh), or generalized (especially trunk, neck, proximal limbs), and may come and go spontaneously (Figs. 15-30 and 15-31). They are papules and nodules, 5 mm to 10 cm in diameter, firm and well-circumscribed or soft and ill-defined. The lesions may or may not be painful, and they may heal with depressed scars. They may become cystic, ulcerating and developing draining tracts that discharge an oily, yellowish-brown to bloody substance (Fig. 15-32). Concurrent constitutional signs (anorexia, depression, lethargy, fever, weight loss, lameness) may be present.° In two horses, blood selenium and vitamin E levels were within normal limits.[47]

Diagnosis

The differential diagnosis includes granulomatous diseases (infectious or sterile), neoplasia (especially lymphoma), and cysts. Definitive diagnosis is based on history, physical examination, cytology, skin biopsy, and culture. Aspirates from intact lesions usually reveal numerous neutrophils and macrophages, occasional multinucleated histiocytic giant cells, and no microorganisms. Macrophages (lipophages) and giant cells contain numerous intracytoplasmic fat droplets (Fig. 15-33). Sudan stains may reveal extracellular and intracellular lipid droplets. Cultures are negative.

The diagnosis of panniculitis can be confirmed only by biopsy, and excisional biopsy is the *only* biopsy technique that is satisfactory for subcutaneous nodules. Punch biopsies fail to deliver sufficient tissue to be of diagnostic value in most cases. Panniculitis may be necrotizing, suppurative, pyogranulomatous, granulomatous, or fibrosing (Figs. 15-34 through 15-36). Special stains are negative for microorganisms, and polarized light examination is negative for foreign material. The sporadic form of generalized panniculitis (steatitis) in foals is characterized by varying degrees of

°References 13, 42, 42a, 43a, 47, 51.

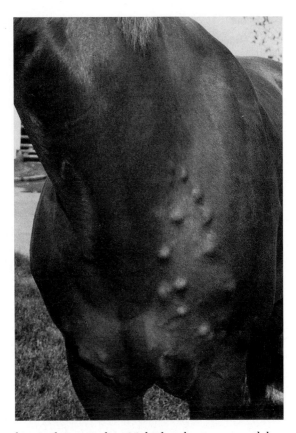

FIGURE 15-30. Idiopathic sterile panniculitis. Multiple subcutaneous nodules on chest.

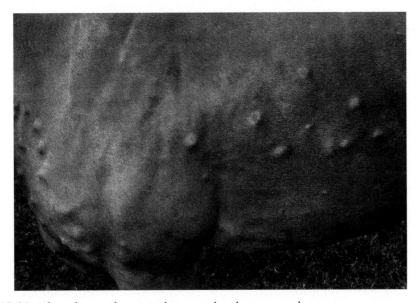

FIGURE 15-31. Idiopathic sterile panniculitis. Annular plaques over thorax.

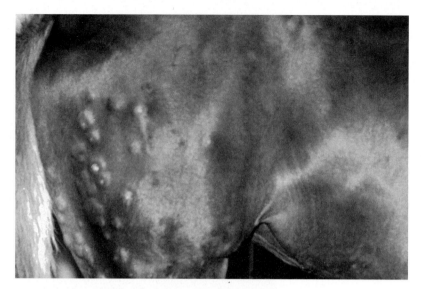

FIGURE 15-32. Idiopathic sterile panniculitis. Draining subcutaneous nodules on thigh.

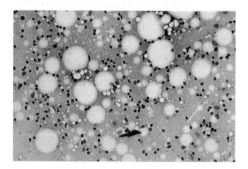

FIGURE 15-33. Idiopathic sterile panniculitis. Granulomatous inflammation with numerous extracellular fat droplets.

noninflammatory fat necrosis and secondary granulomatous panniculitis.[43,50,52] Ceroid is present in lipocytes, macrophages, and interlobular connective tissue septae. Ceroid is a pink-to-yellow homogeneous material in H & E stains and deep crimson in acid-fast stains. Dystrophic mineralization may be prominent.

The rare nodular form of panniculitis is characterized by variable degrees of nodular-to-diffuse, pyogranulomatous-to-fibrosing panniculitis.[42a,43a,47,51] Multiple lymphoid nodules are often present (Fig. 15-37).

Clinical Management

In the sporadic steatitis of foals, no successful therapy has been described. Although deficiencies of selenium and/or vitamin E have been suspected, treatment with these substances has not been successful. There are rare reports of spontaneous recovery.[50]

In the rare nodular form of panniculitis, most horses have been treated with systemic glucocorticoids (2 mg/kg prednisolone or prednisone orally q24h; 0.2 mg/kg dexamethasone orally q24h).[47,51] There has been no consistent pattern of response to glucocorticoids. Some horses have gone into rapid remission (14 to 21 days), with no recurrence after therapy is stopped.[42,47,51] Other

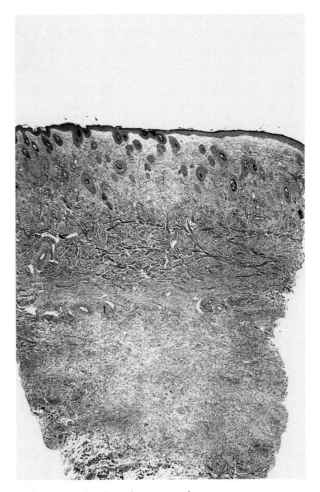

FIGURE 15-34. Panniculitis in sterile idiopathic panniculitis.

horses have responded, suffered recurrences when off medication, and required chronic alternate-day treatment.[42a,47,51] Still other horses have not responded at all.[47] It is not known whether additional immunomodulatory therapy with agents such as azathioprine, inorganic iodides, and omega-3/omega-6 fatty acids would be useful.[4,17] In one horse with a solitary nodule, surgical excision was successful.[49]

• SARCOIDOSIS

Equine sarcoidosis (generalized or systemic granulomatous disease) is a rare disorder characterized by exfoliative dermatitis, severe wasting, and sarcoidal granulomatous inflammation of multiple organ systems. It accounts for 0.44% of the equine dermatoses seen at the Cornell University Clinic.

Causes and Pathogenesis

Although the etiopathogenesis of this disorder is unknown, it has many similarities to human sarcoidosis, which is thought to represent an immunologic reaction to an infectious agent or

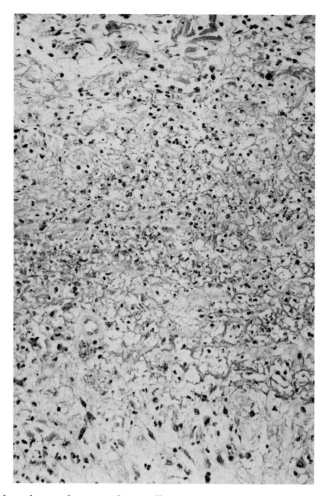

FIGURE 15-35. Idiopathic sterile panniculitis. Diffuse, necrotizing, suppurative panniculitis.

allergen.° It may be that multiple triggering factors are involved in this syndrome. In horses, cultures, electron microscopic examination, and animal inoculation studies have failed to demonstrate an infectious agent.[14,19a,56,59] Direct immunofluorescence or immunoperoxidase testing of affected skin have been negative.[14,56,59]

A condition similar to equine sarcoidosis has been described in a horse infected with *Mycobacterium intracellulare* serotype 8 (see Chapter 4). This is interesting, because equine sarcoidosis, as well as opportunistic mycobacterial infections in dogs and cats, are seen much more commonly in the western United States than in the northeastern United States. Perhaps mycobacterial antigens play a role in equine sarcoidosis.

It has also been suggested that hairy vetch (*Vicia* sp.) toxicosis may be a cause of some cases of equine sarcoidosis (see Chapter 13). Many horses with sarcoidosis have had no exposure to hairy vetch.

In human sarcoidosis, the center of sarcoidal granulomas is composed of macrophages, multinucleated histiocytic giant cells, and helper (CD4+) T lymphocytes, whereas the periphery

---

°References 1, 4, 13-15, 18, 19a, 55, 56, 58, 59.

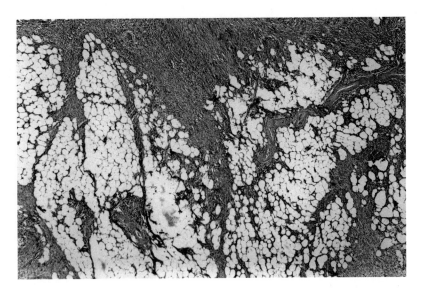

FIGURE 15-36. Septal panniculitis.

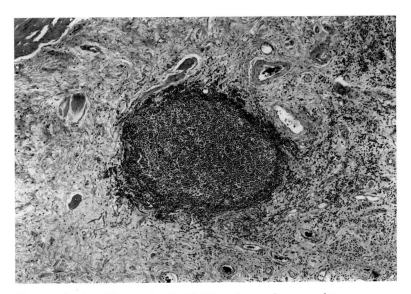

FIGURE 15-37. Lymphoid nodule associated with idiopathic sterile panniculitis.

of the granuloma has a large number of interdigitating macrophages and suppressor (CD8+) T lymphocytes.[5] It is probable that this arrangement of interdigitating macrophage—CD8+ cells on the periphery and the epithelioid cell—CD4+ cells pattern in the center provides an efficient perimeter defense against a persistent, poorly degradable antigen of low potency.

In one horse with pulmonary mineralization, macrophages expressed the hypercalcemic hormone, PTH-related protein.[58a] However, this horse was not hypercalcemic.

Polymerase chain reaction (PCR) technology has shown that mycobacterial (multiple species) DNA is present in most skin lesions in humans with sarcoidosis.[57] Similar studies in equine sarcoidosis are awaited.

In one study, three horses with sarcoidosis had positive titers to *Borrelia burgdorferi*.[58]

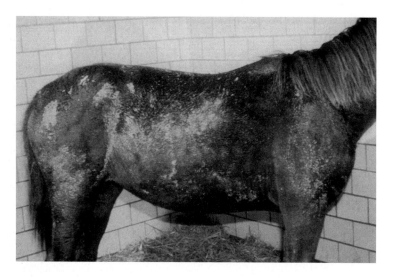

FIGURE 15-38. Sarcoidosis. Generalized exfoliative dermatitis.

Clinical Findings

No age (3 to >20 years), breed, or sex predilections are apparent. The onset is usually insidious, but may be explosive. The dermatosis usually begins as scaling, crusting, and alopecia on the face or legs, and progresses to a multifocal or generalized exfoliative dermatitis (Figs. 15-38 and 15-39, *A*). The mane and tail tend to be spared. Cutaneous nodules are very rarely seen, either alone or in conjunction with the aforementioned skin lesions. In one horse, the skin of the lips and eyelids had blotchy areas of depigmentation.[56] Peripheral lymph nodes may be enlarged. Affected horses usually go on to develop a wasting syndrome characterized by exercise intolerance, poor appetite, weight loss, and persistent low-grade fever. Clinical signs of lung involvement may include exercise intolerance, increased resting respiratory rate, and/or mild dyspnea. Liver and gastrointestinal involvement may cause diarrhea and icterus. Rarely, bone lesions may produce lameness.

Occasional horses develop isolated hyperkeratotic, crusted, alopecic plaques, especially on the legs (Fig. 15-39, *B*). These horses are typically otherwise healthy.

Diagnosis

The differential diagnosis includes dermatophilosis, dermatophytosis, pemphigus foliaceus, systemic lupus erythematosus, drug reaction, contact dermatitis, seborrhea, multisystemic eosinophilic epitheliotropic disease, epitheliotropic lymphoma, and toxicoses (arsenic, iodine, vetch). Definitive diagnosis is based on history, physical examination, and skin biopsy. Histopathologic findings include a nodular-to-diffuse sarcoidal granulomatous dermatitis that may affect all portions of the dermis (Fig. 15-40).[13,55,56,58,59] Multinucleated histiocytic giant cells are numerous (Fig. 15-41). Rarely, the subcutaneous fat may be affected to a lesser degree.[56] Identical lesions are usually found in other organs, in descending order of frequency, especially the lung, mesenteric and thoracic lymph nodes, liver, gastrointestinal tract, spleen, and kidney, bone, central nervous system, heart, adrenal glands, and thyroid glands. Some horses have variable combinations of leukocytosis, mild nonregenerative anemia, hyperfibrinogenemia, hyperglobulinemia, and hypoalbuminemia.[58,58a]

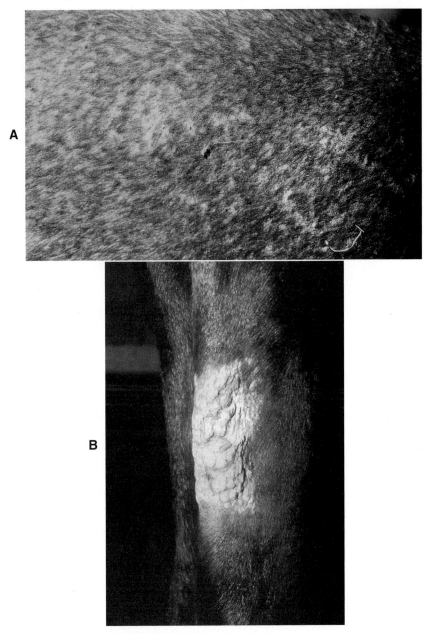

FIGURE 15-39. Sarcoidosis. **A,** Close-up of exfoliative dermatitis. **B,** Solitary hyperkeratotic, crusted, alopecic plaque on leg. (*Courtesy Dr. M. Sloet.*)

Clinical Management

The prognosis varies with the chronicity and severity of the disease.[13,14,59] Some horses resolve spontaneously. Most horses suffer a progressive dermatitis and wasting over the course of weeks to months and are eventually euthanized. Immunosuppressive doses of glucocorticoids (prednisolone or prednisone 2 to 4 mg/kg orally q24h; dexamethasone 0.2 to 0.4 mg/kg orally q24h) may be effective if administered early in the course of the disease—before the onset of the wasting

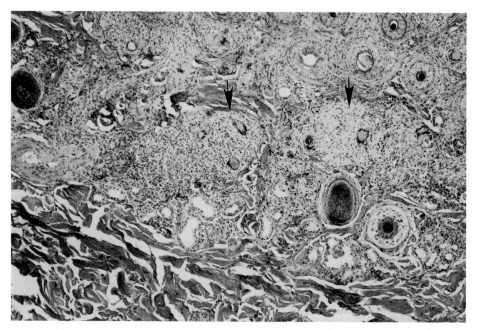

FIGURE 15-40. Sarcoidosis. Sarcoidal granulomatous dermatitis (*arrows*).

syndrome—and continued on an alternate-morning basis for several weeks. Two of four horses in one study were "cured" with prednisolone (no follow-up period stated); the other two horses had only partial responses.[58] One horse was successfully treated with prednisone, relapsed 10 months later, and again responded to treatment with prednisone.[56] Animals experiencing the wasting syndrome usually do not respond. A few horses have experienced spontaneous remissions.

● IDIOPATHIC STERILE PYOGRANULOMA

Sterile pyogranulomas of unknown cause have rarely been recognized in horses (see Preface and Acknowledgments).[15] They account for 0.44% of the equine dermatoses seen at the Cornell University Clinic. Lesions have been asymptomatic, single or multiple, firm, papular-to nodular-to-plaque-like, and scattered on the body. Some lesions are ulcerated (Figs. 15-22, *E* and *F*, and 15-42). Rare cases show polycyclic dermal cords (Figs. 15-43 and 15-44). Affected horses were otherwise healthy. Cytologic examination reveals pyogranulomatous inflammation with no microorganisms (Fig. 15-45). Histopathologic findings included nodular to diffuse pyogranulomatous dermatitis within the dermis (Figs. 15-46 and 15-47). The panniculus was occasionally involved. Special stains and cultures were negative. Two horses were treated with systemic glucocorticoids (2 mg/kg prednisone orally q24h) and went into remission within 3 weeks. However, the two horses with multiple, multifocal lesions relapsed within 6 to 8 weeks after therapy was stopped.

● SCLERODERMA

In humans, scleroderma occurs in localized and generalized forms.[4] The cause and pathogenesis of scleroderma are unknown, with genetic, environmental, and immunologic factors being implicated. Classically, three main theories have emerged: (1) the vascular theory (early endothelial

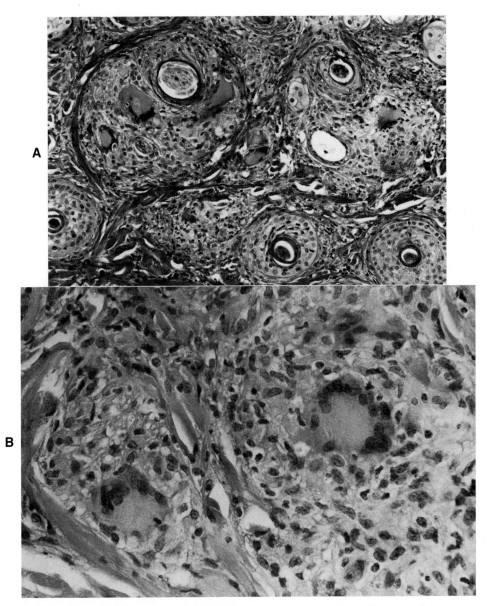

FIGURE 15-41. Sarcoidosis. **A,** Sarcoidal granuloma in sarcoidosis. **B,** Multinucleated histiocytic giant cells.

injury, perivascular fibrosis, hypoxia, and abnormal vascular reactivity); (2) the abnormal collagen metabolism theory (increased production of collagen and reduced collagenase activity); (3) the immunologic theory (humoral and cell-mediated autoimmunity). The possible importance of *Borrelia burgdorferi* infections and early eosinophil-induced pathology are being explored.[4,61] An increased incidence of scleroderma occurs in humans exposed to silica dust and various chemicals and therapeutics.[4,61]

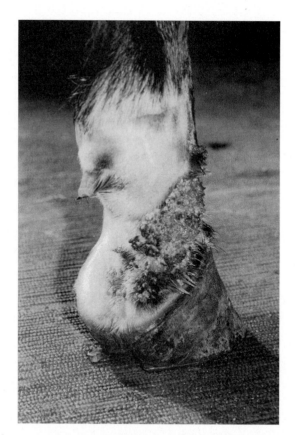

FIGURE 15-42. Sterile pyogranuloma. Ulcerated plaque on distal leg.

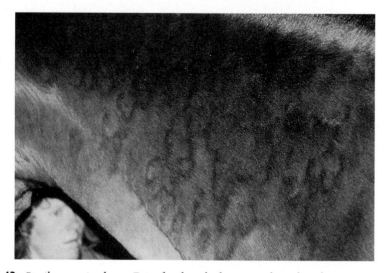

FIGURE 15-43. Sterile pyogranuloma. Raised polycyclic lesions on lateral neck.

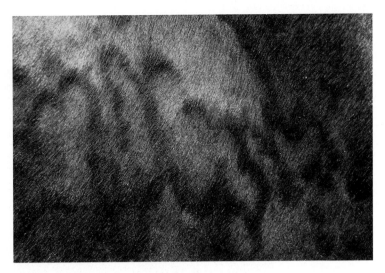

FIGURE 15-44. Close-up of lesions in Fig. 15-43.

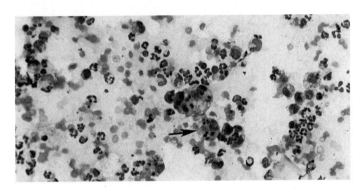

FIGURE 15-45. Sterile pyogranuloma. Pyogranulomatous inflammation with nondegenerate neutrophils and neutrophagocytosis (*arrow*).

Localized Scleroderma

Localized scleroderma (morphea) was reported in a 2-year-old Morgan cross.[60] The horse presented with bilateral, asymmetric, plaques of thickened skin over the rump and hind legs. The lesions varied from 2 to 6 cm in diameter to 10 × 25 cm. Some of the lesions had a raised peripheral rim and a depressed center. In most lesions, the overlying skin and hair coat were normal. Pruritus and pain were absent, and the horse was otherwise healthy. Skin biopsy revealed a markedly thickened deep dermal collagen layer and a mild perivascular accumulation of lymphocytes.

In humans, dogs, and cats, spontaneous remission may occur over a period of several weeks.[4,16] In humans, pentoxifylline has been recommended.[4]

Generalized Scleroderma

In humans, generalized scleroderma (systemic sclerosis) is a rare multisystemic disorder that results in progressive fibrosis and microvascular injury to the skin, lungs, gastrointestinal tract, kidneys, and heart.[4]

Generalized scleroderma was reported in a 9-year-old Paso Fino mare.[61] The animal was depressed and thin, and a large, hard plaque on the ventral abdomen extended from the udder to

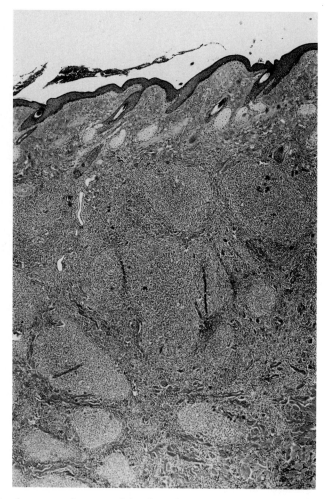

FIGURE 15-46. Sterile pyogranuloma. Nodular deep dermal pyogranulomatous inflammation.

the xiphoid and up one-third of the ventrolateral aspect of the body wall. Histopathologic findings included numerous thick bands of mature fibrous tissue that infiltrated the dermis, subcutis, and skeletal muscle. A mild, perivascular lymphohistiocytic infiltrate was present. At necropsy examination, variably increased amounts of mature fibrous tissue were present in the liver, pancreas, lungs, and kidneys. The 4-year-old daughter of this mare was reported to have a similar condition.

In humans, treatment of systemic sclerosis is usually unrewarding.[4]

● ANHIDROSIS

Anhidrosis is common in horses in hot, humid climates and is characterized by the inability to sweat in response to an adequate stimulus.[11,13,62,75,81-86]

Cause and Pathogenesis

The etiopathogenesis is unknown, but no particular diet, vitamin-mineral supplement or deficiency, or hereditary predilection appears to play a role.[81-86] The onset of the condition is not always associated with poor acclimatization but may be precipitated by heat stress in a humid environment,

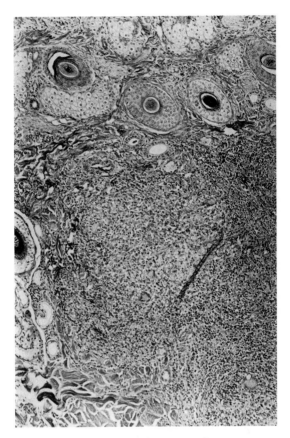

FIGURE 15-47. Pyogranuloma with idiopathic sterile pyogranuloma.

whether previously experienced or not.[67,81-86] Horses can lose up to 45 L of fluid per day via sweat in strenuous exercise, and the major electrolytes lost are chloride, potassium, and sodium.[65]

Equine anhidrosis is believed to result from a conditioned insensitivity of sweat glands to epinephrine.[8,11,13,81-86] Blood epinephrine levels in horses in the tropics are higher than those in horses in temperate climates.[68-71] Blood levels of epinephrine in normal and anhidrotic horses in the tropics are similar,[64,68-71] but anhidrotics have a very poor sweating response to intravenously or intradermally administered epinephrine. Ultrastructural studies of the sweat glands of anhidrotic horses indicate that the condition, which is induced by prolonged stimulation, results from a gradual failure of the mechanism of sweat production, and culminates in secretory cell degeneration.[76,77] Ultrastructural studies also demonstrated that the percentage of degenerate secretory cells remains about the same after the heat stress is relieved and the horse has recovered.[77] Thus, it is likely that susceptible horses suffer a progressive increase in the number of irreversibly damaged secretory cells over a period of years. Areas on the body that may retain the ability to sweat include under the mane, in the saddle and halter regions, and the axillary, inguinal, and perineal regions.[75]

Clinical Features

Equine anhidrosis (dry-coat, nonsweating) has an incidence of up to 20% in some geographic areas (hot, humid climates) and is an economically significant condition in horses in rigorous training for racing, endurance, polo, or show, as well as in brood mares and idle pleasure horses.[66,81-86] In the

United States it is a particular problem in the Gulf Coast states. Horses of all ages, sexes, breeds, and colors may be affected. Adolescents are rarely affected.[81] Native and imported horses are equally affected.

The severity of clinical signs depends on the degree of anhidrosis.[72] Most commonly there is a progressive decline in sweating capacity in response to a similar thermal load. Affected horses exhibit a patchy or inadequate sweating response and are slow to cool out after exercise (hyperthermia and tachypnea may persist for 1 to 2 hours postexercise). Although high-protein diets were reported to be common in anhidrotic horses, others have failed to corroborate this.[75]

Acutely, anhidrosis is characterized by labored breathing, flared nostrils, fever (up to 42° C), and partial or complete lack of sweating. The predominant clinical sign of impending anhidrosis is tachypnea.[75] Interestingly, affected horses are not usually tachycardic and often drink *less* water. Collapse and death may occur. Chronically, a dry hair coat, excessive scaling, and partial alopecia of the face and neck may be seen. Residual areas of sweating may persist under the mane and saddle and in the axillae and groin.[81] The skin is hot and dry. Pruritus, polydipsia, polyuria, poor appetite, and loss of body condition may occur.

Diagnosis

Diagnosis is based on history, physical examination, and response to intradermal injections of epinephrine.[8,11,13,71,82-86] Epinephrine at concentrations of 1:1,000, 1:10,000 1:100,000, and 1:1,000,000 is injected intradermally at a dose of 0.5 ml each. In normal horses, sweating occurs over the injection sites within minutes, at all dilutions. Anhidrotic horses respond to *only* the 1:1,000 dilution, and then only after a period of 5 hours or more.

It has been suggested that epinephrine is not completely suitable for such a diagnostic test because it has both β- and α-adrenergic receptor agonist properties.[75] Salbutamol sulfate, a specific β_2 agonist, has been used in a semiquantitative test for anhidrosis in thoroughbred horses.[74] A control of sterile water and 6 dilutions of salbutamol (10^{-3} to 10^{-8} w/v) were injected intradermally, and results were read 20 minutes later. Horses with long-standing anhidrosis did not sweat at any dilution, normal horses sweated at the 10^{-8} w/v dilution, and partially anhidrotic horses responded to dilutions of 10^{-4} to 10^{-6} w/v.

Anhidrotic horses may have low blood levels of chloride and sodium,[8,11,67,73] but hemograms, serum chemistry panels, and serum electrolytes are frequently normal.[81-86] Serum T_4 and T_3 levels may be low, but return to normal as affected horses recover,[13,81] confirming the existence of the euthyroid sick syndrome (see Chapter 10). Thyroidectomized horses sweat normally.[75] Histopathologic findings are often subtle and consist of thinning of sweat gland secretory epithelial cells and superficial blockage of some glandular ducts.[69,76,77] Ultrastructural studies reveal flattening, degranulation, and degeneration of secretory cells.[76,77]

Clinical Management

No form of medical treatment has any consistent benefit.[13,72,82-66] Medications reported to be occasionally effective include oral and intravenous electrolyte supplements,* 1,000 to 3,000 IU vitamin E per day orally,[8,11,67,82] 15 gm iodinated casein per day orally,[8,11,67,79] feed supplements containing specific amino acids (e.g., tyrosine),[75] and injections of ACTH.[9,87] Anecdotal reports suggest success with α-methyldopa (decrease sympathetic outflow from the central nervous system).[75] Again, the benefit (if any) of such treatments has *not* been demonstrated in controlled studies.

The most logical and effective mode of therapy is to move the horse to a cooler, more arid climate,[8,13,72,75,82-86] whereupon horses recover within 4 to 6 weeks. If this is not feasible, affected

---

*References 8, 11, 62, 66, 67, 81-86.

horses should be kept in air-conditioned, low-humidity stalls and exercised during the cool periods of the day.[8,9,13,72,82-86] Recurrences are to be expected if the horse is returned to a hot, humid climate.[72,75] Active cooling by washing with cold water (15° C) was shown to be a safe, effective means of facilitating heat dissipation in horses after exercise in hot, humid environments.[78]

• HYPERHIDROSIS

Hyperhidrosis is excessive sweating. *Generalized hyperhidrosis* may be seen with high ambient temperatures, vigorous exercise, severe pain (e.g., colic), the administration of certain drugs (epinephrine, acetylcholine, promazine, colloidal silver, prostaglandin $F_{2\alpha}$), hyperadrenocorticism, and pheochromocytoma.[5,8-11,13] *Localized hyperhidrosis* may be associated with local injections of epinephrine, dourine, and Horner's syndrome (hypothalamic, brain stem, or spinal cord lesions; guttural pouch infections; careless intravenous injections).[5,8,9,88]

• HEMATIDROSIS

Hematidrosis is the presence of blood in sweat and has been reported in horses with equine infectious anemia, purpura hemorrhagica, and various bleeding diatheses.[5,11] In addition to blood-tinged or frankly bloody sweat, red to bluish-red vesicles and bullae may be seen.

• PASTERN DERMATITIS

Pastern dermatitis is a common cutaneous reaction pattern in the horse.[13,19a,90]

Cause and Pathogenesis

Pastern dermatitis is *not* a single disease, but rather a cutaneous reaction pattern of the horse. It is essential that the veterinarian realize that this is a multifactorial dermatitis having many potential causes (Table 15-3).

Anecdotal reports indicate that skin biopsy specimens from Shires and Clydesdales with pastern dermatitis are characterized by vasculitis.[90a] It has been hypothesized that pastern dermatitis in these two breeds is an immune-mediated vasculitis with many possible triggering factors (see Chapter 9), wherein genetically determined immunodysregulation plays a key role.[90a]

Some horse owners say that when they take their animal to areas with alkaline soil, pastern dermatitis develops overnight (contact dermatitis?)!

● Table 15-3 **DIFFERENTIAL DIAGNOSIS OF EQUINE PASTERN DERMATITIS**

Staphylococcal folliculitis/furunculosis
Dermatophilosis
Dermatophytosis
Chorioptic mange
Trombiculosis
Vaccinia
Primary irritant contact dermatitis
Contact hypersensitivity
Photosensitization
Vasculitis
Pemphigus foliaceus

Clinical Features

Pastern dermatitis (grease-heel, scratches, cracked heels, mud fever, verrucous pododermatitis, grapes) occurs with no apparent sex predilection in adult horses.[1,8,13,90,91] Although all breeds are affected, it is most commonly seen in draft horses, especially those with feathering.

The dermatitis typically involves the caudal aspect of the pasterns (Fig. 15-48). The hind limbs are most commonly affected, and the condition is usually more-or-less bilaterally symmetric. Initially, there is erythema, edema, and scaling, which progresses to exudation, matting of hair, and crusting. There is variable pain and pruritus. Secondary bacterial infection is a frequent complication and is associated with an intensification of the inflammation and often the development of a foul-smelling discharge. In chronic cases the skin becomes progressively lichenified, hyperkeratotic, and fissured and may develop papillomatous or polypoid areas of hyperplastic to granulomatous to exuberant granulation tissue reaction (verrucous pododermatitis, "grapes") (Fig. 15-49). Limb edema, draining tracts, and lameness may develop.

Diagnosis

The differential diagnosis is lengthy (Table 15-3). Successful management requires *early* specific diagnosis before severe chronic changes intervene. In chronic cases, the etiology may be indeterminable. If so, the diagnosis of chronic, idiopathic pastern dermatitis is rendered.

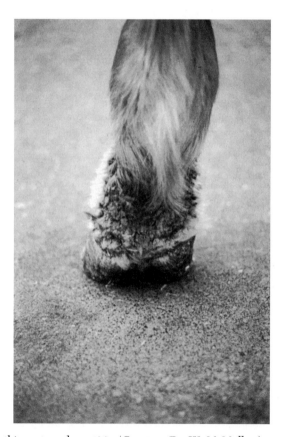

FIGURE 15-48. Idiopathic pastern dermatitis. (*Courtesy Dr. W. McMullen.*)

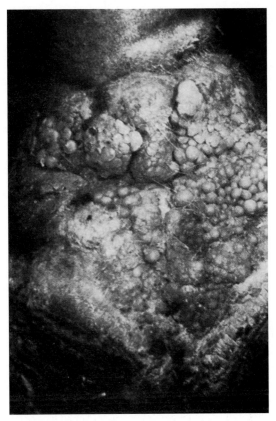

FIGURE 15-49. Chronic idiopathic pastern dermatitis with marked verrucous hyperplasia ("grapes"). (*Courtesy Dr. W. McMullen.*)

Clinical Management

Therapy is most successful when administered specifically and early. General symptomatic care includes:[1,8,13,89-91]

1. Removal of the horse from wet, muddy, unhygienic conditions.
2. Minimized contact with potentially irritating chemicals, dusts, plants, and so forth.
3. Gentle clipping and cleansing.
4. Daily application of shampoos or soaks containing antimicrobial (e.g., benzoyl peroxide, chlorhexidine), astringent (e.g., benzoyl peroxide, aluminum acetate), or hypertonic and drawing (e.g., magnesium sulfate) properties. Lesions that are dry and thickened benefit from the daily application of emollient creams or ointments that contain antimicrobial agents and glucocorticoids (e.g., Animax, Lotrimin-HC, Otomax).
5. Systemic antibiotics, systemic glucocorticoids, or both of these if indicated.

Chronic, medically refractory cases with marked proliferative and exuberant granulation tissue reactions may require surgical excision or cryosurgical intervention.[8,13,91]

Even with conscientious therapy, traditional treatments may fail. Even when therapy is successful, relapses may occur. Owners must be advised of this possibility so that therapeutic reintervention can be initiated rapidly, which minimizes the intensity and cost of treatment.

● Table 15-4	**DIFFERENTIAL DIAGNOSIS OF CORONARY BAND DISORDERS**

Pemphigus foliaceous
Vasculitis
Photodermatitis
Multisystemic eosinophilic epitheliotropic disease
Sarcoidosis
Vesicular stomatitis
Epidermolysis bullosa
Ergotism
Vitamin A deficiency
Dermatophilosis
Hepatocutaneous syndrome
Coronary band dysplasia (dystrophy)

● CORONARY BAND DISORDERS

Disorders of the coronary band are rare in horses. In most instances, the coronary band is involved in addition to other areas of the integument (Table 15-4).[13,92] Multisystemic eosinophilic epitheliotropic disease and sarcoidosis may begin on the coronary bands but progress to other areas of the body within days to weeks. Pemphigus foliaceous and vasculitis may affect the coronary bands only.[13,92]

Clinical Features

Coronitis may be characterized by flaking, crusting, exudation, or ulceration. Vesicles, pustules, and necrosis are rarely seen. A common early observation in coronitis is a "winging out," or uplifting of the hair at the coronary band.[92] Chronic coronary band disease may lead to hoof wall defects.

Coronary band dysplasia (dystrophy) is an uncommon syndrome, perhaps multifactorial in nature, wherein the coronary bands are symmetrically diseased.[92,92a] It accounts for 1% of the equine dermatoses seen at the Cornell University Clinic. Unfortunately, historical information has been sketchy and follow-up has been nonexistent. There are no apparent breed (anecdotes suggest draft horses) or sex predilections, but horses are often affected at an early age (weeks to months old). All coronary bands become abnormal in appearance: scaly, crusty, variably erythematous (Fig. 15-50). The condition causes no apparent discomfort. However, chronic coronary band disease produces hoof wall deformities. Ergots and chestnuts may be affected. Shave biopsy specimens from five horses have shown pronounced parakeratotic hyperkeratosis and epidermal dysplasia (Figs. 15-51 and 15-52) accompanied by varying degrees of neutrophilic and/or eosinophilic exocytosis, microabscessation, and exudative crust formation. The condition is apparently persistent, and no treatment has been successful. Topical or systemic retinoids might be useful but are presently unproven.

The *"hepatocutaneous syndrome"* is a poorly described condition wherein an erosive, ulcerative, and exudative coronitis becomes necrotic and may lead to sloughing of the hoof wall.[92] It is associated with liver pathology. Skin biopsy specimens examined by one of the authors (DWS) revealed marked parakeratotic hyperkeratosis ("red"), pallor of the upper epidermis due to inter- and intracellular edema ("white"), and hyperplasia of the lower epidermis ("blue"), resembling the classic "red, white, and blue" appearance of the hepatocutaneous syndrome (necrolytic migratory erythema) of dogs (Fig. 15-53).[17]

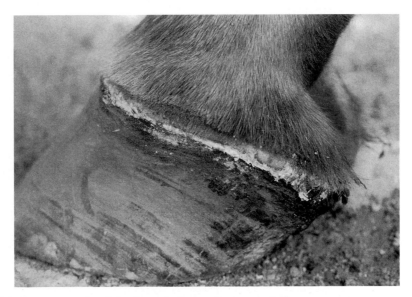

FIGURE 15-50. Coronary band dysplasia. Scaling and crusting of the coronet.

Diagnosis

The diagnosis is based on history, physical examination, cytologic examination, and coronary band biopsy. Cytologic examination may reveal suppurative inflammation with microorganisms (infection), neutrophilic-to-eosinophilic inflammation with acantholysis (pemphigus foliaceous), or eosinophilic inflammation (multisystemic eosinophilic epitheliotropic disease), but often the examination does not clarify the differential diagnosis. Biopsy is the most reliable way of establishing the definitive diagnosis. Unfortunately, biopsy of the coronary band may cause hoof wall defects. Thus, only superficial shave biopsies just to the depth of the dermis can be obtained without adverse consequences.

Clinical Management

The treatment of coronary band disease is obviously most appropriate and most successful when based on a specific diagnosis.

• SELF-MUTILATION SYNDROME

Self-mutilation syndrome, a form of stereotypes, is a rare behavioral disorder of horses.[94,96] It accounts for 0.44% of the equine dermatoses seen at the Cornell University Clinic.

Cause and Pathogenesis

Although several management and environmental factors have been examined, none were consistently related to the expression of this disorder.[94] In one study, 15 of 57 affected horses (26.3%) were known to have relatives that exhibited similar behavior.[94]

Stereotypes are defined as stylized, repetitive, apparently functionless motor responses or sequences.[95,96] Endogenous opioids may be involved in the propagation of stereotypes.[93-96] Their release is facilitated in a stress-primed system, and they may sensitize dopaminergic mechanisms directly involved in repetitive behavior. Some evidence for opioid modulation and opioid-

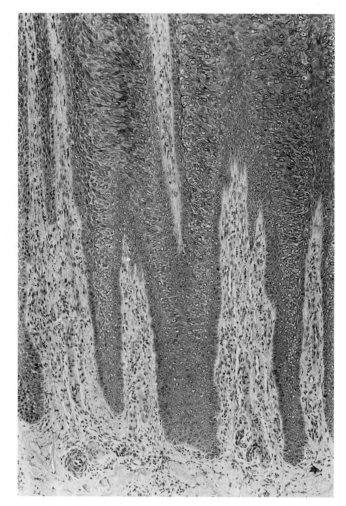

FIGURE 15-51. Coronary band dysplasia. Lymphocytic and neutrophilic inflammation of dermal papillae.

dopamine interaction is suggested by the dramatic reduction of self-mutilative behavior afforded by opioid antagonists and dopamine antagonists.[93,94] Others have suggested that equine self-mutilation syndrome may be similar to obsessive-compulsive disorders or Tourette's syndrome of humans.[94,96]

Clinical Features

In a survey conducted by the Ontario Veterinary College in Canada, the prevalence of self-mutilation was 1.9% in stallions and 0.7% in geldings.[94] No breed predilections have been established, but males and adolescents are predisposed.[94] Affected horses most commonly bite at their flank, then the pectoral, lateral thoracic, tail, and limb regions.[94,96] Most horses (61.4%) bite at both sides of their body. Hypersensitivity to touch is seen in 39% of affected horses.[94] Episodes of self-mutilation last for seconds to hours (median between 1 and 10 minutes), and occur from 25 times/

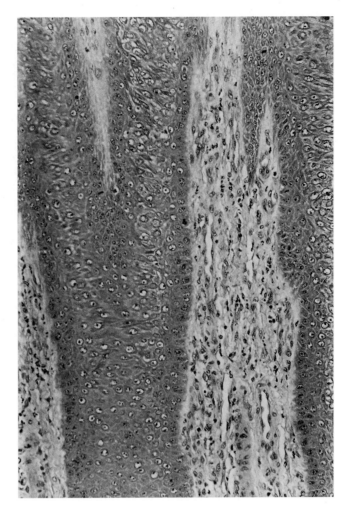

FIGURE 15-52. Close-up of Fig. 15-51. Note disorganized, "jumbled" appearance of lower layers of epidermis.

day to monthly (most horses exhibit the behavior daily).[94] Lesions produced include irregular areas of alopecia, inflammation, erosion, ulceration, and crusting.

Diagnosis

Equine self-mutilation syndrome is clinically distinctive. One must always be sure to rule-out organic causes of pain or pruritus.

Clinical Management

Equine self-mutilation syndrome is undesirable because it can lead to considerable damage to the horse and the owner's property. There is presently no consistently effective treatment.[94-96] Manipulation of the horse's social environment, even if by trial and error, may reduce self-mutilative behavior.[95,96] Occasional horses have been reported to respond to various medicaments: nalmefene

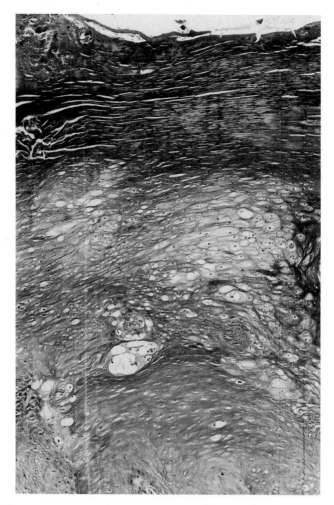

FIGURE 15-53. Hepatocutaneous syndrome. Dense surface parakeratotic hyperkeratosis, subjacent laminar intra- and intercellular edema, and underlying epidermal hyperplasia.

(opioid antagonist),[93] acepromazine or fluphenazine (dopamine antagonists),[94] and megestrol acetate or progesterone in oil (progestins).[95,96] Anecdotally, the most commonly used agent is megestrol acetate, 65 to 85 mg/500 kg orally q24h.[96] Some horses can be maintained with similar doses once or twice weekly. The authors have had good luck with amitriptyline (1 mg/kg q12h PO) in a small number of horses. Improvement was noted following castration in 7 of 10 stallions.[94]

● REFERENCES

General References

1. Barbet JL, et al: Diseases of the skin. In: Colahan PT, et al (eds): Equine Medicine and Surgery IV, Vol II. American Veterinary Publications, Goleta, 1991, p 1569.
2. Fadok VA: Overview of equine papular and nodular dermatoses. Vet Clin N Am Equine Pract 11:61, 1995.
3. Fairley RA: Collagenolysis: "It ain't easy being pink." Vet Pathol 28:96, 1991.
4. Freedberg IM, et al: Fitzpatrick's Dermatology in General Medicine V. McGraw-Hill Book, New York, 1999.
5. Kral F, Schwartzman R M: Veterinary and Comparative Dermatology. J.B. Lippincott, Philadelphia, 1964.

6. Mason KV: Clinical and pathophysiologic aspects of parasitic skin diseases. In: Ihrke, PJ, et al (eds): Advances in Veterinary Dermatology II. Pergamon Press, New York, 1993, p 177.

7. Mathison PT: Eosinophilic nodular dermatoses. Vet Clin N Am Equine Pract 11:75, 1995.

8. McMullen WC: The skin. In: Mansmann RA, et al (eds): Equine Medicine and Surgery III. American Veterinary Publications, Santa Barbara, 1982, p 789.

9. Mullowney PC: Dermatologic diseases of horses, Part V. Allergic, immune-mediated, and miscellaneous skin diseases. Comp Cont Educ 7:S217, 1985.

10. Pascoe RR: Equine nodular and erosive skin conditions: the common and not so common. Equine Vet Educ 3:153, 1991.

11. Radostits OM, et al: Veterinary Medicine. A Textbook of the Diseases of Cattle, Sheep, Pigs, Goats, and Horses VIII. Baillière-Tindall, Philadelphia, 1994.

12. Scott DW: Nodular skin diseases. In: Robinson NE (eds): Current Therapy in Equine Medicine II. W.B. Saunders Co, Philadelphia, 1987, p 634.

13. Scott DW: Large Animal Dermatology. W.B. Saunders Co, Philadelphia, 1988.

14. Scott DW: Unusual immune-mediated skin diseases in the horse. Equine Pract 13(2):10, 1991.

15. Scott DW: Diagnostic des dermatoses inflammatoires équines: analyse de la modalité de réaction histopathologique: étude personnelle portant sur 315 cas. Point Vét 24:245, 1992.

16. Scott DW: Analyse du type de réaction histopathologique dans le diagnostic des dermatoses inflammatoires chez le chat: étude portant sur 394 cas. Point Vét 26:57, 1994.

17. Scott DW, et al: Muller & Kirk's Small Animal Dermatology VI. W.B. Saunders Co, Philadelphia, 2001.

18. Stannard AA: Equine dermatology. Proc Am Assoc Equine Practit 22:273, 1976.

19. von Tscharner C: Lesioni nodulari della pelle del cavallo. Ippologia 2:6, 1991.

19a. von Tscharner C, et al: Stannard's illustrated equine dermatology notes. Vet Dermatol 11:161, 2000.

20. Williams MA, Angarano DW: Diseases of the skin. In: Kobluk CN., et al: The Horse. Diseases and Clinical Management. Vol. 1. W.B. Saunders Co, Philadelphia, 1995, p 541.

21. Williams PD: Lumps, bumps, and swellings—a clinical approach to diagnosis. Equine Vet Educ 7:300, 1995.

Eosinophilic Granuloma

22. Fernandez CJ, et al: Staining abnormalities of dermal collagen in eosinophil- or neutrophil-rich inflammatory dermatoses of horses and cats as demonstrated with Masson's trichrome stain. Vet Dermatol 11:43, 2000.

23. Finnochio EJ: Nodular necrobiosis. Mod Vet Pract 62:76, 1981.

24. Griffin CE: Nodular collagenolytic granuloma (nodular necrobiosis). In: Robinson NE (ed): Current Therapy in Equine Medicine. W.B. Saunders Co, Philadelphia, 1983, p 545.

25. Griffin CE: Dermal nodules in horses. Mod Vet Pract 66:704, 1985.

26. Nicholls TJ, et al: Nodular necrobiosis in a horse. Aust Vet J 60:148, 1983.

27. Pascoe RR: Equine Dermatoses. University of Sydney Post-Graduate Foundation in Veterinary Science, Sydney. Vet Rev No. 22, 1981.

27a. Slovis NM, et al: Injection site eosinophilic granulomas and collagenolysis in 3 horses. J Vet Intern Med 13:606, 1999.

28. Thomsett LR: A nodular skin disease of horses. Vet Dermatol News 3, March 1978.

29. Thomsett LR: Noninfectious skin diseases of horses. Vet Clin N Am Large Anim. Pract 6:57, 1984.

30. Thomsett LR: Skin diseases of the horse. In Pract 1:15, 1979.

Unilateral Papular Dermatosis

31. Rothwell TLW, Birch CB: Unilateral papular dermatitis in a horse. Aust Vet J 68:122, 1991.

32. Walton DK, Scott DW: Unilateral papular dermatosis in the horse. Equine Pract 4(9):15, 1982.

Axillary Nodular Necrosis

33. Scott DW, Fuji RN: Equine "axillary nodular necrosis": What is it? Equine Pract 21(5):14, 1999.

Multisystemic Eosinophilic Epitheliotropic Disease

34. Breider MA, et al: Chronic eosinophilic pancreatitis and ulcerative colitis in a horse. J Am Vet Med Assoc 186:809, 1985.

35. Gibson KT, Alders RG: Eosinophilic enterocolitis and dermatitis in two horses. Equine Vet J 19:247, 1987.

36. Guaguère E, et al: Case clinique: dermatite éosinophilique généralisée et entérocolite éosinophilique chez un cheval. Point Vét 20:863, 1988.

36a. Henson FMD, et al: Multisystemic eosinophilic epitheliotropic disease in a Welsh pony. Equine Vet Educ 14:176, 2002.

37. Hillyer MH, Mair TS: Multisystemic eosinophilic epitheliotropic disease in a horse: attempted treatment with hydroxyurea and dexamethasone. Vet Rec 130:392, 1992.

38. Lindberg R, et al: Clinical and pathophysiological features on granulomatous enteritis and eosinophilic granulomatosis in the horse. Zbl Vet Med Assoc 32:526, 1985.

39. Sanford SE: Multisystemic eosinophilic epitheliotropic disease in a horse. Can Vet J 30:253, 1989.

40. Wilkie JSN, et al: Chronic eosinophilic dermatitis: a manifestation of a multisystemic, eosinophilic, epitheliotropic disease in five horses. Vet Pathol 22:297, 1985.

Linear Alopecia

41. Fadok VA: Update on four unusual equine dermatoses. Vet Clin N Am Equine Pract 11:105, 1995.

Panniculitis

42. Bassage LH II, et al: Sterile nodular panniculitis associated with lameness in a horse. J Am Vet Med Assoc 209:1242, 1996.

42a. Dagleish MP, et al: Serum α1-proteinase inhibitor concentration in 2 quarter horse foals with idiopathic granulomatous panniculitis. Equine Vet J 32:449, 2000.

43. Dodd DC, et al: Muscle degeneration and yellow fat disease in foals. N Z Vet J 8:45, 1960.

43a. Dunstan RW: Sterile nodular panniculitis associated with lameness in a horse. J Am Vet Med Assoc 209:1244, 1996.

44. Dyson S, Platt H: Panniculitis in an aged pony resembling Weber-Christian disease in man. Equine Vet J 17:145, 1985.

45. Foreman JH, et al: Generalized steatitis associated with selenium deficiency and normal vitamin E status in a foal. J Am Vet Med Assoc 189:83, 1986.
46. Hartley WJ, Dodd DC: Muscular dystrophy in New Zealand livestock. N Z Vet J 5:61, 1957.
47. Karcher LF, et al: Sterile nodular panniculitis in five horses. J Am Vet Med Assoc 196:1823, 1990.
48. Kroneman J, Wensvoort P: Muscular dystrophy and yellow fat disease in Shetland pony foals. Neth J Vet Sci 1:42, 1968.
49. Peyton LC, et al: Fat necrosis in a foal. Equine Vet J 13:131,1981.
50. Platt H, Whitwell KE: Clinical and pathological observations on generalized steatitis in foals. J Comp Pathol 81:499, 1971.
51. Scott DW: Sterile nodular panniculitis in a horse. Equine Pract 7(1):30, 1985.
52. Wensvoort P: Morphogenesis of the altered adipose tissues in generalized steatitis in equidae. Tijdschr Diergeneeskd 99:1060, 19974.
53. Wensvoort P: Age-related features of generalized steatitis in equidae. Tijdschr Diergeneeskd 99:10067, 1974.
54. Wensvoort P, Steenbergen-Botterweg WA: Non-extractable lipids in the adipose tissues of horses and ponies affected with generalized steatitis. Tijdschr Diergeneeskd 100:106, 1975.

Sarcoidosis
55. Düll U, et al: Sarkoidose—Eine seltene autoimmunerkrakung bei einem Pferd. Prak Tierärztl 78:486, 1997.
56. Heath SE, et al: Idiopathic granulomatous disease involving the skin in a horse. J Am Vet Med Assoc 197:1033, 1990.
57. Li N, et al: Identification of mycobacterial DNA in cutaneous lesions of sarcoidosis. J Cutan Pathol 26:271, 1999.
58. Rose JF, et al: A series of four cases of generalized granulomatous in the horse. In: Kwochka KW, et al (eds): Advances in Veterinary Dermatology III. Butterworth-Heinemann, Boston, 1998, p 562.
58a. Sellers RS, et al: Idiopathic systemic granulomatous disease and macrophage expression of PTHrP in a miniature pony. J Comp Pathol 125:214, 2001.
59. Stannard AA: Generalized granulomatous disease. In: Robinson NE (ed): Current Therapy in Equine Medicine II. W.B. Saunders Co, Philadelphia, 1987 p 645.

Localized Scleroderma
60. Littlewood JD, et al: Idiopathic fibrosing dermatitis in a horse: a possible case of equine morphea. Equine Vet Educ 7:295, 1995.

Generalized Scleroderma
61. Frank LA, et al: Diffuse systemic sclerosis in a Paso Fino mare. Comp Cont Educ Pract Vet 22:274, 2000.

Anhidrosis
62. Arnold TF: Panting in cattle and nonsweating horses. Vet Rec 62:463, 1950.
63. Barnes JE: "Dry sweating" in horses. Vet Rec 50:977, 1938.
64. Beadle RE, et al: Summertime plasma catecholamine concentrations in healthy and anhidrotic horses in Louisiana. Am J Vet Res 43:1446, 1982.

65. Carlson G, Ocen P: Composition of equine sweat following exercise in high environmental temperatures and in response to intravenous epinephrine administration. J Equine Med Surg 3:27, 1979.
66. Correa JE, Calderin GG: Anhidrosis, dry coat syndrome in the Thoroughbred. J Am Vet Med Assoc 149:1556, 1966.
67. Currie AK, Seagaer SWJ: Anhidrosis. Proc Am Assoc Equine Practit 22:249, 1976.
68. Evans CL, Smith DFG: The relationship between sweating and the catecholamine content of the blood in the horse. J Physiol 132:542, 1956.
69. Evans CL, et al: A histological study of the sweat glands of normal and dry coated horses. J Comp Pathol Ther 67:397, 1957.
70. Evans CL, et al: Physiologic factors on the condition of "dry-coat" in horses. Vet Rec 69:1, 1957.
71. Evans CL: Physiological mechanisms that underlie sweating in the horse. Br Vet J 122: 117, 1996.
72. Geor RJ, McCutcheon LJ: Thermoregulation and clinical disorders associated with exercise and heat stress. Comp Cont Educ 18:436, 1996.
73. Gilyard RT: Chronic anhidrosis with lowered blood chlorides in race horses. Cornell Vet 34:332, 1944.
74. Guthrie AJ: Use of semi-quantitative sweat test in Thoroughbred horses. J So Afr Vet Assoc 63:162, 1992.
75. Hubert JD, Beadle RE: Equine anhidrosis. Comp Cont Educ Pract Vet 20:846, 1998.
76. Jenkinson DM, et al: Ultrastructural variations in the sweat glands of anhidrotic horses. Equine Vet J 17:287, 1985.
77. Jenkinson DM, et al: Effects of season and lower ambient temperature on the structure of the sweat glands in anhidrotic horses. Equine Vet J 21:59, 1989.
78. Kohn CW, et al: Evaluation of washing with cold water to facilitate heat dissipation in horses exercised in hot, humid condition. Am J Vet Res 60:299, 1999.
79. Magsood M: Iodinated casein therapy for the "nonsweating" syndrome in horses. Vet Rec 68:475, 1956.
80. Marsh JH: Treatment of "dry-coat" in Thoroughbreds with vitamin E. Vet Rec 73:1124, 1961.
81. Mayhew IG, Ferguson HO: Clinical, clinicopathologic, and epidemiologic features of anhidrosis in central Florida Thoroughbred horses. J Vet Intern Med 1:136, 1987.
82. Warner AE, Mayhew IG: Equine anhidrosis: a survey of affected horses in Florida. J Am Vet Med Assoc 180:627, 1982.
83. Warner AE: Equine anhidrosis. Comp Cont Educ 4:S434, 1982.
84. Warner A, Mayhew IG: Equine anhidrosis: a review of pathophysiologic mechanisms. Vet Res Commun 6:249, 1983.
85. Warner AE: Anhidrosis. In: Robinson NE (ed): Current Therapy in Equine Medicine. W.B. Saunders Co, Philadelphia, 1983, p 170.
86. Warner AE: Anhidrosis. In: Robinson NE (ed): Current Therapy in Equine Medicine. W.B. Saunders Co, Philadelphia, 1983, p 187.
87. Woods PR: Internal diseases that have skin lesions. Vet Clin N Am Equine Pract 11:111, 995.

Hyperhidrosis
88. Smith TS, Mayhew IG: Horner's syndrome in large animals. Cornell Vet 67:529, 1977.

Pastern Dermatitis
89. Cornes C: Greasy heel. University of Sydney Postgraduate Foundation in Veterinary Science Control and Therapy Series, Mailing 185, 1995, p 806.
90. English M, Pollen S: Pastern dermatitis and unguilysis in two draft horses. Equine Pract 17(8):25, 1995.
90a. Ferraro GL: Pastern dermatitis in Shires and Clydesdales. J Equine Vet Sci 21:524, 2001.
91. McMullen WC: Scratches. In: Robinson NE (ed): Current Therapy in Equine Medicine. W.B. Saunders Co, Philadelphia, 1983, p 549.

Coronary Band Disorders
92. Foil CS, Conroy J: Dermatoses of claws, nails, and hoof. In: von Tscharner C, et al (eds): Advances in Veterinary Dermatology I. Baillière-Tindall, Philadelphia, 1990, p 420.

92a. Menzies-Gow NJ, et al: Coronary band dystrophy in two horses. Vet Rec 150:665, 2002.

Self-Mutilation Syndrome
93. Dodman NH, et al: Use of a narcotic antagonist (nalmefene) to suppress self-mutilative behavior in a stallion. J Am Vet Med Assoc 192:1585, 1988.
94. Dodman NH, et al: Equine self-mutilation syndrome (57 cases). J Am Vet Med Assoc 204:1219, 1994.
95. Houpt KA: Domestic Animal Behavior for Veterinarians and Animal Scientists II. Iowa State University Press, Ames, 1991, p 143.
96. Houpt KA, McDonnell SM: Equine stereotypes. Comp Cont Educ 15:1265, 1993.

Chapter 16

Neoplastic and Non-Neoplastic Tumors

• CUTANEOUS ONCOLOGY

Veterinary oncology has come into its own as a specialty. Detailed information on the etiopathogenesis and immunologic aspects of neoplasia is available in other publications[8,15,16] and is therefore not presented here. This chapter is an overview of equine cutaneous neoplasia as well as non-neoplastic tumors.

Unlike in other domestic animal species, the risk for cutaneous neoplasia in horses does not increase with age.[15,54,64] Saddle horses (a composite of crossbreeds) are at increased risk for cutaneous neoplasia.[64] Male horses appear to be predisposed to develop mast cell tumors.[73] Breed predilections for cutaneous tumors are presented in Table 16-1.

Numerous surveys of skin tumors in horses have been published.* The skin is the most common site of neoplasia in the horse, accounting for about 50% of all equine neoplasms[29,41,65] and most equine cutaneous neoplasms are mesenchymal in origin and biologically benign. The most common cutaneous neoplasms in the horse as reported in the veterinary literature are sarcoids, squamous cell carcinomas, papillomas, and melanocytoma/melanoma. In a retrospective study[74] of skin biopsies submitted over a 16-year period (1978-1994) to the Diagnostic Laboratory at the College of Veterinary Medicine at Cornell University, the most common equine cutaneous neoplasms were sarcoid, melanoma, papilloma, squamous cell carcinoma, mast cell tumor, and fibroma (Table 16-2). In that study, skin neoplasms accounted for 37.5% (703 of 1871) of the equine skin biopsies and 8.8% (703 of 8009) of the total equine biopsies submitted.

The key to appropriate management and accurate prognosis of cutaneous neoplasms is specific diagnosis. This can be achieved only by biopsy and histologic evaluation. Exfoliative cytologic techniques (aspiration and impression smear) are easy and rapid and often provide valuable

● Table 16-1	BREED PREDILECTIONS FOR CUTANEOUS NEOPLASMS AND NON-NEOPLASTIC TUMORS IN THE HORSE
Squamous cell carcinoma	American paint, Appaloosa, Belgian, Clydesdale, Pinto, Shire
Sarcoid	Appaloosa, Arabian, quarter horse
Hemangioma	Arabian
Melanoma	Arabian, Lippizaner, Percheron
Dermoid cyst	Thoroughbred
Linear epidermal nevi	Belgian
Actinic keratosis	American paint, Appaloosa, Belgian, Clydesdale, Pinto, Shire
Calcinosis circumscripta	Standardbred

*References 29-38, 40-46, 48-55, 59, 60, 62, 63, 65, 72, 76-79.

698

● Table 16-2 **CUTANEOUS NEOPLASMS OF THE HORSE IDENTIFIED OVER A PERIOD OF 16 YEARS (1978-1994)[79]**

NEOPLASM	NUMBER	PERCENTAGE
Sarcoid	256	35.3
Melanoma	101	13.9
Papilloma	76	10.5
Squamous cell carcinoma	50	6.9
Mast cell tumor	50	6.9
Fibroma	45	6.2
Melanocytoma	35	4.8
Basal cell tumor	20	2.8
Hemangioma	17	2.3
Lymphoma	16	2.2
Fibrosarcoma	15	2.1
Schwannoma	14	2.0
Undifferentiated sarcoma	8	1.1
Epitrichial sweat gland adenoma	7	1.0
Lipoma	3	0.4
Myxoma	2	0.2
Hemangiosarcoma	2	0.2
Malignant fibrous histiocytoma	2	0.2
Undifferentiated carcinoma	2	0.2
Epitrichial sweat gland carcinoma	1	0.1
Lymphangioma	1	0.1
Leiomyoma	1	0.1
Carcinosarcoma	1	0.1
TOTAL	725	100

information about neoplastic cell type and differentiation. The techniques, methods, and interpretation used in cytologic studies have been beautifully described and illustrated.[18-23] However, exfoliative cytologic evaluation is inferior to and is no substitute for biopsy and histopathologic examination. Historical and clinical considerations often allow the experienced clinician to formulate an inclusive differential diagnosis on a cutaneous neoplasm, but variability renders such "odds playing" unreliable. In short, "a lump is a lump" until it is evaluated histologically.

The detailed histopathologic description of equine cutaneous neoplasms is beyond the scope of this chapter. Only the histopathologic essence of individual neoplasms is presented here. For in-depth information and photomicrographic illustrations, the reader is referred to other texts on cutaneous neoplasia[5a,8,17,78] and the individual references cited for each neoplasm.

The use of markers—enzyme histochemical and immunohistochemical methods for identifying specific cell types—has increased and has facilitated the diagnosis of neoplastic conditions.[5,14,24-27] Examples of these markers are presented in Chapter 2.

Clinical management of cutaneous neoplasms may include surgery, cryosurgery, electrosurgery, laser surgery, radiotherapy, chemotherapy, immunotherapy, radiofrequency hyperthermia, phototherapy, and combinations of these. Detailed information on the various treatment modalities is available in a number of excellent references.° Brief comments are included under clinical management for each tumor.

°References 4, 6, 10, 12, 13a, 15, 16, 28, 46a, 81, 82.

The crucial difference between normal and neoplastic cells stems from discrete changes in specific genes controlling proliferation and tissue homeostasis.[39] More than 100 such cancer-related genes have been discovered. Two principal types of growth-regulating genes have been associated with the pathogenesis of neoplasia: *oncogenes* encode proteins that convey various growth advantages, while *tumor-suppressor genes* encode proteins that restrict cell proliferation and differentiation.

The p53 tumor-suppressor gene is the most striking and well-studied example, and mutations of this gene occur in about 50% of cell cancer types in humans.[39] Tumor-suppressor genes are vulnerable sites for critical DNA damage because they normally function as physiologic barriers against clonal expansion or genomic mutability, and they are able to hinder growth and metastasis of cells driven to uncontrolled proliferation by oncogenes. p53 participates in many cellular functions: cell cycle control, DNA repair, differentiation, genomic plasticity, and programmed cell death. The p53 gene is an important component in a biochemical pathway or pathways central to carcinogenesis, and p53 mutations provide a selective advantage for clonal expansion of preneoplastic and neoplastic cells. Overexpression of p53 is positively associated with gene mutation. Mutations in p53 were found in most equine squamous cell carcinomas.[146]

● EPITHELIAL NEOPLASMS

Papillomas

CAUSE AND PATHOGENESIS

Papillomas are common,[79,83-85] benign, viral-induced epithelial neoplasms of the horse.[*] There are presently two forms of cutaneous viral papillomas recognized in horses. Presumably these two very different clinicopathologic syndromes are caused by different types of equine papilloma viruses (DNA papovaviruses). In addition, two penile papillomas failed to hybridize with a classical equine viral papillomatosis probe, indicating that a third equine papillomavirus type exists.[100] Viral papillomas are transmitted by direct and indirect (fomite) contact.[73] Infection requires damaged skin (e.g., environmental trauma, ectoparasites, ultraviolet light damage).[73]

Classical *equine viral papillomatosis* occurs in young animals, most commonly on the muzzle.[73] Experimentally, the incubation period varies from 19 to 67 days.[87,92] Spontaneous remission usually occurs within 2 to 3 months.[73,85,92]

Equine ear papillomas occur in horses of all ages, most commonly on the pinnae, and they rarely, if ever, spontaneously resolve.[73,86,89,101] Black flies are probably important in transmitting the causative papillomavirus, both through damaging the skin and as mechanical vectors.

No in vitro system for papillomavirus propagation is available. Detection methods differ dramatically in their sensitivity.[97] *Southern blot hybridization* is highly specific and sensitive, but it is time-consuming and does not allow detection of DNA segments of unknown types. *Dot blot* and *reverse blot hybridization* have good sensitivity and reasonable accuracy, but they are also laborious. *In situ hybridization* is less sensitive than Southern blot but does allow identification of cells harboring viral DNA. *Polymerase chain reaction (PCR)* is the most widely used technique, but it is not as sensitive as the others.

Papillomavirus is fairly stable in the environment and can survive for 63 days at 4° to 8° C or for 6 hours at 37° C.[98] Humoral immunity (neutralizing antibodies) protects against viral challenge but does not play a role in clearance of established lesions.[98] Cellular immunity is of key importance in papilloma regression.[98] Papillomavirus vaccines (live or formalin-inactivated) are effective preventives but are of no known therapeutic benefit.[98]

---

*References 9, 10, 15, 25, 44, 50, 56, 60, 73, 79, 83-85, 88, 96, 99, 100, 104.

There is great interest and much research in the role of papillomaviruses and oncogenesis.[97] The viral genome can be divided in parts labeled as *L* (later region), *E* (early region), and *LCR* (long control region). The L1 and L2 genes encode for viral capsid proteins, and the E region consists of genes involved in regulation of viral DNA replication (E1 and E2) or cell proliferation and immortalization (E6 and E7). In addition, E2 protein is an important viral transcription factor regulating expression of E6 and E7 oncogenes. E4 protein binds keratins and facilitates production of virions by disrupting normal cell differentiation. E6 and E7 proteins have oncogene potential and can interfere with cellular factors involved in the control of cell proliferation and the prevention of cell immortalization. E6 and E7 oncogenes are capable of immortalizing cells, inducing cell growth, and promoting chromosomal instability in the host cell. E6 oncoprotein causes degradation of p53 protein by the cellular ubiquitin proteolysis system, leading to unblocking of cell division and host DNA synthesis, which results in chromosomal instability and accumulation of various mutations in affected cells.

CLINICAL FINDINGS

Viral Papillomatosis

Viral papillomatosis (warts, verrucae, "grass warts") occurs in horses younger than 3 years of age and often less than 1 year of age.[*] Congenital papillomas have been reported, but these were probably epidermal nevi (see page 778). Viral papillomatosis is common in the horse,[†] although some surveys indicate that papillomas account for only 0.6% to 10.5% of all equine skin neoplasms.[‡] These surveys are biopsy-based, and since clinicians rarely, if ever, biopsy classical viral papillomas, they clearly underestimate the prevalence of the disorder. There are no apparent breed or sex predilections.

Lesions occur most commonly on the muzzle and lips (Fig. 16-1), less commonly on the eyelid, external genitalia, and distal legs (Fig. 16-2), and rarely elsewhere.[6,44,131,155] They begin as small, 1-mm diameter, raised, smooth, shiny, gray to white papules.[92] A rapid growth and increased number of lesions (2 to over 100) occurs over a 39- to 54-day period. Fully developed papillomas are 0.2 to 2 cm in diameter, 0.5 cm in height, broad-based to pedunculated, gray to pink to white in color, and have a hyperkeratotic surface characterized by numerous keratinous, frond-like projections.

Ear Papillomas

Equine ear papillomas (aural plaque, papillary acanthoma, hyperplastic dermatitis of the ear, "ear fungus") are common and occur with no apparent breed or sex predilections.[§] The condition is seen in horses of all ages, but rarely in animals less than 1 year of age. Lesions begin as small, 1- to 2-mm diameter, well-demarcated, raised, depigmented, shiny papules on the lateral surface of the pinna. The condition is more or less bilaterally symmetric. Lesions enlarge and coalesce to become 1- to 3-cm diameter, white, hyperkeratotic plaques (Fig. 16-3). The surface hyperkeratosis can be scraped off to reveal an underlying shiny, pink, nonulcerated plaque. Similar lesions are occasionally seen around the anus and external genitalia. The condition is asymptomatic but may appear more "active" and symptomatic in summers when the effects of biting flies (especially black flies) complicate matters.

---

*References 9, 10, 15, 47, 58, 61, 73, 85.

†References 42, 47, 50, 57, 65, 73, 74, 84.

‡References 30, 41, 66, 69, 74, 83.

§References 9, 44, 56, 60, 73, 84-86, 89, 101.

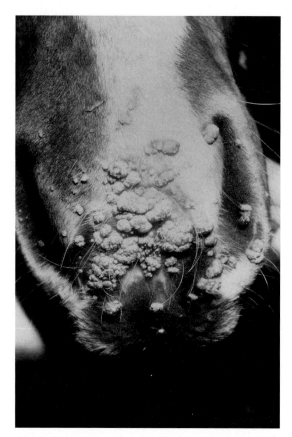

FIGURE 16-1. Typical viral papillomatosis on the muzzle of a young horse.

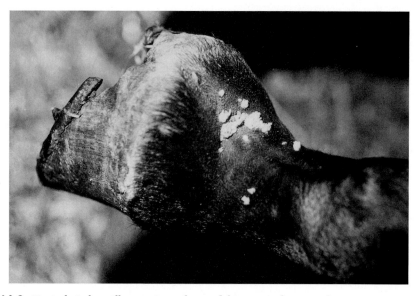

FIGURE 16-2. Typical viral papillomatosis on the caudal pastern of a young horse.

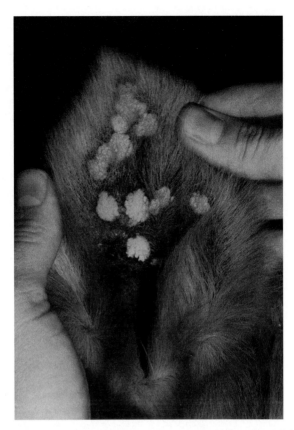

FIGURE 16-3. Typical ear papillomas ("aural plaques") on the lateral surface of the pinna.

DIAGNOSIS

Both types of equine papillomas are visually distinctive and further diagnostic work is rarely indicated. Sarcoid must be considered in the differential diagnosis for any "papilloma" or "wart" in an atypical site in an adult horse.[73]

Equine viral papillomatosis has been the subject of extensive pathologic studies.[90-94] Histologically, three evolutionary phases are seen: growth, development, and regression.[92] The growth phase is characterized by marked hyperplasia of epidermal basal cells, mild to moderate acanthosis and ortho- and parakeratotic hyperkeratosis, and the presence of very few viral inclusion bodies. The development phase is characterized by the classical features of pronounced papillated epidermal hyperplasia and papillomatosis (Fig. 16-4); koilocytosis (Fig. 16-5); increased numbers, size, and clumping of keratohyalin granules; hypomelanosis; numerous mitoses; and hyperplasia and "nesting" of epidermal basal cells. Viral intranuclear inclusion bodies are visualized in about half of the lesions, most commonly in the stratum corneum, and less commonly in the stratum granulosum and stratum spinosum. Older, regressing lesions are accompanied by increased proliferation of fibroblasts and infiltration of lymphocytes. Electron microscopic examination suggested that the hypomelanosis was due to a disturbance in melanin synthesis and melanocyte-keratinocyte interaction in the epidermal melanin unit.[91] Langerhans' cells were reported to decrease significantly in size and number in the development phase, but they markedly increased in number, especially at the dermoepidermal junction, in the regression phase.[94] Cytokeratin expression in viral papillomas was reported to be different from that in normal skin.[93]

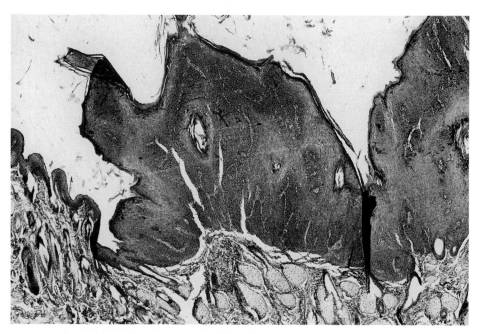

FIGURE 16-4. Viral papilloma. Note pronounced papillated epidermal hyperplasia.

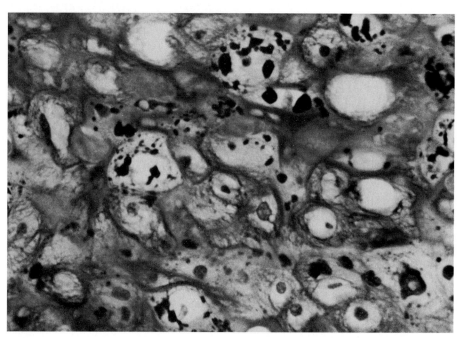

FIGURE 16-5. Viral papilloma. Note koilocytosis ("ballooning degeneration") of keratinocytes and clumping and irregular size and shape of keratohyalin granules.

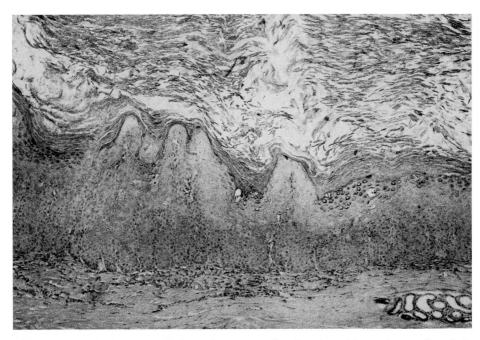

FIGURE 16-6. Ear papilloma ("aural plaque"). Note papillated epidermal hyperplasia and marked ortho-keratotic hyperkeratosis.

Ear papillomas are characterized histopathologically by changes discussed above (Figs. 16-6 and 16-7). However, the epidermal hyperplasia is only mildly papillated, papillomatosis is mild to absent, and hypomelanosis is striking (Figs. 16-7 and 16-8).[70] These lesions are histopathologically analogous to so-called verruca plana or "flat warts" in humans.[5] Electron microscopic studies have revealed intranuclear crystalline arrays of hexagonal viral particles (38 to 42 nm in diameter), identical to those seen in classical equine viral papillomatosis.[89]

Immunohistochemical studies detect papillomavirus antigen in the lesions of both equine viral papillomatosis[95,102] and equine ear papilloma.[89] Expression of lectin binding in equine viral papillomatosis lesions was the same as that found in normal skin, possibly because of the well-differentiated and organized nature of these neoplasms.[107]

CLINICAL MANAGEMENT

The lesions of *equine viral papillomatosis* typically resolve spontaneously within 3 months. Chronically affected animals should be suspected of being immunosuppressed.[73,108] For lesions that must be removed for aesthetic or health reasons, surgical excision or cryosurgery is effective.* It has been anecdotally stated that surgical excision of some larger lesions may encourage the others to regress.[3,50,56,57] However, a controlled study in horses designed to test this hypothesis showed that the duration of other lesions was *not* decreased and, in fact, may have been increased.[103]

Many topical agents have been tried on individual lesions when surgery was impractical.[73,108] The most commonly recommended agents include podophyllin (50% podophyllin; 20% podo-phyllin in 95% ethyl alcohol; 2% podophyllin in 25% salicylic acid), trifluoroacetic acid, and tincture of benzoin.[44,56-58,60,106] These agents were applied once daily until remission occurred. All

---

*References 60, 73, 108, 128, 135, 182, 291.

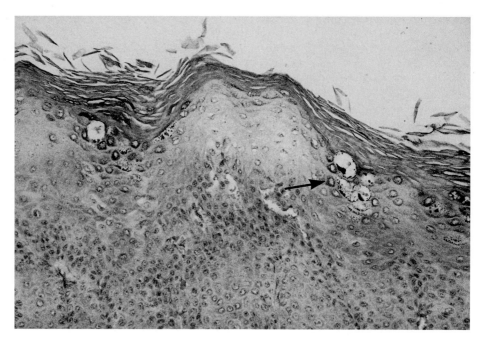

FIGURE 16-7. Ear papilloma. Note koilocytosis and keratohyalin granule irregularities *(arrow)*.

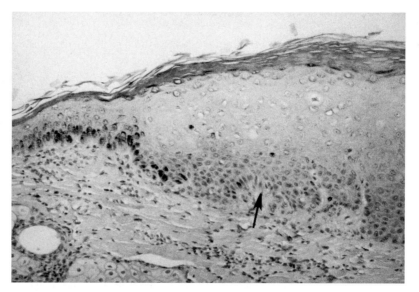

FIGURE 16-8. Ear papilloma. Normal skin *(left)* with melanization of basilar epidermis and sudden transition to papilloma with hypomelanosis *(arrow)*.

such reports are purely anecdotal. Recent anecdotes include the topical application of imiquimod or Eastern blood root in zinc chloride (see Sarcoid). Other treatment anecdotes include the intralesional or intravenous administration of mycobacterial or *Propionibacterium acnes* products as immunostimulants and the intralesional administration of cisplatin or IL-2.[44,108] It must be remembered that any treatment that provokes an inflammatory reaction may cause permanent depigmentation.

Autogenous tumor cell ("wart") vaccines have been reported to be "satisfactory" or "of value" for the treatment of equine viral papillomatosis.[15,56,84] All such reports are purely anecdotal. Studies in cattle[73] and dogs [98] have shown that autogenous and commercial vaccines are effective for the prevention of lesions but not in resolving existing lesions.

With the increasing interest in laser therapy of skin lesions, caution has been urged when using lasers on lesions of suspected viral origin.[105] Papillomavirus antigen has been demonstrated in the vapor of CO_2 laser–treated viral papillomas.

Because viral papillomatosis is contagious, spread of disease may be reduced by isolating affected horses and restricting access of immunologically naive horses to infected premises.[44] Contaminated stalls, feed and water containers, grooming equipment, and bridlery should be cleaned and disinfected using lye or povidone-iodine compounds.[44,108]

Equine ear papillomas rarely, if ever, regress. Effective therapy has not been reported. Anecdotal reports suggested that the topical application of tretinoin (Retin-A, Ortho; 0.025%, 0.05%, 0.1% cream; 0.01%, 0.025% gel) was effective for the treatment of equine ear papillomas, but we have had no success with this form of therapy. Recent anecdotes include the topical application of imiquimod or Eastern blood root in zinc chloride (see Sarcoid). In summer, when ear papillomas might be aggravated by fly bites, it may be reasonable to use fly repellents, fly screens, or insecticidal environmental sprays.[44] Fortunately, these lesions are only a cosmetic problem.

Squamous Cell Carcinoma

CAUSE AND PATHOGENESIS

Squamous cell carcinoma is a common malignant neoplasm of the horse arising from keratinocytes.[*] It is the second most common cutaneous neoplasm of the horse, accounting for 6.9% to 37% of the equine skin neoplasms in many surveys.[†] It is the most common neoplasm of the equine eyelid and external genitalia.[38a,44,67,133a]

Squamous cell carcinoma occurs most frequently in sun-damaged skin and is usually preceded by actinic (solar) keratosis and carcinoma in situ.[15,73,78,133] The prevalence of squamous cell carcinoma increases with increased mean annual solar radiation, increased altitude, increased longitude, decreased latitude, decreased skin and hair pigmentation (white, gray-white, cremello, Palomino), and sparse hair coat.[15,73,115,130,133] The p53 gene is overexpressed in equine squamous cell carcinomas to an extent compatible with gene mutation.[138,146] Rarely, squamous cell carcinoma has been reported to arise from burn scars[141] and nonhealing wounds with chronic infection.[110,119] In humans, dogs, and cats, papillomaviruses have an etiologic role in some squamous cell carcinomas.[5,14] However, papillomavirus antigen was not detected in equine squamous cell carcinomas.[95,102] The irritant and carcinogenic properties of equine smegma have been implicated in the etiology of squamous cell carcinoma of the prepuce.[15,133,140]

CLINICAL FINDINGS

The prevalence of equine squamous cell carcinoma increases with age (mean age of 10 to 12 years; range of 1 to 29 years).[‡] Although any breed can be affected, there is a significant increased prevalence in relatively lightly pigmented draft breeds (Belgian, Clydesdale, Shire), as well as in Appaloosas, American Paints, and Pintos that have been chronically exposed to sunlight.[44,115,130] Sexually intact males and females are significantly less likely (5 to 2 times, respectively) to develop squamous cell carcinoma than castrated males.[115,142]

---

[*]References 6, 9, 15, 29, 30, 34-36, 44, 73, 78, 79, 85, 111, 125, 133, 144, 155.
[†]References 30, 37, 38a, 46, 69, 74, 79, 111, 133, 144, 155.
[‡]References 73, 111, 115, 130, 133, 142, 155.

Squamous cell carcinoma can occur anywhere on the body, especially at mucocutaneous junctions.* The most commonly affected areas are the eyelid (Fig. 16-9), prepuce (Fig. 16-10, *A*), and vulva (Fig. 16-10, *B*).† Periocular squamous cell carcinoma may be bilateral in up to 16% of the horses.[115] Squamous cell carcinomas arising in burn scars and chronically infected, nonhealing wounds become clinically recognizable after 1½ to 8 years.[110,119,141] Lesions are usually solitary, poorly circumscribed, 0.5 to 6 cm in diameter, beginning as nonhealing, enlarging, granulating ulcers or as proliferative, often cauliflower-like masses (Fig. 16-11).[73,83-85] The lesions may be painful. Necrosis and a foul odor are common. In the early stages, persistent, nonhealing, ulcerative lesions appear similar to granulation tissue and may be mistaken for delayed wound healing. Eventually these granulating, ulcerative lesions develop a crater-like appearance with indurated borders. Productive squamous cell carcinomas resemble a papilloma, but with a broader base (cauliflower-like). Precursor lesions (see Actinic Keratosis) are often not observed by owners. Inflammation and secondary infection (bacteria, *Habronema* spp., fungi [*Pythium, Basidiobolus*]) may be complicating factors.[133] Hypercalcemia and pseudohyperparathyroidism were reported in a mare with metastatic vulvar squamous cell carcinoma.[129]

DIAGNOSIS

The differential diagnosis of squamous cell carcinoma includes numerous neoplastic and granulomatous disorders. Cytologic examination is useful for establishing a presumptive diagnosis, showing atypical keratinocytes.[122] Histologically, squamous cell carcinoma consists of irregular masses or cords of keratinocytes that proliferate downward and invade the dermis (Fig. 16-12).[79] Frequent findings include keratin formation, horn pearls, intercellular bridges, mitoses, and atypia. Solar elastosis may occasionally be seen.[112] Squamous cell carcinomas are positive for cyto-keratin, and such examinations may be critical in establishing the true identity of spindle cell and clear cell varieties.

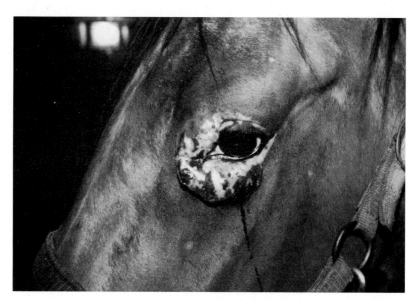

FIGURE 16-9. Squamous cell carcinoma. Ulcerated, depigmented mass involving lower eyelid and medial canthus.

---

*References 6, 15, 29, 37, 44, 58, 73, 79, 109, 130, 155.
†References 30, 41, 46, 83, 110, 115, 120, 125,130, 131, 133, 142, 144, 155.

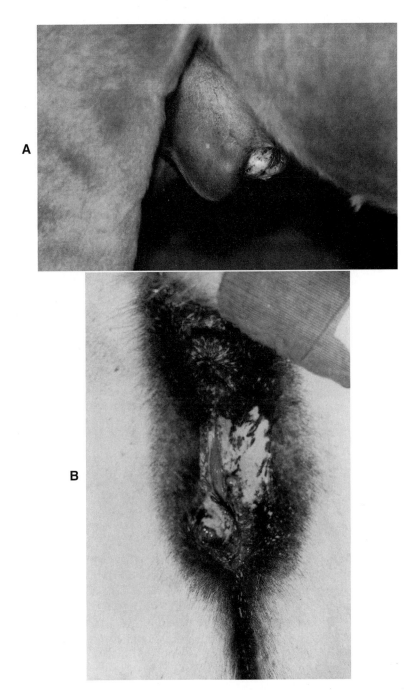

FIGURE 16-10. Squamous cell carcinoma. **A,** Ulcerated mass on prepuce. **B,** Ulcerated, depigmented mass involving vulva.

An intense inflammatory response consisting of numerous CD3+ T lymphocytes, CD79+ B lymphocytes, IgG+ plasma cells, and macrophages is associated with equine squamous cell carcinomas.[139] This response was not correlated with the histologic grade or invasiveness, suggesting that the local antitumor immune response failed to prevent tumor invasion or metastasis.

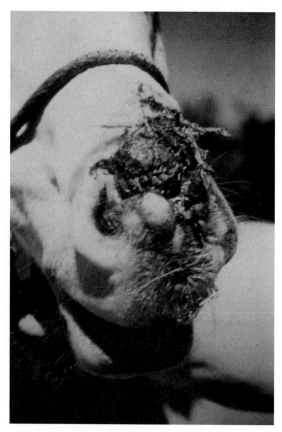

FIGURE 16-11. Squamous cell carcinoma. Ulcerative, necrotizing, proliferative mass on muzzle of white horse.

CLINICAL MANAGEMENT

Squamous cell carcinomas are generally locally invasive but slow to metastasize.° Up to 20% of the lesions will eventually show metastasis to local lymph nodes and, less commonly, to the lungs.[†] Treatment may include surgical excision, cryosurgery, radiofrequency hyperthermia, laser surgery, radiotherapy, chemotherapy, immunotherapy, or combinations of these.[‡] Treatment is most successful when initiated early in the course of the disease and when surgical excision is used in conjunction with other adjunctive therapies.[44]

Treatment of eyelid squamous cell carcinoma depends on the size of the lesion, location of the lesion, success or failure of prior therapy, economics, and availability of therapeutic modalities to the veterinarian or referral center.[67] The prognosis is better for small lesions (<1 cm diameter), and preservation of the functional integrity of the eyelid and eyelid margin is critical. Treatments that preserve as much normal tissue as possible are most appropriate, and surgical excision alone is seldom indicated.

Small lesions (<1 cm diameter and <0.2 cm depth) can be managed successfully by cryosurgery, radiofrequency hyperthermia, carbon dioxide laser ablation, or beta radiation.[67] Lesions

---

°References 15, 73, 78, 111, 133, 155.
[†]References 6, 15, 38, 44, 51, 129, 130, 133, 142.
[‡]References 73, 111, 113, 116, 120, 133, 135, 148.

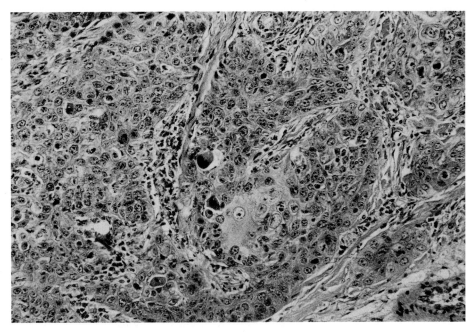

FIGURE 16-12. Squamous cell carcinoma. Malignant proliferation of keratinocytes.

1 to 2 cm in diameter and >0.2 cm in depth can usually be treated by cryosurgery, laser therapy, interstitial radiotherapy, or intratumoral cisplatin injections.[67] Large lesions (>2 cm in diameter and >0.2 cm in depth) require careful consideration of therapeutic options, availability of various options, and a guarded long-term prognosis.[67]

Surgery, Cryosurgery, Radiofrequency Hyperthermia, Laser Surgery

Wide *surgical excision*, where feasible, is the treatment of choice.* In periocular squamous cell carcinoma, the recurrence rate is 30% to 44%.[116,130,142] The median survival time for periocular squamous cell carcinoma was 47 months, with 22% of the horses having died or been euthanized as a result of their disease.[116] Survival time is inversely related to tumor size.[116]

In a small number of cases treated with carbon dioxide *laser ablation,* the recurrence rate is about 22%.[46a,117]

Cryosurgery may be effective in 67% to 87% of the horses treated and is most effective for lesions ≤2 cm in diameter.† Surgical debulking (cytoreduction) should precede the cryosurgical treatment of larger lesions. Leukotrichia and leukoderma should be anticipated. *Radiofrequency hyperthermia* may be effective in up to 75% of the small superficial lesions.[6,44,124] Leukotrichia and leukoderma should be anticipated.

Radiotherapy

Radiotherapy, where available and feasible, can be very useful. *Teletherapy* or *external beam radiotherapy* (orthovoltage or megavoltage) may be effective in 75% to 100% of the horses treated.‡ *Beta-radiotherapy by surface brachytherapy* (plesiotherapy) from strontium 90 may

---

*References 15, 60, 73, 130, 133, 155.
†References 44, 60, 118, 126-128, 133, 192a.
‡References 6, 82, 114, 119, 130, 143, 151, 190.

achieve a 2-year cure rate of 89%, but is only effective for lesions that are less than 0.2 cm in diameter and less than 4 mm in depth.[6,121,151] *Gamma-radiotherapy by interstitial brachytherapy* (using various implants or "seeds" such as gold 198, iridium 192, cobalt 60, cesium 137, or radon 222) may achieve a 2-year cure rate of 70% to 100%.* Complications of radiotherapy include local necrosis, alopecia, and depigmentation; damage to normal structures; corneal opacity; and cataracts. Disadvantages of radiotherapy include extreme expense, limited availability, risks associated with human exposure, prolonged biologic isolation of the patient, and licensing restrictions for their handling. Each state and country has specific radiation hazard laws that must be satisfied.

Chemotherapy

Chemotherapy is useful in some cases. *Cisplatin* (Platinol, Bristol-Meyers) was injected in a water and oil emulsion intratumorally (1 mg/cm^3 of tissue) four times at 2-week intervals following cytoreductive surgery, with a mean relapse-free interval of 41 months and an overall relapse-free survival rate of 92% at 1 year and 77% at 4 years.[147,148] Side effects were not observed. Cisplatin is a broad-spectrum antineoplastic agent that binds to DNA, causing interstrand and intrastrand cross-links, and procedures for proper handling and disposal must be followed.[80a,265]

5-fluorouracil (Efudex, Roche Derm) was applied topically as a 5% cream to squamous cell carcinomas of the external genitalia with or without prior cytoreductive surgery.[120] For males, 5-fluorouracil was applied every 14 days for 2 to 7 treatments (mean 5). In females, the agent was applied daily for 1 to 8 months (mean 4). Complete remissions were achieved in all cases, with no recurrences after follow-up periods of 5 to 52 months. Side effects were not observed. Three horses with superficial, ulcerative squamous cell carcinoma involving the external nares, lip, or muzzle were treated daily for 30 days with 5-fluorouracil cream.[137] Erythema, swelling, blistering, and ulceration occurred during the treatment period, and two of the three horses were still in remission 1 year later. 5-Fluorouracil is a fluorinated pyrimidine that blocks the methylation reaction of deoxyuridylic acid to thymidylic acid, thus interfering with the synthesis of DNA. Adverse reactions to topically administered 5-fluorouracil in humans include pain, pruritus, burning, and hyperpigmentation. Thus, caution is warranted when applying this agent (e.g., wear disposable gloves, avoid applying to normal skin). Intratumoral administration of 5-fluorouracil was not effective in horses.[137]

Intratumoral injections of *bleomycin* are effective.[113,149] A comparison of intratumoral administration of cisplatin versus bleomycin for treatment of periocular squamous cell carcinomas revealed a 1-year local control rate of 93% for cisplatin and 78% for bleomycin.[149] Treatment with bleomycin is much more expensive.[81]

Anecdotal reports indicate that bloodroot extracts may have some value.[38a]

Immunotherapy

Immunotherapy is of unproven benefit in equine squamous cell carcinoma.[6,113] One horse with periocular squamous cell carcinoma and metastasis to the submandibular lymph node was treated with cryotherapy and intratumoral injections of a BCG cell wall emulsion (see Sarcoid).[134] The periocular mass disappeared, the submandibular lymph node returned to normal size, and the horse was normal after a 1½-year follow-up. Other authors have not found BCG to be successful.[9,44]

Preventive measures include routine cleaning of the prepuce and penis and avoiding exposure to sunlight, if possible, from 9 AM to 3 PM (maximum ultraviolet light intensity is from 11 AM to 2 PM).[44,111,115,133] The development of new squamous cell carcinomas is common when ultraviolet light is not avoided.

---

*References 6, 82, 114a, 123, 132, 150-154.

Basal Cell Tumor

CAUSE AND PATHOGENESIS

The term *basal cell tumor* has been used in veterinary literature to classify a large group of neoplasms of domestic animals. Numerous histopathologic "subclassifications" have been applied to these neoplasms: medusa head, garland or ribbon, trabecular, solid, cystic, adenoid, basosquamous, and granular cell.[14,73,78] In general, these various histopathologic types are often found within the same neoplasm and apparently offer no useful clinical, prognostic, or therapeutic information. Most veterinary basal cell tumors are benign and *not* contiguous with the basal cell layer of the epidermis; these lesions generally show differentiation toward follicular structures and have been reclassified in dogs and cats.[14] It is likely that such reclassification would be appropriate in horses as well. However, because the number of basal cell tumors carefully described and illustrated in equine skin is very small, the "basal cell" terminology will be retained for the present.

These tumors are rare, benign neoplasms of the horse that are thought to arise from the basal cells of the epidermis. Although these tumors accounted for 2.8% to 5.7% of the equine cutaneous neoplasms in two surveys,[68,71] they were only briefly mentioned in other surveys* and not even acknowledged in most. The cause of basal cell tumors in horses is unknown. In humans, there is a strong correlation between exposure to ultraviolet light and the development of basal cell tumors.[5] However, the occurrence of these lesions in haired, dark-skinned areas of horses indicates that ultraviolet light exposure is of no etiologic importance in this species.[156,156a]

CLINICAL FINDINGS

Basal cell tumors occur in horses with no apparent breed or sex predilections. The mean age of affected horses is 10.6 years (range 4 to 26 years).[9,156,156a] The lesions are solitary, rounded, firm, well-circumscribed, and 0.5 to 5 cm in diameter. The overlying skin may be normal, hyperpigmented, alopecic, or ulcerated. The lesions can occur anywhere, but are most commonly reported on the distal limbs, trunk, face, and neck (Fig. 16-13).[9,59,156,156a]

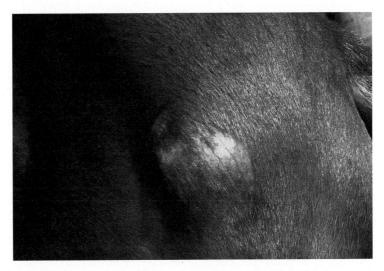

FIGURE 16-13. Basal cell tumor. Partially alopecic mass on the lateral thigh.

---

*References 41, 51, 59, 60, 73, 85.

DIAGNOSIS

Equine basal cell tumors are most commonly misdiagnosed clinically as sarcoid, squamous cell carcinoma, or melanoma.[156,156a] Histopathologically, basal cell tumors are characterized by a well-circumscribed, symmetric proliferation of basaloid cells (Fig. 16-14). The most common reported pattern is solid, followed by adenoid and medusoid.[156,156a] There was no correlation between histopathologic pattern and location on the body. Basal cell tumors are positive for cytokeratin.

CLINICAL MANAGEMENT

Clinical management of basal cell tumors may include surgical excision, cryotherapy, laser therapy, and observation without treatment.[9,73,156,156a] Complete surgical excision resulted in no recurrences after a 3- to 8-year follow-up period.[156]

Trichoepithelioma

CAUSE AND PATHOGENESIS

Trichoepitheliomas are benign neoplasms thought to arise from keratinocytes that differentiate toward all three segments of the hair follicle.[14] They are positive for cytokeratin. The cause of trichoepitheliomas is unknown. In humans, a syndrome of multiple trichoepitheliomas is hereditary.[5]

CLINICAL FINDINGS

The authors have seen only one horse with a solitary trichoepithelioma. A 22-year-old Thoroughbred gelding was presented for a 4-cm diameter, hyperkeratotic nodule over the mandible.

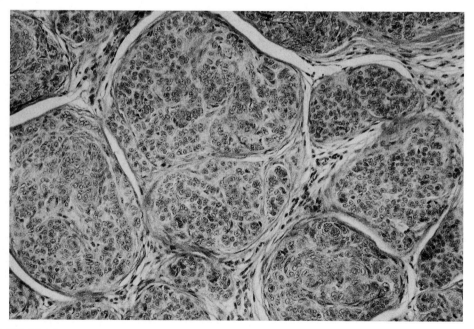

FIGURE 16-14. Basal cell tumor. Nodular proliferations of basal cells. Note retraction spaces separating nodules from surrounding stroma.

DIAGNOSIS

Histopathologically, trichoepitheliomas vary considerably, depending on the degree of differentiation and whether the tumor is primarily related to the follicular sheath or the hair matrix.[14] Frequent characteristics include horn cysts, differentiation toward hair follicle-like structures, and formation of abortive or rudimentary hairs (Fig. 16-15).

CLINICAL MANAGEMENT

Clinical management of trichoepithelioma may include surgical excision, cryotherapy, electrosurgery, and observation without treatment.

Dilated Pore of Winer

CAUSE AND PATHOGENESIS

The cause of this lesion is unknown, although evidence favors a developmental origin arising from the combined forces of obstruction and intrafollicular pressure leading to hair follicle hyperplasia.[14]

CLINICAL FINDINGS

A single case has been described in the horse.[443] The lesion was firm, well-circumscribed, and located caudal to the point of the elbow. Surgical excision was curative.

DIAGNOSIS

Histopathologically, the lesion is characterized by a markedly dilated, keratinized, pilar infundibulum lined by an epithelium that is atrophic near the ostium but increasingly hyperplastic toward the base (Fig. 16-16). The epithelium at the base shows psoriasiform hyperplasia with rete ridges and irregular projections into the surrounding dermis.

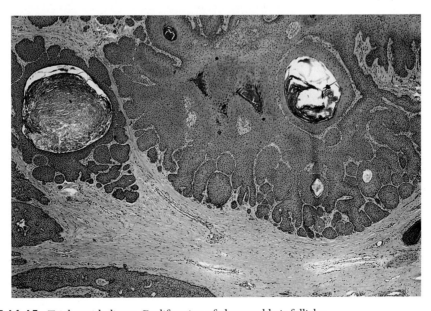

FIGURE 16-15. Trichoepithelioma. Proliferation of abnormal hair follicles.

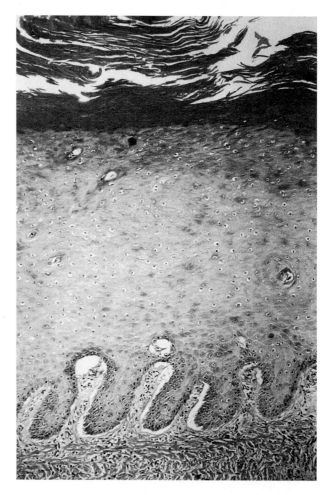

FIGURE 16-16. Dilated pore of Winer. Base of cyst shows psoriasiform hyperplasia and trichilemmal keratinization.

CLINICAL MANAGEMENT

Clinical management of dilated pore of Winer includes surgical excision or observation without treatment.

Sebaceous Gland Tumors

CAUSE AND PATHOGENESIS

Sebaceous gland tumors are very rare skin neoplasms of the horse arising from sebocytes.° Their cause is unknown.

CLINICAL FINDINGS

There is little clinicopathologic information recorded on these neoplasms, since they are typically listed only as "sebaceous adenoma" or "sebaceous gland tumor" in a survey of equine skin

---

°References 2, 9, 30, 51, 65, 73, 85.

tumors.[30,65] A sebaceous carcinoma of the prepuce which metastasized to the peritoneal cavity was reported in one horse.[157]

DIAGNOSIS

Cytologic examination reveals clustering of lipidized sebocytes and a variable percentage of basaloid cells. Histopathologically, sebaceous gland tumors are classified as nodular sebaceous hyperplasia (greatly enlarged sebaceous glands composed of numerous lobules grouped symmetrically around centrally located sebaceous ducts); sebaceous adenoma (lobules of sebaceous cells of irregular shape and size, which are asymmetrically arranged and well demarcated from the surrounding tissue and contain mostly mature sebocytes and fewer undifferentiated germinative cells); sebaceous epithelioma (tumor similar to basal cell tumor but containing mostly undifferentiated germinative cells and fewer mature sebocytes); and sebaceous carcinoma (tumor with pleomorphism and atypia). Sebaceous gland tumors are positive for cytokeratin.

CLINICAL MANAGEMENT

Clinical management of sebaceous gland tumors may include surgical excision, cryosurgery, and observation without treatment.

Sweat Gland Tumors

CAUSE AND PATHOGENESIS

Epitrichial sweat gland tumors are rare neoplasms of the horse arising from the glandular or ductular components of epitrichial sweat glands.[9,59,60,73] They accounted for only 1.1% of the cutaneous neoplasms in one survey.[68] The cause of these tumors is unknown.

CLINICAL FINDINGS

These neoplasms are most commonly benign and most commonly reported on the pinna and vulva (Fig. 16-17).[34,37,59,60,158] Lesions are usually solitary, firm to cystic, well-circumscribed nodules. The overlying skin may be normal, alopecic, or ulcerated.

DIAGNOSIS

Cytologic examination may reveal clusters of epithelial cells containing secretory droplets. Ulcerated lesions may mimic squamous cell carcinomas.[60] Histopathologically, epitrichial sweat gland tumors are characterized by benign[37,59,60] or malignant[34,158] proliferations of epitrichial sweat gland epithelium, which may feature predominantly secretory or ductal epithelium and may be solid or cystic in appearance (Fig. 16-18). Sweat gland tumors are positive for cytokeratin.

CLINICAL MANAGEMENT

Clinical management of epitrichial sweat gland tumors may include surgical excision, cryosurgery, or observation without treatment.

● MESENCHYMAL NEOPLASMS

Tumors of Fibroblast Origin

As a result of the early confusion and controversy over the histologic diagnosis of the equine sarcoid, many of the surveys on equine cutaneous neoplasia published prior to 1980 are misleading.[30,262] Most of these publications indicated that "fibropapillomas," "fibrosarcomas," "fibromas," or "invasive fibromas" were the most common equine cutaneous neoplasm.° In most instances, the

---

°References 2, 29, 34, 41, 65, 68, 71, 153.

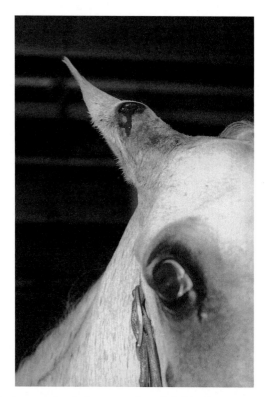

FIGURE 16-17. Epitrichial sweat gland adenoma. Ulcerated, bleeding mass on pinna.

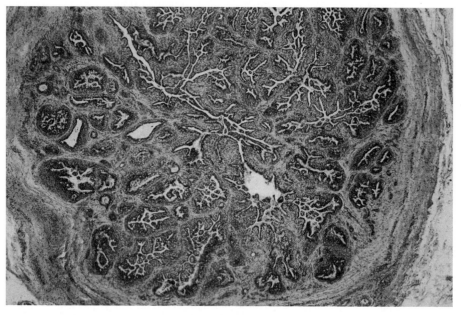

FIGURE 16-18. Epitrichial sweat gland adenoma. Note acinar and ductal differentiation and surrounding desmoplasia.[1]

clinical information provided for these horses was typical for that of sarcoids. The histologic variability of the equine sarcoid is discussed below.

SARCOID
Cause and Pathogenesis

The sarcoid is a common, locally aggressive, fibroblastic cutaneous neoplasm of the horse.[73,79,223] It is the most common skin neoplasm of the horse, accounting for 35.3% to 90% of the total in numerous surveys.[*] Sarcoids accounted for 0.7% to 2% of the equine clinical cases presented to two American and two Swiss university clinics.[161,178,227,232] These tumors adversely affect the material value of horses, and they often compromise the use of the animal because of their location, although they are not life-threatening in most instances. In the United Kingdom, the equine sarcoid is probably the most common cutaneous reason for euthanasia, and the loss to the equine industry is considerable.[207]

The etiology of sarcoids is believed to be viral.[73,172a,223,227] Lesions frequently occur in areas subjected to trauma, and there may be a history of a previous wound 3 to 6 months earlier.[†] The lesions may be spread to other areas on the same horse or possibly to other horses through biting, rubbing, fomites, and insects.[47,60,78,228,266] Epizootics in herds and examples of multiple-case horse families living together are consistent with an infectious origin.[†] Sarcoids have been autotransplanted, but transmission to other sites on donor horses or to other horses by injection of various sarcoid tissue extracts has not been routinely successful.[227,233,237,249,272]

Bovine papillomaviruses (BVP) occur as six subtypes and are divided into two groups (A and B). Viruses in subgroup A can transform fibroblasts and epithelial cells, whereas viruses in subgroup B can transform only epithelial cells. BPV-1 and BVP-2 are members of subgroup A.

Bovine papillomavirus (probably types 1 and 2) was inoculated into horse skin and produced fibroblastic proliferations.[237,244,247,256] Cultured fetal equine fibroblasts were transformed when exposed to BPV-2,[283] and common membrane neoantigens were found on BPV-induced neoplastic cells from cattle and horses.[162] However, (1) BPV-induced lesions in horses were distinguished by a short incubation period and rapid spontaneous regression uncharacteristic of equine sarcoid;[247] (2) the fibroblastic growths produced in equine skin with BPV differed histologically from equine sarcoid by lacking an epidermal component and active fibroblast proliferation at the dermo-epidermal junction;[78,247,262,273] (3) horses with naturally occurring sarcoids do not have antibodies against BPV,[227,246] whereas horses with BPV-induced lesions do;[227,256] and (4) attempts to produce typical papillomas in calves with equine sarcoid extracts were unsuccessful.[249] Attempts to find BPV particles in equine sarcoids by electron microscopy have been unsuccessful.[227] Attempts to detect BPV in equine sarcoids by antibody techniques (e.g., immunohistochemistry) have also been unsuccessful.[102,162,227] These are not unexpected findings, since the horse is not the natural host for BPV and cannot support the vegetative portion of the viral life cycle.[159,227]

More sensitive techniques such as molecular hybridization, restriction enzyme analysis, and polymerase chain reaction have demonstrated BPV-DNA sequences in the vast majority of equine sarcoids.[§] In the majority of lesions, viral sequences identical to or very similar to BPV-1 or BPV-2 are present. It is interesting to note that BPV-1 was most commonly detected in horses from the eastern United States, Belgium, Germany, and Switzerland,[160,226a,238,265] whereas BPV-2 was most commonly detected in horses from the western United States.[172a] Similar BPV-like DNA sequences were also found in normal skin from sarcoid-bearing horses, normal equine skin, and

*References 30, 36, 38a, 46, 48, 52, 57, 59, 60, 66, 68, 74, 79, 179a, 191, 198, 209, 220a, 227, 229, 243, 257, 260.
†References 43, 47, 60, 66, 78, 79, 198, 236, 266, 272.
‡References 84, 167, 189, 200, 220, 227, 245.
§References 159, 160, 172a, 210-212, 221, 226a, 227, 238, 251, 252, 263, 264, 267.

normal equine fetal muscle.[172a,267] The fact that BPV-DNA was detected in 63% of the samples of normal skin in sarcoid-bearing horses suggests the possibility of a latent viral phase and may be one explanation for the high rate of recurrence following surgical excision of sarcoids.[172a] BPV-DNA sequences were not detected in lymphocyte DNA from horses bearing sarcoids[160] or in blood cells of donkeys with sarcoids.[235] There may be variants of BPV that are specific for horses arising through mutational events, or there may be as yet unidentified equine papillomaviruses that are very closely related to some of the BPVs.[227]

A retrovirus was found in sarcoids and a cell line established from a sarcoid[175,176,181] but was subsequently characterized as an endogenous virus unrelated to sarcoids.[183,184,227] Tumor-specific antigens were demonstrated in an equine sarcoid cell line,[275,276] and cell-mediated immune response against sarcoid antigens were demonstrated to occur in affected horses.[166,168,170] Tubulo-reticular inclusions were found in the fibroblasts from naturally occurring sarcoids and in cultured cells from these, but not in normal skin from sarcoid-bearing horses or normal horses.[222] The significance of this finding is presently unknown.

An association between sarcoid susceptibility and the MHC encoded class II allele ELA W13 was reported at the population level in several breeds.[219,227,230] Further studies in multiple-case families and in large half-sibling groups demonstrated that particular ELA haplotypes segregate with susceptibility to sarcoids.[167,189,220] The "sarcoid-susceptible" haplotypes often, but not always, included the W13 MHC class II antigen associated with sarcoid at the population level. The family data suggest the existence of a "sarcoid-susceptibility gene" linked to MHC region. The equine sarcoid may be considered a virus-induced tumor with a variety of manifestations as a result of interactions between the etiologic agent, the environment, and the host genome.[169]

Circumstantial evidence incriminates flies in the pathogenesis and epidemiology of sarcoids.[207] Perhaps the different flies in different geographical areas have some role in the regional variations in numbers and types of sarcoid.[207]

No mutations of the tumor suppressor gene p53 were found in equine sarcoids.[172]

Clinical Findings

The majority of the veterinary literature would indicate that there are no breed or sex predilections.[73,165,198,228] Recent studies have demonstrated that Appaloosas, Arabians, quarter horses, and geldings are at increased risk, and that standardbreds are at decreased risk.[161,228,242,253] Given the etiologic significance of BPVs in equine sarcoids, the increased risk in Appaloosas and quarter horses is interesting, because these are breeds generally found on cattle farms.[232] Although sarcoids may occur in horses of any age, they are extraordinarily rare in horses less than 1 year of age, and the majority of affected animals are ≤7 years of age.[169,198,227-229,266] Coat color, seasonal, and geographic predilections have not been identified.[73,198]

Sarcoids may occur anywhere on the body, but the majority of lesions occur on the head (especially on the pinnae, commissures of the lips [Fig. 16-19], and periocularly [Fig. 16-20]), neck (Fig. 16-21), legs (Fig. 16-22), and ventral body surface.* In northern climates, sarcoids seem to be found primarily on the head and abdomen, whereas in warmer climates they occur most commonly on the limbs.[44,227] Anywhere from 14% to 84% of affected horses have multiple sarcoids.† Referral clinics and veterinary schools tend to see animals with multiple lesions, whereas primary care veterinarians often see animals with solitary lesions. The gross appearance of sarcoids can be quite variable, but four broad categories are recognized: (1) verrucous (wart-like) (see Fig. 16-21), (2) fibroblastic (proud flesh–like) (Figs. 16-22 and 16-23), (3) mixed verrucous and fibroblastic,

---

*References 30, 43, 60, 73, 85, 165, 169, 198, 209, 223, 226a, 227, 228, 257, 266.
†References 36, 66, 73, 83, 169, 178, 213, 227, 228, 266.

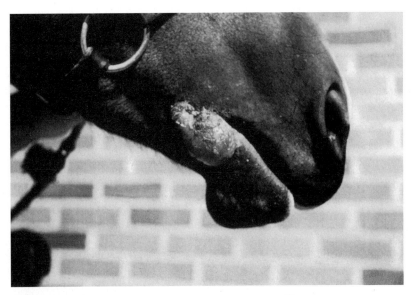

FIGURE 16-19. Equine sarcoid. Fibroblastic mass at commissure of lips.

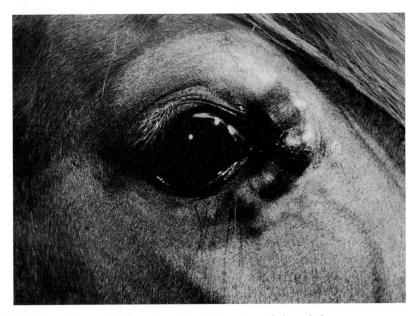

FIGURE 16-20. Equine sarcoid. Multiple nodular lesions in medial canthal area.

and (4) occult (flat) (Fig. 16-24).[66,73,227] Lesions are usually firm and annular, 1 cm to enormous in diameter (Fig. 16-25), and often poorly circumscribed. The overlying skin may appear normal, alopecic, hyperkeratotic, hyperpigmented, ulcerated, or combinations of these. Occult sarcoids begin as annular areas of slightly thickened, scaly to hyperkeratotic skin that becomes progressively alopecic and variably hyperpigmented. All four morphologic types of sarcoids may have smaller satellite lesions around the larger primary lesion (Fig. 16-26). Some authors have suggested two

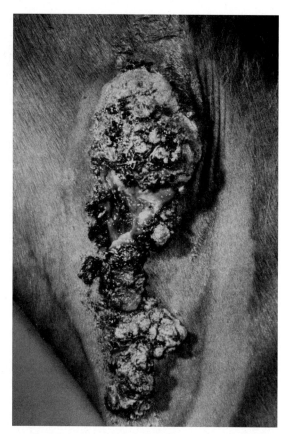

FIGURE 16-21. Equine sarcoid. Verrucous masses on neck.

other forms of equine sarcoid: nodular (entirely subcutaneous with normal overlying skin and hair coat) and "malevolent" (particularly invasive with infiltrated lymphatic vessels resulting in multiple cords of tumor masses).[207]

The type of sarcoid appears to have some geographic variations, with occult and verrucous lesions being unusual in Africa and Australia but particularly common in the United Kingdom.[207]

Some authors have reported that there is a tendency for the different gross forms of sarcoids to occur more frequently on certain body sites: occult sarcoids occurring most commonly on the neck, face, sheath, medial thigh, and shoulder; verrucous sarcoids, on the head, neck, axillae, and groin; nodular sarcoids, on the eyelids, groin, and prepuce; fibroblastic sarcoids, on the axillae, groin, legs, periocular region, previous wound sites, and the sites of other sarcoid types subjected to trauma; "malevolent" sarcoids, on the elbow and jaw.[38a,178,187,207,269] Other authors have not had similar experiences.[266] Many horses have a range of morphologic forms.[198]

Associations between clinical parameters of sarcoids and the ELA system were analyzed in 120 Swedish horses.[169] Lesions at different sites differed in size, and multiple tumors, early onset, long duration, and older age all had an association with large tumor size. There was an association between certain ELA specificities and early onset (A5), increased recurrence rates after surgery (W13), and increased prevalence (A3W13). The largest lesions were found on the distal limbs, which may reflect that certain sites are more frequently exposed to mechanical irritation that both initiates wounds and stimulates tumor growth.

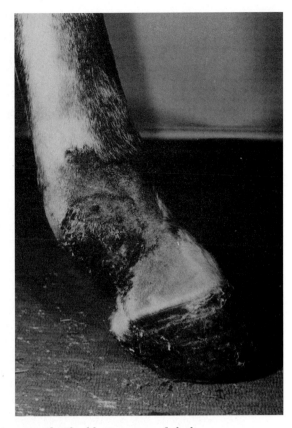

FIGURE 16-22. Equine sarcoid. Fibroblastic mass on fetlock.

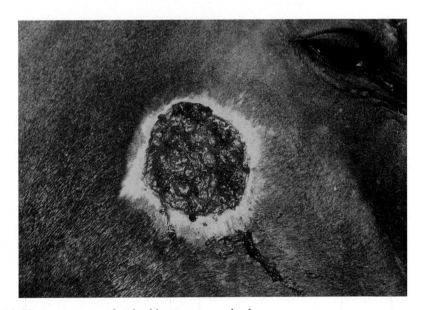

FIGURE 16-23. Equine sarcoid. Fibroblastic mass on cheek.

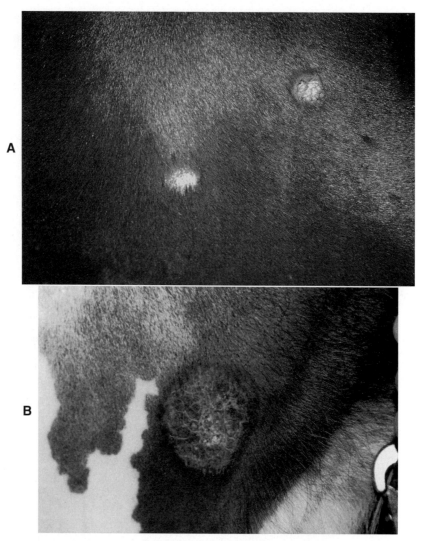

FIGURE 16-24. Equine sarcoid. **A,** Two alopecic, hyperkeratotic plaques on lateral neck. **B,** Hypotrichotic, crusted plaque on shoulder.

Diagnosis

The major differential diagnoses for the various morphologic forms of sarcoid are verrucous (papilloma, squamous cell carcinoma), fibroblastic (squamous cell carcinoma, exuberant granulation tissue, habronemiasis, infectious granulomas), occult (dermatophytosis, dermatophilosis, staphylococcal folliculitis, onchocerciasis), nodular (dermal neoplasms [especially melanocytic neoplasms and mast cell tumors] and granulomas [especially eosinophilic granuloma]). Diagnosis is confirmed by skin biopsy. It is generally accepted that the manipulations used for taking a biopsy or the removal of only part of the neoplasm may stimulate growth of the remaining tissue and include the risk of transforming a quiescent sarcoid into an active proliferating form.° Thus, biopsy of occult, nodular, or small verrucous sarcoids has been discouraged by some clinicians.[38a]

°References 198, 207a, 226b, 243, 248, 262.

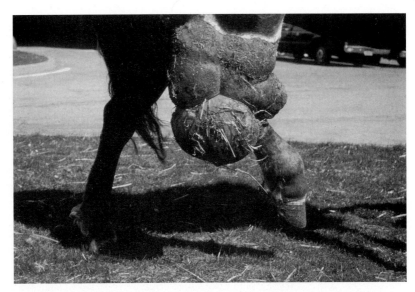

FIGURE 16-25. Equine sarcoid. Enormous recurrent tumor on hind leg. (*Courtesy Dr. J. King.*)

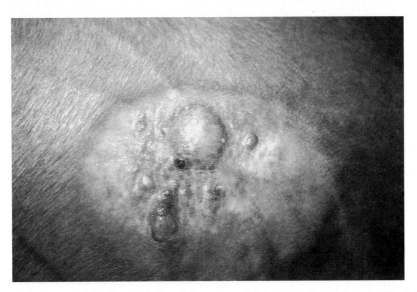

FIGURE 16-26. Equine sarcoid. Original nodule surrounded by several papules ("satellite" lesions) on ventral abdomen.

Equine sarcoids are characterized histologically by fibroblastic proliferation with associated epidermal hyperplasia and dermoepidermal activity (Fig. 16-27).[*] However, in one study[226a] epidermal hyperplasia, rete ridges, and "picket fence" formation at the dermoepidermal junction were absent in 46%, 54%, and 52%, respectively, of the sarcoids studied. These changes were absent more frequently in occult and nodular sarcoids. The dermis shows variable amounts of collagen fibers and fibroblasts in a whorled, tangled, herringbone, criss-cross or linear pattern, or combinations of these. Because of this variability of dermal configuration, a given sarcoid or area

[*]References 43, 44, 66, 78, 262, 273.

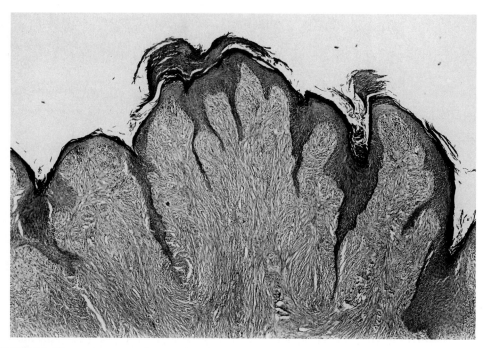

FIGURE 16-27. Equine sarcoid. Attenuated, pointed hair follicles protrude into a subjacent fibrous proliferation.

within a sarcoid could be misdiagnosed as fibroma, fibropapilloma, fibrosarcoma, neurofibroma, neurofibrosarcoma, schwannoma, or exuberant granulation tissue.[67,191,226a] The schwannoma-like appearance of some areas of some equine sarcoids probably resulted in multiple periocular sarcoids being misdiagnosed as schwannomas ("neurofibromas")[9,59,60] (see Schwannoma). Because of this histopathologic overlap, some authors recommend that BPV-DNA must be shown to be absent before one of these much less common mesenchymal neoplasms can be diagnosed.[226a] Neoplastic cells are spindle-shaped or fusiform to stellate, often with hyperchromasia and atypia. Distinct borders separating neoplasm and normal tissue are often absent. The number of mitoses is variable but is usually low (1/HPF). Fibroblasts at the dermoepidermal junction are frequently oriented perpendicularly to the basement membrane zone in a so-called "picket-fence" pattern (Fig. 16-28). The overlying epidermis is hyperplastic and hyperkeratotic. Rete ridges (mostly attenuated hair follicles) are often elongated and pointed (see Fig. 16-27). Occult sarcoids are often overlooked histologically because they are characterized by focal epidermal hyperplasia and hyperkeratosis with underlying junctional fibroblast proliferation. Lesions that historically began as flat sarcoids then suddenly began to enlarge have typically had histologic features of an occult (superficial) and deep sarcoid (Fig. 16-29).

No major qualitative differences were found in the connective tissue composition and organization of equine sarcoids and normal adult equine skin, but sarcoid cells exhibited an increased level of collagen synthesis.[279] The proliferative fraction of sarcoids is low, with only a mean of 1.44% of the cells showing nuclear Ki67 staining.[226a] Immunohistochemical staining for keratins 10 and 16, Ki67, and p53 showed no important differences between five clinical types of sarcoid.[226a]

In situ hybridization studies demonstrated papillomavirus only in dermal spindle cells, not in keratinocytes.[271] In addition, the papillomavirus-positive spindle cells were mostly localized to the subepidermal dermis, while CD11c+ dermal dendrocytes were mostly localized to the deep dermis, where papillomavirus was rarely found.

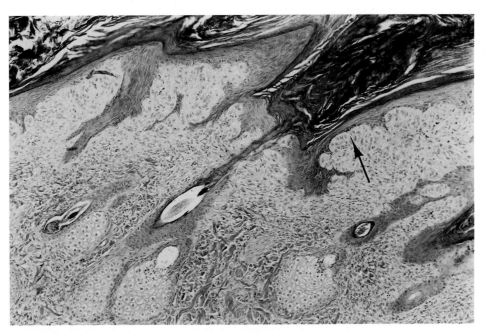

FIGURE 16-28. Equine sarcoid. A hyperkeratotic, hyperplastic epidermis overlies a band-like proliferation of fibroblastic cells. Some fibroblasts at the dermoepidermal junction are oriented perpendicularly to the epidermis in a so-called "picket fence–like" appearance *(arrow)*.

BPV-DNA was detected in 88% and 93%, respectively, of the swabs and scrapings made from equine sarcoids.[226b] Although there is still much to confirm (value in nodular and occult sarcoids, investigation of normal skin from affected horses, and so forth), this technique offers the exciting possibility of a rapid, accurate, and practical test for clinicians.[207a]

Clinical Management

Sarcoids do not metastasize. Some lesions come and go, and some may undergo spontaneous remission, but this may take several years.* About 30% of the horses in two studies showed signs of spontaneous regression of one or more of their sarcoids.[169,226c] Spontaneous regression appeared unassociated with ELA or any clinical parameter. Static occult and verrucous sarcoids may often be best left alone, since the trauma of biopsy or surgical excision may cause sudden increased growth and aggressive behavior.† Treatment may include surgical excision, cryosurgery, radio-frequency hyperthermia, laser therapy, radiotherapy, chemotherapy, immunotherapy, or combinations of these.‡ The choice and success of therapy is dependent on factors such as site, size, aggressiveness, and number of lesions; previous attempts at treatment; clinician experience; and availability of services, equipment, and facilities.§ Lesions on the legs and axillae may be more aggressive and resistant, whereas periocular lesions may be more amenable to therapy. Recurrent lesions tend to be more resistant to therapy.

Sarcoids are treated routinely, and often successfully, by veterinarians in private practice.[191] Common protocols include observation without treatment for small tumors that do not cause the

---

*References 43, 66, 73, 78, 171, 173, 188, 260, 272.
†References 6, 43, 47, 66, 73, 171, 188, 198, 207, 209, 260.
‡References 73, 163, 165, 179a, 191, 198, 224, 225, 227, 229.
§References 6, 163, 179a, 191, 198, 227.

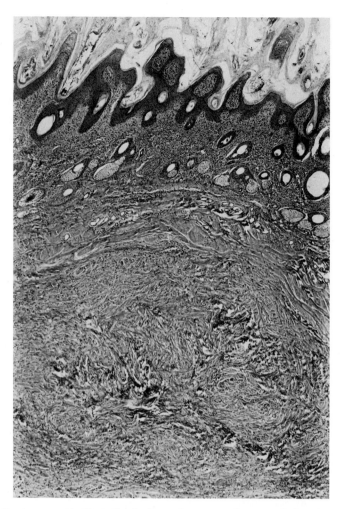

FIGURE 16-29. Equine sarcoid. Clinically, the lesion began as a flat sarcoid, then became nodular 2 years later. Note the typical flat sarcoid appearance superficially, and the deep proliferative sarcoid, which are separated by a zone of normal dermis.

horse discomfort and do not impede its use, and surgical excision with or without various types of immunotherapy for larger sarcoids or those that impede an animal's use. Only limited data on the incidence and prevalence of sarcoids in the field and on the success of these and other treatments are available.

It seems likely that the sarcoid cases referred to large clinics or veterinary schools may not be typical of the overall population.[191] They may represent fast-growing, recurrent, or multiple tumors that have proven refractory to one or more treatments given by practitioners. The reports of treatment of sarcoids have usually been generated using these referred cases. The relevance of these studies to the treatment of primary, often solitary sarcoids is unclear.

• *Surgery, cryotherapy, hyperthermia, laser. Wide surgical excision* is followed by recurrence in 50% to 72% of the cases within 6 months.° If possible, surgical margins should be >1 cm and the practitioner must beware of autotransplantation.† Careful selection of patients, rigorous measures

---

°References 47, 60, 163, 165, 171, 179, 188, 191, 209, 224, 228, 236, 260, 270, 280.
†References 163, 168, 171, 188, 209, 228, 229.

taken to avoid autotransplantation, and wide surgical margins can reduce the postsurgical recurrence rate to 18%.[226c] In one study, early onset, long duration, large size, and localization to the distal limbs all appeared to increase the risk of recurrence after surgery.[169] Cytoreductive surgery should be combined with other treatments; it is commonly used before other modes of therapy to reduce exophytic tumor volume and to improve the killing efficiency of combination therapy.

Cryosurgery is an effective treatment modality, being associated with 1-year cure rates of 42% to 100%.[*] This technique should not be used in tissue with closely underlying, vital soft tissue structures, such as the distal limbs and periorbital area. Frequent complications of cryosurgery include delayed healing, scarring, and depigmentation of hair and skin. When only selected sarcoids in horses with multiple sarcoids were treated by cryosurgery, spontaneous regression of untreated tumors was occasionally observed, perhaps as a result of cryoimmune response to sarcoid cell components.[6,46,213,227]

Radiofrequency hyperthermia has been effective for the treatment of some sarcoids,[163,196] but presently available data do not permit specific recommendations. It seems unlikely that this method will become a practical means of therapy for any but the smallest sarcoids, and the method has no apparent benefit over any other treatments.[207]

Laser therapy (carbon dioxide laser excision and ablation) has been reported to be effective in 62% to 81% of the cases treated with follow-up periods of 6 to 12 months.[†] Dehiscence may occur in 40% of the horses treated.[46a] Animals with multiple sarcoids are more likely to suffer recurrences.

• *Radiotherapy.* Radiotherapy, where available and feasible, can be useful. *Teletherapy* or *external beam radiotherapy* (orthovoltage or megavoltage) is successful in only 10% to 30% of cases.[114,190,195] In contrast, *interstitial brachytherapy* (γ-radiation) using various implants such as gold 198, iridium 192, cobalt 60, or radon 222 have been curative in 50% to 100% of the cases.[†] This method is especially useful for periorbital lesions.[207]

• *Photodynamic therapy.* Photodynamic therapy involves administering a photosensitizing agent, allowing it to accumulate in neoplastic tissue, and activating it afterwards by visible light. Liberated free radicals and singlet oxygen damage vascular endothelium and cell membranes. In a small study, photodynamic therapy caused a reduction in size but did not eliminate sarcoids.[226]

• *Chemotherapy.* Chemotherapy may be useful in some cases. *Bleomycin* (Blenoxane, Bristol-Meyers) was injected intratumorally (15 mg in 20 ml sterile water; 1 ml solution/10 mm diameter lesion) every 1 to 2 weeks for one to five injections.[164] Although 75% of the horses were cured, the follow-up period was only 2 to 4 months. It was recommended that lesions ≤2.5 cm in diameter were the most likely to respond. The solution is stable for several months in the refrigerator, and the injections are not too painful. Side effects were not observed. Other investigators have not found intratumoral bleomycin injections to be very effective in sarcoids.[81] Bleomycin is an antineoplastic antibiotic that inhibits the incorporation of thymidine into DNA and labilizes DNA structure.

Cisplatin (Plantinol, Bristol-Meyers) in a water-and-oil emulsion was injected intratumorally (1 mg/cm^3 of tissue) four times at 2-week intervals following cytoreductive surgery,[80a] with a mean relapse-free interval of 41 months and an overall relapse-free survival rate of 92% at 1 year and 77% at 4 years (see Squamous Cell Carcinoma).[147,148] Side effects were not observed.[191,265]

Topical application of cytotoxic agents may be effective in treating small sarcoids.[§] Daily treatment is required for 30 to 90 days. Examples of such topicals include 50% podophyllin in alcohol,

---

[*]References 60, 113, 118, 128, 135, 163, 171, 179, 182, 187, 188, 192a, 198, 201, 203, 207-209, 213, 218, 224, 226c, 227-229, 270, 291.
[†]References 38a, 46a, 173, 178, 179, 191, 224, 226c, 227, 242, 270.
[‡]References 6, 82, 132, 143, 154, 186, 224, 227-229, 268, 274, 290.
[§]References 56, 58, 59, 163, 194, 206, 225, 231, 254.

1% arsenic pentoxide in DMSO, 50% podophyllin in tincture of benzoin, 5% 5-fluorouracil, and a mixture of 5-fluorouracil, thiouracil, and several heavy metal salts. Results are inconsistent,[171,227] and published information is largely anecdotal. The 5-fluorouracil/thiouracil/heavy metal salts (AW-3-LUDES, University of Liverpool) are said to produce a resolution rate of over 80%.[206] However, if the lesions have received previous therapy (e.g., cryosurgery, BCG), the resolution rate drops to 40% to 50%.

• *Immunotherapy.* Immunotherapy with *mycobacterial products* (commercial whole attenuated bacillus Calmette-Guérin [BCG]; modified mycobacterial cell wall preparation in oil [Regressin-V, Vetrepharm Research Inc.]; mycobacterial cell wall skeleton-trehalose dimycolate combination [Ribigen-E, Ribi Immunochem Research, Inc.]) has been effective in the treatment of sarcoids, especially periocular lesions.[*] Success rates vary from 59% to 100% in several reports.[†] The best results are seen with periocular sarcoids, whereas sarcoids on the limbs and in the axillary region are less responsive.[191,240] Intralesional injections are administered every 2 to 3 weeks, for an average of four treatments. These products are least successful when treating large or multiple lesions, lesions on the legs, and lesions previously treated by cryosurgery.[205,229,240,269] Postinjection inflammatory reactions are common and may lead to necrosis, ulceration, and discharge. Owners must be informed that the lesions usually look worse before healing occurs. Occasional horses show transient malaise, anorexia, lymphadenopathy, pyrexia (up to 40° C), and leukocytosis after injection. Premedication with flunixin meglumine and corticosteroids are recommended. Fatal anaphylaxis has occurred following repeated injections of whole attenuated BCG, and these products are no longer recommended.

Anecdotal information indicates that the intravenous and intralesional administration of heat-killed *Propionibacterium acnes* (Eqstim, Neogen) and the intralesional injection of acemannan (Acemannan Immunostimulant, VPL) are not effective for the treatment of equine sarcoids.[81] Other anecdotal information indicates that Eqstim has given good results (protocols vary widely; intralesional and/or intravenous injections given weekly for 6 to 8 weeks).[38a]

Autogenous sarcoid vaccines and subcutaneous implantation of slabs of tumor tissue at distant sites have met with occasional anecdotal success, but cannot be recommended.[‡] It has been suggested that both the severity and number of lesions may increase dramatically following their use.[207]

Treatment with bovine wart vaccine and various poxvirus vaccines was unsuccessful.[66,254] Twenty horses with an average of four sarcoids per horse were treated sublesionally and perilesionally with a commercial poxvirus immunostimulant (Baypamun) or placebo.[258] Tumor regression was reported in 5 of 10 horses with the placebo, and 3 of 10 horses with the immunostimulant. The authors suggested that all regressions were probably spontaneous.

Two topical agents are currently achieving anecdotal success in the treatment of sarcoids. *Imiquimod* (Aldara, 3M) is an imidazoquinolone amine used as a topical "immune response modifier" for the treatment of humans with viral papillomas on the external genitalia and on the perianal area.[176a] The exact mechanism of action is unknown, and imiquimod apparently has no *in vitro* antiviral activity. It does induce the production of a variety of cytokines (IL-1, IL-6, IL-8, IL-12, IFN-α, TNF-α, MIP-1α) and enhances cell-mediated immunity and cell-mediated cytolytic antiviral activity. In humans, the 5% imiquimod cream is applied 3 times weekly (e.g., Monday-Wednesday-Friday) and removed with mild soap and water after 6 to 10 hours. Treatment is continued until cure is achieved or for a maximum of 16 weeks.

---

[*]References 67, 163, 165, 185, 191, 225, 227, 229, 250.
[†]References 113, 174, 203-205, 217, 226c, 227, 228, 234, 240, 255, 259, 269, 277, 281, 284, 285.
[‡]References 81, 163, 202, 225, 229, 241, 278.

A paste containing Eastern bloodroot and zinc chloride (XXTERRA, Larson Laboratories, Inc., Fort Collins, CO) is not approved for use on horses but is being enthusiastically promoted for the treatment of equine sarcoids. Other similar products ("Indian mud") containing different subspecies and concentrations of blood root are also used. XXTERRA is supplied with a "money back guarantee" and is reported to be "effective in over 90% of the equine sarcoids treated." The product is applied under a Telfa pad and bandaged, if possible. The application is repeated every 4 days until the sarcoid "falls off." The product purportedly does not harm normal skin of the horse or the human applicator. The mechanism of action is unknown but is hypothesized to involve altered antigenicity of the neoplasm.

Another bloodroot extract that contains *Sanguinaria canadensis*, puccoon, gromwell, distilled water, and trace minerals (Animex, NIES Inc.) has been used to treat various kinds of skin lesions, including sarcoids. It is an escharotic salve that penetrates the lesion, killing affected cells while leaving surrounding healthy tissue intact. The lesion usually sloughs in 7 to 10 days. Some authors consider this product to be the treatment of choice for small sarcoids that can be easily bandaged.[38a]

• *Miscellaneous treatments.* *Xanthates* inhibit the replication and transcription of DNA and RNA viruses (including BPV-1) and have antitumor activity, especially when combined with monocarboxylic acids.[239] A small number of equine sarcoids were treated intralesionally with a xanthate compound (tricyclodecan-9-l-xanthogenate with a potassium salt of lauric acid) with and without the simultaneous administration of recombinant human TNF-α.[239] Less than 50% of the lesions regressed.

Various *homeopathic remedies* have been of anecdotal benefit in some equine sarcoids.[225,282]

FIBROMA

Cause and Pathogenesis

Fibromas are uncommon to rare benign neoplasms of the horse arising from dermal or subcutaneous fibroblasts.[°] They account for 2.1% to 17.1% of equine skin neoplasms in various surveys.[†] As indicated previously, the higher percentages almost assuredly are explained by sarcoids being misdiagnosed as fibromas. The cause of fibromas is unknown.

Clinical Findings

Fibromas occur in adult to aged horses with no apparent breed or sex predilections. They can occur anywhere, but most commonly on the periocular area, neck, and legs (Fig. 16-30).[‡] Lesions are usually solitary, well-circumscribed, dermal or subcutaneous in location, firm ("fibroma durum") to soft ("fibroma molle"), and from 0.5 to 7.5 cm in diameter. The overlying skin is usually normal in appearance but may be alopecic, hyperpigmented, or both of these.

Diagnosis

Cytologic examination may reveal small numbers of spindle-shaped fibroblasts. Histopathologically, fibromas are characterized by well-circumscribed whorls and interlacing bundles of fibroblasts and collagen fibers (Fig. 16-31). The neoplastic cells are typically fusiform, and mitoses are rare. Fibromas containing focal areas of mucinous degeneration are sometimes referred to as *fibromyxomas* or *myxofibromas*.[68,79] Fibromas are positive for vimentin.

°References 29, 34, 53, 62, 63, 65, 66, 68, 74, 76.
†References 30, 37, 66, 68, 71, 74, 83.
‡References 9, 34, 47, 59, 60, 62, 68, 73, 83, 131, 153, 155, 286-288.

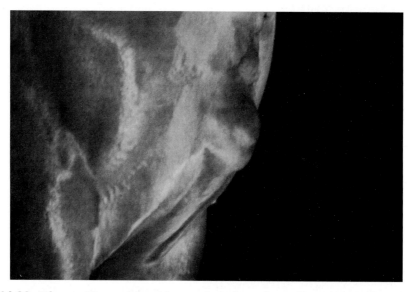

FIGURE 16-30. Fibroma. Firm nodule with normal overlying skin and hair coat on chest. *(Courtesy Dr. S. Fubini.)*

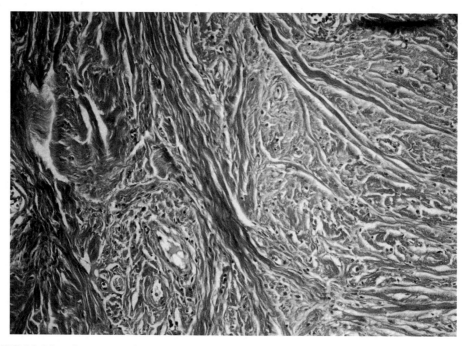

FIGURE 16-31. Fibroma. Interlacing bundles of fibroblasts and collagen bundles.

Clinical Management

Clinical management of fibromas may include surgical excision, cryosurgery, or observation without treatment.[9,73] Some periocular fibromas have been successfully treated with interstitial radiotherapy ([198]Au grains).[153]

FIBROSARCOMA

Cause and Pathogenesis

Fibrosarcomas are rare malignant neoplasms of the horse arising from dermal or subcutaneous fibroblasts.* They account for 0.4% to 5.7% of the equine skin neoplasms in some surveys.[30,51,65,68,71,74] Again, the higher percentages most likely are explained by sarcoids being misdiagnosed as fibrosarcomas. The cause of most fibrosarcomas is unknown. One fibrosarcoma occurred in burn wounds.[141]

Clinical Findings

Fibrosarcomas occur in adult to aged horses with no apparent breed or sex predilections.[†] They can occur anywhere, especially on the eyelid, trunk, and limbs. Lesions are usually solitary, poorly demarcated, firm to fleshy, infiltrative subcutaneous masses that are frequently ulcerated and secondarily infected.

Diagnosis

Cytologic examination reveals pleomorphic, atypical fibroblasts. Histopathologically, fibrosarcomas are characterized by interwoven bundles of immature fibroblasts and moderate numbers of collagen fibers (Fig. 16-32). The neoplastic cells are usually fusiform, mitotic figures are common, and cellular atypia is pronounced. Fibrosarcomas with focal areas of mucinous degeneration have been called *fibromyxosarcomas*.[68] Fibrosarcomas are positive for vimentin.

Clinical Management

The treatment of choice is wide surgical excision, but recurrence is common. Radiotherapy (mainly orthovoltage external beam or interstitial brachytherapy) was reported to be curative in up to 50% of the cases treated.[‡] Cryosurgery may be useful.[291] Chemotherapy is unlikely to be useful, but one horse was apparently cured after surgical excision, intravenous vincristine, and oral razoxin.[293] One horse was unresponsive to surgical excision and intratumoral injections of BCG.[113] A horse with a preputial fibrosarcoma was apparently cured (6 month follow-up) by the topical application of 5-fluorouracil.[293a] The biologic behavior of equine cutaneous fibrosarcomas is not clear. One horse with a tumor in the skin of the flank had metastases to the heart and spinal cord.[292]

FIBROMATOSIS

Fibromatosis was reported in a 15-year-old thoroughbred mare.[294] The condition was initially recognized as a 10-cm diameter, firm, soft tissue mass in the pectoral region. Over the course of a year, the mass enlarged to involve most of the thorax and ventral abdomen. Histologically, thick intertwined bands of collagen dissected diffusely between the dermal and skeletal muscle tissues. The deep location, relationship to a musculoaponeurotic system, diffuse growth, nonencapsulation, and engulfment of muscle fibers fulfilled the criteria for a diagnosis of fibromatosis.

Tumors of Neural Origin

SCHWANNOMA

Cause and Pathogenesis

Schwannomas (neurofibroma, neurilemoma, neurinoma, nerve sheath tumor, or perineural fibroblastoma) are uncommon neoplasms of the horse arising from dermal or subcutaneous Schwann

---

*References 6, 8, 30, 34, 47, 53, 59, 60, 68.
†References 6, 8, 9, 34-36, 113, 292, 293, 293a.
‡References 6, 15, 114, 143, 195, 289, 290.

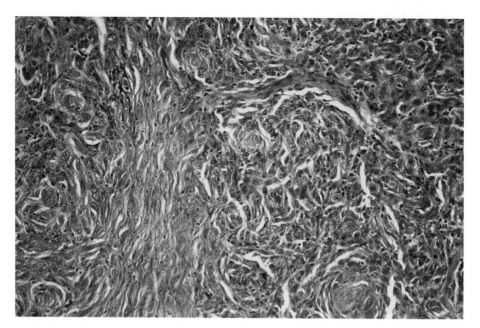

FIGURE 16-32. Fibrosarcoma. Disorganized proliferation of collagen fibers and malignant fibroblasts.

cells (nerve sheath).* They account for 2% to 5% of the equine cutaneous neoplasms in various surveys.[66,68,71,74,83,153] The higher percentages are probably explained by sarcoids being misdiagnosed as schwannomas. The cause of these neoplasms is unknown.

There is much confusion about terminology concerning these neoplasms in the veterinary literature. Schwannoma lesions have been classified as neurinomas, neurilemomas, schwannomas, malignant schwannomas, neurofibromas, and neurofibrosarcomas. Some authors have proposed the term *peripheral nerve sheath tumor* to include those tumors involving peripheral nerves and nerve roots, because of the presumed common cell of origin and similar biologic behavior.[14]

Clinical Findings

Schwannomas are typically seen in adult horses, 3 to 16 years of age, with no apparent breed or sex predilections.[294a] Lesions are usually solitary, firm, 1 to 4 cm in diameter, with the overlying skin and hair coat being normal. There is probably no site predilection. Schwannomas have also been reported to begin as single or multiple, firm, rounded, 2- to 3-mm diameter subcutaneous papules, especially on the eyelids (Fig. 16-33),[59,60,83,153] which may enlarge to 2 cm in diameter, at which point they may become multiloculated, alopecic, and ulcerated. Most of these were probably sarcoids with schwannoma-like areas within the tumors.

Diagnosis

Histopathologically, schwannomas are characterized by three patterns or combinations of these: (1) "neurofibroma" (Fig. 16-34, A)—faintly eosinophilic, thin, wavy fibers lying in loosely textured strands that extend in various directions, with spindle-shaped cells that may exhibit nuclear palisading; (2) "neurilemoma"—areas of spindle-shaped cells exhibiting nuclear palisading and

---

*References 9, 30, 59, 60, 65, 85, 295.

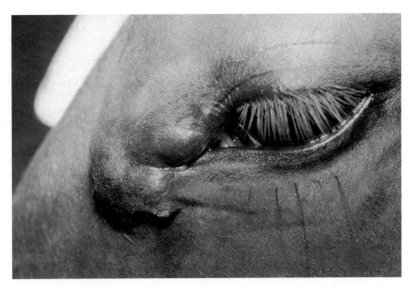

FIGURE 16-33. Schwannoma. Two nodules in medial canthus area. (*Courtesy Dr. R. Pascoe.*)

twisting bands or rows (Antoni Type A tissue) alternating with an edematous stroma containing relatively few haphazardly arranged cells (Antoni Type B tissue), and Verocay bodies (Fig. 16-34, B); and (3) "plexiform"—multinodular neoplastic growth with primitive Verocay bodies within remnants of the perineurium. A fourth histopathologic variety—"fascicular," wherein spindle cells grew in dense interlacing bundles[294a]—was subsequently shown to be a dermal melanocytoma (BA Summers, personal communication, 2001). Schwannomas are positive for vimentin and S-100 protein.

Clinical Management

The treatment of choice is surgical excision. About 50% of periocular schwannomas recur following surgical excision, usually within 6 months.[59,60] Two or more excisions may be necessary to effect a cure. Again, these lesions were probably equine sarcoids. Interstitial radiotherapy with [198]Au has been reported to be effective in a small number of periocular schwannomas.[153] Anecdotal reports indicated that interstitial radiotherapy with iridium-192 is very effective, intralesional cisplatin may be effective, and intralesional BCG is not very effective.[9]

Leiomyoma

Leiomyomas are extremely rare cutaneous neoplasms. They accounted for only 0.1% of the cutaneous neoplasms in one survey.[74] They arise from smooth muscle cells of arrector pili muscles or cutaneous blood vessels.[14] The cause of these neoplasms is unknown. Leiomyomas are positive for vimentin and smooth muscle actin.

A 7-year-old thoroughbred gelding was presented for a firm, well-circumscribed, 2-cm diameter, intradermal nodule over the lateral thorax.[74] Histologic examination of an excisional biopsy revealed interlacing bundles of smooth muscle fibers that tended to intersect at right angles (Figs. 16-35 and 16-36). Cell nuclei were cigar-shaped with blunt rounded ends. The neoplasm appeared to arise from arrector pili muscle.

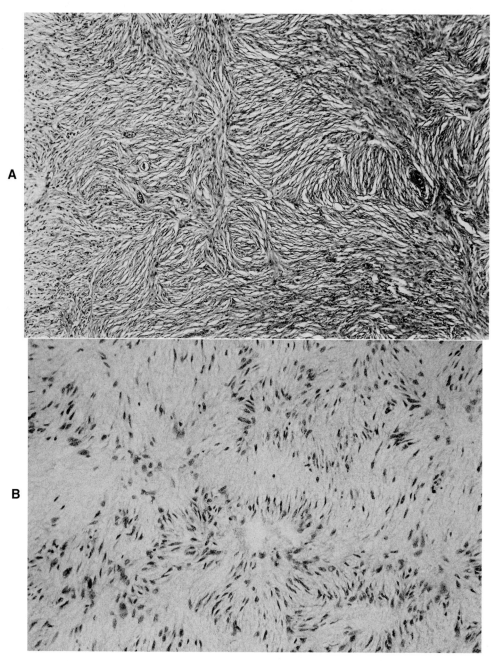

FIGURE 16-34. Schwannoma. **A,** Intermingling and palisading of thin, wavy fibers and Schwann cells. **B,** Palisading of spindle-shaped cells (Antoni type A) alternating with edematous stroma (Antoni type B).

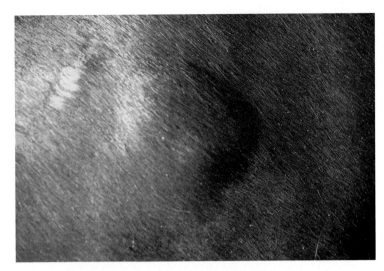

FIGURE 16-35. Leiomyoma. Firm dermal nodule over lateral thorax.

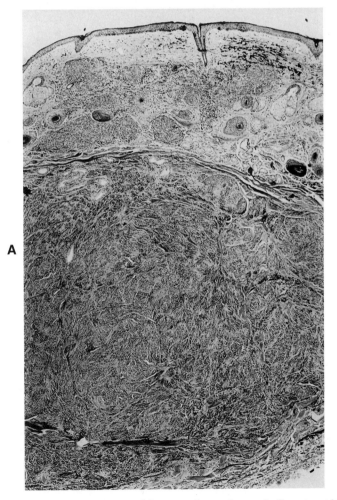

FIGURE 16-36. Leiomyoma. **A,** Nodular proliferation of smooth muscle fibers in middle and deep dermis.

Continued

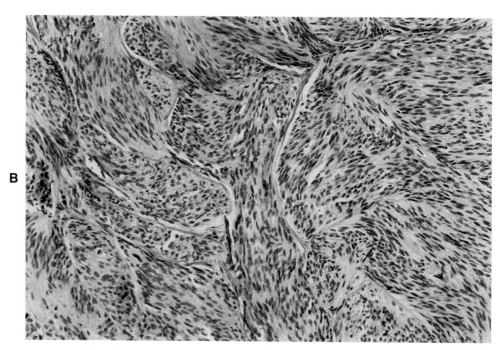

FIGURE 16-36, cont'd. B, Interlacing bundles of smooth muscle fibers and cells.

Tumors of Vascular Origin

HEMANGIOMA

Cause and Pathogenesis

Hemangiomas are uncommon benign neoplasms arising from the endothelial cells of blood vessels.* They account for 1% to 4% of all equine skin neoplasms.[51,53,74,83,301] The cause of most hemangiomas is unknown. It appears that chronic solar damage may be the cause of cutaneous hemangiomas in lightly pigmented, sparsely haired dogs.[14]

Clinical Findings

There are no apparent breed or sex predilections. Although hemangiomas can occur at any age, they are often seen in horses less than 1 year of age and may be congenital (Fig. 16-37).[298-306] Anecdotal reports suggest that congenital hemangiomas are particularly common in Arabians.[9] Equine hemangiomas are usually solitary and may occur anywhere,† but they most commonly affect the distal limbs (metacarpus, metatarsus, hock, fetlock, tibia, coronet) (Figs. 16-38 through 16-40).[29,59,296,301,303-306] The lesions may be (1) well-circumscribed, nodular, firm-to-fluctuant, blush-to-black or (2) well-circumscribed, plaque-like, dark, hyperkeratotic-to-verrucous ("verrucous hemangioma"). Lesions vary from 4 to 30 cm in diameter, and the overlying skin may be normal, alopecic, ulcerated, or infected. Hemangiomas ("vascular hamartomas") were described as solitary, up to 6 cm diameter, firm-to-fluctuant subcutaneous swellings on the dorsal carpal region of three young thoroughbreds.[297] Episodic hemorrhage from hemangiomas may be seen, but blood loss anemia is rare.[9,301]

---

*References 9, 29, 30, 45, 53, 59, 65, 83, 301.
†References 45, 131, 299, 301, 302, 304.

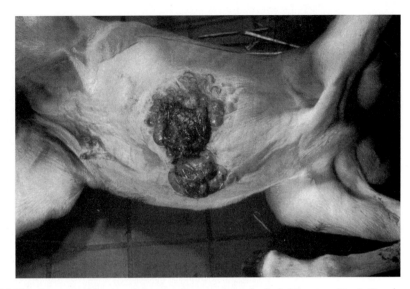

FIGURE 16-37. Congenital hemangiomas on the ventrum of a foal. *(Courtesy Dr. J. King.)*

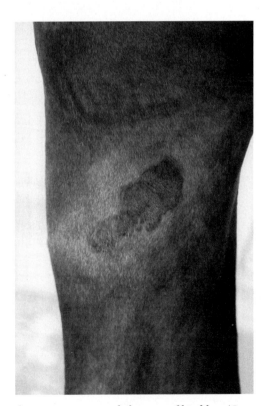

FIGURE 16-38. Verrucous hemangioma on medial aspect of hind leg. *(Courtesy Dr. A. Stannard.)*

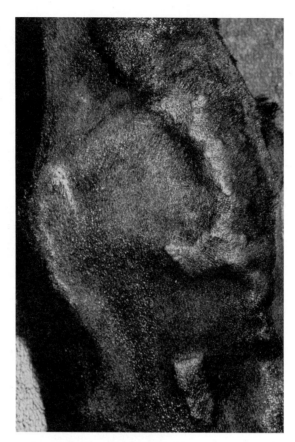

FIGURE 16-39. Verrucous hemangioma on the fetlock of a young equine.

Diagnosis

Histopathologically, hemangiomas are characterized by the proliferation of blood-filled vascular spaces lined by single layers of well-differentiated endothelial cells (Fig. 16-41). They are sub-classified as cavernous, capillary, or both of these depending on the size of the vascular spaces and the amount of intervening fibrous tissue.[301] The verrucous hemangioma is characterized by a multinodular capillary hemangioma with hyperplasia and hyperkeratosis of the overlying epidermis (Figs. 16-42 and 16-43).[73] These multinodular expansive growths have a substantial number of pericytes arranged concentrically around the vascular channels and are consistently associated with well-differentiated muscular arteries and veins.[303]

The subcutaneous hemangiomas on the dorsal carpal region of young thoroughbreds were characterized by abnormal subcutaneous blood vessels that varied greatly in size, wall thickness, and complexity.[297] The vessels sometimes formed very large cavernous structures that were thrombosed.

Electron microscopy may be beneficial in determining the vascular origin of a neoplasm, as Weibel-Palade bodies are a specific cytoplasmic marker for endothelial cells. In addition, immuno-histochemistry may be useful, because vimentin, factor VIII-related antigen (von Willebrand's factor), type IV collagen, laminin, and CD31 are found in blood vascular proliferations.[14,299,304,309,310] Lectins (e.g., *Ulex europaeus* [UEA-1]) are not good markers for vascular neoplasms.

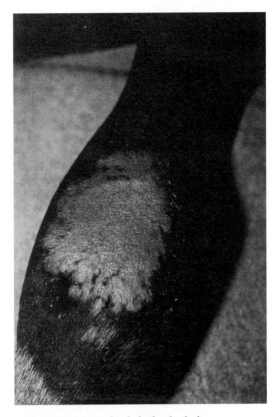

FIGURE 16-40. Verrucous hemangioma on the fetlock of a foal.

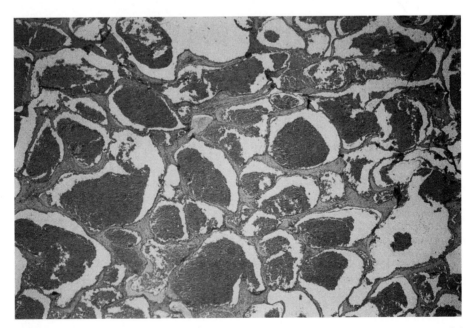

FIGURE 16-41. Cavernous hemangioma. Large, dilated, thin-walled blood vessels separated by thin connective tissue septae.

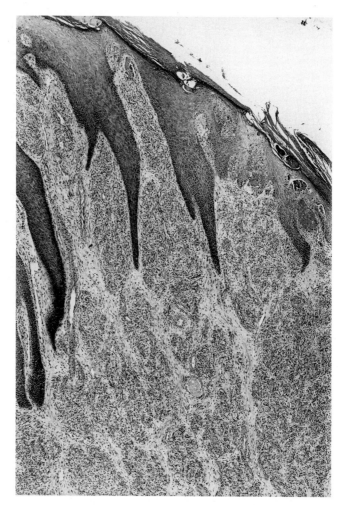

FIGURE 16-42. Verrucous hemangioma. Multinodular capillary hemangioma with overlying irregular to papillated epidermal hyperplasia.

Clinical Management

Clinical management of hemangiomas may include surgical excision, cryosurgery, and observation without treatment. A few cases have recurred following surgical excision and required a second surgery.[297,298,304] Radiotherapy (orthovoltage and interstitial) has been reported to be effective in two cases.[301,302] One congenital hemangioma underwent spontaneous remission after 1 year.[299]

HEMANGIOSARCOMA

Cause and Pathogenesis

Hemangiosarcomas are very rare malignant cutaneous neoplasms arising from the endothelial cells by blood vessels.° They accounted for only 0.2% of the cutaneous neoplasms in one survey.[74] The cause of most hemangiosarcomas is unknown. In humans, they have been associated with exposure

---

°References 30, 51, 83, 301, 307, 308, 311.

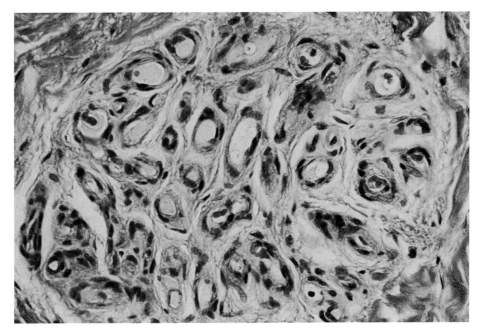

FIGURE 16-43. Verrucous hemangioma. Nodular proliferation of well-differentiated blood vessels.

to thorium dioxide, arsenicals, and vinyl chloride.[5] It appears that chronic solar damage may be the cause of cutaneous hemangiosarcomas in lightly pigmented, sparsely coated dogs and on the pinnae of white-eared cats.[14]

Clinical Findings

There are no apparent breed or sex predilections, and affected horses have ranged from 5 to 12 years of age.[307,308,310] Equine hemangiosarcomas are usually solitary and occur most commonly on the neck, trunk, and proximal limbs.[45,301,307,308,310] The lesions are 1.5 to 25 cm in diameter and vary from firm-to-fluctuant nodules, to ill-defined swellings, to bruise-like, to bleeding ulcers. Intermittent hemorrhage from the lesions may be seen and some horses develop blood loss anemia.[301,307,310] One horse had multiple metastatic subcutaneous nodules affecting the trunk and legs.[310]

The most commonly affected noncutaneous tissues are the lung and pleura, skeletal muscle, and spleen.[311] Anemia, neutrophilia, and thrombocytopenia are common.[311]

Diagnosis

Histopathologically, hemangiosarcomas are characterized by an invasive proliferation of atypical endothelial cells with areas of vascular space formation (Fig. 16-44). They are positive for vimentin, factor VIII–related antigen (von Willebrand's factor), type IV collagen, laminin, and CD31.[14,309,310]

Clinical Management

The therapy of choice for hemangiosarcomas is radical surgical excision. However, after *any* form of therapy, the prognosis for horses with hemangiosarcomas is guarded, with local recurrence and metastasis being possible. Where follow-up information is available, two horses survived 6 and 8

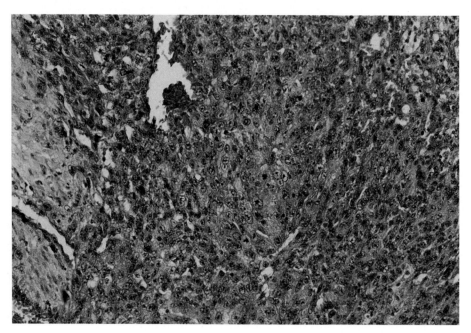

FIGURE 16-44. Hemangiosarcoma. Areas of vascular space formation within proliferation of malignant endothelial cells.

years after radical surgical excision,[301] while three other horses had pulmonary metastasis 2 months to 1 year after their neoplasms were recognized.[307,308]

LYMPHANGIOMA

Cause and Pathogenesis

Lymphangiomas are very rare benign neoplasms of equine skin.* They accounted for only 0.1% of the cutaneous neoplasms in one survey.[74] They arise from the endothelial cells of lymphatic vessels. The terminology used for benign lymphatic vessel lesions is confusing, with congenital lesions being referred to as *congenital lymphangiomas, congenital lymphangiectasis,* and *lymphatic hamartomas*. Acquired lesions are called *acquired lymphangiomas, lymphangiectasis,* or *lymphangiomatosis*. Their cause is unknown.

Clinical Findings

Most lymphangiomas are congenital or are noted within the first 6 months of life. Lesions are multinodular, firm to fluctuant, subcutaneous, and poorly circumscribed. The lesions are often quite large (up to 30 cm in diameter). They may be accompanied by pitting edema and turgid vesicles and may occur on the inguinal and axillary regions and the medial thigh. The size of the swellings may vary over time.

Diagnosis

Histologically, lymphangiomas are characterized by a proliferation of variably sized, cavernous, angular vascular spaces (Fig. 16-45). They are lined by a single layer of endothelial cells and occur within the dermis, the subcutis, or both. Lymphangiomas are positive for vimentin, factor

*References 9, 59, 60, 73, 311a, 312, 313.

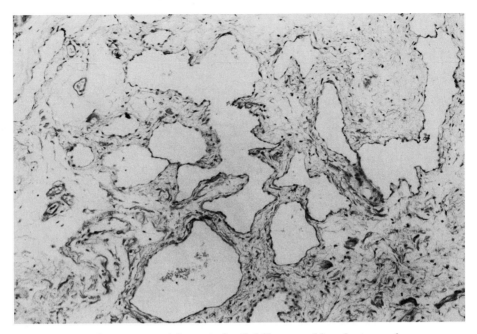

FIGURE 16-45. Lymphangioma. Proliferation of well-differentiated lymphatic vessels.

VIII–related antigen (von Willebrand's factor), and CD31.[311a] However, unlike hemangiomas, lymphangiomas are negative for laminin and type IV collagen. Electron microscopic examination reveals an absence of continuous basement membrane as well as pericytes.[311a]

Clinical Management

Clinical management of lymphangiomas includes wide surgical excision or observation without treatment. In one horse, the mass extended through the left inguinal and femoral canals and involved the kidney, testicle, pelvic inlet, and the lumbar musculature.[313] The animal was euthanized.

Tumors of Adipose Origin

LIPOMA AND LIPOSARCOMA

Cause and Pathogenesis

Lipomas (benign) and liposarcomas (malignant) are rare equine neoplasms arising from subcutaneous lipocytes (adipocytes).[30,59,60,65,79] They accounted for 0.4% to 3% of the equine skin neoplasms in two surveys.[74,79] The cause of these neoplasms is unknown.

Clinical Findings

Lipomas occur most commonly in young adult horses (1 to 3 years old), with no apparent sex or breed predilections.[58-60,68,70-72,74,315] They may be congenital.[316] Obese individuals may be predisposed.[9] Lesions are solitary, well-circumscribed, soft to flabby, and variable in size (2 to 50 cm in diameter). The are usually slow-growing, and the overlying skin is usually normal. Lesions occur most commonly on the trunk (Fig. 16-46) and proximal limbs.° *Infiltrative lipomas* were reported on the lateral neck[314] and flank[318] of young adult horses.

°References 37, 59, 60, 79, 315, 317.

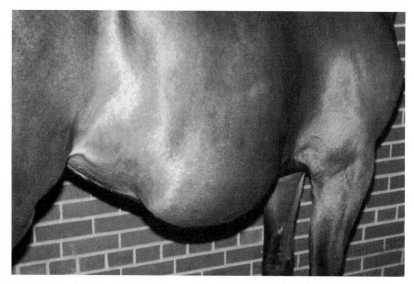

FIGURE 16-46. Lipoma. Huge subcutaneous mass on ventrolateral trunk. (*Courtesy Dr. S. Fubini.*)

Diagnosis

Cytologic examination of lipomas reveals an often acellular preparation containing numerous lipid droplets and occasionally lipocytes (Fig. 16-47, *A*). Histopathologically, lipomas are characterized by a well-circumscribed proliferation of normal-appearing lipocytes (Fig. 16-47, *B*). Some lipomas contain a significant fibrous tissue component and are called *fibrolipomas*.[317] Infiltrative lipomas are characterized by a poorly circumscribed proliferation of normal-appearing lipocytes that infiltrate surrounding tissues, especially muscle and collagen. Liposarcomas are characterized by a cellular, infiltrative proliferation of atypical lipocytes. Lipomas and liposarcomas are positive for vimentin.

Clinical Management

Clinical management of lipomas may include surgical excision or observation without treatment. The therapy of choice for infiltrative lipomas and liposarcomas is wide surgical excision.

MAST CELL TUMOR
Cause and Pathogenesis

Mast cell tumors (mastocytoma, cutaneous mastocytosis) are uncommon, usually benign neoplasms of the horse that arise from mast cells.[*] They accounted for 6.9% of the cutaneous neoplasms in one survey.[74] The cause of mast cell tumors is unknown. It is debatable whether most equine mast cell tumors are truly neoplastic.[44] Attempts to transmit the tumor to newborn foals by subcutaneous or intrathymic injections and to an unborn foal in utero by intramuscular injection were unsuccessful.[320,337]

Clinical Findings

Equine mast cell tumors show no breed predilection and affect horses from 1 to 18 years of age (average 9.5 years).[327] In one study,[336] no cases were seen in thoroughbreds, although this breed

---

*References 6, 9, 47, 60, 73, 79, 319, 327, 329, 337.

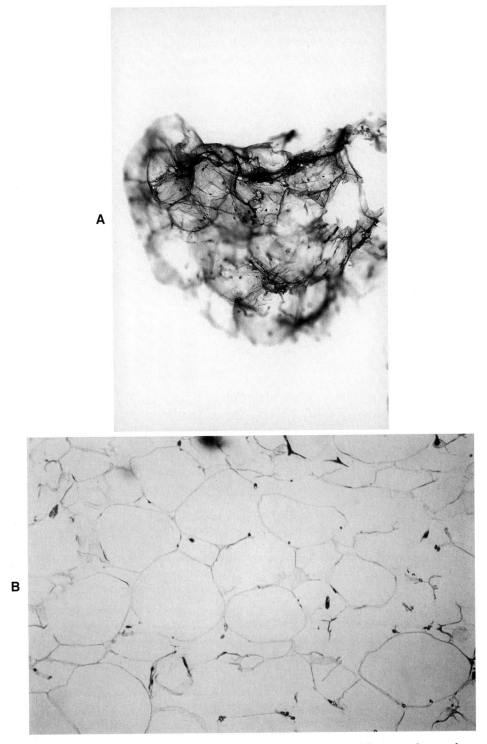

FIGURE 16-47. Lipoma. **A,** Needle aspirate reveals lipocytes. **B,** Proliferation of normal appearing lipocytes.

accounted for 50% of the hospital population. Males are predisposed.[*] The tumors are usually solitary, raised, firm, fairly well-demarcated, and 0.5 to 20 cm in diameter. The overlying skin may be normal, alopecic, hyperpigmented, or ulcerated. Occasional lesions area fluctuant and may sporadically discharge a caseous material. Lesions most commonly affect the head (lip, nostril, jaw, periorbital area) (Fig. 16-48), neck, trunk, and limbs (Figs. 16-49 and 16-50).[†] Limb lesions are often hard, immovable, and in proximity to synovial joints. Rarely, a horse may have two widely separated lesions or a cluster of three lesions.[319,327] Solitary mast cell tumors have also been reported to affect the nasal cavity,[325,327,332] trachea,[339] conjunctiva,[327] sclera,[324,338] nictitans,[325] and globe.[326] Cutaneous tumors usually show slow, progressive growth or become static, even over a course of 2 years.[327] Rarely, a lesion may show sudden rapid growth.[325,327,333] Lesions are typically nonpainful and nonpruritic.

Rarely, widespread multiple mast cell tumors occur in foals.[73,320,330] Lesions are raised, annular, well-circumscribed, and a few millimeters to 3 cm in diameter. Larger lesions develop soft centers and ulcerate. Individual lesions may last only 30 days and may spontaneously resolve, only to be replaced by new ones. Affected foals are otherwise healthy. This condition has been likened to *urticaria pigmentosa* in humans.[5]

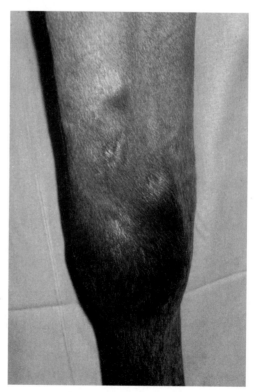

FIGURE 16-48. Mast cell tumor. Two nodules on medial carpal area. (*Courtesy Dr. W. McMullen.*)

---

[*]References 73, 79, 319, 327, 336, 337.
[†]References 6, 44, 319, 321, 327, 328, 333, 335, 340.

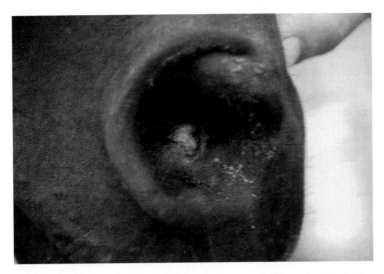

FIGURE 16-49. Mast cell tumor. Ulcerated nodule in right nostril. *(Courtesy Dr. A. Stannard.)*

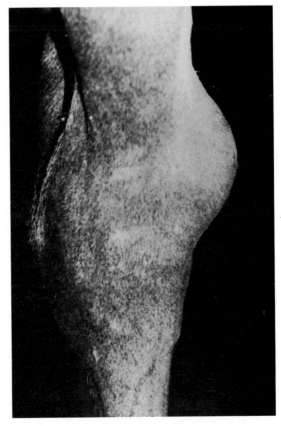

FIGURE 16-50. Mast cell tumor. Firm, poorly demarcated nodule that was adherent to underlying tissue.

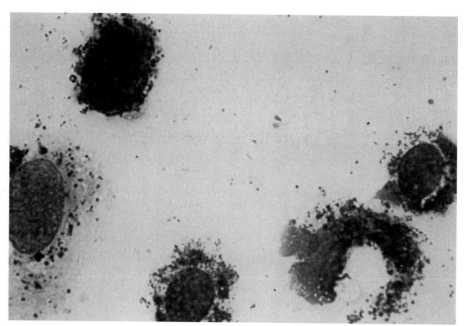

FIGURE 16-51. Mast cell tumor. Needle aspirate reveals mast cells.

Diagnosis

This is one neoplasm in which stained aspirates are useful in establishing an immediate tentative diagnosis (Fig. 16-51). However, this procedure should not replace a complete histologic examination.

Histopathologically, mast cell tumors are characterized by single to multifocal coalescing nodules and sheets of well-differentiated mast cells (Figs. 16-52 and 16-53).[319,327] Mitotic figures are few in number. The subcutis is usually involved, and even the underlying superficial musculature can be infiltrated.[319,327] Most lesions show numerous eosinophils to be scattered diffusely and/or present in aggregates. Accumulations of eosinophils are usually associated with well-circumscribed areas of necrosis (eosinophils and collagen). Older lesions contain variable degrees of fibrosis and palisading granuloma formation (Figs. 16-54 and 16-55). Dystrophic mineralization is frequently seen in areas of collagen degeneration and necrosis. Some old lesions predominantly consist of fibrosis and dystrophic mineralization, with only small packets of mast cells remaining (Fig. 16-56). Such lesions are often misdiagnosed as calcinosis circumscripta.[73]

Radiographic examination reveals a well-demarcated, soft tissue swelling with granular mineralization.[336] There is usually minimal or no periosteal reaction. If heavily mineralized, mast cell tumors can be mistaken for calcinosis circumscripta or eosinophilic granuloma radiographically.

Clinical Management

Complete surgical excision is curative. Even incomplete surgical excision or biopsy have been followed by spontaneous remission.[44,73,327,336,337] Where surgical excision is not an option, sublesional injections of glucocorticoid (5 to 10 mg of triamcinolone acetonide or 10 to 20 mg of methylprednisolone acetate), cryosurgery, or radiotherapy may be effective.[6,73,337] Rarely, a lesion will spontaneously resolve.[9] Anecdotal reports indicate that cimetidine (5 mg/kg q24h, orally, for 3 to 6 weeks) and intralesional injections of distilled water or cisplatin may be useful.[9]

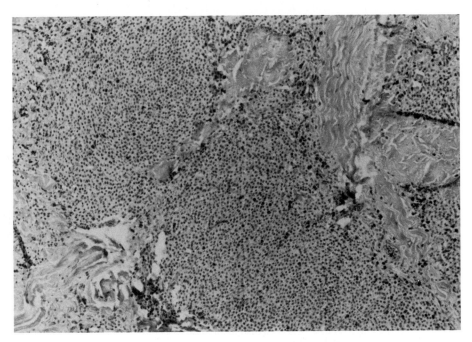

FIGURE 16-52. Mast cell tumor. Multinodular proliferation of mast cells.

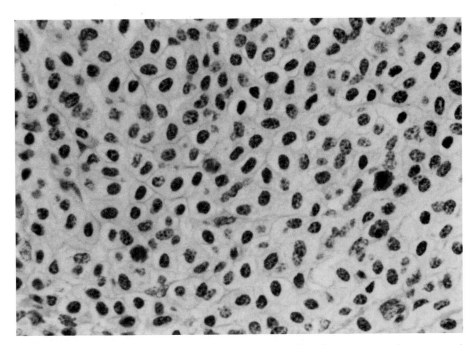

FIGURE 16-53. Mast cell tumor. Well-differentiated mast cells, whose intracytoplasmic granules stain poorly or not at all with H & E.

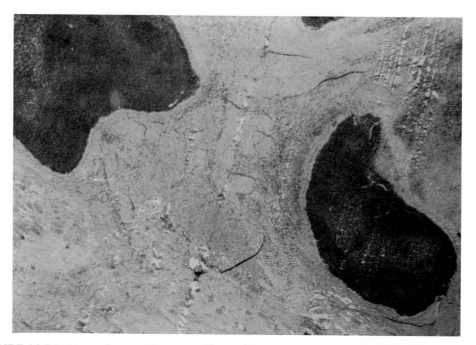

FIGURE 16-54. Mast cell tumor. Two areas of eosinophilic necrosis surrounded by eosinophilic inflammation and fibrosis.

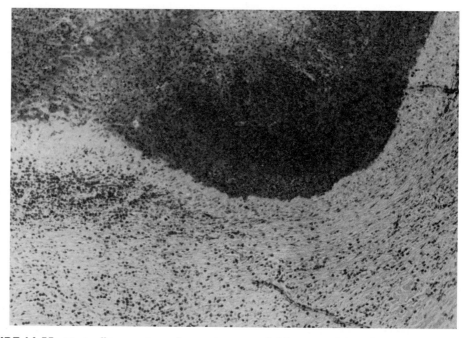

FIGURE 16-55. Mast cell tumor. Area of necrosis surrounded by eosinophils and histiocytes.

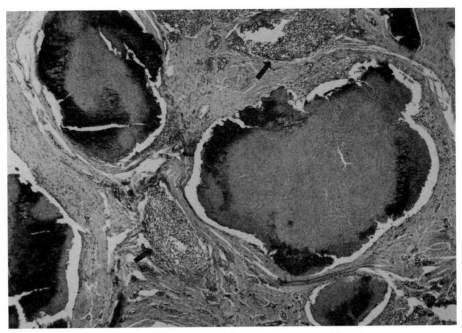

FIGURE 16-56. Mast cell tumor. Multifocal areas of dystrophic mineralization and surrounding fibrosis. Unless the small residual nodules of mast cells are noted (*arrow*), this lesion could be misdiagnosed as calcinosis circumscripta.

Equine cutaneous mast cell tumors are benign and widespread metastasis has not been reported. Four purportedly "malignant" mast cell tumors have been reported.[325,331,333] In one horse, the diagnosis of malignancy was based on the histopathologic finding of numerous mitoses. However, the horse was cured following surgical excision. The other three horses had an enlarged regional lymph node, which was histopathologically identical to the skin tumor. These horses were euthanized, and no other organ systems were involved.

● LYMPHOHISTIOCYTIC NEOPLASMS

Tumors of Lymphocytic Origin

LYMPHOMA

Cause and Pathogenesis

Cutaneous lymphoma (lymphosarcoma, malignant lymphoma, reticulum cell sarcoma) is a rare malignant neoplasm of horses arising from lymphocytes.[*] It accounts for 0.6% to 3% of the equine skin neoplasms in various surveys.[†] From 4% to 35% of the horses with lymphoma in various studies have cutaneous lesions.[15,347,356,358,362] The cause of these neoplasms is unknown.

The histiolymphocytic form of equine cutaneous lymphoma has been the subject of some interesting studies. No retroviral virions were found by electron microscopy in tumor tissue or in cells cocultivated with tissue culture cell lines.[345,367] No reverse transcriptase activity was demonstrated in tumor cell suspensions. Coryneform bacteria were found extracellularly and intracellularly within histiocytes and lymphocytes of impression smears and biopsy specimens.[345,367]

---

*References 15, 29, 30, 34, 41, 42, 65, 66, 79, 85.
†References 29, 30, 43, 66, 74, 79.

The bacteria were gram-positive and variably acid-fast. They replicated after 14 days in cell culture medium, but did not grow in solid media under aerobic or anaerobic environments. This bacterium produced no clinical effects when given subcutaneously to three normal horses (follow-up period of 8 months).[331] The coryneform bacteria in these cases were hypothesized to be an equine saprophytic bacterium that grows in an immunosuppressed host.[345]

Histologically, lymphoma can be divided into nonepitheliotropic and epitheliotropic forms.[5,14] The epitheliotropic lymphomas are typically of T lymphocyte origin. Mycosis fungoides and its associated leukemia, the Sézary syndrome, are two subsets of cutaneous T cell lymphoma. Nonepitheliotropic cutaneous lymphomas involve the dermis and subcutis and are a heterogenous group with respect to immunophenotype.

Clinical Findings

• *Nonepitheliotropic lymphoma.* Nonepitheliotropic cutaneous lymphoma usually occurs in adult to aged animals (but with a range of 2 months to 23 years old), with no sex or breed predilections.* Most horses have concurrent systemic illness, including depression, poor appetite, weight loss, anemia, leukemia, and peripheral lymphadenopathy. However, some horses, especially those with the histiolymphocytic phenotype, can have multiple skin lesions for months to years before systemic involvement occurs.† The lesions in the histiolymphocytic type of lymphoma are typically subcutaneous and may be widespread or regionally clustered (e.g., shoulder, lateral thigh). Horses with lymphoma may be immunosuppressed[346] and may develop immune-mediated hemolytic anemia or thrombocytopenia or both of these.[346,364]

Cutaneous lesions are typically multiple and widespread,‡ although lesions may be solitary or multiple and localized (especially eyelids) (Fig. 16-57).[346,357,359] These lesions are typically firm, well-circumscribed papules and nodules, 0.5 to 10 cm in diameter, and dermoepidermal to subcutaneous in location. The head, neck (Fig. 16-58), trunk (Fig. 16-59), and proximal extremities are typically involved. Eyelid lesions may be unilateral or bilateral, and involve the upper lid, lower lid, or both of these.[363] Less commonly, urticarial-like lesions, large plaques, or diffuse areas of thickened, hard skin are present. Generalized paraneoplastic pruritus and alopecia has been reported in a horse with diffuse lymphoma.[346a]

• *Epitheliotropic lymphoma.* Rarely, horses may have a multifocal to generalized exfoliative dermatitis (alopecia, marked scaling and crusting) (Figs. 16-60 and 16-61) with or without pruritus and focal areas of nodules (2 to 8 cm) or ulceration (especially over pressure points) (Fig. 16-62).[346,352,361,362,372] These horses have an epitheliotropic lymphoma (so-called "mycosis fungoides").

Sézary's syndrome is an epitheliotropic T cell lymphoma characterized by erythroderma, pruritus, peripheral lymphadenopathy, and the presence of Sézary, or Lutzner, cells (8 to 20 µm) lymphocytes that have marked hyperconvoluted or "cerebriform" nuclei) in the cutaneous infiltrate and in the peripheral blood.[5,14] A horse with multiple 0.5- to 2-cm subcutaneous lymphomas on the neck and thorax and lymphocytic leukemia (43.4×10^9 lymphocytes/L) had numerous Sézary-like cells in the peripheral blood.[360] However, the lymphoma was shown to be B cell in origin, thus failing to fulfill all the criteria for Sézary's syndrome.

Diagnosis

This is one neoplasm in which stained aspirates are useful in establishing an immediate tentative diagnosis (Fig. 16-63). However, this procedure should not replace a complete histologic examin-

---

*References 15, 49, 356, 358, 362, 363, 365, 370.
†References 342, 353, 356, 359, 365, 367.
‡References 15, 341, 344, 348, 349, 351-356, 358, 359, 365, 367-371.

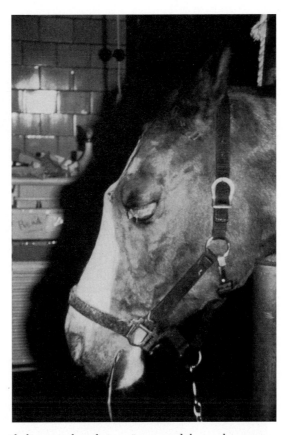

FIGURE 16-57. Nonepitheliotropic lymphoma. Large nodule involving upper eyelid. *(Courtesy Dr. S. Fubini.)*

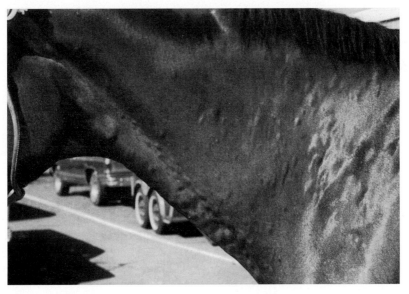

FIGURE 16-58. Nonepitheliotropic lymphoma. Multiple dermal and subcutaneous papules, plaques, and nodules over the neck and shoulder.

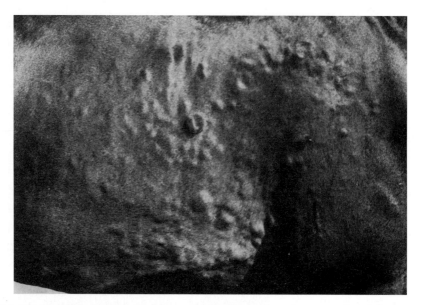

FIGURE 16-59. Nonepitheliotropic lymphoma. Multiple papules, plaques, and nodules over the trunk. *(Courtesy Dr. W. Rebhun.)*

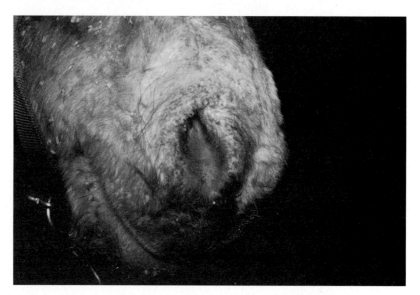

FIGURE 16-60. Epitheliotropic lymphoma. Marked scaling and crusting on muzzle.

ation. Histopathologically, equine cutaneous lymphoma is usually characterized by nodular-to-diffuse infiltration of the deep dermis and subcutis, sometimes with finger-like projections into the underlying skeletal muscle (Figs. 16-64 and 16-65).[359,367] Phenotypic types include histio-lymphocytic, lymphoblastic, plasmacytic, and lymphoma with follicular development.[359] Rarely the lymphomatous infiltrate will be epitheliotropic, involving epidermis, hair follicles, and epitrichial sweat glands (Figs. 16-66 and 16-67).[74,351,352,361,372] Pautrier microabscesses are seen. Electron microscopic examination of two cases of epitheliotropic lymphoma revealed neoplastic lymphoid cells with convoluted ("cerebriform") nuclei.[361,372]

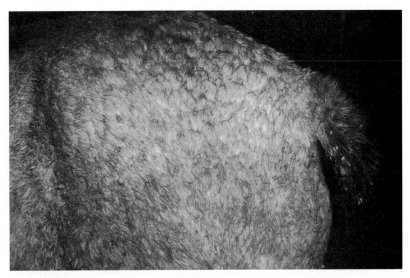

FIGURE 16-61. Epitheliotropic lymphoma. Severe crusting, scaling, and alopecia over the rump and tail.

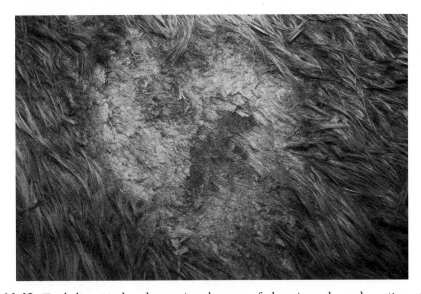

FIGURE 16-62. Epitheliotropic lymphoma. Annular area of alopecia, scale, and crusting with central ulceration.

Studies on the histiolymphocytic form have seemingly been confusing and contradictory. Some investigators report that the cellular proliferation consists of pleomorphic lymphocytes and pleomorphic histiocytes that are often binucleated or multinucleated histiocytic giant cells (Fig. 16-68).[345,359,367] Mitotic figures are usually sparse. Electron microscopic studies reveal the presence of unusual mitochondrial crystalline inclusions.[345] Lectin histochemical studies suggest that the histiocytic cells are reactive rather than neoplastic, and that the lymphocytic cells are the primary neoplastic component.

However, recent studies indicated that there were typically two cell populations: (1) small, mature T lymphocytes (CD3+, CD5+) that were non-neoplastic (PNCA-, Ki-67-) and were the

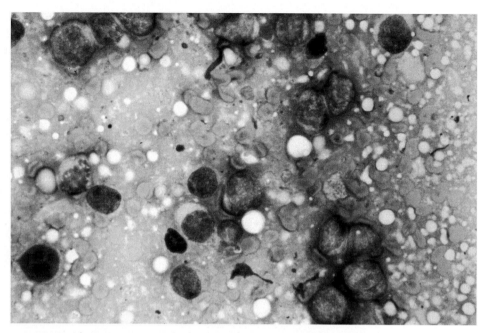

FIGURE 16-63. Lymphoma. Needle aspirate reveals malignant lymphocytes.

predominant cell type, and (2) large, pleomorphic, mitotic B lymphocytes (BLA.36+) that were the neoplastic cell type (PNCA+, Ki-67K+).[349,353] A third cell population was occasionally present in small numbers: epithelioid macrophages and multinucleated histiocytic giant cells. Amyloid was occasionally present. Regional lymph nodes and underlying skeletal muscle could be involved. The investigators proposed the name "T cell–rich, large B cell lymphoma" for these lesions. Whether these two different interpretations represent two different entities or not awaits clarification.

In general, equine noncutaneous lymphomas are either B cell or T cell in origin.[343,353] Equine cutaneous lymphomas, be they nonepitheliotropic or epitheliotropic, are usually of T cell origin.*

Clinical Management

Many horses with lymphoma are systemically ill and die or are euthanized within weeks to months.[†] One horse was treated with methotrexate (100 mg intravenously q24h) and dexamethasone (40 mg intravenously q24h) and experienced significant reduction in size of its skin tumors and lymph nodes, but died in 2 weeks.[371] Palliative temporary reduction in skin tumor size can be achieved with glucocorticoids.[15,44,366]

Specific antineoplastic drugs have not been used extensively, nor have they been scientifically evaluated and reported for equine lymphoma. One recommended protocol (multiple agent chemotherapy) for the treatment of equine lymphoma is the combination of cytosine arabinoside (200 to 300 mg/m^2 subcutaneously or intramuscularly once every 1 to 2 weeks), chlorambucil (20 mg/m^2 PO q2wk, alternated with the cytosine arabinoside), and prednisone (1 to 2 mg/kg PO q48h).[44,366] Other drugs that have been used singly or in combination to treat equine lymphoma include L-asparaginase (10,000 to 40,000 IU/m^2 IM q2-3wk), cyclophosphamide (200 to 300 mg/m^2 IV q2-3wk), and cytosine arabinoside-prednisone or cyclophosphamide-prednisone.[44]

---

*References 348, 349, 352, 353, 355, 366.
†References 15, 356, 358, 359, 362, 370.

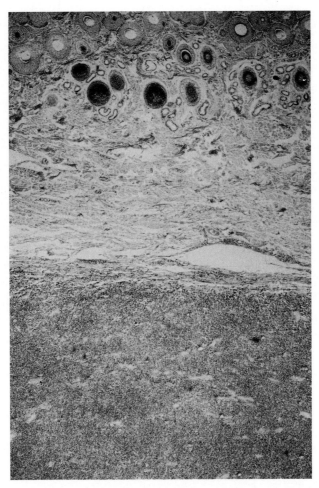

FIGURE 16-64. Nonepitheliotropic lymphoma. Diffuse infiltration of subcutis with malignant lymphocytes.

These treatment protocols are expensive, associated with possible complications, and of unproven benefit.

Horses with the histiolymphocytic form often remain healthy for years before they become ill or are lost to follow-up.* Some horses have waxing and waning lesions or may spontaneously resolve and recur.[15,342,355] It is hard to believe that horses that survive 4[359] and 11 years[355] have true lymphoma. These horses may have a pseudolymphoma.[5,14]

Horses with cutaneous lymphoma (pseudolymphoma?) unaccompanied by systemic illness have rarely received treatment. One horse was treated with megestrol acetate (0.2 mg/kg orally for 8 days) and a sublesional injection of betamethasone (20 mg).[355] The cutaneous lesions markedly decreased in size, but the horse subsequently died and no necropsy was performed. Another horse was given cyclophosphamide (300 mg/m[2] intravenously on day 1 and 36) and an autogenous tumor cell vaccine (0.5 ml intramuscularly at four sites on day 4, 21, and 39).[350] There was a marked reduction in the size of the skin lesions, and the horse remained stable for a subsequent 19 months.

*References 9, 349, 355, 356, 359, 365, 367.

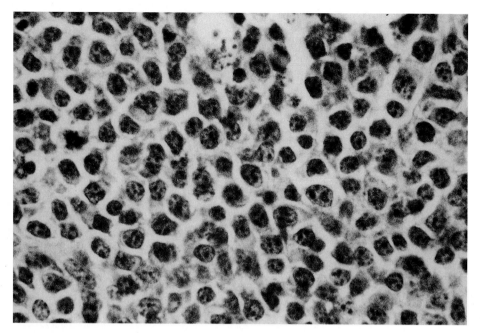

FIGURE 16-65. Nonepitheliotropic lymphoma. Proliferation of malignant lymphocytes.

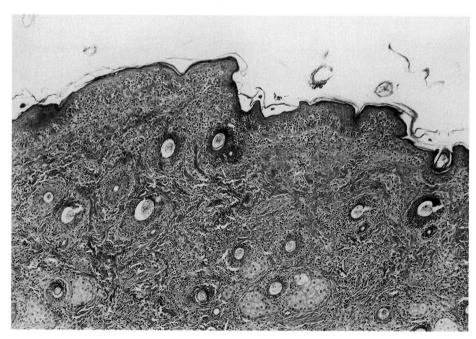

FIGURE 16-66. Epitheliotropic lymphoma. Neoplastic lymphocytes are infiltrating epidermis and outer root sheath of hair follicles.

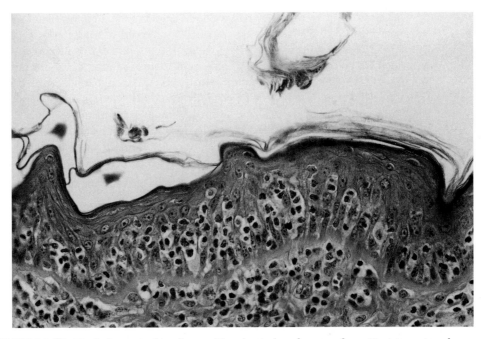

FIGURE 16-67. Epitheliotropic lymphoma. Neoplastic lymphocytes form Pautrier microabscesses in epidermis.

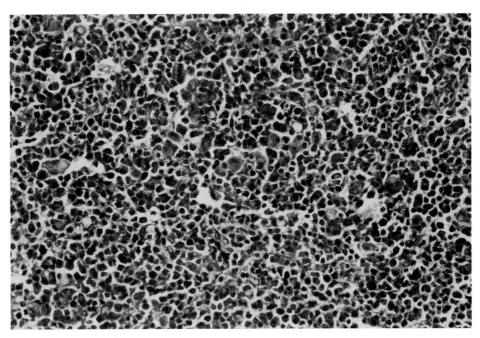

FIGURE 16-68. Histiolymphocytic lymphoma. Pleomorphic lymphocytic and histiocytic cells in the dermis. This horse spontaneously resolved after 2 years.

One horse with a T cell–rich, large B cell lymphoma had multiple nodules for years but was otherwise healthy.[349] The horse had previously received a 10-day course of treatment with a synthetic progestin (attrenogest 0.044 mg/kg orally) based on anecdotal reports that some cutaneous lymphomas in horses had undergone remission after progesterone therapy or during pregnancy.[9] The skin lesions temporarily regressed. After a 1-year history of disease, the horse had a granulosa-theca cell ovarian tumor surgically removed, whereupon the lesions regressed within 1 month. During the following 11 months, the lesions recurred and regressed twice, presumably related to fluctuations in hormone concentrations with the estrous cycle. Progesterone receptors were demonstrated on the lymphoma cells. Anecdotal reports indicate that "a significant number of cases" of cutaneous histiolymphocytic lymphoma/T cell–rich, large B cell lymphomas are associated with ovarian granulosa cell tumors in mares and that removal of the ovarian tumor is curative.[9] Again, these observations cause one to wonder whether the "histiolymphocytic lymphomas" and "T cell–rich, large B cell lymphomas" are truly malignancies, or fascinating pseudolymphomas.

PLASMACYTOMA
Cause and Pathogenesis

Cutaneous plasmacytomas (cutaneous extramedullary plasmacytomas) are thought to be extremely rare in horses. However, some investigators have suggested that all reports of so-called "cutaneous amyloidosis" in horses were actually plasmacytomas wherein the amyloid deposits (AL-type) overshadowed the neoplastic tissue.[375] The cause of cutaneous plasmacytomas is unknown. They may occur in association with chronic B lymphocyte stimulation, but they rarely occur in association with multiple myeloma.[14]

Clinical Findings

A 17-year-old horse developed numerous cutaneous and subcutaneous nodules over the entire body.[373] Lymph nodes, joint capsules, muscles, the right eye, and the nasal mucosa were also involved. A similar case was reported by other investigators.[374]

Diagnosis

Histologically, plasmacytomas are characterized by sheets, packets, and cords of variably differentiated plasma cells infiltrating the dermis and subcutis. Immunohistochemically, amyloid is present as light-chain amyloid of the AL-type.

Clinical Management

Successful treatment has not been reported.

PSEUDOLYMPHOMA
Cause and Pathogenesis

Pseudolymphomas have been defined as disorders in which a histologic picture suggesting lymphoma stands in sharp contrast to benign biologic behavior.[5,14] In humans, dogs, and cats, pseudolymphomas have been associated with reactions to sunlight, drugs, arthropods, contactants, and idiopathy.

Clinical Findings

Pseudolymphomas have occasionally been recognized in horses.[73] Lesions are seen in late summer and fall, are usually solitary, and occur most frequently over the head and trunk (Fig. 16-69). The nodules are firm, well-circumscribed, and asymptomatic, and the overlying skin is usually normal. The authors wonder whether the reported "histiolymphocytic" and "T–cell rich, large B cell" lymphomas in horses are actually pseudolymphomas (see Lymphoma).

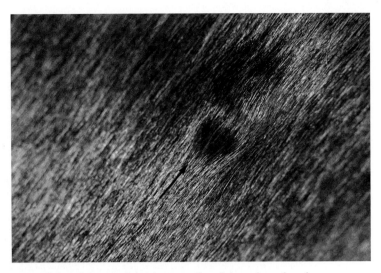

FIGURE 16-69. Pseudolymphoma (tick bite). Dermal nodule on lateral neck.

Diagnosis

Histologic examination reveals a nodular-to-diffuse dermal and, occasionally, subcutaneous infiltrate consisting of lymphocytes, histiocytes, plasma cells, and eosinophils (Figs. 16-70 and 16-71).

Clinical Management

Clinical management may include surgical excision or observation without treatment.

Tumors of Histiocytic Origin

MALIGNANT FIBROUS HISTIOCYTOMA

Cause and Pathogenesis

Malignant fibrous histiocytomas (extraskeletal giant cell tumors, giant cell tumors of soft tissues, or dermatofibrosarcomas) are rare malignant neoplasms.[9,376-379] They accounted for only 0.2% of the cutaneous neoplasms in one survey.[74] They are believed to arise from undifferentiated mesenchymal cells. The cause of these neoplasms is unknown.

Clinical Findings

No breed or sex predilections are evident. Age of affected horses has ranged from 3 to 12 years. Although these neoplasms can occur anywhere, the majority affect the neck, thigh, and stifle (Fig. 16-72).[378,379] Lesions are solitary, raised, firm, poorly circumscribed, and 1 cm to several centimeters in diameter.

Diagnosis

Histopathologically, malignant fibrous histiocytomas are characterized by an infiltrative mass composed of varying mixtures of pleomorphic histiocytes, fibroblasts, and multinucleated tumor giant cells (Fig. 16-73). Mitotic figures and a storiform ("cartwheel") arrangement of fibroblasts and histiocytes are common features. Malignant fibrous histiocytomas are positive for vimentin, lysozyme, and α_1-antichymotrypsin.

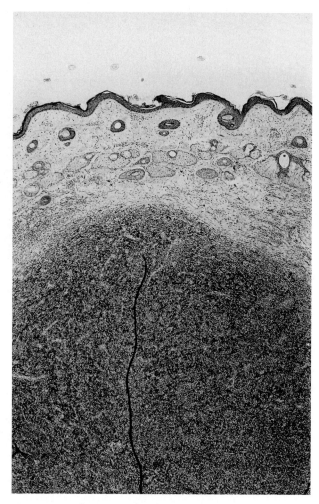

FIGURE 16-70. Pseudolymphoma (tick bite). Deep dermal and subcutaneous nodular accumulation of predominantly lymphocytes, histiocytes, and eosinophils.

Clinical Management

The treatment of choice is radical surgical excision. Recurrence after surgical excision is common (50% of cases in one study),[379] but metastasis has not been reported.

• MELANOCYTIC NEOPLASMS

The nomenclature for melanocytic tumors is complex and confusing, with terms such as *melanoma* (benign or malignant), *melanosarcoma, melanocytoma, melanosis, melanomatosis, melanocytic nevus, nevocellular nevus, acquired nevus,* and *congenital nevus* having uncertain meaning in different contexts.* The so-called nevus cell, which makes up the pigmented nevi of humans, is now known to be a melanocyte with slight histopathologic and biochemical alterations. On this basis, it has been suggested that all noncongenital, benign proliferations of melanocytes be

---

*References 387, 391, 395, 404, 408, 409, 413, 414, 426, 427.

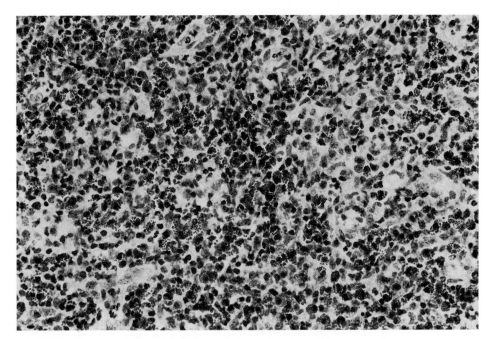

FIGURE 16-71. Pseudolymphoma (tick bite). Lymphocytes, histiocytes, and eosinophils.

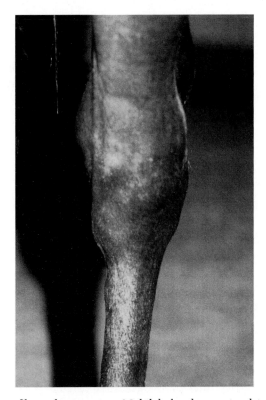

FIGURE 16-72. Malignant fibrous histiocytoma. Multilobulated tumor involving hock.

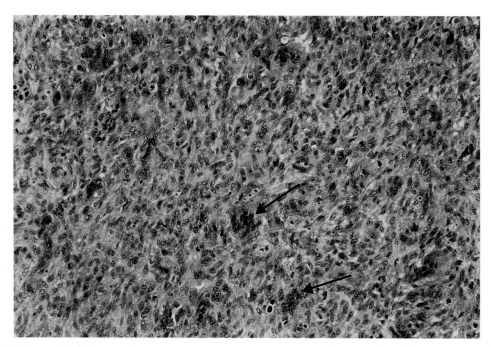

FIGURE 16-73. Malignant fibrous histiocytoma. Proliferation of pleomorphic histiocytes, fibroblasts, and multinucleated tumor giant cells *(arrows)*.

designated *melanocytoma*.[14] The term *melanoma* is used in this text as synonymous with a malignant proliferation of melanocytes.

Melanocytic neoplasms are reported to account for 3.8% to 18.7% of all equine neoplasms.[30,44,74,79] These figures are based on biopsy reports and likely significantly underestimate the true incidence, since most clinicians do not biopsy classical melanocytic neoplasms.

Melanocytoma

CAUSE AND PATHOGENESIS

Melanocytomas (benign melanomas, melanocytic nevi) are uncommon benign skin neoplasms of the horse arising from melanocytes.[388,428] They accounted for 4.8% of the cutaneous neoplasms in one survey.[74] The cause of these lesions is unknown.

CLINICAL FINDINGS

Melanocytomas occur most frequently in young horses (prior to 2 years of age) with no apparent breed, sex, or coat color predilections.[388,408,420a,428] Occasionally, melanocytomas may be congenital,[385,388] and they have been previously reported as "malignant melanomas," even though surgical excision was curative.[386] Solitary melanocytomas are occasionally seen in older horses.[428] The lesions in young horses are usually solitary and most commonly occur on the legs or trunk. They rarely occur in the perineal, genital, or tail (Fig. 16-74) areas. Lesions are usually firm, well-circumscribed, and 1 to 5.5 cm in diameter. The overlying skin may be normal, alopecic, hyperpigmented, hyperkeratotic, or ulcerated. A giant congenital melanocytoma was present at birth in one horse.[385] The lesion was a large patch of thickened, nodular skin in the saddle region. The associated hair was darker in color.

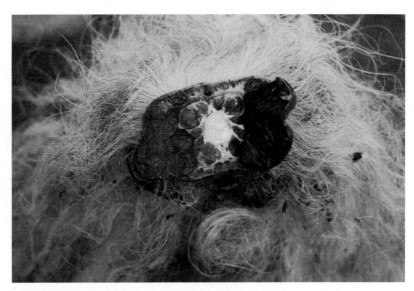

FIGURE 16-74. Solitary melanocytoma on tail of young horse.

DIAGNOSIS

Cytologic examination reveals variably shaped melanocytes. Histopathologically, melanocytomas are characterized by a variety of cell patterns ranging from sheets, to streams, or nests of melanocytes (Fig. 16-75).[388] Cell morphology ranges from epithelioid (Fig. 16-76), to spindle (Fig. 16-77), to a mixture of these (Fig. 16-78). Cellular pleomorphism and binucleate cells are often seen. Mitotic activity is generally low. Melanin pigmentation varies from mild to heavy, and melanophages are admixed with the tumor cells or in the adjacent tissue. Marked involvement of the epidermis and hair follicle epithelium with nests of neoplastic melanocytes may be seen (Fig. 16-79). Melanocytomas are positive for vimentin and S-100.

CLINICAL MANAGEMENT

Complete surgical excision is curative.[386,388,420a]

Melanoma

CAUSE AND PATHOGENESIS

Melanomas (malignant melanomas, melanosarcomas, melanomatosis) are common malignant skin neoplasms of the horse arising from melanocytes.° They accounted for 13.9% of the cutaneous neoplasms in one survey.[74] The true prevalence of melanomas is probably greatly underestimated in such biopsy-based surveys, since clinicians rarely biopsy classical equine melanomas. The cause of melanomas is unknown. They are thought to arise in older gray horses as a consequence of perturbed melanin metabolism leading to either formation of new melanoblasts or increased activity of resident melanoblasts, resulting in focal areas of overproduction of melanin.[44] In time, hyperplastic melanoblasts undergo malignant transformation. In humans, there is a correlation between exposure to ultraviolet light and the development of melanoma.[5] However, given the sun-protected areas of occurrence of the vast majority of equine melanomas (underside of tail, perianal

---

°References 9, 30, 44, 380, 381, 389, 390, 396, 398, 402, 407, 408, 410, 420-421, 423a, 428, 429.

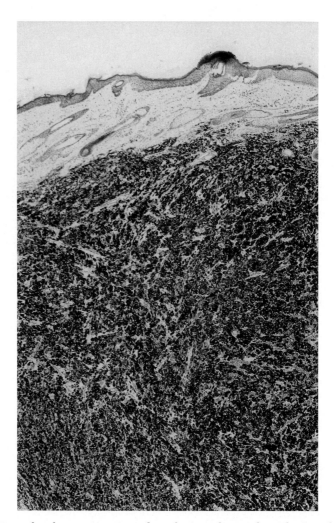

FIGURE 16-75. Dermal melanocytoma. Deep dermal accumulation of neoplastic melanocytes.

area), this is unlikely to be an important factor in the horse.[387b] Chronic exposure to insecticides may also be a risk factor in humans.[384]

The results of large clinicopathologic studies on equine cutaneous melanoma have been very contradictory. One opinion—based on histopathologic appearance and proliferation indices (Ki-67) in Spanish purebred horses in Spain—is that the cutaneous lesions (and the "metastases"!)—consist of benign melanocytes and melanophages.[423a] These authors suggest that this condition is a non-neoplastic pigmentary disorder, perhaps due to a failure of melanin degradation as the animals' hairs become progressively less pigmented with increasing age. In another extensive histopathologic study of cutaneous melanomas in Camarque-type gray horses in France, the melanocytes were described as being remarkably atypical and malignant.[387a] These two interpretations are clearly diametrically opposed. The studies were, however, conducted on two different breeds.

In a recent study,[420a] no differences were found in growth fraction (Ki67), S-phase index (PCNA), or DNA configuration between metastatic melanomas and surgically excised and cured melanocytomas. Thus, in contrast to dogs, cats, and humans, proliferation markers and DNA

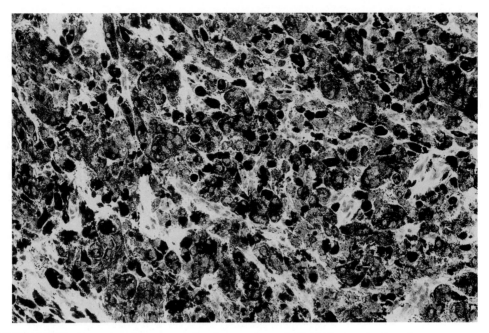

FIGURE 16-76. Dermal melanocytoma. Predominantly epithelioid-like neoplastic melanocytes.

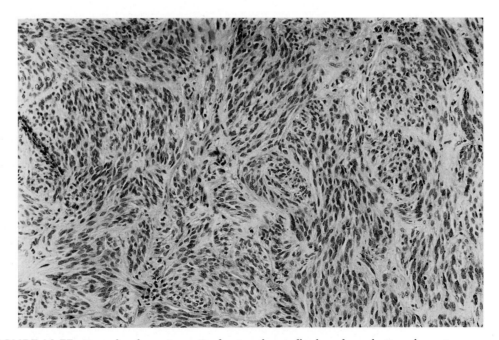

FIGURE 16-77. Dermal melanocytoma. Predominantly spindle-shaped neoplastic melanocytes.

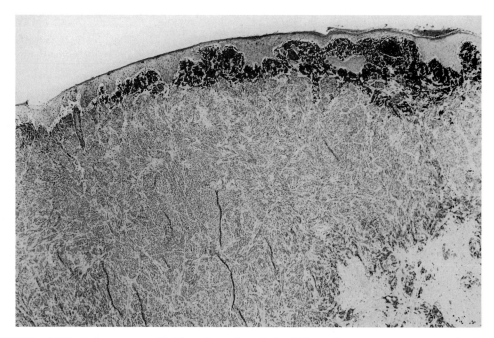

FIGURE 16-78. Melanocytoma. Highly melanized epithelioid-like melanocytes are present at the dermo-epidermal junction, while sparsely-to-nonmelanized spindle-shaped melanocytes comprise the deeper areas of the tumor.

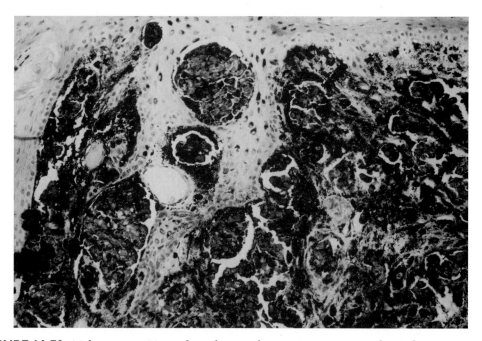

FIGURE 16-79. Melanocytoma. Nests of neoplastic melanocytes are present in the epidermis.

changes (index and ploidy) seem to be of no use for evaluating the behavior of melanocytic neoplasms in horses.

CLINICAL FINDINGS

Classical multiple melanomas (melanomatosis) typically occur in horses over 6 years of age, with no sex predilection.* Congenital melanomas are very rare.[388,399] These multiple melanomas occur most commonly, but not exclusively, in gray or white horses, especially Arabians, Percherons, Lippizaners, and specifically bred subsets of these genetic stocks.[†] Typically, these horses are born with a dark hair coat that fades with age. It has been estimated that about 80% of gray horses over 15 years of age have multiple melanomas.[73,79,409,387a,423a] The lesions occur most commonly on the undersurface of the tail and the perianal region (Fig. 16-80).[387a] Less commonly, tumors may be seen on the lips, at the base of the ear (parotid region), periorbitally (Fig. 16-81), on the distal legs, and virtually anywhere.[‡] The tumors are usually firm, nodular to plaque-like, and may or may not be alopecic, hyperpigmented, or ulcerated. Some lesions discharge a thick, black, tarry substance. Coalescing nodules may give the skin a cobblestone appearance. Some tumors are pedunculated or verrucous in appearance. In one study,[387b] the number and size of lesions was significantly related to the age of the horses. The appearance of multiple melanomas may be heralded by the appearance of vitiligo.[407,426]

Less commonly, melanomas may occur as solitary lesions.[428] The lesions are firm, 0.5 to 12 cm in diameter, and may occur in the classical perineal/genital/ventral tail area or in various "atypical" areas: leg, tip of tail, foot, neck, and ear.[§]

Three growth patterns are described for equine cutaneous melanomas: (1) slow growth for years without metastasis, (2) slow growth for years with sudden rapid growth and metastasis, and (3) rapid growth and malignancy from the onset.[78] Approximately two-thirds of the horses have metastatic disease at necropsy, often without clinical signs referable to the metastases.[¶] However, some horses do develop clinical signs (especially lameness) referable to their primary tumor[401,406] or clinical signs (especially neurologic) associated with their metastases.[Π]

DIAGNOSIS

Cytologic examination reveals pleomorphic and atypical melanocytes. Histopathologically, melanomas are characterized by atypical melanocytes in sheets, packets (nests or theques), and cords.[78,389,428,429] The melanocytes may be predominantly epithelioid, spindle, or a combination of these. The tendency for these lesions to begin in close association with hair follicles[423a] or epitrichial sweat glands[387a] and to not involve the epidermis and dermoepidermal junction[387a,423a] is quite different from what is usually seen in humans, dogs, and cats.[5,14] Melanomas are positive for vimentin and IMB45 and variably positive for S-100 and neuron-specific enolase.

CLINICAL MANAGEMENT

Wide surgical excision may be curative for solitary melanomas, but is impractical or impossible for multiple melanomas. Cryosurgery may be useful in some cases.[291,394] Some authors have noted that rapid recurrence is very common following surgical excision or cryotherapy.[6,9,44] Incomplete elimination of melanomas by either surgical excision or cryosurgery may increase the risk of

---

*References 29, 34-37, 41, 59, 60, 79, 83, 387b, 390, 408.
†References 67, 73, 380, 395, 396, 398, 407, 415, 419, 421, 423, 423a, 428.
‡References 67, 131, 381, 387a, 397, 401, 405, 406, 408, 416-418, 421, 422, 423a, 424, 425, 428.
§References 401, 405, 406, 411, 421, 428.
¶References 29, 44, 73, 79, 396, 397, 403, 405, 406, 409, 409a, 411, 420, 423, 424, 428, 429.
ΠReferences 382, 397, 405, 409a, 415a, 420, 422, 425.

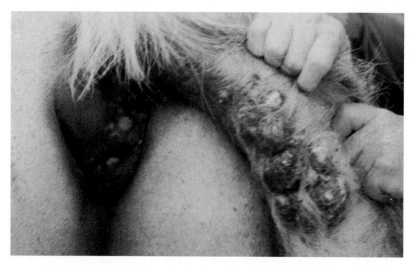

FIGURE 16-80. Melanoma. Multiple melanotic-to-amelanotic papules, nodules, and plaques on the ventral surface of the tail and perianal area. *(Courtesy Dr. J. King.)*

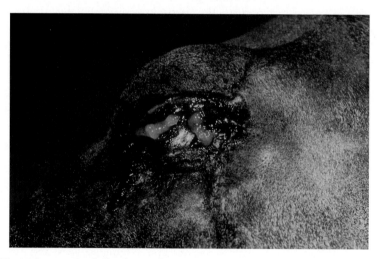

FIGURE 16-81. Melanoma (eyelid). Ulcerated periocular mass.

aggressive tumor regrowth.[44] Radiotherapy, traditional chemotherapy, and immunotherapy with BCG have not been beneficial.[6,44,394]

Cimetidine (2.5 mg/kg q8h or 5 mg/kg q12h orally for at least 3 months), an H_2-blocker antihistamine with immunomodulatory effects, was reported to be effective for treating equine multiple melanomas.[392,393] The drug was reported to cause complete remissions or, most commonly, stop the progression of the disease while reducing the size and number of tumors by about 50%. However, other investigators were *not* able to document the clinical efficacy of cimetidine.* Some investigators suggest that cimetidine is more apt to be useful in actively growing tumors,[9,44] but this was *not* substantiated in one study.[400]

---

*References 9, 44, 383, 400, 409a, 423a, 430.

Intratumoral chemotherapy with cisplatin in oily emulsion is often effective for small lesions (<3 cm diameter).[9,38a,44,80a,147,394]

Anecdotal reports indicate that a relatively crude whole-cell melanoma vaccine may be useful,[403] but others have not had success with such products.[38a,409a]

● MISCELLANEOUS CUTANEOUS NEOPLASMS

There are anecdotal, undocumented reports of other cutaneous neoplasms in the horse. These include hemangiopericytoma,[65] histiocytoma,[29] myxoma,[30,74] myxosarcoma,[45] and osteoma cutis.[65]

Carcinosarcoma

Cutaneous carcinosarcoma was reported in a 14-year-old Arabian mare.[158] A well-circumscribed, firm-to-cystic, 5-cm diameter mass was present in the right flank. Histopathologically, two discrete populations of neoplastic cells were present. One cell type was pleomorphic, elongated, and mesenchymal and was supported by variably dense bands of connective tissue stroma. The other cell type was pleomorphic, rounded, and epithelial and occurred in dense sheets and formed irregular glandular acini.

● PARANEOPLASTIC SYNDROMES

The symptoms produced by neoplasia can be due to the direct effect of the neoplasm on the body, or they can be caused indirectly by seemingly unrelated processes. These indirect systemic effects of neoplasia are known as *paraneoplastic syndromes*.[5,14] Presently recognized dermatologic examples of paraneoplastic syndromes include pemphigus (see Chapter 9), vasculitis (see Chapter 9), and pruritus (see Lymphoma). In addition, severe generalized pruritus has been seen by the authors and others[14a,85a] in association with visceral neoplasia (especially carcinomas and lymphomas). A cause-and-effect relationship has not been established in these cases.

● NON-NEOPLASTIC TUMORS

Cutaneous Cysts

A *cyst* is a non-neoplastic, simple sac-like structure with an epithelial lining. Classification of cysts depends on identification of the lining epithelium or the preexisting structure from which the cyst arose.

DERMOID CYSTS

Cause and Pathogenesis

Dermoid cysts are uncommon in the horse.* They are developmental anomalies and are often congenital and, possibly, hereditary.

Clinical Findings

Dermoid cysts are usually recognized at birth or within the first year of life. No sex predilection exists. One author suggested that thoroughbreds were predisposed,[59,60] but another report indicated no breed predilection.[443] The majority of dermoid cysts occur on the dorsal midline in the thoracic and lumbar areas (Fig. 16-82). Lesions may be solitary or multiple (up to 17), firm to fluctuant, well-circumscribed, rounded, and 2 mm to several centimeters in diameter. The overlying skin is usually normal.

---

*References 9, 47, 59, 60, 73, 431, 443.

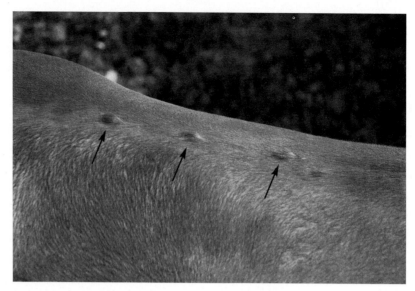

FIGURE 16-82. Dermoid cysts. Three firm, well-circumscribed dermal nodules on dorsal midline of the back (*arrows*).

Diagnosis

On cut section, dermoid cysts contain a seromucoid fluid, yellowish to grayish greasy/caseous/cheesy material and coiled hairs. Needle aspiration typically reveals numerous squames, occasionally cholesterol crystals, and an oily background. Histopathologically, the cyst wall undergoes epidermal differentiation and contains well-developed small hair follicles, sebaceous glands, and occasionally epitrichial sweat glands (Fig. 16-83). The cyst cavity is filled with keratin and hair shafts.

Clinical Management

Clinical management of dermoid cysts may include surgical excision or observation without treatment.

FOLLICULAR CYSTS

Cause and Pathogenesis

Follicular cysts are uncommon in the horse.[443] They are classified according to the differentiation of their epithelial lining into infundibular, isthmus-catagen (trichilemmal), matrical, and hybrid forms.[14] Infundibular cysts have been previously called "epidermoid" or "epidermal inclusion" cysts. The cause of these cysts is unknown.

Clinical Findings

Follicular cysts occur in horses 7 to 19 years of age, with no apparent breed or sex predilections.[436,443] Most lesions occur on the head or distal limbs (Fig. 16-84). Lesions are solitary, well-circumscribed, round, firm to fluctuant, and 7 mm to 3 cm in diameter. The overlying skin is usually normal.

Diagnosis

On cut section, follicular cysts contain a yellow to gray mucus-like substance. Needle aspiration typically reveals numerous squames, occasionally cholesterol crystals, and an oily background. Histopathologically, the cyst wall undergoes epidermal differentiation; the cyst cavity contains

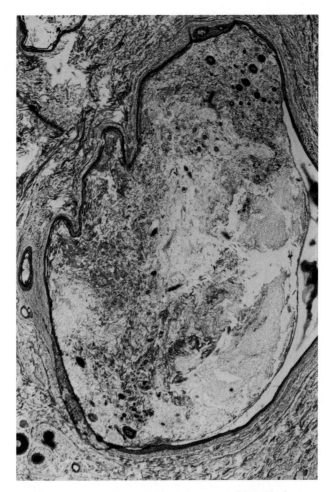

FIGURE 16-83. Dermoid cyst. Cyst cavity is filled with keratin and hair shafts.

lamellar, often concentrically arranged keratin (Figs. 16-85 and 16-86); and a connection to a rudimentary hair follicle may be seen if serial sections are employed.

Clinical Management

Clinical management of follicular cysts includes surgical excision or observation without treatment.

HETEROTOPIC POLYODONTIA

Cause and Pathogenesis

Heterotopic polyodontia (conchal fistula, cyst, or sinus; dentigerous cyst; temporal teratoma or odontoma; ear fistula; ear tooth) is rare in the horse.[435,436,438] It is a developmental anomaly caused by misplaced tooth germ of the first branchial arch, usually displaced toward the ear with the first branchial cleft. The misplaced tooth is generally attached to the temporal bone and is associated with a secretory membrane that forms a fistulous tract that leads to a sinus opening on the cranial border of the pinna. The tooth may form as a pedunculated mass enclosed by skin and attached by a pedicle to the head, or it may be intracranial.

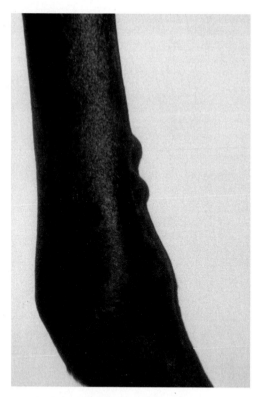

FIGURE 16-84. Follicular cyst (leg). Two dermal nodules on distal leg.

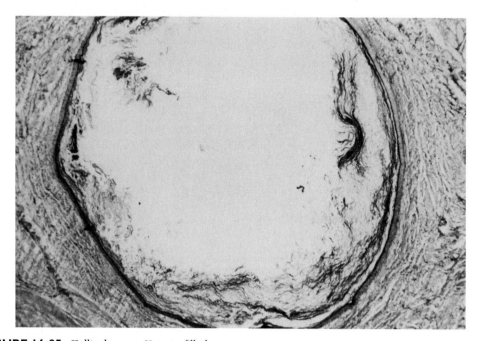

FIGURE 16-85. Follicular cyst. Keratin-filled cyst.

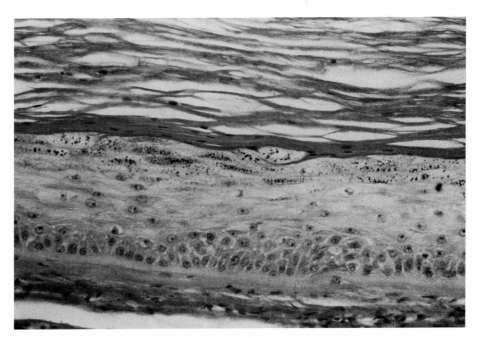

FIGURE 16-86. Follicular cyst. Epithelial wall of cyst undergoes normal epidermal differentiation.

Clinical Findings

There are no breed or sex predilections. The lesions may be present at birth or may not be noticed until the horse is 7 years old.° Lesions are usually solitary, slow-growing, and located at or near the base of the ear. Uncommonly, the lesions may be bilateral.[9] An occasional lesion may occur on the forehead. Early lesions are firm and nodular. Later lesions become cystic and may or may not develop sinuses that discharge a grayish, mucoid, or slightly milky material.

Diagnosis

Radiography may or may not reveal a tooth-like structure within the mass.[439] Histopathologically, heterotopic polyodontia is characterized by a fistulous tract, its lining (epidermis, dermis, hair follicles, glands) and one or more ectopic teeth or tooth-like structures.

Clinical Management

Clinical management includes surgical excision or observation without treatment. Complications of surgery include excessive hemorrhage, fracture and concussion, incomplete removal of the cyst and its lining, damage to the external auditory meatus, and damage to the surrounding neuro-vascular bundles.[437]

Heterotopic Salivary Tissue

A weanling colt had a draining wound in the temporal region since birth.[433] A swollen area with a palpable, hair-lined, draining fibrous tract was present caudoventral to the zygomatic process and extended toward the base of the ear. A clear, seromucoid fluid could be expressed. Surgical excision was curative. Histopathologically, connective tissue surrounded deep, well-delineated, mixed-type salivary gland tissue.

°References 60, 432, 434, 435, 437-440, 442.

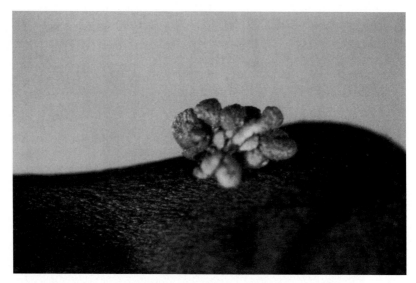

FIGURE 16-87. Epidermal nevus. Congenital papillomatous lesion on distal leg of a foal. *(Courtesy Dr. J. King.)*

Nevi

A nevus (hamartoma) is a circumscribed developmental defect of the skin, characterized by hyperplasia of one or more skin components.[5,14] They may or may not be congenital. The mechanism of nevus formation is not understood. A failure in the normal orderly embryonic inductive process has been theorized.

EPIDERMAL NEVI

Cause and Pathogenesis

Several cases of so-called "congenital papilloma" have been reported in newborn foals and fetuses.[9,34,61,444-450] These animals have had solitary lesions, typical viral papillomatosis has not been reported on the premises, and histopathologic findings have not included evidence of viral infection. It is highly likely that these foals had epidermal nevi. In addition, so-called "linear keratosis" is most likely another form of epidermal nevus in horses: a linear epidermal nevus (see Chapter 11). Linear epidermal nevi were reported in a family of Belgian horses.[448]

Clinical Findings

No breed or sex predilections are apparent for solitary epidermal nevi. Lesions are solitary, present at birth, and occur on the head (forehead, lips, nostrils), neck, back, rib cage, rump, and leg (Fig. 16-87). They are usually hyperpigmented, hyperkeratotic (villous projections from the surface), soft to rubbery in consistency, and plaque-like or pedunculated. Some lesions are rounded and up to 8 cm in diameter. Others are linear or L-shaped (0.6 × 3 cm to 5 × 33 cm).

Linear epidermal nevi appear to be a genodermatosis of Belgian horses.[448] Lesions are first noticed between 6 months and 1 year of age in either sex. Bilateral, linear, vertically oriented bands of hyperkeratosis and alopecia are seen on the caudal aspect of the rear cannon bone areas (Figs. 16-88 and 16-89). Lesions are approximately 14 cm long by 3 cm wide.

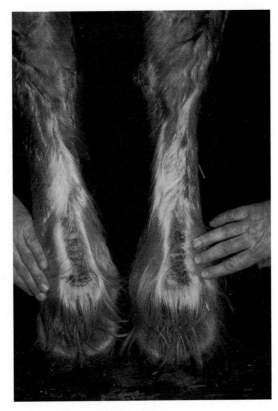

FIGURE 16-88. Linear epidermal nevus. Bilateral, linear, vertically oriented bands of hyperkeratosis and alopecia on the caudal aspect of the rear cannon bone area. (*Courtesy Dr. M. Paradis.*)

Diagnosis

Histopathologically, the lesions are characterized by marked hyperkeratosis (predominantly orthokeratotic), marked papillated epidermal hyperplasia, and papillomatosis (Figs. 16-90 and 16-91). Inflammation is absent or minimal. Evidence of viral infection (inclusion bodies, koilocytosis, clumping and irregularities of keratohyalin granules) is not seen.

Clinical Management

Clinical management of solitary lesions includes surgical excision or observation without treatment. In one case,[444] the lesion sloughed after the topical application of podophyllin for a few days.

Linear epidermal nevi in Belgians are improved, but not cured, by the daily application of 50% propylene glycol or 0.1% tretinoin cream.[448]

Keratoses

Keratoses are firm, elevated, circumscribed areas of keratinocyte proliferation and excessive keratin production.[5,14,67,451] Keratoses are rarely reported in horses.

ACTINIC KERATOSIS

Actinic (solar) keratoses are caused by excessive exposure to ultraviolet and occur more commonly in sunny areas of the world. Actinic keratosis may be single or multiple, appear in lightly haired and lightly pigmented skin, and vary in appearance from ill-defined areas of erythema, hyper-

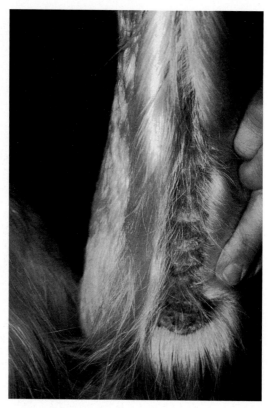

FIGURE 16-89. Linear epidermal nevus. Close-up of hyperkeratotic, alopecia, linear, vertically oriented lesion. (*Courtesy Dr. M. Paradis.*)

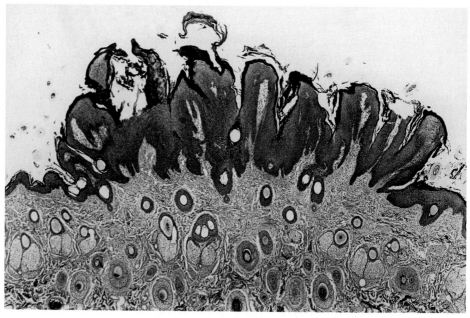

FIGURE 16-90. Congenital epidermal nevus. Focal papillated epidermal hyperplasia and papillomatosis.

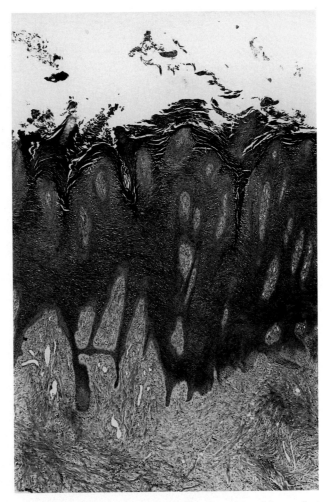

FIGURE 16-91. Linear epidermal nevus. Marked papillated epidermal hyperplasia, papillomatosis, and hyperkeratosis.

keratosis, and crusting to indurated, crusted, hyperkeratotic plaques varying from 0.2 to 2 cm in diameter. Many middle-aged to older horses with nonpigmented eyelid margins have actinic keratoses present as small plaques that owners are not aware of.[67] Actinic keratoses are the precursors of many equine cutaneous squamous cell carcinomas (see Squamous Cell Carcinoma). Histopathologically, they are characterized by atypia and dysplasia of the epidermis and superficial hair follicle epithelium, hyperkeratosis (especially parakeratotic), and occasionally solar elastosis of the subjacent dermis (Fig. 16-92, *A*). Clinical management includes avoidance of sunlight and photoprotection, cryosurgery, and surgical excision.

LINEAR KERATOSIS

Linear keratosis is a visually distinctive equine dermatosis (see Chapter 11) that is probably an epidermal nevus (see page 778).

CANNON KERATOSIS

Cannon keratosis is a visually distinctive equine dermatosis of unknown etiology (see Chapter 11).

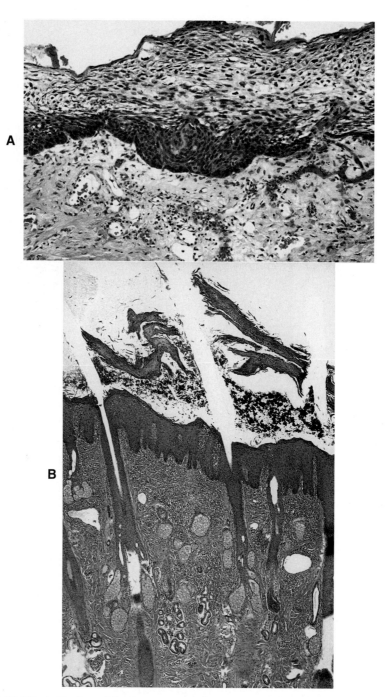

FIGURE 16-92. A, Epidermal dysplasia in actinic keratosis. Note how keratinocytes vary in staining intensity, size, and shape, and how their polarity is totally disrupted. **B,** Lichenoid keratosis. Interface dermatitis with overlying dense parakeratotic hyperkeratosis.

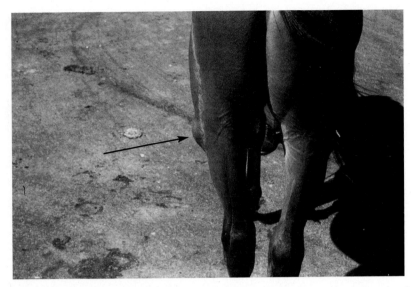

FIGURE 16-93. Calcinosis circumscripta. Large, firm nodule adherent to overlying tissue on lateral aspect of the left stifle *(arrow). (Courtesy Dr. J. Baird.)*

LICHENOID KERATOSIS

Lichenoid keratoses are rarely described in dogs and humans.[5,14] The authors have seen only one horse with lichenoid keratoses. A 13-year-old Appaloosa gelding was presented for asymptomatic bilateral hyperkeratotic plaques affecting the skin of the anterior nares. Histologically, an irregular epidermal hyperplasia with overlying parakeratotic hyperkeratosis and an underlying interface dermatitis were seen (Fig. 16-92, *B*). The twice daily topical application of 0.1% fluocinolone acetonide and 60% DMSO (Synotic, Fort Dodge) resulted in marked shrinkage of the lesions.

Calcinosis Circumscripta

CAUSE AND PATHOGENESIS

Calcinosis circumscripta (tumoral calcinosis, synovial osteochondromatosis) is a rare dermatosis of the horse.° The cause and pathogenesis are unknown. Although prolonged and chronic trauma to localized areas has been suggested, the condition frequently occurs in young horses and usually in horses with no history of trauma. Calcium and phosphorus serum concentrations are typically within normal limits.

CLINICAL FINDINGS

Although many breeds have been affected, 50% of reported cases have occurred in standard-breds.[452-455,457] The majority of affected horses have been $1^1/_2$ to 4 years of age, and 85% have been males. Lesions have occurred over the lateral stifle area in 90% of the cases (Fig. 16-93), and 30% have had bilateral stifle involvement. Rarely are any symptoms (e.g., lameness and local pain) attributable to the lesions. In rare cases, lesions may be seen on the carpus or tarsus.[9] The lesions are hard, well-circumscribed, subcutaneous, and 3 to 20 cm in diameter. The overlying skin is usually normal.

°References 9, 73, 452, 453, 455-458.

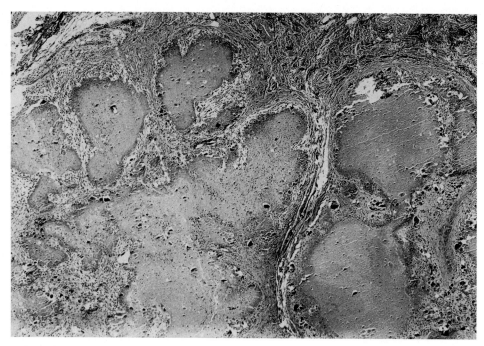

FIGURE 16-94. Calcinosis circumscripta. Large foci of mineral separated by fibrous trabeculae and granulomatous inflammation.

DIAGNOSIS

Skin biopsy reveals a multinodular deposition of mineral separated by variable degrees of fibrosis and granulomatous inflammation (Fig. 16-94). The surrounding tissues should be carefully examined for evidence of mast cell tumor or eosinophilic granuloma, both of which can exhibit marked degrees of dystrophic mineralization.[73,456,457] Radiographically, localized deposits of radiopaque material are seen within soft tissues. Here, again, the differential diagnosis includes mast cell tumor and eosinophilic granuloma.

CLINICAL MANAGEMENT

Because equine calcinosis circumscripta is (1) rarely symptomatic, (2) rarely progressive, and (3) only treatable by surgical excision, treatment is not usually recommended. When therapy is required for symptomatic relief or for cosmetic reasons, surgical excision is the only effective treatment. However, postoperative wound dehiscence and septic arthritis can occur as surgical complications.

● REFERENCES

General Textbook Sources

1. Bone JF, et al: Equine Medicine and Surgery I. American Veterinary Publications, Inc, Wheaton, 1963.
2. Bostock DE, Owen LN: Neoplasia in the Cat, Dog, and Horse. Year Book Medical Publishers, Chicago, 1975.
3. Catcott EJ, Smithcors JF: Equine Medicine and Surgery II. American Veterinary Publications, Inc, Wheaton, 1972.
4. Colahan PT, et al: Equine Medicine and Surgery IV. American Veterinary Publications, Inc, Goleta, 1991.

5. Freedberg IM, et al: Fitzpatrick's Dermatology in General Medicine V. McGraw-Hill, Inc, New York, 1999.

5a. Goldschmidt MH, et al: Histological Classification of Epithelial and Melanocytic Tumors of the Skin of Domestic Animals. Armed Forces Institute of Pathology, Washington, D.C., 1998.

6. Kobluk CN, et al: The Horse. Diseases and Clinical Management. W.B. Saunders Co, Philadelphia, 1995.

7. Mansmann RA, et al: Equine Medicine and Surgery III. American Veterinary Publications, Inc, Santa Barbara, 1982.

8. Moulton JE: Tumors in Domestic Animals III. University of California Press, Berkeley, 1990.

9. Pascoe RRR, Knottenbelt DC: Manual of Equine Dermatology. W.B. Saunders Co, Philadelphia, 1999.

10. Radostits OM, et al: Veterinary Medicine. A Textbook of the Diseases of Cattle, Sheep, Pigs, Goats and Horses VIII. Baillière-Tindall, Philadelphia, 1994.

11. Robinson NE: Current Therapy in Equine Medicine. W.B. Saunders Co, Philadelphia, 1983.

12. Robinson NE: Current Therapy in Equine Medicine II. W.B. Saunders Co, Philadelphia, 1987.

13. Robinson NE: Current Therapy in Equine Medicine III. W.B. Saunders Co, Philadelphia, 1992.

13a. Robinson NE: Current Therapy in Equine Medicine IV. W.B. Saunders Co, Philadelphia, 1997.

14. Scott DW, et al: Muller & Kirk's Small Animal Dermatology VI. W.B. Saunders Co, Philadelphia, 2000.

14a. Sloet van Oldruitenborgh-Oosterban MM, Knottenbelt DC: The Practitioners Guide to Equine Dermatology. Uitgeverij Libre BV, Leeuwarden, Holland, 2001.

15. Theilen GH, Madewell BR: Veterinary Cancer Medicine II. Lea & Febiger. Philadelphia, 1987.

16. Withrow SJ, MacEwen EG: Clinical Veterinary Oncology II. W.B. Saunders Co, Philadelphia, 1996.

17. Yager JA, Scott DW: The skin and appendages. In: Jubb KVF, et al (eds): Pathology of Domestic Animals IV. Vol I. Academic Press, New York, 1993, p 531.

Cytology

18. Alleman AR, Bain PJ: Diagnosing neoplasia: the cytologic criteria for malignancy. Vet Med 95:204, 2000.

19. Barton CL: Cytologic analysis of cutaneous neoplasia: an algorithmic approach. Comp Cont Ed 9:20, 1987.

20. Carter RF, Valli VEO: Advances in the cytologic diagnosis of canine lymphoma. Semin Vet Med Surg (Small Anim) 3:167, 1988.

21. Hall RL, MacWilliams PS: The cytologic examination of cutaneous and subcutaneous masses. Semin Vet Med Surg (Small Anim) 3:94, 1988.

22. Stirtzinger T: The cytologic diagnosis of mesenchymal tumors. Semin Vet Med Surg (Small Anim) 3:157, 1988.

23. Thrall MA: Cytologic examination of cutaneous and subcutaneous lumps and lesions. Vet Med 95:224, 2000.

Immunohistochemistry

24. Desnoyers MM, et al: Immuno-histochemical detection of intermediate filament proteins in formalin fixed normal and neoplastic tissues. Can J Vet Res 54:360, 1990.

25. Elias JW: Immunohistopathology: A Practical Approach to Diagnosis. American Society of Clinical Pathologists, Chicago, 1990.

26. Doherty MJ, et al: Immunoenzyme techniques in dermatopathology. J Am Acad Dermatol 20:827, 1989.

27. Wick MR, et al: The immunohistology of cutaneous neoplasia: a practical perspective. J Cutan Pathol 20:481, 1993.

Survey Articles and Chapters

28. Adams R, et al: Excision of cutaneous tumors in the horse using histologic guidance. Vet Surg 17:241, 1988.

29. Baker JR, Leyland A: Histological survey of tumors of the horse, with particular reference to those of the skin. Vet Rec 96:419, 1975.

30. Bastianello SS: A survey of neoplasia in domestic species over a 40-year period from 1935 to 1974 in the Republic of South Africa. IV. Tumours occurring in Equidae. Onderstepoort J Vet Res 50:91, 1983.

31. British Equine Veterinary Association Survey of Equine Diseases. Vet Rec 77:528, 1965.

32. Canderé JL, et al: Les principales tumeurs cutanées du cheval: actualités et perspectives. Point Vét 27:935, 1996.

33. Cotchin E: Neoplasms of the Domesticated Mammals. Commonwealth Agricultural Bureaux, England, 1956.

34. Cotchin E: Tumours in farm animals: a survey of tumours examined at the Royal Veterinary College, London, during 1950-60. Vet Rec 72:816, 1960.

35. Cotchin E, Baker-Smith J: Tumours in horses encountered in an abattoir survey. Vet Rec 97:339, 1975.

36. Cotchin E: A general survey of tumours in the horse. Equine Vet J 9:16, 1977.

37. Damodaran S, Ramachandran PV: A survey of neoplasms in Equidae. Indian Vet J 52:531, 1975.

38. Feldman WH: Neoplasms of Domesticated Animals. W.B. Saunders Co, Philadelphia, 1932.

38a. Foy JM, et al: Common equine skin tumors. Comp Cont Ed 24:242, 2002.

39. Harris CC: p53: at the cross roads of molecular carcinogenesis and molecular epidemiology. J Invest Dermatol Symp Proc 1:115, 1996.

40. Head KW: Skin diseases: neoplastic disease. Vet Rec 65:926, 1953.

41. Head KW: Some data concerning the distribution of skin tumours in domestic animals. In: Rook A, Walton GS (eds): Comparative Pathology and Physiology of the Skin. Blackwell Scientific Publications, Oxford, 1965, p 615.

42. Hopes R: Skin diseases in horses. Vet Dermatol News 1:4, 1976.

43. Jackson C: The incidence and pathology of tumours of domesticated animals in South Africa. Onderstepoort J Vet Res Anim Sci Ind 6:3, 1936.

44. Johnson PJ: Dermatologic tumors (excluding sarcoids). Vet Clin N Am Equine Pract 14:625, 1998.

45. Kerr KM, Alden CL: Equine neoplasia—a ten-year survey. Proc Am Assoc Vet Lab Diagn 17:183, 1974.

46. Krawiecki JM: A propos des tumeurs cutanées du cheval. Point Vét 22:839, 1990.

46a. McCauley CT, et al: Use of a carbon dioxide laser for surgical management of cutaneous masses in horses: 32 cases (1993-2000). J Am Vet Med Assoc 220:1192, 2002.

47. McMullan WC: The skin. In: Mansmann RA, et al (eds): Equine Medicine and Surgery III. American Veterinary Publications, Santa Barbara, 1982, p 789.

48. Miller RI, Campbell RSF: A survey of granulomatous and neoplastic diseases of equine skin in North Queensland. Aust Vet J 59:33, 1982.

49. Moulton JE: Occurrence and types of tumours in large domestic animals. Ann NY Acad Sci 108:620, 1963.

50. Mullowney PC, Fadok VA: Dermatologic diseases of horses. Part II. Bacterial and viral skin diseases. Comp Cont Educ 6:516, 1984.

51. Mullowney PC: Dermatologic diseases of horses. Part IV. Environmental, congenital, and neoplastic diseases. Comp Cont Educ 7:522, 1985.

52. Murray DR, et al: Granulomatous and neoplastic diseases of the skin of horses. Aust Vet J 54:338, 1978.

53. Murray M: Neoplasms of domestic animals in East Africa. Br Vet J 124:514, 1968.

54. Nobel TA, et al: Neoplasms in domestic animals in Israel (1959-1969). Refuah Vet 27:115, 1970.

55. Nobel TA, et al: Neoplasms in domestic animals in Israel (1969-1979). Refuah Vet 36:23, 1979.

56. Page EH: Common skin diseases of the horse. Proc Am Assoc Equine Practit 18:385, 1972.

57. Panel Report. Skin diseases in horses. Mod Vet Pract 67:43, 1986.

58. Pascoe RR: The nature and treatment of skin conditions observed in horses in Queensland. Aust Vet J 49:35, 1973.

59. Pascoe RR, Summers PM: Clinical survey of tumors and tumor-like lesions in horses in southeast Queensland. Equine Vet J 13:235, 1981.

60. Pascoe RR: Equine Dermatoses. University of Sydney Post-Graduate Foundation in Veterinary Science, Veterinary Review No 22, Sydney, 1981.

61. Pascoe RR: Infectious skin diseases of horses. Vet Clin N Am Large Anim Pract 6:27, 1984.

62. Plummer PJG: A survey of sixty tumours from domesticated animals. Can J Comp Med 15:234, 1951.

63. Plummer PJG: A survey of six hundred and thirty-six tumours from domesticated animals. Can J Comp Med 20:239, 1956.

64. Priester WA, Mantel N: Occurrence of tumors in domestic animals. Data from 12 United States and Canadian Colleges of Veterinary Medicine. J Natl Cancer Inst 47:1333, 1971.

65. Priester WA: Skin tumors in domestic animals. Data from 12 United States and Canadian Colleges of Veterinary Medicine. J Natl Cancer Inst 50:457, 1973.

66. Ragland WL, et al: Equine sarcoid. Equine Vet J 2:168, 1970.

67. Rebhun WC: Tumors of the eye and ocular adnexal tissues. Vet Clin N Am Equine Pract 14:579, 1998.

68. Runnells RA, Benbrook EA: Connective tissue tumors of horses and mules. Am J Vet Res 2:427, 1941.

69. Runnells RA, Benbrook EA: Epithelial tumors of horses. Am J Vet Res 3:176, 1942.

70. Sastry GA: Neoplasms of animals in India. Indian Vet J 42:332, 1957.

71. Sastry GA: Neoplasms in animals in India. Vet Med 54:428, 1959.

72. Sastry GA, Tweihaus HJ: A study of the animal neoplasms in Kansas State. IV. Others. Indian Vet J 42:332, 1965.

73. Scott DW: Large Animal Dermatology. W.B. Saunders Co, Philadelphia, 1988.

74. Scott DW, Miller WH Jr: Unpublished observations. College of Veterinary Medicine, Cornell University, Ithaca, NY.

75. Seiler RJ, Punita I: Neoplasia of domestic mammals: review of cases diagnosed at University Pertanian, Malaysia. Kajian Vet 11:80, 1979.

76. Singh P, et al: A survey of tumours in domestic animals. Indian Vet J 68:721, 1991.

77. Smit JD: Skin lesions in South African domestic animals with specific reference to the incidence and prognosis of various skin tumors. J S Afr Vet Med Assoc 33:363, 1962.

78. Stannard AA, Pulley LT: Tumors of the skin and soft tissues. In: Moulton JE (ed): Tumors in Domestic Animals II. University of California Press, Berkeley, 1978, p 16.

79. Sundberg JP, et al: Neoplasms of Equidae. J Am Vet Med Assoc 170: 150, 1977.

80. Teifke JP, Löhr CV: Immunohistochemical detection of p53 overexpression in paraffin wax-imbedded squamous cell carcinomas of cattle, horses, cats, and dogs. J Comp Pathol 114:205, 1996.

80a. Théon A: Cisplatin treatment for cutaneous tumors. In Robinson NE (ed): Current Therapy in Equine Medicine IV. W.B. Saunders, Philadelphia, 1997, p 372.

81. Théon AP: Intralesional and topical chemotherapy and immunotherapy. Vet Clin N Am Equine Pract 14:659, 1998.

82. Théon AP: Radiation therapy in the horse. Vet Clin N Am Equine Pract 14:673, 1998.

83. Thomsett LR: Skin diseases of the horse. In Pract 1:15, 1979.

84. Thomsett LR: Noninfectious skin diseases of horses. Vet Clin N Am Large Anim Pract 6:59, 1984.

85. Thomsett LR: Dermatology. In: Hickman J (ed.): Equine Surgery and Medicine. Academic Press, New York, 1985, p 297.

85a. Thomsett LR: Pigmentation and pigmentary disorders of the equine skin. Equin Vet Edu 3:130, 1991.

Papilloma

86. Binninger CE, Piper RC: Hyperplastic dermatitis of the equine ear. J Am Vet Med Assoc 153:69, 1968.

87. Cook RH, Olson C: Experimental transmission of cutaneous papillomas of the horse. Am J Pathol 27:1087, 1951.

88. Douville P: De la papillomatose chez le cheval et le chien. Rev Vét (Toulouse) 99:145, 1948.

89. Fairley RA, Haines DM: The electron microscopic and immunohistochemical demonstration of a papillomavirus in equine aural plaque. Vet Pathol 29:79, 1992.

90. Fulton RE, et al: The fine structure of equine papillomas and equine papilloma virus. J Ultrastruct Res 30:328, 1970.

91. Hamada M, Itakura C: Ultrastructural morphology of hypomelanosis in equine cutaneous papillomas. J Comp Pathol 103:200, 1990.

92. Hamada M, et al: Histopathological development of equine cutaneous papillomas. J Comp Pathol 102:393, 1990.

93. Hamada M, et al: Keratin expression in equine normal epidermis and cutaneous papillomas using monoclonal antibodies. J Comp Pathol 102:405, 1990.

94. Hamada M, et al: Langerhan's cells in equine cutaneous papillomas and normal skin. Vet Pathol 29:152, 1992.

95. Junge RE, et al: Papillomas and squamous cell carcinomas of horses. J Am Vet Med Assoc 185:656, 1984.

96. Lancaster WD, Olson C: Animal papillomaviruses. Microbiol Rev 46:191, 1982.

97. Majewski S, Tablonska S: Human papillomavirus-associated tumors of the skin and mucosa. J Am Acad Dermatol 36:659, 1997.

98. Nicholls PK, Stanley MA: Canine papillomatosis—a centenary review. J Comp Pathol 120:219, 1999.

99. O'Banion MK, et al: Equine papillomavirus: partial characterization and presence in common equine skin tumors. J Cell Biochem 9(Suppl):73, 1985.

100. O'Banion MK, et al: Cloning and characterization of an equine cutaneous papilloma virus. Virology 152:100, 1986.

101. Stannard AA: Some important dermatoses in the horse. Mod Vet Pract 53:31, 1972.

102. Sundberg JP, et al: Immunoperoxidase localization of papilloma virus in hyperplastic and neoplastic epithelial lesions of animals. Am J Vet Res 45:1441, 1984.

103. Sundberg JP, et al: Equine papillomatosis: is partial resection of lesions an effective treatment? Vet Med 80:71, 1985.

104. Sundberg JP, O'Banion MK: Animal papillomaviruses associated with malignant tumors. Adv Viral Oncol 8:55, 1989.

105. Sundberg JP: Urges caution with use of lasers on lesions of suspected viral origin. J Am Vet Med Assoc 196:1007, 1990.

106. Vaughan JT, et al: Condyloma acuminata. J Cutan Pathol 3:244, 1976.

107. Whiteley HE, Sundberg JP: Expression of lectin binding in cutaneous papillomas of animals. J Comp Pathol 99:86, 1988.

108. Williams MA: Papillomatosis: warts and aural plaques. In: Robinson NE (ed): Current Therapy in Equine Medicine IV. W.B. Saunders Co, Philadelphia, 1997, p 389.

Squamous Cell Carcinoma

109. Akerejola OO, et al: Equine squamous-cell carcinoma in northern Nigeria. Vet Rec 103:336, 1978.

110. Baird AN, Frelier PF: Squamous cell carcinoma originating from an epithelial scar in a horse. J Am Vet Med Assoc 196:1999, 1990.

111. Burney DP, et al: Identifying and treating squamous cell carcinoma of horses. Vet Med 87:588, 1992.

112. Campbell GA, et al: Solar elastosis with squamous cell carcinoma in two horses. Vet Pathol 24:463, 1987.

113. Desbrosse AM, et al: Tumeurs oculaires et périoculaires chez le cheval: étude rétrospective de six cas. Point Vét 24:59, 1992.

114. Dixon RT: Radiation therapy in horses. Aust Vet J 43:508, 1967.

114a. Dixon RT: Results of radon-222 gamma-radiation therapy in an equine practice. Aust Vet J 48:279, 1972.

115. Dugan SJ, et al: Epidemiologic study of ocular/adnexal squamous cell carcinoma in horses. J Am Vet Med Assoc 198:251, 1991.

116. Dugan SJ, et al: Prognostic factors and survival of horses with ocular/adnexal squamous cell carcinoma: 147 cases (1978-1988). J Am Vet Med Assoc 198:298, 1991.

117. English RV, et al: Carbon dioxide laser ablation for the treatment of limbal squamous cell carcinoma in horses. J Am Vet Med Assoc 196:439, 1990.

118. Farris H, et al: Cryosurgery of equine cutaneous neoplastic and non-neoplastic lesions. Proc Am Assoc Equine Pract 21:177, 1975.

119. Fessler JF, et al: Squamous cell carcinoma associated with a chronic wound in a horse. J Am Vet Med Assoc 202:615, 1993.

120. Fortier LA, HacHarg MA: Topical use of 5-fluorouracil for treatment of squamous cell carcinoma of the external genitalia of horses: 11 cases (1988-1992). J Am Vet Med Assoc 205:1183, 1994.

121. Frauenfelder HC, et al: ^{90}Sr for treatment of periocular squamous cell carcinoma in the horse. J Am Vet Med Assoc 180:307, 1982.

122. Garma-Aviña A: The cytology of squamous cell carcinomas in domestic animals. J Vet Diagn Invest 6:238, 1994.

123. Gavin PR, Gillette EL: Interstitial radiation therapy of equine squamous cell carcinoma. J Am Vet Radiol Soc 19:138, 1978.

124. Grier RL, et al: Treatment of bovine and equine ocular squamous cell carcinoma by radiofrequency hyperthermia. J Am. Vet Med Assoc 177:55, 1980.

125. Guaguère E, et al: Cas clinique. Epithelioma spinocellulaire de la vulve chez une jument. Point Vét 23:97, 1991.

126. Harling DE, et al: Excision and cryosurgical treatment of five cases of squamous cell carcinoma in the horse. Equine Vet J (supp 12):105, 1983.

127. Hilbert BJ, et al: Cryotherapy of periocular squamous cell carcinoma in the horse. J Am Vet Med Assoc 170:1305, 1977.

128. Joyce JR: Cryosurgical treatment of tumors of horses and cattle. J Am Vet Med Assoc 168:226, 1976.

129. Karcher LF, et al: Pseudohyperparathyroidism in a mare associated with squamous cell carcinoma of the vulva. Cornell Vet 80:153, 1990.

130. King TC, et al: Therapeutic management of ocular squamous cell carcinoma in the horse: 43 cases (1979-1989). Equine Vet J 23:449, 1991.

131. Klein WR, et al: Penis-und Preputiumtumoren beim Pferd. Prakt Tierärztl 72:192, 1991.

132. Lewis RE: Radon implant therapy of squamous cell carcinoma and equine sarcoid. Proc Am Assoc Equine Practit 10:217, 1964.

133. MacFadden KE, Pace LW: Clinical manifestations of squamous cell carcinoma in horses. Comp Cont Educ Pract Vet 13:669, 1991.

133a. Mair TS, et al: Surgical treatment of 45 horses affected by squamous cell carcinoma of the penis and prepuce. Equine Vet J 323:406, 2000.

134. McCalla TL, et al: Immunotherapy of periocular squamous cell carcinoma with metastasis in a pony. J Am Vet Med Assoc 200:1678, 1992.

135. Miller R: Treatment of some equine cutaneous neoplasms: a review. Aust Vet Practit 10:119, 1980.

136. Orenberg EK, et al: Implant delivery system: intralesional delivery of chemotherapeutic agents for treatment of spontaneous skin tumors in veterinary patients. Clin Dermatol 9:561, 1992.

137. Paterson S: Treatment of superficial ulcerative squamous cell carcinoma in three horses with topical 5-fluorouracil. Vet Rec 141:626, 1997.

138. Pazzi KA, et al: Analysis of the equine tumor suppressor gene p53 in the normal horse and in eight cutaneous squamous cell carcinomas. Cancer Lett 107:125, 1996.

139. Pérez J, et al: Immunohistochemical study of the inflammatory infiltrate associated with equine squamous cell carcinoma. J Comp Pathol 121:385, 1999.

140. Plaut A, Kohn-Speyer AC: The carcinogenic action of smegma. Science 105:391, 1947.

141. Schumacher J, et al: Burn-induced neoplasia in two horses. Equine Vet J 18:410, 1986.

142. Schwink K: Factors influencing morbidity and outcome of equine ocular squamous cell carcinoma. Equine Vet J 19:198, 1987.

143. Silver IA, Cater DB: Radiotherapy and chemotherapy for domestic animals. I. Treatment of malignant tumors and benign conditions in the horse. Acta Radiol 2:226, 1964.

144. Strafuss AC: Squamous cell carcinoma in horses. J Am Vet Med Assoc 168:61, 1976.

145. Szilvassy IP, et al: Preputial carcinoma in a horse. Vet Med. Small Anim Clin 67:1329, 1972.

146. Teifke JP, Löhr CV: Immunohistochemical detection of P53 overexpression in paraffin wax-embedded squamous cell carcinomas of cattle, horses, cats, and dog. J Comp Pathol 114:205, 1996.

147. Théon AP, et al: Intratumoral chemotherapy with cisplatin in oily emulsion in horses. J Am Vet Med Assoc 202:261, 1993.

148. Théon AP, et al: Perioperative intratumoral administration of cisplatin for treatment of cutaneous tumors in Equidae. J Am Vet Med Assoc 205:1170, 1994.

149. Théon AP, et al: Comparison of intratumoral administration of cisplatin versus bleomycin for treatment of periocular squamous cell carcinomas in horses. Am J Vet Res 58:431, 1997.

150. Théon AP, Pascoe JR: Iridium-192 interstitial brachytherapy for equine periocular tumours: treatment results and prognostic factors in 115 horses. Equine Vet J 27:117, 1995.

151. Walker MA, et al: Two-year nonrecurrence rates for equine ocular and periorbital squamous cell carcinoma following radiotherapy. Vet Radiol 27:146, 1986.

152. Wilkie DA, Burt JK: Combined treatment of ocular squamous cell carcinoma in a horse, using radiofrequency hyperthermia and interstitial [198]Au implants. J Am Vet Med Assoc 196:1831, 1990.

153. Wyn-Jones G: Treatment of periocular tumours of horses using radioactive gold[198] grains. Equine Vet J 11:3, 1979.

154. Wyn-Jones G: Treatment of equine cutaneous neoplasia by radiotherapy using iridium[192] linear sources. Equine Vet J 15:361, 1983.

155. Zanichelli S, et al: Observations on squamous cell carcinoma in the horse. Pferdeheilk 10:219, 1994.

Basal Cell Tumor

156. Schuh JCL, Valentine BA: Equine basal cell tumors. Vet Pathol 24:44, 1987.

156a. Slovis NM, et al: Equine basal cell tumors: 6 cases (1985-1999). J Vet Intern Med 15:43, 2001.

Sebaceous Gland Tumors

157. McMartin DN, Gruhn RF: Sebaceous carcinoma in a horse. Vet Pathol 14:532, 1977.

Sweat Gland Tumors

158. Anderson WI, et al: Two rare cutaneous neoplasms in horses: Apocrine gland adenocarcinoma and carcinosarcoma. Cornell Vet 80:339, 1990.

Sarcoid

159. Amtmann E, et al: Equine connective tissue tumors contain unintegrated bovine papillomavirus DNA. J Virol 35:962, 1980.

160. Angelos JA, et al: Characterization of BPV-like DNA in equine sarcoids. Arch Virol 119:95, 1991.

161. Angelos JA, et al: Evaluation of breed as a risk factor for sarcoid and uveitis in horses. Anim Genetics 19:417, 1988.

162. Barthold SW, Olson C: Common membrane neoantigens on bovine papillomavirus-induced fibroma cells from cattle and horses. Am J Vet Res 39:1643, 1978.

163. Bertone AL, McClure JJ: Therapy for sarcoids. Comp Cont Educ Pract Vet 12:262, 1990.

164. Boure L, et al: Essai de traitement des sarcoïdes du cheval par injections intra-tumorales de bléomycine. Point Vét 23:199, 1991.

165. Brandt K, et al: Equine Sarkoide-Vorkommen und Behandlung. Pferdeheilk 12:739, 1996.

166. Broström H, et al: Cell-mediated immunity in horses with sarcoid cells in vitro. Am J Vet Res 40:1701, 1979.

167. Broström H, et al: Association between equine leukocyte antigens (ELA) and equine sarcoid tumors in the population of Swedish halfbreds and some of their families. Vet Immunol Immunopathol 19:215, 1988.

168. Broström H, et al: Surface antigens on equine sarcoid cells and normal dermal fibroblasts as assessed by xenogeneic antisera. Res Vet Sci 46:172, 1989.

169. Broström H: Equine sarcoids. A clinical and epidemiological study in relation to equine leucocyte antigens (ELA). Acta Vet Scand 36:223, 1995.

170. Broström H, et al: Generation of in vitro natural cytotoxicity of horse lymphocytes against sarcoid-derived tumors cells not expressing major histocompatibility complex antigens. Am J Vet Res 57:992, 1996.

171. Brown MP: Surgical treatment of equine sarcoid. In: Robinson NE (ed): Current Therapy in Equine Medicine. W.B. Saunders Co, Philadelphia, 1983, p 537.

172. Bucher K, et al: Tumour suppressor gene P53 in the horse: identification, cloning, sequencing, and a possible role in the pathogenesis of equine sarcoid. Res Vet Sci 61:114, 1996.

172a. Carr EA, et al: Bovine papillomavirus DNA in neoplastic and non-neoplastic tissues obtained from horses with and without sarcoids in the western United States. Am J Vet Res 62:741, 2001.

173. Carstanjen B, et al: Carbon dioxide laser as a surgical instrument for sarcoid therapy—a retrospective study on 60 cases. Can Vet J 38:773, 1997.

173a. Carstanjen B, Lepage OM: Equines Sarkoid (Teil II): Therapiemöglichkeiten und Prognosen. Prak Tierheilk 79:730, 1998.

174. Chambery C: Deux cas de sarcöides de la paupière traités par le BCG. Pract Vét Equine 14:157, 1983.

175. Cheevers WP, et al: Isolation of a retrovirus from cultured equine sarcoid tumor cells. Am J Vet Res 43:804, 1982.

176. Cheevers WP, et al: Spontaneous expression of an endogenous retrovirus by the equine sarcoid-derived MC-1 cell line. Am J Vet Res 47:50, 1986.

176a. Dahl MV: Imiquimod: an immune response modifier. J Am Acad Dermatol 43(suppl):S1, 2000.

177. de Groot R, de Groot E: Radiotherapy for "equine sarcoid" and other superficial lesions in the horse. Vet Radiol 25:92, 1984.

178. Diehl M, Gerber H: Traitement de la sarcöide équine au Laser à gaz carbonique. Schweiz Arch Tierheilk 130:113, 1988.

179. Diehl M, et al: Spezifische Methoden zur Entfernung des Equinen Sarkoides. Prakt Tierärztl Prax 7:14, 1987.

179a. Dionne R, Vrins A: Le sarcöide équin. Où en sommes-nous? Méd Vét Québec 30:50, 2000.

180. Dubath ML: Recherche d'association entre le système ELA et une prédisposition aux sarcöides équins. Schweiz Arch Tierheilk 129:41, 1987.

181. England JJ, et al: Virus-like particles in an equine sarcoid cell line. Am J Vet Res 34:1601, 1973.

182. Farris H, et al: Cryotherapy of equine sarcoid and other lesions. Vet Med Small Animal Clin 71:325, 1976.

183. Fatemi-Nainie S, et al: Identification of a transforming retrovirus from cultured equine dermal fibrosarcoma. Virol 120:49, 1982.

184. Fatemi-Nainie S, et al: Cultural characteristics and tumorigenicity of the equine sarcoid-derived MC-1 cell line. Am J Vet Res 45:1105, 1984.

185. Fleming DD: BCG therapy for equine sarcoid. In: Robinson NE (ed): Current Therapy in Equine Medicine. W.B. Saunders Co Philadelphia, 1983, p 539.

186. Frauenfelder HC, et al: ^{222}Rn for treatment of periocular fibrous connective tissue sarcomas in horse. J Am Vet Med Assoc 180:307, 1982.

187. Fretz PB, Barber SM: Prospective analysis of cryosurgery as the sole treatment for equine sarcoids. Vet Clin N Am 10:847, 1980.

188. Genetzky RM, et al: Equine sarcoids: causes, diagnosis, and treatment. Comp Cont Educ 5:S416, 1983.

189. Gerber H, et al: Association between predisposition to equine sarcoid and MHC in multiple-case families. In: Powell DG (ed): Equine Infectious Diseases V. University Press of Kentucky, Lexington, 1988, p 272.

190. Gillette EL, Carlson WD: An evaluation of radiation therapy in veterinary medicine. J Am Vet Radiol Soc 5:58, 1964.

191. Goodrich L, et al: Equine sarcoids. Vet Clin N Am Equine Pract 14:607, 1998.

192. Gorman NT: Equine sarcoid—time for optimism. Equine Vet J 17:412, 1985.

192a. Hanson RR: Cryotherapy for equine skin conditions. In: Robinson NE (ed): Current Therapy in Equine Medicine IV. W.B. Saunders, Philadelphia, 1997, p 370.

193. Harman KS: A case of equine sarcoid. Cornell Vet 39:432, 1949.

194. Hesselholt M, Ingerslev H: Equine sarcoid. Dansk Dyrlaeg Med 57:9, 1974.

195. Hilmas DE, Gillette EL: Radiotherapy of spontaneous fibrous connective-tissue sarcomas in animals. J Natl Cancer Inst 56:365, 1976.

196. Hoffman KD, et al: Radio-frequency current-induced hyperthermia for the treatment of equine sarcoid. Equine Pract 5:24, 1983.

197. Houlton JEF: Treatment of periocular equine sarcoids. Equine Vet J 2(suppl. 1):117, 1983.

198. Howarth S: Sarcoids: the story so far. Vet Ann 30:145, 1990.

199. Ivascu I, et al: Clinical and pathological observations on five cases of equine sarcoidosis identified in Romania. Zbl Vet Med A21:815, 1974.

200. James VS: A family tendency to equine sarcoids. Southwest Vet 21:235, 1968.

201. Joyce JR: Cryosurgery for removal of equine sarcoids. Vet Med Small Anim Clin 70:200, 1975.

202. Kinnunen R, et al: Bio-immunoterapialla hoidettu hevosen sarkoidi—Tapausselostus. Suomen Eläin 97:197, 1991.

203. Klein WR, et al: Equine sarcoid. BCG immunotherapy compared to cryosurgery in a prospective randomized clinical trial. Cancer Immunol Immunother 21:133, 1986.

204. Klein WR: BCG-Immunotherapie für das Sarkoid beim Pferd. Prakt Tier 69:17, 1988.

205. Klein WR: Immunotherapie van het plaveiselcelcarcinoom bij het runderoog en het sarcoïd bij het paard. Tijdschr Diergeneesk 115:1149, 1990.

206. Knottenbelt DC, Walker JA: Topical treatment of the equine sarcoid. Equine Vet Educ 6:72, 1994.

207. Knottenbelt DC, et al: Diagnosis and treatment of the equine sarcoid. In Pract 17:123, 1995.

207a. Knottenbelt DC, Mathews JB: A positive step forwards in the diagnosis of equine sarcoid. Vet J 161:224, 2001.

208. Krahwinkel DJ, et al: Cryosurgical treatment of cancerous and noncancerous diseases of dogs, horses, and cats. J Am Vet Med Assoc 169:201, 1976.

209. Krawiecki JM, et al: Le sarcoïde du cheval. Point Vét 22:843, 1991.

210. Lancaster WD, et al: Bovine papilloma virus: presence of virus-specific DNA sequences in naturally occurring equine tumors. Proc Natl Acad Sci 74:524, 1977.

211. Lancaster WD, et al: Hybridisation of bovine papillomavirus type 1 and type 2 DNA from virus-induced hamster tumours and naturally occurring equine tumours. Intervirol 11:227, 1979.

212. Lancaster WD: Apparent lack of integration of bovine papillomavirus DNA in virus-induced equine and bovine tumour cells and virus-transformed mouse cells. Virol 180:251, 1981.

213. Lane JG: The treatment of equine sarcoids by cryosurgery. Equine Vet J 9:127, 1977.

214. Laursen BA: Behandling of equine sarcoider med kryokirurgi. Dansk Vet Tidsskr 70:97, 1987.

215. Lavach JD, Severin GA: Neoplasia of the equine eye, adnexa, and orbit: a review of 68 cases. J Am Vet Med Assoc 170:202, 1977.

216. Lavach JD, et al: Immunotherapy of periocular sarcoids in horses. Vet Clin N Am Large Anim Pract 6:3, 1984.

217. Lavach JD, et al: BCG treatment of periocular sarcoid. Equine Vet J 17:445, 1985.

218. Lawsen ABA: Behandling af equine sarcoider med kryokirurgi. Dansk Vet Tidsskr 70:97, 1987.

219. Lazary S, et al: Equine leukocyte antigens in sarcoid-affected horses. Equine Vet J 17:283, 1985.

220. Lazary S: Untersuchungen über die Anfälligkeit für die Erkrankung am equinen Sarkoid. Prakt Tier 69:12, 1988.

220a. Lepage MF, et al: Equines Sarkoid (Till I): Ursach, Diagnose, Differentialdiagnose. Prak Tierheilk 79:627, 1998.

221. Lory S, et al: In situ hybridization of equine sarcoids with bovine papilloma virus. Vet Rec 132:132, 1993.

222. Madewell BR, Mann RJ: Tubuloreticular inclusions in equine connective tissue neoplasms. J Comp Pathol 100:449, 1989.

223. Martens A, DeMoor A: Sarcoïden bij het paard deel I: Klinische vormen, voorkomen, epidemiologie, etiologie en pathogenese. Vlaams Diergeneeskd Tijdschr 65:10, 1996.

224. Martens A, DeMoor A: Sarcoïden bij het paard deel II: Chirurgische excisie, laser therapie, hyperthermie, cryo-en radiotherapie. Vlaams Diergeneeskd Tijdschr 65:18, 1996.

225. Martens A, DeMoor A: Sarcoïden bij het paard deel III: Chemotherapie, homeopathie en biologische therapie. Vlaams Diergeneeskd Tijdschr 65:25, 1996.

226. Martens A, et al: In vitro and in vivo evaluation of hypericin for photodynamic therapy of equine sarcoids. Vet J 159:77, 2000.

226a. Martens A, et al: Histopathological characteristics of five clinical types of equine sarcoid. Res Vet Sci 69:295, 2000.

226b. Martens A, et al: PCR detection of bovine papilloma virus DNA in superficial swabs and scrapings from equine sarcoids. Vet J 161:280, 2001.

226c. Martens A, et al: Evaluation of excision, cryosurgery and local BCG vaccination for the treatment of equine sarcoids. Vet Rec 149:665, 2001.

227. Marti E, et al: Report of the first international workshop on equine sarcoid. Equine Vet J 25:397, 1993.

228. McConaghy FF, et al: Management of equine sarcoids: 1975-93. NZ Vet J 42:180, 1994.

229. McConaghy FF, et al: Equine sarcoid: a persistent therapeutic challenge. Comp Cont Educ Pract Vet 16-1022, 1994.

230. Meredith D, et al: Equine leukocyte antigens: relationship with sarcoid tumors and laminitis in two pure breeds. Immunogenetics 23:221, 1986.

231. Metcalf JW: Improved technique in sarcoid removal. Proc Am Assoc Equine Practit 17:45, 1971.

232. Mohammed HO, et al: Factors associated with the risk of developing sarcoid tumours in horses. Equine Vet J 24:165, 1992.

233. Montpellier JR, et al: Greffe d'une tumeur schwannienne chez le mulet. Bull Acad Vét Fr 12:91, 1939.

234. Murphy JM, et al: Immunotherapy in ocular equine sarcoid. J Am Vet Med Assoc 174:269, 1979.

235. Nasir L, et al: Screening for bovine papillomavirus in peripheral blood cells of donkeys with and without sarcoids. Res Vet Sci 63:289, 1997.

236. Olson C: Equine sarcoid: a cutaneous neoplasm. Am J Vet Res 9:333, 1948.

237. Olson C, Cook RH: Cutaneous sarcoma-like lesions of the horse caused by the agent of bovine papilloma. Proc Soc Exp Biol Med 77:281, 1951.

238. Otten N, et al: DNA of bovine papillomavirus type 1 and 2 in equine sarcoids. PCR detection and direct sequencing. Arch Virol 132:121, 1993.

239. Otten N, et al: Experimental treatment of equine sarcoid using a xanthate compound and recombinant human tumour necrosis factor alpha. J Vet Med A41:757, 1994.

240. Owen R, Jagger DW: Clinical observations on the use of BCG cell wall fraction for treatment of periocular and other equine sarcoids. Vet Rec 120:548, 1987.

241. Page EH, Tiffany LW: Use of an autogenous equine fibrosarcoma vaccine. J Am Vet Med Assoc 150:177, 1967.

242. Palmer SE: Carbon dioxide laser removal of a verrucous sarcoid from the ear of a horse. J Am Vet Med Assoc 195:1125, 1989.

243. Piscopo SE: The complexities of sarcoid tumors. Equine Pract 21:14, 1999.

244. Ragland WL, et al: Experimental viral fibromatosis of the equine dermis. Lab Invest 14:598, 1965.

245. Ragland WL, et al: An epizootic of equine sarcoid. Nature 210:1399, 1966.

246. Ragland WL, Spencer GR: Attempts to relate bovine papilloma virus to the cause of equine sarcoid: immunity to bovine papilloma virus. Am J Vet Res 29:1363, 1968.

247. Ragland WL: Attempts to relate bovine papilloma virus to the cause of equine sarcoid. Equidae inoculated intradermally with bovine papilloma virus. Am J Vet Res 30:743, 1969.

248. Ragland WL, et al: Equine sarcoid. Equine Vet J 2:2, 1970.

249. Ragland WL, et al: Attempts to relate bovine papilloma virus to the cause of equine sarcoid: horses, donkeys, and calves inoculated with equine sarcoid extracts. Equine Vet J 2:168, 1970.

250. Rebhun WC: Immunotherapy for sarcoids. In: Robinson NE (ed): Current Therapy in Equine Medicine II. W.B. Saunders Co Philadelphia, 1987, p 637.

251. Reid SWJ, Smith KT: The equine sarcoid: detection of papillomaviral DNA in sarcoid tumours by use of consensus primers and the polymerase chain reaction. In: Plowright W, et al (eds): Equine Infectious Diseases. R&W Publications, Newmarket, 1991, p 297.

252. Reid SWJ, et al: Detection, cloning, and characterization of papillomaviral DNA present in sarcoid tumours of Equus asinus. Vet Rec 135:430, 1994.

253. Reid SWJ, Mohammed HO: Longitudinal and cross-sectional studies to evaluate the risk of sarcoid associated with castration. Can J Vet Res 61:89, 1997.

254. Roberts D: Experimental treatment of equine sarcoid. Vet Med Small Anim Clin 65:67, 1970.

255. Schwartzman SM, et al: Immunotherapy of equine sarcoid with cell wall skeleton (CNS)-trehalose dimycolate (TDM) biologic. Equine Pract 6:13, 1984.

256. Segre D, et al: Neutralization of bovine papillomavirus with serum from cattle and horses with experimental papillomas. Am J Vet Res 16-517, 1955.

257. Strafuss AC, et al: Sarcoid in horses. Vet Med Small Anim Clin 68:1246, 1973.

258. Studer U, et al: Zur Therapie des Equinen Sarkoids mit einem unspezifischen Immunostimulator-Beitrag Zur Epidemiologie und zur spontanen Regression des Sarkoids. Schweiz Arch Tierheilk 139:385, 1997.

259. Sullins KE, et al: BCG treatment of periocular sarcoid. Equine Vet J 17:445, 1985.

260. Sullins KE, et al: Equine sarcoid. Equine Pract 8:21, 1986.

261. Tallberg TH, et al: Equine sarcoid successfully treated by bioimmunotherapy. Deutsch Z Onkol 26:34, 1994.

262. Tarwid JN, et al: Equine sarcoids: a study with emphasis on pathologic diagnosis. Comp Cont Educ 7:S293, 1985.

263. Teifke JP, Weiss E: Nachweis boviner Papillomavirus DNA in Sarkoiden des Pferdes mittels der Polymerase-Kettenreakton (PCR). Berl Münch Tierärztl Wschr 104:185, 1991.

264. Teifke JP: Morphologische und molekularbiologische Untersuchungen zur Ätiologie des equinen Sarkoids. Tierärztl Prax 22:368, 1994.

265. Théon AP, et al: Comparison of perioperative versus postoperative intratumoral administration of cisplatin for treatment of cutaneous sarcoids and squamous cell carcinomas in horses. J Am Vet Med Assoc 215:1655, 1999.

266. Torrontegui BO, Reid SWJ: Clinical and pathological epidemiology of the equine sarcoid in a referral population. Equine Vet Educ 6:85, 1994.

267. Trenfield K, et al: Sequences of papillomavirus DNA in equine sarcoids. Equine Vet J 17:449, 1985.

268. Turrel JM, et al: Iridium[192] interstitial brachytherapy of equine sarcoid. Vet Radiol 26:20, 1985.

269. Vanselow BA, et al: BCG emulsion immunotherapy of equine sarcoid. Equine Vet J 20:444, 1988.

270. Vingerhoets M, et al: Traitement de la sarcoïde équine au Laser à gaz carbonique. Schweiz Arch Tierheilk 130:113, 1988.

271. von Tscharner C, et al: Involvement of dermal dendritic cells in the pathogenesis of equine sarcoids. In: Kwochka KW, et al (eds): Advances in Veterinary Dermatology III. Butterworth-Heinemann, Boston, 1998, p 561.

272. Voss JL: Transmission of equine sarcoid. Am J Vet Res 30:183, 1969.

273. Walker D: Defining the equine sarcoid. Vet Rec 96:494, 1975.

274. Walker M, et al: Iridium-192 brachytherapy for equine sarcoid, one and two year remission rates. Vet Radiol 32:206, 1991.

275. Watson RE, et al: Cultural characteristics of a cell line derived from an equine sarcoid. Appl Microbiol 24:727, 1972.

276. Watson RE, Larson KA: Detection of tumor-specific antigens in an equine sarcoid cell line. Infect Immunol 9:714, 1974.

277. Webster CJ, Webster JM: Treatment of equine sarcoids with BCG. Vet Rec 116-131, 1985.

278. Wheat JD: Therapy for equine sarcoids. Mod Vet Pract 45:62, 1964.

279. Williams IF, et al: Connective tissue composition of the equine sarcoid. Equine Vet J 14:305, 1982.

280. Wilson DG, et al: Immediate split thickness autogenous skin grafts in the horse. Case reports on the treatment of equine sarcoids in three horses. Vet Surg 16-167, 1987.

281. Winston M, et al: Treatment of equine sarcoids. J Am Vet Med Assoc 175:775, 1979.

282. Wolter H: Die homöopathische Behandlung des equinen Sarkoids. Prakt Tierärztl 69:19, 1988.

283. Wood AL, Spradbrow PB: Transformation of cultured equine fibroblasts with a bovine papillomavirus. Res Vet Sci 38:241, 1985.

284. Wyman M, et al: Immunotherapy of equine sarcoid: a report of two cases. J Am Vet Med Assoc 171:449, 1977.

285. Zeldner N, Bracken F: Immunotherapy for periocular sarcoid in a mule. Mod Vet Pract 66:891, 1985.

Fibroma

286. Hartog JH: Een omvangrijk subcutaan fibroom aan het achterbeen bij een paard. Tijdschr Diergeneesk 69:305, 1942.

287. Hobday F: Case of fibroma in the prepuce. J Comp Pathol Ther 5:272, 1892.

287a. Maiti SK, et al: Bilateral multiple knee fibroma durum in a horse. Indian Vet J 76:243, 1999.

288. Nakamura Y, et al: Tumor of the neck of a Thoroughbred. J Vet Med Tokyo 608:138, 1974.

Fibrosarcoma

289. Dixon RT: Radiation therapy in horses. Aust Vet J 43:508, 1967.

290. Dixon RT: Results of Radon[222] γ radiation therapy in an equine practice. Aust Vet J 48:279, 1972.

291. Podkonjak KR: Veterinary cryotherapy-2. Vet Med Small Animal Clin 77:183, 1982.

292. Reinertson EL: Fibrosarcoma in a horse. Cornell Vet 64:617, 1974.

293. Riggott JM, Quarmby WB: Treatment of fibrosarcoma in a horse. Equine Vet J 12:193, 1980.

293a. Roels S, et al: Successful treatment of an equine preputial fibrosarcoma using 5-fluorouracil/ evaluation of the treatment using quantitative PCNA and Ki67 (MIB1) immunostaining. J Vet Med A 45:591, 1998.

Fibromatosis

294. Ihrke PJ, et al: Fibromatosis in a horse. J Am Vet Med Assoc 183:1100, 1983.

Schwannoma

294a. Fernandez CA, et al: Equine dermal schwannoma. Vet Pathol 33:607, 1996.

295. Jones SA, Strafuss AC: Scanning electron microscopy of nerve sheath neoplasms. Am J Vet Res 39:1069, 1978.

Hemangioma

296. Cannon SRL, Loh H: Treatment of a cavernous haemangioma-like lesion in a polo pony. Equine Vet J 14:254, 1982.

297. Colbourne CM, et al: Vascular hamartomas of the dorsal carpal regions in three young Thoroughbred horses. Aust Vet J 75:20, 1997.

298. Drolet R, et al: Cutaneous hemangioma in two foals. Equine Pract 19:12, 1997.

299. Gröndahl AM, Jansen JH: Juvenile (capillary) hemangioma in a Standardbred foal. Equine Pract 13:7, 1991.

300. Gutberlet K, Brehm W: Vaskuläres Hamartom der lilnken Geskhtshälfte bei einem 7-jährigen Vollbluthengst. Pferdeheilk 13:47, 1997.
301. Hargis AM, McElwain TF: Vascular neoplasia in the skin of horses. J Am Vet Med Assoc 184:1121, 1984.
302. Humphrey K: Haemangioma in a horse. Postgrad Comm Vet Sci Univ Sydney Control and Therapy Series, #3546, 1994, p 662.
303. Jabara AG, et al: A congenital vascular naevus in a foal. Aust Vet J 61:286, 1984.
304. Johnson GC, et al: Histological and immunohistochemical characterization of hemangiomas in the skin of seven young horses. Vet Pathol 33:142, 1996.
305. Sartin EA, Hodge TG: Congenital dermal hemangioendothelioma in two foals. Vet Pathol 19:569, 1982.
306. Scott DW, Hackett RP Jr: Cutaneous hemangioma in a mule. Equine Pract 5:8, 1983.

Hemangiosarcoma
307. Collins MB, et al: Haemangiosarcoma in the horse: three cases. Aust Vet J 71:296, 1994.
308. Jean D, et al: Cutaneous hemangiosarcoma with pulmonary metastasis in a horse. J Am Vet Med Assoc 204:776, 1994.
309. Katayama Y, et al: An autopsy case of malignant hemangioendothelioma in the Thoroughbred horse—Histological, immunohistochemical, and lectin—Histochemical observations. Bull Equine Res Inst 29:6, 1992.
310. Katayama Y, et al: Clinical and immunohistochemical observation of hemangiosarcoma in a racing Thoroughbred. Equine Pract 18(3):24, 1996.
311. Southwood LL, et al: Disseminated hemangiosarcoma in the horse: 35 cases. J Vet Intern Med 14:105, 2000.

Lymphangioma
311a. Gehlen H, Wohlsein P: Cutaneous lymphangioma in a young Standardbred mare. Equine Vet J 32:86, 2000.
312. Hartog JH: Subcutaan lymphangioom bij een paard. Tijdschr Diergeneesk 68:207, 1941.
313. Turk JR, et al: Cystic lymphangioma in a colt. J Am Vet Med Assoc 174:1228, 1979.

Lipoma and Liposarcoma
314. Blackwell JG: Unusual adipose tissue growth in a colt. J Am Vet Med Assoc 161:1141, 1972.
315. Bristol DG, Fubini SL: External lipomas in three horses. J Am Vet Med Assoc 185:791, 1984.
316. Dunkerley SAC, et al: Lipoma in a foal. J Am Vet Med Assoc 210:332, 1997.
317. Hartog JH: Een fibrolipoom op de kruin bij een paard. Tijdschr Diergeneesk 68:374, 1941.
318. Lepage OM, et al: Infiltrative lipoma in a quarter horse. Cornell Vet 83:57, 1993.

Mast Cell Tumor
319. Altera K, Clark L: Equine cutaneous mastocytosis. Pathol Vet 7:43, 1970.
320. Cheville NF, et al: Generalized equine cutaneous mastocytosis. Vet Pathol 9:394, 1972.
321. Doran RE, et al: Mastocytoma in a horse. Equine Vet J 18:500, 1986.
322. Frese K: Mastzellentumoren beim Pferd. Berl. Munch Tierärztl Wschr 18:342, 1969.
323. Hani H, von Tscharner C: Mastocytoma beim Pferd. Schweiz Arch Tierheilk 121:269, 1979.
324. Hum S, Bowers JR: Ocular mastocytosis in a horse. Aust Vet J 66:32, 1989.
325. Malikides N, et al: Mast cell tumors in the horse: four case reports. Equine Pract 18(7):12, 1996.
326. Martin CL, Leipold HW: Mastocytoma of the globe in a horse. J Am Anim Hosp Assoc 8:32, 1972.
327. McEntee MF: Equine cutaneous mastocytoma: morphology, biological behavior and evolution of the lesion. J Comp Pathol 104:171, 1991.
328. Nyrop KA, et al: Equine cutaneous mastocytoma. Comp Cont Educ 8:757, 1986.
329. Nyrop KA: Cutaneous mastocytosis. In: Robinson NE (ed): Current Therapy in Equine Medicine III. W.B. Saunders Co, Philadelphia, 1992, p 702.
330. Prasse KW, et al: Generalized mastocytosis in a foal, resembling urticaria pigmentosa of man. J Am Vet Med Assoc 166:68, 1975.
331. Reppas GP, Canfield PJ: Malignant mast cell neoplasia with local metastasis in a horse. NZ Vet J 44:22, 1996.
332. Richardson JD, et al: Nasopharyngeal mast cell tumor in a horse. Vet Rec 134:238, 1994.
333. Riley CB, et al: Malignant mast cell tumours in horses. Aust Vet J 68:346, 1991.
334. Ritmeester AM, et al: Primary intraosseous mast cell tumour of the third phalanx in a Quarter Horse. Equine Vet J 29:151, 1997.
335. Sabrazès J, Lafon CH: Granulome de la lèvre à mastzellen et à eosinophiles chez un cheval. Folia Haematol 6:3, 1908.
336. Samii VF, et al: Radiographic features of mastocytosis in the equine limb. Equine Vet J 29:63, 1997.
337. Stannard AA: Equine dermatology. Proc Am Assoc Equine Practit 22:273, 1976.
338. Ward DA, et al: Scleral mastocytosis in a horse. Equine Vet J 25:79, 1993.
339. Wenger IE, Caron JP: Tracheal mastocytosis in a horse. Can Vet J 29:563, 1988.
340. Whitler WA, et al: Equine mast cell tumor. Equine Pract 16:16, 1994.

Lymphoma
341. Adams R, et al: Malignant lymphoma in three horses with ulcerative pharyngitis. J Am Vet Med Assoc 193:674, 1988.
342. Anderson RG: A peculiar case of subcutaneous round-celled sarcoma in the horse. J Comp Pathol 26:52, 1913.
343. Asahina M, et al: An immunohistochemical study of an equine B-cell lymphoma. J Comp Pathol 111:445, 1994.
344. Craig JF, Davies GO: Multiple subcutaneous round-celled sarcomata in a Thoroughbred mare. Vet Rec 50:270, 1938.
345. Detilleux PG, et al: Ultrastructure and lectin histochemistry of equine cutaneous histiolymphocytic lymphosarcomas. Vet Pathol 26:409, 1989.
346. Dopson LC, et al: Immunosuppression associated with lymphosarcoma in two horses. J Am Vet Med Assoc 182:1239, 1983.
346a. Finley MR: Paraneoplastic pruritus and alopecia in a horse with diffuse lymphoma. J Am Vet Med Assoc 213:102, 1998.
347. Fujimoto Y, et al: Pathological observations on equine leukemia complex in Japan. Bull Equine Res Inst 19:69, 1982.

348. Gerard MP, et al: Cutaneous lymphoma with extensive periarticular involvement in a horse. J Am Vet Med Assoc 213:391, 1998.
349. Henson KL, et al: Regression of subcutaneous lymphoma following removal of an ovarian granulosa-theca cell tumor in a horse. J Am Vet Med Assoc 212:1419, 1998.
350. Gollagher RD, et al: Immunotherapy of equine cutaneous lymphosarcoma using low dose cyclophosphamide and autologous tumor cells with vaccinia virus. Can Vet J 34:371, 1993.
351. Gupta RN, et al: Cutaneous involvement of malignant lymphoma in a horse. Cornell Vet 62:205, 1972.
352. Hilbe M, et al: Ein Fall eines malignen epitheliotropen kutanen lymphoms (mycosis fungoides) bei eingen Pferd. Berl Münch Tierärztl Wschr 110:86, 1997.
353. Kelley LC, Mahaffey EA: Equine malignant lymphomas: morphologic and immunohistochemical classification. Vet Pathol 35:241, 1998.
354. Kofler J, et al: Cutaneous multilocular T-cell lymphosarcoma in a horse-clinical, ultrasonographic, and pathological findings. J Vet Med A 45:11, 1998.
355. Littlewood JD, et al: Equine cutaneous lymphoma: a case report. Vet Dermatol 6:105, 1995.
356. Mair TS, Hillyer MH: Clinical features of lymphosarcoma in the horse: 77 cases. Equine Vet Educ 4:108, 1991.
357. Murphy CJ, et al: Bilateral eyelid swelling attributable to lymphosarcoma in a horse. J Am Vet Med Assoc 194:939, 1973.
358. Neufield JL: Lymphosarcoma in the horse: a review. Can Vet J 14:129, 1973.
359. Platt H: Observations on the pathology of non-alimentary lymphomas in the horse. J Comp Pathol 98:177, 1988.
360. Polkes AC, et al: B-cell lymphoma in a horse with associated Sézary-like cells in the peripheral blood. J Vet Intern Med 13:620, 1999.
361. Potter, K, Anez D: Mycosis fungoides in a horse. J Am Vet Med Assoc 212:550, 1998.
362. Rebhun WC, Bertone A: Equine lymphosarcoma. J Am Vet Med Assoc 184:720, 1984.
363. Rebhun WC, DelPiero F: Ocular lesions in horses with lymphosarcoma: 21 cases (1977-1997). J Am Vet Med Assoc 212:852, 1998.
364. Reef VB, et al: Lymphosarcoma and associated immune-mediated hemolytic anemia and thrombocytopenia in horses. J Am Vet Med Assoc 184:313, 1984.
365. Rutgers HC, et al: Huidleukose bij een paard. Tijdschr Diergeneesk 104:511, 1979.
366. Schneider DA: Lymphoproliferative and myeloproliferative disorders. In: Robinson NE (ed): Current Therapy in Equine Medicine IV. W.B. Saunders Co, Philadelphia, 1997, p 296.
367. Sheahan BJ, et al: Histiolymphocytic lymphosarcoma in the subcutis of two horses. Vet Pathol 17:123, 1986.
368. Stewart WL, et al: Subcutaneous sarcoma in the horse. Vet Rec 56:96, 1944.
369. Theilen GH, Fowler ME: Lymphosarcoma (lymphocytic leukemia) in the horse. J Am Vet Med Assoc 140:923, 1962.
370. Vanden Hoven R, Franken P: Clinical aspects of lymphosarcoma in the horse: a clinical report of 16 cases. Equine Vet J 15:49, 1983.
371. Ward JM, Whitlock RH: Chemotherapy of equine leukemia with amethopterin. Vet Med Small Animal Clin 62:1003, 1967.
372. Walder E, Ferrer L: Pathogenesis and histopathology of newly recognized dermatoses. In: von Tscharner C, Halliwell REW (eds): Advances in Veterinary Dermatology I. Baillière-Tindall, Philadelphia, 1990, p 441.

Plasmacytoma
373. Geisel O, et al: Kutane Amyloidose vom Immunglobulin-Ursprung bei einen Pferd. Pferdeheilk 5:299, 1989.
374. Linke RP, et al: Equine cutaneous amyloidosis derived from an immunoglobulin γ-light chain. Immunohistochemical, immunochemical, and chemical results. Biol Chem Hoppe-Seyler 372:835, 1991.
375. Platz SJ, et al: Identification of γ-light chain amyloid in eight canine and two feline extramedullary plasmacytomas. J Comp Pathol 116:45, 1997.

Malignant Fibrous Histiocytoma
376. Danks AG, Olafson P: Giant-cell sarcoma. Cornell Vet 29:68, 1939.
377. Ford GH, et al: Giant cell tumor of soft parts: a report of an equine and a feline case. Vet Pathol 12:428, 1975.
378. Hamir AN: Equine giant cell tumor of soft tissues. Cornell Vet 79:173, 1989.
379. Render JA, et al: Giant cell tumor of soft parts in six horses. J Am Vet Med Assoc 183:790, 1983.

Melanocytic Neoplasms
380. Ajello P: Contribute allo studio dei tumori melanotici nei cavalli a mantello scuro. Nuova Vet 15:368, 1937.
381. Ajello P: Beitrag zum Studium der melanotischen Tumoren bei dunkelhaarigen Pferden. Wien Tierärztl Mschr 24:513, 1937.
382. Arnett RH: Rupture of the liver from melanosis. Cornell Vet 10:48, 1920.
382a. Bonesi GL, et al: Melanoma em equídeos de pelagem branca-freqüência, distribuiçao e lesões em carcaças. Anais Bras Dermatol 73:533, 1998.
383. Bowers JR, et al: Efficacy of cimetidine for therapy of skin tumours of horses—10 cases. Aust Equine Practit 12:30, 1994.
384. Burkhart CG, Burkhart CN: Melanoma and insecticides: is there a connection? J Am Acad Dermatol 42:302, 2000.
385. Calderwood-Mays MB, et al: A giant congenital pigmented nevus in a horse. Am J Dermatopathol 6(suppl):325, 1984.
386. Cox JH, et al: Congenital malignant melanoma in two foals. J Am Vet Med Assoc 194:945, 1989.
387. Dick W: Melanosis in men and horses. Lancet, 1932, p 192.
387a. Fleury C, et al: The study of cutaneous melanomas in Camarque-type gray-skinned horses (1): clinical-pathological characterization. Pigment Cell Res 13:39, 2000.
387b. Fleury C, et al: The study of cutaneous melanomas in Camarque-type gray-skinned horses (2): epidemiological survey. Pigment Cell Res 13:47, 2000.

388. Foley GL, et al: Congenital and acquired melano-cytomas (benign melanomas) in eighteen young horses. Vet Pathol 28:363, 1991.

389. Garma-Avina A, et al: Cutaneous melanomas in domestic animals. J Cutan Pathol 8:3, 1981.

390. Gebhart W, Neibauer GW: Beziehungen Zwischen Pigmenschward und Melanomatose am Beispeil des Lippizanerschimmels. Arch Dermatol Forsch 259:29, 1977.

391. Gessard C: Sur la formation du pigment mélanique dans les tumeurs du cheval. Compt Rend Acad Sci (Paris) 136:1086, 1903.

392. Goetz TE, et al: Clinical management of progressive multifocal benign and malignant melanomas of horses with oral cimetidine. Proc Am Assoc Equine Practit 35:431, 1989.

393. Goetz TE, et al: Cimetidine for treatment of melanomas in three horses. J Am Vet Med Assoc 196:449, 1990.

394. Goetz TE, Long MT: Treatment of melanomas in horses. Comp Cont Educ 15:608, 1993.

395. Goldberg SA: The differential features between melanosis and melanosarcoma. J Am Vet Med Assoc 56:140, 1919.

396. Gorham S, Robl M: Melanoma in the gray horse: the darker side of equine aging. Vet Med 81:446, 1986.

397. Grant B, Lincoln S: Melanosarcoma as a cause of lameness in a horse. Vet Med Small Animal Clin 67:995, 1972.

398. Hadwen S: The melanomata of gray and white horses. Can Med Assoc J 25:519, 1931.

399. Hamilton DP, Byerly CS: Congenital malignant melanoma in a foal. J Am Vet Med Assoc 164:1040, 1974.

400. Hare JE, Staempfli HR: Cimetidine for the treatment of melanomas in horses: efficacy determined by client questionnaire. Equine Pract 16-18, 1994.

401. Honnas CM, et al: Malignant melanoma in the foot of a horse. J Am Vet Med Assoc 197:756, 1990.

402. Jaeger A: Die Melanosarkomatose der Schimmel-pferde. Virchows Arch Pathol Anat 198:1, 1909.

403. Jeglum KA: Melanomas. In: Robinson NE (ed): Current Therapy in Equine Medicine IV. W.B. Saunders Co, Philadelphia, 1997, p 399.

404. Keye H: Ueber die natürliche Abwanderung des Pigments aus der Haut in die Lymphotrüsen bei Pferden. Zbl Allg Pathol Anat 34:57, 1923.

405. Kirker-Head CA, et al: Pelvic limb lameness due to malignant melanoma in a horse. J Am Vet Med Assoc 186:1215, 1985.

406. Kunze DJ, et al: Malignant melanoma of the coronary band in a horse. J Am Vet Med Assoc 188:297, 1986.

407. Lerner AB, Case GW: Melanomas in horses. Yale J. Biol. Med. 46:646, 1973.

408. Levene A: Equine melanotic disease. Tumori 57:133, 1971.

409. McFadyean J: Equine melanomatosis. J Comp Pathol Ther 46:186, 1933.

409a. McGillivray KC, et al: Metastatic melanoma in horses. J Vet Intern Med 16:452, 2002.

410. Mangrulkar MY: Melanomata in domesticated animals. Indian J Vet Sci 14:178, 1944.

411. Markel MD, Dorr TE: Multiple myeloma in a horse. J Am Vet Med Assoc 188:621, 1986.

412. Montes LF, et al: Equine melanoma. J Cutan Pathol 6:234, 1979.

413. Morel T: Mécanisme de la pigmentation dans la mélanose et les tumeurs mélaniques chez le cheval. Bull Assoc Fr Cancer 7:454, 1918.

414. Morel T: Mélanose et tumeurs mélaniques chez le cheval. Bull Assoc Fr Cancer 7:340, 1918.

415. Mostafa MSE: A case of malignant melanoma in a bay horse. Br Vet J 109:201, 1953.

415a. Patterson-Kane LC, et al: Disseminated metastatic intramedullary melanoma in an aged horse. J Comp Pathol 125:204, 2001.

416. Petit G: Enorme sarcome mélanique de la cuisse chez un cheval. Rec Méd Vét 10:597, 1903.

417. Petit G: Mélanose de la parotide chez le cheval. Bull Assoc Fr Cancer 7:325, 1918.

418. Petit G: Courte note sur un curieux cas de mélanose mammaire. Bull Assoc Fr Cancer 7:328, 1918.

419. Peyronny L: La mélanose du cheval blanc. Rev Gén Méd Vét 2:113, 1903.

420. Rodriquez F, et al: Metastatic melanoma causing spinal cord compression in a horse. Vet Rec 142:248, 1998.

420a. Roels S, et al: Proliferation, DNA ploidy, p53 over-expression, and nuclear DNA fragmentation in 6 equine melanocytic tumors. J Vet Med A 47:439, 2000.

421. Runnels RA, Benbrook EA: Malignant melanomas of horses and mules. Am J Vet Res 2:340, 1941.

422. Schott HC, et al: Melanoma as a cause of spinal cord compression in two horses. J Am Vet Med Assoc 196:1820, 1990.

423. Shokry M, Lotfi MM: Malignant perianal melanoma in a horse. Mod Vet Pract 65:226, 1984.

423a. Rodríguez M, et al: Grey horse melanotic condition: a pigmentary disorder. J Equine Vet Sci 17:677, 1997.

424. Traub JL, Schroeder WG: Malignant melanoma in a horse. Vet Med Small Animal Clin 75:261, 1980.

425. Traver DS, et al: Epidural melanoma causing posterior paresis in a horse. J Am Vet Med Assoc 170:1400, 1977.

426. Tuthill RJ, et al: Equine melanotic disease: a unique animal model for human dermal melanocytic disease. Lab Invest 46:85A, 1982.

427. Tuthill RJ, et al: Pilar neurocristic hamartoma: its relationship to blue nevus and equine melanotic disease. Arch Dermatol 118:592, 1982.

428. Valentine BA: Equine melanocytic tumors: a retrospective study of 53 horses (1988 to 1991). J Vet Int Med 9:291, 1995.

429. Valentine B, Graham M: Equine melanocytic tumors. Vet Pathol 29:439, 1992.

430. Warnick LD, et al: Evaluation of cimetidine treatment for melanomas in seven horses. Equine Pract 17:16, 1995.

Cysts

431. Abraham CG Jr, Genetzky RM: Diagnosing dermoid cysts in a horse. Vet Med 90: 72, 1995.

432. Bello TR: Surgical removal of a dentigerous cyst from a horse. Southwest Vet 21:152, 1962.

433. Dahlgren LA, et al: Heterotopic salivary tissue in a weanling colt. J Am Vet Med Assoc 201:303, 1992.

434. Elkins AD, Walter PA: Managing a dentigerous cyst in a Hackney pony. Vet Med 79:1294, 1984.

435. Fessler JM: Heterotopic polyodontia in the horse: nine cases (1969-1986). J Am Vet Med Assoc 192:535, 1988.

436. Gordon LR: The cytology and histology of epidermal inclusion cysts in the horse. J Equine Med Surg 2:371, 1978.

437. Hunt RJ, et al: Intracranial trauma associated with extraction of a temporal ear tooth (dentigerous cyst) in a horse. Cornell Vet 81:103, 1991.

438. Lindsay WA, Beck KA: Temporal teratoma in a horse. Comp Cont Educ 8:S168, 1986.

439. Mariën T, et al: Temporal teratomas in two horses. Vlaams Diergeneesk Tijdschr 67:66, 1998.

440. Mason BJE: Temporal teratoma in the horse. Vet Rec 95:226, 1974.

441. Pascoe RR: Conchal fistula in two horses. Aust Vet Practit 11:109, 1981.

442. Watrous BJ, Rendano VT: Radiographic interpretation—a case report. Mod Vet Pract 61:188, 1980.

443. Wellington JR, Scott DW: Equine keratinizing cutaneous cysts. Equine Pract 13:8, 1991.

Nevi

444. Atwell RB, Summers PM: Congenital papilloma in a foal. Aust Vet J 53:229, 1977.

445. Garma-Avina A, et al: Equine congenital cutaneous papillomatosis: a report of 5 cases. Equine Vet J 13:59, 1981.

446. Kohn FG: Akanthom mit Physalidenbildung beim Pferde foetus. Mb Prakt Tierheilk 22:376, 1911.

447. Njoko CO, Burwash WA: Congenital cutaneous papilloma in a foal. Cornell Vet 62:54, 1972.

448. Paradis M, et al: Linear epidermal nevi in a family of Belgian horses. Equine Pract 15(7):10, 1993.

449. Schueler RL: Congenital equine papillomatosis. J Am Vet Med Assoc 162:640, 1977.

450. Trolldenier W: Angeborenes Papillom beim Pferde foetus. Mb Prakt Tierheilk 15:202, 1904.

Keratoses

451. Hargis AM: A review of solar-induced lesions in domestic animals. Comp Cont Educ Pract Vet 3:287, 1981.

Calcinosis Circumscripta

452. Dodd DC, Raker CW: Tumoral calcinosis (calcinosis circumscripta) in the horse. J Am Vet Med Assoc 157:968, 1970.

453. Goulden BE, O'Callaghan MW: Tumoral calcinosis in the horse. NZ Vet J 28:217, 1980.

454. Hutchins DR: Tumoral calcinosis in the horse. Aust Vet J 48:200, 1972.

455. O'Connor JP, Lucey MD: Tumoral calcinosis (calcinosis circumscripta) in the horse. Irish Vet J 31:173, 1977.

456. Scott DW: Nodular skin disease in the horse. In: Robinson NE (ed): Current Therapy in Equine Medicine II. W.B. Saunders Co Philadelphia, 1987, p 634.

457. Stone WC, et al: The pathologic mineralization of soft tissue: calcinosis circumscripta in horses. Comp Cont Educ 12:1643, 1990.

458. Youssef HA, et al: Kalzinose beim Pferd. Prakt Tierärztl 73:302, 1992.

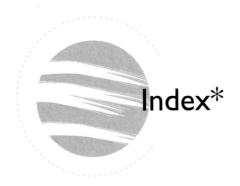

Index*

---

*NOTE: Page numbers followed by *f* indicate figures; *t*, tables.